ADVANCE PRA

Psychopathology and phenomenology are central to our un[ ] volume brings readers an updated knowledge of the field, addr[ ] nomenology, psychopathology, clinical practice, and the patient's lived experience of mental disorders. It provides an insight into the complex phenomenon of psychopathology. The book is impressive in scope and diverse in content and the contributors are all experienced professionals working in this area. Anyone who wants to understand more about these topics needs to read this book. This is indeed "a must" read for all those interested in this subject.

Afzal Javed, Consultant Psychiatrist, UK and President Elect,
World Psychiatric Association

This book is a welcome antidote to reductionism and oversimplification in the research and clinical approach to mental disorders. A treasure of information and reflection - which has been available up to now only to a very small circle of scholars proficient in German and French and having access to rich libraries - has been collected in a single volume. It should become a must-read in psychiatric education and continuing professional development.

Mario Maj, Professor of Psychiatry and Chairman of the
Department of Psychiatry of the University of Naples, Italy
and Past President, World Psychiatric Association

Phenomenology is fundamental for identifying psychopathology and is the first step in understanding mental disorders. This is lost in a field where brief assessment is common and psychopathology targets for scientific discovery are shallow. This Handbook provides essential reading addressing an unmet need for depth in psychopathology concepts. Implications for clinical care and research are substantial.

William T. Carpenter, Jr., MD, Professor of Psychiatry,
The University of Maryland School of Medicine, USA

A tour de force of breadth, depth and expertise, this volume provides the most detailed mapping of phenomenological psychopathology to date. Written and edited by major scholars from multiple disciplines, this volume systematically covers the field with unprecedented detail and richness of approaches, authors, and ideas.

Havi Carel, Professor of Philosophy,
University of Bristol, UK

There has not, to date, been a book with such ambition. The framing of phenomenological and existential psychopathology, its anthropology, the definition of theoretical basis and origins, the addition of a psychodynamic corpus, the exposure of major pathologies and situations of pain in the existence, the confrontation of it with neurosciences and cognitive sciences: this is what is at stake here. The book gathers remarkable contributions from all parts of Europe, the US and the AngloSaxon world. This is what enables phenomenological psychopathology to reach an unprecedented status, which is both global, and at the heart of contemporary scientific, anthropologic and philosophical life.

Georges Charbonneau MDR, HDR, *Le Cercle
Herméneutique* édi. et Université Paris VII Denis Diderot.

OXFORD
HANDBOOKS
IN PHILOSOPHY
AND PSYCHIATRY

SERIES EDITORS: K.W.M. FULFORD, LISA BORTOLOTTI, MATTHEW R. BROOME, KATHERINE MORRIS, JOHN Z. SADLER, AND GIOVANNI STANGHELLINI

Volumes in the Series:

The Oxford Handbook of Philosophy and Psychiatry
Edited by K.W.M. Fulford, Martin Davies, Richard Gipps, George Graham, John Sadler, Giovanni Stanghellini, and Tim Thornton

The Oxford Handbook of Psychiatric Ethics
Edited by John Z. Sadler, Werdie (C.W.) Van Staden, and K.W.M. Fulford

The Oxford Handbook of Philosophy and Psychoanalysis
Edited by Richard Gipps and Michael Lacewing

The Oxford Handbook of Phenomenological Psychopathology
Edited by Giovanni Stanghellini, Matthew R. Broome, Anthony Vincent Fernandez, Paolo Fusar-Poli, Andrea Raballo, and René Rosfort

THE OXFORD HANDBOOK OF

PHENOMENOLOGICAL PSYCHOPATHOLOGY

Edited by

GIOVANNI STANGHELLINI

MATTHEW R. BROOME

ANTHONY VINCENT FERNANDEZ

PAOLO FUSAR-POLI

ANDREA RABALLO

and

RENÉ ROSFORT

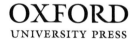

OXFORD

UNIVERSITY PRESS

OXFORD

UNIVERSITY PRESS

Great Clarendon Street, Oxford, OX2 6DP,
United Kingdom

Oxford University Press is a department of the University of Oxford.
It furthers the University's objective of excellence in research, scholarship,
and education by publishing worldwide. Oxford is a registered trade mark of
Oxford University Press in the UK and in certain other countries

First published 2019
First published in paperback 2021

Published in the United States of America by Oxford University Press
198 Madison Avenue, New York, NY 10016, United States of America

British Library Cataloguing in Publication Data
Data available

Library of Congress Cataloging in Publication Data
Data available

ISBN 978–0–19–880315–7 (Hbk.)
ISBN 978–0–19–289592–9 (Pbk.)

Printed and bound by
CPI Group (UK) Ltd, Croydon, CR0 4YY

Summary Table of Contents

OXFORD HANDBOOK OF PHENOMENOLOGICAL PSYCHOPATHOLOGY

Editors

G. Stanghellini

M.R. Broome

A.F. Fernandez

P. Fusar Poli

A. Raballo

R. Rosfort

International Advisory Board

A. Ballerini (Psychiatry)

M. Ballerini (Psychiatry)

H. Carel (Philosophy)

G. Di Petta (Psychiatry)

T. Fuchs (Psychiatry, Philosophy)

K.W.M. Fulford (Psychiatry, Philosophy)

S. Gallagher (Philosophy)

V. Gallese (Neurosciences)

P. Lysaker (Clinical Psychology)

L. Madeira (Psychiatry)

M. Mancini (Psychology)

A. Mishara (Psychiatry)

M. Musalek (Psychiatry)

G. Owen (Psychiatry)

F. Oyebode (Psychiatry)

J. Parnas (Psychiatry)

M. Ratcliffe (Philosophy)

M. Rossi Monti (Psychiatry)

L.A. Sass (Clinical Psychology)

M.A. Schwartz (Psychiatry)

D. Zahavi (Philosophy)

TABLE OF CONTENTS

SECTION TWO: FOUNDATIONS AND METHODS

SECTION EDITORS: ANTHONY VINCENT FERNANDEZ AND RENÉ ROSFORT

SECTION THREE: KEY CONCEPTS

SECTION EDITORS: MATTHEW R. BROOME AND GIOVANNI STANGHELLINI

SECTION FOUR: DESCRIPTIVE PSYCHOPATHOLOGY

SECTION EDITORS: MATTHEW R. BROOME AND ANDREA RABALLO

SECTION FIVE: LIFE-WORLDS

SECTION EDITORS: ANTHONY VINCENT FERNANDEZ
AND GIOVANNI STANGHELLINI

SECTION SIX: CLINICAL PSYCHOPATHOLOGY

SECTION EDITORS: MATTHEW R. BROOME AND
PAOLO FUSAR-POLI

SECTION SEVEN: PHENOMENOLOGICAL PSYCHOPATHOLOGY

SECTION EDITORS: MATTHEW R. BROOME AND PAOLO FUSAR-POLI

LIST OF CONTRIBUTORS

Claire Ahern, Brain and Psychological Sciences Research Centre, Swinburne University of Technology, Melbourne, Australia

Kevin Aho, Department of Communication and Philosophy, College of Arts and Sciences, Florida Gulf Coast University, USA

Angela Ales Bello, Faculty of Philosophy, Pontifical Lateran University, Italy

Massimiliano Aragona, Crossing Dialogues Association, Rome, Italy

Arnaldo Ballerini (deceased), President Società italiana per la Psicopatologia Fenomenologica

Massimo Ballerini, Department of Mental Health, USLCENTRO Florence, Italy and School of Dynamic Phenomenological Psychotherapy, Florence, Italy

Francesco Barale, Department of Brain and Behavioral Sciences, University of Pavia, Italy

Marco O. Bertelli, CREA (Research and Clinical Centre), San Sebastiano Foundation, Florence, Italy

Allan Beveridge, Consultant Psychiatrist, Queen Margaret Hospital, Dunfermline, UK

Ilaria Bonoldi, Institute of Psychiatry, Psychology and Neuroscience, King's College London, UK and Department of Brain and Behavioral Sciences, University of Pavia, Italy

Matthias Bormuth, Institute of Philosophy, Carl von Ossietzky University Oldenburg, Germany

Anna Bortolan, School of Philosophy, University College Dublin, Ireland

Francesca Brencio, Department of Aesthetics and History of Philosophy, University of Seville, Spain

Davide Broglia, Psychiatrist, Italy

Matthew R. Broome, Professor of Psychiatry and Youth Mental Health and Director of the Institute for Mental Health, University of Birmingham, UK; Distinguished Research Fellow, Oxford Uehiro Centre for Practical Ethics, University of Oxford, UK; Honorary Consultant Psychiatrist, Oxford Health NHS Foundation Trust and Birmingham Women's and Children's NHS Foundation Trust, UK

Martin Bürgy, Klinikum Stuttgart, Germany

Sergio Carmenates, North Lisbon Hospital Center, EPE, Portugal

Giovanni Castellini, Psychiatric Unit, Department of Health Sciences, University of Florence, Italy

Richard A. Cohen, University at Buffalo (SUNY), USA

Cristina Costa, North Lisbon Hospital Center, EPE, Portugal

John Cutting, Institute of Psychiatry, Psychology & Neuroscience, King's College London, UK

Alessandra D'Agostino, Department of Humanities, Carlo Bo University of Urbino, Italy

Johan De Groef, VZW Zonnelied, Roosdaal, Belgium

Sanneke de Haan, Department of Culture Studies, Tilburg University, The Netherlands

Roberta de Monticelli, Faculty of Philosophy, Vita-Salute San Raffaele University, Italy

Giulia Zelda De Vidovich, Department of Brain and Behavioral Sciences, University of Pavia, Italy

Katerina Deligiorgi, Department of Philosophy, University of Sussex, UK

Gilberto Di Petta, Mental Health Department of, ASL Naples, Italy and School of Dynamic Phenomenological Psychotherapy, Florence, Italy

Otto Doerr-Zegers, Centre for Studies on Phenomenology and Psychiatry, Diego Portales University, Santiago, Chile

Jérôme Englebert, University of Liège, Belgium

Daniel B. Fassnacht, Research School of Psychology, ANU College of Health and Medicine, Australian National University, Canberra, Australia

Anthony Vincent Fernandez, is Assistant Professor in the Department of Philosophy at Kent State University, USA, and Postdoctoral Research Fellow in the Faculty of Philosophy at University of Oxford, UK.

Francesca Ferri, Department of Psychology, University of Essex, UK

Maria Luísa Figueira, Faculty of Medicine, University of Lisbon, Portugal

Adam Fishman, Department of Clinical Psychology, GSAPP, Rutgers University, New Jersey, USA

John Foot, School of Modern Languages, University of Bristol, UK

Thomas Fuchs, Psychiatric Clinic, University of Heidelberg, Germany

K. W. M. (Bill) Fulford, St Catherine's College, Oxford, UK

Paolo Fusar-Poli, is Reader in Psychiatry and Youth Mental Health at the Department of Psychosis Studies, Institute of Department of Brain and Behavioral Sciences, King's College London and Associate Professor at the Department of Behavioural Sciences, University of Pavia, Italy.

Shaun Gallagher, Department of Philosophy, University of Memphis, USA and Faculty of Law, Humanities and the Arts, University of Wollongong, Australia

Vittorio Gallese, Unit of Neuroscience, Department of Medicine and Surgery, University of Parma, Italy and Institute of Philosophy, School of Advanced Study, University of London, UK

Grant Gillett, Division of Health Sciences, University of Otago, Dunedin, New Zealand

Richard Gipps, Associate of Faculty of Philosophy, University of Oxford, UK and Clinical Psychologist in private practice

Lewis R. Gordon, University of Connecticut, USA

Anthony Hatzimoysis, Department of History and Philosophy of Science, National and Kapodistrian University of Athens, Greece

Sara Heinämaa, Department of Social Sciences and Philosophy, University of Jyväskylä

Martin Heinze, Brandenburg Medical School, Clinic for Psychiatry and Psychotherapy, Immanuel Klinik, Rüdersdorf, Germany

Mads Gram Henriksen, Department of Media, Cognition and Communication, Center for Subjectivity Research, University of Copenhagen, Denmark

Christoph Hoerl, Department of Philosophy, University of Warwick, UK

Klaus Hoffmann, Center for Psychiatry Reichenau, Clinic of Forensic Psychiatry and Psychotherapy, Germany

Julian C. Hughes, Bristol Medical School, University of Bristol, UK

Clara S. Humpston, School of Psychology, Cardiff University, UK and Institute of Psychiatry, Psychology and Neuroscience, King's College London, UK

Eduardo Iacoponi, King's College London, UK

Jake Jackson, Department of Philosophy, Temple University, Pennsylvania, USA

Lennart Jansson, Department of Clinical Medicine, University of Copenhagen, Denmark

Roman Knorr, Center for Psychiatry Reichenau, Clinic of Forensic Psychiatry and Psychotherapy, Germany

Allan Koster, Postdoctoral Researcher in the Department of Communication and Psychology at Aalborg University.

Joel Krueger, Department of Sociology, Philosophy and Anthropology, University of Exeter, UK

Michael Kyrios, College of Education, Psychology and Social Work, Flinders University, Bedford Park, Adelaide, Australia

Roberta Lanfredini, Department of Literature and Philosophy, University of Florence, Italy

Dorothée Legrand, Archives Husserl, CNRS, Ecole Normale Supérieure, Paris Sciences and Letters Research University, Paris, France

Federico Leoni, Department of Human Sciences, University of Verona, Italy

María Inés López-Ibor, Faculty of Medicine, Complutense University, Madrid, Spain and Juan José López-Ibor Foundation, Spain

Luís Madeira, Faculty of Medicine, University of Lisbon, Portugal

Milena Mancini, Department of Psychological, Humanistic and Territorial Sciences, G. d'Annunzio University of Chieti, Italy

Eric Matthews, School of Divinity, History and Philosophy, University of Aberdeen, UK

Franz Mayr, University of Portland, USA

Guilherme Messas, School of Medical Sciences, Santa Casa de São Paulo, Brazil

Stefano Micali, Centre for Phenomenology and Continental Philosophy, KU Leuven, Belgium

Aaron Mishara, Chicago School of Professional Psychology, USA

Dermot Moran, Boston College, USA and University College Dublin, Ireland

Marcin Moskalewicz, Department of Social Sciences, Poznan University of Medical Sciences, Poland and Oxford Research Centre in the Humanities (TORCH), University of Oxford, UK

Shannon M. Mussett, Department of Philosophy, Utah Valley University, USA

Barnaby Nelson, Orygen, National Centre of Excellence in Youth Mental Health, University of Melbourne, Australia

Julie Nordgaard, Mental Health Center Amager and University of Copenhagen, Denmark

Georg Northoff, Mind, Brain Imaging and Neuroethics Research Unit, Institute of Mental Health Research, University of Ottawa, Canada

Søren Overgaard, Department of Media, Cognition and Communication, Center for Subjectivity Research, University of Copenhagen, Denmark

Gareth S. Owen, Department of Psychological Medicine, Institute of Psychiatry, Psychology and Neuroscience, King's College London, UK

Femi Oyebode, University of Birmingham, UK

Josef Parnas, Faculty of Health Sciences and Faculty of Humanities, Center for Subjectivity Research, University of Copenhagen, Denmark

Lorenzo Pelizza, Department of Mental Health and Addiction, Reggio Emilia Public Health Centre, Italy

James Phillips, Yale School of Medicine, USA

Andrea Raballo, Division of Psychiatry, Department of Medicine, University of Perugia, Italy

Matthew Ratcliffe, Department of Philosophy, University of York, UK

Valdo Ricca, Psychiatric Unit, Department of Health Sciences, University of Florence, Italy

Elisa Rondini, CREA (Research and Clinical Centre), San Sebastiano Foundation, Florence, Italy; Opera Don Orione, Rome, Italy; Department of Philosophy, Social Sciences and Education (FISSUF), University of Perugia, Italy

René Rosfort, is Associate Professor of Ethics and Philosophy of Religion at the Søren Kierkegaard Research Centre, University of Copenhagen, Denmark.

Mario Rossi Monti, Department of Humanities, Carlo Bo University of Urbino, Italy and School of Dynamic Phenomenological Psychotherapy, Florence, Italy

Louis Sass, Department of Clinical Psychology, GSAPP, Rutgers University, New Jersey, USA

Paolo Scudellari, University of Bologna, Italy

Patrick Seniuk, Centre for Theory of Practical Knowledge, Södertörn University, Sweden

Maxine Sheets-Johnstone, Department of Philosophy, University of Oregon, USA

Giovanni Stanghellini, Professor of Dynamic Psychology, G. d'Annunzio University, Chieti, Italy, Chair School of Dynamic Phenomenological Psychotherapy, Florence, Italy and Adjunct Professor, D. Portales University, Santiago, Chile.

Anthony Steinbock, Department of Philosophy and Phenomenology Research Center, Southern Illinois University, USA

Robert D. Stolorow, Institute of Contemporary Psychoanalysis, California, USA

Joona Taipale, Department of Social Sciences and Philosophy, University of Jyväskylä

Melissa Tamelini, Institute of Psychiatry, Clinics Hospital, Faculty of Medicine of the University of São Paulo, Brazil

Stefania Ucelli di Nemi, Department of Brain and Behavioral Sciences, University of Pavia, Italy

Gabor S. Ungvari, Department of Psychiatry, School of Public Health, Chinese University of Hong Kong

Annick Urfer-Parnas, Department of Psychiatry, University Hospital of Amager, Denmark

Harvey Wickham, King's College London, UK

Andrzej Wiercinski, University of Warsaw, Poland

Dan Zahavi, Center for Subjectivity Research, University of Copenhagen, Denmark and Faculty of Philosophy, University of Oxford, UK

Julia Picazo Zappino, Faculty of Medicine, Complutense University, Madrid, Spain

Yuliya Zaytseva, Department of Applied Neurosciences and Brain Imaging, National Institute of Mental Health, Klecany, Czech Republic

Rafaela Zorzanelli, Rio de Janeiro State University, Brazil

CHAPTER 1

....

INTRODUCTION

....

GIOVANNI STANGHELLINI, MATTHEW R. BROOME,
ANTHONY VINCENT FERNANDEZ, PAOLO FUSAR-
POLI, ANDREA RABALLO, AND RENÉ ROSFORT

WHAT IS PSYCHOPATHOLOGY?

....

THIS volume brings together cutting-edge research arising from the fertile relationship among phenomenology, psychopathology, clinical practice, and the patient's lived experience of mental disorders. Perhaps unsurprisingly, a rebirth of interest in conceptual and philosophical issues in psychiatry followed closely on the heels of "the decade of the brain" and advances in neurosciences (Fulford et al. 2003). With empirical scientific advancements comes the obligation to think critically about their broader significance, their impact on advancing knowledge, their place within current conceptual frameworks, and how these new findings can help us better understand mental suffering and improve care for persons living with mental disorders. This historical moment, just over one hundred years after the publication of the first edition of Karl Jaspers's *General Psychopathology*, is similar to the conceptual terrain of the "first biological psychiatry" in which Jaspers found himself in the early twentieth century (Shorter 1997). We are in the heyday of a new reductionistic wave propelled, in part, by the US National Institute of Mental Health's Research Domain Criteria (RDoC) project, which aims to provide a new research classification founded on the assumption that mental disorders are disorders of brain circuitry (Insel and Cuthbert 2015; Akram and Giordano 2017). However, psychiatry is not only a biological discipline. It must maintain an intense concern with the quality of our patients' experiences (Broome 2009; Ratcliffe and Broome 2011; Stanghellini and Broome 2014; Fernandez and Stanghellini in press). In fact, the primary focus of psychiatry is the "psyche" and not the brain, which is of interest to psychiatry only insofar as it helps us to better understand the relevant psychic phenomena. Thus, we must investigate the relationship between these subjective experiences, the brain, and the way we classify psychiatric disorders. Phenomenological psychopathology is increasingly central to these discussions (Stanghellini and Rossi 2014).

However, it's not enough simply to acknowledge that psychiatry's primary domain of investigation is the psyche. At present, the psychiatric study of psyche and subjectivity is defined mainly by changes in experience and behavior—not (or, at least, not uncontroversially) in terms of biological abnormalities. In fact, to date, there are no established and validated biomarkers for clinical use in psychiatry (Kapur, Philips, and Insel 2012; Fusar-Poli and Meyer-Lindenberg 2016). Therefore, psychopathology, the discipline that assesses and makes sense of the suffering psyche, is at the heart of psychiatry (Galderisi and Falkai 2018). In contemporary usage, the term "psychopathology" is employed in a number of different ways (Stanghellini 2009). It is commonly conflated with *symptomatology*—the study of isolated symptoms in view of their clinical, that is, diagnostic and aetiological, significance. Assessing symptoms allows for the identification of specific diagnostic categories that, in turn, facilitate clinical care. Psychopathology certainly includes the study of symptoms, but it is not reducible to this kind of study. Whereas symptomatology is strictly disease- or illness-oriented, psychopathology is also *person*-oriented since it attempts to describe a patient's experience and her relationship to her experiences and to the world. Biomedical science was built on the transformation of a complaint into a symptom. This allowed medical science to see in a complaint—for example, exhaustion—the effect of a cause situated in the human body—for example, an anatomical anomaly or biochemical imbalance. This may overshadow the fact that a complaint has not only a *cause*, but also a *meaning*, which expresses a question or desire. A person may seek not only the resolution of her complaint, but also the fulfillment of her aspiration to understand how this complaint fits into her existence. Biomedical science—with all its authority and success—risks excluding the subjectivity of patients and the meaning that their symptoms hold for them. A phenomenological approach to psychopathology does not exclude the possibility or utility of viewing abnormal phenomena as symptoms caused by a dysfunction to be treated or ameliorated. However, the phenomenological approach explores lived experience and personal meaning alongside the hunt for causes. The patient, as a person, should be acknowledged as an active partner in the diagnostic process, capable of interpreting her own complaints. On this approach, symptoms are taken as the outcome of a mediation between a vulnerable self and the sick person trying to cope and make sense of her complaints (Stanghellini 2016).

"Psychopathology" has also been used as a synonym of *nosography*. The latter outlines provisional and conventional characteristics of a syndrome (i.e. a combination of symptoms empirically and statistically aggregated) and thereby serves the goal of classification which is essential to formulating a clinical diagnosis. However, psychopathology is not only about diagnosis and is not, therefore, reducible to nosography. To psychopathology, what matters most is that the "chaos of phenomena" should stand out in an evident way and in multiple connections. Psychopathology aims to make sense of, or comprehend, that which at first seems incomprehensible (Fernandez and Stanghellini in press). It promotes explicit attention to the person's whole field of experience, rather than a restricted focus on symptoms selected according to their putative diagnostic *relevance*. The existing classifications of mental illnesses are provisional diagnostic conventions. Since no extraclinical (e.g. biological) indexes of putative nosological discontinuities are available, our current taxonomy is based exclusively on psychopathologically defined syndromes. Hence psychopathology is still the primary method of linking symptoms and diagnosis in psychiatry. Yet, if psychopathology is conflated with nosography, then only those symptoms that are assumed to have diagnostic value will be investigated. We stand in a sort of nosography-focused twilight state where we wear clinical blinkers structured by contemporary classificatory systems (Andreasen 2006). The dominant focus on diagnosis covers over many of the actual experiences of people suffering from mental disorders. As a consequence, clinical utility is confined to ad hoc bits of information useful for clinical decision-making. By confining our study to the phenomena that we have already deemed relevant to diagnosis, we neglect the diverse elements of the patients' experience—thus limiting our capacity to understand the worlds they live in and closing us off to the discovery of new psychopathological knowledge (Lawrie et al. 2016; First et al. 2018; Maj 2018; Reed et al. 2018).

PHENOMENOLOGICAL PSYCHOPATHOLOGY AS THE BASIC SCIENCE OF PSYCHIATRY

There are at least six reasons why phenomenological psychopathology is a the heart of psychiatry (Stanghellini and Fiorillo 2015):

1) Psychiatry is an interdisciplinary field adopting multiple languages to deconstruct the complexity of the suffering psyche. Practitioners approach their discipline from many different angles, including neuroscience, sociology, genetics, epidemiology, dynamic or cognitive psychology, etc., each of which has its own language, methodology, and practice. Psychiatrists therefore need a common ground and a shared language if they want to understand each other. Phenomenological psychopathology is not one of numerous approaches aiming to conceptualize mental disorders—such as psychoanalysis or the cognitive sciences. Phenomenological psychopathology develops a framework for approaching mental illness in which theoretical assumptions are minimized and the forms and contents of the patient's subjective experience are prioritized. Although the emphasis on subjectivity looks like a theoretical commitment, that commitment is the product of a stance that seeks to respect the phenomenon rather than impose upon it. Thus, phenomenological psychopathology can be understood as *psychopathologia prima* and the basic science of psychiatry—it is the shared language that allows clinicians with different theoretical backgrounds to understand each other when dealing with mental disorders.

2) Psychiatry aims to establish *rigorous diagnoses*. Phenomenological psychopathology plays a central role in a field where the major disorders cannot be neuroscientifically defined as disease entities, but are exclusively syndromes that can be defined only in terms of symptoms. Neurophysiological, biochemical, endocrinological, neuroanatomical, cognitive, or behavioral measures (i.e. endophenotypes) help to improve the diagnosis of mental disorders. But we also need a phenomenological clarification of experiential traits and constructs (i.e. pheno-phenotypes). Even if we aim for a neuroscientific classification, we must accurately delineate the experiential phenomena that we want to explain or reduce to neuroscientific terms. As an example, "delusion" is a heterogeneous category that must be split into more specific sub-categories to successfully identify its neurobiological correlates (Stanghellini and Raballo 2015). In addition, the use of the "phenomenological razor" (Rossi Monti and Stanghellini 1996) is particularly useful in sorting out "psychopathological receptors." Even therapeutic decision-making, including accurately targeted pharmacological intervention, requires fine-grained distinctions among the abnormal phenomena that we aim to

treat (Stanghellini and Ramella Cravaro 2015). Phenomenology provides tools that can facilitate successful clinical diagnosis as well as the revision of our diagnostic categories (Fernandez 2016; Fernandez 2019).

3) Psychiatry is about *understanding* disturbed human experience, in addition to assessing, diagnosing, and classifying it. Phenomenological psychopathology functions as a bridge between human sciences and clinical sciences within psychiatric knowledge, thus providing the basic tools to make sense of mental suffering. The dominant focus on diagnosis and on those symptoms deemed relevant for nosographical diagnosis disregards the complexity and diversity of people's experiences. Moreover, it excludes the scrutiny of what is relevant *from the patient's perspective*—the way in which one's vulnerability and suffering is distinctly personal. In mainstream practice, interviewing is seen as a technique that should conform to the technical-rational paradigm of natural sciences (namely laboratory techniques in biological sciences) in which psychiatry as a branch of biomedicine is positioned. Interview techniques are typically designed to reduce information variance and to elicit only "diagnostic-relevant" answers. Standard assessment procedures are devised in such a way that the patient's symptomatology needs to fit pre-existing diagnostic criteria, overlooking the subtle experiential differences and their meaning for the patient. Phenomenological psychopathology, on the contrary, wants to "give the word" to the patients, instead of merely assessing their abnormalities according to pre-structured interviews. This is the essential precondition to understand their wounded existence, and to open up to the discovery of new psychopathological knowledge (Nordgaard, Sass, and Parnas 2013).

4) Phenomenological psychopathology attempts to describe the diversity of experiential alterations and differences and to bracket common sense, socio-political, and scientific views about what is abnormal. Mainstream diagnostic concepts, for example, typically appeal to "social and occupational dysfunction," which is defined strictly in behavioral and quantitative terms (less than n social contacts per time unit) rather than being conceived as a consequence of typical and specific motivations, peculiarities of intersubjectivity, and of the values held by persons with a diagnosis of mental disorder. Phenomenological psychopathology is also about grasping what is human in apparently alienating (e.g. irrational or nonsensical) phenomena. We should remember that we, as clinical psychiatrists, do not usually sit in front of a broken brain—we sit in front of a suffering person. Indeed, mental disorders are primarily disorders of the human psyche. If the crucial task of psychiatry is understanding mental suffering, then its project should be to articulate the life-world of each person and identify the *conditions of possibility* for the emergence of pathological phenomena in human existence. This can shed light on the structure, meaning, and importance of the phenomenon at issue. Phenomenological psychopathology can help us rethink the meaning of psychopathological conditions.

5) Psychiatry is also about caring for troubled human existence, rather than judging, marginalizing, punishing, or stigmatizing it. Phenomenological psychopathology connects understanding with caring, and endeavors to establish an epistemological as well as ethical framework for this. This framework is a *dialogical* one. In some countries, phenomenological approaches have dramatically improved the care of psychiatric patients leading through the development of modern mental health models of care (Barbui et al. 2018). The kind of clinical practice promoted by phenomenological

psychopathology is fundamentally a quest for meaning. It encourages the patient to unfold his experiences and his personal horizon of meaning, helping him to reflect upon them and take a position on them. In this framework, the clinician promotes a reciprocal exchange of perspectives with his patient. The clinician and patient cooperate in the co-construction of a meaningful narrative that includes and, if possible, integrates contributions from both original perspectives. And, when it is not possible to establish consensus, the clinician should facilitate coexistence of apparently conflicting values and beliefs, embracing a diversity of perspectives (Stanghellini and Mancini 2017; Broome 2009).

6) Psychiatry looks for a way to connect first-person experience with brain functioning. Phenomenological psychopathology aims to bridge understanding (*Verstehen*) and causal explanation (*Erklären*) in research as well as in clinical settings. As the science of abnormal subjectivity, psychopathology relies both on explanations based on deductive and inductive methods, and on understanding that is achievable only by immersing oneself in a singular situation. Phenomenological psychopathology in itself is prior to any causal accounts of subpersonal mechanisms. At least some of the inconsistent and heterogeneous results in neuroscience research are perhaps the result of insufficient knowledge in descriptive psychopathology. Basic psychopathological knowledge is a prerequisite for research in explanatory psychopathologies and it can help clarify fundamental concepts in biological psychiatry. We must accurately describe the phenomenon before we can arrive at a satisfying explanation. This is not a new agenda. It was Karl Jaspers's principal aim when he founded psychopathology as the basic science for psychiatry in the early twentieth century (Broome 2013; Stanghellini and Fuchs 2013).

Section Outlines

The Handbook is Divided into Seven Sections. Section One—*History*—is edited by Anthony Vincent Fernandez and René Rosfort. This section includes intellectual biographies of leading figures of the phenomenological movement, including philosophers such as Husserl, Stein, Heidegger, Gadamer, Sartre, Beauvoir, Merleau-Ponty, Ricoeur, and Levinas, as well as psychiatrists and psychologists such as Jaspers, Binswanger, Boss, Fanon, Laing, Minkowski, Straus, Kretschmer, Tellenbach, Blankenburg, Kimura, and Basaglia. This section provides a broad historical and intellectual background, which highlights two key points. First, it illustrates the variety of research methods and topics that fall under the label of "phenomenology." Second, it demonstrates that psychiatric and psychopathological research has had an intimate and fruitful relationship with philosophical phenomenology.

Section Two—*Foundations and Methods*—is edited by Anthony Vincent Fernandez and René Rosfort. Phenomenology is often characterized by its method or approach, rather than by its subject matter. However, whereas most phenomenologists agree that method is key to the identity of phenomenology, they rarely agree on what, exactly, phenomenology's methods are and should be. This situation is made even more complex when phenomenology is applied to interdisciplinary contexts, such as psychopathology. Once phenomenology enters into conversation with the needs of clinical practice and scientific, empirical approaches to psychiatric research, its methodological identity needs to be clarified and adapted. This section addresses these issues. First, it provides accounts of phenomenology's broad approach—including descriptive, transcendental, and hermeneutic methods—its subject matter, and its focus on the temporal and intersubjective aspects of experience, such as phenomenological notions of normality and abnormality. Second, it provides accounts of phenomenology's relationship with naturalism, the cognitive sciences, and introspective methods.

Section Three—*Key Concepts*—is edited by Matthew Broome and Giovanni Stanghellini. This section includes the definition of key theoretical concepts, for example, self, emotion, consciousness, the unconscious, intentionality, personhood, values, embodiment, autonomy, alterity, *Beflindlichkeit*, time, moral conscience and explanation and understanding. The contributors show how the meanings of these terms came about through phenomenological work, and how they can be used in clinical and research settings. Each term is briefly defined in light of its use in the standard psychiatric, psychological, and neuroscientific literature. Then each chapter offers some accounts of the ways phenomenologists have reconceived these notions. This section's main aim is to show how phenomenological reconceptualization of notions used in psychiatry, psychology, and the sciences offers clarification and insight into what sometimes were previously ambiguous concepts.

Section Four—*Descriptive Psychopathology*—is edited by Andrea Raballo and Matthew Broome. This section includes an account of basic abnormal psychic phenomena and each chapter provides descriptions, definitions, and vignettes of a type of abnormal phenomenon. These areas of psychopathology include consciousness and its disorders, the experience of time and its disorders, disorders of attention, concentration, and memory, thought, speech, and language and associated disorders, affectivity and its disorders, selfhood and associated disorders, vital anxiety, phenomenal consciousness and hallucinations, disorders of bodily experience, catatonia, eating disorders, grief, gender dysphoria, the psychopathology of hysteria, dissociation, conversion and somatization, obsessions and phobias, and thought passivity.

Section Five—*Life-Worlds*—is edited by Giovanni Stanghellini and Anthony Vincent Fernandez. Whereas Section Three deals with particular abnormal phenomena, this section takes a more holistic approach. By "life-world" we mean the reality as it appears and is self-evident from the perspective of a given person. This approach provides accounts of how psychopathological phenomena are organized into a coherent gestalt, with core disturbances in one aspect of subjectivity motivating disturbances and alterations across the full scope of one's experience. As lived experience is always situated within the grounds of body, time, space, and others, each kind of psychopathological life-world can be described through an investigation of each of these features of lived experience. This section includes the description of the life-worlds of persons affected by hysteria, phobias, obsessions, borderline personality disorder, feeding and eating disorders, melancholia, mania, schizophrenia, and addictions.

Section Six—*Clinical Psychopathology*—is edited by Matthew Broome and Paolo Fusar-Poli. This section includes chapters discussing the connection between symptoms and current categorical diagnosis in mainstream diagnostic manuals, and how phenomenological psychopathology may be able to improve this. The "phenomenological razor" is used to sharpen the clinician's capacity to establish a valid and reliable classification through symptom assessment. The associations between particular abnormal phenomena and particular kinds of life-worlds are also discussed, figuring out what kinds of life-worlds the patients inhabit when particular abnormal phenomena are expressed. Topics discussed in this section include first-rank symptoms, schizophrenic delusions, paranoiac delusions, delusional mood, auditory verbal hallucinations, affective temperaments, schizophrenic autism, dysphoria and borderline condition, high-risk psychosis, psychopathology and the law, the clinical significance of atmospheres, psychopathy, and trauma.

Section Seven—*Phenomenological Psychopathology: Present and Future*—is edited by Paolo Fusar-Poli and Matthew Broome. This section demonstrates how phenomenological psychopathology can contribute to a variety of disciplines that are partially embedded in psychiatric knowledge and that deal with abnormal human subjectivity. And, reciprocally, it demonstrates how these disciplines can and should inform phenomenological investigations. The topics covered include neuroscience, the bodily self in phenomenology and neuroscience, qualitative research, quantitative research, psychotherapy, ethics, politics and society, clinician training, classification, clinical decision-making, psychoanalysis, autobiography, and neurodiversity.

BIBLIOGRAPHY

Akram F. and Giordano J. (2017). "Research Domain Criteria as Psychiatric Nosology: Conceptual, Practical and Neuroethical Implications." *Cambridge Quarterly of Healthcare Ethics* 26: 592–601.

Andreasen N. C. (2006). "DSM and the Death of Phenomenology in America: An Example of Unintended Consequences." *Schizophrenia Bulletin* 33(1): 108–112. doi:10.1093/schbul/sbl054

Barbui C., Papola D., and Saraceno B. (2018). "Forty Years Without Mental Hospitals in Italy." *International Journal of Mental Health Systems* Jul 31;12: 43. doi: 10.1186/s13033-018-0223-1. eCollection 2018 PMID: 30079100.

Broome M. R. (2009). "Philosophy as the Science of Value: Neo-Kantianism as a Guide to Psychiatric Interviewing." *Philosophy, Psychiatry, & Psychology* 15(2): 107–116. doi:10.1353/ppp.0.0172

Broome M. R. (2013). "Jaspers and Neuroscience." *Oxford Medicine Online.* doi:10.1093/med/9780199609253.003.0009

Fernandez A. V. (2016) "Phenomenology, Typification, and Ideal Types in Psychiatric Diagnosis and Classification." In R. Bluhm (ed.), *Knowing and Acting in Medicine*, pp. 39–58. Lanham: Rowman & Littlefield International.

Fernandez A. V. (2019) "Phenomenology and Dimensional Approaches to Psychiatric Research and Classification." *Philosophy, Psychiatry & Psychology.*

Fernandez A. V. and G. Stanghellini (in press). "Comprehending the Whole Person: On Expanding Jaspers' Notion of Empathy." In A. L. Mishara, P. Corlett, P. Fletcher, A. Kranjec, and M. A. Schwartz (eds.), *Phenomenological Neuropsychiatry: How Patient Experience Bridges Clinic with Clinical Neuroscience.* New York: Springer.

First M. B., Rebello T. J., Keeley J. W., et al. (2018). "Do Mental Health Professionals Use Diagnostic Classifications the Way We Think They Do? A Global Survey." *World Psychiatry* 17(2): 187–195.

Fulford K. W. M., Morris K. J., Sadler J. Z., and Stanghellini G. (2003). "Past Improbable, Future Possible: The Renaissance in Philosophy and Psychiatry." In K. W. M. Fulford, K. J. Morris, J. Z. Sadler, and G. Stanghellini (eds.), *Nature and Narrative: An Introduction to the New Philosophy of Psychiatry*, pp. 1–41. Oxford: Oxford University Press. doi:10.1093/med/9780198526117.003.0001

Fusar-Poli P. and Meyer-Lindenberg A. (2016). "Forty Years of Structural Imaging in Psychosis: Promises and Truth." *Acta Psychiatrica Scandinavica* 134(3): 207–224. doi: 10.1111/acps.12619 Epub 2016 Jul 12. Review. PMID: 27404479.

Galderisi S. and Falkai P. (2018). "Psychiatry and Psychiatrists: Fourteen Core Statements." *European Psychiatry* 52: 136–138. doi: 10.1016/j.eurpsy.2018.05.013 PMID: 29914673

Insel T. and Cuthbert B. N. (2015). "Brain Disorders? Precisely: Precision Medicine Comes to Psychiatry." *Science* 348(6234): 499–500.

Kapur S., Phillips A. G., and Insel T. R. (2012): "Why Has It Taken So Long for Biological Psychiatry to Develop Clinical Tests and What To Do About It?" *Molecular Psychiatry* 17(12): 1174–1179. doi: 10.1038/mp.2012.105 Epub 2012 Aug 7. PMID: 22869033.

Lawrie S. M., O'Donovan M. C., Saks E., Burns T., and Lieberman J. A. (2016). "Improving Classification of Psychoses." *Lancet Psychiatry* 3(4): 367–374.

Maj M. (2018). "Why the Clinical Utility of Diagnostic Categories in Psychiatry is Intrinsically Limited and How We Can Use New Approaches to Complement Them." *World Psychiatry* 17(2): 121–122.

Nordgaard J., Sass L. A., and Parnas J. (2013). "The Psychiatric Interview: Validity, Structure, and Subjectivity." *European Archives of Psychiatry and Clinical Neuroscience* 263: 353–364.

Ratcliffe M. and Broome M. R. (2011). "Existential Phenomenology, Psychiatric Illness, and the Death of Possibilities." In S. Crowell (ed.), *The Cambridge Companion to Existentialism*, pp. 361–382. Cambridge: Cambridge University Press. doi:10.1017/CCOL9780521513340.018

Reed G. M., Sharan P., Rebello T. J., et al. (2018). "The ICD-11 Developmental Field Study of Reliability of Diagnoses of High-Burden Mental Disorders: Results Among Adult Patients in Mental Health Settings of 13 Countries." *World Psychiatry* 17(2): 174–186.

Rossi Monti M. and Stanghellini G. (1996). Psychopathology: An Edgeless Razor? *Comprehensive Psychiatry* 37(3): 196–204.

Shorter E. (1997). *A History of Psychiatry*. New York: Wiley.

Stanghellini G. (2009). "The Meanings of Psychopathology." *Current Opinion in Psychiatry* 22(6): 559–564. doi:10.1097/YCO.0b013e3283318e36

Stanghellini G. (2016). *Lost in Dialogue*. Oxford: Oxford University Press.

Stanghellini G. and Fuchs T. (2013) *One Century of Karl Jaspers' General Psychopathology*. Oxford: Oxford University Press.

Stanghellini G. and Broome M. R. (2014). "Psychopathology as the Basic Science of Psychiatry." *The British Journal of Psychiatry* 205(3): 169–170. doi:10.1192/bjp.bp.113.138974

Stanghellini G. and Rossi R. (2014). "Pheno-Phenotypes: A Holistic Approach to the Psychopathology of Schizophrenia." *Current Opinion in Psychiatry* 27(3): 236–241. doi:10.1097/YCO.0000000000000059

Stanghellini G. and Fiorillo A. (2015). "Five Reasons for Teaching Psychopathology." *World Psychiatry* 14(1): 107–108. doi:10.1002/wps.20200

Stanghellini G. and Raballo A. (2015). "Differential Typology of Delusions in Major Depression and Schizophrenia: A Critique to the Unitary Concept of 'Psychosis'." *Journal of Affective Disorders* 171: 171–178. doi:10.1016/j.jad.2014.09.027

Stanghellini G. and Ramella Cravaro V. (2015). "The Phenomenological Dissection in Psychopathology." *Journal of Psychopathology* Feb 20: 345–350.

Stanghellini G. and Mancini M. (2017). *The Therapeutic Interview in Mental Health*. Cambridge: Cambridge University Press.

SECTION ONE

....

HISTORY

....

SECTION EDITORS: ANTHONY VINCENT
FERNANDEZ AND RENÉ ROSFORT

CHAPTER 2

....

EDMUND HUSSERL

....

ROBERTA DE MONTICELLI

THE "FUNCTIONARY OF HUMANITY"

....

PHENOMENOLOGY, as a method of philosophical research, a style of thinking, and an intellectual and moral attitude toward the world, is better identified by its living exercise than by the doctrines of its classics, including those of its recognized founder, Edmund Husserl (1859–1938). Yet when it comes to such a complex, diverse—and dramatic—object as the variety of mental disorders and psychic suffering, a grasp of the very spirit of "the founder" becomes essential. More than being the founder of a philosophical movement, Husserl was tireless in pursuing meaning, order, value, and coherence within ordinary experience and everyday life. This approach allowed him to shed a powerful light on what life and experience can be like when lacking such qualities.

Husserl sees himself as a pupil of Socrates and, like him, as a "beginner" in philosophy. He never tires of repeating it: that recurrent sophistic attitude which "deprives life of any rational sense" and lived experience of any relation to truth and value, and first motivated Socratic questioning, rekindles even now a need for philosophy and "the examined life" (Husserl 1956: 11). Husserl, the "functionary of humanity," had a caring, almost medical attitude toward pathogenic obstacles to the growth of individuation, inner freedom, moral responsibility, and cognitive plasticity of which personal flourishing ideally consists (Husserl 1976: 15).

There are many themes in Husserl's thought that are inspiring sources for phenomenological psychopathology. We shall reconstruct Husserlian phenomenology out of six of them, relating them to some major issues and authors in the literature on psychopathology.

FROM STUMPF'S LAB AND CANTOR'S PARADISE TO THE LIFE-WORLD

....

Husserl's intellectual career starts at the University of Halle, where the young mathematician, psychologist, and philosopher defended his postdoctoral Dissertation *On the Concept of Numbers* on June 28, 1887, with two great innovators, respectively, of mathematics and experimental psychology, Georg Cantor and Carl Stumpf, on his examining board (Schumann 1977: 17). Husserl had already been an assistant to Carl Weierstrass, another major figure in that "foundational crisis" which originated set theory, formal mathematics, and modern symbolic logic. In Vienna, Franz Brentano had introduced him to the new discipline of empirical psychology. There he would work out the key concept of intentionality he famously took over from Brentano, the basic conceptual tool for a phenomenological theory of consciousness. But it is in Stumpf's lab where they collaborated on what they called *experimental phenomenology* (Albertazzi 2013), a pioneering set of research projects on perception that Husserl continued while preparing his *Philosophy of Arithmetic* (Husserl 1970) and later his *Logical Investigations* (Husserl 1975, 1984). Husserl's thought was born at the crossroads of two scientific revolutions: one in the world of ideal objects and a priori thought and the other in the world of experience and a posteriori knowledge. The generating core of phenomenology is made up of these two ingredients that in Husserl's thought give rise to a radically new conception of both worlds—the ideal and the empirical, abstractness and concreteness—and of their intimate link (Husserl 1977a: 7–18). Focusing on this point should allow us to grasp the unity and coherence of Husserl's thought throughout his career, for it is the very same point he made in the first and last pages of his corpus: *Philosophy of Arithmetic* and the *Crisis* (Husserl 1976). As we shall see, this point is also the very foundation of what is specific to *phenomenological* psychopathology in many of its varieties and to its corresponding clinical attitude toward the patient.

Back to the Things Themselves

Let's turn our attention to the very motto of phenomenologists: "Back to the things themselves." This dictum expresses a basic principle of phenomenology, that is, *the principle of priority of the given over the construed.* Of course, in itself there is nothing uniquely phenomenological about this principle. It is a typical feature of empiricism. What phenomenology rejects about empiricism is the idea of sensory atomism, that is, a lack of structure in the given (the phenomenal world) *as such.* That is, contrary to Kant's formless "manifold of the intuition," any phenomenal object has form or structure *as given to the senses.*

This discovery—let's call it the gestalt principle—may well be the common ("Stumpfian") heritage of phenomenology and gestalt theory. Husserl advances beyond this principle through two important steps. The first step is a generalization from ordinary *perceptual* objects to all sorts of *intuitively given* ones, including ideal objects. The idea of a "figural moment" (a line of trees, a school of fish, a swarm of birds, etc.) is generalized into that of a structure with any content whatsoever. We do have structural intuitions: a letter-type, a geometric figure, the logical form of a proposition, such as $p \mathbin{\&} \neg p$. To be "self-given," in any modality of intuitive presence—be it sensory perception, emotional feeling, empathy, logical or mathematical intuition—is to be given as a structured, internally differentiated, organized whole, or as a part of it.

The second step is Husserl's rigorous foundation for an anti-reductive ontology of everyday life, rejecting physicalism as well as psychological atomism. He achieved this by generalizing the idea of gestalt into the idea of a structure with any content whatsoever, "keeping together" or "containing" partial contents. Is there a way of being "together" which is tighter than that of an arbitrary collection, or a mereological sum? Take a melody, and consider what you can't do if you don't want to disrupt it. You cannot change a note arbitrarily, without changing other notes accordingly. What you can change and how depends on the "contents" of the parts, not just as parts, but based on their function in the whole.

Eidos and the Irreducible Richness of the Life-World

The key notion of Husserl's mereology is that of Unity of Containment (or "unitary foundation"—*Einheitliche Fundierung*—in Husserl's terminology. This term refers to a bond on possible (co)variations of contents. This definition spells out what we saw in the case of the melody: for each part of the melody there are constraints on free variation relative to the other parts. You cannot vary a note and keep the others unchanged. In Husserl's terms, the part is not an independent or separable *bit*, but a dependent or inseparable *moment*. These constraints are "rooted in the contents" of the melody (Husserl 1984: 235–236).

We have in this way reached the most central notion of Husserlian phenomenology, and one of the most disputed in the Husserlian corpus: *eidos* or essence or material a priori. The *eidos* of a thing is not a separate universal: it is nothing but a bond or constraint on possible variations of the thing's contents, beyond the limits of which that thing ceases to exist or to be a "good" instance of that "kind of thing."

The results of these advancements can be summarized in three points: the principle of priority of the self-given over the construed, "saving" the phenomena or the richness of the sensible world, with all its secondary and tertiary qualities, all the colors and values of things; the principle of eidetic structure, providing empirical reality with intrinsic bounds or limits that any thing of a given sort—a mountain, a piece of music, a human being, a human civilization—must comply with or risk ceasing to exist; and, finally, the holistic principle forbidding reduction of a given entity to the sum of its component parts (of a melody to its tones, of a person to her or his parts such as body and mind). These principles come together, as three facets of the ontology of the concrete everyday world where the phenomenological philosopher is at home. In the *Crisis*, this is called the life-world: it is the world of all encounters, stimulating our cognitive curiosity and emotional responses, and in which our interests, choices, actions, culture, and institutions are rooted.

HUSSERLIAN ISSUES RELEVANT TO PHENOMENOLOGICAL PSYCHOPATHOLOGY

One can easily see the relevance of these principles to the clinical approach to the patient—and first of all to the appraisal of the patient's "melody." No version of the *Diagnostic and Statistical Manual of Mental Disorders*, including the current one, gives us an account of how the various symptoms of each disorder hang together in a concrete individual case. The differential diagnostics based on the presence of any sum of a minimal number of symptoms would not by itself be sufficient to grasp the "invariant style" (Binswanger 1923) or the "living plot" of the symptoms' bearer (Minkowski 1933). The problem with this operational approach is that the very "contents" of the individual case are missed. The classics of phe-nomenological psychopathology did in fact produce a sort of eidetic, not so much of the varieties of mental disease, as of the varieties of persons with mental suffering. Their study cases are sometimes paradigms of the method of eidetic variation on—and beyond—the bounds of normality, which end up with "gestalten," ideal-typical cases, which, at the same time, bear the mark of a personal individuality as required by the "inseparability of matter of fact and essence"(Husserl 1977a: 12, English translation at 8).

Naturalistic and Personalistic Attitudes—and the Epoché

A medical doctor in the exercise of her profession has to keep switching from a "personal-istic" to a "naturalistic" attitude toward her patient. This crucial conceptual distinction is introduced by Husserl as part of the description of the "world of the natural attitude," that is, the pre-theoretical everyday stance we find ourselves in when pursuing our habitual activi-ties in the surrounding world, dealing with things, encountering people, and taking their ex-istence for granted in our commitments and daily work routines (Husserl 1977a: 50–62). The "personalistic" attitude (*Einstellung*) is the one we *naturally*, pre-theoretically adopt when encountering persons: it is the right position (*Stellung*) corresponding to the *phenomenon* of personhood, that is, the "mode of presence" of another person. This is altogether different from the mode of presence of a thing. A person is perceived as such, as a center of spon-taneous action and affection, as a being endowed with sensibility and power, whose gaze can make me feel ashamed or move me to tears. "Empathy" is the technical phenomenolog-ical term to denote those modes of consciousness, or experience, in which another subject is (immediately, preconceptually) given *as* a person. The personalistic attitude qualifies the "subjective pole" of any mode of consciousness whose "objective pole" is another person: its "position" is right if it is adequate to the *Seinsinn* or "noema," the apparent "meaning" of the presented being, often an adult, morally autonomous and self-responsible human being. The personalistic attitude is the "natural" intersubjective attitude, as opposed to the "naturalistic" attitude, or the scientific and technical one the medical doctor has to adopt when operating on my stomach. She will have to switch back to the personalistic one when consulting my will or informing me about her diagnosis.

Note that the preceding description has been made possible by focusing on our pre-theoretical attitude, and its "naive," uncritical confidence in the solid ground of reality we are immersed in and surrounded by. Doing this means "bracketing" the overall commitment to reality built into the natural attitude or "suspending" this natural attitude to allow philo-sophical reflection on it: an exercise of "epoché," the gateway to phenomenology.

The peculiarity of phenomenological psychiatry, as opposed to the rest of the medical pro-fession, is that the personalistic attitude seems to become the appropriate one even at the spe-cifically clinical level, beyond the natural pre-theoretical phases of the clinical relation. The conceptualization of this difference is the legacy of Karl Jaspers. Both in clinical theory and therapeutic practice he conceives of psychopathology as a bold extension of folk psychology, which is what we engage in when trying to "understand" other people's motivations on the basis of the direct, "empathic" understanding we gather of their emotions and intentions through interpersonal communication. Yet this extension famously finds its limit at the very heart of the world of mental disorders with the apparent disruption of the "normal" motivational connections in typical cases of schizophrenia. Here empathic understanding (*Verstehen*) must be replaced by causal explanation (*Erklären*), and the psychiatrist's attitude becomes a "naturalistic" one (Jaspers 1959).

Reason and Normality

The exclusion of the personalistic attitude in the clinical relationship exactly where the very "drama of insanity" bursts out distinguishes the weak from the strict sense of phenomeno-logical psychopathology (Minkowski 1966). Overcoming Jaspers's limit, making sense even of delusions, is the first achievement of a phenomenologically inspired psychiatry.

While any state of consciousness is a lived experience (*Erlebnis*), not all lived experi-ence is an encounter with reality (*Erfahrung*), or, in Husserl's terminology, an "originarily presenting" consciousness, presenting reality "in flesh and bones" (Husserl 1977a: 11; Spiegelberg 1972: xliv). Sensory perception is the paradigm of *Erfahrung*, not its only form. Emotional feeling presents the value-qualities of reality; empathy presents the embodied subjective aspects of it. The mark of an encounter with reality is fallibility—and corrigibility.

The major innovation of Husserl's concept of intentionality with respect to Brentano's lies in the ability to distinguish among the different intentional structures of different modes of consciousness, particularly of the modes which are susceptible to encounters with reality. This is no longer just the "aboutness" or direction toward an object characteristic of most mental states. No classical phenomenologist has been as aware as Husserl of the importance of *both* poles of the intentional relation. Perception, as we have seen, can get reality wrong and correct itself. It would not be able to do this if it were just a function of the causal impact of reality on the sensory organs. Perception has a claim of validity built into it, expressed by its "positional" subjective pole. It tacitly claims that the perceived thing is there and transcends the actually present side of it, like a cube seen by its front face. This further virtu-ally infinite source of information, which is given as the horizon of any perceptual certainty, is exactly what we call "reality." We could not "learn from experience" if we could not further explore that horizon, turning false positions of certainty into perplexity, doubt, conjecture. Because of its veridicality claim, perception is "under the jurisdiction of reason" (Husserl 1977a: 259). But *any* experience reveals itself to be under this "jurisdiction," for any experi-ence has a positionality of its own. An emotion can be inappropriate; a desire, misguided; a decision, bad; a judgment, false. Any intentional state is subject to questioning with regard to its "positional" validity claim. This, according to Husserl, is Socrates's wonderful discovery about consciousness, and it leads to the birth of philosophy.

This is also the reason why phenomenology, as a study of consciousness, cannot be reduced to descriptive psychology, as Brentano thought. For consciousness, even at its most basic level of embodiment in the sensible and social world, is "under the jurisdiction of reason" (Husserl 1977a: 259). Note that the limited concept of intentionality inherited from Brentano is also the current one in most contemporary analytic philosophy of mind. In fact, intentionality is usually explained as "directedness" or "aboutness," or the property that a mental state usually has to be "about" an object (Searle 1983: 1; Chalmers 1996: 19; Crane 2001: 13). In contrast, Husserl's theory of intentionality as involving positionality as well at its subjective pole, and hence potentially a quest for adequacy or *reason*, provides the key concept for a fine-grained analysis of the ways this quest is escaped through illusion, self-deception, biased and uncritical thinking, or irrationality. "Man is a normative animal," as Husserl has it (Husserl 1988: 59), and a pretty reluctant one.

How does this all concern psychopathology? It does so by helping it to disambiguate its basic category, that of "normality/abnormality." "Normality" has a statistical/factual sense and a normative one. The most significant when thinking of mental disorders is the latter. Yet fear of undue interference of morality in the realm of medicine keeps mainstream psychiatry clinging to the former. This does not do justice to what we consider real impairment of free will and agency, often significant enough to excuse psychotic patients from penal and moral responsibility—not to mention failures to adequately address the difference between "madness" and dissent from social conventions, ignorance of which can lead to the worst abuses of medical power.

Variations of Global Motivational Structures

The impact of Husserl's fine-grained analysis of embodied normality on psychopathology goes even deeper. It gives rise to two main conceptual advances: the typology of (deviant) norms and forms of being-in-the-world (Binswanger 1960; Straus 1966; von Gebsattel 1954), each corresponding to a deep and characteristic alteration of the whole personality more than to nosographic categories (Minkowski 1933); and the identification of the basic and global nature of pathogenic deviation from normality, the "loss of natural evidence" (Blankenburg 1971). The link between the two can be found in a quote Binswanger famously comments upon, from Husserl's *Formal and Transcendental Logic*: "The real world *is* only under a presumption, constantly renewed, that experience ought to always unfold in the same constitutive style" (Binswanger 1960: 24). Now, as Husserl constantly shows through his "constitutive" analyses, the ordinary "constitutive style" of reality depends on at least four covariant variables: the structures of lived space, those of lived time, those of inter-subjectivity, and those of basic self-constitution. A major alteration of the norm can occur along any of these axes, issuing in a different "constitutive style" of lived experience—and yielding the phenomenology of psychiatric alienation as described by phenomenological psychopathologists.

The Loss of Natural Evidence

"Negative" symptoms (such as affective flattening, impoverishment of speech and language, anhedonia, attentional impairment) can underlie major positive symptoms of schizophrenia such as hallucinations and delusions, but can also subsist without them, as in chronic difficulty in a person's relationship toward reality and other people. Husserl's constitutive analysis offers a powerful frame for understanding this difficulty. It is as if the "presumption" concerning the customary style of evidence had gone missing—as if the familiarity of the common world had been disrupted. It is as if that *epoché* with which a phenomenologist "brackets" all tacit assumptions of common sense had fallen upon a person like a spell, dissolving the bedrock of normal interaction and linguistic communication, the "background" of tacit rules (Wittgenstein 2001) or the "underground" (Schneider 1950) of such rules that provide the "continuous consistency [*Kontinuerliche Einstimmigkeit*]" of ordinary experience (Husserl 1977b: 206). Wolfgang Blankenburg famously called this condition "a loss of natural evidence" (Blankenburg 1971). As a consequence, nothing in the life-world can be taken for granted, no fluid habit of action can be acquired—"common sense" falls apart.

Levels of Self-Constitution: The Lived Body

Self-constitution is the basic, pre-reflective experience we have of ourselves. Selfhood is normally "given" with the ordinary experience of other things and persons as the living, subjective pole of this experience, "taking positions," being passively motivated, "struck" by all salient qualities of the surrounding world. Mainstream cognitive research considers typical schizophrenic delusions of thought insertion, "voices," etc., to be effects of a dysfunction in the self-monitoring mechanism of the brain (Frith 1992). Yet far from being a second-order supplement to basic experience, pre-reflective self-awareness is *constitutive* of embodied perception, as Husserl has shown by describing the spatial horizon of action-and-perception, where objects occupy positions in a self-centered system of coordinates structured by gravity and kinaesthesia (Husserl 1952: 144–161). The key concept of this domain of analysis is the *Leib/Körper* distinction, that is, the distinction between the organism that obviously supports all mental life but is only given as an object, in a naturalistic attitude, from a third-person perspective; and our lived body, or the body experienced from a first-person perspective, as the origin of this perspective, "flagged up" by pain and pleasure, lived through one's sense of agency and power (Straus 1969). After Husserl, different ingredients of basic self-awareness—sense of agency, sense of ownership, cenesthesia (Schneider 1950; Jaspers 1959; Gallagher 2005), tactile sensibility (Merleau-Ponty 1942), and emotional sensibility (Scheler 1980; Ratcliffe 2008; Fuchs 2013) have been identified and made available to the psychopathology of selfhood (Stanghellini 2006). For example, Josef Parnas, Dan Zahavi, and colleagues have designed EASE, a psychometric tool which has already been translated into nine languages and is used to measure disorders of self-experience in patients at risk of developing schizophrenia (Parnas et al. 2005; Zahavi 2000).

Common Sense and Social Interaction and Cognition

It is a phenomenological fact, demonstrated by Husserl's research and by that of his collaborators on social interaction and cognition (Husserl 1973; Stein 2008), that both the constitution of a common, intersubjective world and the constitution of oneself depend on primary intersubjectivity, the foundation of which is the mother–child pair. Italian phenomenological psychopathology in particular has underlined the importance of this fact, which grounds the very possibility of interpersonal therapeutics, where the psychiatrist can offer his "patient consciousness" (Calvi 2013) as a mirror and resource for completion of a partially failed or distorted self-constitution (Calvi 1996). The discovery of mirror neurons as the neurobiological foundations of primary intersubjectivity (Gallese 2006; Rizzolatti and Sinigaglia 2006) have revived the rich phenomenology of pre-reflective attunement, encounter, primary socialization, and interaction which animated early phenomenology by updating it through criticism of alternative models of social cognition such as theory of mind and simulation theory (Zahavi 2011). This revival of empathy research has had a significant impact on contemporary psychopathological research on autism (Ballerini et al. 2006).

BIBLIOGRAPHY

Albertazzi L. (ed.) (2013). *Handbook of Experimental Phenomenology*. Oxford: Wiley Blackwell.

Binswanger L. (1992–1994). *Ausgewählte Werke in 4 Bänden*. Heidelberg: Roland Asanger.

Binswanger L. (1923). *Über Phänomenologie*. "Zschr. Ges. Neur. u. Psychiat." In Binswanger L. (1947). *Ausgewählte Vorträge und Aufsätze*, Bd I: 13–49. Bern: Francke.

Binswanger L. (1960). *Melancholie und Manie. Phänomenologische Studien*. Pfullingen: Neske.

Blankenburg W. (1971). *Der Verlust der natürlichen Selbstverständlichkeit. Ein Beitrag zur Psychopathologie symptomarmer Schizophrenien*. Stuttgart: Enke.

Ballerini A., Barale F., Ucelli S., and Gallese V. (eds.) (2006) *Autismo. L'umanità nascosta*. Torino: Einaudi.

Ballerini A. and Callieri B. (eds.) (1996). *Breviario di psicopatologia*. Milano: Feltrinelli.

Calvi L. (1996). Il fremito della carne e l'anancastico. *Contributo alla comprensione degli ossesivi e dei fobici*. in Ballerini A. and Callieri B. (eds.) (1996), pp. 51–58.

Calvi L. (2013). *La coscienza paziente. Esercizi per una cura fenomenologica*. Roma: Giovanni Fioriti Editore.

Chalmers D. J. (1996). *The Conscious Mind*. Oxford: Oxford University Press.

Crane T. (2001). *Elements of Mind—An Introduction to the Philosophy of Mind*. Oxford: Oxford University Press.

Frith C. D. (1992). *Cognitive Neuropsychology of Schizophrenia*. Sussex: Psychology Press.

Fuchs T. (2013). "The Phenomenology of Affectivity." In K. W. M. Fulford, M. Davies, R. G. T. Gipps, G. Graham, J. Z. Sadler, G. Stanghellini, and T. Thornton (eds.), *The Oxford Handbook of Philosophy and Psychiatry*, pp. 612–631. Oxford: Oxford University Press.

Husserl E. (1952). *Ideen zur einer reinen Phänomenologie und phänomenologischen Philosophie*. Zweites Buch: *Phänomenologische Untersuchungen zur Konstitution*. HUA 4. The Hague: Martinus Nijhoff.

Husserl E. (1956). *Erste Philosophie (1923/4)*. Erste Teil: Kritische Ideengeschichte. HUA 7. The Hague: Martinus Nijhoff.

Husserl E. (1970). *Philosophie der Arithmetik*. Mit ergänzenden Texten (1890–1901). HUA 12. The Hague: Martinus Nijhoff.

Husserl E. (1973). *Cartesianische Meditationen und Pariser Vorträge*. HUA 1. The Hague: Martinus Nijhoff.

Husserl E. (1975). *Logische Untersuchungen*. Erster Teil. Prolegomena zur reinen Logik. Text der 1. und der 2. Auflage. HUA 18. The Hague: Martinus Nijhoff.

Husserl E. (1976). *Die Krisis der europäischen Wissenschaften und die transzendentale Phänomenologie*. Eine Einleitung in die phänomenologische Philosophie. HUA 6. The Hague: Martinus Nijhoff.

Husserl E. (1977a). *Ideen zu einer reinen Phänomenologie und phänomenologischen Philosophie*. Erstes Buch: *Allgemeine Einführung in die reine Phänomenologie 1*. Halbband: Text der 1.-3. Auflage—Nachdruck HUA 3-1. The Hague: Martinus Nijhoff. (English translation (1982). *Ideas Pertaining to a Pure Phenomenology and to a Phenomenological Philosophy, First Book. General Introduction to a Pure Phenomenology*, trans. Fred Kersten).

Husserl E. (1977b). *Formale und Transzendentale Logik*. Band I: Versuch einer Kritik der Logischen Vernunft. Dordrecht: Kluwer Academic Publishers.

Husserl E. (1984). *Logische Untersuchungen*. Zweiter Teil. Untersuchungen zur Phänomenologie und Theorie der Erkenntnis. In zwei Bänden. HUA 19. The Hague, Netherlands: Martinus Nijhoff.

Husserl E. (1988b). "Formale Typen von Kultur in Menschheitsentwicklung (1923)." In E. Husserl, *Aufsätze und Vorträge. 1922–1937*, pp. 59–94. The Hague: Kluwer Academic Publishers.

Gallagher S. (2005). *How the Body Shapes the Mind*. Oxford: Oxford University Press.

Gallese V. (2006). "Intentional Attunement: A Neurophysiological Perspective on Social Cognition and its Disruption in Autism." *Brain Research* 1079: 5–24.

Jaspers K. (1959). *Allgemeine Psychopathologie*, 7. unveränderte Auflage. Heidelberg: Springer Verlag.

Merleau-Ponty M. (1942). *La structure du comportement*. Paris: Presses Universitaires de France.

Minkowski E. (1933). *Le temps vécu: études phénoménologiques et psychopathologiques*. Paris: Collection de l'évolution psychiatrique.

Minkowski E. (1966). *Traité de psychopathologie*. Paris: Presses Universitaires de France.

Parnas J., Møller P., Kircher T, Thalbitzer J., Jansson L., Handest P., and Zahavi D. (2005). "EASE. Examination of Anomalous Self-Experience." *Psychopathology* 38: 236–258.

Ratcliffe M. (2008). *Feelings of Being: Phenomenology, Psychiatry and the Sense of Reality*. Oxford: Oxford University Press

Rizzolatti G. and Sinigaglia C. (2006). *So quel che fai*. Milano: Cortina.

Scheler M. (1980). *Der Formalismus in der Ethik und die materiale Wertethik*. Bern: Francke Verlag.

Schneider K. (1950). *Klinische Psychopathologie*. Stuttgart: Thieme.

Schumann K. (1977). *Husserl-Chronik—Denk- und Lebensweg Edmund Husserls*. Den Haag: Martinis Nijhoff.

Searle J. R. (1983), *Intentionality*. Cambridge: Cambridge University Press

Spiegelberg H. (1972). *Phenomenology in Psychology and Psychiatry: A Historical Introduction*. Evanston: Northwestern University Press.

Stanghellini G. (2006). *Psicopatologia del senso comune*. Milano: Raffaello Cortina.

Stein E. (2008). *Zum Problem der Einfühlung*. Gesamtausgabe, Bd. 5. Freiburg: Herder.

Straus E. W. (1966). *Phenomenological Psychology*. London: Tavistock Publications.

Straus E. W. (1969). *Psychiatry and Philosophy*. Berlin: Springer Verlag.

von Gebsattel V. E. (1954). *Prolegomena einer medizinischen Anthropologie. Ausgewählte Aufsätze*. Berlin: Springer Verlag.

Wittgenstein L. (2001). *Philosophical Investigations*, trans. G. E. M. Anscombe. Oxford: Blackwell.

Zahavi D. (2011). "Empathy and Direct Social Perception: A Phenomenological Proposal." *Review of Philosophy and Psychology* 2: 541–558.

Zahavi D. (ed.) (2000). *Exploring the Self: Philosophical and Psychopathological Perspectives on Self-Experience*. Amsterdam: John Benjamins.

CHAPTER 3

THE ROLE OF PSYCHOLOGY ACCORDING TO EDITH STEIN

ANGELA ALES BELLO

INTRODUCTION

EDITH Stein (1891–1942) was one of Husserl's most talented students in Göttingen. In her dissertation on empathy from 1916, *On the Problem of Empathy*, composed under Husserl's guidance in Freiburg im Breisgau (Stein 2008), she applied his method to inter-subjective relations. During that time she also helped him with the transcriptions of his manuscripts, particularly the second volume of *Ideas Pertaining to a Pure Phenomenology and to a Phenomenological Philosophy* (Husserl 1989). Regarding the question of the phenomenological method, in her 1922 long essay entitled "Philosophy of Psychology and the Humanities" (Stein 1970), which I shall deal with later, she resumed some of the themes that Husserl had developed in his *Ideas* by placing the accent on consciousness as a flow of lived experiences (*Erlebnisstrom*), obtained after a change in the natural attitude (*epoché*). Through the Husserlian method it was possible to better describe how a human being is constituted starting from inside. She distanced herself from Heidegger, whom she would later criticize, kindly but robustly, and was closer to two of Husserl's other students: Hedwig Conrad-Martius and Gerda Walther.

Then her philosophy assumed a new intellectual course linked to her conversion from Judaism to Catholicism. The critical confrontation with the ideas of Husserl and Thomas Aquinas marked the beginning of a vast project of inquiry that involved Greek thought passing through medieval and modern philosophy to reach contemporary thought. Her intention was not to return to the past, but to seek the truth, and both phenomenology and the medieval philosophers—not only Aquinas, but also Augustine and Duns Scotus—were helpful in this attempt. She felt the need to get to grips with the traditional metaphysical questions, that is, the meaning of the human being, of the world, and of God. Her last and most important book was *Finite and Eternal Being* (Stein 2004), written while she was already a nun in the Carmel of Köln. In any case as regards the analysis of the human being, both in his/her individuality and inside the communities, she remained faithful to the phenomenological approach (Ales Bello 2002). The topic, in which she showed the originality of her approach, is represented, in fact, by the analysis of the human beings in their psychic and spiritual manifestations (Stein 2006a), in their gender differences (Stein 2000a), and in their community life (Stein 2006b). Because of the Nazis' persecution of Jews, she left Germany and entered into the Carmel in Echt Holland; while staying there she wrote *The Science of the Cross* on the mystical writings of St. John of the Cross (Stein 2003). However, the Nazis soon reached Holland too, and she was captured and sent to Auschwitz, where she died in 1942.

She was interested not only in philosophy but also in the development of the sciences, particularly the human sciences, and she dedicated a great deal of attention to the relationship between body and soul, challenging the conclusions of experimental psychology, which was still in its formative stages at the beginning of the twentieth century.

In 1922, Stein published a long essay, "*Beiträge zur philosophischen Begründung der Psychologie und der Geisteswissenschaften*" (Stein 1970; English translation: "Philosophy of Psychology and the Humanities" (Stein 2000b)) in the fifth volume of the *Jahrbuch für Philosophie und phänomenologische Forschung* (1922), edited by Husserl. This essay must be read against the background of the lively discussions at the time about the significance of psychology as a science; discussions in which Husserl, under the influence of his teachers, Franz Brentano and Wilhelm Maximilian Wundt, had participated as a young scholar.

In this work, she examines in a phenomenological manner the structures that experimental psychology employs and the claim that it is a scientific discipline. She argues that psychology fails to grasp the essential significance of psychic phenomena. The essay represented the realization of Husserl's project and, in Edith Stein's characteristic style, dealt with the matter with great clarity and analytical acuity.

PSYCHE AND CAUSALITY

Edith Stein begins with a question that recurs throughout the history of philosophy, but which became particularly important in the age of positivism: Is the human being subject to the bonds of causality that characterize the physical nature of which it is an integrated part?

Stein begins by examining a common and daily experience: I feel cold, but I can deceive myself as to the content of this sensation that I describe as "cold," and I can be deceived by my consciousness of this lived experience. Certainly, I feel when I am aware of the sensation; I feel cold and nothing else when I have this sensation, but it is possible that I feel cold without really being cold, and I may subsequently realize this. In the case of feelings regarding myself (*Gefühle*) (feeling cold, for example) an external condition (cold) and an internal property or capacity both present themselves. In the case of the *Gefühle*, we can speak of a life force (*Lebenskraft*) that nevertheless must not be confused with the pure I as the flow of lived experiences (*Erlebnisse*) (Stein 1970: 19–20).[1]

This is an important distinction between psychology and phenomenology; it is also a clarification of the relationship between psyche and consciousness. Here, we find the earlier distinction made by Husserl, who stressed that the causes that determine psychic life must not

---

[1] All translations from German are the author's own.

be sought in life feelings (*Lebensgefühle*), but in the "modes" of a life force (*Lebenskraft*) that is announced in them (Stein 1970: 20).

Changes in life conditions reflect a greater or lesser life force; this means that causality has nothing to do with the sphere of lived experiences. No pure lived experience can form part of a causal event; rather, as has already been said, lived experiences concern the life force insofar as both life feelings and lived experiences are only manifestations of the real causality of the psyche.

It is important to note, however, that psychic causality is different from physical causality; the psyche of an individual is a world of its own just like material nature is its own world. Even force manifests itself differently in the two cases. Whereas in physical nature, force can be observed as the result of a material event, in the psychic sphere it can be grasped only through its lived modes. A distinction has to be made between the sphere of lived experiences (*Erlebnisse*) and that of the life sphere (*Lebenssphäre*), which constitutes a substratum of the flow of lived experiences (Stein 1970: 22).

The relationship between the two spheres can be better understood if one notes that consciousness and the flux of its lived experiences can be imagined as devoid of life feelings. In this case we find ourselves faced with a flow of data of a different kind, that is, quality and intensity without "colouring" and tension, namely, the tension peculiar to the life sphere. One has to note the presence of life feelings, of a "field" that has its characteristics, but which "colours" all the data of the flow; this flow cannot be brought to a halt (Stein 1970: 30).

According to Stein, there does not exist any kind of determinism in psychic life, even though we can note some connections and, therefore, some "causal" relationships. Indeed, these enable us to note the presence in the psychic life of a "causality" that is completely different from the exact causality characteristic of scientific thought. Likewise, a quantitative determination of psychic states is out of the question, because we are here concerned with a flow of qualitative states *that* can be recognized only in their essential structure.

There is also present in the I another series of phenomena that are characterized by their representing an intentional moving toward something; these are "acts" (*Akte*) or intentional lived experiences (*intentionale Erlebnisse*) with which spiritual life commences. Even in psychic life it is possible to trace a first form of intentionality, but this is no more than outlined. If we examine some acts that we perform in everyday life, we shall realize the meaning of intentionality. With the meticulousness and clarity that distinguish her style, Stein gives us very precise indications to pinpoint them. Our eyes may be turned inward to discover the acts present there and this, in turn, is important, because it enables us to understand others' acts, as in the case of empathy (Stein 2008), and also ourselves. Here we have the act of reflection. Assuming a reflective or meditative attitude, we can begin to describe these acts. If we are concerned with an external object that presents itself as "transcendent," we have an act that places us in a relationship with what is outside ourselves. One could describe it, even though Stein does not use this term, as an act of "perception." In the case of external objects, moreover, we can relate their various aspects in such a manner that they are no longer merely one beside the other; rather, they form part of a connection, before and after, for example, as is the case for "apperception." We can also put them all together, and here we have a "synthesis." We can even concern ourselves with the particular act that is the "setting in motion of what comes after through what there is before" (*in-Bewegung-gesetzt-werden der späteren durch die früheren*), which is "motivation" (*Motivation*) (Stein 1970: 34–35).

MOTIVATION

Motivation presents itself as the type of link that exists between acts. We are here neither concerned with a co-penetration of simultaneous or successive phases nor with the associative connection; rather, we are dealing with an issuing of the one lived experience from the other, a manner in which the one completes itself or is so completed by virtue of the other. Given this relationship, the structure of lived experiences where a relationship of motivation is established becomes configured as acts that have their origin in the pure I. The I performs one act because it has already performed the other. This can happen either consciously or unconsciously; an explicit motivation exists in the case in which one proceeds from the premises to the consequences, while an implicit motivation exists when, like in a mathematical proof, we make use of a theorem without demonstrating it *ex novo*. It is clear that every explicit motivation becomes sedimented as implicit and that every implicit motivation is capable of being made explicit (Stein 1970: 35–36).

Implicit motivations occur in the ambit of perception. When we examine the knowledge of a thing that can be sensed, it becomes clear that having sensations is a first form of motivation. But we have a motivation relationship in the proper sense of the term when, face to face with some physical thing of which we can see only a part, we deem the existence of the other parts to be equally true, and this comprehension can eventually motivate a free movement that pushes us to a verification through actual perception. In the same way, something that is perceptively given may be the motive for believing in the existence of a thing and the belief in its existence may be what motivates our judgment regarding its existence. In the ethical sphere, similarly, grasping a value may be the motive for the will and for acting (Stein 1970: 36).

The relationship between act and motivation can be understood as follows: when consciousness turns to an object, it does not intend a void X, but something that has a content of determinate sense, as a bearer of a unitary consistency of being that is enclosed within it. Little by little, the content gives itself, filling out the sense of the object. This is true not only of physical things, but also of our knowledge of propositions and the state of things. In the latter case, a state of things may form part of different logical connections, for that is what rational motivation consists of. The ambit of possibilities, however, is limited and when the knowing subject oversteps this ambit, we come face to face with the irrational (Stein 1970: 37–38).

The passage from one act to another takes place thanks to motivation, and it is for this same reason that the flow of lived experiences becomes configured as the sum total of acts and motivations that underlie lived experiences. Motivation, therefore, serves to justify a series of acts that in the cognitive ambit regard the "turning to," the taking of position, and consequently accepting and negating as "free" acts.

In spite of the distinction between causality and motivation, there is a connection between the two. Offering an example that is particularly dear to her, Stein shows how causal factors and motivations can both come into play. The joy that somebody gives me motivates me to form the intention to return the joy, but a feeling that suddenly gets the better of me prevents me from carrying out something that would be motivated in a reasonable manner (Stein 1970: 69).

The life of the psyche, therefore, seems to be the combined action of several forces: the sensible force, which presents itself in relation to the apprehension of sense data and in our sense impulses, and the spiritual force, which is a force that is wholly new and different from the sense force, manifesting itself in spiritual activities and capacities. Spiritual activity can only be realized, however, within the collaboration of the sense force. The latter has its roots in nature and this justifies its psychophysical connection, that is, the link between psyche, body, and material nature. Through the spiritual force, the psyche opens to the objective world and can acquire new impulses. The nourishment of the spiritual force of the individual psyche may derive from an "objective" spiritual world, a world of values, or from the spiritual force of other subjects and from the divine spirit. In any case, it is necessary to locate a personal core (*Kern*) subtracted from all physical and psychic conditioning that is constituted by the capacity of willing, the sphere of free acts (Stein 1970: 106).

By way of conclusion, we can ask which kind of science is psychology, according to Stein. Arguing against, above all, the positivist claim, she underscores the impossibility of founding psychology as an exact science in conformity with a scientific model bound up with physics. This scientific model is present in contemporary psychology, particularly in cognitivism. In this sense psychology is linked with anatomy, neurophysiology, and the neurosciences, which use technical instruments to explore the human body and brain. That shows the actuality of Edith Stein's contribution in favor of a humanistic approach to psychology and to psychopathology (Ales Bello 2016).

BIBLIOGRAPHY

Ales Bello A. (2002). "Edith Stein's Contribution to Phenomenology." In A. T. Tymieniecka (ed.), *Phenomenology World–Wide. Foundations—Expanding Dynamics—Life-Engagement. A Guide for Research and Study*, pp. 232–240. Dordrecht: Kluwer.

Ales Bello A. (2016). *Il Senso dell'Umano. Tra fenomenologia, psicologia e psicopatologia*. Roma: Castelvecchi.

Husserl E. (1989). *Ideas Pertaining to a Pure Phenomenology and to a Phenomenological Philosophy, Second Book: Studies in the Phenomenologicy of Constitution*, trans. R. Rojcewicz and A. Schuwer. The Hague: Kluwer.

Stein E. (1970). *Beiträge zur philosophischen Begründung der Psychologie und der Geisteswissenschaften* [1922]. Tübingen: Max Niemeyer Verlag.

Stein E. (2000a). *Die Frau. Reflexionen und Fragestellungen* [1928–1930]. Gesamtausgabe, Band 13. Freiburg im Breisgau: Verlag Herder.

Stein E. (2000b), *Philosophy of Psychology and the Humanities*, trans. M. C. Baseheart and M. Sawicki. The Collected Works of Edith Stein. Washington, D.C.: ICS Publications.

Stein E. (2003). *Kreuzeswissenschaft: Studie über Johannes vom Kreuz* [1916]. Gesamtausgabe, Band 18. Freiburg im Breisgau: Verlag Herder.

Stein E. (2004). *Der Aufbau der menschlichen Person: Vorlesung zur philosophischen Anthropologie* [1932]. Gesamtausgabe, vol. 14. Freiburg im Breisgau: Verlag Herder.

Stein E. (2006a). *Endliches und ewiges Sein. Versuch eines Aufstiegs zum Sinn des Seins* [1936]. Gesamtausgabe, Band 11/12. Freiburg im Breisgau: Verlag Herder.

Stein E. (2006b). *Eine Untersuchung über den Staat* [1925]. Gesamtausgabe, Band 7. Freiburg im Breisgau: Verlag Herder.

Stein E. (2008). *Zum Problem der Einfühlung* [1916]. Gesamtausgabe, Band 5. Freiburg im Breisgau: Verlag Herder.

CHAPTER 4

....

MARTIN HEIDEGGER

....

ANTHONY VINCENT FERNANDEZ

INTRODUCTION

....

MARTIN Heidegger (1889–1976) is one of the most influential philosophers of the twentieth century. His magnum opus, *Being and Time*, was a catalyst for French existentialism, philosophical hermeneutics, and even deconstruction and poststructuralism. Many of the central works of twentieth-century continental philosophy—including Jean-Paul Sartre's *Being and Nothingness*, Maurice Merleau-Ponty's *Phenomenology of Perception*, Simone de Beauvoir's *The Second Sex*, and Hans-Georg Gadamer's *Truth and Method*—are deeply indebted to Heidegger's philosophical project.

Today, Heidegger's influence extends beyond philosophy. His account of Dasein,[1] or human existence, permeates the human and social sciences, including nursing, psychiatry, psychology, sociology, anthropology, and artificial intelligence. This broad influence owes much to his rich account of everyday life. Rather than starting from a detached intellectual or scientific perspective, Heidegger starts from our "average everydayness." He explores what it means to be human, which requires that he address everything from the nature of tool use to the challenges of maintaining a social identity to our inevitable confrontation with death.

In this chapter, I outline Heidegger's influence on psychology and psychiatry, focusing especially on his relationships with the Swiss psychiatrists, Ludwig Binswanger and Medard Boss. The first section outlines Heidegger's early life and work, up to and including the publication of *Being and Time*, in which he develops his famous concept of being-in-the-world. The second section focuses on Heidegger's initial influence on psychiatry via Binswanger's founding of Daseinsanalysis, a Heideggerian approach to psychopathology

---

[1] The German *Dasein* is often left untranslated in the English editions of Heidegger's texts. The term translates simply to "being-there." It serves as what Heidegger calls a "formal indication," a way of pointing at the phenomenon one wants to study without our presuppositions leading us astray. In this case, Heidegger wants to avoid problematically framing his study with concepts like "human," "person," "subjectivity," "mind," or "consciousness," all of which come with extensive historical and conceptual baggage. *Dasein* allows him to point to what he wants to study—what it's like for us to "be-there"— without determining the direction of his study in advance (Heidegger 2008: 61–62; see also Burch 2013; O'Rourke 2018).

and psychotherapy. The third section turns to Heidegger's relationship with Boss, including Heidegger's rejection of Binswanger's Daseinsanalysis and his lectures at Boss's home in Zollikon, Switzerland.

HEIDEGGER'S EARLY LIFE AND WORK: 1889–1927

Martin Heidegger was born in Messkirch, Germany, to Friedrich and Johanna Heidegger, and grew up with his younger brother, Fritz. Friedrich was a master cooper and sexton of the local Catholic church. Martin was therefore brought up in the Catholic tradition and his education, beginning from the age of fourteen, was supported by the church. This support was, however, both a blessing and a curse. The church financed educational opportunities far beyond his family's means. But it provided these opportunities on the condition that he enter the priesthood. Therefore, when his faith waned, he found himself in a difficult position: Leave the church and forfeit the opportunity to continue his studies or remain faithful and limit himself to topics that the church would support? (Safranski 1999: chapter 1).

Heidegger struggled with this dilemma for years. In 1909, he entered the novitiate with the intention of becoming a priest but was discharged two weeks later when he complained of heart trouble (Safranski 1999: 15). In 1911, while studying at the seminary, he was again discharged for heart trouble. At this time, it was determined that he did not have the physical constitution to serve the church. After a period at home in Messkirch, Heidegger decided to end his studies of theology. He enrolled at the University of Freiburg in the winter semester 1911–1912 to study mathematics, science, and philosophy. In the absence of the Catholic church's financial support, he managed to raise enough funds with a loan, a small grant from the university, and private tutoring. In 1913, he received his doctorate under the supervision of Professor Arthur Schneider, Chair of Catholic Philosophy (Safranski 1999: 43).

Shortly after completing his doctorate, Heidegger began his habilitation. Despite no longer pursuing the priesthood, he was able to secure a grant from a Catholic institution to support three years of study. The following year, 1914, saw the outbreak of the First World War. Owing to his heart condition, Heidegger was able to defer military service and continue working on his habilitation, which he submitted in 1915. Later that year he was once again recruited for military service but he was hospitalized a few weeks later, then transferred to a postal supervision center where he censored letters sent to non-allied countries (Safranski 1999: 67).

In 1916, Heidegger met Edmund Husserl, the founder of phenomenology. Husserl, who had just moved from Göttingen to take up a chair at Freiburg, immediately acquired a close circle of acolytes and assistants, including Edith Stein and Heidegger himself. His phenomenology shared much in common with strands of neo-Kantianism active at the time, but it promised a radical new method for understanding human experience. The phenomenologist was said to be a perpetual beginner, bracketing out her previous beliefs and prejudices in order to attend not only to the objects of experience but to the way we experience, or to the experiencing itself. Heidegger, enamored with this new approach, quickly caught Husserl's attention. Soon, Husserl treated Heidegger not only as an acolyte and assistant, but as a near equal. Even when Heidegger was sent off for active military duty in 1918—joining the frontline meteorological service—the two remained in close correspondence (Safranski 1999: chapter 5).

However, as Heidegger's thinking developed, he merged his own scholastic and Aristotelian training with Husserl's new method, developing a radically new approach to ontology. To appreciate the radical nature of Heidegger's ontological project, we first need a general understanding of what ontology is, according to Heidegger. Most of our inquiries, including most of our scientific investigations, philosophical studies, and everyday questions, are *ontic*—they ask about concrete beings or entities. However, some of our philosophical questions are *ontological*, rather than ontic—they ask about what it means to be, rather than about concrete beings. We can clarify this distinction with a classic phenomenological example: a coffee mug. If I investigate a coffee mug ontically, there are a variety of questions that I might ask: What is it made of? How much liquid does it hold? Who made it? What is its monetary value? These are all questions about the coffee mug itself—questions about its concrete characteristics, history, value, and so on. But I can also study a coffee mug ontologically, in which case I would ask a different set of questions: What does it mean to *be* a coffee mug? What are the features that something must have in order to count as a coffee mug? What makes a coffee mug different from a teacup? This distinction between the ontic and the ontological is what Heidegger calls the "ontological difference" (see e.g. Heidegger 1962: 83; 1988: 227–229; 2001: 116). This difference is key to his philosophical program and its proper interpretation was a major point of contention in psychological and psychiatric applications of his work.

How, then, did Heidegger transform the field of ontology? One of Heidegger's key insights is that ontology isn't just a philosophical program. Ontology permeates everyday life. Every time I engage with an ontic being—such as a coffee mug, a writing desk, or my colleague—I operate with a tacit sense of what it means to *be* this being. This doesn't mean that I can list off necessary and sufficient criteria. Rather, I demonstrate my understanding through my successful engagement. I demonstrate that I understand what it means to be a coffee mug by pulling one out of the cabinet, filling it with coffee, and taking a sip as I sit down at my desk. This is what Heidegger calls a "pre-ontological" understanding. We may not operate with a well-formulated ontological theory. But we always have a sense of what it means to be.

This insight into the everydayness of ontology grounds Heidegger's approach in his 1927 magnum opus, *Being and Time*.[2] Here, he argues that ontology must begin with an investigation of the being for whom "Being is an *issue*," the being who asks the question of being in the first place: the human being (Heidegger 1962: 32). Who we take ourselves to be is always a project, a challenge, a process of becoming. Whether I consider myself to be a friend, a carpenter, an American, or a tourist, there are certain norms and obligations that I must fulfill. If I don't conform to these norms, then I risk losing this possibility for being. In some cases, this loss is trivial. Today I'm a tourist; tomorrow I'm a professor. But, in many cases, the loss of who we take ourselves to be is traumatic. Whether the source of loss is a divorce, a layoff, a fight with a friend, or a political collapse, we lose the possibility for being who we were. In such cases, we realize that our being or identity is fundamentally tied to our social and environmental relations. We become who we are through our interactions with others and

---

[2] For an accessible introduction to Heidegger's philosophy, see Richard Polt (1999). For a detailed account of the development of *Being and Time*, see Theodore Kisiel (1995).

the way we take up what our environment offers us. This is why Heidegger says that Dasein, or human existence, is not an isolated subject or a Cartesian mental substance: Dasein is "being-in-the-world." Human existence is always embedded in a world, in a concrete history and community, and can only understand itself as such.

Our being-in-the-world is a complex and multifaceted phenomenon but, as Heidegger argues, its essence is "care" (*Sorge*)—or what he sometimes refers to as "disclosedness" (Heidegger 1962: 235–241). Dasein is the being that discloses, or opens up, a world of sense and meaning. The coffee mug, for instance, never shows up to me as a brute object. It shows up as the gift that my mother gave me when I moved away for college or as the thing that I need to wash in the kitchen sink so that I can use it again in the morning. Everything that I experience has its sense and meaning within a web of relations, which are ultimately tied to both my cultural context and my particular aims and projects.

Heidegger argues that a world is opened up, or disclosed, through "thrown projection." We find ourselves already thrown into a world—we are constrained by our culture, language, class, religious upbringing, and even our previous life choices. But we also project possibilities—we might become a friend, a father, a carpenter, or a professor, or perhaps we'll continue to be who we already are. The world we find ourselves thrown into both opens and constrains our potentialities-for-being, the range of possibilities that we can project. According to Heidegger, this tension of thrownness and projection discloses a meaningful world.

The particular meaning that something has for me emerges from the tension between my concrete thrownness and the particular possibilities that I project for myself. In a classroom, for example, the whiteboard has a substantially different meaning for the students, the professor, and the custodian. How we engage with the whiteboard depends on who we take ourselves to be. For the students it is the thing to look at when taking notes. For the professor it is a way to supplement her lecture and illustrate her point. For the custodian it is an object to clean in preparation for the next day of classes. But, of course, none of us are fixed in these roles or possibilities. The custodian might also be a student in that very classroom. And one of the students—perhaps working toward his PhD—might lecture to undergraduates in this classroom before attending his evening graduate seminar. Our identities are neither stable nor uniform. They are always in flux, and each possibility that we take up shifts how we experience and make sense of our world.

But this interchangeability of our possibilities—the simple fact that you might take my place and I might take yours—suggests that they are not really our own. The possibilities we take up are simply given to us by our society and circumstances, and we fulfill them in the way anyone would fulfill them. If I take myself to be a professor, then this means that I teach, mentor students, attend conferences, and publish papers. If I fail to do some or all of these things, then I risk losing my possibility for being a professor—not only in the sense that I might lose my job, but in the sense that no one will recognize me *as* a professor. However, in my day-to-day life, who I take myself to be isn't something that I reflect upon. I simply fulfill the social norms required for maintaining my possibilities without much thought. Heidegger calls this mode of existence "inauthentic" (*uneigentlich*) and he contrasts it with an "authentic" (*eigentlich*) mode of existence. By employing these terms, Heidegger isn't necessarily disapproving of our everyday way of life. Rather, his primary aim is to distinguish two different modes of comportment. In an inauthentic comportment, we take up our possibilities without explicit reflection. But, in an authentic comportment, we actively choose our possibility for being—even if we simply choose the possibility that we find ourselves already thrown into.

These features of human life make up the core of Heidegger's ontology of human existence. With the publication of *Being and Time*, Heidegger established himself as one of the foremost philosophers of the twentieth century. But he probably hadn't expected that it would inspire generations of psychiatrists, providing a foundation for a new approach to psychopathology and psychotherapy.

HEIDEGGER'S FIRST CONTACT WITH PSYCHIATRY: 1928–1947

While Heidegger had a long-standing relationship with the philosopher and psychiatrist, Karl Jaspers, it was Ludwig Binswanger who first saw the importance of Heidegger's work for psychopathology and psychotherapy. Heidegger and Binswanger met in 1929 following a brief correspondence regarding the celebration of Husserl's seventieth birthday (Frie 1999: 246). Binswanger—a student of Eugen Bleuler and Carl Jung, and a close friend of Sigmund Freud—was steeped in the psychoanalytic tradition. However, unsatisfied with the philosophical foundations of psychoanalysis, he found in Heidegger's *Being and Time* a promising new way of thinking about human existence.

Binswanger established a psychiatric approach that he called "Daseinsanalysis" (*Daseinsanalyse*).[3] On this approach, mental illness is not the product of innate drives or an inherent tension between id, ego, and superego, but a pathological way of projecting one's possibilities for being. Binswanger found that many of his patients operated with a profoundly limited capacity for self- and world-interpretation, often as the result of traumatic life events. When confronted with especially distressing events, they resorted to a narrow repertoire of interpretive concepts to make sense of themselves and their situations, resulting in a pathological rather than a healthy response. To restore the mental health of his patients, Binswanger helped them broaden their scope of possibilities for being (see e.g. Binswanger 1958).

Initially, Binswanger clearly distinguished his own aims from those of Heidegger. He characterized his project as an ontic application of Heidegger's ontology of Dasein. In other words, Heidegger's ontological account of human existence provided a framework for Binswanger's ontic studies of particular human pathologies. Over time, however, Binswanger became more critical of Heidegger's approach. He argued that Heidegger mischaracterized the social dimension of human existence and, therefore, failed to understand the nature of the face-to-face, I–Thou relationship, which is key to effective psychotherapy (Binswanger 1993; see also Frie 1999: 249).

---

[3] The German *Daseinsanalyse* is translated either as "Daseinsanalysis"—maintaining the tradition of not translating "Dasein"—or as "existential analysis." While the latter translation is less awkward, it risks confusing Binswanger's approach with other existential approaches to psychology and psychiatry, such as Sartre's existential psychoanalysis (Sartre 1993).

Binswanger's goal was to help his patients achieve an authentic existence. But, on Heidegger's account, authenticity seems to be something one achieves alone. As Roger Frie says, "Binswanger argues that for Heidegger, authentic existence is a private world, structured by Dasein's concern for its own Being; Dasein as care achieves its authenticity in essential isolation from others" (Frie 1999: 249). In light of Heidegger's allegedly solipsistic characterization, Binswanger sought to revise both our understanding of what authenticity is and how it's achieved. He argues that genuine authenticity emerges from a relationship of dialogue, openness, and mutual engagement—and, moreover, this relationship must be founded on love, not care. Only through a fundamental attunement of love can the therapist help her patient achieve authenticity (Frie 1999: 248).

Throughout the 1930s and into the 1940s, Binswanger established his new approach to psychotherapy, helping patients overcome their limited possibilities for being and achieve genuine authenticity. During this time, Heidegger underwent a crisis of possibilities in his own life. Because he had joined the Nazi party and served, briefly, as rector of the University of Freiburg in the early 1930s, he faced denazification proceedings after the Second World War.[4] Based largely on Jaspers's expert opinion, he was barred from teaching for four years (Safranski 1999: 339). Heidegger, suddenly stripped of his possibility for being a professor, experienced a mental breakdown. He entered a sanitorium in Badenweiler where he was treated by Victor Baron von Gebsattel, a psychiatrist working in Binswanger's now influential school of Daseinsanalysis (Safranski 1999: 351). The following year, 1947, Heidegger read Binswanger's *Grundformen und Erkenntnis menschlichen Daseins* (*Basic Forms and Knowledge of Human Existence*), which he had received from Binswanger in 1944 (Frie 1999: 250). Upon reading the book, he wrote a supportive and encouraging letter to Binswanger, who had been anxiously awaiting Heidegger's assessment.

HEIDEGGER, BOSS, AND THE ZOLLIKON SEMINARS: 1947–1976

That same year, Heidegger received a letter from another psychiatrist, Medard Boss, who read *Being and Time* while serving as a battalion doctor in the Swiss army during the war. The two met shortly after and, over the next three decades, developed a close friendship. But Heidegger's relationship with Boss cast a dark shadow over Binswanger and his Daseinsanalytic project. Despite his initial enthusiasm for Binswanger's work, he found in Boss a more formidable representative of his project, eventually rescinding his approval of Binswanger's work altogether.

The friendship between Heidegger and Boss culminated in a series of seminars held at the University of Zurich Psychiatric Clinic and at Boss's home in Zollikon, Switzerland,

---

[4] For a time, there was considerable debate over the nature of Heidegger's anti-Semitic views and his service to the Nazi party. It was well known that he referred to the "inner truth and greatness" of National Socialism, but later criticized the movement for its attempt to mobilize the German people into an organized machine, a mere resource for military domination—what Heidegger refers to as "standing reserves" (Heidegger 1993). However, in light of the publication of Heidegger's *Black Notebooks*, his anti-Semitic sentiments are undeniable (see Cesare 2018).

from 1959 to 1969 (K. Aho 2018a). Heidegger lectured to a group of psychiatrists on ontology, hermeneutics, the nature of embodiment, time and temporality, and—of course—a Heideggerian approach to psychiatric research and practice. In light of the wide-ranging nature of Heidegger's lectures, I focus here on two of his contributions to psychology and psychiatry: his characterization of the relationship between Daseinsanalysis and ontology, as clarified through his critique of Binswanger, and his general theory of health and illness, developed in collaboration with Boss.

While Heidegger was enthusiastic about the application of his work in psychology and psychiatry, he did have some reservations about the way in which his insights were being applied. In particular, he was concerned that some of these applications involved a misunderstanding of the ontological difference—and he attributed the source of this misunderstanding to Binswanger. To illustrate the misunderstanding, Heidegger returned to Binswanger's critique, in which he argued that Heidegger's ontology—which established care as the being, or essence, of Dasein—left no space for love, which is essential to the therapeutic relationship that leads one out of illness and into authenticity. Heidegger claimed that this critique is not only unwarranted, but is grounded in a fundamental misunderstanding of the ontological difference:

> Binswanger's misunderstanding consists not so much of the fact that he wants to supplement "care" with love, but that he does not see that care has an existential, that is, *ontological* sense. Therefore, the analytic of Da-sein asks for Dasein's basic *ontological* (*existential*) constitution [*Verfassung*] and does not wish to give a mere description of the ontic phenomena of Dasein.
>
> (Heidegger 2001: 116)

As Heidegger characterizes it, care refers to our basic openness to the world, our basic capacity to find the world meaningfully articulated. It is therefore an ontological structure of Dasein, an essential structure that grounds all particular modes of existence. Love, on the other hand, is one of these particular, ontic modes. Love is just one of the many ways in which we might relate to others. Properly understood, Heidegger's notion of care leaves ample room for love, even if Heidegger never produced a study of love himself.

Despite Binswanger admitting his "productive misunderstanding" in the wake of this critique, Heidegger suggested that Binswanger's misunderstanding permeated his entire project and, therefore, undermined its legitimacy. He claimed that if Daseinsanalysis is to be successfully employed, it must respect the ontological difference: Daseinsanalysis is merely an ontic application of the ontological analysis of human existence—the insights of Daseinsanalysis cannot, therefore, challenge the insights of Heidegger's own ontology.[5]

This brings us to the second element of Heidegger's contribution to psychology and psychiatry: his theory of health and illness. If pathology does not touch the ontological constitution of Dasein, but only its ontic ways of being, then how should we understand the nature of health and illness? Heidegger argues that illness should be understood as a specific

---

[5] I've argued elsewhere that Binswanger's confused understanding of the ontological difference actually provides a more accurate depiction of both human existence and mental illness. Heidegger denied that mental illness could involve alterations of the ontological structure of human existence. However, in some cases, appealing to alterations in the ontological structure itself provides a more illuminating, and accurate, account of the condition in question (Fernandez 2018).

kind of negation, which he calls "privation." To say that the ill person is "deprived of health" implies that health is his proper mode of being—that it, in some sense, belongs to him. As Heidegger says,

> It is a remarkable fact that your whole medical profession moves within a negation in the sense of a privation. You deal with illness. The doctor asks someone who comes to him, "What is wrong with you?" The sick person is *not healthy*. This being-healthy, this being-well, this finding oneself well is not simply absent but is disturbed. Illness is a phenomenon of privation. Each privation implies the essential belonging to something that is lacking, which is in need of something.
>
> (Heidegger 2001: 46)

According to Heidegger, illness is not simply the privation of some natural biological function. It is the privation of possibilities: "Each illness is a loss of freedom, a constriction of the possibility for living" (Heidegger 2001: 175). In this respect, illness is what Heidegger calls a "deficient mode" of existence. This concept, employed throughout *Being and Time*, refers to any instance in which one is not open to the full or genuine range of possibilities. It is a particular, ontic way of being open to the world—a way of being open that, nevertheless, constrains the possibilities that one is open to.

This is the foundation upon which Boss constructed his new Daseinsanalytic approach.[6] While he investigated the nuances of various mental illnesses, he construed each illness as a reduction of one's freedom for possibilities. The therapist's goal is, therefore, to help her patient maximize his openness toward possibilities for being (Kouba 2015: 104). Boss went so far as to argue—in *Existential Foundations of Medicine and Psychology*—that this characterization of illness applies not only to mental illness, but to somatic illness as well. Building upon his earlier work on psychosomatic conditions, he characterized all forms of illness as an impairment of our potentialities and freedom for possibilities (Boss 1979: 199–200). Therefore, while Heidegger's influence on conceptions of health and illness began with psychiatric conditions, it eventually extended to the full range of illness.

CONCLUSION: HEIDEGGER'S INFLUENCE TODAY

Today, Heidegger's work influences not only the philosophical and theoretical literature on health and illness, but medical research and practice itself—especially approaches to psychiatry and nursing. One of the most direct applications is found in the phenomenology of depressive disorders, in which Heidegger's theory of mood and attunement is used to articulate the affective disturbance characteristic of depressive episodes (K. Aho 2013; Fernandez 2014a, 2014b; Ratcliffe 2015; Svenaeus, 2007). But his account of human existence provides a foundation for understanding a broad range of conditions—from acute, life-threating illness to chronic disabilities (Abrams 2016; J. Aho and K. Aho 2009; K. Aho 2018b; Carel 2016; Svenaeus 2000).

---

[6] To distinguish Binswanger's and Boss's approaches, they are sometimes referred to as "psychiatric Daseinsanalysis" and "therapeutic Daseinsanalysis," respectively (see e.g. Kouba 2015).

BIBLIOGRAPHY

Abrams T. (2016). *Heidegger and the Politics of Disablement*. New York: Palgrave Pivot.

Aho J. and Aho K. (2009). *Body Matters: A Phenomenology of Sickness, Disease, and Illness*. Lanham: Lexington Books.

Aho K. (2013). "Depression and Embodiment: Phenomenological Reflections on Motility, Affectivity, and Transcendence." *Medicine, Health Care and Philosophy* 16(4): 751–759.

Aho K. (2018a). "Existential Medicine: Heidegger and the Lessons from Zollikon." In K. Aho (ed.), *Existential Medicine: Essays on Health and Illness*, pp. xi–xxiv. Lanham: Rowman & Littlefield International.

Aho K. (ed.) (2018b). *Existential Medicine: Essays on Health and Illness*. Lanham: Rowman & Littlefield International.

Binswanger L. (1958). "The Existential Analysis School of Thought." In R. May, E. Angel, and H. F. Ellenberger (eds.), *Existence: A New Dimension in Psychology and Psychiatry*, pp. 191–213. New York: Basic Books.

Binswanger L. (1993). *Grundformen und Erkenntnis menschlichen Daseins*. Heidelberg: Asanger.

Boss M. (1979). *Existential Foundations of Medicine and Psychology*, trans. S. Conway and A. Cleaves. New York: Jason Aronson.

Burch M. I. (2013). "The Existential Sources of Phenomenology: Heidegger on Formal Indication." *European Journal of Philosophy* 21(2): 258–278.

Carel H. (2016). *The Phenomenology of Illness*. New York: Oxford University Press.

Cesare D. D. (2018). *Heidegger and the Jews: The Black Notebooks*. Medford: Polity Press.

Fernandez A. V. (2014a). "Depression as Existential Feeling or De-Situatedness? Distinguishing Structure from Mode in Psychopathology." *Phenomenology and the Cognitive Sciences* 13(4): 595–612.

Fernandez A. V. (2014b). "Reconsidering the Affective Dimension of Depression and Mania: Towards a Phenomenological Dissolution of the Paradox of Mixed States." *Journal of Psychopathology* 20(4): 414–420.

Fernandez A. V. (2018). "Beyond the Ontological Difference: Heidegger, Binswanger, and the Future of Existential Analysis." In K. Aho (ed.), *Existential Medicine: Essays on Health and Illness*, pp. 27–42. Lanham: Rowman & Littlefield International.

Frie R. (1999). "Interpreting a Misinterpretation: Ludwig Binswanger and Martin Heidegger." *Journal of the British Society for Phenomenology* 30(3): 244–257.

Heidegger M. (1962). *Being and Time*, trans. J. Macquarrie and E. Robinson. New York: Harper Perennial Modern Classics.

Heidegger M. (1988). *The Basic Problems of Phenomenology*, trans. A. Hofstadter. Bloomington: Indiana University Press.

Heidegger M. (1993). "The Question Concerning Technology." In D. F. Krell (ed.), *Martin Heidegger: Basic Writings*, pp. 311–341. New York: HarperCollins Publishers.

Heidegger M. (2001). *Zollikon Seminars: Protocols—Conversations—Letters*, trans. F. Mayr and R. Askay. Evanston: Northwestern University Press.

Heidegger M. (2008). *Ontology—The Hermeneutics of Facticity*, trans. J. van Buren. Bloomington: Indiana University Press.

Kisiel T. (1995). *The Genesis of Heidegger's Being and Time*. Berkeley: University of California Press.

Kouba P. (2015). *The Phenomenon of Mental Disorder: Perspectives of Heidegger's Thought in Psychopathology*. Switzerland: Springer.

O'Rourke J. (2018). "Heidegger on Expression: Formal Indication and Destruction in the Early Freiburg Lectures." *Journal of the British Society for Phenomenology* 49(2): 109–125.

Polt R. (1999). *Heidegger: An Introduction.* Ithaca: Cornell University Press.

Ratcliffe M. (2015). *Experiences of Depression: A Study in Phenomenology.* Oxford: Oxford University Press.

Safranski R. (1999). *Martin Heidegger: Between Good and Evil,* trans. E. Osers. Cambridge, MA: Harvard University Press.

Sartre J.-P. (1993). *Being and Nothingness,* trans. H. E. Barnes. New York: Washington Square Press.

Svenaeus F. (2000). *The Hermeneutics of Medicine and the Phenomenology of Health: Steps Towards a Philosophy of Medical Practice.* Dordrecht: Springer.

Svenaeus F. (2007). "Do Antidepressants Affect the Self? A Phenomenological Approach." *Medicine, Health Care and Philosophy* 10(2): 153–166.

CHAPTER 5

....

JEAN-PAUL SARTRE

....

ANTHONY HATZIMOYSIS

BIOGRAPHICAL SKETCH
....

THE most famous French philosopher of the twentieth century, Jean-Paul Sartre, observed with an unflinching eye the moving generosity and the common duplicity, the existential revelations and the mundane self-deceptions, the intriguing varieties of the ordinary, and the pathological engagement with the world. Born in Paris in 1905, he entered the *École Normale Supérieure* in 1924, where he majored in philosophy, while showing systematic interest in psychology: he paid regular visits to patients at St Anne's Psychiatric Hospital, studied Jaspers's *General Psychopathology*, and volunteered as a subject in psychology experiments whose results formed the backdrop of his 1927 dissertation on "The Image in Psychological Life: Its Role and Nature."

Initially drawn to philosophy as a resource of ideas for his fiction writing, he dedicated himself to phenomenological research at the prompting of Raymond Aron, who arranged for Sartre's visit at the *Institut français* in Berlin: from September 1933 to June 1934, Sartre studied Husserl's major works, expanded the draft of his philosophical novel, *Nausea* (Sartre 2000), and composed his seminal essay on "Intentionality" (Sartre 1970). There follows a decade of phenomenological writings, including *The Transcendence of the Ego* (2004a), *The Sketch for a Theory of the Emotions* (2004b), and *The Imaginary* (2004c), characterized by the originality of Sartre's critique of idealism, as well as by the novelty of the topics he chose to explore.

With the outbreak of the Second World War, Sartre was posted in the meteorological corps of the French army, and then incarcerated as a prisoner of war from early 1940 until his escape in the summer of 1941—during which he kept a diary that bears clear witness to the existentialist turn of his phenomenological thinking (Sartre 1984). 1943 sees the publication of Sartre's *magnum opus, Being and Nothingness*, which culminates his involvement with phenomenological ontology and sets the context for the political, aesthetic, and broadly construed psychoanalytic projects he undertook until his death in 1980: he wrote the script for a cinematic biography of Freud (Sartre 1984), participated in public debates over the status of psychoanalysis (Cannon 1991), and concluded his career with a voluminous exploration of the formative years in the life of a concrete individual, Gustav Flaubert (Sartre 1981). However, even the most abstract of his philosophical works involve vivid psychological portraits delivered with magisterial strokes which make a lasting impression in the reader's mind.

CRITIQUE OF THE REIFICATION
OF PSYCHIC STATES

For Sartre, consciousness is a movement of fleeing oneself: to be conscious is to transcend oneself toward something. The world encountered in experience is value-laden: "it is things which abruptly unveil themselves to us as hateful, sympathetic, horrible, loveable" (Sartre 1970: 5). Accordingly, our sentiments are attuned to changes because they are a kind of perceptual state of those aspects of reality relevant to our concerns; they are "ways of discovering the world" (Sartre 1970: 5).

Consciousness is primarily a *positional* consciousness of a certain object, in the sense that consciousness sets before itself the object as a target of its intentional activity. When one is positionally conscious of an object, one is also *non-positionally* conscious of being conscious of that object. Pre-reflective consciousness is thus non-positionally aware of itself as being directed toward its objects. On the ground of those distinctions, Sartre raises a forceful critique on the traditional conception of the "Ego," a cover-term for the referent of the first-person pronoun. For Sartre, the "I" could not be residing inside consciousness since consciousness has no inside. If the "I" exists, it can only exist "outside, *in the world*" (Sartre 2004a: 1; emphasis in the original).

Sartre asserts that the "I" appears in reflection, it presents itself to us, it is given to our intuition; hence, it could not be easily dismissed as an accident of our grammar, or a figment of cultural imagination. He effectively undermines, though, the view that the ego is always present in our mental life, lurking behind every conscious move: the "I" arises when consciousness turns its attention to its acts, and thinks of a particular being as the locus of certain passions or actions. The overall point of his discussion is that if consciousness is to be a genuine transcendence toward the world, then the ego of philosophical tradition ought to be transcended. The unity of our consciousness as a whole is found not in an ego, but in the temporal interplay of our sensations, thoughts, and affects: "consciousness refers constantly back to itself, whoever says 'a consciousness' means the whole of consciousness" (Sartre 2004a: 39).

When it is narrated, our experience is considered under certain headings, such as "qualities of character," "acts," and "states." A psychic state appears when a reflective consciousness turns its attention on past conscious activities and surveys those consciousnesses under the heading of particular concepts. However, in a reversal of actual priorities, the reflectively created state is taken to underlie one's feelings, thoughts, and actions. The state misleadingly appears as the principle that ties together various activities of consciousness, and holds the meaning of one's relation to the world. The analysis of that relation becomes an exploration of the allegedly hidden meaning of conscious experience. Our feelings, thoughts, and actions provide clues to the mechanics of each psychic state that acts on the agent as a physical force, accounting for her past attitude and conditioning her future stance. Hence, the alleged aim of the scientist is to uncover the meaning of the state through the psychoanalysis of verbal and physical behavior. On this point, cognitive psychology and classical psychoanalysis concur in their view of psychic states as entities to which the agent can have only restricted access, and over which she may enjoy very limited control. The vocabulary of passivity that permeates much of the folk and scientific discourse on emotions reflects a conception of human beings as governed by entities dwelling somewhere between the spontaneous activities of the stream of consciousness, and the bodily constitution of our interaction with the world. That space in between the mental and the physical is that of the psychological, whose dual character speaks to the paradoxical nature of psychic states: passive yet purposive, involuntary but intentional, evaluative no less than physiological. A further, and even deeper problem, for Sartre, is that zooming in on psychic states produces theoretical short-sightedness: psychic states cannot be studied independently of human nature and the world, since the psychic facts that we meet in our research are never prior: "they, in their essential structure, are reactions of man to the world: they therefore presuppose man and the world, and cannot take on their true meaning unless those two notions have first been elucidated" (Sartre 2004b: 7–8).

THE PHENOMENOLOGY OF EMOTIONAL EXPERIENCE

Sartre's critique of the reification of psychic states paves the way for his original account of emotional experience. An emotion is not a clog of mental machinery, but how the whole of consciousness operates in a certain situation. During an emotional episode, one's relation to the world is "magically" transformed by means of one's body. The world is understood as a totality of phenomena linked by a complex network of references to each other. In the world of daily activity, we experience reality as a combination of demands and affordances; the link between them is experienced as ruled by deterministic processes between causes and effects. The "instrumental world" of action is captured in the "pragmatic intuition" of the situation that makes certain moves available for the subject, while denying her others. For Sartre, the world encountered in emotional experience—what we characterize as a "hateful," "joyful," or "bleak" world—is distinguished from the instrumental world. The agent's response in an emotional episode engages the overall stance and physiology of the body not to effect material changes in the world, but to alter her perception of reality, and, through that, her relation to the world: "during emotion, it is the body which, directed by the consciousness, changes its relationship to the world so that the world should change its qualities" (Sartre 2004b: 41).

To appreciate the significance of Sartre's phenomenological approach to emotions, it is important to grasp Sartre's argumentation against two prominent alternative accounts, on the one hand, the James-Lange reductively naturalistic model and, on the other, the classical psychoanalytic view of emotional phenomena.

CRITIQUE OF REDUCTIVE NATURALISM ABOUT EMOTIONS

Sartre conceives of his sketch for a theory of the emotions as an experiment in phenomenological psychology. Its subject matter is the human being in her situation, and its objective is to identify the essence of emotional phenomena by showing how embodied consciousness constitutes their meaning.

The meaning of an emotion is the main casualty in the first classic theory Sartre examines. The "Peripheric" theory is thus called because it locates the source of the emotion in the periphery of mental activity, namely in the body. According to the reductionist version of that theory, as put forward by William James and Carl Lange, the feeling of somatic changes as they occur is the emotion. The reductionist theory maps emotions to bodily feelings. However, the model is subject to the charge of irrelevance: even if the bodily changes occurring in feeling jealous, for instance, are a synthesis of all the bodily changes occurring in feeling angry, sad, disgusted, and afraid, it is not on the basis of being (positionally) aware of such bodily changes that one is (non-positionally) aware of feeling jealous. Rather it is by focusing on the manifest features of the world—the smirk in her face, her unpersuasive excuses—that one is attributing betrayal to the other, and jealousy to oneself. If jealousy should be identified with perception it would be the perception of her dismissive gesture, not of the change in the location of your diaphragm.

The distinction between the two types of awareness shows the force and the subtlety of the Sartrean critique. Sartre's complaint is not that, for example, in feeling jealous one is not undergoing any bodily processes. His criticism is that when one is focusing on an emotion, one finds "something *more* and something *else*" than mere physiological processes (Sartre 2004b: 15; emphasis in the original). Something *more*, since however much information one accumulates about the mechanics of bodily events, one is none the wiser as to which, if any, of the emotions these events pick out, in the absence of any information about how the agent perceives, evaluates, or responds to the salient features of a situation. And something *else*, since however much a bodily state is perturbed in an emotional occurrence, the physiological disturbance cannot account for the disturbing character of emotional experience. For instance, part of the explanation for the discrepancy between a (positional) awareness of pulse rate, and a (non-positional) awareness of terror is that the former is exhausted by the perception of modifications in one's body, while the latter denotes a "relation between our psychic being and the world." That relation is not an arbitrary product of "quantitative, continuous modifications of vegetative states," but the realization of an "organised and describable structure" that involves the human being in a situation (Sartre 2004b: 17).

The Peripheric theory locates emotion on the inner side of bodily experience, at the cost of leaving the agent's relation to the world outside the theory's preview. Cut off from the rest of reality, emotion becomes a self-enclosed, private, internal affair of someone who is subject to bodily perturbations. Hence, emotion is deprived of its significance: the theory accounts neither for what the emotion indicates for the life of the person who is angry, jealous, or joyous, nor for what his anger, jealousy, or joy is really about (Hatzimoysis 2011: 41–77).

CRITIQUE OF THE CLASSICAL PSYCHOANALYTIC METATHEORY

Sartre's phenomenological discourse is opposed to a major principle of classical psychoanalysis: the postulation of unconscious emotions, or other non-conscious states, as explanatory entities of human phenomena. The importance of interpretations generated during the psychoanalytic process is not questioned by Sartre. What he doubts is the validity of the metapsychological interpretation of the practice. As Sartre understands it, the psychoanalytic theory dissociates the phenomenon analyzed from its signification. What the phenomenon allegedly signifies is the repressed state that, unbeknownst to the subject, produces the behavior under consideration. The relation between the behavior and its signification is supposed to be that between an effect and its cause. The former depends on the latter for its production, but, like all causally related items, they are distinct things that may exist separately from each other. It is claimed by classical psychoanalysts that the repressed desire that causes the behavior lies outside the domain of conscious engagement with the world. Accordingly, an examination of how an agent experiences a situation will not enable us to understand her behavior without invoking a metatheory of causal connections that designates fixed relations between the events under consideration and their alleged sources.

Whatever the metaphysical credentials of a theory of psychic causality, the problem is that it undermines the very practice that it is supposed to sustain. Viewing human conduct as passively produced by forces that lie outside the domain of meaningful activity is in clear tension with the analytic practice of looking into the particular features of a situation, as these are conveyed by the analysand's communication, in order to interpret her behavior. And it is precisely this tension, between the practitioner's search for meaning and the theoreticians' postulation of fixed causal relations that erodes the foundations of the psychoanalytic approach to emotions: "The profound contradiction in all psychoanalysis is that it presents at the same time a bond of causality and a bond of understanding between the phenomena that it studies. These two types of relationship are incompatible" (Sartre 2004b: 32–33).

Meaningful behavior cannot be interpreted satisfactorily by an appeal to unconscious causes, not so much because they are unconscious, but because they are causes. However, casting doubts about the unconscious need not be followed by a declaration of mental transparency. Sartre only asserts that the signification of an emotional phenomenon should be sought in our engagement with the world. This does not mean that "the signification must be perfectly explicit. There are many possible degrees of condensation and of clarity" (Sartre 2004b: 31–32).

EXISTENTIAL PSYCHOANALYSIS

Bringing our ever present, yet non-thematized, self-awareness into the light, articulating our pre-reflective consciousness into an explicit narrative about how we view the world, is a task for existentialist psychoanalysis, that is, Sartre's invention of a therapeutic method grounded on his ontology of conscious being (Sartre 2003: part IV).

Consciousness is non-positionally conscious of itself, it is a "being-for-itself," a being that is a presence to itself, and thus, a being that is always at a distance from itself; that distance is impossible to cross, precisely because—not being some physical distance—it is nothing. That *nothingness* is the hallmark of our way of being, which—contrary to the reifying metaphors of both idealist and materialist metaphysics—is not a thing, but a consciousness *of* things. A being-in-itself, such as a table or a chair, is a plenitude of being, identical to itself, always being what it is; a conscious being, marked by a distance to itself, is a lack of being, non-identical to what it is (Hatzimoysis 2011: 23–39).

The constant striving of acquiring identity, of becoming one with oneself, not as an inert object, but as a free agent, marks each conscious being's unique way of being, and constitutes her fundamental project—what she makes herself to be in and through the way she responds to the world. Each person's fundamental project is a unique and freely chosen way of becoming oneself, in her unceasing attempt to solve the problem of how to be something complete and at one with oneself, while being a free agent, always throwing herself out of her past toward the future.

The responsibility that comes with the realization that we are free, that even not to choose, in certain circumstances, is just the choice to not choose, is for many people too much to bear, and is thus masked through attempts to live in bad faith. Often assimilated to the epistemic phenomenon of self-deception, bad faith could be better understood as a project of falsely identifying oneself either with one's *facticity*—whatever about one's past, one's body, or one's historical reality cannot be otherwise—or with one's *transcendence*—the ability to constantly move beyond one's present being, toward an as yet unformed self. Identifying with one's facticity allows one to think of oneself not as an agent, but as an overdetermined subject, thus rescinding any responsibility for how one lives. Alternatively, identifying oneself with pure transcendence allows one to pretend that one's choices are unrelated to the economic, social, political, or cultural facts of one's actual situation.

Existentialist psychoanalysis aims to help the analysand grow out of her immersion into bad faith, and toward an authentic way of being (Sartre 2003: 94n). As a therapeutic method, it purports to help the patient move away from impure reflection—that is, the common tendency to conceive oneself as an object, with fixed properties, which supposedly determine the course of one's life, and toward a purifying reflection that makes the agent recognize the network of rationalizations, convenient oversights, and deliberate exculpations, which have led the patient to gradually trap herself into a distorted self-image.

We have to acknowledge that we are normative beings, that our identities are formed by the commitments we undertake to act, think, or respond affectively in certain ways—to acknowledge that a conscious being "*has to be* what it is" (Sartre 2003: 21; emphasis in the original). We also have to face up to the particular commitments each one of us has, as these can be revealed by an opening to our own experience of the phenomena, to the way the world—with its challenges, affordances, and rewards—appear to ourselves, given the projects in which our situated freedom unfolds (Webber 2009).

That opening to the phenomena forms the ground of existentialist psychoanalysis, which, according to Sartre, differs from traditional psychoanalysis in at least three respects: it encourages flexibility, as it denies that there is a fixed therapeutic protocol, serviceable for all types of patients, irrespective of the particularities of their situation; it promotes the collaboration of analyst and analysand, so as to undermine the myth of the patient's passivity, while increasing awareness of the shared responsibility for what transpires in a therapeutic context; and, finally, as the therapy progresses over time, it gives the subject's own "intuition" of her experience an important role, over the ready-made interpretations supplied in the analyst's textbooks (2003: 594).

Training in existential psychoanalysis is itself a demanding process, requiring no less than a secure grasp of phenomenological analysis of the concrete existence, that is, the embodied "human being-in-situation," in its three ontological dimensions of being-in-itself, being-for-itself, and being-for-others (Sartre 2003: 27).

The overall principle of existential psychoanalysis is that each agent is a totality and not a collection, and thus she expresses herself even in the most insignificant or superficial of her behaviors: "there is not a taste, a mannerism, or a human act which is not revealing . . . A gesture refers to a *Weltanschauung* and we sense it" (2003: 479). Its goal is to decode and interpret the behavioral patterns, so as to articulate them conceptually. Its point of departure is the pre-reflective awareness of lived experience. And its overall goal is to reach not some past psychic complex, but the choice that renders meaningful how one lives—so that the analysand achieves authenticity, owning up to the projects through which she, as a situated freedom, is making herself into the person she is (Sartre 2003: 589–593).

BIBLIOGRAPHY

Cannon B. (1991). *Sartre and Psychoanalysis*. Lawrence: University Press of Kansas.

Hatzimoysis A. (2011). *The Philosophy of Sartre*. Durham: Accumen.

Sartre J.-P. (1970). "Intentionality: A Fundamental Idea in Husserl's Phenomenology" [1933], trans. J. Fell. *Journal of the British Society of Phenomenology* 1(2): 4–5.

Sartre J-P. (1981). *The Family Idiot: Gustave Flaubert, 1821–1857* vol. 1 [1971], trans. C. Cosman. Chicago: Chicago University Press.

Sartre J.-P. (1984). *War Diaries: Notebooks from a Phoney War 1939–40*, trans. Q. Hoare. London: Verso.

Sartre J.-P. (2000). *Nausea* [1938], trans. R. Baldick. London: Penguin Classics.

Sartre J.-P. (2003). *Being and Nothingness* [1943], trans. H. Barnes. London: Routledge.

Sartre J.-P. (2004a). *The Transcendence of the Ego* [1937], trans. A. Brown. London: Routledge.

Sartre J.-P. (2004b) *Sketch for a Theory of the Emotions* [1939], trans. P. Mariet. London: Routledge.

Sartre J-P. (2004c). *The Imaginary: A Phenomenological Psychology of the Imagination* [1940], trans. J. Webber. London: Routledge.

Webber J. (2009). *The Existentialism of Jean-Paul Sartre*. New York: Routledge.

CHAPTER 6

MERLEAU-PONTY, PHENOMENOLOGY, AND PSYCHOPATHOLOGY

MAXINE SHEETS-JOHNSTONE

A BRIEF BIOGRAPHY OF MERLEAU-PONTY

MERLEAU-PONTY was born on March 14, 1908, in Rochefort-sur-Mer, France. He was raised by his mother, his father having died when Merleau-Ponty was five years old. After completing his secondary schooling and studies at the Lycée Louis-le-Grand in Paris, Merleau-Ponty was a student at the École Normale Supérieure where he met Jean-Paul Sartre and Simone de Beauvoir. He attended the "Paris Lectures" of Edmund Husserl in 1929 and received his agrégation in philosophy in 1930. In 1934, he was given a permanent professorship at a lycée in Chartres and had his first article—"Christianity and *Ressentiment*"—published in 1935. He was conscripted in 1939 and served briefly as a lieutenant in an infantry regiment. In 1940 he returned to teaching at a lycée in Paris and later that year married Suzanne Berthe Jolibois. Their only child, Marianne Merleau-Ponty, was born in June 1941. In 1945, Merleau-Ponty defended his major doctoral thesis, "Phenomenology of Perception," and, with Sartre, Beauvoir, and others, founded *Les temps modernes*. In 1949 he was appointed Professor of Child Psychology and Pedagogy at the Université de Paris, Sorbonne, and in 1952 was elected Chair of Philosophy at the College de France. From 1935 onward, in addition to writing several books, he wrote a number of articles, many of which are included in *The Primacy of Perception* and *Sens et Non-sens*. He continued teaching as well as writing, teaching in particular courses on Nature, until his death on May 3, 1961. He died of coronary thrombosis. Several of his writings, including *The Visible and the Invisible*, were published posthumously.

Assessing Merleau-Ponty's Writings
in Psychopathology

Merleau-Ponty's writings in psychopathology were both exceptional and non-exceptional. They were exceptional in bringing scientific research into phenomenology. Husserl had written from time to time on the abnormal—for example, in *Ideas II*, Husserl considers what transpires when a particular sense organ no longer functions normally while others continue to do so (Husserl 1989: 71ff.)—but he did not delve into the psychopathological. Heidegger too might be cited: the "they" might be viewed as metaphysically abnormal, the "they" being those who repress recognition of their own mortality, who see death as happening only to others, and whom Heidegger deems "inauthentic" (Heidegger 1962). Merleau-Ponty, in contrast, delved into contemporary studies of psychopathology, in particular, the extensive studies of Kurt Goldstein and Adhémar Gelb. He also based his own psychopathological analyses on the writings of Sigmund Freud even as he diverged from them. Thus one might say that he devoted himself assiduously to available contemporary literature in the then burgeoning fields of neuropsychiatry and psychoanalysis.

The writings of Merleau-Ponty were non-exceptional in that Merleau-Ponty was not the only philosopher to take up the studies of Gelb and Goldstein. Indeed, Merleau-Ponty drew on the writings of Ernst Cassirer in his own investigations, sometimes without due citation. A remarkable difference exists between the two philosophers. While Merleau-Ponty read the writings of Gelb and Goldstein, Cassirer visited the Frankfurt Neurological Institute where Gelb and Goldstein conducted their research. He observed patients at the Institute and even had "frequent conversations" with a patient (unnamed, but quite likely Schneider, a patient whose spatial sense of his own body, including its orientation, was severely damaged, and whose capacities and lack thereof were at the time taken to be basic to phenomenological understandings of the body and space) (Cassirer 1957: 239). It is not surprising, then, that Goldstein cites Cassirer substantively in his own writings (Goldstein 1939, 1940). Cassirer's citations of Goldstein and Gelb in support of his differentiating "active space" and "symbolic space" are of particular interest insofar as they mirror Goldstein and Gelb's original distinction, and in turn, Merleau-Ponty's distinction, between concrete movement and abstract movement. Cassirer states, "Certain experiments dealing with pathological modifications in the spatial consciousness . . . show that many persons[,] whose ability to recognize spatial forms and to interpret them objectively is gravely impaired[,] can perform highly complex spatial tasks if these can be approached in another way, through certain movements and 'kinesthetic' perceptions" (Cassirer 1957: 153 n. 10). Cassirer's conclusion in which he cites studies of blind persons—"we must conceive the 'space' of the blind not as a representative image-space but primarily as a dynamic 'behavior space', a definite field of action and movement" (1957: 153 n. 10)—reads in its structure and "must" as if it could have come from the later hand of Merleau-Ponty (see e.g. 1962: xvi, 254; 1968: 134). Merleau-Ponty in fact echoes Cassirer's recognition of "movements and 'kinesthetic' perceptions," and a "'behavior space'" when he introduces the idea of "the body in face of its task" (1962: 100), though without giving prominence to kinesthesia. The sensory modality to which Merleau-Ponty attaches primary significance is vision, and this not only in taking up Gelb and Goldstein's specifications of concrete and abstract movement and in his own specification of "the spatiality of the situation" (1962: 100) with respect to Schneider, the patient on whom he focuses, but in his later writings in *The Visible and the Invisible* in which he draws far more extensively on Freud.

CEZANNE'S DOUBT AND MERLEAU-PONTY'S DOUBT

Merleau-Ponty's article "Cezanne's Doubt" is a blueprint of Merleau-Ponty's own doubt, and in turn, a blueprint of his philosophy of existence. In other words, what Merleau-Ponty construes in his psychoanalytic diagnosis of Cezanne and how he construes it are reflected in his own personally tinged psychoanalytic philosophy. Psychoanalytic diagnosis and philosophy are indeed intertwined. For example, Merleau-Ponty states, "My point of view: a philosophy, like a work of art, is an object that can arouse more thoughts than those that are 'contained' in it. . . . [Like a work of art, a philosophy] retains a meaning outside of its historical context, even *has* a meaning only outside of that context" (1968: 199). Merleau-Ponty's chosen title, "Cezanne's Doubt," exemplifies this "point of view." While Descartes's famous methodological doubt is epistemologically oriented, Cezanne's methodological doubt is artistically oriented. The doubts, however, are essentially and existentially intertwined: both Descartes and Cezanne broke away from tradition, Descartes with respect to philosophy, Cezanne with respect to art. What may surely be termed Merleau-Ponty's doubt, as evidenced in *Phenomenology of Perception*, centers in part on Sartre's ontological *Being and Nothingness*, on what Sartre describes as the in-itself and the for-itself, or in other words, on what Merleau-Ponty sees as divisionary thinking that admits no middle ground, and on what he proceeds to centralize in *ambiguity*. His specific *methodological* doubt, however, is tethered exclusively to Husserl. As Albert Rabil points out, "Merleau-Ponty's method was drawn from a variety of sources among which he made few distinctions" (Rabil 1967: 164). He earlier astutely observes, "It is interesting that the preface to *Phenomenology of Perception* can be read independently of the body of that book. There is no attempt to apply the phenomenological method as it is outlined to the descriptions of experience which abound there" (1967: 62). Phenomenologist and phenomenological historian Herbert Spiegelberg makes a similar observation:

> How far can Merleau-Ponty's writings be considered to be demonstrations of the phenomenological method? This is not an easy question to answer. Few if any of his texts read like protocols of phenomenological research. The reason is not only that he usually starts out from a critical discussion of the traditional views. Most of the presentation of his own position takes the form of simple assertions of findings that he seems to have made long before. Rarely does he carry out the analysis before our very eyes or invite us to look with him at the phenomena

by a methodical and painstaking investigation. Instead, he gives us his results ready-made, leaving it to us to do our own verifying.

(Spiegelberg 1971: 559)

Merleau-Ponty's methodological insistence on finding and describing a reversibility (chiasm, *Ineinander*, intertwining) that sustains ambiguity is readily evident in "Cezanne's Doubt":

> There is a rapport between Cezanne's schizoid temperament and his work because the work reveals a metaphysical sense of the disease: a way of seeing the world reduced to the totality of frozen appearances, with all expressive values suspended. Thus illness ceases to be an absurd fact and a fate and becomes a general possibility of human existence. It becomes so when this existence bravely faces one of its paradoxes, the phenomenon of expression. In this sense to be schizoid and to be Cezanne come to the same thing. It is therefore impossible to separate creative liberty from that behavior . . . already evident in Cezanne's first gestures as a child and in the way he reacted to things. (1964: 20–21)

This same intertwining describes sexuality and existence.

MERLEAU-PONTY'S AMBIGUOUS WAY OF LIFE

Merleau-Ponty writes of the "interfusion between sexuality and existence" (1962: 169). He states, "[A]s an ambiguous atmosphere, sexuality is co-extensive with life. In other words, ambiguity is of the essence of human existence, and everything we live or think has always several meanings" (1962: 169). A puzzling and at the same time highly suggestive remark concerning sexuality follows. Merleau-Ponty observes, "A way of life—an attitude of escapism and the need of solitude—is perhaps a generalized expression of a certain state of sexuality" (1962: 169). That "certain state of sexuality" remains unelucidated, though Merleau-Ponty proceeds to remark:

> In thus becoming transformed into existence, sexuality has taken upon itself so general a significance, the sexual theme has contrived to be for the subject the occasion for so many accurate and true observations in themselves, of so many rationally based decisions, and it has become so loaded with the passage of time that it is an impossible undertaking to seek, within the framework of sexuality, the explanation of the framework of existence. The fact remains that this existence is the act of taking up and making explicit a sexual situation, and that in this way it has always at least a double sense. (1962: 169)

"[A]n attitude of escapism" and "the need of solitude" are a striking "way of life" in light of commentaries about Merleau-Ponty. At the very beginning of his Preface to Merleau-Ponty's *Signs*, Richard McCleary states, "[Merleau-Ponty] was well enough known in the cosmopolitan world he comments on in *Signs*, but the studied wall of solitude he built about him made it hard for even intimates to know him" (McCleary 1964: ix). In fact, McCleary states, "He kept his distance," though "from that distance he made men wonder . . . [h]is studied anonymity became at times intensely personal" (1964: ix). He furthermore remarks on what Merleau-Ponty himself would designate as his personal "style": Merleau-Ponty's "stage is a shifting world, which he sees according to his own lights"; Merleau-Ponty "is simply trying to express more clearly the experience he shares with other men, who cannot put it into words and yet are vital to his effort"; Merleau-Ponty is "searching for himself by questioning his world. We hear him learning 'to speak with his own voice'" (1964: x). A comment by Spiegelberg runs along similar lines:

> Usually the writings of Merleau-Ponty avoid the first person singular. This is hardly [an] accident. The focus of his thought is not on the ego, but on the phenomenon ahead, the *Sache*. It is therefore not surprising that Merleau-Ponty has not yet given any autobiographical statement nor has any formulation of his comprehensive plans or guiding motifs appeared. . . . Perhaps the most revealing among the titles of Merleau-Ponty's books to appear thus far is that of the collection of his essays, *Sens et non-sens*.
>
> (Spiegelberg 1971: 524).

It is notable that Spiegelberg goes on to point out, "Merleau-Ponty's thought has been called a 'Philosophy of Ambiguity'" (1971: 524–525). Does a certain "way of life" with its "attitude of escapism and the need of solitude" constitute the "thought" that personally motivates a philosophy of ambiguity?

SEXUALITY AND AMBIGUITY

We see across the whole of Merleau-Ponty's developing existential analyses the conceptual bond between intertwining and ambiguity that is everywhere descriptive of life. A novelistic biographer might interpret this conceptual bond psychoanalytically. Merleau-Ponty's focal concern with Freud's sexually based psychoanalytic and Freud's notion of overdetermination (discussed particularly in Freud's writings on dreams) might add to the hypothetical interpretive sketch. In particular, a novelistic biographer might interpret Merleau-Ponty's elaborations of Freud's sexually based psychoanalytic and notion of overdetermination together with his own existential analyses that anchor our lives in an interfusion of sexuality and existence, in ambiguity, in a prepersonal I, and in the anonymous—all of them central concepts in Merleau-Ponty's writings—as living in the challenge of a bisexual orientation, what might be described as an inescapable *Ineinander*, surely a challenge given the time and the academic contexts in which he lived. The dialectic of sexuality that he describes as "the tending of an existence toward another existence which denies it, and yet without which it is not sustained," and his claim that "Sexuality conceals itself from itself beneath a mask of generality, and continually tries to escape from the tension and drama which it sets up" (1962: 168) lend a certain credence to the hypothetical sketch. Moreover taking up Freud's notion of overdetermination, Merleau-Ponty writes, "The 'associations' of psychoanalysis are in reality 'rays' of time and of the world. . . . there is no association that comes into play unless there is overdetermination, that is, a relation of relations, a coincidence that cannot be fortuitous, that has an *ominal* [presumably meaning 'portentous'] sense. The tacit Cogito 'thinks' only overdeterminations" (1968: 240).

   If one were to take up the novelistic biographer's hypothetical sketch, not to convince anyone of its truth, but to show that one's quest to be true to the truths of experience may well be shadowed by one's own life challenges, and indeed in a way precisely as Merleau-Ponty details in his conception of the invisible and of the unconscious—the "tacit Cogito"—one might furthermore bring out in illuminating ways how historical limitations play into one's conceptual and theoretical perspectives and have the possibility of skewing one's analyses. Lacan's notion of the "mirror image," for example, is front and center in Merleau-Ponty's developmental writings on infants and children; the term "body image" (from neurologist Henry Head's original writings) is front and center in Merleau-Ponty's elucidation of pathological bodies. As Martin Dillon astutely notes, "The term 'image' is ill suited for its function insofar as it suggests an exclusively visual or representation form of awareness" (Dillon 1978: 98 n. 6; see also Sheets-Johnstone 2005). As noted earlier, a visual awareness predominates in Merleau-Ponty's writings. It is in fact central throughout his analyses, a fact that explains not simply the prominence of the invisible, but the chiasm of the visible and the invisible and their ambiguous relationship.

In brief, Merleau-Ponty anchors our lives in ambiguity, in a prepersonal I, in the anonymous, and in an overdetermined tacit Cogito's thinking by which "any entity can be *accentuated* as an emblem of Being" (1968: 270), in which the unconscious "[is] to be understood on the basis of the flesh" (1968: 270), in which "every analysis that "*disentangles* renders unintelligible" (1968: 268), and in an overarching "interfusion of sexuality and existence, which means that existence permeates sexuality and *vice versa*, so that it is impossible to determine in a given decision or action, the proportion of sexual to other motivations, impossible to label a decision or act 'sexual' or 'non-sexual'" (1962: 169).

FREUDIAN INFLUENCES AND MERLEAU-PONTY'S EXISTENTIAL ANALYSES

To an interesting degree, Merleau-Ponty's developmental journey within his discipline follows that of Freud within his. Both Merleau-Ponty and Freud were thoroughly cognizant of the existing knowledge and goals of their respective disciplines, but wanted to develop that knowledge and those goals not along further lines but along different lines. As psychiatrist Edward Nersessian notes in his essay on the concept of signal anxiety, Freud "boldly broke new ground in his attempts to understand human suffering both scientifically and imaginatively" (Nersessian 2013/2015: 173/827). Nersessian points out specifically that:

> As a medical doctor and neuro-pathologist, Freud's primary goal was the advancement of science. . . . At a certain point, however, around 1923, he found the science of his day to be too limiting and restrictive, and he moved beyond the confines of that body of knowledge, creating his own anatomy of the mind as an alternative to the established functional anatomy of the brain. This break allowed his imagination to move freely with little constraint. (2013/2015: 173/ 827)

In a similar way, Merleau-Ponty wanted to advance phenomenological studies that he found limited and restrictive, particularly with respect to Husserl's phenomenological methodology and Sartre's ontology, and in turn moved to create his own existential analyses that were initially fortified by scientific studies of behavior and of psychopathology. Just as Freud "forged his way forward undeterred by what we today call confirmation bias" (ibid.), so Merleau-Ponty forged his way forward undeterred by the fact that no method existed by which his studies and conclusions could be confirmed. Indeed, as we have seen with respect to *Phenomenology of Perception*, "There is no attempt to apply the phenomenological method as it is outlined to the descriptions of experience which abound there" (Rabil 1967: 62).

Not only are Merleau-Ponty's analyses methodologically akin to Freud's self-analysis in their idiosyncratic line of thought, but his basic concepts are offshoots of Freud's and in some instances even grounded in Freud's. For example, after remarking on how "much remains to be done to draw from psychoanalytic experience all that it contains," and after giving as an example the fact that "In order to account for that osmosis between the body's anonymous life and the person's official life which is Freud's great discovery, it was necessary to introduce something *between* the organism and our selves considered as a sequence of deliberate acts and express understandings," Merleau-Ponty states, "This was Freud's *unconscious*" (1964: 229).

Merleau-Ponty does not leave the concept of the unconscious intact, but declares, "we still have to find the right formulation for what he intended by this provisional designation" (1964: 229). He reformulates Freud's notion in a way that strikingly accords with his own philosophy: "In an approximative language, Freud is on the point of discovering what other thinkers have more appropriately named *ambiguous perception*" (1964: 229).

Merleau-Ponty's Analysis of Schneider

Merleau-Ponty takes up Schneider's pathological condition, his ability to execute "[c]oncrete movements and acts of grasping," such movements and acts "enjoy[ing] a privileged position," and his inability to execute abstract movements such as pointing (1962: 103). The patient, Merleau-Ponty concludes, is aware "neither of the stimulus nor of his reaction: quite simply he is his body and his body is the potentiality of a certain world" (1962: 106). This world-centered body is actually "the body in face of its tasks," the body that Merleau-Ponty terms the prepersonal phenomenal everyday body. Thus in spite of his disclaimer that the normal is not deduced from the abnormal, Merleau-Ponty deduces the normal from the abnormal. In particular, possible bodily variations—a body that is "without hands, feet, head ... and, *a* fortiori a sexless man," and more broadly, a man lacking "all human 'functions', from sexuality to motility and intelligence" (1962: 170)—variations that Dillon points out in clarifying Merleau-Ponty's troubled assertion in the context of his examination of "the case of Schneider" that "[e]verything in man is a necessity" (1962: 170), all these variations allow Merleau-Ponty "to reveal the normal through departures from it" (Dillon 1980: 78). In fact, Dillon remarks, "In a later essay, 'Phenomenology and the Sciences of Man' . . ., Merleau-Ponty makes this very point about the correlation between Husserlian eidetics [essences] and the 'inductive' methodology of the empirial sciences" (1980: 78).

Notable in Merleau-Ponty's linking of Schneider's spontaneous concrete movement with normal everyday movement is not only his deduction of the normal from the pathological, but his passing over of any recognition of learning. We are not born with all those everyday adult abilities specified and described in terms of concrete movement—for example, the very basic capacity to grasp. As normal human infants, we all learn our bodies and learn to move ourselves (Sheets-Johnstone 1999/exp. 2nd edn. 2011). Following remarks on abstract movement—"The patient, like the scientist, verifies mediately and clarifies his hypothesis by cross-checking facts, and makes his way blindly toward the one which co-ordinates them all" (1962: 131)—Merleau-Ponty goes on to affirm a "world-centered body," hence the difference between concrete and abstract movement in terms of perception: "This procedure [that patient and scientist go through] contrasts with, and by so doing throws into relief, the spontaneous method of normal perception, that kind of living system of meanings which makes the concrete essence of the object immediately recognizable, and allows its 'sensible properties' to appear only the through that essence" (1962: 131).

Puzzles about the Touching and the Touched

In *The Visible and the Invisible*, Merleau-Ponty links seer and seen with touching and touched. The example he gives of the reversibility of seer and seen is rooted in tactility: "We must habituate ourselves to think that every visible is cut out in the tangible"; "we know that . . . vision is a palpation with the look" (1968: 134). He goes on to affirm that "the thickness of flesh between the seer and the thing is constitutive for the thing of its visibility as for the seer of his corporeity," and further, that "What we call a visible is . . . a quality pregnant with a texture, the surface of a depth" (1968: 136). In all his descriptions and examples of the visible, a distinctively I–world relationship obtains. In striking contrast, an I–world relationship is absent in his singular example and description of tactility. In its stead is the left hand touching the right hand: "a veritable touching of the touch, when my right hand touches my left hand while it is palpating the things, where the 'touching subject' passes over to the rank of the touched" (1968: 133–134). What is odd and even puzzling is that there is not an intercorporeity example of touching and touched—a handshake, a pat on the back, even a kiss. What is odd and even puzzling too is that there are no definitive "things" that the left hand is "palpating," and even why it is necessary to bring in "the things" since it is a question of the reversibility of touching and touched hands. An embrace would indeed seem a more everyday life example of the reversibility of touching and touched than what amounts to an I–I reversible relationship. We might in fact recall the remark of philosopher Marjorie Grene, an otherwise avowed aficionado of Merleau-Ponty: "Every time I read him, I have, once more, the sense that his approach to philosophical problems is entirely, overwhelmingly right. . . . As with no other thinker, I say, yes, so it is—but what about that hand trick? Alas, I cannot make it work" (Grene 1976: 619).

Back to Cezanne

Is Merleau-Ponty's diagnosis of Cezanne a self-diagnosis as well, a divergence from tradition that engenders a new perspective and that seeks expression? Is there thus "a rapport" between Merleau-Ponty's "schizoid temperament and his work" as there is between Cezanne's "schizoid temperament and his work"? In short, is Merleau-Ponty's "creative liberty" akin to that of Cezanne? In support of this possibility, consider that what Merleau-Ponty states as true of speech and expression is equally true of writing and expression: "The analysis of speech and expression brings home to us the enigmatic nature of our own body even more effectively than did our remarks on bodily space and unity" (1962: 197).

BIBLIOGRAPHY

Cassirer E. (1957). *The Phenomenology of Knowledge*, vol. 3. New Haven: Yale University Press.

Dillon M. C. (1978). "Merleau-Ponty and the Psychogenesis of the Self." *Journal of Phenomenological Psychology* 9: 84–98.

Dillon M. C. (1980). "Merleau-Ponty on Existential Sexuality: A Critique." *Journal of Phenomenological Psychology* 11: 67–82.

Goldstein K. (1939). *The Organism*. New York: American Book Company.

Goldstein K. (1940). *Human Nature in the Light of Psychopathology*. Cambridge: Harvard University Press.

Grene M. (1976). "Merleau-Ponty and the Renewal of Ontology." *Review of Metaphysics* 29: 605–625.

Heidegger M. (1962). *Being and Time*, trans. J. Macquarrie and E. Robinson. New York: Harper & Row.

Husserl E. (1989). *Ideas Pertaining to a Pure Phenomenology and to a Phenomenological Philosophy (Ideas II)*, trans. R. Rojcewicz and A. Schuwer. Boston: Kluwer Academic.

McCleary R. (1964). *Preface to Signs*, trans. R. McCleary. Evanston: Northwestern University Press.

Merleau-Ponty M. (1962). *Phenomenology of Perception*, trans. C. Smith. New York: Routledge & Kegan Paul.

Merleau-Ponty Maurice. (1964). *Signs*, trans. R. McCleary. Evanston: Northwestern University Press.

Merleau-Ponty M. (1968). *The Visible and the Invisible*, ed. C. Lefort, trans. A. Lingis. Evanston: Northwestern University Press.

Nersessian E. (2013/2015). "Psychoanalytic Theory of Anxiety: Proposals for Reconsideration." In S. Arbiser and J. Schneider (eds.), *On Freud's "Inhibitions, Symptoms and Anxiety,"* pp. 172–184. London: Karnac Press. Eine Überprüfung des Konzepts der Signalangst. In V. W. Bohleber (ed.) *Angst. Neubetrachtungen Eines Psychoanalytischen Konzepts. Psyche* 69: 826–845.

Rabil A. (1967). *Merleau-Ponty: Existentialist of the Social World*. New York: Columbia University Press.

Sheets-Johnstone M. (2005). "What Are We Naming?" In H. D. Preester and V. Knockaert (eds.), *Body Image and Body Schema: Interdisciplinary Perspectives on the Body*, pp. 211–231. Philadelphia: John Benjamins.

Sheets-Johnstone M. (2011). *The Primacy of Movement*, expanded 2nd edn. Philadelphia: John Benjamins.

Spiegelberg H. (1971). *The Phenomenological Movement*, vol. 2, 2nd edn. The Hague: Martinus Nijhoff.

CHAPTER 7

SIMONE DE BEAUVOIR

SHANNON M. MUSSETT

BIOGRAPHY

SIMONE de Beauvoir was a French existentialist, author, and activist who produced her most important works from the mid- to late-twentieth century. Influenced by earlier thinkers such as Edmund Husserl, Henri Bergson, Martin Heidegger, Immanuel Kant, and G. W. F. Hegel, she developed a unique approach to phenomenology through her ongoing concern with issues of tyranny, oppression, and liberation. Although she often eschewed the title, "philosopher," preferring instead to be considered a literary figure (her most famous novel, *The Mandarins*, won the *Prix Goncourt* in 1954), she remains one of the most important philosophers of the twentieth century.

BEAUVOIR'S LIFE

Born on January 9, 1908, Beauvoir quickly proved to be intellectually motivated. She excelled at school, passing the *baccaluaréat* exams in philosophy and mathematics in 1925. At the Sorbonne she engaged in a wide range of disciplines, including history, logic, ethics, sociology, and psychology, concluding her study with a graduate *diplôme* on Leibniz written under Léon Brunschvig. She went on to complete her teacher training at the lycée Janson-de-Sailly with fellow students, Maurice Merleau-Ponty and Claude Lévi-Strauss, both of whom played significant roles in Beauvoir's philosophical development. Beauvoir took second place in the philosophy *agrégation* exam (at twenty-one years of age, she was the youngest student ever to pass) losing to Jean-Paul Sartre, for whom it was the second attempt. Beauvoir was not an official student at the elite *École Normale Superiour*, but she attended lectures there. During this time, she met a group of students, including Paul Nizan and Sartre, who invited her to study with them because of her intellectual acuity. Thus began her lifelong involvement, intellectually and often romantically, with Sartre. Despite their relationship, Beauvoir and Sartre never married and had numerous other romantic commitments. Beauvoir herself had relationships with women and men, most notably, Jacques Bost, Nelson Algren, Claude Lanzmann, and Olga Kosakievicz, all of whom impacted her work in significant ways.

Beauvoir taught briefly but was dismissed from teaching in 1943 due to a complaint about student corruption. In the 1940s, she began publishing fiction, much of which provides a literary framework for the themes developed in her philosophy. During this decade, she also wrote two important works on existential ethics, *Pyrrhus and Cineas* (1944) and *The Ethics of Ambiguity* (1947), both of which underscore her lifelong dedication to questions of morality.

Her engagement with phenomenology came to fruition in her 1949 book, *The Second Sex*. This work is often considered the bedrock of modern philosophical feminism and a significant advance in the area of phenomenology. Beauvoir was also active in founding and running the journal, *Les temps modernes*, with Sartre and Merleau-Ponty. She remained a prolific novelist, essayist, autobiographer, philosopher, and political activist (against French colonialization and in favor of women's reproductive rights) until the end of her life. In 1970, she published another significant work in existential phenomenology, *Old Age*.[1] Beauvoir died on April 14, 1986.[2]

BEAUVOIR'S RELATIONSHIP TO PHENOMENOLOGICAL PSYCHOPATHOLOGY

Beauvoir's relationship to phenomenological psychopathology revolves around her method—which is itself deeply phenomenological in most of her work—as well as her nuanced understanding of and relationship to psychology and psychoanalysis. Unlike psychoanalysis, which seeks out the causes of abnormal symptoms, Beauvoir's work is at its finest when she allows the so-called "abnormal" to speak for itself, and in so doing, to show that atypical behaviors are more often than not systematically produced and misunderstood, rather than markers of individual psychological aberration.

Despite her interest in psychology and psychoanalysis, as well as her learned treatment of many thinkers in these traditions, she did not claim to diagnose disorders in any fashion, but rather to understand how various groups and individuals become marginalized and oppressed by dominant philosophical and political systems. Unlike Sartre, who early on rejects the unconscious as a strategy of bad faith, Beauvoir finds that psychoanalysis is not always a problematic discipline in providing descriptions of complex human behaviors. This admiration is most evident in her depictions in *The Second Sex* of Jacques Lacan's notion of identity as largely formed through reflection and distortion through the other, and in her adoption of Freud's conception of the fundamentally sexed nature of human experience (even as she staunchly opposes his sexism).

Beauvoir admires how psychoanalysis shows how "no factor intervenes in psychic life without having taken on human meaning; it is not the body-object described by scientists that exists concretely but the body lived by the subject" (Beauvoir 2010: 49). She has in mind

---

[1] The book, *La vieillesse* is translated as *The Coming of Age* in the English edition. However, this less accurate translation fails to capture the starkness of the title in French.

[2] See Mussett 2003 for a more detailed biographical account.

the particular role that sexuality plays in embodiment. For her, our experience is not determined by our unconscious libidinal drives; rather, it is constituted by our more basic desire "to connect concretely with existence through the whole world, grasped in all possible ways," (2010: 56) which is not originally sexual in nature (although sexuality is one of the primary ways in which experience is concretized).

But psychoanalysis is not without its major shortcomings. In *The Second Sex*, Beauvoir lambastes Freud for his lack of concern for the differences between men and women and his general grafting of the female to the masculine model of sexuality and personhood. She notes that Freud's woman is merely a "modified man," thus insufficiently describing her experience as a differently sexed being (Beauvoir 2010: 50). Beauvoir expands this problematic to the general rigidity evident in psychoanalysis regarding individual differences and free choice. She explains that psychoanalysts maintain an intractable dedication to deterministic forces which prevail unhindered regardless of individual and cultural vicissitudes. If action is determined by epic psychic structures and largely unknowable and unchangeable libidinal energies, then psychoanalysis must ultimately be rejected by existentialism with its emphasis on freedom and choice. True existential choice necessarily requires a direct confrontation with the drives and prohibitions that lurk in the intersections of mind and body, not a kind of fatalism regarding their power over human action. Thus, we must recover "the original intentionality of existence . . . Without going back to this source, man [*sic*] appears a battlefield of drives and prohibitions equally devoid of meaning and contingent" (2010: 55). Here we can see Beauvoir's links to phenomenological psychopathology very clearly. Looking for the causes of drives and symptoms without taking into account the way in which human beings make meaning of the world in general only leads to unfounded metaphysical assumptions that obscure individual lived experience.

Beauvoir is drawn to literature and autobiography precisely because they allow us to speak of a kind of experience that is out of reach to philosophy and science. Literature, often more so than philosophy, taps into aspects of living in the world that are far from conscious and yet belong to all of us as human beings. Her belief that fictional and autobiographical narratives have the potential to reveal deep truths about human experience that other disciplines lack, makes her a detailed and innovative practitioner of existential phenomenology.

THE PATHOLOGIZING OF WOMEN AND THE ELDERLY

Despite the central role literature and autobiography play in her theoretical framework, the clearest access that we have into Beauvoir's relationship to the development of phenomenological psychopathology can be found in her two studies, *The Second Sex* and *Old Age* [*La Vieillesse*]. Both of these works follow similar structures—the first half of the book explores various interpretive lenses employed in understanding the phenomena in question: in the case of women in the West, how they appear as the "Other" to the masculine subject through multiple theoretical and scientific perspectives (biology, psychoanalysis, literature, historical materialism, history, etc.). In the case of the elderly, how they appear as outcasts through the perspectives of biology, ethnology, and history. In both books, Beauvoir shows how women and the elderly come to be pathologized as aberrant from the perspective of the dominant culture. This notion of finding the feminine or the elderly somehow *abnormal* may seem un-usual, given that the former constitute half of the population, and the latter are the inevitable terminus for all human beings who survive past middle age. Beauvoir's reliance upon the self–other dynamic is helpful in comprehending this important move in her work.

Utilizing the phenomenological method of Hegel, but also some basic tenants of struc-turalism, such as those found in Lévi-Strauss's anthropology and Lacan's psychoanalysis, Beauvoir conceives of a fundamental self–other dynamic operative in identity formation and interpersonal relationships, both on the individual and social levels. As she explains, "the category of *Other* is as original as consciousness itself. The duality between Self and Other can be found in the most primitive societies, in the most ancient mythologies" (Beauvoir 2010: 6). Instead of an originary belongingness (what Heidegger would refer to as *Mitsein*, or being-with) she instead emphasizes a more Hegelian framework wherein "a fundamental hostility to any other consciousness is found in consciousness itself; the subject posits it-self only in opposition; it asserts itself as the essential and sets up the other as inessential, as the object" (2010: 7). This critical claim comes to play a role in her later analysis of how the elderly—consciousness sets itself up as essential (one could say, as the primary meaning-bestowing subject) only by distinguishing itself from the other, to which it immediately puts itself in opposition. This opposition, as found in Hegel's master–slave dialectic, is conten-tious and often results in the oppression of the other by the subject, at least until their shared humanity is recognized by both. Mutual recognition, when it is achieved out of this conflic-tual psychic structure, initiates a move away from inequality, psychic violence, and tyranny, and toward relationships of respect, generosity, and freedom.

Woman as the absolute Other serves a vital role in a patriarchal structure insofar as she becomes a repository for all that threatens human power. Thus, she becomes associated with birth and death (nature in general), and finitude and mortality—all of the aspects of human existence which give it meaning, but which also mark it as doomed to death and decay. In the second half of *The Second Sex*, titled "Lived Experience," Beauvoir provides rich phenome-nological descriptions of women's lives in order to track the pervasiveness of the feminine as Other. The section opens with her most famous quote: "One is not born, but rather becomes, woman" (2010: 283). Throughout this volume, she emphasizes the societal structures that impose alterity (otherness) on women from the moment of birth until death. Beginning in childhood, girls and women must adopt and navigate their status as the absolute Other to the masculine subject. Using literary accounts and sociological and psychological studies, Beauvoir often allows women to speak for themselves. Throughout the work she references analysts and psychologists such as Freud, Lacan, Carl Jung, Jean Piaget, Karen Horny, Alfred Kinsey, Helene Deutsch, Alfred Adler, Albert Ellis, and Wilhelm Stekel, as well as writers such as Henry de Montherlant, Violette Leduc, Leo Tolstoy, Richard Wright, Colette Audrey, Honoré de Balzac, and Henrik Ibsen, among many others. She provides multiple first-person accounts and case studies from women describing what it is like to undergo puberty, sexual initiation, maternity, aging, lesbianism, love, and work in order to give a multiperspectival account of the lived experiences of women as Other. Her choices range from the words of the women and girls undergoing the experiences to writings by men about them in order to show the often tremendous gulf evident between what women say they experience and what men claim is the meaning of these experiences. In some ways, the collection of experiential descriptions that suffuse the second half of *The Second Sex* continues decades later in her similar study on the alienation and pathologization of the elderly in Western culture.

Following the same phenomenological method employed in *The Second Sex*, Beauvoir titles the first half of *Old Age*, "Old Age Seen from Without," and juxtaposes it with the second part, "The Being-in-the-World." Again, she first focuses on theoretical, anthropological, literary, and scientific interpretations of the elderly, followed by numerous personal accounts of their lived experiences. As with women, the elderly undergo a social exclusion by younger populations who define their own subjectivity through being *not* other, in this case, old. Beauvoir argues that the elderly individual suffers even more radically than woman because [he is] "to a far more radical extent than a woman, a mere object. She is necessary to society whereas he is of no worth at all. He cannot be used in barter, nor for reproductive purposes, nor as a producer: he is no longer anything but a burden" (Beauvoir 1996: 89). As a result, the elderly suffer even more extreme pathologization than women; because they are, in effect, "useless" in modern capitalist society; they are shunned, silenced, forgotten, and abused, resulting in lives filled with boredom, sadness, and vulnerability.[3] Such an observation is alarming because whereas women compose half of the population, old age is something that befalls all human beings if they live long enough. In her phenomenological descriptions of the experiences of the aged, she notes how age comes upon us as a surprise, and from the judgment of others. The subject does not call herself old, those individuals and social structures around her do. Even more so than she does in *The Second Sex*, Beauvoir finds that the othering of the aged is never chosen by them (for there are no benefits in an advanced capitalist society to being old) but are forced upon the elderly by institutions and public opinion.

Beauvoir describes in detail what it *feels* like to age both from a philosophical and an autobiographical perspective. In *Old Age* she notes that "For the aged person death is no longer a general, abstract fate: it is a personal event, an event that is near at hand" (Beauvoir 1996: 440). Such an insight parallels the phenomenological descriptions of her own experiences of aging as depicted in one volume of her collected autobiography, *Hard Times*. This work concludes with dark ruminations on the approaching horrors of old age and death. At only fifty-four years of age, Beauvoir laments the inevitable waning of passions, faculties, and social standing. Describing the lived experience of bodily decline and diminished intellectual passion, she observes: "My powers of revolt are dimmed now by the imminence of my end and the fatality of the deteriorations that troop before it; but my joys have paled as well. Death is no longer a brutal event in the far distance; it haunts my sleep. Awake I sense its shadow between the world and me: it has already begun" (Beauvoir 1992: 378–379). The feminine is abject to the masculine insofar as it carries with it all that smacks of mortality, finitude, and natural growth and decay. The elderly are abject because of their temporal nearness to the absolute limit—death itself. Beauvoir's work masterfully explores this relationship between aging and death from multiple angles thus giving voice to the voiceless and socially discarded.

Beauvoir's approach, which involves listening to the marginalized and alienated groups of society, provides an invaluable perspective in the field of phenomenological psychopathology. By allowing the socially pathologized and oppressed to speak for themselves, her writings continue to impact philosophical and psychological discussion in profound and illuminating ways.

---

[3] See Mussett 2006.

BIBLIOGRAPHY

Beauvoir S. de. (1992). *Hard Times: The Force of Circumstance, Vol. II: The Autobiography of Simone de Beauvoir*, trans. R. Howard. New York: Paragon House.

Beauvoir S. de. (1996). *The Coming of Age [Old Age]*, trans. P. O'Brian. New York: W. W. Norton & Company.

Beauvoir S. de. (1997). *The Ethics of Ambiguity*, trans. B. Frechtman. Seacaucus: Citadel Press.

Beauvoir S. de. (1999). *The Mandarins*, trans. L. Friedman. New York: W.W. Norton & Co.

Beauvoir S. de. (2004). *"Pyrrhus and Cineas,"* trans. M. Timmermann. In M. Simons (ed.), *Simone de Beauvoir: Philosophical Writings*. Urbana: University of Illinois Press.

Beauvoir, S. de. (2010). *The Second Sex*, trans. C. Borde and S. M. Chevallier. New York: Knopf Doubleday.

Mussett S. M. (2003). *Simone de Beauvoir. Internet Encyclopedia of Philosophy*. http://www.iep.utm.edu/beauvoir/#H1

Mussett S. M. (2006). "Ageing and Existentialism: Simone de Beauvoir and the Limits of Freedom." In C. Tandy (ed.), *Death and Anti-Death. Volume 4: Twenty Years after de Beauvoir. Thirty Years After Heidegger*, pp. 231–255. Palo Alto: Ria University Press.

CHAPTER 8

··

MAX SCHELER

··

JOHN CUTTING

Biographical Sketch
···

MAX Scheler (1874–1928) was born in Munich in 1874 and died in Frankfurt in 1928. He was only fifty-four. He lived through some of the most turbulent decades ever—the First World War, hyperinflation, revolutions of right and left. His personal life was also torrid—three marriages, a psychopathic son, dismissal from a university post for alleged sexual impropriety. His religious affiliations were unconventional, bordering on the bizarre—his mother was an orthodox Jew, his father Lutheran, he became a Catholic, then lapsed, then rejoined the faith, and latterly renounced all forms of theism in favor of an idiosyncratic "panentheism," which holds that human beings are partners with some absolute Being with the purpose of producing a God-like entity. There are two biographies: *Max Scheler* (Staude 1967) and *Max Scheler* (Mader 1995).

He was an intensely charismatic man, single-handedly responsible for converting the philosopher and martyr Edith Stein to Catholicism, captivating all manner of audiences in formal lectures or impromptu get-togethers, once even holding the attention of the German High Command in a four-hour lecture on, of all subjects, pacifism. His contemporary philosophical colleagues revered him. Heidegger, Hartmann, and Ortega y Gasset, for example, wrote movingly about him after his death. In short, he was *primus inter pares*.

His corpus of writings, fifteen volumes in *The Collected Works*, is wide-ranging (Scheler 1954–1997). He took an interest in all the nascent disciplines of his time—sociology, psychology, psychopathology, and the new physics of relativity. He had a cosmopolitan sense of new directions in philosophy, championing Bergson and the American pragmatists. He was exquisitely attuned to the contemporary political scene: he lent support to the intellectual justification of German war aims at the start of the First World War; he then offered himself as a diplomat at the end of the war to heal the wounds; he was a friend of Walter Rathenau, the Weimar foreign minister who was assassinated by Nazis in the early 1920s; he was the most high-ranking intellectual to warn of the evils of National Socialism long before Hitler came to power. All in all, he was what the Jewish call a *Mensch*, a "man for all seasons."

He was extremely knowledgeable about psychopathology, too, and influenced one of the greatest psychopathologists of the twentieth century, Kurt Schneider, who had been his student (Cutting et al. 2016). Schneider went on to produce breakthrough formulations of . depression (Schneider 2012) and schizophrenia (Schneider 1939). Scheler himself wrote an article on compensation neurosis (Scheler 1984).

PHILOSOPHICAL DEVELOPMENT

His philosophical trajectory begins with his undergraduate and postgraduate theses on some of the various realms of knowledge available to the human being—logic, ethics, psychology, and the transcendental approach of Kant. (This sets down markers for his life-long preoccupation with epistemology.) In 1901 he met Husserl, whose phenomenological philosophy was to play a significant role in the field of non-Anglo-American intellectual debate for most of the twentieth century. Quite what happened in that meeting has never been satisfactorily established. Spiegelberg gives Scheler's account of it: Scheler had already worked out what Husserl referred to as "categorical intuition"—the ability of the human mind to grasp categories or essences prior to any sensory appreciation of some matter (Spiegelberg 1994). What matters, from a general overview of Scheler's philosophy, is that from that point forth Scheler saw in Husserl's phenomenological philosophy something that provided the answer to what had been troubling him about psychology and philosophy for several years, namely that the human being could grasp the essence of something, which Husserl called "categorical intuition," quite independently of their ability to pick up on the elements of that experience. Heretofore it had been axiomatic in psychology and much of philosophy that achieving a meaningful view of anything was a step-wise process—sensation converted to perception converted to apperception, that is, meaning. Scheler and Husserl both realized that this was wrong. Husserl later backtracked on the very insight that had inspired Scheler, and reverted to a view of cognition whereby categories could only be understood if their elemental constituents had been previously perceived. To add to Scheler's preoccupation with knowledge, in all its various forms, we can say that his appreciation that human beings can grasp the essence of things independently of any empirical calculation or abstraction was also a philosophical principle that he never renounced.

PHENOMENOLOGY OF EMOTION AND VALUE

In 1913 came the publication of two of his most celebrated works. The first was *Zur Phänomenologie und Theorie der Sympathiegefühl und vom Liebe und Hass* (*On the Phenomenology and Theory of the Feeling of Sympathy and of Love and Hate*). This ran through five editions and was retitled *Wesen und Formen der Sympathie* (*The Nature of Sympathy*) from the second edition onwards. The second treatise—*Der Formalismus in der Ethik und die materiale Wertethik* (*Formalism in Ethics and Non-Formal Ethics of Values*) (Scheler 1973b)—was published in Husserl's journal of phenomenology, a second part being published in the same journal in 1916.

We can discuss both together as they jointly constitute the bulk of Scheler's phenomenology of emotion and value. He planned a comprehensive, if not exhaustive, treatment of the entire area, and there are additional articles in his *Collected Works* on shame (Scheler 1987), and on *ordo amoris* (the order of the heart) (Scheler 1973a). The outstanding notion developed in the first book is an answer to the "question of our knowledge of other minds." We know these exist, Scheler says, not by logical analogy from our knowledge of ourselves and not by means of empathy, that is, transferring something of ourselves into the other, *but by sympathy, direct knowledge of what is there.* In the second treatise he elaborates on what it is that is grasped in such a task, how it is done, and how the entire moral and emotional make-up of a human being originates in a similar way through direct knowledge of a hierarchical order of objective values. The overall theme in both books is the postulation of a special faculty in human beings, some of which is shared with other animals, for "perceiving" an entire realm of values and discriminating between levels of these, a faculty moreover which is independent of cognition and whose structural variations in the population makes for a different moral tenor in different people, and whose "valueception," as he calls it, is registered by a correlative hierarchy of emotion. We can now add to our developing picture of Scheler's philosophy his delineation of an entire realm of emotional life in humans, with its own laws, its own perceptual apparatus, and its consequences for human nature itself.

KNOWLEDGE AND THE REALMS OF EXISTENCE

Some commentators refer to three phases in Scheler's philosophical development (Frings 1965). The works on emotion and value just discussed are deemed part of the first phase. A second phase is considered to be the books and book-length articles he brought out in the early and mid-1920s. This was an immensely prolific phase, but two books stand out, *Vom Ewigen im Menschen* (*On the Eternal in Man*) published in 1921 (Scheler 1972), and *Die Wissensformen und die Gesellschaft* (*Forms of Knowledge and Society*) from 1926 (Scheler 1926). Both deal with knowledge but in a wider and more profound framework than hitherto. The first covers philosophical and religious knowledge, the second mainly practical knowledge. Both, however, do something barely touched on before, and that is to trace knowledge back to its origin, to ask, in brief, what *is* knowledge?

I can only give a taste of the range and depth of his answers. He was writing now like a man possessed. He had a premonition of his approaching death. His wife recalled him philosophizing from the moment he woke up, scribbling things down on menus and train tickets; Heidegger (1984) writes of "day-and-night-long conversations with him" and of a man driven to "powerlessness and despair" in his search for answers.

Knowledge, as he argues, "is a relationship between entities . . . in which one entity acquires part of the nature of another entity without in any way altering the nature of this second entity. The 'known' becomes part of he or she who knows" (Scheler 1926: 247). Knowing something therefore assumes there is something there to be known, and any entity is potentially knowable. This means, for instance, that because at least some human beings possess knowledge about a religious entity—God—then God must exist for that knowledge to have been conveyed to human beings, however few. Knowledge, however, differs radically according to the realm in which the entity exists, and the way some entity exists differs across such realms. According to Scheler there are about nine realms of fundamentally different sorts—for example, absolute, external world, internal world, environment. Therefore the manner in which God exists—in the absolute realm—is not the same as the way things exist in the external world, and neither is the knowledge form appropriate to participating in the nature of God—faith—the same as the knowledge form which allows participation in things in the external world—perception. Over time, chiefly in early childhood, the continual participation of the knower in the objects falling within the jurisdiction of their correlative knowledge moulds the way the knower treats subsequent objects of the same kind, even distorting them. "How you are loved is how you will love," he writes, which means that if you are hated and not loved as a child you will grow up a hateful person, and the same goes for other realms. He calls this process whereby an object influences subjective appraisal, "functionalisation." Finally, though we could pick out numerous other pearls, what starts the knowledge process going is "love." Why should anyone "stretch out," he writes, to another being and want to know it in the first place anyway? The answer is "love": this was already identified by Plato as the hallmark of the spur to philosophical knowledge, and it is inherent in all new sorts of knowledge which are pursued by amateurs (lovers) before professionals take over (Scheler 1972). To continue our cumulative summary of Scheler's philosophy we can now say that he was developing a middle road between idealism and realism, where there was indeed "not nothing" out there but only through our *various* facilities of knowledge could this be objectified and made actual.

Anthropology and Metaphysics

The last few years of his life constitute a third phase in his philosophy when he turned more and more to anthropology and metaphysics. Much of his writings from this period were published posthumously, having been collated and saved for posterity by his third wife through all the years of the Nazi regime when he was a proscribed person. Again we are spoilt for choice, but we can single out *Die Stellung des Menschen im Kosmos* (*The Human Place in the Cosmos*) (Scheler 2009), published in 1927, as a concise summary of his philosophical anthropology, and volumes 10 to 15 of his *Collected Works*, of which I have translated several essays from volumes 11 and 12 under the title *The Constitution of the Human Being*, as the draft for a book on metaphysics that he never lived to complete (Scheler 2008b). My own favorite is the long treatise—*Idealismus—Realismus* (*Idealism and Realism*)—partly translated in 1973.

His philosophical anthropology is an attempt to answer the question, "What is the human being and what is his place in being?" His answer is that the human being shares much with the higher non-human animals—for example, intelligence, a certain emotional repertoire—but differs from such animals in possessing *Geist* (spirit and reason) which allows it to stand back and criticize and objectivize the very properties that it does share with other animals. The human is unique in the cosmos, uniquely separate from other animals in having *Geist* and uniquely separate from God in being an animal. Its achievements and woes all stem from this fact.

As for his metaphysics this is truly unique vis-à-vis any other philosopher. His notion of what metaphysics is—in short, the superordinate of all knowledges and that includes theology, science, and art—and his metaphysical method—essentially thought experiments akin to Husserl's phenomenological reduction but more radical and in both directions, imagining a human being without its animality and imagining it without its spiritual and rational component—are magnificent. We can finish perhaps with a few quotes from his *Idealismus—Realismus*:

> Reality is transintelligible for every possible knowing mind. Only the *what* of the being, not the *being* of the what is intelligible.
>
> (Scheler 1973c: 312)

> Reality is the resistance to our continually active, spontaneous, but at the same time completely involuntary impulsive life.
>
> (Scheler 1973c: 325)

> Knowledge first becomes conscious knowledge [*Bewusstsein*], that is comes out of its original ecstatic form of simply "having" things, in which there is no knowledge of the having of that through which and in which it is had, when the act of being thrown back on the self, probably only possible for men, comes into play.
>
> (Scheler 1973c: 294)

BIBLIOGRAPHY

Cutting J., Mouratidou M., Fuchs T., and Owen G. (2016). "Max Scheler's Influence on Kurt Schneider." *History of Psychiatry* 31: 1–9.

Dunlop F. (1991). *Thinkers of our Time: Scheler*. London: The Claridge Press.

Frings M. S. (1965). *Max Scheler: A Concise Introduction into the World of a Great Thinker*. Pittsburgh: Duquesne University Press.

Heidegger M. (1984). *The Metaphysical Foundations of Logic* [1978], trans. M. Heim. Bloomington: Indiana University Press.

Mader W. (1995). *Max Scheler*. Bonn: Bouvier Verlag.

Scheler M. (1926). *Die Wissensformen und die Gesellschaft*. Leipzig: Der Neue-Geist Verlag.

Scheler M. (1954–1997). *Gesammelte Werke*, Band 1–15. Bonn: Bouvier Verlag.

Scheler M. (1972). *On the Eternal in Man* [1921], trans. B. Nobel. Hamden: Archon Books.

Scheler M. (1973a) "Ordo amoris" [1933]. In *Max Scheler: Selected Philosophical Essays*, trans. D. R. Lachterman, pp 98–135. Evanston: Northwestern University Press.

Scheler M. (1973b). *Formalism in Ethics and Non-Formal Ethics of Values [1913-1916]*, trans. M. S. Frings and R. L. Funk. Evanston: Northwestern University Press.

Scheler M. (1973c). "Idealism and Realism" [1927]. In *Max Scheler: Selected Philosophical Essays*, trans. D. R Lachterman, pp. 288–356. Evanston: Northwestern University Press.

Scheler M. (1984) "The Psychology of So-Called Compensation Hysteria and the Real Battle against Illness" [1915], trans. E. Vacek. *Journal of Phenomenological Psychology* 15: 125–143.

Scheler M. (1987) "Shame and Feelings of Modesty" [1933]. In *Max Scheler, Person and Self-Value, Three Essays*, trans. M. S. Frings, pp. 1–85. The Hague: Martinus Nijhoff.

Scheler M. (2008a). *The Nature of Sympathy* [1948], trans. P. Heath. New Brunswick: Transaction Publishers.

Scheler M. (2008b). *The Constitution of the Human Being* [1926-1928], trans. J. Cutting. Milwaukee: Marquette University Press.

Scheler M. (2009). *The Human Place in the Cosmos* [1928], trans. M. S. Frings. Evanston: Northwestern University Press.

Schneider K. (1939). *Psychischer Befund und Psychiatrische Diagnose*. Leipzig: George Thieme.

Schneider K. (2012). "The Stratification of Emotional Life and the Structure of Depressive States" [1920]. In M. R. Broome, R. Harland, G. Owen, and A. Stringaris (eds.), *The Maudsley Reader of Phenomenological Psychiatry*, pp 203–214. Cambridge: Cambridge University Press.

Spiegelberg H. (1994). *The Phenomenological Movement*. Dordrecht: Kluwer Academic Publishers.

Staude, J. R. (1967). *Max Scheler*. New York: The Free Press.

CHAPTER 9

....

HANS-GEORG GADAMER

....

ANDRZEJ WIERCINSKI

INTRODUCTION

....

HERMENEUTICS as the art of understanding does not deal only with interpretation of texts but concerns the totality of being a human being-in-the-world. Its task is to contribute to the understanding of human experience, particularly by helping to unveil meanings that are hidden in the different aspects of the human realities. In the foreword to the Second Edition of his *Truth and Method*, Gadamer, a hermeneutic philosopher par excellence, explains that the way hermeneutics breaks with the instrumental mind is a truly scientific commitment to the integrity of all understanding, which is, following Heidegger, not merely one of the human faculties, but a mode of being a human being. Thus, to be a human being means to live an interpretive existence: *existentia hermeneutica*. Gadamer's hermeneutic concern is philosophical: "Not what we do or what we ought to do, but what happens to us over and above our wanting and doing" (Gadamer 2006: xxvi). Since all understanding is interpretation, hermeneutics places in the very center of the event of understanding what happens to us when we understand. Not the conditions of possibility of knowledge, not the methods of acquiring certain knowledge, but the transformation of the subject who interprets is the core of the hermeneutic task as the event of truth and the event of sense. The meaning of what wants to be understood is not simply there; it shows itself as different from a thing and at the same time as something indistinguishable. This aesthetic non-differentiation in the process of a total mediation can be perceived as a happening indifference (Gadamer 2006: 110–119). Gadamer's notion of aesthetic non-differentiation is fundamental for understanding how the original life significance can be transformed into the reflected experience. Its indispensability for the interpretation of a personal condition in a conversation with the other highlights the important consequence of understanding Gadamer's phenomenological hermeneutics not as the immanence of consciousness, not even disclosedness of Dasein, but as the truth of language.

INTELLECTUAL BIOGRAPHY

Hans-Georg Gadamer, born in 1900 in Marburg, inaugurated the century of hermeneutics as a new discourse not only in philosophy and the humanities but across the disciplines (Di Cesare 2013; Grondin 2003). Since the essence of tradition is to exist in the medium of language that expresses itself like a Thou, Gadamer's phenomenological hermeneutics is lingually oriented.[1] Language as conversation is a medium through which the world discloses itself to human Dasein. Gadamer places the idea of conversation at the very center of hermeneutics, reformulating the old tradition of a dialectics of question and answer through the perspective of the history of its effects. By prioritizing the role of conversation in the event of understanding, he contributes to the culture of dialogue. In continuation with Heidegger's *Being and Time*, Gadamer's *opus magnum* on temporality and historicity of human understanding, *Truth and Method* (1960), uncovers the phenomenon of understanding. Gadamer's main concern is not to elaborate on the rules of interpretation but to address the question of what happens when we understand. Each time we understand, "we understand in a *different way, if we understand at all*" (Gadamer 2006: 296). Gadamer's notion of historically effected consciousness as a stream in which we actively participate when we understand helps to recognize tradition as the source of meaning that is relevant for us and underlines the centrality of the subject matter in the interpretive process. We are the tradition that we want to understand as human beings who are historical, lingual, and finite beings: "To be historically means that knowledge of oneself can never be complete" (Gadamer 2006: 301). Since understanding happens within horizons that are permeable and open to other horizons, "understanding is always the fusion of these horizons supposedly existing by themselves" (Gadamer 2006: 305). The fusion of horizons not only respects the difference but puts the interpreter in the in-between of familiarity and strangeness. By highlighting the role of prejudices in the process of understanding, Gadamer questions the wish of achieving total transparency regarding the conditions of understanding.

Critical engagement with Jürgen Habermas, Jacques Derrida, and Paul Ricoeur, inspired Gadamer to rethink the scope of philosophical hermeneutics by accentuating the in-between of tradition and critique. Gadamer's interest in Platonic dialectic as the art of carrying on a conversation allowed for his passionate engagement with art, medicine, and social sciences, and highlighted the relevance of hermeneutics for society and social life. His essays in *The Enigma of Health* (Gadamer 1996) critically engage with the prevailing view of medical practice in an age of science and create space for medicine as the art of healing. Gadamer not only cautions against a too simplistic pathologization of the human condition but invites us to embrace difficult aspects of human behavior in the gesture of hermeneutic hospitality.

As one of the most famous students of Heidegger and the inheritor of his thinking, Gadamer became internationally famous after his retirement from the University of Heidelberg, where he was Jaspers's successor for almost two decades. His long and

---

[1] Linguality (*Sprachlichkeit*) is the essential trait of Gadamerian hermeneutics, emphasizing the lingual (and not linguistic) character of human understanding. I prefer the translation "linguality/lingual" over "linguisticity/linguistic," since the latter translation might erroneously suggest a relationship to the field of linguistics (*Linguistik/Sprachwissenschaft*).

accomplished life as a hermeneutic philosopher extends beyond his death in 2002 and continues to inspire thinkers to participate in the event of understanding in and through which the world opens itself to us.

HEALTH AS UNSTABLE EQUILIBRIUM: A HERMENEUTIC APPROACH TO MEDICAL PRACTICE

With Karl Jaspers's pioneering 1913 book *General Psychopathology*, phenomenological description of the patient's life experience became crucial for psychiatric assessment aiming at scientific precision, attempting to free itself from all theoretical and habitual presuppositions. Such a static understanding in psychopathology was supposed to allow for the unprejudiced access to mental phenomena by opposing descriptive to explanatory psychopathology. Though Gadamer was certainly indebted to Jaspers, for whom every understanding is interpretation, he claims that there is no presuppositionless access to what wants to be understood. In fact, the task of understanding is to disclose how prejudices and prejudgments condition our understanding. The self is not a disengaged individual but exists in a concrete sociocultural surrounding. As Gadamer argues:

> Long before we understand ourselves through the process of self-examination, we understand ourselves in a self-evident way in the family, society, and state in which we live. The focus of subjectivity is a distorting mirror. The self-awareness of the individual is only a flickering in the closed circuits of historical life. *That is why the prejudices of the individual, far more than his judgments, constitute the historical reality of his being.*
>
> (Gadamer 2006: 278)

Gadamer's major contribution to psychopathology lies not in offering ground-breaking discoveries about the *how* of concrete medical diagnosis and treatments, but in emphasizing the essential importance of understanding what it means to be a human being-in-the-world. This understanding calls for readiness and openness to learning, predominantly about ourselves, in the challenging condition, which we call illness. The role of medical professionals is not to validate their scientific understanding while engaging the patient, but to learn together *with* the patient about our self-understanding by thinking about and dealing with the medical condition. The real necessity of facing our life while being ill drives doctors and patients toward the task of thinking. This existential inescapability discloses to us something essential about our self-understanding.

Gadamerian phenomenological hermeneutics of medicine thematizes health in its unstable equilibrium (Svenaeus 2001: 74, 80). Illness is not a simple lack of health that needs to be restored but demonstrates itself in different forms far beyond the experience of sickness. The task of medicine as the art of healing is to contribute to living this unstable equilibrium in the totality of human experience of being-in-the-world. Following Plato's understanding of disturbed equilibrium, Gadamer stresses that the body can heal only if the care of the soul is not overlooked (Plato 1995: 270b ff.). The equilibrium means that the successful care of the human being depends on various activities always in the right measure and at the right time.

The right measure, what is appropriate or fitting, is an interior measure of a human being, which takes into account a totality of lived experience. This right measure is not a question of a quantitative measuring, but of a qualitive self-reflexive lived experience:

> Modern science has come to regard the results of [its] measuring procedures as the real facts which it must seek to order and collect. But the data provided in this way only reflect conventionally established criteria brought to the phenomena from without. They are always our own criteria that we impose on the thing we wish to measure. The living body and life are things that cannot simply be measured.
>
> (Gadamer 1996: 32)

Essential for Gadamer is to argue that the art of healing which tends to care about restoring the hidden and unstable equilibrium is a qualitative deliberation on the issue in question of the doctor together with the patient rather than a quantitative calculation of contemporary medicine.

A hermeneutic approach to medical practice offers a richer understanding of health and illness with reference to the human being's mode of being-in-the-world rather than to a particular medical disorder that can be scientifically defined and professionally treated. In *The Enigma of Health*, Gadamer emphasizes illness as the fundamental rupture in human beings' mode of being, which prompts the thematization of health: "Health is not a state that one introspectively feels in oneself;" it is rather "the rhythm of life" (Gadamer 1996: 113–114). Gadamer offers a hermeneutic alternative to the predominantly scientific modes of understanding health and illness by embracing the truth of lived experience in its totality without silencing what seems to be incomprehensible, unpredictable, and in-explicable. Critically assessing the potential of contemporary medicine in eliminating the disruptive consequences illness has on the life world of the ill person, Gadamer calls for a close introspection into uniquely personal life-history. The positivistic notion of objectivism reduces human experience to aspects, which can be formally investigated by instrumental rationality. By problematizing instrumental notions of rationality and the positivistic notion of objectivism, Gadamer warns against monolithic biological explanations of an observable pathology that fits into diagnostic categories (Gadamer 1996: 42). Instead, Gadamer advocates listening to the life-story of the patient to decipher together with the patient the meaning of the patient's existential experience without expurgating uncertainty, ambiguity, and complexity of the human condition. Gadamer calls for being thoughtful of the tension between understanding of health as an existential and individual experience of being a human being and disease as the manifestation of a disturbance of a personal condition.

What seems to be crucial in medical practice is not so much specific knowledge content, but dialectical understanding as an ability to act wisely in a particular situation. For Gadamer, hermeneutics is the art of conversation, a path of experiencing, which is open to the dialogical engagement with the other. This path of experiencing, which recognizes the possibility of superiority of the partner, who might be right, is the only way we can live our life in a constant search for the truth about ourselves. When Gadamer speaks about the openness to the conversation as the only kind of integrity of the philosopher, we can extend it to the existential principle of every human being. Hence, the importance of the conversation in medical practice, when reaching an understanding of the issue in question happens as a fusion of horizons of patient and doctor. Describing the fusion of horizons, Gadamer writes: "We can now see that this is what takes place in conversation, in which something is expressed that is not only mine or my author's, but common" (Gadamer 2006: 390).

UNDERSTANDING ILLNESS: THE TASK OF INTERPRETATION

Understanding psychopathological conditions requires being situated between description and interpretation in doctors and patients alike. Phenomenological hermeneutics challenges core assumptions in medicine by readdressing the understanding of the human being as the self, which grows as thrown into the world and is shaped by the sociohistorical conditions (Gadamer 1996: 81). The art of healing puts at the very center an individual life project and the medical professionals search together *with* the patient for the modes of care that can assist the patients with living their life. Such an art as a care practice favors the persons in their existence instead of being predominantly concerned with the physiological manifestations of a disease.

Gadamer's phenomenological hermeneutics of medicine assigns the ontological primacy to health as a state of equilibrium and understands illness as a lack of equilibrium. Even a diseased person experiences some equilibrium (Wiercinski 2013: 19–28). Thus, illness can be defined only in a negative sense as the lack of equilibrium which needs to be restored while facing the unpredictability of the human condition. The relationship between hermeneutic insight and clinical discourse proves to be medically promising, especially while facing the increasing medicalization and pathologization of the human condition. Hermeneutics helps to promote an understanding of the art of healing, which overcomes the tendency in contemporary medicine to interpret phenomenological descriptions of the human condition into the language of clinical and pathophysiological processes that call for pharmacological intervention. Clinical medicine can be practiced as hermeneutics by addressing the phenomena of health and illness as the first-person human experience which calls for understanding. The healing process is a transformation of the relationship of a human being's being-in-the-world to one's embodied lived experience. Understanding a disease presents us with an almost incomprehensible challenge of facing something that shows itself as outrageously different and obscure and yet as something that wants to be understood. Gadamer's phenomenological hermeneutics accentuates the importance of disclosure of what was uncovered in the understanding of the phenomenon in question:

> As a phenomenon of lived experience insight into one's own illness is clearly not simply insight in the sense of knowledge of a true state of affairs, but rather, like all insight, it is something which is acquired with great difficulty and by overcoming significant resistance. We know the important role which concealment of the awareness of ill-health plays in certain human illnesses and, above all, what an important role this concealment can play in the lived existence of a person.
>
> (Gadamer 1996: 52)

The phenomenon of illness needs to be interpreted within the meaning structures of human experience. To unveil meanings hidden in illness, it is essential to address the impact illness has on human life. The singularity of this experience calls for prudent assessment of the experience of illness and serves as a warning against premature formalization of the effects illness can have on human life, both from the scientific objectivized medical perspective and from the particular experience of the affected person: "Medicine is the only science which, ultimately, does not make or produce anything. Rather, it is one which must participate in the wonderful capacity of life to renew itself, to set itself aright" (Gadamer 1996: 89).

Instead of reducing medicine to observing and fixing problems identified as pathology, phenomenological hermeneutics calls for paying attention to the world of the patient by listening to the patient's experience. In order to make it happen, the notion of the patient needs to be transformed from a dysfunctional object in need of medical treatment into an irreplaceable existence, which unfolds while living one's life. The individuality of being-in-the-world cannot be reduced to a common experience of being a human being. This causes obvious difficulties for medicine, since it allows a human being to experience the world in one's own way and to make sense of this personal experience. Gadamer stresses the unavoidability of suffering in a process of self-education. Suffering cannot be reduced to a biological condition that can be fixed with medical technology (Gadamer 1996: 21). Stressing the delicate borderline between suffering as a mode of being a human being-in-the-world and pathological disorder, prompts medicine to be aware of premature medicalization of the human condition.

GADAMER'S PHENOMENOLOGICAL HERMENEUTICS OF MEDICINE

An important but also a difficult task of medical practice is not to see a singular medical problem but to engage critically and constructively the totality of lived experience in an exchange between patient and doctor. The overemphasis of the relevance of medical technology for diagnosis and treatment of the patient reduces illness to a case of physiological imbalance and leads undoubtedly to the growing estrangement of the doctor and the patient. Even for the treating doctor, it often poses a significant challenge of trusting the machinery rather than one's own judgment. Gadamer stresses the inescapable personal responsibility of the doctor and also of the patient, who needs to respond to her or his own condition in a unique way. Hence, the importance of the doctor–patient conversation in all stages of their engagement (Gadamer 1996: 128).

Gadamer's phenomenological hermeneutics of medicine stresses the priority of the question. It is an experience of asking questions, while we need to clarify our understanding of ourselves, particularly when the health equilibrium is broken. We ask questions because we know that we do not know what is happening to us. In a conversation, we wish to arrive at understanding of ourselves by engaging the other and by searching for understanding *with* the other (Gadamer 2006: 385). A medical encounter discloses not only a possible understanding of a dis-ease, but different ways of seeing the world, which is the result of the fusion of the horizons of the doctor and the patient mediated by the use of language and tradition. This encounter, in which neither participants of the conversation knows what will "come out" of it, leads not only to an enlargement of understanding of the medical condition, but to the enlarged self of the doctor and the patient alike.

Medicine, for Gadamer, is "withdrawing itself and helping to set the other person free" (Gadamer 1996: 43). This means that the successful medical treatment cannot be the result of the competence of health professionals but must include the personal engagement of the patient in understanding her or his own condition and in a dynamic involvement in acting toward recovery. Gadamer emphasizes that it is important to see two sets of judgments, one which leads to diagnosis that needs to be done by negotiating and the other which leads to treatment. Here, it is important to distinguish between the understanding of the medical condition from the understanding of the person, which is essentially needed to create a connection with the patient. This connection is not only needed as the bonus of the interpersonal interaction between the doctor and the patient but is essential for the healing process. It is a question of working together on the common task (Gadamer 1996: 38). Working toward a shared understanding happens as the fusion of horizons: Understanding in the medical context comes into being as the effect of interaction between the doctor and the patient.

In a conversation between the doctor and the patient it is crucial to be open and to listen to each other in order to understand. However, what happens very often is rather the opposite: "Instead of learning to look for illness in the eyes of the patient or to listen for it in the patient's voice, [the doctor] tries to read off the data provided by technologically sophisticated measuring instruments" (Gadamer 1996: 98). This listening to each other has a powerful transformative effect. The transformation of the person means that one becomes another person and "that what existed previously exists no longer" (Gadamer 2006: 111).

In his phenomenological hermeneutics of medicine, Gadamer reminds us that as human beings we inhabit a shared world. This means that to be a human being is to be an ethical being. A medical encounter is a meeting of human beings who bear responsibility for each other. It is exactly the reciprocity of responsibility, which revolutionizes the understanding of medical practice. The doctor and the patient are mutually responsible for each other. If, for Gadamer, the practice of hermeneutics means the participation in an ongoing dialogue with others, the art of healing can be practiced only in a dialogical horizon. An encounter between doctor and patient is in its essence a dialogical encounter and it happens as thinking in action. The active role of the doctor and the patient is essential to understanding of the disease and necessary for treatment.

Gadamer highlights the importance of hermeneutic imagination, which allows one to understand and to deal with the intricacies of the human condition (Gadamer 2006: 555, 572). This calls for attention to what it means to be a human being and thus to what counts and matters for an individual in a way which is not only unique for each person, but to a large extent also incommunicable. Gadamer emphasizes the importance of insight while dealing with illness, and particularly with mental illness, when a patient is often unable to experience her- or himself as ill. The ambiguity implicit in the understanding of mental health highlights the tension in human existence. An increasingly biological interpretation of mental illness and medicalization of a mental condition that can be treated with a particular drug reduces medicine to measurable variables. Therefore, Gadamer's hermeneutics of medicine calls for overcoming the reduction of health sciences to physiopathology and for inclusive care of human beings in their being-in-the-world (Gadamer 1996: 77). Gadamer warns against giving up responsibility for one's own well-being, particularly with reference to mental disorders, and depending too heavily on decision-making by the doctor. He welcomes the rapid advancements of psychoanalysis without overlooking its substantial problems (Wiercinski 2014: 311–313).

For Gadamer, mental illness is characterized by not feeling at home (*unheimlich*) in the world. His understanding calls for moving beyond a scientific explanation of mental illness in terms of neurobiological processes without neglecting the contribution of specific medical sciences:

> In mental illness the twofold manner of "being at home" which is constitutive of human life, being at home in the world and being at home with oneself, is no longer successfully accomplished. Mental illness does not so much involve the loss of specific abilities as the failure to meet a challenge with which we are all permanently confronted, that is of sustaining the equilibrium between our *animalitas* and that in which we identify our vocation as human beings. When suffering from mental illness our condition does not simply fall into an animal-vegetative state; the deforming loss of equilibrium is rather something which peculiarly affects the mind.
>
> (Gadamer 1996: 60)

If mental health is perceived as a state of equilibrium, mental illness is a rupture of this equilibrium caused by the inability of dealing with the possibilities surrounding us, and by our understanding of these possibilities (Gadamer 1996: 58).

CONCLUSION

The fundamental task of being a human being is self-understanding in the world, in which the self is thrown into the variety of languages that cannot be reduced to one language. To understand oneself in the world means understanding the self and the other. To understand the other, one needs to listen to the other with a strong conviction that the other might be right. To help a human being find itself at home in this complex world can be seen as a genuine goal of a phenomenological hermeneutics of medicine and, in fact, medicine itself. The task of medicine is to help uncover the phenomenon of being a human being in the adequacy of one's own vocation without a premature pressure to solve all the difficult problems that the self experiences. If medicine wishes to be an art of healing, it must be a dialogical science, an art of healing that assists in finding one's own way to live one's life.

Gadamer problematizes the understanding of the nature of the professional medical practice. Participating in the act of healing is, in itself, a hermeneutic enterprise. The understanding of the doctor is happening in the medical encounter while engaging the medical problem and the patient. It discloses not only the matter to be understood but, predominantly, who the self is as a person who is involved.

Gadamer's contribution to psychopathology is particularly important at the level of inescapable interpretation of the primordial lived experience of the human being as a finite, lingual, temporal, and historical agent in a concrete life-world (*Lebenswelt*). Interpreting the manifestation of human suffering in the world requires, from both the patient and the doctor, an attentiveness to the lived experience and a willingness to search together for an understanding and its creative productivity for the patient. Suffering discloses something essential about our way of being-in-the-world and cannot be reduced to a medical problem in need of being controlled or overcome. It can help to uncover what it means to be a human being. This uncovering is happening as a hermeneutic logic of question and answer and leads to an understanding. This is not merely a reconstruction (reproduction) of meaning, but a truly creative and productive engagement in which we re-cognize what has been cognized in that which needs to be understood.

Gadamer's hermeneutic contribution to psychopathology reminds us that no one methodological approach to understanding human psyche could possibly claim dominance. Psychopathology is an interdisciplinary field and as such needs to be open to the infinite task of interpretation. Medicine in the scientific age is not able to deal with the enigma of health, which, by its illusive and enigmatic nature cannot be measured. Understanding health as a condition of an engaged being-in-the world with others does not follow the traditional health–illness dichotomy but calls for re-humanization of medicine in its self-understanding beyond scientifically determined processes of rationalization, automatization, and specialization.

BIBLIOGRAPHY

Di Cesare D. (2013). *Gadamer: A Philosophical Portrait*, trans. N. Keane. Bloomington: Indiana University Press.

Gadamer H.-G. (1996). *The Enigma of Health: The Art of Healing in A Scientific Age*, trans. J. Gaiger and N. Walker. Stanford: Stanford University Press.

Gadamer H.-G. (2006). *Truth and Method*, 2nd rev. ed., trans. J. Weinsheimer and D. G. Marshall. New York: Crossroad.

Grondin J. (2003). *Hans-Georg Gadamer: A Biography*, trans. J Weinsheimer. New Haven: Yale University Press.

Plato. (1995). *Phaedrus*, trans. A. Nehamas and P. Woodruff. Indianapolis: Hackett.

Svenaeus F. (2001). *The Hermeneutics of Medicine and the Phenomenology of Health: Steps towards a Philosophy of Medical Practice*, 2nd rev. ed. Dordrecht: Kluwer.

Wiercinski A. (2013). "Hermeneutics of Medicine: The Phronetic Dimension of Medical Ethics." In A. Bobko (ed.), *Etyka wobec współczesnych wyzwań: Wybrane aspekty [Ethics Facing Contemporary Challenges: Selected Aspects]*, pp. 19–28. Rzeszów: Uniwersytet Rzeszowski.

Wiercinski A. (2014). "Questioning the Limits of Interpretation: The Intrinsic Challenges to Hermeneutics and Psychoanalysis." In H. Lang, P. Dybel, and G. Pagel (eds.), *Grenzen der Interpretation in Hermeneutik und Psychoanalyse*, pp. 295–315. Würzburg: Königshausen & Neumann.

CHAPTER 10

....

PAUL RICOEUR

....

RENÉ ROSFORT

PHILOSOPHICAL DEVELOPMENT

PAUL Ricoeur (1913–2005) was a protagonist of the first generation of French phenomenology. As is the case with his phenomenological contemporaries in France, his approach
to Husserlian and Heideggerian phenomenology is characterized by a productive combination of appropriation and critical development. Ricoeur's work extends over more than
half a century and deals with a remarkable variety of themes and interlocutors that is singular among the major phenomenologists of the twentieth century. He is perhaps the most
comprehensive thinker in the phenomenological tradition. His authorship includes careful
engagements with major cultural phenomena of the twentieth century such as psychoanalysis, existentialism, hermeneutics, structuralism, poststructuralism, narrative theory, and
even neuroscience. Moreover, throughout his long career he published numerous essays
on the questions of politics and institutions of his day. Ricoeur was a practicing Christian
and, while maintaining strict separation between his philosophical and theological work,
he contributed with books and a vast amount of articles on religion and in particular the
Christian tradition, which he considered to be one of the principal sources of Western
philosophy. Despite the span and variety of his work, Ricoeur still managed to maintain a
consistent theoretical core throughout the development of his philosophy. His principal theoretical interest is concerned with the question of selfhood and personal identity, and his
life-long mottos—"a philosophy of detour" and "the long way of interpretation"—capture his
hermeneutical approach to these questions (e.g. Ricoeur 1992: 16–23; Ricoeur 2004a: 255–
260; Ricoeur 2008: 83–85).

Ricoeur develops his philosophy in dialogue with primarily three major philosophical
traditions: French reflexive philosophy, German phenomenology, and Anglophone philosophy. The three traditions shape his philosophical development marking various stages
of his intellectual life.[1] Ricoeur was trained in reflexive philosophy, which was one of the

----

[1] For thorough accounts of Ricoeur's life and intellectual development, see Dosse 2008; Greisch 2001.
For accessible and concise introductions to his life and work in English, see Reagan 1996; Simms 2003;
Pellauer 2007; Pellauer and Dauenhauer 2016.

dominant traditions in French philosophy in the first half of the twentieth century, and this tradition remained an active, albeit increasingly subdued element in his philosophy. The tradition of reflexive philosophy originated in the eighteenth century with Maine de Biran, was continued by Félix Ravaisson in the nineteenth century, and developed further by Léon Brunschvicg, Jean Nabert, and Gabriel Marcel in the first half of the twentieth century. This tradition is concerned with investigating how the subject becomes aware of itself as a self through the lived experience of thinking. It is a critical development of Descartes's cogito, which is the primacy of reflection that emphasizes the lived and embodied character of re-flection. Ricoeur's work with the tradition of reflexive philosophy is enriched and devel-oped through his encounter with German phenomenology during the Second World War, which Ricoeur was spent as a prisoner of war in various camps. The years of imprisonment were foundational for his philosophical development. His status of officer provided him with several privileges, among which were long hours for study and the possibility of giving lectures on various philosophical topics to his fellow prisoners. Jaspers and Husserl were the philosophers that he spent most time on during the prison years. The immediate fruits of these studies are his first two books on Jaspers (Dufrenne and Ricoeur 1947; Ricoeur 1947), a translation of Husserl's *Ideas I* published in 1950, and several dense articles on Husserl's phenomenology in the 1950s (Ricoeur 1967b). While Jaspers subsided into the background of his work, phenomenology remained the principal methodological tool throughout his ca-reer, and, as we shall see, his major contribution to philosophy is his hermeneutical develop-ment of phenomenology. From 1971 to his retirement in 1991 Ricoeur was the John Nuveen professor of divinity at the University of Chicago. The American years were extremely productive, and the encounter with Anglophone philosophy left a substantial imprint on Ricoeur's late works. Ricoeur enters into critical discussions with prominent Anglophone philosophers, in particular concerning philosophy of language, philosophy of mind, and ethics. The result of these discussions is the development of his hermeneutical phenome-nology into an influential narrative theory (Ricoeur 1984, 1985, 1988), and a complex theory of selfhood revolving around the normative challenges involved in personal identity (1992, 2004b, 2005).

Ricoeur's contribution to phenomenological psychopathology is still to be fully appreciated and explored. Although Ricoeur does not engage directly with psychopa-thology, he has published a seminal, and controversial, book on Freud and a great number of articles on psychoanalysis (Ricoeur 1970, 2012). Moreover, the central themes of Ricoeur's authorship, in particular the conflictual character of selfhood and the normative challenges of personal identity, provide a fecund phenomenological foundation for psychopathology (Stanghellini and Rosfort 2013). In what follows, I will explicate Ricoeur's hermeneutical phenomenology and narrative theory, concluding with an outline of how his ethics of iden-tity can contribute to phenomenological psychopathology.

HERMENEUTICAL PHENOMENOLOGY

Ricoeur's approach to phenomenology engages with the history of phenomenology before and after Husserl and deals in particular with the philosophical limits of Husserl's phenom-enology. As he writes in one of his surveys of Husserl's phenomenology: "[P]henomenology is a vast project whose expression is not restricted to one work or to any specific group of works. It is less a doctrine than a method capable of many exemplifications of which Husserl exploited only a few" (Ricoeur 1967b: 4). This historical perspective on phenomenology and his critical approach to Husserl's project leads Ricoeur to develop a Kantian version of phenomenology that exploits the limits of a phenomenological description to establish a normative theory of subjectivity. The entanglement of descriptive and normative aspects of human experience is central to his first major phenomenological works on the challenges of human freedom (Ricoeur 1966, 1967a, 1986a), and remains a central theme throughout his works.

Ricoeur's argument is that the difficulty of human freedom is caused by the conflictual character of human subjectivity. In fact, human beings experience themselves first and foremost through the fallible character of their will, and this affective experience of our own limits results in a troubled sense of self that Ricoeur calls "a wounded Cogito [*un Cogito blessé*]" (1970: 439). Our sense of being a self is constantly troubled by a sense of otherness, and Husserl, on Ricoeur's account, did not acknowledge this affective dialectics of self and otherness at the core of human experience nor did he explore the normative complexity involved in human emotional experience (Ricoeur 1967a: 175–201; Ricoeur 1986b: 266–270). The troubled sense of self prompts a constant self-questioning, which in turn makes interpretation fundamental to Ricoeur's hermeneutical development of phenomenology.

The focus on affectivity and interpretation would make Heidegger an obvious choice for Ricoeur. However, Ricoeur criticizes Heidegger's hermeneutical development of Husserlian phenomenology for its exclusive focus on in the ontological depths of existence. Heidegger's quest for a fundamental ontology, Ricoeur argues, blinds him to ethical challenges of human existence that Ricoeur himself made the foundation of his hermeneutical phenomenology (Ricoeur 1986a: 47–79; Ricoeur 2004a: 9–11). It is this insistence on the experiential primacy of ethics that makes Ricoeur argue that "Husserl did phenomenology, but Kant limited and founded it" (Ricoeur 1967b: 201). In other words, the limits to Husserl's descriptive analysis of experience, and to Heidegger's normative hermeneutics of experience, become visible through Ricoeur's adoption of a Kantian ethics of personhood.

To be a self is to become a person. This is the fundamental ethical challenge that constitutes the heart of Ricoeur's hermeneutical phenomenology. The human self experiences itself through thinking, and this thinking is always "wounded" in the sense that it is characterized by affective disturbances caused by an inescapable otherness that troubles the sense of selfhood. This dialectics of selfhood and otherness accounts for the non-coinciding, conflictual character of human experience of being a self. Our sense of being a self is fragile and constantly disturbed, for better or worse, by an otherness that we cannot control. In order to live with this basic fragility of being a self we need to reappropriate ourselves through the ethical task of becoming a person (Ricoeur 1986a: 69). Personhood is a normative ideal in the sense that it is a particular way to see, understand, and treat a human being—oneself as well as the other. Although it is an ideal, it is Ricoeur's argument that we cannot make descriptive sense of human subjectivity without it. The ideal of personhood allows us to make sense of the dialectics of self and otherness that is disclosed by our phenomenological investigation of human subjectivity. The self is never at rest with itself. To be a self is to exist through the otherness that makes the self a human self. This basic otherness makes itself known in and through the passivity that we experience through our body, our being situated in the world, through language, and most incisively through the encounter with the other person. This otherness is, as mentioned, responsible for the fragile character of human self-awareness and that which makes human identity a task rather than a fact. Because human selfhood is constituted by an otherness that we cannot control our identity cannot be understood in terms of our sense of being ourselves. To be a self is more than being myself. Or as Ricoeur succinctly puts it: "To say self is not to say myself" (Ricoeur 1992: 180). In other words, we need the notion of personhood to make sense of the dialectics of self and otherness in our troubled sense of self, and to reappropriate our identity through this dialectics. Ricoeur proposes a narrative approach to this task of becoming the person who we are.

Narrative Identity

Ricoeur's narrative approach to human identity is shaped by his exploration of Freud's work with the conflicts of the human mind (Ricoeur 1970). Ricoeur is particularly interested in Freud's interpretative approach and his emphasis on the weight of the past. Freud taught us to be suspicious of human consciousness, and this suspicion brings out one of the limits of a phenomenological analysis, namely, the idea that we can make sense of human experience in terms of the pre-reflective experiential structures of human self-awareness. Central to Freud's groundbreaking account of human identity is that human self-awareness is never transparent, but fraught with suppressed memories and unconscious desires that constantly disrupt our sense of identity and complicate our existence. For Ricoeur, however, this seminal idea is also Freud's weakness. The preoccupation with the weight of the past and with the archaeology of libidinal desires blinds Freud to the significance of the future in our understanding of human identity. There is more to human identity than the traumas of past and the obscurity of our desires, so Ricoeur argues that we need a hermeneutical phenomenology that combines Freudian archaeology with Hegelian teleology to make sense of challenges to human identity (Ricoeur 1970: 460). While the former is concerned with a phenomenological description of the conflictual structure of identity, the latter is a hermeneutical endeavor to reconcile this conflict by finding a meaning or telos in our particular human existence.

Human selfhood is not merely marked by the constant disturbance of an otherness that we cannot control. Our sense of self is also characterized by an effort or a desire to find a meaning that can secure an existential continuity from past to future, and thus enable us to be reconciled with the otherness that disrupts our identity. The principal argument of Ricoeur's hermeneutical approach to human identity is that this dialectics of disrupting archaeology and reconciling teleology is articulated in and through human language. To reappropriate our identity we have to engage with the complexity of the words, symbols, and metaphors that constitute our existence. Language, and in particular symbols and metaphors, brings out the dialectics of past and future by embedding us firmly in a cultural history that is not of our making, while at the same time allowing us to shape the future of our common culture through our individual words (Ricoeur 1967a, 2003). Ricoeur's work with language allows him to develop his account of human freedom, in particular, the normative demand of human autonomy and the involuntary aspects of this autonomy. Language manifests this ambiguity of autonomy. We express ourselves in words that we have not created, and we cannot control the meaning of these words or how they are perceived and understood by those with whom we talk. Language is the manifestation of an evolving surplus of meaning (Ricoeur 1976). We cannot escape the problem of interpretation—our own as well as that of the other:

> The man who speaks in symbols is first of all a narrator [*un récitant*]; he transmits an abundance of meaning over which he has little command and thus makes him think. This thickness of manifold meaning is what solicits his understanding [*intelligence*]; interpretation consists less in suppressing ambiguity than in understanding it and in explicating its richness!
>
> (Ricoeur 1970: 49; translation modified)

Our identity is entangled with and partly constituted by the stories that we tell ourselves and others. Our story-telling is, on Ricoeur's account, a way to make sense of the aporetics of temporality. This aporetics consists in the fact that human temporality cannot be reduced to our personal experience of time nor to the impersonal cosmic time that governs the universe. Human temporality is a "third kind of time" (Ricoeur 1988: 245) that is made up by the "discordant concordance" of impersonal cosmic time and lived phenomenological time, that is, by the way time affects us involuntarily and by how we voluntarily understand and shape time.

This third kind of time, proper human time, is configured through narratives, and these narratives constitute the fragile sense of personal identity that makes possible a human life. This narrative identity is fragile because the stories that we tell about ourselves, about *who* we are, are interwoven with the inarticulate otherness of *what* we are (e.g. our biology, our parents, our culture, our loved ones). Our words are that which secure continuity between our past and our future, but our identity cannot be reduced to the stories that we tell about ourselves. On the contrary, Ricoeur's theory of narrative identity is concerned with the various forms of otherness that challenge our identity. These are the aspects of our identity that we have not chosen and cannot extricate ourselves from. It is a theory that is meant to help us become the person who we are, that is, to reappropriate ourselves through the dialectics of selfhood and otherness that Ricoeur explored in his early works.

The fragility of our narrative identity becomes most manifest in our encounter with the other person, which is also why the key notion of Ricoeur's understanding of personal identity is "keeping one's word" (Ricoeur 1992: 113–139; Ricoeur 2005: 99–109). Many aspects of our identity are simply a matter of physiological and psychological inertia through time. We grow older minute-by-minute, year by year, and innumerable aspects of our life are the result of more or less mindless habits. This means that in a certain sense our identity is secured by our sheer physical existence. Ricoeur categorizes these fundamental aspects of human identity under the notion of "sameness" or "idem," and he has dedicated hundreds of pages to meticulous phenomenological analyses of these involuntary aspects of our identity throughout his career (e.g. Ricoeur 1966, 1970, 1988, 1992). Although he acknowledges the importance of the "sameness" of our identity, he is still convinced that our identity depends on our conscious struggle against the inertia, against "the most perfidious of passions, the passion to become a thing again" (Ricoeur 1966: 297). In other words, our identity is more than the mere fact of our existence; it is a normative challenge. We are responsible for *who* we are, even though so many aspects of *what* we are out of our control. Our identity becomes *personal* through the responsible reappropriation of ourselves in and through the disruptive changes of time. Ricoeur captures this normative aspect of our identity with the notion "keeping one's word" or "ipse" (Ricoeur 1992: 118–119).

Ricoeur's theory of narrative identity is the culmination of his hermeneutical phenomenology that combines a Husserlian emphasis on a descriptive approach to the concrete givenness of the world with a Kantian insistence on the normative character of being a human person. Moreover, it testifies to the persistent dialectical character of Ricoeur's thinking. Narrative identity is constituted by the dialectics of a description of "the sameness" or "the idem" of *what* we are and the normative demand to become ourselves or "the ipse" of *who* we are by "keeping our word." It is this dialectical aspect of his conception of narrative identity that provides perhaps the most promising contribution to phenomenological psychopathology.

THE DIALECTICAL MODEL OF SUFFERING

Karl Jaspers played, as mentioned, a foundational role in Ricoeur's philosophical development. Jaspers's philosophy of existence was the topic of his first two books, and particularly the dialectical character of Jaspers's thinking has left an enduring mark on Ricoeur's work. The dialectical approach to the human person pervades Jaspers's psychopathology and is central to his work with the patient's attitude or position-taking (*Stellungnahme*) toward her illness (Jaspers 1997: 414–427). Jaspers's argument is that understanding mental illness requires an account of how the person reflectively responds to and makes sense of her suffering. A psychopathological account of a person's suffering must begin with the acknowledgment that there is always "an awareness of one's awareness" at play in suffering, and that this awareness shapes the illness that we seek to understand psychopathologically (Jaspers 1997: 400). Mental suffering, in other words, is dialectical in the sense that the brute fact of suffering is always complicated by the person's interpretation of her suffering. This dialectical model of mental illness has had a significant bearing on the theories of major phenomenological psychopathologists in the twentieth century such as Eugène Minkowski, Wolfgang Blankenburg, and Kimura Bin (Stanghellini and Rosfort 2015a).

Ricoeur's account of narrative identity can be used as a tool to develop this dialectical model and to articulate the problem of autonomy as a major factor in mental illness. The patient of a mental illness is always an agent who relates herself to her illness, and she exists with and tries to make sense of her suffering through narratives. Ricoeur's theory of narratives can help us bring out the autonomy at work in the passivity of suffering. The experience of suffering is passive in the sense that we experience suffering as something that happens to us, as an involuntary disturbance of our sense of being a self. This passivity enhances the suffering involved in a mental illness because of the undermining effect it has on our autonomy (Stanghellini and Rosfort 2015b). Suffering makes us feel incapacitated, vulnerable, and at times utterly helpless. Narratives can be used a way to cope with this sense of passivity because, as Ricoeur argues, "[w]hat sedimentation has contracted, the narrative can redeploy" (1992: 122; translation modified). Narratives redeploy the fact of suffering as the normative task of regaining our sense of autonomy. This is not to say that narratives make suffering less painful or disturbing. On the contrary, the phenomenological character of Ricoeur's theory of narratives articulates the various experiential aspects of suffering, while providing a hermeneutical account of how to help the patient reappropriate her sense of autonomy in and through this experience of suffering.

Bibliography

Dosse F. (2008). *Paul Ricoeur. Les sens d'une vie* (1913–2005), édition revue et augmentée. Paris: La Découverte.

Dufrenne M. and Ricoeur P. (1947). *Karl Jaspers et la philosophie de l'existence*. Paris: Seuil.

Greisch J. (2001). *Paul Ricoeur. L'itinérance du sens*. Grenoble: Millon.

Jaspers K. (1997). *General Psychopathology*, trans. J. Hoenig and M. W. Hamilton [1959]. Baltimore: The Johns Hopkins University Press.

Pellauer D. (2007). *Ricoeur: A Guide for the Perplexed*. New York: Continuum.

Pellauer D. and Dauenhauer B. (2016). Paul Ricoeur. *The Stanford Encyclopedia of Philosophy* (Summer 2016 edition), Edward N. Zalta (ed.), http://plato.stanford.edu/archives/sum2016/entries/ricoeur/.

Reagan C E (1996). *Paul Ricoeur: His Life and His Work*. Chicago: Chicago University Press.

Ricoeur P. (1947). *Gabriel Marcel et Karl Jaspers. Philosophie du mystère et philosophie du paradoxe*. Paris: Temps Present.

Ricoeur P. (1966). *Freedom and Nature: The Voluntary and the Involuntary* [1950], trans. E. Kohak. Evanston: Northwestern University Press.

Ricoeur P. (1967a). *The Symbolism of Evil*, trans. E. Buchanan. Boston: Beacon Press.

Ricoeur P. (1967b). *Husserl: An Analysis of His Phenomenology*, trans. E. G. Ballard and L. E. Embree. Evanston: Northwestern University Press.

Ricoeur P. (1970). *Freud and Philosophy: An Essay on Interpretation* [1965], trans. D. Savage. New Haven: Yale University Press.

Ricoeur P. (1976). *Interpretation Theory: Discourse and the Surplus of Meaning*. Fort Worth: Texas Christian University Press.

Ricoeur P. (1984). *Time and Narrative*, vol. 1 [1983], trans. K. McLaughlin and D. Pellauer. Chicago: University of Chicago Press.

Ricoeur P. (1985). *Time and Narrative*, vol. 2 [1984], trans. K. McLaughlin and D. Pellauer. Chicago: University of Chicago Press.

Ricoeur P. (1986a). *Fallible Man* [1960], trans. C. A. Kelbley. New York: Fordham University Press.

Ricoeur P. (1986b). "Sympathie et respect. Phénoménologie et ethique de la seconde personne [1954]." In Paul Ricoeur, *A l'école de la phénoménologie*, pp. 266–283. Paris: Vrin.

Ricoeur P. (1988). *Time and Narrative*, vol. 3 [1985], trans. K. Blamey and D. Pellauer. Chicago: University of Chicago Press.

Ricoeur P. (1992). *Oneself as Another* [1990], trans. K. Blamey. Chicago: University of Chicago Press.

Ricoeur P. (2003). *The Rule of Metaphor: The Creation of Meaning in Language* [1975], trans. R. Czerny, K. McLaughlin, and J. Costello. London: Routledge.

Ricoeur P. (2004a). *The Conflict of Interpretations: Essays in Hermeneutics* [1969], trans. W. Domingo, et al. London: Continuum.

Ricoeur P. (2004b). *Memory, History, Forgetting* [2000], trans. K. Blamey and D. Pellauer. Chicago: University of Chicago Press.

Ricoeur P. (2005). *The Course of Recognition* [2004], trans. D. Pellauer. Chicago: University of Chicago Press.

Ricoeur P. (2008). *From Text to Action: Essays in Hermeneutics II* [1986], trans. K. Blamey and J. B. Thompson. London: Continuum.

Ricoeur R. (2012). *On Psychoanalysis* [2008], trans. D. Pellauer. Cambridge: Polity Press.

Simms K. (2003). *Paul Ricoeur*. London. Routledge.

Stanghellini G. and Rosfort R. (2013). *Emotions and Personhood: Exploring Fragility—Making Sense of Vulnerability*. Oxford: Oxford University Press.

Stanghellini G. and Rosfort R. (2015a). "Disordered Selves or Persons with Schizophrenia?" *Current Opinion in Psychiatry* 28: 256–263.

Stanghellini G. and Rosfort R. (2015b). "The Patient as an Autonomous Person." In J. Z. Sadler, K. W. M Fulford, and W. van Staden (eds.), *Oxford Handbook of Psychiatric Ethics*, pp. 319–335. Oxford: Oxford University Press.

CHAPTER 11

....

EMMANUEL LEVINAS

....

RICHARD A. COHEN

INTRODUCTION

EMMANUEL Levinas (1906–1995) is a phenomenological philosopher of ethics. His great originality and importance derives from two elements or dimensions of his thought. One, and no doubt central, the primacy of ethics: an argument that intelligibility, sense, and significance, originate not in knowing but in moral responsibility and justice. Two, scientific contributions: rigorous phenomenological investigations conducted in various regions of signification such as sensibility, worldliness, eros, and temporality. The latter have the additional virtue, or ambition, of contesting and correcting the earlier and more celebrated phenomenological studies of Martin Heidegger in *Being and Time* (1927). Levinas is at once one of the masters of the rigorous science of phenomenology, in France having been one of the first and leading expositors of Husserl and Heidegger, having engaged in and published many fundamental and original phenomenological studies of his own. And then, as well, he moved beyond the borders of phenomenology, outside the limits of noetic-noematic "intentionality," and through many lectures and publications proposed what is perhaps the most original and outstanding twentieth-century continental philosophy of ethics, an ethics which profoundly makes sense of the "humanity of the human." Each of these by itself is an extraordinary accomplishment; together they place Levinas in the top tier of world philosophers. Two basic ideas orient his thought: first, knowledge, to be knowledge, must acknowledge its roots in moral responsibility; and second, moral responsibility means helping others, putting the other first, and such solicitousness is the highest priority of all the exigencies which compete for human attention. To be human is to aid others. Thus Levinas breaks with both monadic and totalizing philosophies: the self, to be itself, must be for-the-other.

BIOGRAPHICAL SKETCH

Levinas was born in 1906 in Kaunas, Lithuania, into a traditional Jewish home. In 1923 he left for university studies in Strasbourg, France. During 1928 to 1929 he studied under Edmund Husserl and Martin Heidegger in nearby Freiburg, Germany. In 1930 he published

The Theory of Intuition in Husserl's Phenomenology, the first book in French on Husserl's phenomenology. "It is," Levinas wrote, "precisely the method by which we are going back to concrete man" (1973: 146). He also became a French citizen, married, and became a teacher at the Alliance Israelite Universelle in Paris. In 1939 he was conscripted into the French army, served as a translator of German and Russian, in 1940 became a prisoner-of-war and spent the duration of the war in Germany in a labor camp, part of a Jewish section. After the war, he returned to his job, was made Director in 1947, and re-engaged in Parisian intellectual life. In two short books of 1947, *Existence and Existent* and *Time and the Other*, Levinas began articulating his own ethical philosophy utilizing the phenomenological method. Breaking new philosophical ground by finding the roots of intelligibility not in knowing but in moral responsibility and justice, the primacy of ethics became the central claim of all his subsequent thought, including his two magisterial books, *Totality and Infinity* (1961), and *Otherwise than Being or Beyond Essence* (1974). Each year from 1957 to 1989 Levinas delivered the keynote address, known as a "Talmudic Reading," at the annual Colloquium of Jewish Intellectuals which he helped to establish. In 1961 he was made Professor of Philosophy at Poitiers; in 1967 at Paris-Nanterre; and finally, from 1973 to 1976, at Paris-Sorbonne. To the end of the 1980s, Levinas, in lectures, articles, and collections, continued to elaborate, refine, and deepen his original ethical philosophy. Following several years of dementia, he died in 1995.

ETHICS AND PHENOMENOLOGY

Though his outlook is comprehensive, Levinas's contributions to philosophy and to psychopathology can be analytically sorted under two headings: phenomenological and ethical. Both appear throughout his writings, especially insofar as Levinas's ethics is not abstract but concrete, the singular requirements of the other and others impinging on and arousing the singular moral and juridical responsibility of the self. Indeed, the inextricable relationship between knowledge (ordinary, scientific, and phenomenological), and goodness, is an explicit and central topic of Levinas's thought. In the following, where I turn to three key elements—body, world, and time—of Levinas's thought, I focus primarily on his *magnum opus*, *Totality and Infinity* (1961). Here Levinas's phenomenological studies are original and well-developed and here so too is his ethics. Not surprisingly his second major work, *Otherwise than Being or Beyond Essence* (1974), deepens many of his earlier themes, especially regarding the character and significance of moral agency and language. Nonetheless all the major themes of Levinas's philosophy are already found in *Totality and Infinity*. A second reason I will draw from *Totality and Infinity* is because its phenomenological studies are so clearly worked out and, while pursuing a path opened up by Heidegger, do not flinch from rejecting the primacy Heidegger accords to ontology and contesting the results of Heidegger's earlier phenomenological studies.

Also the arrangement of the text of *Totality and Infinity* lends itself to our interests. Subsection two, entitled "Interiority and Economy," is primarily phenomenological; and subsection three, entitled "Exteriority and the Face," is primarily ethical. Thus *Totality and Infinity* lends itself to seeing the multi-layered and complex meanings of subjectivity and worldliness and then appreciating more clearly and precisely the impact of the otherness of the other person on such worldly subjectivity. Thus, to use terms taken from grammar, we begin with the nominative, and see how it is put into the accusative. To be sure, ethics does not come "after" ontology in a chronological sense. Indeed, ethics has priority, it "comes first" in the sense that its imperatives trump the imperatives to know and to will. Nevertheless, this analytical division between phenomenology and ethics is illuminating.

One of Heidegger's great insights, building on Edmund Husserl's notion of "intentionality," was that subjectivity is not monadic, not a *cogito* or substance in opposition to the world. Rather, humans are always already "in-the-world," they are in this sense "ecstatic" beings, projected not self-contained. For this reason Heidegger drops the very term "subject" and replaces it with the term "*Dasein*," which in ordinary German means "existence," but in Heidegger's usage refers to "being there" out in the world. Humans are thus worldly beings in their very essence. To be and to be there, in the world, is the same thing for humans. So Heidegger's phenomenological question is not "How do we know there are other minds?" but "What is the character of the worldly being which we are?" His answer is twofold. First, the world is what he calls an "instrumental totality." That is to say, the world is not first something we know, but something we use, an instrumental engagement. A hammer, for instance, is a hammer not when I cognize it, but when I hammer away at something, that is, when I use it. The second feature of the world, to which we will turn shortly, is that it is historical, that we are permeated by a meaningfulness that comes from and through historical development.

Levinas agrees that human subjectivity is not a monad or substance. Nevertheless, regarding Heidegger's first point, that the world is an instrumental totality, Levinas's phenomenological investigations discover something important which, Levinas argues, Heidegger's analyses overlooked and left out. And this is that the world is not first a tool; it is something *enjoyed*. The hammer, then, is not simply what it is when one is hammering, but it is even more primitively something one enjoys handling. The world is first, then, sensational rather than instrumental. The sun is not just for light; one enjoys its warmth on one's arms; one enjoys the brilliance of colors. While this difference may not seem to be particularly important, it is actually the basis for the entire disagreement between Heideggerian ontology and Levinasian ethics. This is because Levinas's philosophy starts not with technology, but with sensibility, with the flesh-and-blood person. While in his later thought Heidegger's major worry is the dehumanization effected by modern technology, Levinas's major worry is always the suffering of flesh-and-blood human beings, the suffering of pain, mental anguish, deprivation, hunger, illness, as well as the suffering caused by injustice. Because Levinas begins with the body as sensibility, in considering the meaning of being-in-the-world he never overlooks, as Heidegger did, the moral imperatives that arise to alleviate concrete sensible suffering.

Regarding the second point about worldliness, its historical character, here again Levinas parts company from Heidegger. The meaning of human being-in-the-world does not, for Levinas, come from the world as a historical formation, does not come—contrary to German Idealism—from History personified, *Geist*, or world Epochs. Or to put this in another way: transcendence for Levinas is not a function of history. Rather, it is a function of the other person. History, for Levinas, is not sufficiently "other," does not free the self from the circuits of immanence. On first sight this may appear to be quite an odd claim. All of history immanent to subjectivity, it seems so unlikely. But the real issue at stake is the source of meaning. Does meaning come to humans from History, like a modern substitute for God, or are humans the makers of history, history being a human project? And if history is a human project, in what way is history genuinely transcendent, genuinely other? For Levinas, the greatest, indeed the only, absolute alterity is the alterity of the other person. This is what he calls "the face of the other." "This infinity, stronger than murder, already resists us in his face, is his face, is the primordial *expression*, is the first word: 'you shall not commit murder.'"[1] The face is neither an ontological nor an historical alterity, but the perspective from which being and history can be evaluated. It is a moral force, the force of weakness, of vulnerability, a call to my own responsibility to and for the other as other. "There is here a relation not with a very great resistance, but with something absolutely *other*: the resistance of what has no resistance—the ethical resistance."[2] The only genuine escape from narcissism, conceived broadly—or one could invoke such terms as "projection," "cathexis," "identification," or even "co-dependence"—the only relation whose terms cannot be assimilated to one another, contained, or integrated, is the infinite obligation toward and aroused by the other person. This relation—which Levinas calls a "relation without relation,"[3] because the self is not destroyed or obliterated in it, but rather exists as "turned inside out" for the other—is from the first a moral one, responsibility to and for the other. Such is each person's highest vocation, to alleviate the suffering of the other, and of all others. So it is not from history that the self finds the highest meaning of its life, but from service to the other person, and in relation to such service history itself must be judged.

Finally, Levinas will propose an entirely new notion of time. Perhaps nothing has been more radical in contemporary philosophy than time, because the overcoming of classical thought has only been achieved by overturning its illusory exit from time to "eternity," its *sub specie aeternitatis*. Heidegger in *Being and Time* (notice the title), following Henri Bergson and Husserl, made an "ecstatic" theory of time fundamental to all signification. Dasein's being-in-the-world was a projection into the future and a retrieval from the past, personally in being-toward-death, and ontologically in the unfolding of history's dispensations. No doubt ecstatic theories of temporality, including Heidegger's, represent a great advance over the previously prevalent "clock" theory of time, time as a series of instants, which Bergson had exposed as the measure of space rather than the flow of duration. But Levinas, while accepting this advance up to a point, is not content. What he discovers, and it is a remarkable discovery, is that the futurity of the future, the "not yet" which cannot be brought into the present, cannot be sustained through projection. Rather, such transcendence, if it is to retain its alterity, must depend on that which is truly transcendent, namely, the face of the other. Time, then, is neither objective nor subjective, but intersubjective.

Levinas's insights into time are so original that they are difficult to understand let alone appreciate at first glance. Yet his argument is compelling. The future cannot be truly future, truly novel and "not" yet, if it is a projection. The past cannot be truly past if it is a retrieval. For a genuine future and past, a genuine temporality, time must be bound to the transcendence of the other person, the only genuinely absolute transcendence, and that transcendence, as we have seen, arises only as morality and justice. Levinas, as a philosopher, will take this step: time is intersubjective, hence time is a function of morality and justice. So what is truly future, not yet, novel, is not some distant project of mine or of history's, but the unachieved world of *justice*. So also what is truly past, gone, immemorial, irretrievable, cannot be

[1] Levinas (1961: 199).   [2] Levinas (1961: 199).   [3] Levinas (1961: 80).

a function of human memory or appropriation, but is rather the lateness, the "too late" of my moral obligation to alleviate the suffering of the other. The moral subject is always too late on the scene, and always too early for the world of justice, which is humanity's ultimate aspiration. Time, then, is a matter of ethics, not ontology, not memory, not history. It is an radical insight, and these few pages cannot do it full justice.

IMPORTANCE FOR PSYCHOTHERAPY

In the last few decades Levinas's philosophy—despite the difficulty, its enormous erudition and catholic range, uncompromising rigor, profundity, and an originality bursting in catachrestic style—is increasingly being recognized, discussed, and appropriated by psychologists and psychotherapists. Two recent collections attest to this: *Psychotherapy for the Other: Levinas and the Face-to-Face Relationship*,[4] whose contributors are all practicing psychotherapists; and *Psychology for the Other: Levinas, Ethics and the Practice of Psychology*,[5] whose contributors are professors of psychology and professors of philosophy.

Yet Levinas has written no explicit therapies. Nor has he written much explicitly about psychology, psychoanalysis, psychopathology, or psychotherapy. Indeed, his attitude toward psychoanalysis, once a fashion of Parisian and European intellectuals following Jacques Lacan, has been dismissive.[6] The great interest and importance of Levinas for psychopathologists (and for other theoreticians and practitioners in psychology), however, derives from grasping the character and significance of his philosophy, however, and more specifically from an appreciation for the meaning and consequences of his central idea that the human is defined not by knowledge, nor by feeling, for that matter, and even less by self-interest or self-esteem,[7] but rather through the exigencies of moral responsibility. In other words, psychology and psychopathologists can learn and improve their self-understanding and their therapeutic work by grasping Levinas's *philosophy*, as a philosophy that is at once and fundamentally an *ethics*, a philosophy for which *morality* counts most.

Inasmuch as psychopathology's idea of health depends, as it must, on a more or less well-defined self-understanding of what it means to be a flourishing human being, then Levinas is important, accordingly, because he articulates with depth and precision a philosophical anthropology. But more specifically Levinas's philosophical anthropology is conceived through the lens of ethics, of good and evil, justice and injustice, in contrast to the pre-eminence philosophy usually accords to knowledge and truth claims. It is not to criticize or denigrate knowledge and truth, however, that Levinas turns to ethics, but precisely the reverse, for, so he argues, it is in ethics that science finds its proper and necessary ground, lacking which science distorts its own purview, for instance as one finds in all forms of positivism. Thus for Levinas

---

[4] Krycka, Kunz, and Sayre (2015). Here let us also add: Fryer (2004); Kunz (1998); Marcus (2008, 2010). A monograph which deals with Levinas's relation both to psychoanalysis and to politics, especially the Frankfurt School: Alford (2002).

[5] Gantt and Williams (2001).

[6] For a different reading, which sees Levinas and Lacan as fellow travelers in their shared critique of Sigmund Freud, see Fryer (2004).

[7] On the question of self-esteem, see Cohen (2001: 283–325).

the distinctions between "reality and appearance" and "true and false," whose coordination so many philosophies have presented as ultimate, turn out to be dependent on the deeper and conditioning distinction between "is and ought." Instead of conceiving that latter distinction subject to the rule of being or knowledge, as philosophers are wont to do, Levinas conceives morality *morally*, as it were, finding the orientation and priority of the "ought," the imperatives of morality, as all deriving from the priority of the other person's needs as my moral commands.

Levinas reconceives "selfhood" in terms of a being-for-the-other initiated not in the self by itself but through obligation and responsibility to and for the other person. Thus the self, through responsibility, is not an "identity," like a fortress, but a "non-identity," "de-posed," or "an-archic," in the etymological sense of the latter term (i.e. not finding its "principle" within itself), a being-for-the-other, the singularizing of a moral self hood—a self-emptying rather that a self-aggrandizement—across its obligations and responsibilities to and for the other person. Levinas goes so far as to call the moral self "maternal,"[8] taking the image of the pregnant woman bearing the other within herself, and appropriates the term "trauma" to indicate the full extent of the other's impact on my moral agency: my "I" is introjected as a "for-the-other," but a for-the-other that makes sense beyond the understanding of being or knowledge, but in the singularity of moral responsibility. In Levinas's own words: "The proximity of the neighbor in its trauma does not only strike up against me, but exalts and elevates me, and, in the literal sense of the term, inspires me. Inspiration, heteronomy, is the very pneuma of the psyche. . . . The for-the-other characteristic of the subject can be interpreted neither as a guilt complex (which presupposes an *initial* freedom), nor as a natural benevolence or divine 'instinct,' nor as some love or some tendency to sacrifice."[9]

The self is thus centered in its decentering: for-the-other before being-for-itself. Its "before" can only be maintained, and can only find its true sense, as a moral orientation, the moral priority of aiding the other person, which takes precedence over all the willfulness and self-interest of the self by itself. Or as Levinas succinctly writes: "No one is good voluntarily," and completes the sentence, from the other side, as it were, "no one is enslaved to the Good."[10] Its center—or decenter—is thus a self-for-the-other prior to being-for-itself, a self as moral responsibility elicited by the priority of the *vulnerability* not of itself but of the other, the other's needs, the other's suffering, and built upon this priority it is decentered toward everyone's responsibility to contribute to the making of a society of justice for all.

Here, then, the human being, and per implication mental health, is no longer defined by self-interest or self-satisfaction, or even by self-enrichment or self-fulfillment, all the usual ways by which the self's quest for ontological or existential wholeness have so often been justified, especially by psychology. Rather, the human self—the humanity of the human—arises as goodness, compassion, the elevation of a responsibility to and for the other, in facing the neighbor morally, and in facing all others through the labors of justice and its institutions. We must keep in mind, in order to quiet the carping voices of instrumental reason which are raised everywhere today, not to mention the narrowmindedness of positivism, cost–benefit analysis, and a ubiquitous commodification, that Levinas wrote neither self-help manuals nor inspirational spiritual literature. His is a rigorous philosophy, but in an ethical key. In the full rigor of his difficult philosophical works, based on strict and clear phenomenological

---

[8] See Cohen (2002: 32–64).   [9] Levinas (1998: 124).   [10] Levinas (1998: 11).

intuitions, strength of argumentation, and the most careful attention to the meaning and status of *importance*, the importance of importance, he refused to reduce the meaningful to the knowledge requirements of a quantitative objectivity. Thus he is neither a positivist nor a dreamer, but a philosopher determined—despite the great difficulties—to give fair hearing to the primacy demanded by ethical imperatives.

The achievement of mental health, from such a perspective, would depend not on repairing the stressed or broken defenses of a stronghold self. It would depend not on a re- treat into the safety and closure of an insular thing-like solidity. But rather mental health would demand raising the self to the dignity which arises through respect for the other person *as moral obligation*, and respect for all others through the tasks of *creating a just so- ciety*. These are not expendable glosses. Ethics is not a luxury. *Nothing is more important*, nothing closer to our true being, than alleviating the suffering of others. "Nothing," Levinas writes, "is more grave, more august, than responsibility for the other."[11] "The word *I* means *here I am*, answering for everything and for everyone."[12] Thus health—to be a flourishing human being—comes not in the proud independence of an impossible self-sufficiency, not in the fortress ego, but in the *weakness*, as it were, the pacific non-fulfillment and vulnera- bility, the *self-sacrifice* of moral striving. *To serve the other is each person's highest vocation.* True humanity, and hence mental health, comes in realizing and rising to the command that nothing is better than helping others. Mental health comes in helping others, through com- passion and giving, for in giving to others one gives of the self, and that self, the self that gives, for-the-other, is our better being.

Conclusion

What should be evident is that Levinas's philosophy, if taken seriously by psychology and psychopathology, represents a significant paradigm shift, a breakthrough, conceiving the human not in objective or subjective terms, but more deeply, or higher, in the ethical terms which represent what is noblest about humans, their humanity. Truth, and health, lies not in being or non-being, but in what is more precious, what is best, for you and for all of us.

BIBLIOGRAPHY

Alford C. F. (2002). *Levinas, the Frankfurt School and Psychoanalysis*. Middletown: Wesleyan University Press.

Cohen R. A. (2001). "Ricoeur and the Lure of Self-Esteem." In R. A. Cohen, *Ethics, Exegesis and Philosophy: Interpretation After Levinas*, pp. 283–325. Cambridge: Cambridge University Press.

Cohen R. A. (2002). "Maternal Psyche." In *Psychology for the Other*, ed. Edwin E. Gantt and Richard N. Williams, pp. 32–64. Pittsburgh: Duquesne University Press.

Fryer D. R. (2004). *The Intervention of the Other: Ethical Subjectivity in Levinas and Lacan*. New York: Other Press.

---

[11] Levinas (1998: 46).   [12] Levinas (1998: 114).

Gantt E. E. and Williams R. N. (eds.) (2001). *Psychology for the Other: Levinas, Ethics and the Practice of Psychology.*

Krycka K. C., Kunz G., and Sayre G. C. (eds.) (2015). *Psychotherapy for the Other: Levinas and the Face-to-Face Relationship.* Pittsburgh: Duquesne University Press.

Kunz G. (1998). *The Paradox of Power and Weakness: Levinas and an Alternative Paradigm for Psychology.* Albany: State University of New York Press.

Levinas E. (1961). *Totality and Infinity.* Pittsburgh: Duquesne University Press.

Levinas E. (1998). *Otherwise than Being or Beyond Essence,* trans. Alphonso Lingis. Pittsburgh: Duquesne University Press.

Marcus P. (2008). *Being for the Other: Emmanuel Levinas, Ethical Living and Psychoanalysis.* Milwaukee: Marquette University Press.

Marcus P. (2010). *In Search of the Good Life: Emmanuel Levinas, Psychoanalysis, and the Art of Living.* London: Karnac Books.

CHAPTER 12

CRITIQUES AND INTEGRATIONS OF PHENOMENOLOGY

Derrida, Foucault, Deleuze

FEDERICO LEONI

INTRODUCTION

PHENOMENOLOGY is a vast philosophical movement that played a central role in the philosophical debates of the first half of the twentieth century. From the second half of the twentieth century onwards, many alternative philosophical movements gradually emerged. However, despite their often radical criticism of the phenomenological approach, these movements regularly touched upon themes or adopted perspectives that had been originally propounded or developed by phenomenology. This is true of Jacques Derrida (1930–2004), Michel Foucault (1926–84), and Gilles Deleuze (1925–95): three protagonists of late twentieth-century French thought and three still extremely influential alternatives to phenomenological thinking (but whose contribution to phenomenology may well prove fruitful). We could give a preliminary definition of phenomenology, obviously a very partial and questionable one. If we define phenomenology as the study of the most general and profound structures of human experience, as the study of the transcendental structure of perception, of affection, of imagination, of desire, and so on, then we could say that there is a shared question at the basis of the approach to phenomenology taken by Derrida, Foucault, and Deleuze. This is the question of a new version of the transcendental, a version in which the desubjectivization, the historicization, the dissemination, in one word the impurity of the transcendental, are placed in the foreground.

JACQUES DERRIDA

Jacques Derrida began his career as a scholar of Husserl, to whom he devoted at least three important works of his early period: a large study, *The Problem of Genesis in Husserl's*

Philosophy, written in the early 1950s, but published only in 1990 (Derrida 2003); the *Introduction to Husserl's Origin of Geometry* (Derrida 1989), a detailed and compelling interpretation of the appendix to Husserl's *The Crisis of European Sciences* (a text that had soon begun to circulate widely as an independent excerpt); and *Voice and Phenomenon* (Derrida 2011), which was literally an anticipation of all the topics later developed by Derrida, once again in the form of an intense, careful, and original dialogue with the philosophy of Husserl. This particular text can be seen as a general introduction to Derrida's overall interpretation of Husserl's thought. On the one hand, Derrida's criticism was aimed at showing simply the impossibility of phenomenology; on the other, his interpretation revived a perspective that Husserl himself had in part foreseen or at least adumbrated. If the main area of focus of Husserl's phenomenology was human experience in its living presence, and if the great ambition of phenomenology was a first-hand description of that same living and immediate presence, then the objection advanced by Derrida was simple: the living presence doesn't exist and a fortiori cannot be the object of a phenomenological description.

Derrida not only argued for this impossibility, but also showed that the very descriptions and concepts elaborated by Husserl implied such an outcome. The element identified by Derrida in the text of Husserl was precise: it was the notion of "retention," which Husserl had placed at the center of his phenomenology of temporality. According to Husserl, the living present "retains" in itself what is no longer present, what has just happened, which in turn had retained in itself what had just happened, and so on. The present, according to Husserl's famous imagery, is like the "comet tail" of retentions (Husserl 1991). Without retention, therefore, there would be no present. The very meaning of present depends on this relationship with the past and on the directionality established by this relationship. However, if this is true—and here lies precisely Derrida's objection—then nothing is ever really present and the present is never an original given: in the beginning there was not presence, but retention, or, better, a trace of presence and origin. This means, for example, that there is no such thing as perception or a truly living body: perception is always the deciphering of an enigma, a relationship not with an object but with something similar to a text. The living body is invariably a web of otherness and intermittency, a body not actually alive but tainted by a foreign element, by a sort of mortality constitutive of life. Again, if the transcendental is understood as a pure and foundational principle, if every purity is intrinsically tainted by something foreign, if every foundation always redirects to something else and a sign always mars every origin, then there is no longer a subject or transcendental subjectivity. The transcendental is replaced by a senseless and indiscernible mechanism in which an absence is also a presence or vice versa.

Psychiatry and phenomenological psychopathology do not seem to have assimilated all the possible consequences of Derrida's position. However, his idea of a presence always mingled with an absence and of a body essentially tainted by otherness could perhaps allow us to understand that there is something structurally unstable and ungraspable in the Husserlian or Merleau-Pontian *Leib*. A kind of psychotic destiny seems to be consubstantial to the body. For this reason, the notion of madness in the broadest sense of the term should be—not simply on the basis of a humanistic appeal to understanding and universal acceptance—fully reintroduced in the concept of humanity, and more precisely in the transcendental structure of the human dimension that phenomenology has always tried to grasp. Compared to the psychopathological approach, which has often placed at the basis of its investigation this transcendental structure as a kind of theme where the variations or alterations are the psychopathological experiences, Derrida's approach is the inverse: the variations precede the theme, and the alteration is coextensive with the living presence. In other words: madness is the structural foundation of experience, not its occasional collapse.

MICHEL FOUCAULT

Michel Foucault's first major work, *Madness and Civilization*, published in 1961, proved to be immensely influential. Early on, Foucault had devoted a number of important studies to the history of psychology, to German philosophy of medicine, and to phenomenological psychology and psychiatry (he had written a large and original introduction to Ludwig Binswanger's *Dream and Existence*). *Madness and Civilization*, which was to be followed by an extensive course entitled *Abnormal* (1974–75), marked a first major shift. For Foucault it was no longer a matter of reflecting on the experience of madness, but rather to show that madness had a history, and that this was not a history of the idea of madness and its treatments, but rather a history of madness itself, which is not a natural given but a cultural construct.

According to Foucault, what today is called madness was in the Middle Ages a vague and heterogeneous territory that included the most diverse forms of social and anthropological marginalization. What has happened, according to Foucault, is not that we have identified a properly medical and psychiatric problem by disentangling it from highly diverse and poorly assorted phenomena. Rather, a medical–psychiatric form of *knowledge* has gradually emerged by extricating itself from *other* forms of knowledge, whether traditional, theological, philosophical, or medical. This new knowledge managed to persuade us of the existence of its object (madness), an object clearly distinguishable from the others and endowed with a kind of essence, be it moral, neurological, or otherwise. Foucault did not believe that psychiatry as a particular form of knowledge identified its specific object by separating it from other objects. Rather, he thought that all forms of knowledge constructed their objects by carving out, each time according to an equally legitimate or arbitrary criterion, a specific portion of the infinitely rich tapestry of reality. Medieval knowledge was perfectly consistent and absolutely objective in its application when it interned beggars together with criminals, visionaries, prostitutes, and people infected with tuberculosis. Equally consistent and objective was nineteenth-century knowledge when it preserved or expunged some of those categories of people and introduced new ones, grouping together, for example, criminals and visionaries but not beggars and tuberculosis-stricken people. Again, with equal legitimacy, the criterion of social marginalization was replaced by that of behavioral abnormality, which required also some attention to its statistical and demographic measurability, some investigation into its possible histological correlates, and so on.

After his controversial study of madness, Foucault explored other territories. By adopting what he called an "archaeological" and "genealogical" perspective, Foucault addressed somewhat interconnected issues, such as medicine (Foucault 1973), penal institutions (Foucault 1977), and sexuality (Foucault 1988–90). In relation to the variegated field of phenomenology and phenomenological psychopathology, at least two consequences of Foucault's work deserve mention. The first is evidently ethical–political and sounds like an invitation—implicit in *Madness and Civilization*—to relativize psychiatric knowledge and its claims of objectivity.

This applies even to psychiatry's seemingly more neutral, objective, and scientifically up-to-date versions, such as statistical–diagnostic or biological–pharmacological ones. It was an invitation to reflect on the fact that often such objectivity concealed unexplored theoretical options, unconscious metaphysical assumptions, and more or less violent and repressive ideological tenets. This is the sense in which Foucault's work was received and understood by the anti-psychiatry movements. These critical reactions to psychiatry emerged in parallel with *Madness and Civilization* (and lasted for about two decades) in several European countries, and it was a movement that took different forms, such as those influenced by R. D. Laing in the United Kingdom and Franco Basaglia in Italy. The second consequence, more theoretical and philosophical in nature, is a relativization of the category of the subject, a category that phenomenological psychiatry and philosophical phenomenology had often brandished against, respectively, the most biologically oriented forms of psychiatry and the most diverse forms of biological and historical–social–economic reductionism. What was claimed, in such confrontation, was the irreducibility of experience and subjectivity to their material conditions and premises. Again, Foucault exhorted his readers to cultivate doubt and to suspect that under the actual subjective experience supposedly grounded in an irreducible individuality or in a transcendental subjectivity as identified by a certain tradition of thought, perhaps quite a different reality might be at work, something deeper and more elusive: an inextricable web of social practices, anonymous and pervasive discourses and cultural constructs that combine knowledge and power in accordance with specific rules and specific effects of meaning, truth, and repression. For Foucault, this web is perhaps the only transcendental dimension that is worth addressing (Foucault 1981; Foucault 1994).

GILLES DELEUZE

Gilles Deleuze (1925–95) was one of the most important French poststructuralist thinkers. He wrote major works such as *Difference and Repetition* (Deleuze 1994), *The Logic of Sense* (Deleuze 1990), and (with Félix Guattari) *Anti-Oedipus* (Deleuze and Guattari 1977) and *A Thousand Plateaus* (Deleuze and Guattari 1987). However, it was in the first of his two famous books dedicated to the cinema, *The Movement-Image* (Deleuze 1986), which was followed two years later by *The Time-Image* (Deleuze 1989), that Deleuze engaged more explicitly and more critically with phenomenology. The context for this criticism may seem odd, but in hindsight it was not. If it is true that cinema is a Bergsonian form of art, then the background of Deleuze's criticism of phenomenology lay precisely in an overall interpretation of the philosophy and culture typical of the twentieth century. According to Deleuze, the twentieth century began by pointing to a dual path or, better, to a grand theoretical alternative, namely, that between Bergson and Husserl. In these pages, Deleuze clearly and openly opted for Bergson and against Husserl. Phenomenology and Bergsonism have often been compared or grouped together on the basis of their common attention to experience and their similar attempt to capture experience in its immediate manifestations. In the *Movement-Image*, however, Deleuze strongly contrasted these two approaches. He argued that while Husserl's battle cry was that every consciousness is consciousness of something, Bergson's was that every consciousness *is* a thing: this was the abyss separating the two positions and their profoundly different treatment of the same problems. Every consciousness is consciousness of something: according to this slogan, Husserlian phenomenology emphasized intentionality, to the point where the intentionality of consciousness and its subjective orientation toward its objects was seen as the basis of experience itself. All consciousness is a thing: according to this slogan, Bergsonism emphasized a subjectless experience, whose primary source of meaning did not lie in the activity of consciousness; rather, consciousness was seen as simply one of the available, but not mandatory and, even less, fundamental modes of organization of experience.

It is perhaps difficult to recognize Husserl's and Bergson's ideas point by point in the slogans coined by Deleuze. It is certainly easier to identify in the Husserlian slogan a classical definition of intentionality. It is less easy, however, to identify in the Bergsonian slogan an authentic position actually espoused by Bergson, despite the fact that he often entertained similar claims (Bergson 2004). However, the Deleuzian formula could also be criticized from the opposite angle. The sentence that should describe the phenomenological position is literally more accurate, but in fact less faithful to Husserl's thought. No doubt for Husserl all consciousness is consciousness of something, and therefore is an intentional consciousness. However, the object of intentionality is in fact never external to intentionality itself: it is never a naturalistically understood object. The polarity is always completely intrinsic to the intentional act—always a noematic rather than an objective polarity. The Bergsonian slogan coined by Deleuze, on the other hand, is literally less accurate, but (not surprisingly) more in tune with the spirit of Bergson's philosophy. The idea that consciousness is not consciousness of something, but a thing among other things floating on the surface of experience, means for Bergson that experience is not a ray of light going from one place to another, from a subject to an object, but is primarily a non-generated dimension deprived of a subject. The immediate experiential evidence is not that a subject is targeting an object, but that experience is simply given: a landscape announces and offers itself, and somehow "is seen," that is, sees itself through itself. Only at a later time, Bergson believes, this subject-less and object-less experience is constructed as a subjective experience and is restructured and endowed with a perspective: the result is that such perspective begins to be seen as a subject, and the content of the experience begins to count as the object of experience.

Deleuze's sketch has, if nothing else, the merit of fully clarifying, through his treatment of Bergson, Deleuze's own position. The battle between Husserl and Bergson is, for Deleuze, one between the strategy of transcendence and the strategy of immanence. The first turns experience into an "exiting from" and a "heading to" something; all the necessary distinctions being made, this is indeed Husserl's position. The second strategy turns experience into a permanent "motion" within a non-transcendable dimension that knows no outside or alterity; in other words, this is a monistic or immanent theory of experience, which refuses to start from dualistic premises and to oppose a subject to an object and consequently to postulate the transcendence and the transcendental as the foundation of the possibility of experience. Deleuze's thought is therefore characterized by a radical anti-conscious and anti-transcendental stance. In other words, confronted with the Cartesian spectrum, Deleuze firmly resorted to a Spinozian option, which in terms of philosophy of experience involved the idea of an original, perfectly auto-immanent, absolutely anonymous, and totally impersonal experience—something that, one might argue, phenomenology itself, with not too dissimilar language, had often adumbrated, especially when confronting the more or less hidden legacy of Cartesianism. One might think, in this regard, of Merleau-Ponty's phenomenology of the flesh (Merleau-Ponty 1968), Jan Patocka's phenomenology of movement

(Patocka 1998), Michel Henry's material phenomenology (Henry 1973), or Renaud Barbaras's phenomenology of life (Barbaras 2006).

A text written in the 1970s, *Anti-Oedipus* (which Deleuze co-authored with Félix Guattari in 1972) represents the most interesting result, but also the most difficult to decipher, of Deleuze's immanentism. The target of the book, as evident from the title, is the psychoanalytic concept of the Oedipus complex. In the normal development and full resolution of such complex, classic Freudianism and Kleinianism saw the path that ensured the emergence of a subject capable of adapting to social life with its inevitable and necessary discontents (Freud 1962) as well as the success of the psychoanalytic treatment. According to this view, this treatment allowed the subject to come to terms with the renunciation of instincts required by society in exchange for protection.

In the eyes of Deleuze and Guattari, Oedipus appeared as the emblem of an entire theoretical discourse, according to which the construction of a subject is dependent on its renunciation of a part of pleasure and on the replacement of a full, primal, anarchist, and uncontrollable pleasure with a void, a lack, a fundamental resistance on the part of external objects. As a consequence, in this view, desire is a relationship entertained with absence or through absence, and the true nature of the desiring subject lies in its tendency to negate its immediate object of desire in order to cut across it and reach for a never fully graspable "beyond." Against all this, Deleuze and Guattari wanted to construct an immanent and positive notion of desire rather than a transcendent and negative one. They saw this as a chance to disentangle psychoanalysis and psychiatry itself from what appeared to them as an essentially ideological function.

Conclusion

Derrida shows that the transcendental is broken, that its powers of constitution are intermittent, that intermittence is the structure of sense itself. Foucault shows that the transcendental is a set of apparatuses which give birth to the subject as a subjected subject, that there is no meaning outside of the apparatuses, and that apparatuses are absolutely contingent and meaningless. Deleuze and Guattari show that if Oedipus is a symbol of disorder, the true alternative is nevertheless not the one which opposes order to disorder, but the one which opposes order and disorder on the one side, and the never-ending creation of new couplings of order and disorder on the other side, that is, the metamorphic and fractal movement or event of what they call chaosmos. The three different positions are three different concepts of difference as a sort of non-transcendental structure of the transcendental itself. It is difficult to say whether a non-transcendental phenomenology would still be phenomenology, and this philosophical question is still open. Phenomenological psychiatry, or phenomenological psychopathology, could nevertheless draw some useful insights and instruments from this ongoing debate: e.g. a more subtle transcendentalism; a more continuous view of the range of psychopathological experiences; a more exact comprehension of the different temporal and spatial structures of psychopathological worlds as the internal possibilities and infinitesimal variations of the transcendental, much more than the crisis or fracture of its functioning; and a more critical way of thinking the structure of institutions, the epistemology of their therapeutical vocation, the archaeology of the subjectivity, or the normativity they assume as a directive principle of the treatments they dispense. In brief, at the very convergence between this kind of subtle transcendentalism and this sort of anti-institutional but not anti-psychiatric psychiatry, what we could find is an idea of treatment which is not the route from disease to health but from vulnerability to singularity.

BIBLIOGRAPHY

Barbaras, R. (2006). *Desire and Distance* [1999], trans. P. B. Milan. Stanford: Stanford University Press.

Bergson H. (2004). *Matter and Memory* [1896], trans. N. M. Paul and W. Scott Palmer. New York: Dover Publications.

Deleuze, G. (1986). *Cinema 1. The Movement-Image* [1983], trans. H. Tomlinson and B. Hammerjam. Minneapolis: University of Minnesota Press.

Deleuze, G. (1989). *Cinema 2. The Time-Image* [1985], trans. H. Tomlinson and R. Galeta. Minneapolis: Minnesota University Press.

Deleuze, G. (1990). *The Logic of Sense* [1990], trans. M. Lester with C. Stivale. New York: Columbia University Press.

Deleuze, G. (1994). *Difference and Repetition* [1968], trans. P. Patton. New York: Columbia University Press.

Deleuze, G. and Guattari, F. (1977). *Anti-Oedipus. Capitalism and Schizophrenia* [1972], trans. R. Hurley, M. Seem, and R. H. Lane. New York: Viking Press.

Deleuze, G. and Guattari, F. (1987). *A Thousand Plateaus* [1980], trans. B. Massumi. Minneapolis: University of Minnesota Press.

Derrida, J. (1989). *Edmund Husserl's Origin of Geometry, An Introduction* [1962], trans. John P. Leavey. Lincoln: Nebraska University Press.

Derrida, J. (2003). *The Problem of Genesis in Husserl's Philosophy* [1990], trans. M. Hobson. Chicago: Chicago University Press.

Derrida, J. (2011). *Voice and Phenomenon. Introduction to the Problem of the Sign in Husserl's Phenomenology* [1967], trans. L. Lawlor. Evanston: Northwestern University Press.

Foucault, M. (1973). *The Birth of the Clinic* [1963], trans. A. Sheridan. New York: Pantheon.

Foucault, M. (1977). *Discipline and Punish* [1975], trans. A. Sheridan. New York: Pantheon.

Foucault, M. (1981). "The Order of Discourse" [1970], trans. I. McLeod. In R. Young (ed.), *Untying the Text: A Post-Structuralist Reader*, pp. 51–78. London: Routledge and Paul Keagan.

Foucault, M. (1988–90). *History of Sexuality I-III* [1976–84], trans. R. Hurley. New York: Vintage Books.

Foucault, M. (1994). *The Order of Things. An Archaeology of Human Sciences* [1966], trans. A. Sheridan. New York: Vintage Books.

Foucault, M. (2001). *Madness and Civilization. A History of Insanity in the Age of Reason* [1962], trans. R. Howard. New York: Vintage Books.

Foucault, M. (2003). *Abnormal. Lectures at the Collège de France* [1997], trans. G. Burchell. New York: Picador.

Freud, S. (1962). *Civilization and its Discontents* [1930], trans. J. Strachey. New York: Norton and Co.

Henry, M. (1973). *The Essence of Manifestation* [1963], trans. G. Etzkorn. Den Haag: Nijhoff.

Husserl, E. (1991). *For the Phenomenology of Inner Consciousness of Time (1893–1917)*, trans. J. B. Brough. Dordrecht: Kluwer Academic Publishers.

Merleau-Ponty, M. (1968). *The Visible and the Invisible* [1964], trans. A. Lingis. Evanston: Northwestern University Press.

Patocka, J. (1998). *Body, Community, Language, World* [1995], trans. E. Kohak. Chicago: Open Court.

CHAPTER 13

....

KARL JASPERS

....

MATTHIAS BORMUTH

INTRODUCTION

....

KARL Jaspers (1883–1969) became one of the founding fathers of phenomenological thinking by publishing his *General Psychopathology* in 1913. International conferences around the globe celebrated the 100th anniversary of his "psychiatric *opus magnum*." One esteemed his leading purpose: "to bring order into the chaos of abnormal psychic phenomena by rigorous description, definition, and classification, and to empower psychiatry with a valid and reliable method to assess and make sense of abnormal human subjectivity."[1]

Although Jaspers's method of understanding differs greatly from those who followed strictly Edmund Husserl's insights, Jaspers shared the ambition to understand the inner world of the patient and its dynamics with colleagues like Ludwig Binswanger at that time. But he relied more on the psychology of understanding conceptualized and exercised in the humanities ("Geisteswissenschaften") by Wilhelm Dilthey, Max Weber, and Georg Simmel.

In later editions of his book Jaspers restricted his concept of understanding to pure descriptions and observed genealogical speculations with great doubts pointing at vague psychological or philosophical premises. Jaspers called these leading ideas "psycho-myths" primarily with Freud and his school in mind. Moreover he criticized all biological attempts as "brain-myth" which pretended to be able to solve the riddle of psychiatric illnesses.

Jaspers's strict critique of speculative theories in the field of psychiatry arose from his increasingly widespread philosophical horizon. The fourth and last edition of his *General Psychopathology*, which was written during the Second World War when Jaspers had been withdrawn from public life in Nazi Germany and was not allowed to publish, philosophically contained a completely new section built up on philosophical grounds which intended to reflect on "The Human Being as a Whole." Jaspers wrote about this part of the book and its "fundamental philosophical questions": "It is no longer part of the field of psychopathological science as such but has a general relevance."[2]

This chapter begins by sketching the biographical and intellectual background without which it would not have been possible for Jaspers to give birth to his famous concept of

[1] Cf. Stanghellini and Fuchs (2013: xiii).   [2] Jaspers (2013: 747–822, 747).

understanding. Then the focus will be more closely directed on its methodological frame. The chapter finishes by directing attention to the question of what philosophical considerations motivated Jaspers to draw the "limits of understanding" more closely and strictly in the last, and nowadays internationally read, edition of the *General Psychopathology*. The thesis is that these limits can be determined as an existential application of Kant's idea and antinomy of freedom.

THE INTELLECTUAL BIOGRAPHY OF JASPERS AS A PSYCHIATRIST

The fact that Jaspers was able to write his psychiatric classic before turning thirty has two more reasons than his great talent to shed methodological lights on the psychopathological appearances. First his personal situation and secondly his favorable circumstances in which he found himself at the Psychiatric and Neurological Clinic of Heidelberg helped him to accomplish this lucid overview of the material.

Due to a severe, chronic lung disease the young assistant was relieved from his usual clinical duties. This meant that Jaspers could spend much more time on research than his colleagues, exploring individual patients and studying psychiatric literature. These conditions made it possible to work as an engaged observer in the sciences. The young psychiatrist had time enough to get to know the phenomena empirically and a sufficient amount of hours to reflect on them in the horizon of historic psychiatric literature.

His elder and more experienced colleagues Karl Wilmanns and Hans W. Gruhle introduced him into their psychology of understanding, while Franz Nissl, the head of the clinic, exercised biological psychiatry at a high level, working with Alois Alzheimer on the histological exploration of dementia. Therefore both ways of approaching psychiatric diseases—the psychological understanding and the biological explanation—were represented prominently at that time in Heidelberg. In his *Philosophical Autobiography* Jaspers summed up the methodological conviction that each way had a limited right on its own: "Whenever (man) becomes known, something of his appearance becomes known, not he himself. Every knowledge of man as a whole proves to be a deception which arises from the fact that one way of inquiry is elevated to the rank of being the only one, one method is made a universal one."[3]

Although Jaspers always admired researchers who made use of the natural sciences in psychiatry his personal affinity was, from early on, directed toward the method of psychological understanding. Already his doctoral thesis on "Eifersuchtswahn," written in 1909, was influenced by the desire to describe psychologically certain psychopathological phenomena and to contextualize them culturally as far as possible. In 1912 Jaspers published a methodological paper, the title of which underlined the significance of Edmund Husserl.[4] But a close reading of "The Phenomenological Approach in Psychopathology," which, in 1968, was the only one of Jaspers's early papers to be translated into English,[5] reveals clearly

---

[3] Jaspers (1957: 20f.).   [4] Jaspers (1912: 391–408), later in (1963: 314–328).
[5] Jaspers (1968: 1313–1325).

that already at this early stage of his intellectual becoming, Jaspers did not belong to the phe-nomenological school as such. In his view it could only provide a descriptive knowledge of the symptomatology of a patient. Therefore Jaspers withdrew from the Husserlian core of the method writing with respect and distance in his recollection: "As method I adopted Husserl's phenomenology, which, in its beginnings, he called descriptive psychology; I retained it al-though I rejected its further development to insight into essences (Wesensschau)."[6]

The possibility of exploring the human subjectivity even in its pathological appearances was, at its core, a scientific claim for which Jaspers never had great sympathy. Looking back on such an ambition he wrote critically: "Never can the balance, so to speak, be struck by sci-entific means. Every sick person is, like any other person, inexhaustible. Never does know-ledge reach a point where the personality with its hidden mysteriousness cannot at least be sense—be it even as mere possibility, as still reflected in wondrous leftovers (of the original personality)."[7]

Much more than to Husserl's phenomenology, Jaspers was attached to the cultural sci-ences which were discussed in the circle that existed in Heidelberg around Max Weber. His colleague and friend Hans Gruhle had paved the way to Max Weber in 1909 and since then Jaspers had exchanged thoughts with the historian, economist, and founder of soci-ology. After the premature death of his intellectual hero, in 1920 Jaspers told the astonished academic world:

> If Max Weber was a philosopher, perhaps he was the only philosopher of our times and was a philosopher in a sense in which no one else could be termed as such today.[8]

Thus it hardly comes as a surprise that in 1949, when Jaspers was at the zenith of public rec-ognition as a philosopher and psychiatrist, he should look back and acknowledge the de-cisive role which Max Weber had played for him throughout his lifetime as a scientist and philosopher: As he writes, "I am indebted to Max Weber not only for my *Psychopathology* of young years, but also for providing me with the means to formulate my philosophy."[9]

Max Weber is connected with the Neokantian school of thinkers around 1900 whose center was—at least for some time—Heidelberg. Wilhelm Windelband and Heinrich Rickert, both colleagues of Weber, were leading figures in the methodological discussion which was being carried on in the humanities ("Geisteswissenschaften") around 1900. The approach of the natural sciences was determined as a "nomothetic" and the own one was called "ide-ographic." This Neokantian dichotomy became decisive for Jaspers. He was convinced that natural events can only be explained externally with the help of logical regularities which have been achieved by using inductive reasoning, whereas inner meaning-making processes can only be grasped by individual empathy. So he took up the popular polarization of "objec-tive causal connections" on "explaining" ("Erklären") and "understanding of psychic events 'from within' as 'understanding' ('Verstehen')."[10]

This short overview of the main influences on the early Jaspers would not be complete without a word concerning the important role of Sigmund Freud. His psychoanalytic ap-proach toward the inner world was widely discussed among his clinical colleagues and in the Weber circle. Heidelberg was one of the few places next to Munich and Zurich where the

---

[6] Jaspers (1957: 18).   [7] Jaspers (1957: 21).   [8] Jaspers (1988: S. 32).
[9] Jaspers (2016: 190).   [10] Jaspers (2013: 14), quoted from Jaspers (1998: 28).

academic world and some psychiatrists were open to the provocative ideas on the genealogy of diverse psychic illnesses. Psychoanalysis was practiced by the assistants by analyzing each other and sometimes certain patients. In the first edition of his *General Psychopathology* Jaspers called Freud one of the most outstanding psychologists next to the philosophers Søren Kierkegaard and especially Friedrich Nietzsche. The second edition of 1920 already takes a more critical position, saying that Freud demonstrated a peculiar lack of intellect in his understanding ascriptions. Now any praise of his outstanding intellectual had vanished and Jaspers states clearly that Freud cannot match the achievements of those two great searchers and confessors of the human self.

This early affinity toward the thoughts of Kierkegaard and Nietzsche, whom Jaspers had already studied in his psychiatric years, can be taken as a sign of his calling as a philosopher. Encouraged by his illness which did not allow him to take up a permanent position in psychiatry, Jaspers decided after five successful years to become a philosopher. Jaspers described enthusiastically his lifelong passion for the life of the mind in his autobiography: "From early youth on I had been philosophizing. Actually I had taken up medicine and psychopathology from philosophical motives."[11]

He published his *Psychology of Worldviews* in 1919, an interdisciplinary work between psychology and philosophy which was pivotal in the decision to invite Jaspers to take up a chair of philosophy at Heidelberg University in 1922. The book became the "earliest writing in the later so-called modern Existentialism" with all the "fundamental questions," as Jaspers recollected over three decades later, "about the world, what it is for man; about the situation of man and about his ultimate situations ("Grenzsituation") from which there is no escape (death, suffering, chance, guilt, struggle); about time and the multidimension nature of its meaning; about the movement of freedom in the process of creating one's self."[12] The challenge of human freedom became the leading idea of Jaspers's philosophical work and also for the last revision of the *General Psychopathology*, as we will see below.

JASPERS'S METHODOLOGICAL HORIZONS OF UNDERSTANDING PSYCHOLOGY

In his formative years as a psychiatrist Jaspers provided a well-received distinction for the phenomenological method of understanding. He introduced three forms of understanding; discerning between "static," "rational," and "genetic" understanding. During the hermeneutic process the first two forms were feeding the third so that at the end a diagnostical judgment could be possible. First the psychopathologist combines the "rational" and "static" approach of isolated psychic phenomena, then he constitutes "genetically" associative understanding and reaches finally a classification of symptoms according to ideotypical entities. In this Weberian approach one can only offer "ideotypical connections," making one's findings only "inherently evident" or "more or less understandable," for which reason the method of understanding cannot compete with the explanatory disciplines.

---

[11] Jaspers (1957: 24).   [12] Jaspers (1957: 29).

The static and rational ways of understanding are necessary elements in creating a genetic synthesis of the psychopathological phenomena. Without doubt, Nietzsche's hermeneutics of unconscious feelings, as developed in his *Genealogy of Morals*, was a decisive inspiration for Jaspers. His *General Psychopathology* reflects on the evidence Nietzsche gave of the genealogy of Jewish-Christian values by focusing on the unconscious resentments against their powerful enemies and oppressors. Probably Max Weber's and William James's reception of Nietzsche's genealogical claim inspired Jaspers's certain openness. Thereby his beginning was connected to Freud's since the founder of psychoanalysis counted among Nietzsche's earliest readers while studying medicine in Vienna more than three decades before.

While Jaspers was initially very open to genealogical suggestions, in psychiatry, his student Kurt Schneider viewed Nietzsche very critically. In his philosophical dissertation—written with Max Scheler in Cologne—Schneider rejected the genealogical end of understanding as proclaimed in the topos of resentment and proclaimed the psychological independence of the values of love, empathy, and justice instead.[13]

But besides this reception of Nietzsche Jaspers did not follow his teacher Weber in the desire to articulate clear suggestions and make aetiological claims. He did not employ the concept of the "ideotype" to make any definite statements as Weber had done in the polemically discussed *The Protestant Ethics and the "Spirit" of Capitalism*. Jaspers's idea of genealogical evidence remained rather vague. The reason was his great, never outspoken, affinity with Wilhelm Dilthey's concept of empathy ("Einfühlung") which provided more literary views on inner dynamics. Jaspers's pathographical studies on van Gogh and especially the poet Hölderlin can be seen as examples of this certain vagueness and the direct reception of Dilthey's essayistic interpretations.[14] Therefore Jaspers spoke of the art of psychological understanding, which allowed an "unprejudiced, direct comprehension of psychic events" and the "irreducible quality of psychic phenomena." As he contends, by means of "comparison, repetition, verification of the results of empathy," the "direct comprehension of expression phenomena" could almost reach the empirico-objective status of natural sciences.[15]

Jaspers argues that the obtainable degree of psychological evidence would depend on the interpreter's subjective ability to understand and the quality of the given material. Therefore he exercised mostly a methodological dualism which mirrored Dilthey's famous polarization between causally compelling, generally valid "science" and the very subjective "adeptness and art" of understanding.[16] As Jaspers argues, the natural scientific connections of psychiatry can be theorized, whereas psychological moments of understanding cannot be grasped systematically and have to be described in the literary-essayistic forms of depiction.[17] According to this, the "instinctive adeptness" of the interpreter constitutes a vague tool of insight prone to error.[18] In his eyes, psychological hermeneutics was only capable of rudimentarily sounding out and connecting unconscious motivations without ever reaching the unfathomable depths of the sea of unconsciousness.

One can resume Jaspers's limited concept of understanding: The deeper causes of pathogenesis were not to discern by psychological and hermeneutical means. He illustrated his notion from early on by a model of disease in which the symptoms correspond to the layers of an onion. The innermost ones stand for the causes of psychic disorder and

---

[13] More details are given in Bormuth (2009).   [14] See Bormuth (2013a, 2013b).
[15] Jaspers (1988: 318f.).   [16] Jaspers (1913: S. 2).
[17] Jaspers *Gesammelte Schriften zur Psychopathologie* (1963: 336).   [18] Jaspers (1913: 2).

are, pathogenetically speaking, the decisive ones, even if the disease phenomena can be influenced pathoplastically by biographic experience of the outer layers. Jaspers sketches the pathogenetic core as constituting "extra conscious dispositions, predispositions, psychic constitutions and extra-conscious-mechanisms,"[19] which, as an "extremely complicated biological process," eludes our knowledge "to an immeasurable degree," thus permitting no direct correlations between changes in brain activity and psychic disorders.[20]

When Jaspers later developed his existence philosophy he insisted even more strongly on the limits of understanding. Having been forced to retire from his philosophical chair due to his Jewish wife Gertrud, he took the opportunity to revise the *General Psychopathology*. The existential root of his thinking deepened in this personal border situation. And the idea of undetermined freedom in circumstances which seem to determine man became entirely the beacon of his thoughts.

As we will see, this focus on the existential possibilities became an important reason why, in the last edition of his book, Jaspers postulated even more strongly the limits of understanding. Not only biological facts but also cultural decisions limit our ability to understand the other and our wish to enlighten the deepest grounds of our convictions, deeds, failings, and psychopathologies. This created a broad gap between Jaspers and all other phenomenological, anthropological, psychoanalytical, and psychosomatic attempts of genetic understanding.

SELF-REFLECTION AND PHENOMENOLOGICAL PSYCHIATRY

Jaspers's ambition of limiting the possible achievements of understanding is strongly correlated with his growing philosophical enthusiasm and profile. The early affinity with Dilthey's idea of the individual incommensurability which lies in the unfathomable unconscious affords turned more and more into the concept of freedom of self-determination. Thereby the perspective of autonomous dynamics—which cannot be determined scientifically—stands in its own right, confronted with the duty to be as well aware of all rationally recognizable causes of biological, social, and psychological kind. Jaspers legitimizes the existential perspective by introducing Kant's critical thoughts on the antinomy of freedom.[21] The postulate of freedom breaks up the original polarization between understanding and explaining psychiatric phenomena. Jaspers goes beyond Dilthey's concept.

Therefore only the last edition of his *General Psychopathology* refers to the philosophical language of critical idealism which can be seen in his exemplary claim: "So far as the human being is empirically explorable as an object of knowledge he is unfree. But in so far as we ourselves experience, act and investigate we are free in our own self-certainty and hence more than we can ever discover."[22] For Jaspers, existence-philosophical self-reflection constitutes a necessary supplement to psychotherapy, which in his eyes no longer belongs

---

[19] Jaspers (1913: 49).   [20] Jaspers (1913: 192).   [21] See Bormuth (2013c).
[22] Jaspers (1998: 754f.).

in any way to the realm of psychiatry. The existential hermeneutics in the Kantian horizon is the decisive means in order to enlighten the individual's personality even with its pathological aspects.

For the Kantian philosopher of existence, Freud, Adler, and Jung are all deeply guilty of being ideological ("weltanschaulich") schools of inner knowledge. One reads in his autobiographical sketch: "For the totality of man lies way beyond any conceivable objectifiability. He is incompletable both as a being-for-himself and as an object of cognition. He remains, so to speak, 'open'. Man is always more than what he knows, or can know, about himself."[23]

The consequences of this attitude can be observed in Jaspers's polemical criticism on Viktor von Weizsäcker and Alexander Mitscherlich, exercised in Heidelberg in the first years after the Second World War. The two were establishing together and very successfully a psychosomatic and psychoanalytical institute. Without too much of a self-critical attitude they claimed to be able to help the patients to find the inner meaning of life which lays hidden in the psychic crisis.[24]

Jaspers's critique of the phenomenological approach of the so-called "Daseinsanalyse" is more benevolent; at least he recognizes it in the *General Psychopathology* as an "intellectual movement" in the psychiatric world. In contrast to the main spokespersons of his time, Viktor von Gebsattel and Ludwig Binswanger, who are now seen as the founding fathers of "anthropological psychiatry," Jaspers raises the fundamental objection that their philosophical ambition in the name of psychiatry goes too far: "The totality of human life and its ultimate origin cannot be the object of any scientific research."[25] He appreciates their descriptive powers but dismisses their aetiological explanations. As Jaspers does not recognize any connection between aetiological and psychological hermeneutics, he ironically designates the psychologico-philosophical interpretations offered by the representatives of the "Daseinsanalyse" as attempts at understanding which create an unspecifically human climate without doing any real damage. One can appreciate the irony in the sentence: "Interpretations are soothing yet interpretations are nothing but interpretations."[26]

In summary then: Whenever it comes to final questions of life conduct which are connected to psychopathological phenomena the self-critical physician should elucidate the subjective character of his judgment. Those philosophical aspects of psychotherapy cannot be legitimized theoretically or rationally. So the communication between the doctor and patient might become an existential one in the sense depending on the willingness of both to think beyond the limits of scientific knowledge. Jaspers writes: "One questions and gropes one freedom to another within the concreteness of the actual situation, taking no responsibility for the other nor making any abstract demands.... Doctor and patient are both human beings and as such fellow-travelers in destiny. The doctor is not a pure technician nor pure authority, but existence for its own sake...."[27]

[23] Jaspers (1957: 19).
[24] Bormuth (2006) focuses on the controversy especially in the chapter "Critique of Psychoanalytic Psychosomatics 1949–1953" (107–125).
[25] Jaspers (1998: 543).   [26] Jaspers (1998: 546).   [27] Jaspers (1998: 798f.).

BIBLIOGRAPHY

Bormuth M. (2006). *Life Conduct in Modern Times*. New York: Springer.

Bormuth M. (2009). "On Psychodynamics of Personal-judgments—Nietzsche's Theory of Resentment and its Reception by Karl Jaspers and Kurt Schneider." *Acta Neuropsychiatrica* 21 (Suppl 2): 10–14.

Bormuth M. (2013a). "Psychopathology in the Modern Age. Karl Jaspers Reads Hölderlin." In T. Fuchs, T. Breyer, and C. Mundt (eds.), *Karl Jaspers' Philosophy and Psychopathology*, pp. 3–17. New York: Springer.

Bormuth M. (2013b). "Karl Jaspers the Pathographer." In G. Stanghellini and T. Fuchs (eds.), *One Century of Karl Jaspers' General Psychopathology*, pp. 133–149. Oxford: Oxford University Press.

Bormuth M. (2013c). "Freedom and Mystery: An Intellectual History of Jaspers' General Psychopathology." *Psychopathology. International Journal of Descriptive and Experimental Psychopathology, Phenomenology and Psychiatric Diagnosis* 46: 281–289.

Jaspers K. (1912). "Die phänomenologische Forschungsrichtung in der Psychopathologie." *Zeitschrift für die gesamte Psychiatrie und Neurologie* 9: 391–408 (later in *Gesammelte Schriften zur Psychopathologie*. Heidelberg: Springer 1963, pp. 314–328).

Jaspers K. (1913). *Allgemeine Psychopathologie*. Berlin: Springer.

Jaspers K. (1957). "Philosophical Autobiography." In P. A. Schilpp (ed.), *The Philosophy of Karl Jaspers*, pp. 1–94. New York: Tudor Publishing Company.

Jaspers K. (1968). "The Phenomenological Approach in Psychopathology." *The British Journal of Psychiatry* 114: 1313–1325.

Jaspers K. (1988). *Max Weber. Gesammelte Schriften*, ed. Hans Saner. München: Piper.

Jaspers K. (2013). *General Psychopathology*, trans. from the German J. Hoenig and M. W. Hamilton (with a new Foreword by P. R. McHugh). Baltimore: Johns Hopkins University Press.

Jaspers K. (2016). "Letter to Willy Hellpach, April 22, 1949." In K. Jaspers, *Korrespondenzen Psychiatrie—Medizin—Naturwissenschaften*, ed. M. Bormuth and D. v. Engelhardt. Göttingen: Wallstein Publishing House.

Stanghellini G. and Fuchs T. (2013). "Editors' Introduction." In G. Stanghellini and T. Fuchs (eds.), *One Century of Karl Jaspers' General Psychopathology*, pp. xiii–xxviii. Oxford: Oxford University Press.

CHAPTER 14

EUGÈNE MINKOWSKI

ANNICK URFER-PARNAS

BIOGRAPHY

EUGÈNE Minkowski (1885–1972) was born in a Polish Jewish family in Warsaw. He began his studies in medicine in Poland, but finished them, for political reasons, in Germany. He obtained the Russian equivalent of an MD and emigrated before the First World War to France where he felt at home. Minkowski trained as a resident in Burghølzli under the supervision of Eugen Bleuler. He volunteered with the French army during the First World War. After the war, he worked for several years as a clinical psychiatrist in a public hospital as a resident until he became Chief Psychiatrist at the Saint-Anne Hospital in Paris. He never achieved an academic position. He was professionally active with many important publications and participated in international conferences. In 1925, he co-founded a psychopathological journal, *L'Evolution Psychiatrique*. During the Nazi occupation of Paris, he refused for ethical reasons to wear the Star of David and decided not to flee the city. He stayed in Paris with his family and helped other colleagues and patients in difficulties (Pilliard-Minkowski 2009).

Minkowski published several important articles and four books: *La Schizophrénie* (1927), *Le temps vécu* (1933), *Vers une cosmologie* (1936), and *Traité de psychopathologie* (1966). Only the second of these books has been translated into English under the title *Lived Time* (1970). However, he was introduced to Anglophone psychiatry in the 1960s by R. D. Laing (1963) and later by Cutting (Cutting and Shepherd 1987). It is only in the last twenty-five years that interest in Minkowski's work has gained momentum in France, leading to many new editions of his published work (Granger 1999). He has also found a place in a recent book about phenomenological psychiatry (Broome et al. 2012).

PSYCHOPATHOLOGICAL ORIENTATION

Minkowski was always attracted by philosophy and his reading of Henri Bergson, especially *Essai sur les données immédiates de la conscience* (*Time and Free Will: An Essay on the Immediate Data of Consciousness*) (Bergson 1889). This work had a profound impact on his view of consciousness and mental disorders. Another influential figure was the phenomenologist Max Scheler, especially his book on the nature of sympathy (Scheler 1913). Minkowski's psychiatric interest was formed by Bleuler's concept of schizophrenia (Bleuler 1911) and especially his conception of autism. In fact, Minkowski introduced Bleuler's nosological concepts of schizophrenia into French psychiatry. However, Minkowski elaborated Bleuler's intuition in a highly original phenomenological manner, pointing to disorders of the structure of consciousness. Without exaggeration, Minkowski must be considered a dominant figure in phenomenological psychiatry due to his success of translating theoretical and abstract philosophical notions into ordinary clinical work. He was not attracted to psychoanalysis because of its exclusive focus on mental content. Rather, his emphasis was on the structure of consciousness underlying manifest symptomatology. He was skeptical about the anatomo-clinical (biological) model of mental illness, pointing out our inability to grasp a transition from organic changes to the richness of psychopathological manifestation (Minkowski 1933).

THE NOTION OF SCHIZOPHRENIA

Minkowski considers schizophrenia to be a spectrum disorder (syndrome), which includes milder forms of schizoïdia (corresponding to the current diagnosis schizotypal disorder) as the most basic constitutionally determined condition. Schizophrenia as a psychosis only emerges due to noxious developmental influences and upon the vulnerability of schizoïdia (Minkowski 1927: 51). Minkowski thus anticipated the more contemporary diathesis-stress model of schizophrenia. Following Bleuler and Kretschmer, he subscribed to a view of two basic existential orientations of human personality, schizoïdia and syntonia, which are implicated in the articulation of psychosis. Schizoïdia is a dimension of interpersonal withdrawal, solitude, and a tendency to indulge private cognitions. On the other hand, syntonia is an extroverted world-oriented sociable attitude. Schizophrenia is characterized by the domination of the schizoid dimension. Bipolar disorder on the other hand is typically a disorder with clear syntonic features. In other words, Minkowski, in contrast to many other researchers, considered bipolar illness not only in terms of disorders of temporality, but also in terms of interpersonal relatedness. The combination of these two dimensions may contribute to the formation of a mixed and atypical clinical picture.

THE VITAL CONTACT WITH REALITY

A basic mode of human presence in the world is referred to by Minkowski as vital contact with reality, designating "a certain *mode of relatedness* between a person and her *inner* and outer *ambient* world" (Urfer 2001: 282) and harmonious attunement to the dynamically changing world. It is not a mental faculty or a physiological function. It is an immediate attunement and resonance with the world and with others. It is a sense of significance, relevance, proportion, and adequacy. It resembles Blankenburg's notion of common sense

(Blankenburg 1971) and Janet's function of reality (Janet 1909). In current psychopathology, it is considered to be based on pre-reflective, automatic bounds between the individual, the world, and the others. In a phenomenological sense, it is based on passive syntheses of operative intentionality (Merleau-Ponty 1945). Vital contact with reality is a structural-dynamic feature of consciousness and an expression of the so-called *Élan vital*, a term borrowed from Bergson (Bergson 1927). There is no adequate translation of *élan vital* into English. It may be described as an intrinsic openness to the world, an energetic vital impulse throwing us outside ourselves, adapted to the ambient becoming (*devenir*) yet at the same time anchored in our inner self. It is not a question of physical relatedness, but spiritual lived synchrony with the situation and other people (Minkowski 1933). There is here a remarkable resemblance with Binswanger's use of Heidegger's notion of *Dasein* (Binswanger 1963) where the terms self and world are not independent but are always unified in a single whole. Minkowski considered that disorders of *élan vital* was the core structural feature of schizophrenia.

Autism

As is well known, Bleuler defined schizophrenic autism as a withdrawal from the external world into the private realm of fantasy (Parnas and Bovet 1991). While agreeing with the central role of autism in the clinical picture of schizophrenia, Minkowski modified the concept in a radical way. Autism is not primarily a withdrawal, but rather a deficiency in the vital contact with reality, leading to ideas, expressions, and behaviors that are somehow inadequate to their context. It is characterized by impoverished interpersonal reciprocity of contact, excessive tendencies to spatialize and objectify phenomena that are not spatial, and an arrest of existential temporality, which manifests by diminishing the guiding role of the future. Second, autism is not, on Minkowski's account, invariably marked by a rich life of phantasy, and Minkowski distinguished between "poor (pure) autism" characterized by poverty of ideation and emotion and "rich autism" with well-developed delusional ideas. A typical instance of the poor autism is given in the following vignette:

> There is immobility around me. Things present themselves in a disconnected way . . . they are understood rather than experienced. They are like pantomimes performed around me, but which I am not able to join, I stay outside . . . Everything around me is motionless and congealed . . . I see the future only as a repetition of the past; there is no flow between me and the world. I can no longer give myself away to the world.
>
> (Minkowski 1927: 99–100, quoted in Urfer 2001: 283)

This division of two forms of autism illustrates Minkowski's claim that in mental illness we need to distinguish between a disorder of structure and a disorder of content (ideo-affective factors). Poor autism exemplifies the structural change in the vital contact with reality. In rich autism, the affective factors play perhaps a compensatory role and contribute to the richness of positive symptomatology. The notion of phenomenological compensation is crucial here: "the individual tries to fill up the lacuna which is emerging in him by seizing the possibilities which he still possess. In this way, he tries to preserve his human existence" (Lanteri-Laura, quoted in Granger 1999: 33). Phenomenological compensation is not an instance of coping, that is, it is not just a cognitive attitude, but also a more global existential endeavor. The notion of phenomenological compensation is associated with Minkowski's general view of the processes of mental causation. Autism, as Minkowski uses the term, "is an anthropological notion that describes nothing less than the entire human person. In 'a progressive extinction of life,' certain schizophrenic patients complain of not being able to feel. The patient is 'in contradiction with the flow and dynamism of life,' and this contradiction is manifest in a sentiment of emptiness, in a disaggregation of personality, and in the predominance of static, immobilized elements" (Urfer 2001: 284). The clinical picture of autism comprises the lack of vital contact with reality with an ensuing distortion of behavior, thinking, and interpersonal relation, and is the expression of the attempt of phenomenological compensation. These are the so-called autistic attitudes, which comprise morbid rationalism, geometrism, and morbid regrets (Minkowski 1997). It is an attitude comprising an effort to submit some or all aspects of life under schematic and often algorithmic rules, typically associated with focus on irrelevant details, neglect of proportion, and deviating from a common sense attitude. The patient may fall victim to constant ruminations, which are however always ego-syntonic. On the surface, such patients may resemble obsessional patients, but the latter rarely go beyond the bounds of common sense.

To illustrate this critical distinction, Minkowski presented a patient at the age of sixteen who becomes preoccupied with all sorts of constructions. He worries about the solidity of his school and thinks that all the buildings are held up only thanks to the terrestrial attraction. He then becomes obsessed by the concept of symmetry, particularly for his body. He strives for a perfect body symmetry, taking up certain positions in front of the mirror and asking himself if the human body does not come down only to symmetry. Eventually, his entire reasoning, thinking, and speech are nothing more than geometry and construction, until this patient ends up by saying "The plan is my whole life," "I will absolutely not upset my plan I'd rather upset my life than the plan" (Minkowski 1927: 116–119).

Morbid regret consists in a tendency toward repetitive and stereotypic complaining about events, situations, and personal features in the past and present. Such complaints may superficially resemble depressive features, but upon closer inspection they appear empty of affective charge, are stereotypic, and perhaps point to an inability to temporalize and access one's own feelings and thoughts. Minkowski coins the notion "travel without goal" to describe autistic activities that are completely out of bounds with what will normally be expected in a situation. This concept corresponds closely to Conrad's notion of "crazy action" (Conrad 1958): "A patient decides to protest against the death sentence of two American anarchists. He writes a letter in his own name, unknown though he is to the world, and decides to deliver it personally to the American ambassador himself. He is surprised when he is firmly conducted to the Police Station and fined" (Minkowski 1927: 156; translation by the author).

Trouble Générateur

Autism or lack of contact with reality is, according to Minkowski, a generative disorder of schizophrenia. *Trouble générateur*, that is, generative (generating) disorder, is one of Minkowski's most original concepts, constituting one of his most significant contributions to contemporary psychiatry (Sass and Parnas 2003). Generative disorder is a pattern of change in the fundamental structure of personality (in the contemporary sense of the term subjectivity), for example, selfhood, spatiality, temporality, and relatedness to the world. These structural changes influence the formation of psychopathological manifestations and single symptoms. It is not a disturbance of an isolated cognitive function or mental faculty, but rather a global affection of our presence in the world.

One can say that psychopathological manifestations or symptoms are incarnations of the trouble générateur. The causal relation between the *trouble générateur*, on the one hand, and the symptomatic manifestation, on the other, should not be articulated in terms of physiological or mechanistic terms. Rather these relations are of mental or psychological nature, comprising meaning, motivation, entailment, and implication. As already mentioned, all psychopathological manifestations have a formal structure and a psychological content. The generative disorder influences the structural aspect of the symptom, whereas contextual ideo-affective factors influence the content of the symptoms. Another aspect of the *trouble générateur* is the epistemological implication. The clinical picture that the patient presents is a certain gestalt or prototype entailed by the trouble générateur. In other words, the diagnosis of schizophrenia cannot be reduced to an additive enumeration of single symptoms, but depends on the perception of this global gestalt and its structural modification:

> The hypochondriac preoccupations of an anxious patient and similar ideas of a schizophrenic patient are different in their nature because the mental states are of a different nature; we do not even dare to say that they are very preoccupied by their health. There is *superficial resemblance* between the ideo-verbal expressions of these two "troubles générateurs," which however have nothing in common. It is the same principle when looking for megalomaniac ideas in a schizophrenic patient and a general paralytic or true obsession in a neurotic and pseudo-obsession in a schizophrenic patient.
>
> (Minkowski 1997: 96–97; translation by the author)

In appreciating the way of being of the patients, we cannot be satisfied by describing and listing the symptoms that the patients present. Rather, we have to engage our entire personality to confront it with the particular pattern that comes out of the patient's entire reaction (Minkowski 1933: 65). In Minkowski's view, the diagnostic process is not just a third-person observation, but crucially involves a second-person dimension in which the subjectivity of the patient and the subjectivity of the psychiatrist are in an intimate relation:

> Sitting face to face with my patient, I am meticulously writing down his utterances, and then suddenly one of his sentences illuminates everything with a particular clarity, and I have a feeling of having seized a complex living whole, of having grasped the "trouble générateur", which now appears as the touchstone of the whole clinical picture. Here we can speak of an example of Bergsonian intuition.
>
> (Minkowski 1948: 145; translation by the author)

This illustrates the nature of gestalt, which is constituted by part–whole interaction, and not by a sum of single elements. Examples of such illumination and insight point to the situation where a change in a single aspect suddenly confers the gestalt with a new meaning.

Psychological states, according to Bergson, are not fragments of the self. They are expressions of the self, because each psychological state reflects and expresses the entire self of the person (Minkowski 1933: 209).

Here Minkowski expresses the concept of diagnosis by penetration, which relies on the second-person grasp of the psychological structure of the patient. This epistemic act is not only cognitive, but involves a global sentiment or affective impact. This is not an inferential process, but rather an instance of direct grasp or intuition (intuition in the sense of direct perception).

The objective approach of psychiatry is insufficient and only allows us to analyze the mental illness by isolating artificially each feature from each other and on which one confers their own autonomous reality (Minkowski 1933: 209). Minkowski argues that we need to complement the objective third-person's approach of listing symptoms with more global acts of "an intellectual sympathy" (diagnosis "*par pénétration*") to grasp the organizing psychological structure of the patient or, in other words, to grasp the gestalt.

CONTEMPORARY RELEVANCE

Almost all of the psychopathological ideas of Minkowski have survived the test of time and are still relevant today. First of all, Bleuler's, Kretschmer's, and Minkowski's idea of spectrum disorder is now well established. Second, the view of schizotypal disorder (schizoïdia) as a more basic expression of the illness is also accepted and institutionalized in the diagnostic manual. Moreover, Minkowski's concept of generative disorders has been revived by contemporary phenomenological psychiatry (Sass and Parnas 2003; Parnas 2011; Nordgaard et al. 2013). Minkowski's view of diagnosis as being based not only on an enumeration of symptoms, but also on a gestalt and pattern recognition is being increasingly revived by a new emphasis on prototypical aspect of psychiatric diagnosis (Parnas and Bovet 2015). Finally, in view of psychiatry's increasingly dehumanizing practice by the mechanic diagnostic and therapeutic approaches, Minkowski's ideal of clinical work as an essentially humanistic endeavor is more needed than ever.

BIBLIOGRAPHY

Bergson H. (1927). *Essai sur les données immédiates de la conscience* [1889]. Paris: Presses Universitaires de France.

Binswanger L. (1963). *Being-in-the-world: Selected Papers*, ed. and trans. J. Needleman. New York: Basic Books.

Blankenburg W. (1971). *Der Verlust der natürlichen Selbstverständlichkeit. Ein Beitrag zur Psychopathologie symptomarmer Schizophrenien*. Stuttgart: Enke.

Bleuler E. (1911). "Dementia Praecox oder Gruppe der Schizophrenien." In G. Aschaffenburg (ed.), *Handbuch der Psychiatrie* (Ger). Leipzig: Deuticke.

Broome M. R., Harland R., Owen G. S., and Stringaris A. (2012). *The Maudsley Reader in Phenomenological Psychiatry*. Cambridge: Cambridge University Press.

Conrad K. (1958). *Die beginnende Schizophrenie. Versuch einer Gestaltanalyse des Wahns*. Stuttgart: Thieme.

Cutting J. and Shepherd M. (1987). *The Clinical Roots of the Schizophrenia Concept*. Cambridge: Cambridge University Press.

Granger B. (1999). *Eugène Minkowski, Une oeuvre philosophique, psychiatrique et social*. Levallois-Perret: Interligne S.A.

Janet P. (1909/1939). *Les névroses*. Paris: Flammarion.

Laing R. D. (1963). "Minkowski and schizophrenia." *Review of Existential Psychology and Psychiatry* 3: 195–207.

Merleau-Ponty M. (1945/1962). *Phénoménologie de la perception*. Paris: Gallimard/ *Phenomenology of Perception*, trans. C. Smith. London: Routledge & Kegan Paul.

Minkowski E. (1927). *La schizophrénie. Psychopathologie des schizoïdes et des schizophrénes*. Paris: Payot.

Minkowski E. (1933/1995). *Le Temps vécu. Etudes phénoménologiques et psychopathologiques*. Paris: Presses Universitaires de France.

Minkowski E. (1936/1999). *Vers une cosmologie*. Paris: Editions Payot & Rivages.

Minkowski E. (1948). "Phénoménologie et analyse existentielle en psychopathologie." *L'évolution Psychiatrique* 11: 137–185.

Minkowski E. (1966/1999). *Traité de psychopathologie*. Le Plessis-Robinson: Institut Synthélabo pour le progrès de la connaissance.

Minkowski E. (1970) *Lived Time: Phenomenological and Psychopathological Studies*, trans. N. Metzel. Evanston: Northwestern University Press.

Minkowski E. (1997). *Au-delà du rationalisme morbide*. Paris: Ed L'Harmattan.

Nordgaard J., Sass L. A., and Parnas J. (2013). "The Psychiatric Interview: Validity, Structure, and Subjectivity." *European Archives of Psychiatry and Clinical Neuroscience* 263: 353–364.

Parnas J. 2011. "A Disappearing Heritage: The Clinical Core of Schizophrenia." *Schizophrenia Bulletin* 37: 1121–1130.

Parnas J. and Bovet P. (1991). "Autism in Schizophrenia Revisited." *Comprehensive Psychiatry* 32: 7–21.

Parnas J. and Bovet P. (2015). "Psychiatry Made Easy: Operation(al)ism and Some of Its Consequences." In K. S. Kendler and J. Parnas (eds.), *Philosophical Issues in Psychiatry III: The Nature and Sources of Historical Change*, pp. 190–212. Oxford: Oxford University Press.

Pilliard-Minkowski J. (2009). *Engène Minkowski 1885–1972, Francoise Minkowska 1982–1950*. Paris: L'Harmattan.

Sass L. A. and Parnas J. (2003). "Schizophrenia, Consciousness, and the Self." *Schizophrenia Bulletin* 29: 427–444.

Scheler M. (1913). *Zur Phänomenologie und Theorie der Sympathiege Gefühle und von Liebe und Hass*. Halle: Niemeyer.

Urfer A. (2001). "Phenomenology and Psychopathology of Schizophrenia: The Views of Eugene Minkowski." *Philosophy, Psychiatry, & Psychology* 8: 279–289.

CHAPTER 15

LUDWIG BINSWANGER

KLAUS HOFFMANN AND ROMAN KNORR

The Binswanger Family and the Bellevue Sanatorium

BINSWANGER's grandfather, bearing the same name, Ludwig Binswanger (1820–80), was born into a Jewish South German country family of small factory owners. He studied medicine in Munich, becoming a general practitioner and psychiatrist, but could not enter the government medical service in Bavaria because he was Jewish. He took an active part in the 1848 revolution in Munich, fighting especially for equal rights for Jews, and got himself into even more difficulties than before. As he was already known as a skilled psychiatrist, Wilhelm Griesinger (1817–68), one of the most influential psychiatrists of the time, recommended him for the post of director of the new cantonal mental hospital in Münsterlingen, Switzerland, near Constance. In 1857 Binswanger bought the sumptuous Bellevue Villa in Kreuzlingen, Switzerland, near the German border town Constance, and founded a private asylum for mentally affected patients. Under his son Robert Binswanger (1850–1910), director from 1880 to 1910, Bellevue Sanatorium grew, more villas were built, the clientele became more and more upper-class, the site increasingly well known. In 1881 Breuer sent Bertha Pappenheim, known as Sigmund Freud's case Anna O., to Bellevue for a morphine withdrawal treatment during the following years; Freud used to send patients who needed long-term treatment to Bellevue.

Ludwig Binswanger (1881–1966) was born into this rich family tradition, in the sanatorium, and he grew up there alongside the patients. After his medical studies in Lausanne, Heidelberg, and Zurich he entered the Burghölzli Clinic in Zurich (as Karl Abraham's successor), then presided over by Eugen Bleuler and his advisor Carl Gustav Jung. Jung supervised his dissertation and joined him in carrying out association experiments. It was together with Jung that he visited Freud for the first time in 1907. In 1907 and 1908 Ludwig Binswanger worked under his uncle, the famous psychiatrist and neurologist Otto Binswanger (1852–1929) at Jena University hospital, becoming familiar mainly with organic psychoses.

In 1908, he returned to Kreuzlingen and went to work for his father. Upon his father's death in 1910, Ludwig took over the sanatorium, which he led until his retirement in 1956.

Over these more than forty years, Bellevue Sanatorium became one of the centers of Central European cultural life and one of the very few if not the only psychiatric sanatorium where psychoanalysis became the main method for treating psychoses. Well-known personalities like the Russian dancer Vaslav Nijinsky; the painter Ernst Ludwig Kirchner, who created twenty-two of his most important wood engravings at Kreuzlingen; the sociologist Max Weber; and the actor and director Gustav Gründgens were treated there. The Bellevue guestbook and the list of correspondents contain recognized artists, scientists, and philosophers like Freud, Edmund Husserl, Max Scheler, Martin Heidegger, Karl Löwith, Martin Buber, Kurt Goldstein, Rudolf Alexander Schröder, Wilhelm Furtwängler, and Werner Bergengrün among others. For Binswanger, psychoanalysis and philosophy were important means for understanding his patients. Binswanger always saw himself as a clinician.

Although he worked closely with Jung in 1907, Binswanger stayed in contact with Freud after the 1914 split with the Zurich group. Despite their differences, mainly regarding philosophical issues, Freud and Binswanger remained good friends. This is evident in the Freud–Binswanger letters (Fichtner 1992). Undoubtedly, Binswanger's contacts with other psychoanalysts became less frequent than his relations with philosophers like Husserl, Heidegger, Buber, and Wilhelm Szilasi. Binswanger became an honorary doctor of the philosophical faculty of the University of Basel in 1941.

Until today, only few of Binswanger's important publications have been translated into English (Needleman 1963). His main oevres, "Einführung in die Probleme der allgemeinen Psychologie" (1922) and "Grundformen und Erkenntnis menschlichen Daseins" (1942), are only available in German and Italian.

Binswanger's Contributions to Phenomenological Psychopathology

Binswanger (like Husserl) refused to follow the split between "Erklären" (explaining) and "Verstehen" (understanding) which was foundational for Karl Jaspers's psychopathology and has contributed to the biologistic ideology of classical psychiatry until the present day. Already in 1913 Binswanger criticized, in the *Internationale Zeitschrift für ärztliche Psychoanalyse*, Jaspers's work on causal and "understandable" connections between destiny and psychosis in dementia praecox "from the standpoint of the psychoanalyst," basing his argument on the phenomenological theory of knowledge of Theodor Lipps. Causality, in Binswanger's words, exists also in the realm of subjective experiences and cannot be restricted to mental phenomena caused by biological processes. He writes:

> Jaspers' causal explanation in psychology is a psychophysical one, as we see; he seems only to admit a psychophysical causality next to physical or natural causality, but not causality in the purely psychic domain. But Jaspers has not succeeded in proving that there is no psychic causality or no causality in the psychic domain. "Every causal connection", says Lipps, "is a regular dependence relationship between judgments made by the thinking mind." All regularity or causality in the world that I know of is only this regular order, taking place in the thinking mind or in consciousness, consisting in this: When one thing, the so-called "cause",

is recognized as real, another thing, the so-called "effect", must be recognized by the thinking
mind as real; and the latter may not be recognized as real if the former has not had to be so
recognized. Now it is not evident why this regular order, taking place in consciousness, should
and cannot extend to the "psychological facts".

(Binswanger 1913: 385)[1]

For the first time, Binswanger showed himself here clearly as a psychiatrist and psychoanalyst who made use of the phenomenological philosophy as the basis of psychoanalysis, that is, he rejected a cleavage. There were other phenomenological psychiatrists who
later followed Jaspers's views but in psychoanalysis, Binswanger's position was shared, for
example, by the Swiss psychoanalyst and protestant minister Oskar Pfister and by the phenomenological psychiatrist Alfred Storch. Freud himself had also rejected Jaspers's view by
stressing that biographical experiences are the cause of mental problems—not neglecting
what he called constitution, that is, biological (including genetic) factors. Jaspers's so-called
"Schichtenlehre" (theory of levels) argues that organic factors are the most determinative,
then follow so-called endogenic factors (manic-depressive illness or schizophrenia), and
on top of that "neurotic symptoms" as variations of the personality (Jaspers 1997: 564–617).
Until recently, this view influenced academic psychiatry much more than Binswanger's and
Freud's view that life circumstances and traumatizations as well as good bonding experiences
can causally influence mental illness and symptoms. Recent findings in neurobiology, however, turn this picture around and now strongly support Freud's and Binswanger's view
that bonding and traumatizations directly influence the biological level or brain function,
indicating that there is no general hierarchy of the organic—endogenic—neurotic.

On Binswanger's account, when a patient with schizophrenia recounts experiences which
we regard as psychotic, these communications, considered phenomenologically, are not
simply symptoms of hallucinatory mental illness, but rather they tell about the sick person's
world of experience. We can see the patient as a person before us, having a relation to dark
mental powers, moving in a mental sphere quite different from our own:

The essential thing . . . in the phenomenological consideration of such psychopathological
phenomena is that they are never an isolated phenomenon; the phenomenon always plays
against the backdrop of an ego, a person; in other words, we always see it as an expression of
a revelation about a particular person. In the particular phenomenon the respective person
reveals something about himself, and conversely we see through the phenomenon into the
person.

(Binswanger 1994a: 68)

For the contemporary discussion, this text retains important implications. Interpersonal
psychoanalysis and attachment theory in particular stress that the human being is orientated
from the beginning toward relation and encounter, that an intentionality exists on both
sides, and that this is a genetically determined need. This is reality-related, directed toward
comprehending the quality of the relationship in its historical development.

Let us turn to Binswanger's important book Über Ideenflucht from 1933 (On the Flight of
Ideas) (Binswanger 1992a). It starts with historical remarks about mania and melancholy
and emphasizes Griesinger, who already showed that diseases are mainly diseases of wishes.
Binswanger sees the wish as an anthropological design of human beings encompassing

---

[1] All translations of Binswanger's works are by the authors.

psychological, logical, and ethical issues which cannot be reduced to biological questions. Referring to Søren Kierkegaard, Heidegger, and Jaspers, Binswanger stressed the self as the existential principle (Binswanger 1992a: 132). All psychiatric symptoms are, according to Binswanger, anthropological modes of existence which can also be examined from the scientific point of view as brain disorders. The phenomenological view not only allows, but requires, that we deal with these symptoms in a psychotherapeutic way, by talking with the patient and by interpreting the symptoms in terms of the interpersonal encounter. The patient is at least partly responsible for his symptoms—not only as contemporary psychiatry sometimes claims by taking his medication, but also by understanding his symptoms in the biographical context.

Psychotic Illness

Binswanger fought to find a sense in illness, especially in psychotic illness. Illness is not only a defect or the symbol of a defect, but also a hermeneutic way of finding a new sense in individual as well in collective life (Binswanger 1992a: 20).

Binswanger draws on European philosophy at length, reaching his conclusion—also formulated by Buber—that love and the basis of existence are rooted in the Other, in the Thou. Here, he also draws a clear line against Heidegger's thinking and stresses his stand in dialogical philosophy, even more radical than Buber but well in line with contemporary interpersonal psychoanalysis and group analysis:

> We see ever more clearly what Heidegger is getting at here, namely the selfness of Dasein (existence) in acting. He glimpses in this—as he says once in passing in "Von Wesen des Grundes" ["On the Essence of Ground"]—the heart of existence. We too, even though in an entirely different sense, speak of the heart of existence or—better—of existence as heart. But we do not glimpse this "heart" in the selfness of existence in acting but in the We-ness of existence in loving. That this is not a matter of a mere difference of opinion, but rather of an ontologically based difference, becomes evident from the fact that no (ontological) way leads to the We-ness of existence in loving from the selfness of existence in acting, but the other way round: from the We-ness in loving to selfness in acting.
>
> (Binswanger 1993: 126)

> I can entertain or busy myself with an image or an idea, but only in a one-sided way, in monologue. But you answer me. I don't just imagine you, but above all you yourself— with every look and every word—imagine yourself to me (and vice-versa). We-ness in loving is a wave, a greeting, a cry, a demand, an embrace of existence with itself, in one word: encounter. This encounter can no more be unilaterally 'brought about' and planned than it can be thought out and "presented": it is—as both Ur-encounter and as factual Thou-encounter—a gift of existence to itself: grace.
>
> (Binswanger 1993: 157)

The texts might sound mystical. They are written in a language no longer familiar to psychoanalysts of today, but lead back to the anthropological dimension of every psychotherapy, because "in a true psychotherapy an I-Thou-relationship must crystallize" (Binswanger 1993: 208). Psychosis has—in Binswanger's view—to do with the loss of the ethical, the dimension of responsibility toward fellow human beings: What we in psychiatry label with such clear moral expressions as irresponsibility or non-committal speech, as "un-restrained" chattering and, depending on the other characteristics, diagnose as a symptom of feeble-mindedness or dementia, a schizophrenic process or a manic flight of ideas, concerns the moral no less than the intellectual sphere and is based in each case on a par-ticular form of existential perception of time and history (Binswanger 1993: 295–296). Through love, through good new object relations, psychotic patients can become healthier again. Love is not just meant as empathy or sympathetic feeling, but as a deep involvement by the care-taker with the patient's subjectivity in the past and present and with his existential dimensions, his relations with other people including the therapist.

After 1945, Binswanger became widely known in German psychiatry and psychoa-nalysis. Gustav Bally acknowledged in his *Introduction to Freud's Psychoanalysis* (Bally 1961) that Binswanger brought a philosophical approach into psychoanalysis. In contrast to Heidegger, Binswanger always stayed in contact with Husserl and with his wife, and he had a close relationship with the Jewish philosopher Buber who for some time had questioned Heidegger's extreme emphasis of the single human being. In Switzerland, first Medard Boss and then his colleague Gion Condrau became interested in Heidegger's philosophy in the 1950s and later, on the basis of Heidegger's philosophy, they devel-oped a form of psychoanalysis which they called Dasein (existence) analysis. Heidegger was often in Switzerland in the 1950s, and Binswanger, who had introduced Boss and Heidegger to each other, lost influence. He never wanted to found a psychoanalytic school, and not at all one based on Heidegger's work.

In his late work *Drei Formen mißglückten Daseins* (*Three Forms of Failed Existence*) (Binswanger 1992b), psychosis is once again seen as an existential human possibility and phenomenon, not only as a disease. The three basic terms "Verstiegenheit" (extravagance), "Verschrobenheit" (eccentricity), and "Manieriertheit" (affectation) are presented as funda-mental forms of being, present in everybody, but becoming dominant in different forms of psychosis. "Verstiegenheit" can never be characteristic of the individual as such; it always exists in relation to the other, to the world:

> What we call psychotherapy is basically nothing else than bringing the sick person to where he can "see" how the overall structure of human existence or "being-in-the-world" is constructed and at which point he has climbed onto difficult terrain. That means: to bring him back from extravagance "down to earth", to the only place from which a new start and a new ascent are possible, into the interhuman encounter.
>
> (Binswanger 1992b: 247)

Binswanger refers to the German philosopher Friedrich Wilhelm Josef Schelling, for whom mental illness was identical with pure reflection (Binswanger 1992b: 305). "Verschrobenheit" also means unawareness of the historical dimension. Love and encounter are the remedies against this (Binswanger 1992b: 316). Only by situating oneself in history, can one detect one's true self—to use Donald W. Winnicott's term (Winnicott 1965)—or "Selbstigung" (selfing) as it is called by Binswanger. Binswanger often comes quite close to a materialistic con-cept of the human psyche which is, according to Karl Marx, the ensemble of the economic conditions of humankind. The true self means to be aware of one's situation and condition in the present society in relation to others as well as to other societies and to the world in its condition. By love and encounter, autism can be changed; not autism, but love, is primary (contrary to Freud's primary autism) (Binswanger 1992b: 418).

In his last major study *Wahn (Paranoia)*, published in 1965 (Binswanger 1994b), Binswanger advocates a phenomenological understanding of psychopathological phenomena that proceeds from a pathology in the area of overall intentionality (not a pathology exclusively limited to the thought functions, as Jaspers argues). The essential feature of mental illness is the exclusive relation to one's own ego, which Binswanger emphasizes with an impressive string of sentences by a woman with delusions, going on to observe that:

> Nowhere do we find a (dual) We, an Us or an Our, not to speak of a Thou or a Thee. Aline exhausts herself fully in the *plural* mode: *I and the Others, the Others and I.* This mode still experiences a decisive expansion, insofar as the communication possibilities here far exceed the usual measure and also make use of electricity, magnetism, telegraphy, telepathy, thought reading, hearing thoughts, mediums, etc.
>
> (Binswanger 1994b: 475)

CONCLUSION

This emphasis on the interpersonal character of mental illness remains one of Binswanger's lasting contributions to mental health care. Mental illness is clearly a deficient mode of transcending "characterized in the first instance by the fact that creation of images is strongly impoverished, namely mechanized, that a fixed scheme takes the place of their variability and mobility" (Binswanger 1994b: 471). But also decisive is the answer of the other, encounter and relation as a new, therapeutic offer. Not only the psychiatrist or the individual psychotherapist are important for this answer, but the whole therapeutic community of the institution which treats the patient, the other patients, the patient's family, friends and work colleagues, etc. Binswanger's view of psychiatry and psychoanalysis is open to society's influence, but also to the multiprofessional settings that he organized in his Bellevue Sanatorium in Kreuzlingen. Inter-human encounter takes place many hours a day, therefore the culture of the institution is central for the healing encounter. Verbal therapies are important, but also arts, sports, common games, and culture. Patients whose deep psychotic regression does not allow extensive talks might be reached by non-verbal methods. Binswanger's work remains relevant today for a phenomenological and psychotherapeutic approach for severely regressed patients, in inpatient as well as in outpatient conditions. Not only academic medical or psychological staff, but also nurses, art therapists, ergotherapists, and sports therapists can benefit from his approaches, as they are all involved in personal encounters with their patients. Binswanger's theory and practice are relevant particularly in therapeutic community and group analysis and in the psychoanalytic approach with severely disturbed patients.

BIBLIOGRAPHY

Bally G. (1961). *Einführung in die Psychoanalyse Sigmund Freuds.* Reinbek: Rowohlt.
Binswanger L. (1913). "Bemerkungen zu der Arbeit Jaspers': Kausale und 'verständliche' Zusammenhänge zwischen Schicksal und Psychose bei der Dementia praecox (Schizophrenie)." *Internationale Zeitschrift für ärztliche Psychoanalyse* 1: 383–390.

Binswanger L. (1992a). "Über Ideenflucht [1933]." In M. Herzog (ed.), *Ludwig Binswanger: Ausgewählte Werke in vier Bänden*, Vol. 1, pp. 1–232. Heidelberg: Asanger.

Binswanger L. (1992b). "Drei Formen mißglückten Daseins [1956]." In M. Herzog (ed.), *Ludwig Binswanger: Ausgewählte Werke in vier Bänden*, Vol. 1, pp. 233–417. Heidelberg: Asanger.

Binswanger L. (1993). "Grundformen und Erkenntnis menschlichen Daseins [1942]". In M. Herzog and H.-J. Braun (eds.), *Ludwig Binswanger: Ausgewählte Werke in vier Bänden*, Vol. 2, pp. Heidelberg: Roland Asanger.

Binswanger L. (1994a). "Über Phänomenologie [1923]." In M. Herzog (ed.), *Ludwig Binswanger: Ausgewählte Werke in vier Bänden*, Vol. 3, pp. 35–69. Heidelberg: Asanger.

Binswanger L. (1994b). "Wahn [1965]." In A. Holzhey-Kunz (ed.), *Ludwig Binswanger: Ausgewählte Werke in vier Bänden*, Vol. 4, pp. 429–539. Heidelberg: Asanger.

Fichtner G. (ed.) (1992). *Sigmund Freud—Ludwig Binswanger. Briefwechsel 1908–1938.* Frankfurt am Main: Fischer.

Jaspers, K. (1997). *General Psychopathology*, trans. J. Hoenig and M. W. Hamilton. Baltimore: Johns Hopkins University Press.

Needleman, J. (1963) *Being-in-the-World: Selected Papers of Ludwig Binswanger*. New York, London: Basic books.

Winnicott, D. W. (1965). "Ego Distortion in Terms of True and False Self [1960]." In D. W. Winnicott (ed.), *The Maturational Process and the Facilitating Environment: Studies in the Theory of Emotional Development*, pp. 140–157. London: Hogarth Press.

CHAPTER 16

MEDARD BOSS

FRANZ MAYR

"We are unknown to ourselves, we men of knowledge" (Nietzsche)

BIOGRAPHY OF MEDARD BOSS (1903–1990)

BORN in St. Gallen, Switzerland, on October 4, 1903, Boss earned his medical degree from the University of Zürich in 1928. During his studies, he traveled to Paris and Vienna. In Vienna's famous medical school he studied under Sigmund Freud and was analyzed by Freud himself. Furthermore he became acquainted with Vienna's philosophical and psychological schools. The Viennese philosopher-psychologist Franz Brentano (1838–1917) was a great influence upon the young Freud and upon Husserl, and indirectly upon Heidegger. After four years as an assistant to Eugen Bleuler (1857–1939) at the Burghölzli hospital (Zürich) Boss continued to study in Berlin and London under earlier disciples of Freud, such as Karen Horney and Kurt Goldstein who opposed Freud's explanation of human behavior by instincts rather than by the total human personality.

Beginning in 1938 Boss became associated with Carl Gustav Jung (aniveres-amima) and his analytical psychology. Jung, who formerly split from the Viennese Freud circle, taught Boss an alternative to Freud's psychoanalysis and interpretation of dreams. At the same time he started to read the works of Ludwig Binswanger who not only worked out an "existential psychotherapy" inspired by Heidegger, but introduced Boss to Heidegger's philosophical work, especially during the Second World War when he served as a military doctor in the Alpine Swiss Army.

In the preface to the first German edition of Martin Heidegger's *Zollikon Seminars*, later edited by Boss, Boss very bluntly tells us of his troubled first encounter with Heidegger's *opus magnum, Being and Time* (1962 [1927]), during his military service:

> For the first time in my life I was occasionally gripped by boredom. In the midst of it what we call "time" became problematic for me. . . by chance I came across a newspaper item about Heidegger's book *Being and Time*. I plunged into it but I discovered that I understood almost none of its content. The book opened up question after question which I had never encountered before in my entire scientifically oriented education. . . Disappointed I laid the

book aside only half-read, but strangely it gave me no rest. I would pick it up again and again and begin studying anew. This first conversation with Heidegger outlasted the war.

(Heidegger 2001: vii–viii)

After much trepidation, Boss had a first meeting with Heidegger in 1946, which started a twenty-five-year friendship with Heidegger. Boss slowly realized that modern psychology and medicine was based upon the Hippocratic medical model (P. Lain Entralgo 1970), the subjectivist philosophy of Descartes and the Newtonian physics, both of which adhered to a mechanistic interpretation of the human being which Heidegger radically questioned (Heidegger 1993). Boss started to lay a new systematic existential foundation for medicine and psychology, in particular psychotherapy. His existential psychotherapy is critical of Freud's so-called "scientific" metapsychology without in any way questioning the greatness of Freud in the "praxis" of psychotherapy from which Boss himself learned so much (Boss 1963: 61–74).

There is no doubt that Boss revered Freud and adored the genius of Heidegger "between good and evil" (Safranski 1998). Boss knew that Freud's psychoanalysis was the newest result of the diverse periods of European Enlightenment. It started with the Greek knowledge of the mortal "self" ("*Gnothi Seauton*," know thyself) and with the Socratic "The unexamined life is not worth living for a human being" (Plato, *Apology*).

Throughout his life, Boss defended Freud's pioneering work in *psychotherapy* despite his abandonment of Freud's *metapsychology* such as the theories of the "unconscious," "repression," the "libido theories," the functions of the *Ego, Id,* and *Superego*. Boss wrote among other things about Freud's fundamental therapeutic rule (absolute honesty and truthfulness between the patient and the therapist), but also on the contradiction between Freud's strong emphasis on human *freedom* and the strongly *deterministic* view (the "psychic apparatus") in his theoretical works (Boss 1979: 277). Finally, Boss agreed with Freud's original idea of the "meaningfulness" not only of dreams but of all human phenomena in mental health and illness (Freud 1953a [1900]; Boss 1963).

One of the first influences upon Boss was his mentor and friend, the Swiss psychiatrist Ludwig Binswanger (1881–1966) who in addition to Jaspers and Bleuler was one of the founders of classical "phenomenological psychopathology" in which Heidegger's *Being and Time* (1927) became the basis of his own psychiatric *Daseinsanalysis*. Binswanger, a lifelong friend but theoretical opponent of Freud, shared many views with Boss's *Daseinsanalysis*. In contrast, Heidegger's relationship with Binswanger's *Daseinsanalysis* (Binswanger 1975: 206–221; Boss 1979: 71) ended up with his critique of Binswanger's (a) *ontical*, subject-oriented psychic "projection" of the world in contrast to Heidegger's circumspective *ontological* being-in-the-world, and (b) Heidegger's critique that Binswanger supplemented Heidegger's ontological *care* with his own ontical *love* which later Binswanger admitted as a "productive misunderstanding" of Heidegger's Analytic of Dasein (Heidegger 2001: 115–116, 190–192, 203–207, 304, 307).

BOSS AND PHENOMENOLOGY

In his main work, Boss did not refer explicitly to Husserl's phenomenology although Husserl's work is presupposed in the *Zollikon Seminars* where Heidegger (and Boss) took a critical stance toward Husserl's "transcendental phenomenology." For Heidegger, Husserl's phenomenology was the last descendant of modern philosophy since Descartes's dualism of the internal "subject" (*res cogitans*) and the external "object" (*res extensa*) (Descartes 1993 [1641]; Heidegger 2001: 105–110, 146–147). Even Husserl called his phenomenology "the secret nostalgia of all modern philosophy" (Husserl 1982: 142; see also Safranski 1998: 79).

The most decisive difference and critique of Husserl's *noesis–noema* dualism as "a pure construct" (Heidegger 2001: 208) can be stated by comparing the two respective terms of Husserl (*subjectivity*) and Heidegger (*being*) (Husserl 1970; Heidegger 2001: 146; Zahavi 2003; Figal 2012). In the 1962 *Preface* to Richardson's book, *Heidegger: Through Phenomenology to Thought*, Heidegger stated:

> The Being-question, unfolded in *Being and Time*, parted company with this [i.e., Husserl's] philosophical position, and that on the basis of what to this day I still consider a more faithful adherence to the principle of phenomenology.
>
> (Heidegger 1963; Richardson 1963: xiv)

First and foremost, "Being" is "hidden" (Heidegger 1962: 36, 56) as a phenomenon and has to be explicated as the unthematic background ("horizon") of all other "beings," inclusive of human Dasein as the "guardian" and "shepherd" of Being (Heidegger 1962: 22–35; Heidegger 1993: 245).

In Husserl's phenomenology, the question of the *Being of beings* (Heidegger 1962: 2–35) was reduced to the being ("objectivity") as intuited essence and "object" (*noema*) which Heidegger called the mere "*vorhanden*" (*present-at-hand*) reality of "things" (Boelen 1975: 93–114; Watanabe 1993). Thus, the early Husserl's intuition of "essence" became in Heidegger the ec-static, *temporal*, that is, *the unfolding essence* (Heidegger 1993: 424) within the primordial pre-understanding of Being. Similarly, in Heidegger's perspective Husserl's (transcendental) consciousness and its "intentionality" presupposes the contextual, "field-like" "*Dasein*" (Heidegger 2001: 207) of a shared historical world (Boelen 1975: 108–114; Ricoeur 1970). Dasein as being-in-the-world and its pre-reflective "mineness" is prior (Heidegger 2001: 129–132, 142) to any epistemological dualism of the "given" and "concepts" in the Kantian or early Husserlian sense ("*hyletic data*") (Heidegger 2001: 142).

Boss gave more attention to Merleau-Ponty's phenomenology of the human body (Boss 1979: 130; Heidegger 2001: 231–234) than to Sartre's frequently overlooked phenomenology of the pre-reflective "self" or Sartre's "gaze" and "mirror" scene in his *Nausea* (2007). Merleau-Ponty's *Phenomenology of Perception* (1962) was influenced—as later Levinas(insomnia, alterity, traumatism)(1961)—by Husserl and Heidegger. With his sensitivity to language (Boss 1979: 125, 133–134), Boss pointed out that Merleau-Ponty, whose work he admired, changed the Sartrean dualistic translation of Heidegger's *being-in-the-world* (*être-dans-le-monde*) into his being-of-the-world (*être-du-monde*) (Sartre 1956). By introducing the concept of the "dwelling" (*Wohnen*) of the soul in the body Merleau-Ponty sets himself (without total success) the special task of transcending Cartesian dualism (Boss 1979: 129). He still cannot overcome the Cartesian heritage (Merleau-Ponty 1945/1962: 198; Boss 1979: 92–97, 130; Heidegger 2001: 157) which is entirely different from Heidegger's "dwelling"—the human being's *ec-static relation to "Being"* as "clearing" in the openness of his "being-in-the-world" (Heidegger 1993: 343–363; Boss 1979: 128–130).

PHENOMENOLOGICAL ASPECTS OF
BOSS'S PSYCHOPATHOLOGY

Boss's psychopathology is not conceived from Husserl's pure phenomenology of "transcendental subjectivity," but rather from Heidegger's "Being," as process of the revealing-concealing *Ereignis* (disclosing Event), "*Dasein*," and "being-in-the-world." Boss's psychopathology, following Heidegger (Heidegger 2001: 153), discussed among other things (against Freud's metapsychology) such psychiatric symptoms as *hysteria, psychosomatic disturbances* (migraines, etc.), *obsessional neuroses, narcissistic neuroses, sadistic perversions, transference and countertransference*, "*acting out*," *guilt feelings*, and the modern depressive neurosis of *boredom* (Boss 1963: 131–284; Heidegger 2001: 208). Heidegger's ontological *Being-with* (*Mitsein*) is, next to the human being's existential *Thrownness* (*Geworfenheit*), *understanding* (*Verstehen*), and *being-unto-death* (Boss 1979: 119–122; Heidegger 2001: 139), the tacit background of all psychopathologies and their existential cures (Boss 1979: 275; Heidegger 2001: 157–211). This does not exclude the importance of the present, and still developing, neurosciences and brain research nor some of Freud's developmental insights (bi-sexuality, Oedipus, Überdetermination of dreams and texts) (Churchland 1986; Panksepp 2004; Sass et al. 2011; Trupp 2000: 56–84) with some of Freud's psychological developmental insights.

It was the French psychiatrist and philosopher, Jacque Lacan, who understood the "unconscious" as "*structured like a language*" (Muller and Richardson 1982; Richardson 1983). After Lacan's (Lacan 1978: 130; Richardson 1993: 50–63) interpretation of the Freudian "unconscious" in terms of the "symbolic" language, Boss pointed out that Freud's initial linguistic use of the term "unconscious" for a psychic "*process*" ended up in a "*substantial*" usage (Boss 1979: 135–136; Heidegger 2001: 153, 216).

Lacan's new interpretation of the unconscious in terms of a special "language" provided a new *non-objectified* understanding of the unconscious. The unconscious is the ultimate "Other" (Being) for the "subject." Nevertheless, Lacan's (subjectivistic-Saussurian) and finally "mathematical" linguistic interpretation of the unconscious could not be integrated into Heidegger's *being-in-the-world* (Saussure 1915; Richardson 1993: 58) or into later Heidegger's view of language as "saying" and "hearing" (Heidegger 2001: 96–97; Mayr 2001).

Boss reinterpreted the Freudian "unconscious" as an a priori construction after the failure of Freud's "natural scientific," *causal* explanation (Heidegger 2001: 224; see also Wittgenstein 1968; Boss 1977: 2–3; Monk 2005: 73–77) of the "gaps" between conscious awareness and the unexplained phenomena of dreams and parapraxes (faulty actions)—such as sudden forgetting, sudden insights, slip of the tongue, *posthypnotic behavior*, etc. (Boss 1963: 86–91; Freud 1995: 572–584; Heidegger 2001: 182, 187). For Boss the unconscious belongs like the conscious to the experience of Dasein's being-in-the-world (Boss 1977: 175–215), which opens up to the "*hiddenness*" of Being itself (Boss 1979: 135–146). Lacan said about "Being": "This last word that is not accessible to us . . . in the scientific attitude" (Lacan 1978: 130). In Heidegger, this "hiddenness" of Being makes itself manifest *as* the inaccessible "mystery" in the human being's conscious *and* "unconscious," temporal being-in-the-world (Heidegger 2001: 183). By contrast, the Freudian *reified* unconscious—as if belonging "to someone else" (Freud 1995a: 575)—with its repressed material is *timeless* and *spaceless* (Freud 1995a: 579).

Removed from the Heideggerian *temporality* and *spatiality* of Dasein's being-in-the-world (Boss 1979: 80–100, 182–183; Freud 1995a). Additionally, Freud's causal "(instinctual) explanation of *dreams* as unconscious wish fulfillment" ("Desire" in Lacan; Richardson 1983: 152–153) censored or repressed by the intrapsychic [Cartesian] Ego, were by Heidegger integrated into the equiprimordial aspects of *holistic* "wakening" *and* "dreaming" of Dasein's existential "being-in-the world" (Heidegger 2001: 245) and understanding of *Being*.

> The dream world cannot be separated as an object domain into itself, but rather the dream world belongs in a certain way to the continuity of being-in-the-world. It is likewise a being-in-the-world.
>
> (Heidegger 2001: 228–231)

Boss applied these insights in his own dream-book "I dreamt last night . . ." (Boss 1979: 45–48, 61–62, 167–169, 179–215) without considering also the linguistic character of the remembered dream world (see Richardson 1993: 57–60).

The most important psychiatrists influential on Boss are the following:

(a) Jaspers: Boss referred to Jaspers's difficulty defining "consciousness" in the Cartesian view of an introspective consciousness (Boss 1979: 133; Heidegger 2001: 225–226). Jaspers applied a broader "phenomenological method" which was earlier also used by the influential philosopher-psychologist Wilhelm Dilthey, with his distinction between scientific "explanation by causes" (*Erklären*) and historical-philosophical "understanding of meaning" (*Verstehen*). Despite Jaspers's originality in understanding some aspect of *schizophrenia*, he still adhered in a *rationalistic* way to the ultimate logical incomprehensibility of schizophrenia instead of the impairment of the pre-reflective, lived life itself. Jaspers's doctrine became the questionable criterion of "poor reality testing" and of a "cognitive error and a false belief" of the schizophrenic mind (Sass 1992: 125–132).

(b) Minkowski: The French-Polish psychiatrist *Eugene Minkowski* (1885–1972) was the author of the famous *Le temps vécu: Etudes phénoménologiques et psychopathologiques* (Paris 1933). In his discussion of "*lived time*" versus the "scientific" clock-time, Minkowski wanted to recover our lost sense of lived time, which played such a great role in Husserl's Augustine-inspired "inner time-consciousness" (Husserl 1966a) but which was critiqued as "subjectivistic" in Heidegger's "existential temporality" of Dasein's being-in-the-world (Ricoeur 1970; Boss 1979: 213; Heidegger 2001: 38–42).

(c) Blankenburg: Equally, Heidegger criticized the phenomenological anthropologist Wolfgang *Blankenburg* (Heidegger 2001: 204, 275) who analyzed the spatial and temporal structures of the world of the schizophrenic (Blankenburg 1971). To Blankenburg's misunderstanding of the "ontological difference," Heidegger remarked:

> In contrast to Binswanger, Blankenburg indeed sees the ontological difference [between Being and beings], but he misinterprets it because he also takes Being (Sein) as *a* being [Seiendes] which must then be mediated with the other.
>
> (Heidegger 2001: 204)

(d) Plügge: Among the anthropological psychiatrists, Heidegger and Boss discussed Herbert Plügge within the context of an *existential* notion of (modern) "*stress*"

(Heidegger 2001: 141–143, 275; Boss 1979: 206–210) and other illnesses in modern technological, post-Marxist society (Marx 1953: 246; Boss 1979: 286–297; Heidegger 2001).

(e) Tellenbach: The psychiatrist Hubertus Tellenbach researched the distortion of the spatial world of the "melancholic" and epileptic (Boss 1979: 37) similar to the disturbance of time observed by Minkowski (1933) and Straus (1956/1963). Boss has shown that many traditional, so-called "organic psychoses" may be causally related to a *biophysical* frontal lobe damage but are (originally) to be *understood* (*Verstehen*) from Dasein's pathological impairment of its ec-static, holistic relation to *Being* and *being-in-the-world*.

According to Boss, Plügge, Blankenburg, and Tellenbach applied mostly an empirical-ontical phenomenology, like Jaspers had done (Spiegelberg 1972: 105; Boss 1979: 213–219). Boss discussed at length illnesses, especially *schizophrenia*, which are phenomenological encroachments on the openness and *existential* freedom of Dasein (Boss 1979: 223–235).

In conclusion, similar to Socrates and Hippocrates, so in our times, Heidegger and Boss had emphasized a) the basic distinction between philosophy, science, the art of medicine and healing, and b) the entirely new "ontological difference" between *Being* and *beings*, always threatened by the abyss of passions and the mystery of suffering (Gr. *Pathos*) of our human time- and death-bound existence.

Bibliography

Binswanger L. (1975). *Being-in-the-world: Selected Papers of Ludwig Binswanger*, trans. J. Needleman. London: Souvenir Books.

Blankenburg W. (1971). *Der Verlust der natürlichen Selbstverständlichkeit: Ein Beitrag zur Psychopathologie symptomarmer Schizophrenien*. Stuttgart: Enke.

Boelen B. (1975). "Martin Heidegger as a Phenomenologist." In P. J. Bossert (ed.), *Phenomenological Perspectives: Historical and Systematic Essays in Honor of Herbert Spiegelberg*, pp. 93–114. Nijhoff: The Hague.

Boss M. (1963). *Psychoanalysis and Daseinanalysis*, trans. L. B. Lefebre. New York: Basic Books.

Boss M. (1977). *I dreamt last night . . .*, trans. S. Conway. New York: Gardner Press.

Boss M. (1979). *Existential Foundation of Medicine and Psychology*, trans. S. Conway, and A. Deaves. New York: Apronson.

Churchland P. S. (1986). *Neurophilosophy*. Cambridge, MA: MIT Press.

Descartes R. (1993). *Meditations on First Philosophy* [1641]. Indianapolis, IN: Hackett Publishing Company.

Figal G. (2012). "Hermeneutical Phenomenology." In D. Zahavi (ed.), *The Oxford Handbook of Contemporary Phenomenology*, pp. 525–542. Oxford: Oxford University Press.

Freud S. (1953a [1900]). *The Interpretation of Dreams*, trans. J. Strachey. *The Standard Edition of the Complete Psychological Works of Sigmund Freud*, vol. 4. London: The Hogarth Press.

Freud S. (1953b). *The Psychopathology of Everyday Life*, trans. J. Strachey. *The Standard Edition of the Complete Psychological Works of Sigmund Freud*, vol. 5. London: The Hogarth Press.

Freud S. (1955). "The Uncanny," trans. J. Strachey. In J. Strachey (ed.), *The Standard Edition of the Complete Psychological Works of Sigmund Freud*, vol. 17, pp. 217–252. London: The Hogarth Press.

Freud S. (1995). "Beyond the Pleasure Principle." In P. Gay (ed.), *The Freud Reader*, pp. 594–626. New York: Norton.

Freud S. (1995a). "The Unconscious." In P. Gay (ed.), *The Freud Reader*, pp. 572–836. New York: Norton.

Heidegger M. (1956). "Logos (Heraclit, Fragment 50)," trans. J. Lacan. *La Psychoanalyse* 1: 59–79.

Heidegger M. (1962). *Being and Time* [1927], trans. J. Macquarrie and E. Robinson. New York: Harper and Row.

Heidegger M. (1963). *Preface*. In W. J. Richardson, *Heidegger: Through Phenomenology to Thought*, pp. xiv–xv. The Hague: Martinus Nijhoff.

Heidegger M. (1993). *Basic Writings* ed. D. F. Krell. San Francisco: Harper.

Heidegger M. (1993a). *Grundprobleme der Phänomenologie (1919–1920). Gesemtausgabe*, vol. 58. Frankfurt am Main: Kloster mann.

Heidegger M. (2001). *Zollikon Seminars: Protocols—Conversations, Letters*. Edited by Medard Boss, trans. F. Mayr and R. Askay. Evanston: Northwestern University Press.

Husserl E. (1966). *Cartesian Meditations: An Introduction to Phenomenology*, trans. D. Cairns. The Hague: Martinus Nijhoff.

Husserl E. (1966a). *Zur Phänomenologie des Inneren Zeitbewusstseins (1893–1917) Husserliana 10*. Den Haag: Martinus Nijhoff.

Husserl E. (1970). *The Crisis of European Sciences and Transcendental Phenomenology*, trans. D. Carr. Evanston: Northwestern University Press.

Husserl E. (1982). *Ideas Pertaining to a Pure Phenomenology and to a Phenomenological Philosophy. First Book. General Introduction to a Pure Phenomenology*, trans. F. Kersten. The Hague: Martinus Nijhoff.

Kant, I. (1998). *Critique of Pure Reason*, trans. P. Guyer and A. W. Wood. Cambridge: Cambridge University Press.

Lain Entralgo P. (1970). *The Therapy of the Word in Classical Antiquity*, ed. and trans. L. J. Rather and J. M. Sharp. New Haven: Yale University Press.

Levinas E. (1961, 1969). *Totality and Infinity: an Essay on Exteriority*, trans. A. Lingis. Pittsburgh: Duquesne University Press.

Lacan J. (1977). *Ecrits. A Selection*, trans. A. Sheridan. New York: Norton.

Lacan J. (1978). *Le Seminaire: Livre II: Le moi dans la Theorie de Freud et dans la technique de la psychoanalyse*. Paris: Seuil.

Marx K. (1953). *Die Frühschriften*. Stuttgart: Kroner.

Mayr F. (1966). *Geschichte der Philosophie I. Antike*. Kevelaer: Butzon-Bercker.

Mayr F. (2001). "The Question of Being, Language and Translation." In M. Heidegger, *Zollikon Seminars: Protocols—Conversations, Letters. Edited by Medard Boss*, trans. F. Mayr and R. Askay, 317–336. Evanston: Northwestern University Press.

Merleau-Ponty M. (1945/1962). *Phenomenologie de la perception*. Paris: Edition Gallimard/ *Phenomenology of Perception*. London: Routledge.

Minkowski E. (1933/1970). *Le Temps vécu: Etudes phénoménologiques et psychopathologiques*. Paris: d'Artrey/*Lived Time: Phenomenological and Psychopathological Studies*, trans. N. Metzel. Evanston: Northwestern University Press.

Monk R. (2005). *How to Read Wittgenstein*. New York: Norton.

Muller J. P. and Richardson W. (1982). *Lacan and Language. A Reader's Guide to Ecrits*. New York: International Universities Press.

Panksepp J. (2004). *Affective Neuroscience*. New York: Oxford University Press.

Richardson W. J. (1963). *Preface.* In W. J. Richardson, *Heidegger: Through Phenomenology to Thought*, pp. xxv–xxix. The Hague: Martinus Nijhoff.

Richardson W. J. (1983). "Psychoanalysis and the Being-question." In J. H. Smith and W. Kerrigan (eds.), *Interpreting Lacan*, pp. 139–159. New Haven: Yale University Press.

Richardson W. J. (1993). "Heidegger Among the Doctors." In J. Sallis (ed.), *Reading Heidegger*, pp. 57–63. Bloomington: Indiana University Press.

Ricoeur P. (1970). *Freud and Philosophy: An Essay on Interpretation.* New Haven: Yale University Press.

Safranski R. (1998). *Martin Heidegger. Between Good and Evil.* Cambridge, Mass: Harvard University Press.

Sartre J. P. (1956). *Being and Nothingness*, trans. H. E. Barnes. New York: Philosophical Library.

Sartre J. P. (2007). *Nausea*, trans. L. Alexander. New York: New Directions.

Sass L. (1992). "Heidegger, Schizophrenia, and the Ontological Difference." *Philosophical Psychology* 5: 109–132.

Sass L., Parnas J., and Zahavi D. (2011). "Phenomenological Psychopathology and Schizophrenia: Contemporary Approaches and Misunderstandings." *Philosophy, Psychiatry, & Psychology* 18: 1–23.

Saussure F. (1915). *Course in General Linguistics*, trans. W. Baskin. New York: McGraw Hill.

Spiegelberg H. (1972). *Phenomenology in Psychology and Psychiatry.* Evanston: Northwestern University Press.

Straus E. (1956/1963). *Vom Sinn der Sinne. Ein Beitrag zur Grundlegung der Psychologie, 2nd edn./The Primary World of Senses: A Vindication of Sensory Experience*, trans. J. Needleman. Glencoe, Il: Free Press.

Trupp M. (2000). *On Freud.* Belmont, CA: Wadsworth.

Watanabe J. (1993). "Categorial Intuition and the Understanding of Being in Husserl and Heidegger." In J. Sallis (ed.), *Reading Heidegger*, pp. 109–117. Bloomington: Indiana University Press.

Wittgenstein L. (1968). *Vorlesungen und Gespräche über Aesthetic, Psychologie, und Religion.* Göttingen: Vandenhoeck.

Zahavi D. (2003). *Husserl's Phenomenology.* Standford, CA: Stanford University Press.

CHAPTER 17

ERWIN STRAUS

THOMAS FUCHS

INTRODUCTION

ERWIN Straus (1891–1975), the neurologist, psychiatrist, psychologist, philosopher, and contemporary of Binswanger, von Gebsattel, and Minkowski, is regarded among the leading representatives of phenomenological and anthropological psychiatry during the period before and after the Second World War. His works on the phenomenology of sensory experience and the *Psychology of the Human World*, which bear the hallmarks of an original mind and a lively writing style, belong to the classic works in this field. As Spiegelberg noted, "few phenomenologists have combined so much of the artist with the scientist" (Spiegelberg 1972: 278).

BIOGRAPHY

Born in Frankfurt in 1891, Erwin Straus qualified as a medical doctor at Berlin University where he started his career and practice as a neurologist and psychiatrist. In 1927, he completed the professorial *Habilitation* and, from 1931 to 1935, he was Extraordinary Professor of Psychiatry at Berlin University. In 1928, he was a co-founding editor of *Der Nervenarzt* (still an internationally recognized journal today), and his co-editorship lasted until 1935. Despite his impressive career, as a Jew, Straus felt forced to emigrate to the United States in 1938. Initially, he was a lecturer in philosophy and psychiatry at Black Mountain College in North Carolina. From 1946 until 1961, he was Director of the Veterans Administration Hospital in Lexington, Kentucky, where he continued lecturing until 1956. He never returned to Germany; nonetheless, he remained firmly associated with the researchers and scholars here, and for many years he maintained close friendships with Victor Emil von Gebsattel, Eugène Minkowski, and Ludwig Binswanger. From 1963 to 1972, he convened the five "Lexington Conferences on Phenomenology, Pure and Applied," which fostered an intensive dialogue between American and European phenomenology. Straus died in Lexington in 1975.

PHENOMENOLOGICAL PSYCHOLOGY

In his early works, for example, *Geschehnis und Erlebnis* (*Event and Experience* (1930)), Straus critically examined the epistemological foundations of Freud's psychoanalysis and behaviorism. He acutely delimited the sphere of psychic experience from abstracted, quasi-physical "arousals," "drives," or stimulus-reaction schemes. According to Straus, experience is formed through a sense-making perception (*Sinnentnahme*) which is stimulated by a given situation, yet nonetheless implies a preconceptual understanding of this situation along with an active, enquiring relationship to it. Since each experience is thus grounded on preceding individual experiences, it is withdrawn from empirical generalizability.

Straus was familiar with Edmund Husserl's phenomenology, which he studied in Munich and Göttingen, and his works were particularly influenced by Husserl's thought, even if he remained skeptical about his turn to transcendental phenomenology. For Straus there is no absolute consciousness beyond the human world—his phenomenology is basically anthropological, meaning that it is always concerned with the experience of the individual as a living organism, his bodily existence, and his life-world. Here, Straus was particularly searching for the "basic axioms of everyday life" which go largely unnoticed because they are intrinsic to our experience.

Erwin Straus's phenomenological psychology is based primarily on his analyses of sensory experience, as he himself emphasized: "In my work I have tried to 'save' sensory experience from theoretical misinterpretation and then to apply the regained understanding of the norm to pathological manifestations" (quoted in Spiegelberg 1972: 269). In 1935, he published his major work *Vom Sinn der Sinne* (*The Primary World of Senses*), in which he concentrated on the study of modern cognitive sciences and psychology since Descartes, Locke, and Hume (Straus 1956). It starts again with a rigorous refutation of behaviorism, including a meticulous account of the framework of Pavlov's famous experiments with dogs, and an analysis of the contradictions inherent to Pavlov's own interpretations of these experiments. In Straus's view, theories tracing back perception and cognition entirely to sensory stimuli are not even adequate to determine the unity and wholeness of an object because sensory data are always given only in isolation. In contrast, Straus demonstrates that the individual pre-history and the secondary qualities of experience fundamentally determine how stimuli are experienced and reacted to as meaningful signals. Straus further disputes that perception and experience occur *within* an organism: their place is the world itself in which human beings and animals move and behave.

On this basis, Straus develops his own theory of animal and human sensing (*Empfinden*) and experience as a "sympathetic communication" with the world that is always linked with the potential for movement (Barbaras 2004). The following aspects form his basic assumptions: the experiencing subject is neither a physiological reaction mechanism nor pure consciousness, but rather a temporalizing, living, and moving organism which experiences events in the context of his life-history and attributes meaning to them accordingly. Moreover, sensory experience is part of the individual's "becoming," meaning that it is never repeated identically but rather each phase points to others that precede and follow it. From this starting point, Straus reconstructs the formation of the unity of experiential space and time.

Straus consistently develops this conceptual scheme in critical delimitation from objectifying psychology that suggests the reduction of the phenomenal world to physical processes including those of the central nervous system. "It is man who thinks, not the brain" is his critical maxim that still applies today (Straus 1956). He therefore vehemently opposes any separation of the neuronal processes from the context of the living, experiencing human subject. According to Straus, physiological analysis only explains the conditions, yet not the reality of human experience and action. In a later essay, Straus proved to be far ahead of his time:

> The physiologist, who in the everyday world relates behavior and brain, actually makes three kinds of things into objects of his reflection: behavior, the brain as macroscopic formation, and the brain in its microscopic structure and biophysical processes. From the whole—the living organism—the inquiry descends to the parts: first of all to an organ—the brain—and finally to its histological elements. Statements concerning the elementary processes acquire their proper sense only in reference back to the original whole.
>
> (Straus 1982: 145)

Thus, the neurosciences with their analyses and findings are referred back to the super-ordinate unity of the living, experiencing organism in its environment—an insight that anticipates the central elements of the current concepts of embodied and enactive cognition.

AESTHESIOLOGY OF THE SENSES

We have already demonstrated how sensory experience is vitally important not only for Straus's psychology but also for his psychopathological works and this should be examined in greater detail. Straus coined his approach of investigating sensory experience as *aesthesiology*, which will now be examined in greater detail (Straus 1958).

According to Straus, perception is constituted by a sentient, bodily, or "pathic" moment on the one hand, and an active, intentional, or "gnostic" (recognizing) moment on the other (Straus 1966a: 11ff.). The first conveys the affective, physiognomic, and expressive properties of the perceptual field, thus establishing a basic connection or attunement between the bodily subject and the world. The second means objectifying perception, that is, grasping the object as such. It may also be understood as the intersubjective constitution of reality through shared concepts which structure perception and turn it into a *sensus communis* or "common sense." It is thus also responsible for the normativity inherent in perception.

Pathic sensing can be understood as a form of sympathetic communication, as a living connection between "I" and "world" analogous to Minkowski's "contact vitale avec la réalité." This not only incorporates bodily sensations as the basis of every perception, but also the unity of sensing and motility, which Straus analyzed, in particular, by referring to the example of dance: animate of movement doesn't occur in physical space as an inert frame; rather, it is always self-movement within a spatial field of the body comprising near and far, rhythmical dynamic qualities, temporal patterns (*Zeitgestalten*), and anticipated possibilities or bodily protentions. This unity of sensing and moving results in the communication of subject and world, "a reaching out beyond oneself, thus attaining to the Other; "it" is the basic phenomenon of sensory experience, a relationship that cannot be reduced to anything in the physical world" (Straus 1958: 147).

On the other hand, in *gnostic* objectifying perception the subject disengages itself from the immediacy of feeling. "A simple perception, which may be expressed by the sentence 'This is an oak,' determines and emphasizes" (Straus 1956: 348; author's trans.). In this determination the continuous flow of feeling is interrupted; we proceed from the uniqueness of the lived moment to the repeatability and the generality of knowledge. According to Straus, man's upright posture is uniquely linked with gnostic cognition for it is associated with:

- distance from the ground, which allows us to move about more freely, yet also imposes a condition of precarious balance;
- distance from the objects that permits us to identify them as such; and
- distance from others, thus distinguishing them as their own centers of perspectivity so that, in common with them, we can constitute the meanings of things (Straus 1966b).

The pathic and gnostic moments are involved in differing relations in every sensory perception. The pathic aspect dominates in the oral senses (smell, taste), while the gnostic or perceptual aspect is prevalent in the far senses (hearing, seeing). The sense of touch falls most of all in the middle of this polarity, since it constitutes the feeling of self and other (Straus 1930: 48). To a certain extent, both aspects are also antagonistic to one another: the gnostic aspect, by intending the object as such, tends to objectify the perceived, and thus to inhibit the pathic aspect, that is, the expressive or affective qualities to which the lived body is susceptible.

The unity of both aspects in perception now results in the dialectical relationship to the world: "Our relation to the Allon is a dialectical one, a contraposition or connection in separation" (Straus 1969a: 33). Within the perceptual field we grasp the *Allon*, the Other, as Straus also defines the world of the subject; yet we grasp it in relationship to us, and ourselves in relation to it. Sensory experience is essentially bipolar, though not only as a relation of perceiver and the *Allon*, but also as the polarity of the pathic and the gnostic aspect within this relationship. "Whether the world is set more distant to us, in sharply contoured objectivity, or whether it approaches us by a loosening of boundaries . . . both, the specified and the blurred objectivity are alterations of communication" (Straus 1956: 218f.; author's trans.).

LANDSCAPE AND GEOGRAPHICAL SPACE

Different spatialities of experience correspond to the pathic and gnostic relationship with the world that Straus defines as "landscape" and "geographical" space (Straus 1956: 335ff.). *Landscape* implies what is a direct way of experiencing: it is centered on me and my body and sub-divided into near and far regions, centripetal and centrifugal directions, surrounded by the horizon and pervaded by references, impressions, and physiognomies. Pathic sensing is tied to the present relationship of the body with the impressions of the landscape; it "never ceases to be perspectival existence. The sensing does not gain a standpoint outside of the world of appearances" (Straus 1956: 207f.; author's trans.).

This original, perspectivist-subjective spatiality is suspended by the *geographical space* of aperspectival, objectifying knowledge: "If I want to recognize, to reach the things as they are in themselves, I have to break through my perspectival boundedness. I must gain distance from myself, dissolve the now, become identifiable within a general order, that is, I must step out from the center, as it were, in which I am positioned in sensing, and become alienated to myself" (Straus 1956: 331; author's trans.). Geographical space is abstracted from the bodily center; it forms in it only one position among many. We release ourselves in it from the direct relationship with that which is sensed and recognize it under a general aspect, namely, one that is accessible to others as well. Nevertheless, this objectifying act is not merely reflective cognition, rather as the gnostic moment it merges with perception itself and becomes inherent to it. For that reason alone can we perceive things *as such*, and moreover, communicate with others about them within a shared context and thus participate in the common world.

As becomes clear, Straus's emphasis on sensory-sympathetic communication does not imply an undifferentiated pre-reflective unity with the world: the human capacity for reflection also incorporates the potential to project oneself in an imaginary position out of the primary bodily standpoint. Straus subsequently referred to this in an essay as "excarnation" or "ekbasis" (stepping out) (Straus 1969b).

Phenomenological Psychopathology

Applying these conceptions to psychopathology, we may distinguish two basic disturbances which are both caused by an *uncoupling* of the pathic and the gnostic component of perception. As Straus notes, "the boundaries of the Allon are displaceable between the poles of intimacy and strangeness, of belonging and distance, of grasping and being grasped, of mastering and being overpowered. Such shifts of boundaries are experienced in the extreme pathological case, as derealization or depersonalization, as inspiration or alien influence" (Straus 1969a: 47).

On the one hand, a lack or loss of the *pathic* aspect leads to a growing alienation from the perceived world, leaving the subject as a pure, detached observer; this amounts to a more or less severe derealization and depersonalization. According to Straus, this emerges due to a loss of sympathetic communication with the world. Without the pathic aspect what is perceived appears empty, unsubstantial, or dead. On the other hand, a disturbance of the *gnostic* moment results in a subjectivization of perception, marked by a preponderance of expressive, overwhelming qualities in the perceptual field. This is the case, for example, in the threatening environments of agoraphobia, in drug intoxication, or in the initial stages of schizophrenia: here, the surroundings change into a puzzling, mysterious, and stage-like scenery, and the patient becomes the "center of the world." The intersubjective constitution of reality is thus replaced by a radically subjectivist or idiosyncratic experience.

According to Straus, every relation to the *Allon* already implies the possibility to be influenced, overwhelmed, or pursued. This possibility is inhibited due to the distance that gnostic perception entails. "If and when distantiation fails, then we are delivered up to the Allon, experiencing its power physiognomically as a growing menace" (Straus 1969a: 77). In the state of psychosis there is a failure of gnostic-determining distance, and the expressive characters of the surroundings come to the fore. The Other now becomes "a realm of the hostile, in which the patient finds himself all alone and defenceless, surrendered to a power which threatens him from all sides. The voices point at him, they have singled out and separated him from all others. He is certain that they mean him and no one else, he is not puzzled that his neighbour does not hear anything . . . In this world, there is no community, no discursive explanation" (Straus 1958). Intersubjective communication requires "the possibility to detach oneself from the impression, to reflect upon oneself, to place oneself within a general order, in which places are convertible" (Straus 1958 l.c.). With the pathic aspect becoming autonomous, the possibility of changing perspective and thus, the intersubjectivity of perception is lost.

In normal experience the pathic and gnostic moments of perception are not separable from one another. The table is not only seen, but also felt, its color and form are sensed in bodily resonance. Yet, it is equally perceived *as* a table in terms of its generally attributable meaning which we have learnt from others. The *common sense* merges as practical meaningfulness with the specific senses. Thus, it becomes possible that perception, *through* its merely subjective or pathic aspect, is oriented to the objects themselves. However, in the case of a weakening or disturbance of the gnostic-intersubjective aspect, perception can no longer present the object as such and instead gives us only its impression, its subjective appearance. It then lacks the solidity of the *object*, the character of the *Allon* or reality. Thus, the surroundings are transformed into a stage-like scenery, an uncanny array of unreal, apparitional things that have questionable meaning. This uncanniness is the characteristic of the schizophrenic *delusional mood (Wahnstimmung)* at the onset of acute psychosis (Jaspers 1963; Fuchs 2005).

According to Straus, it is no longer possible for patients in psychosis to classify their experiences in the general, intersubjective, or geographical space:

> When, for example, a psychotic girl reports that while shopping she noticed the glance of someone who she believed to be following her, yet without being able to tell where the person stood . . . then such experiences no longer have anything to do with discursive, intelligible, geographical space. . . . [The patients'] being-in-the-world is so modified that a bridge between the psychotic experience of space and geographical space can no longer be built, nor can a return be effected that would lead from geographical space to the spatial conditions in which the psychotic experience takes place. In such cases of psychotic alteration it is characteristic for the hallucinations to appear in sensory fields for which normally the pathic moment of affection is essential.
>
> (Straus 1969a: 359)

Hence, the psychotic patient no longer arrives at the general, intersubjectively constituted object, or the *Allon* as a real counterpart. On the contrary, he or she remains enclosed in a subjectified, solipsistic perception. However, this psychopathological alteration of experience can only be explained on the basis of a phenomenological analysis of everyday perception.

CONCLUSION

This short exposition of Erwin Straus's elaborate work can certainly not offer a substitute for an in-depth reading of his major works. Nevertheless, it should have become obvious that for Straus an understanding of psychopathological phenomena is always grounded upon the anthropological analysis of human experience: namely, in the forms of sensing, perception, self-movement, and communication that characterize the human life-world and its "basic axioms of everyday life" (Straus 1958). Accordingly, his fundamental analysis of temporality in depression (Straus 1928/1966: 290ff.) is also based on an examination of the relationship of subjective or immanent and objective or world time: the slow-down of the subjective time of "becoming" up to a point of standstill leads to a decoupling from world time and conditions the superiority of the past in the depressive experience of guilt. This analysis subsequently became the starting point for numerous phenomenological studies on the depressive experience of time (von Gebsattel 1954; Tellenbach 1980; Kimura 1992; Fuchs 2001; Fuchs 2013; Stanghellini et al. 2016).

Straus's comprehensive analyses and results derived from the dialogue between his phenomenological, anthropological, and clinical questions and research. And it was out of this dialogue "that Straus developed and elaborated his most comprehensive theoretical conception: the structure of the norm and pathology of I-World relations" (Titelman 1976: 19). Seen in this light, psychiatry is never to be restricted to a medical model, either in terms of its knowledge or its action: "The object of psychiatric action is not primarily the brain, the body, or the organism; it should be integral man in the uniqueness of his individual existence as this discloses itself—independently of the distinction between health and sick—in existential communication" (Straus 1969a: 2). To illuminate this fundamental communication with the world in its pre-reflective forms, and also to analyze its disorders, represents a common thread that runs through Straus's work as a whole, through his lifelong searches and enquiries. Consequently, his basic attitude as a psychiatrist, researcher, lecturer, and as a person is perhaps most appropriately summarized by the title of his own essay, "Man—A Questioning Being" (Straus 1966a: 166–187).

BIBLIOGRAPHY

Barbaras R. (2004). "Affectivity and Movement: The Sense of Sensing in Erwin Straus." *Phenomenology and the Cognitive Sciences* 3: 215–228.

Fuchs T. (2001). "Melancholia as a Desynchronization. Towards a Psychopathology of Interpersonal Time." *Psychopathology* 34: 179–186.

Fuchs T. (2005). "Delusional Mood and Delusional Perception—A Phenomenological Analysis." *Psychopathology* 38: 133–139.

Fuchs T. (2013). "Temporality and Psychopathology." *Phenomenology and the Cognitive Sciences* 12: 75–104.

Jaspers K. (1963). *General Psychopathology*, trans. J. Hoenig and M. W. Hamilton. Chicago: University of Chicago Press.

Kimura B. (1992). *Ecrits de psychopathologie phénoménologique*, trans. J. Bouderlique. Paris: Presses Universitaires France.

Spiegelberg H. (1972). *Phenomenology in Psychology and Psychiatry: A Historical Introduction*. Evanston: Northwestern University Press.

Stanghellini G., Ballerini M., Presenza S., Mancini M., Northoff G., and Cutting J. (2016). "Abnormal Time Experiences in Major Depression. An Empirical Qualitative Study." *Psychopathology* 42: 45–55.

Straus E. (1928/1966). "Das Zeiterlebnis in der endogenen Depression und in der psychopathischen Verstimmung." *Monatsschrift für Psychiatrie und Neurologie* 68: 640–656. Eng. trans. "Disorders of Personal Time in Depressive States." In E. Straus, *Phenomenological Psychology*, pp. 290–295. New York: Basic Books.

Straus E. (1930). *Geschehnis und Erlebnis*. Berlin: Springer.

Straus E. (1956/1963). *Vom Sinn der Sinne*, 2nd edn. Berlin: Springer. Eng. trans. *The Primary World of the Senses: A Vindication*, trans. J. Needleman. Glencoe/Ill: Free Press.

Straus E. (1958). "Aesthesiology and Hallucinations." In R. May, E. Angel, and H. F. Ellenberger (eds.), *Existence: A New Dimension in Psychiatry and Psychology*, pp. 139–169. New York: Basic Books.

Straus E. (1960). "Die Ästhesiologie und ihre Bedeutung für das Verständnis der Halluzinationen." In E. Straus (ed.), *Psychologie der menschlichen Welt*, pp. 236–269. Berlin: Springer.

Straus E. (1966a). *Phenomenological Psychology*. New York: Basic Books.

Straus E. (1966b). "The Upright Posture." In E. Straus (ed.), *Phenomenological Psychology*, pp. 137–165. New York: Basic Books.

Straus E. (1969a). *Psychiatry and Philosophy*, trans. E. Eng. New York: Springer.

Straus E. (1969b). "Embodiment and Excarnation." In M. Greene (ed.), *Toward a Unity of Knowledge, Psychological Issues* 6, pp. 217–250. New York: International University Press.

Straus E. (1982). *Man, Time, and World: Two Contributions to Anthropological Psychology*. Pittsburgh: Duquesne University Press.

Tellenbach H. (1980). *Melancholy: History of the Problem, Endogeneity, Typology, Pathogenesis, Clinical Considerations*, trans. E. Eng. Pittsburgh: Duquesne University Press.

Titelman P. (1976). "A Phenomenological Approach to Psychopathology: The Conception of Erwin Straus." *Journal of Phenomenological Psychology* 7: 15–33.

von Gebsattel E. (1954). "Zeitbezogenes Zwangsdenken in der Melancholie." In E. von Gebsattel (ed.), *Prolegomena einer medizinischen Anthropologie*, pp. 1–18. Berlin: Springer.

CHAPTER 18

ERNST KRETSCHMER

MARIO ROSSI MONTI

BIOGRAPHICAL SKETCH

THE son of a pastor, Ernst Kretschmer (1888–1964) was born in Wüstenrot, Germany, on October 8, 1888. After studying philosophy, history, and medicine at the universities of Munich, Hamburg, and Tübingen, in 1913 he became an assistant to Professor Robert Gaupp in Tübingen. Gaupp, who was also Kurt Schneider's teacher, represented for Kretschmer a fundamental point of reference and left a profound mark on his thought and training. For some, Kretschmer's behavior during the Nazi period was ambivalent. On the one hand, in 1933, three years after his election to the presidency of the General Medical Society for Psychotherapy, he decided to resign as a form of protest, and his place was taken by Carl G. Jung. The psychiatrist Oswald Bumke recalled a telling remark made by Kretschmer in those years: "It's a funny thing with psychopaths. In normal times we render expert opinions on them; in times of political unrest they rule us" (Cocks 1985: 101). He also firmly rejected the idea of a pure Arian race and made use of a narrow definition of schizophrenia in order to oppose the programs of compulsory sterilization implemented by the Nazi regime. On the other side, however, Kretschmer was among the signatories of the *Vow of Allegiance of the Professors of German Universities and High Schools to Adolf Hitler* and appears to have made compromises with the regime (Klee 2005; Müller 2001). In his autobiography *Characters and Thoughts* (*Gestalten und Gedanken*) (Kretschmer 1963), Kretschmer wrote that during the rise of Nazism he held out until the end. After the war, in 1946, Kretschmer was offered a professorship at the University of Tübingen where he remained as professor of psychiatry until 1959. He died in Tübingen in 1964.

CONTRIBUTIONS TO PSYCHOPATHOLOGY

Kretschmer's contributions to the field of psychopathology can be schematically reduced to two main themes: the first consists in the analysis of a particular form of delusion called "sensitive delusion of reference," developed in his book *Der Sensitive Beziehungswahn* (*The*

Sensitive Delusion of Reference) (Kretschmer 1918); the second concerns the construction of a constitutional typology (Kretschmer 1921), which attempts to identify, on the basis of the temperamental and physical-constitutional characteristics of the subjects, all possible degrees and steps leading to the two major psychoses: manic-depressive psychosis and schizophrenia.

The name of Robert Gaupp, Kretschmer's teacher, is linked to an event of extraordinary interest—the criminal case of the elementary school teacher Ernst Wagner who was tormented by feelings of deep humiliation caused by his alleged acts of zoophilia, a persecutory delusion involving his fellow countrymen. This delusion led him in 1913 to set the entire village of Müllhausen on fire, burning down houses and barns and killing eight men. Earlier that same night Wagner had killed his wife and four children in their sleep. Gaupp's report, based on a thorough reconstruction of the psychopathological experience of the patient, led to the diagnosis of "paranoia" and to the resulting possibility of commuting the death sentence to imprisonment for life. The psychopathological analysis conducted by Gaupp revolved around the idea that it was possible to reconstruct how, over the years, Wagner had *developed* his paranoid delusion. The idea of a "development" of personality, brilliantly expounded by Karl Jaspers in his *Allgemeine Psychopathologie* (Jaspers 1959), had allowed Gaupp to reach an understanding of the psychopathological pathways that had brought Wagner to delusion. Ernst Kretschmer's contribution to the growth of psychopathological knowledge is based precisely on the possibility of extending Jaspers's concept of "development" (and therefore of comprehensibility) also to the field of "real" delusions, namely to the primary delusions which—according to Jaspers's theory—were impossible to comprehend in their genesis.

This is precisely the challenge that Kretschmer took up in order to contrast his views (and that of the Tübingen School) with those of Karl Jaspers and Kurt Schneider, the most authoritative representatives of the Heidelberg School, which had been the cradle of German psychopathology. With the publication of *Der Sensitive Beziehungswahn* in 1918, Kretschmer attacked the nosology of psychoses. The sensitive delusion of reference is a particular clinical form of delusion characterized by systematized, non-bizarre, and non-hallucinatory delusions, which coincide with the paranoia described by Kraepelin (1915). It is based on a "concentric relationship" in which the subject feels at the center of a threatening experience that envelops him, making his or her thoughts revolve around a key event that acts as a pivot for the emergence of the delusion. It is a key event (*Schlüsselerlebnis*) that, as Kretschmer puts it, "unlocks" the character, triggering the onset of psychosis. When a key event touches a particular point of a sensitive personality, the subject experiences feeling of inadequacy, failure, humiliation, and shame. This, on Kretschmer's view, is the real turning point for the onset of delusion. This key experience connects the sensitive personality with the emergence of delusion, which in order to take place requires two other ingredients in addition to the key event: a particular type of personality (the sensitive personality) and a particular environment.

The sensitive personality is characterized by a dialectic relationship between two contradictory tendencies: on the one hand, a sthenic disposition of character (ambition, pride, sense of superiority and power) and, on the other, an asthenic disposition (timidity, a hypersensitivity that can develop into social hyperesthesia, meticulousness, hesitation, shame, sense of inferiority and guilt, inhibition, secretiveness, and rigid morality). In the sensitive person, Kretschmer specifies, the asthenic tendency prevails. The asthenic side, however, is counteracted by a sthenic tendency. As a result, on the one hand, these subjects display an extraordinary weakness of mind and a delicate vulnerability, while, on the other, they nurture grand ambitions and show presumptuousness and stubbornness. They typically refrain from expressing their feelings and remain in a state of permanent tension, perhaps afflicted by the tormenting memories of a painful experience. The third ingredient of the triad is the environment. Due to their weakness and strong tendency toward introspection, these people tend to live an isolated life. When their suffering is intense or their constitution particularly unstable, a process of inversion takes place by which their anxieties and fears are projected onto the outside world, thereby taking the form of delusional beliefs. The sensitive person, for example, becomes convinced that his or her feeling of shame is universally known, and he or she is the object of derision and ridicule. The character of Hans Kohlhaas, depicted by Heinrich von Kleist in a famous novella, is analyzed by Kretschmer to illustrate how an honest sixteenth-century merchant, having suffered a series of injustices, could turn a state of shameful failure into a furious rage that induced him to terrorize for years the entire region of Saxony—in a manner similar to that which Gaupp described in the case of the elementary teacher Ernst Wagner.

The fact is that in the clinical cases described by Kretschmer it is possible to identify primary delusional experiences in Jaspers's sense or of typical delusional perceptions in Schneider's sense. From this point of view, there is no longer any clear demarcation between the development of secondary delusion in abnormal personalities and primary delusion in paranoid schizophrenia. According to Kretschmer, in place of this clear distinction, a *continuity* between personality, primary delusions, and schizophrenia can be identified. Therefore, there is not a gap between personality and psychosis, as the School of Heidelberg had argued, but, on the contrary, a series of gradual steps. Thanks to Kretschmer's careful clinical discussions and analyses, the sensitive delusion of reference has become the prototype for the psychological comprehension of some cases of paranoid psychoses. This comprehension requires a prolonged and systematic relationship with the patient. Kretschmer followed his paradigmatic cases for years, pushing Jaspers's method of "genetic understanding" to the extreme. This type of understanding does not aim at reliving an isolated significant experience (*Erlebnis*), but rather at identifying an evolutionary path, a chain of concatenated experiences and meanings that run through the entire history and existential world of the patient.

KRETSCHMER'S CONSTITUTIONAL TYPOLOGY

Kretschmer's constitutional typology was influenced by Bénédict Morel's theory of "degeneration" (Morel 1857) and by the French anthropological tradition (Magnan 1885) which was based on the attempt to identify the bodily marks of the psychic involution supposedly occurring in the transition from one generation to the other. Kretschmer, however, was not so much interested in the identification of the stigmata of "degeneration," but rather in the transitional steps, at the bodily level, between character and psychosis. In *Körperbau und Character* (*Physique and Character*) (Kretschmer 1921) and in *Medizinische Psychologie* (*Medical Psychology*) (Kretschmer 1922), Kretschmer described in parallel the two sequences leading from a normal character to the two major psychoses: on the one side, cyclothymic and cycloid mental constitutions and eventually manic-depressive psychosis; on the other, schizothymic and schizoid mental constitutions and eventually schizophrenia. The two major psychoses could be considered as the extreme development of certain normal types of character or as a sort of caricature of them. From this point of view, psychoses would not arise as something completely new and unexpected since between normality and pathology there would be a whole spectrum of gradual steps and nuances.

Kretschmer's attempt to identify these transitional steps led him to formulate a constitutional typology based on the identification of two types of normal constitutions: a cyclothymic constitution and a schizothymic constitution. These two broad biotypological entities, combined in various proportions, include the great mass of ordinary varieties. A third type is represented by individuals of athletic and muscular constitution who are characterized by a tenacious and sticky temperament. This group was later brought in the leptsomic constitutional type.

Each constitutional type, however, is not characterized by a single temperament, but by a contrasting pair of features. As a result, individuals with a mental schizothymic constitution are physically "leptosomic" (cylindrical trunk, elongated figure, thin chest, thin shoulders, long neck, slender bones and muscles), while, psychologically, they are characterized by what Kretschmer calls "psychaesthetic proportion," that is, a balanced relationship between two contradictory tendencies: hyperesthesia and sensitivity on the one hand, and affective anaesthesia and coldness-dullness on the other. These two tendencies coexist side by side without eliminating each other. Individuals with a cyclothymic constitution are physically "pyknic" (stocky, with short extremities, rotund figure, vivid complexion, large circumference of the head, trunk and abdomen, thin and narrow shoulders, tendency to develop early baldness), while, psychologically, they are characterized by a "diathetic proportion," that is, a balance between two antinomic affective tendencies: euphoric exaltation and joviality-enthusiasm on the one hand, sadness and despair-discouragement on the other. The athletic type is physically robust (muscular, trapezoidal trunk, broad shoulders, slender legs) and, psychologically, he is characterized by an affective viscosity centered on the antinomic couple torpidity-explosiveness.

The above characteristics gradually emerge along the path that leads from cyclothymic constitution to manic-depressive psychosis, and from schizothymic constitution to schizophrenia. For example, the schizoid person, writes Kretschmer (Kretschmer 1921, 1922), is not alternately hypersensitive or cold, but is *both* at the same time and in different degrees, so much so that it is possible to outline a continuous line running from what he calls the Hölderlin type (hypersensitive, fragile, excitable) up to those cold, hard subjects that have fallen prey to a real dementia praecox (schizophrenia) and wander in a corner of the asylum like obtuse beasts. The "psychaesthetic proportion" is defined precisely by the degree in which hypersensitivity and coldness mingle in the individual subject. Such proportion, however, should not be taken as static or fixed once and for all, since it undergoes significant fluctuations in relation to age and the vicissitudes of life.

The conclusions drawn by Kretschmer's constitutional studies could not be accepted by Jaspers, who believed in a clear-cut differentiation between the area of normal psychic life and that of psychotic mental life. If a relationship exists between schizoid personality and schizophrenia, Jaspers argued, this relationship is to be understood in terms of a gap rather than a gradual shift (Jaspers 1959: 645). Kretschmer's descriptions—Jaspers wrote—are beautifully wrapped in a pseudo-exact scientific coating that creates confusion because it stems from a mixture of different methods. Kretschmer's fundamental error, according to Jaspers, lay in his hypostatization, namely in the automatic transformation of ideas into entities. It is intuitively correct to argue that a thin body with long extremities and narrow chest is not inhabited by a jovial and cheerful soul, or that a large body with short extremities is not inhabited by an arid and virtuous one. This is a matter of intuitive physiognomic thinking about human nature and, as such, it does not require further investigation. However, to turn this insight into a scientific law of causality is quite a different matter. In fact, many counterexamples refute it. At most, one could speak of a correlation, as it happens with many phenomena that have no real affinity with each other. Moreover, Jaspers concluded, physiognomics is, after prophecy, the most fallacious art ever invented by an eccentric mind (Jaspers 1959: 268).

Empirical research has subsequently proved Jaspers right and demonstrated the unsustainability of Kretschmer's constitutional typology. However, beyond this particular aspect, the fact remains that even in Kretschmer's constitutional typology it is possible to detect a dialectical principle privileging the understanding of the transitional forms and the paths leading to psychosis over the study of the rigid clinical forms established by nosology. Kretschmer's psychodynamic approach (which, however, does not draw on psychoanalysis) represents a fundamental contribution to the understanding of the path to psychosis.

Beyond Primary Delusions

In conclusion, Kretschmer's analysis of the sensitive delusion of reference has been, in the words of Martin Roth (Roth 1982), the first authoritative challenge to the dichotomy between comprehensible phenomena and "developments" on the one side, and incomprehensible phenomena and "processes" on the other. In this sense, Kretschmer's dynamic (but not psychoanalytic) pathogenetic model has fractured—like a Trojan horse—the dogma of the incomprehensibility of delusions and has set an example for the study of a wider range of delusions. Nonetheless, Kretschmer has been widely criticized and accused of daring too much and, at the same time, too little. He dared too little in the sense that he excluded any reference to psychoanalytic approaches (despite its model being highly dynamic) and confined to one specific form of delusion the challenge to the dogma of incomprehensibility. On the other hand, he dared too much in the eyes of those who, like Jaspers and Schneider, embraced the assumption of primary incomprehensibility of delusions and considered the clinical situations he described as personality developments. These criticisms, however, were oblivious to the fact that in the cases of sensitive delusion of reference described by Kretschmer many primary delusions and many first-rank Schneiderian symptoms had been amply documented. What has happened—we may ask—to Kretschmer's contributions to psychopathology? While the somatic-based constitutional type now belongs to the history of psychiatry, the attention to the comprehensibility of the paths leading to the area of major psychoses remains an unavoidable point of reference for those who refuse to give up the attempt to introduce the dimension of subjectivity and understanding into the area of psychosis. This attempt is particularly important at a time when mainstream psychiatry is struggling to get rid of any dimension that cannot be described in objective terms and measured quantitatively or behaviorally. Kretschmer's contribution was immediately picked up by another great psychopathologist, Eugène Minkowski, and elaborated further in close relationship with the approach taken in the same years by Wimmer and by the Scandinavian school of psychiatry in the development of the concept of psychogenic psychosis (Wimmer 2003; Strömgren 1974; Retterstøl 1978; Wimmer 2003). The Open Dialogue method in the treatment of psychoses, developed by Jaakko Seikkula (Seikkula and Olson 2003; Seikkula and Arnkil 2006) in the past decades in Finland and now widespread across the globe, represents a tentative therapeutic application of Kretschmer's dynamic-comprehensive approach to psychosis. In addition, the "basic symptoms model," developed in Germany since the 1970s, has successfully adopted the idea of a continuum in the development of schizophrenic psychoses in particular. After Klosterkötter (1988) successfully developed the serial connections model in order to explain the first-rank Schneiderian symptoms, one could argue—in homage to Kretschmer's sensitive delusion of reference—that every primary delusion is now largely understandable.

ACKNOWLEDGMENT

This entry should have been written together with Professor Arnaldo Ballerini who, unfortunately, passed away before we could get to work. In illustrating Kretschmer's thought, I can only gratefully recall the passion and the clinical and methodological rigor with which Arnaldo Ballerini introduced me to the study of psychiatry and psychopathology.

BIBLIOGRAPHY

Cocks G. (1985). *Psychotherapy in the Third Reich: The Göring Institute*. Oxford: Oxford University Press.

Jaspers K. (1959). *Allgemeine Psychopathologie*, 7. unveränderte Auflage [1913]. Heidelberg: Springer.

Klee E. (2005). *Das Personenlexikon zum Dritten Reich. Wer war was vor und nach 1945*, 2. Auflage [2003]. Frankfurt am Main: Fischer Verlag.

Klosterkötter J. (1988). *Basissymptome und Endphaenomene der Schizophrenie*. Heidelberg: Springer.

Kraepelin E. (1915). *Psychiatrie*. Leipzig: Barthes.

Kretschmer E. (1918). *Der sensitive Beziehungswahn*. Berlin: Springer.

Kretschmer E. (1921). *Körperbau und Character*. Berlin: Springer.

Kretschmer E. (1922). *Medizinische Psychologie*. Stuttgart: Thieme.

Kretschmer E. (1963). *Gestalten und Gedanken*. Stuttgart: Thieme.

Magnan V. (1885). *Des anomalies, des aberrations et des perversions sexuelles*. Paris: A. Delahaye, E. Lecrosnier.

Morel V. B. (1857). *Traité des Dégénérescences*. Bailliére: Paris.

Müller R. (2001). *Wege zum Ruhm. Militärpsychiatrie im Zweiten Weltkrieg. Das Beispiel Marburg*. Köln: PapyRossa.

Retterstøl N. (1978). "The Scandinavian Concept of Reactive Psychosis, Schizophreniform Psychosis and Schizophrenia." *Psychiatria clinica* 11: 180–187.

Roth M. (1982). "New and Old Concepts in Psychiatric Diagnosis and Classification: A Commentary of Recent Developments." *Neurologia, psichiatria, scienze umane. Atti Congresso Nazionale della Società Italiana di Psichiatria* 1: 21–38.

Seikkula J. and Olson M. (2003). "The Open Dialogue Approach to Acute Psychosis: Its Poetics and Micropolitics." *Family Process* 42: 403–418.

Seikkula J. and Arnkil T. (2006). *Dialogical Meetings in Social Networks*. London: Karnac.

Strömgren E. (1974). "Psychogenic Psychoses." In S. Hirsch and M. Shepherd (eds.), *Themes and Variations in European Psychiatry*, pp. 97–120. Bristol: John Wright and Sons.

Strömgren E. (1986). "Psychogene Psychosen." *Nervenarzt 57*: 88–95.

Wimmer A. (2003). *Psychogenic Psychoses*. Adelaide: Adelaide Academic Press.

CHAPTER 19

....

HUBERTUS TELLENBACH

....

STEFANO MICALI

INTRODUCTION

....

THERE are authors belonging to the tradition of phenomenological psychopathology who have had a major impact on psychiatric research: Karl Jaspers, Ludwig Binswanger, and Eugène Minkowski are probably the first names that come to mind. Yet, there are also authors in this tradition who have not received the attention their outstanding work deserves. Hubertus Tellenbach belongs to the latter category. Despite the fact that his most important work—*Melancholy*—has been translated into more than twelve languages (Tellenbach 1980)—for example, Italian, French, and Japanese—the appreciation of the richness of his work is still inadequate. Furthermore, Tellenbach's research remains to be discovered in the English-speaking world. Tellenbach's most important contributions to psychiatry are to be found in four different areas of research: 1) the methodology of the psychopathological approach (Tellenbach 1968, 1980); 2) the study of melancholia (Tellenbach 1956, 1960, 1969, 1980); 3) the phenomenology of atmosphere and mood (Tellenbach 1968); and 4) an intercultural investigation of fatherhood (Tellenbach 1976, 1978, 1979). In this chapter, I will focus primarily on the first two areas, although some aspects related to the third area will also be mentioned.

Hubertus Tellenbach, born in Cologne in 1914, studied medicine and philosophy from 1933 to 1938 in Mönchengladbach, Königsberg, and in Freiburg im Breisgau. In Freiburg, he attended Martin Heidegger's courses, which had a profound influence on his approach to psychopathology. He received a doctoral degree in both philosophy and medicine. In 1956, he started working at the University of Heidelberg where he became a professor in the Department of Psychiatry. Tellenbach was clinical director of the Department of Psychopathology from 1971 until his retirement in 1979. He continued working and publishing material until he died in 1994.

METHODOLOGICAL REFLECTIONS:
THE FIELD OF ENDOGENEITY

A basic assumption of phenomenological psychiatry is that no mental illness can be described or treated without a thorough analysis of subjective experience. Phenomenological descriptions of psychopathological disturbances remain the irreplaceable reference point of all empirical studies. Psychopathological disturbances cannot, for example, be reduced to subpersonal, biological symptoms. German and French phenomenological psychopathology even questions the legitimacy of the term "symptom" with respect to psychiatric disorders (Tellenbach 1968; Tatossian 1979; Kraus 1991). The term "symptom" in a medical context has a specific semiotic status: it is a sign referring to an occurring process that is not immediately visible or accessible. It implies an inferential process: we can infer the objective existence of a disease in terms of a pathological dysfunction to which we have no direct access from the manifestations of several symptoms. According to Tellenbach, psychopathological appearances are *sensu stricto* not symptoms (Tellenbach 1968). They do not refer to anything else. The feeling of a lack of feeling cannot be conceived as a symptom of depression; it is rather a primal manifestation of the disturbance, that is, an essential characteristic (*Merkmal*) of the phenomenon as such. The fundamental categorical distinction between symptoms and characteristics should not be overlooked in the psychiatric context since it reveals an implicit reductionism. Furthermore, there is no "single" manifestation that can be clearly isolated from the other disturbances in psychopathological disorders. Of course, it is not only legitimate, but also necessary, to distinguish between single manifestations for diagnostic purposes. However, this distinction is not rooted in separable aspects of the phenomena as such. The globality of the transformation cannot be reduced to a single psychological aspect or to a physical disturbance. Each manifestation of melancholia is always representative of an overall alteration of the human being.

Tellenbach introduces the notion of endogeneity in order to analyze the specific characteristics of psychopathological disturbances. The study of endogeneity aims at overcoming the classical paradigm of understanding the relationship between mind and body. Psychoanalysis insists on the psychogenic relevance of unconscious dynamics causing changes at the bodily level. Biological psychiatry emphasizes the dependence of mental states on somatic processes of biochemical nature. Tellenbach introduces the notion of endogeneity in order to escape this rigid alternative between two opposite and reverse forms of causality. The notion of endogeneity intends to address a field of phenomena concerning the globality of subjective life: "it is the human being *in toto* which is transformed" (Tellenbach 1980: 28). Bin Kimura's concept of *Ki* (Kimura 1966) refers precisely to the global alteration that marks the atmospheric character of the encounter with a person with schizophrenia. It is noteworthy that endogeneity is not related only to pathological phenomena. The sphere of the endogenous can find its paradigmatic exemplification in the different stages of life: infancy—childhood—adolescence—adulthood—old age. These stages are neither attributable to the personal, psychological characteristics nor could they be reduced to subpersonal, biological processes. Each critical phase of maturation is a turning point of the whole human being. Each phase is incomparable with the other and constitutes a global configuration. The notion of "endon" refers to this global configuration. The transformation of this dimension is therefore defined as endokinesis. As Blankenburg writes: "Neither as the personal moment of an inwardness nor the apersonal moment of the apersonal biological, does it (the endon) unfold in the essential lawful regularities of life" (Blankenburg 1964: 184). Psychopathological disturbances like the melancholic or schizophrenic condition can be fully understood only in light of the notion of endogeneity. But other experiences too, such as the spiritual encounter in religion or art, can signify the beginning of a new life: they can transform the person radically.

Another crucial aspect of endogenity is to be found in the "kinesis" or the inner motion. This endogenous aspect of kinesis is particularly visible in the inhibition of the *élan vital* emphasized by Gebsattel with regard to the melancholic condition: a vital retardation of both the subjective flow and bodily movements occurs in melancholia with a loss of the affective resonance of the surroundings (Gebsattel 1954). The rhythm of life tends to be suspended. The self is just a witness to a frozen life. The melancholic patient is not able to feel anything, not even sadness. He is also incapable of entering in relation to his own inner death: "This suffering is endogenously inflected, is strange, incomprehensible, monstrous, deformed, even perverted suffering, a pathic apathy as it were" (Tellenbach 1980: 26). That melancholia has an endogenous character is shown by the fact that it does not leave traces in the inner life, once it has disappeared (Tellenbach 1980: 26).

Tellenbach emphasizes the affinity between the concept of endogeneity and Heidegger's notion of thrownness (*Geworfenheit*) developed in *Being and Time* (Heidegger 1996). At first sight it seems legitimate to conceive of research on endogeneity as a more detailed analysis of Heidegger's notion of facticity. On further examination, this interpretation becomes problematic. The concept of endogeneity is different from Heidegger's notion of *Geworfenheit* given its ecological and cosmic character: endogeneity refers to a vivid experience of a lived body in an ecological and social context within the life-world. Tellenbach stresses the intertwinement between endogeneity and the rhythms of nature, the impact of the rhythms of the day, of the months on our life, the "incorporation of the human life in his environment" (Tellenbach 1980: 23). A typical character of endogeneity manifests itself in the rhythm of vital activities. The positive manifestations of vital rhythms are the periodic processes of waking, sleeping, being active, resting, regularity of eating, drinking, suckling or nursing, the menstrual cycle, etc. The notion of endogeneity is conceived as the root of all structures that constitute us as living organisms, such as sexual orientations, temperaments, or predispositions of character as influenced by inheritance factors. The dimension of endogeneity goes beyond the categorical framework articulated in *Being and Time* where the organism is considered only in negative terms, and the embodied aspects are not adequately considered. Tellenbach's ecological paradigm—in his terminology, endo-cosmo-genetic paradigm—is closer to holistic approaches developed by Kurt Goldstein (1939) or Viktor von Weiszäcker (1940). Endogeneity is prior to the spiritual and existential dimension, but it is also strongly influenced by our projects, decisions, emotional responses, and spiritual attitudes to the situation. Furthermore, social interaction can have a crucial impact on the endogenous dimension. It is not possible to find in Tellenbach's analysis any negative or dismissive approach to common sense or to daily life in the life-world, which is reduced to inauthenticity in forms of dejection in *Being and Time*. The value of Tellenbach's integrative approach is particularly apparent in clinical diagnosis. It allows one to detect the complex interplay between biological processes, endogenous modifications, and existential attitudes. His research on *typus melancholicus* is an exemplary expression of his integrative approach.

THE *TYPUS MELANCHOLICUS*

The constellation of includence and remanence are the essential features for under-standing the pathogenesis of the endogenetic transformation in the melancholic condition. These constellations are not causes of depression but they could rather be conceived as its precondition.

Let us first explain the fundamental notion of includence. The melancholic type tends to-ward an over-identification with fixed social roles: "The melancholic's conscience is, in the first instance, a guardian of the established orders" (Tellenbach 1980: 122). Not measure and proportion, but orderliness "prevails" in the melancholic type. Everything has to be in the right place according to pre-established standards: "Nothing is allowed to interfere that would change the course of things, nothing unexpected, unforeseen" (Tellenbach 1980: 123). Everything has to go as expected. "It is characteristic when a woman, who later became mel-ancholic, reports that the morning after her husband's death she took her laundry and began ironing—'for the sake of order'" (Tellenbach 1980: 123). No contingency, chance, or ambi-guity is allowed. Invasive anxiety is connected with each novelty. The self-enclosure within a fixed order allows the subject to avoid the confrontation with everything out of the or-dinary: the accident and the possibility of guilt are in this sense particularly threatening. The person identifies him/herself with a specific environment (such as his/her own house), with specific activities (e.g. work performance), or with a symbiotic relation with the other. This exclusive "self-inclusion-into and self-understanding-out of a given order" (Tellenbach 1980: 120) is a constitutive feature of the melancholic type: Includence. The patient is self-enclosed within orders whose boundaries he/she is no longer able to transcend. Once unex-pected circumstances, such as moving houses or a disease, interrupt the routine of the given order, a crisis leading to severe depression can appear.

Remanence signifies the inescapable feeling of remaining behind oneself, especially with regard to one's own duties, tasks, and performances. The core of remanence is being in debt: "The essential form of such a condition of being in default to the self-demand is invariably being in debt: being in default to one's own demand for performance, or being in debt with regard to ethical and religious orders" (Tellenbach 1980: 148). Each unfinished task is felt as a mistake and source of guilt: "*debet* is already culpa" (Tellenbach 1980: 149). If the melancholic type accomplishes a good performance with a small imperfection, he tends to experience this imperfection as a personal catastrophe: "The melancholic type resembles a person who wishes to eradicate in advance all possible guilt, who pays as it were before-hand for what he has not yet taken, who sees himself as already in default when it is not even possible" (Tellenbach 1980: 151). He simply tries to accomplish the impossible. Human existence entails an ineradicable excess of possibilities over our capacity to actualize them, which implies a difficult confrontation with the finitude of one's own resources, time, and talents. The melancholic type is not able to live with the sense of indebtedness inherent to the human condition. He tries to eradicate all sense of indebtedness. Guilt becomes om-nipresent in an existence that wants nothing more than to avoid this guilt. Even fate—like unexpected sickness—is experienced as guilt or, at least, is an occasion for asking about the person's own wrongdoing: "Wherever anything fateful impinges on his order, the question occurs to him: How am I to blame for that?" (Tellenbach 1980: 153; translation modified).

A typical situation in which the constellation of includence and remanence can emerge is work performance. A sense of debt and guilt with regard to one's performance is the most common feature in this sense:

> Includence is the situation of constriction, within which the *melancholic type* is no longer able to surpass himself in the mode of his possible achievement, although for him, in terms of his order, everything depends on this—and this is the situation too in which he cannot on the other hand remain. Let us sketch once more the model of such situational change: a typological melancholic succeeds in some outstanding accomplishment. What happens when demands are unduly increased or his powers diminish? He wants by all means to get the job out of the way because his norm of responsibility requires that he does not remain obligated; but at the same time he is controlled by emphasis on accuracy because of his predisposition on orderliness.
>
> (Tellenbach 1980: 146)

Such a situation is not bearable in the long term: it leads to a crisis. He has to change himself—reducing the accuracy in order to match the new requirements. This example paradigmatically shows the interrelation between includence and remanence. The two constellations always appear together although remanence (or includence) can alternately be the dominant one in the specific case.

Tellenbach's approach can be termed kinetic typology, since it considers the genesis and the development of several situational experiences lived by the person. The investigation of the sequence of the situations detects the pathogenetic aspects. Even if the theme of the self-accusation remains the same, a radical change of the way of experiencing can occur: "the self no longer manages its theme but is rather managed by it," "the self no longer has or possesses its theme, but is possessed by it" (Tellenbach 1980: 173). These strange formulations tend to do justice to the strangeness of the phenomena. They intend to refer to the coherent deformation of the experience according to which the self is not capable of intentionally addressing the theme in a coherent and consistent way. The theme has become so overwhelming that no intentional content can emerge. The pathological aspect lies in the affective disproportion and exaggeration of a single event in the life-story, which results in an unknown despair. Despair is not to be understood as a lack of hope. It is rather a situation in which the subject oscillates between different possibilities without being able to make a decision. It is stuck with a self-contradiction with no way out. Despair is in this sense "remaining trapped in the doubt" (1980: 165). The self is no longer able to bear the self-contradictory tendencies inherent to the constellation of includence and remanence.

Conclusion

I wish to conclude by emphasizing the importance of Tellenbach's analyses of the *typus melancholicus* in order to understand the alarming relevance of depression in our contemporary liquid society (Micali 2010; Ambrosini et al. 2011). Subjectivity forms itself in social interaction, in specific matrices of praxis, discourses, gestures, and power-relations. Foucault introduces the term "dispositif" to refer to this kind of matrix (Foucault 1977; Deleuze 1990). Tellenbach's research concerning the *typus melancholicus* can shed light on an essential feature of our liquid society: the cult of performance. The cult of performance has in itself the seed of depression (Ehrenberg 1998; Micali 2010). Liquid society requires an infinite malleability and flexibility. The individual cannot adjust himself to the given conditions since these conditions change "faster than it takes the ways of acting to consolidate into habits and routines" (Bauman 2005: 2). The principle of perpetual training imposes itself in all areas: "One is never finished with anything" (Deleuze 1990: 23).

The liquid society combines and enhances the two tendencies of *typus melancholicus* (includence and remanence) in a particular way. On the one hand, a minute-by-minute plan of the entire process of work performance is required. The time schedule is defined in increasingly specific detail. No deviation is tolerated. On the other hand, the individual has to show initiative, open-mindedness, and creativity. He or she is required to be innovative, ready to develop new approaches, improving the efficiency of the process. According to the infinite process of capitalistic self-optimization, work performances always have to go beyond the previous outcomes. Hartmut Rosa considers the notion of acceleration as a key concept for understanding essential features of our post-disciplinary society (2010). The acceleration concerns the whole dimension of social interaction: the consumption of commodities, the telematic communication, performance at work, leisure activities, and so on. Under such circumstances the individual can easily feel inadequate. Deleuze argues that the contemporary human being is no longer the enclosed human being, but "the human being in debt [*l'homme endetté*]" (Deleuze 1990: 247). Recent sociological and philosophical research from different areas confirms this conclusion (Bauman 2005; Deleuze 1990; Ehrenberg 1998; Gorz 2010).

Tellenbach's research on the melancholic type can contribute to clarifying the connections between our society based on performance and optimatization and the phenomenon of depression (Haubl et al. 2013). The attitudinal constellation of remanence and includence is internal to the *dispositif* of the cult of performance typical of our liquid society where each person "must become for him or herself a business" (Gorz 2010: 21). Each person has to become "a form of fixed capital that needs to be continually reproduced, modernized, broadened, and recapitalized. . . . She/he must be her/his own producer, her/his own employer and her/his own seller, imposing upon herself/himself whatever constraints are necessary in order to ensure the viability and competitiveness of the business which she/he is" (Gorz 2010: 21). Being bound, almost condemned, to high performativity leads to the feeling of being left behind. If under specific negative circumstances the feeling of being left behind reaches a threatening intensity, it can easily become pathogenic.

Bibliography

Ambrosini A., Stanghellini G., and Langer A. I. (2011). "Typus Melancholicus from Tellenbach up to the Present Day." *Actas Españolas de Psiquiatría* 39: 302–311.
Bauman Z. (2005). *Liquid Life*. Malden, MA: Polity Press.
Blankenburg W. (1964). "Persönlichkeitstruktur." *Confinia Psychiatrica* 8: 183–198.
Deleuze G. (1990). *Pourparlers*. Paris: Editions Minuits.
Ehrenberg A. (1998). *La fatigue d'être soi*. Paris: Odile Jacob.
Foucault M. (1977). "The Confession of the Flesh." In G. Hemel (ed.), *Power/Knowledge*, pp. 194–228. Hempstead: Harvester Wheatsheaf.

Gebsattel V. E. von. (1954). *Prolegomena einer medizinischen Anthropologie*. Berlin, Göttingen, Heidelberg: Springer.

Goldstein K. (1939). *The Organism*. New York: American Book Company.

Gorz A. (2010). *The Immaterial*. Chicago: Chicago University Press.

Haubl R., Hausinger B, and Voss G. G. (eds.) (2013). *Riskante Arbeitswelten*. Frankfurt am Main: Campus.

Heidegger M. (1996). *Being and Time*, trans. J. Stambaugh. Albany: State University of New York Press.

Kimura, B. (1966). "Schulderlebnis und Klima (Fuhdo)." *Nervenarzt* 37: 160–199.

Kraus A. (1991). "Phänomenologische und symptomatologisch-kriteriologische Diagnostik." *Fundamenta Psychiatrica* 5: 102–109.

Micali S. (2010). "The Capitalistic Cult of Performance." *Philosophy Today* 54: 379–391.

Rosa H. (2010). *Alienation and Acceleration*. Aarhus: Aarhus Universitetsforlag.

Tatossian A. (1979). *Phénoménologie des psychoses*. Paris: Masson.

Tellenbach H. (1956). "Räumlichkeit der Melancholischen." *Nervenarzt* 27: 12–18.

Tellenbach H. (1960). "Gestalten der Melancholie." *Jahrbuch für Psychologie, Psychotherapie und medizicnische Anthropologie* 7: 39–133.

Tellenbach H. (1966). "Sinngestalten des Leidens und des Hoffens. Eine Untersuchung an den Confinien der Psychopathologie." In W. von Baeyer and Richard M. Griffith (eds.), *Conditio humana: Erwin W. Straus on his 75th Birthday*, pp. 307–318. Berlin: Springer.

Tellenbach H. (1968). *Geschmack und Atmosphäre. Medien menschlichen Elementarkontaktes*. Salzburg: Otto Müller Verlag.

Tellenbach, H. (1969). "Die Freilegung des melancholischen Typus im Rahmen einer kinetischen Typologie." In H. Hippius and H. Selback (eds.), *Das depressive Syndrom*, pp. 173–181. Müinchen: Urban u. Schwarzenberg.

Tellenbach H. (ed.) (1976). *Das Vaterbild in Mythos und Geschichte*. Stuttgart: Kohlhammer.

Tellenbach H. (ed.) (1978). *Das Vaterbild im Abendland*. Stuttgart: Kohlhammer.

Tellenbach H. (ed.) (1979) *Vaterbilder in Kulturen Asiens, Afrikas und Ozeaniens. Religionswissenschaft, Ethnologie*. Stuttgart: Kohlhammer.

Tellenbach H. (1980). *Melancholy*. Pittsburgh: Duquesne University Press.

von Weizsächer V. (1940). *Der Gestaltkreis. Theorie der Einheit von Wahrnehmen und Bewegen*. Leipzig: Thieme.

CHAPTER 20

KIMURA BIN

JAMES PHILLIPS

INTRODUCTION

KIMURA Bin (1931–) (in Japan the family name is placed first) is a Japanese psychiatrist who combined a phenomenological approach to psychiatry with traditional Japanese concepts. Although preoccupied in his early development with music theory, Kimura became, at the age of twenty, the thirty-sixth physician in his family (Pélicier 1992; Sass 2001). In his medical studies he discovered a book by a Japanese psychiatrist, M. Murakami, that introduced him to the theoretical work on schizophrenia by Western figures such as Minkowski, Binswanger, Janet, and Kronfeld. Noting his interest, Murakami invited him to participate in a translation of Binswanger's *Schizophrenia*. This intense experience of Binswanger's ideas made him decide on a career in psychiatry. In the following years he pursued a reading of the literature of phenomenological psychiatry, an intense study of Heidegger's *Being and Time*, further reading in music theory, and a new interest in Japanese Zen Buddhism. In his professional life he was a professor of psychiatry in the city of Nagoya and then in Kyoto. During his training he spent two years at the university clinic in Munich (1961–1963) and later he returned to Germany as a visiting professor in Heidelberg (1969–1970). In a study of depersonalization written while in Munich he made a distinction between the self or I as acting agent and the self as object of reflection—a distinction he would pursue for many years. Throughout his career he has published much in the area of phenomenological psychiatry, often making the connection with Japanese Zen Buddhism. He has also translated into Japanese works by psychiatrists and philosophers such as Heidegger, Binswanger, Frankl, von Weizsäcker, Tellenbach, Blankenburg, and Ellenberger.

Although Kimura wrote on many aspects of psychiatry and psychopathology, his work on schizophrenia is his most intense, original, and widely known. It is on that work that I will focus in this chapter.

EVERYDAY EXPERIENCE

Inasmuch as in his study of the self-disturbance of schizophrenia Kimura focuses on certain dimensions of normal self-experience, and in fact understands schizophrenia as a pathology of such experience, it will be fruitful to begin with a description of everyday self-experience (Zahavi 2001). First, there is a distinction between the self in action and the self as object of reflection. If I am engaged in an activity, my awareness of myself *while* doing something is different from my thinking about that activity after it has been completed. In Merleau-Ponty's terms, this is the distinction between pre-reflective or operative consciousness and reflective consciousness. Of course in normal experience we constantly veer from one to the other. A tennis player readily alternates between being totally involved in the play at one moment and quickly reflecting on it a moment later (e.g. "I should have pulled that serve more to his backhand"). We can think of the same distinction in the language of narrative theory of the self. The developed narrative is a product of reflection, but there is also the narrative quality of life as lived. If, for instance, part of my life narrative is my life as a parent, I might be implicitly and non-reflectively aware of this while doing something with my child.

A second distinction in everyday self-experience is that between oneself as an individual subject and oneself as a member of a community of selves. This plays out in many ways. First, even if I am in a private train of thought, I am not thinking in a private language; I am participating in a language that is shared by millions of others. And further, this private thought is often a private *conversation*, peopled by many imagined others, some of my direct acquaintance, others not. And finally, in real contacts with other people, I am more clearly involved in a shared consciousness of my contemporaries, whether that is a conversation with a few or with a community.

Finally, we must attend to the bodily self, the manner in which, whatever I am doing, I am acting as an embodied self. The tennis player is a perfect example of an embodied self—less aware of his body when his game is going well, more aware of it when a sprain interferes with his play.

We take our embodiment and the other dimensions of selfhood so much for granted that we are usually unaware of them. In this range of normal self-experiences, we automatically keep track of the fact that these various selves are all oneself. Whether I am engaged in an activity or thinking about it, whether I am engaged in private thought or having a conversation, whether I am solving a mathematical problem in my head or absorbed in physical, sexual activity—in all of these manifestations of my selfhood I am effortlessly aware that they are all me. I take their integration for granted and generally don't give it a second's thought.

There are occasions when I am made aware of one or another aspect of selfhood. I trip on the tennis court and am aware that my bruised knee interferes with my play. My conversation partner reminds me that I am not listening to him because I'm absorbed in my own thought.

There are also occasions when an aspect of myself feels like not me, feels other. I look in the mirror and for an instant think, is that me? I overhear another person talking about me and struggle to accept that the person she's talking about is really me.

These are minor breaks in the seamless continuity of selfhood. What Kimura will tell us is that in schizophrenia such breaks are not minor, they define schizophrenic experience. What we observe in schizophrenia is a failure of self-integration.

A CENTRAL THEME

Kimura investigates schizophrenia from a variety of perspectives. There is, however, a central theme that permeates the texts, a distinction between what he calls the subjective, noetic self and the objective, noematic self, and the failure in schizophrenia to maintain the balance between the two. The terms are those of Edmund Husserl, noema (and noematic) referring to the object of consciousness (in perception, e.g. a tree), noesis (and noetic) referring to the process of knowing or perceiving (I actually see the tree from a particular angle, in a particular "profile"). Kimura cautions that his use of these Husserlian categories is not necessarily faithful to Husserl:

> That which I call the noetic-noematic relationship is different from what Husserl describes with these same terms. The noetic qualifies for me as mode of experience that cannot be limited to the subjective or objective. It is in no way a matter of a substance. It resembles an atmosphere, but with the difference that it can't be understood as a quasi-object. Our real I is experienced as a noetic event, it is not visible as an object. In contrast, the image of the I or self that is the object of consciousness, as all that which is constituted as an intentional object of consciousness, is noematic.
>
> (Pélicier 1992: 188)

In what follows we will trace Kimura's elaboration of this distinction and its disturbance in schizophrenia from a variety of perspectives. The first I will label a Husserlian perspective because it develops his use of the noetic dimension as just described—a reflective moment within the subjective self.

HUSSERLIAN PERSPECTIVE

In his "Reflection and Self in the Schizophrenic" (Kimura 1992a) Kimura, citing a Japanese colleague Nagai Mari, invokes Husserlian terminology to distinguish two types of reflection: the first, a reflection after the act, in which the subject's reflection makes of the act a noematic object; the second, a simultaneous reflection that accompanies the act, and that remains entirely within the noetic sphere. The second would be like the tennis player observing his play *while* engaging in it. "One could say that a subjective self here accompanies another self no less subjective and observes it constantly 'from behind'. There is no objective, noematic self involved here; a sole noetic self splits into two simultaneous 'moments' which occupy alternatively the places of seeing and seen, and which nonetheless remain subjective-noetic" (Kimura 1992a: 118). Kimura points out that simultaneous reflection is quite difficult for the average person, and carried out only with great effort and some confusion (the tennis player would lose track of his play if reflecting on it *while* playing).

Kimura suggests that while simultaneous reflection is rare in normal experience, it is common in schizophrenic experience (and in that way makes it hard for the person with schizophrenia to pay attention to what he is doing). For this to result in disturbed self-experience, Kimura speculates on another feature of simultaneous reflection. Recall that in simultaneous reflection there are two moments within the noetic sphere: the observing subject and the observed subject. It may happen that one or the other of these may be experienced as alien, at which point the individual drifts into delusional psychosis. If the reflecting self is experienced as foreign, the result is paranoia ("I'm being looked at"); if the reflected-upon self is experienced as foreign, while still within the subject, the result is a delusion of one's mind being occupied by a foreign source ("I'm controlled by the computer planted in my head"). In describing a patient's confusion about what is inside and what is outside his mind, Kimura writes of one patient:

> This patient's words clearly suggest that the "I" or "self" as an entity remains identifiable from outside and recognizable as an object (I'm so and so, he says; he speaks of things being "into me," "with me," and "within myself"; he refers to "my hand"). By contrast, the personal subject or agent of this I-for-myself is no longer itself but has been altered by what he refers to as a "topological translocation," a "psycho-making" and manipulation by "Dr. M."
>
> (Kimura 2001: 332)

LINGUISTIC PERSPECTIVE

In another paper, "Pathology of the Immediate" (Kimura 1992b), Kimura reflects on schizophrenic disturbance from a linguistic perspective. Here he returns to the basic distinction between the subjective (noetic) I and the objective (noematic) self. He now distinguishes the self in action—the subjective I—pre-linguistic and unmediated through language, from the reflected-upon self, mediated through language. The acting I is immediate and fugitive in a manner that escapes articulation but at the same time, very readily flows into a secondary reflection that exists only as a mediated, articulated, noematic self.

Kimura begins the paper with a recognition that daily experience is almost entirely mediated through language: "[I]n daily life we experience everything as such or such thing. Thus the structure of language infiltrates itself profoundly into that 'as such'" (Kimura 1992b: 129). Importantly, we experience ourselves in the same mediated manner. When the I of immediate experience becomes aware of itself as I, it has already been transformed into an objective I or self, mediated through language. Kimura writes: "As for the I, which seems apparently the most immediately given, this also, when it becomes conscious of itself as 'I,' is constituted equally as an experience mediated by a negative differentiation that inserts itself between the 'I' that is in the process of becoming conscious and the 'I' that can be articulated in language, which latter is only the non-I for the immediate I" (Kimura 1992b: 132).

Kimura at times describes the subjective, unmediated I as an openness to the world prior to a separation of I and world, and at other times as function or action, a force that Bergson calls "*l'élan vital*" and Nietzsche "the Will to Power." Kimura refers to it as "the subject itself as the *vital ground* of . . . self-consciousness," in contrast to "the I that is *represented* in human consciousness" (Kimura 2001: 335), a corresponding objective, noematic sense of self. The subjective, vital I functions correctly, however, only when it is associated with the mediated, objective I. I act spontaneously, but always with a background sense that it is I, this particular self, that is acting. This need for the symbolized, mediated I does not imply a limitation or contamination of subjective experience but rather a need of the subjective I for its objectivized companion. The course of normal, everyday experience requires a balance between the two I's, the purely subjective I and its objectification in a symbolized, verbalized self—in Kimura's words, that "ordinary spontaneity is determined as a noetic I under the influence of the noematic self" (Kimura 1992b: 134). An ordinary statement such as "I'm going to the store" implies that balance—"I am going to the store," and "it is I and not another who is going to the store."

The person with schizophrenia is not able to balance the two senses of self, the unmediated I and the objective self. Each needs the other, and when either is disordered, the other will also be disordered. A failure of unmediated vital activity will affect the ability to develop an adequate mediated, objective sense of self, and a failure to develop the latter will prevent the person with schizophrenia from feeling any strength or confidence in his ability to act or function adequately in the world.

In this situation there is a failure in bridging the gulf between immediacy and mediation. When the natural split in the I is not mastered, a gulf remains between the subjective and objective selves. A person with schizophrenia may experience this gulf as difference. The unity of the self is broken and, as described in the previous section, one dimension of the self may be experienced as *other* than the self. Kimura discusses this experience of otherness further in describing Blankenburg's patient, Anne (Blankenburg 1971). Unable to experience her own subjectivity, and confusing the other person with the other within her, "the intrusion (*Eingriff*) of the *other* in her self-consciousness takes with her the form of a consciousness of being other than the others" (Kimura 1992a: 124). Kimura expands on the notion of otherness:

> One could draw the conclusion that the specific trouble-point in schizophrenic reflection resides precisely in the fact that it is not "the other" (*der Andere*), but rather alterity or otherness (*das Andere*), that appears as another self in self-consciousness of the patient. Consequently, the essential change in the schizophrenic himself is found in the constant questioning that defines him, of which one of the moments, alterity or otherness, is not integrated into the identity of the self, but remains as such naked.
>
> (Kimura 1992a: 127)

Kimura suggests that this sense of otherness may go beyond a personalized other and be experienced as an otherness at the core of the schizophrenic self—what he terms "a transcendent otherness ... transcendental other ... the absolute non-I, the absolutely other ... the principle of absolute extraneousness at the core of the self" (Kimura 1992b: 138).

Entangled in this confusion over who she is, the person with schizophrenia is unable to experience real spontaneity in her actions. Rather than just act, she halts with questions such as "who is acting?" and "who am I?" And with a sense of otherness at the center of herself, it is not hard to imagine her developing delusions of influence, that someone or something else inside or outside her mind is causing her activity.

INTERPERSONAL PERSPECTIVE

For Kimura problems in interpersonal relations do not simply follow from the self-disturbance described above. Rather, he places self-disturbance and disturbed interpersonal relations together in the foundation of schizophrenia. He begins his discussion of the interpersonal with the Japanese concept *aïda* (Kimura 1992a). This concept, related to the concept of openness described above, expresses a primary bond between self and world, as well as a primary bond between oneself and others, and also the relation between dimensions of oneself. In the Japanese sensibility we do not start as monads but rather as members of a community of others. One develops oneself as an individual self out of an initial state of unity with others.

In a normal relationship that flows out of a fundamental bond of *aïda*, each individual must experience herself as the complex of the subjective and objective, the unmediated and mediated described above; and each must experience the other as the same complex interiority, one subjectivity meeting another. According to Kimura, this does not happen in schizophrenia. The altered state of the patient's *aïda* doesn't allow it. For Kimura ". . . it is the intersubjective constitution of the world itself that is disturbed in the foundation of schizophrenia" (Kimura 1992a: 125).

In schizophrenia the interpersonal world (*aïda*) and the intrasubjective world collapse together. We have already seen how the intrasubjective world breaks down in schizophrenia. Unable to manage the balance between the spontaneous, immediate I and the objectivized, mediated self, the person with schizophrenia experiences the otherness of the mediated self as *an other*, an other that attacks her from outside, as in paranoia, or an other that dwells within her mind as a foreign source or agent. From the interpersonal perspective, the patient is unable to participate in *aïda*.

The interior process of finding one's bond with others—subject to subject—is called *jikaku*. In the encounter with a schizophrenic patient the psychiatrist experiences the strangeness in the patient that prevents the usual flow of interpersonal *aïda*, as well as a disruption in one's own *jikaku*. "As Japanese we try to overcome individuality in flowing from our personal self to find the common *aïda*. It's in that manner that I encounter schizophrenics in my *jikaku*" (Pélicier 1992: 188). In describing further this experience of the patient's schizophrenia, Kimura writes:

> I search for the key to schizophrenia in my own interiority where the schizophrenic provokes an abnormal noetic atmosphere that comes from his effort to avoid contact with others at a noetic level. The alteration which the schizophrenic encounter provokes in *aïda* blocks one's usual consciousness of oneself. This difficulty particular to schizophrenia corresponds to a deficiency in the noetic level of individualization that makes impossible development at the noematic level.
>
> (Pélicier 1992: 188)

TEMPORAL PERSPECTIVE

In a paper entitled "Temporality in Schizophrenia: Contrast between Schizophrenia Temporality and the Temporality of Non-schizophrenic Delusional Psychoses" (Kimura 1992c), Kimura proposes to erect a psychopathology based on temporality, on the idea that temporality is experienced differently in the various psychoses. He invokes Heidegger's three "ecstases" of past, present, and future to lead his discussion and, in contrast to melancholy that is rooted in guilt over the past, he considers schizophrenia as a psychopathology of the future. Quoting Heidegger, he points out that the self (*Dasein*) is always ahead of itself (*sich vorweg*) and always coming to itself (*auf-sich-selbst zukommen*) (Kimura 1992c: 141). In the balance between the noetic I and the noematic self, the self is not a fixed, developed entity. It is a self always in formation throughout one's life. In the Heideggerian terminology just cited, the self is always ahead of itself and always coming back to itself. And as we saw above, the subjective, noetic I acts only in relation to the objective, noematic self. If the latter is not developing properly, the operative I will not function correctly, and the core schizophrenic disturbance will persist through the passage of time.

Conclusion: Between *Onozukara* and *Mizukara*

It is fitting to conclude this chapter with a discussion of "Between *Onozukara* and *Mizukara*: Pathology of the Ego from a Traditional Japanese Perspective" (Kimura 1992d), in which Kimura reflects on his understanding of schizophrenia in the context of traditional Japanese concepts. The first is *aïda*, which we have seen above, and which represents the bond or "between" that unites just about anything—for example, the *aïda* between Sunday and Monday—but more importantly includes the "between" in interpersonal relations, and even the "between" in dimensions of the self. Moreover, the unity of *aïda* is so basic that it precedes individuation—individuation in the interpersonal sphere and individuation in the intrapersonal sphere. The latter implies that "everyone of us has to constitute himself as a self on the basis of this 'interior' *aïda*" (Kimura 1992d: 37).

How this is accomplished requires an excursus into ancient Japanese etymology. In traditional Japanese the word *mizukara* meant oneself or myself. With the introduction of Chinese characters or ideograms the Chinese character *ji* was introduced to translate *mizukara* (*kara* = "my own body," and *mi* = "my own flesh"). The problem was the same character was used to translate another Japanese word *onozukara* ("in itself" in an impersonal sense). "Japanese thus used these two words to differentiate these two notions: *ji-ko* or *ji-bun* for 'myself' (*mizukara*) and *ji-nen* for 'in itself' (*onozukara*)" (Kimura 1992d: 38). Over time *ji-nen* ("in itself" or *onozukara*) came to mean nature.

Kimura explains the seemingly confusing fact that *mizukara* and *onozukara* are represented by the same Chinese character in the following manner. The *ji* in both concepts means to arise spontaneously out of an origin. "*Ji-ko, ji-nen/shi-zen, mizukara onozukara* are in other words different modes of the auto-articulation or auto-manifestation of the spontaneous, universal movement out of an originary point" (Kimura 1992d: 39). Consequently, in Japanese thought the concept of "self" covers both nature and the individual self. In this sense an authentic self implies participation in the universal process of nature. "The 'self' is, one might say, 'interiorized nature', and nature is in some manner 'exteriorized self'" (Kimura 1992d: 39). Thus self and nature, *mizukara* and *onozukara*, have the same origin.

We can now say that there is an interpersonal *aïda* (oneself and others) and an intrapersonal *aïda* (*mizukara* and *onozukara* within the self). The latter implies that an authentic self includes a transcendent principle of nature (*onozukara*) within the self. Kimura refers to this intrapersonal *aïda* as the *arch-aïda*.

Relating these concepts to what we have covered earlier in the chapter, we can say that these Japanese concepts of intrasubjective *aïda*, *mizukara*, and *onozukara* represent Kimura's deepened, Japanese understanding of what he has described in Western terminology. *Mizukara* and *onozukara* are loosely the equivalents of the noetic, unmediated I and the mediated, noematic self. In more familiar language, the mediated, noematic, *onozukara* dimension of the self implies a principle of *otherness* at the center of the self.

Continuing his analysis of intrasubjective *aïda*, Kimura turns finally to schizophrenia, stating that "the fundamental problematic of schizophrenic disturbances, as a failure of interpersonal relations, can now be understood entirely in terms of pathologic changes in the constitution of the *arch-aïda*" (Kimura 1992d: 41). To the question, is the schizophrenic disturbance a self-disturbance or an interpersonal disturbance, the answer is that there is no difference. As I wrote on another occasion: "Following Kimura's analysis, the self is constituted in a double relation, a relation to itself and a relation to the other. And the two relations are themselves related" (Phillips 2001: 344). There is an "interpersonal" split at the center of the intrapersonal self. Kimura reminds us that ordinary intercourse with others, interpersonal *aïda*, involves the meeting of two subjective selves—two intrasubjective *aïdas*—each with a principle of otherness at the center of itself. "Encountering another subject means relating one's interior self to a completely other interior self, that is to say, to the absolutely unknown interior *aïda* of another, who himself also relates himself to himself in a radically strange interior world that remains inaccessible to any imaginary projection of the first subject" (Kimura 1992d: 43). If the schizophrenic, or pre-schizophrenic, individual has not developed her own subjective self, with its basis in interior otherness, the interpersonal relation will collapse into a confusion of what is self and what is non-self. Unable to recognize her own interior otherness as herself, the schizophrenic confuses it with the otherness of the other and concludes that her mind has been taken over by an alien source.

Kimura concludes this text, and I will conclude the chapter, with his recommendations for treatment of schizophrenic individuals. Aside from what can be accomplished with antipsychotic medications, he says that the only way the psychotherapist can help the patient develop a full self is through presenting himself or herself as a real person with an adequately developed sense of self, trying to reach the patient as subject to subject. "[T]he therapist becomes, above all, that authentic 'other' whom we have described as an internal contradiction between a finite individuality and a transcendental infinite, or again, as an internal difference between *mizukara* and *onozukara*" (Kimura 1992d: 45).

BIBLIOGRAPHY

Blankenburg W. (1971). *Der Verlust der Natürlichen Selbstverständlichkeit. Ein Beitrag zur Psychopathologie Symtomärmer Schizophrenien*. Stutgart: Ferdinand Enke Verlag.

Kimura B. (1992a). "Réflexion et soi chez le schizophrène." In B. Kimura, *Ecrits de Psychopathologie Phénoménologique*, pp. 117–128. Paris: Presses Universitaires de France.

Kimura B. (1992b). "Pathologie de l'immédiateté." In B. Kimura, *Ecrits de Psychopathologie Phénoménologique*, pp. 129–164. Paris: Presses Universitaires de France.

Kimura B. (1992c). "Temporalité de la schizophrénie." In B. Kimura, *Ecrits de Psychopathologie Phénoménologique*, pp. 65–92. Paris: Presses Universitaires de France.

Kimura B. (1992d). "Entre onozukara et mizukara: Pathologie de l'ego à partir d'un point de vue traditionnel japonais." In B. Kimura, *Ecrits de Psychopathologie Phénoménologique*, pp.35–47. Paris: Presses Universitaires de France.

Kimura B. (2001). "Cogito and I: A Bio-logical Approach." *Philosophy, Psychiatry, & Psychology* 8(4): 331–336.

Pélicier Y. (1992). "Autobiographie résumée de Kimura." In B. Kimura, *Ecrits de Psychopathologie Phénoménologique*, pp. 183–194. Paris: Presses Universitaires de France.

Phillips J. (2001). "Kimura Bin on Schizophrenia." *Philosophy, Psychiatry, & Psychology* 8(4): 343–346.

Sass L. (2001). "Self and World in Schizophrenia: Three Classic Approaches." *Philosophy, Psychiatry, & Psychology* 8(4): 251–270.

Zahavi D. (2001). "Schizophrenia and Self-awareness." *Philosophy, Psychiatry, & Psychology* 8(4): 339–341.

CHAPTER 21

....

WOLFGANG BLANKENBURG

....

MARTIN HEINZE

Biographical Sketch

WOLFGANG Blankenburg (b.1928, Bremen, Germany, d. 2002, Marburg, Germany) studied philosophy and psychology from 1947 and, from 1950, also medicine at the University of Freiburg, Germany. In 1956 he received his doctorate. The topic of his dissertation was the study of a patient with paranoid schizophrenia, using a Dasein-analytical approach that took its lead from psychoanalysis as well as from Heidegger's account of Dasein, or human existence. The schizophrenic condition remained a major focus of his future research. In 1957 he began internal medicine and psychosomatic training at Heidelberg University Hospital. Two years later, he became an assistant researcher, and in 1963 senior physician at the Psychiatric University Clinic in Freiburg. There he completed his habilitation thesis in 1967. In 1969 Blankenburg went back to the Psychiatric University Hospital in Heidelberg. After Walter von Baeyer's retirement, he took over the position of acting director of the clinic. From 1975 he was director of the Psychiatric Clinic I at the hospial Bremen-Ost. In 1979 he was appointed to the chair of psychiatry at the University of Marburg, a position he kept until his retirement in 1993. Blankenburg was a member of many national and international psychiatric and research societies and was invited to lecture around the world, having strong connections to Japan, Italy, France, and South America. He was appointed honorary member of the Berlin-based "Gesellschaft für Philosophie und Wissenschaften der Psyche" whose foundation and structure he helped to shape. He strongly supported this society's approach to understanding psychic phenomena out of the heterodisciplinarity of all scientific disciplines dealing with them, and to arguing that one's approach to such phenomena should be open-minded and never seen as completed. With his vast experience he became a spiritual rector for younger colleagues and an indispensable interlocutor. He was married to Ute Blankenburg, née Hägele, and had three children.

Blankenburg only published one monograph. He wrote more than 170 essays which are spread through anthologies, psychiatric journals, as well as sometimes remote journals in other fields. Thus the oeuvre is not easy to access. The publication of his most important essays in the edition by Martin Heinze (Blankenburg 2007, 2017) is helpful and includes a bibliography of all his writings. His monograph was translated into nearly all major languages, including Japanese and recently Chinese. Unfortunately this book was never translated into English, and neither were his essays. This task is still to be undertaken.

CONTRIBUTIONS TO PSYCHOPATHOLOGY

Blankenburg made an indispensable contribution to the advancement of not only phenomenological psychopathology, but also psychopathology in general. The period of his writing was shaped by the still existing vitality of the tradition of anthropological psychiatry on the one hand, and by the already incipient reform psychiatry and the second biological psychiatry on the other. In these conflicting fields he formed a psychiatric thought which includes a variety of mediations between the poles of empiricism and theory, clinical and social psychiatry, and philosophy and psychotherapeutic practice.

Blankenburg writes in the tradition of those psychiatrists for whom phenomenology constituted an essential basic science for psychopathology. In his earlier works he made use of phenomenology in order to create an understanding of schizophrenia not only as a dysfunctional set of symptoms but as a different way of personal existence (for his attitude toward phenomenology compare Wiggins 2001). The attitude toward valuing psychiatric conditions not only as negative constraints on a person's way of living but positively as belonging to the set of human possibilities still holds today and is reflected in contemporary discussions about empowerment and resilience.

In his later works he remained open to the methodological alternatives that could be provided by different schools of philosophy and expanded the philosophical, and later sociological, foundation for his own work. Unlike many other authors of anthropological psychiatry, he adopted not only theories of phenomenological provenance, but also critical theory and structuralism, giving the social reality of human beings its proper place. He also granted empiricism, in particular the specific patient-related practice, a larger space and used it as a critical corrective to older theoretical work that was more centered on the individual rather than on his or her relationships. Nevertheless, Blankenburg did remain a phenomenologist in his own sense: to regard all human experiences and actions as important and analyzing them in detail without being restrained by an overly narrow notion of phenomenology in a Heideggerian or even Husserlian sense.

Being devoted to openness meant that Blankenburg was repeatedly correcting his own concepts through the reception of empirical research and new conceptual ideas. This resulted in the wide range of topics that characterize his work. There are contributions to the relationship between philosophy and psychiatry, to the mind–body problem, to a critique of Daseinsanalysis, and not least to a dialectical approach fostering the idea of a psychopathology of freedom. The clinical essays deal with themes such as illusion, common sense, suffering, and the facilitation of therapy through taking over a future-II-perspective, that is, allowing a patient to view his life as it could be seen from his position in the future and thus opening a realm for change and activities.

Altogether, Blankenburg created a philosophically informed link between clinical psychiatry, anthropology, and sociology, which makes his texts of continuing interest to psychiatrists and philosophers alike. With his writings, Blankenburg proves himself to be a sustainable thinker, and a "quiet" one in the sense that he did not foster a general theory of psychopathology but remained open to diverse phenomena in all their details. He unfolds no dramatic thesis, but critically appropriates the best of the tradition and pursues the concrete and precise tasks of mediating theoretical knowledge and the practice of psychiatry and psychotherapy.

PSYCHIATRIC ANTHROPOLOGY

In his earliest writings, Blankenburg follows an approach adopted from previous authors of phenomenological psychiatry, especially Binswanger, Tellenbach, Boss, and Zutt: the deduction of general aspects of human existence or fundamental anthropological situations out of the analysis of individual cases. In particular, the phenomenon of delusion is a priority for him. One example of this is an essay on becoming independent of the content of a delusion, published in 1965. In this essay, Blankenburg summarizes delusion as "a possibility of a processual modification of the world-self-relation" (1965a: 139).[1] The subject of delusion, "chosen" by the patient, will be understandable from the analysis of his biography and life situation, but above all from the constitution of meaning which emerged for the individual patient within his biographical development and was converted through the disease process.

From the investigation of Daseinsanalysis in his dissertation grows a body of work, in which characteristic features of psychiatric disorders are developed out of individual case studies. Another text of the same year about the differential phenomenology of delusional perception is of significance, since contents of the special meaning of the abnormal delusional experience for the individual can be made concretely intelligible from the subject's biographical background. Thus, starting from the phenomena, interpretation succeeds. Here, phenomenology and hermeneutics are the tools for the psychopathologists (1965b). In another essay Blankenburg then defines what "anthropological" means in psychiatric science: The "anthropological" refers to both a human being as a research subject and at the same time to a method appropriate to study this subject. Pathological deviations should be understood in general not only along the line of "healing" and "wholeness" of the human condition, but positively out of the nature of the human being. Important here is the adjective "positive." Psychopathology would be understood in a much more superficial way if malfunction were only to be regarded negatively (1967).

For his own idea of psychopathology, Blankenburg uses the keyword "dialectical." In an essay from 1981 on the reach of the dialectical approach in psychiatry, he determines dialectic as dealing with the negative per se. At the same time, he also points out that there is something "ambivalent" in the basic constitution of human beings which can be grasped only with such large oppositions as body and soul or growth and decay. Thus, dialectical thinking is a method adequate for understanding a human being as subject. More than that, the methodological approach of dialectics also has practical meaning because in the broadest sense Blankenburg wants "every regular change of standpoint" to be understood out of a dialectical attitude "that allows us to systematically set aside limited horizons" (1981: 47).

---

[1] All quotations of Blankenburg are translated into English by the author.

The symptoms expressed in psychopathology become apparent only after being seen as possibilities of human existence. The point is to understand the reality of each individual disturbance, its history, and its developmental opportunities comprehensively. The methodology of individual case analysis as a basis for general understanding culminates in Blankenburg's habilitation thesis on schizophrenia simplex, his renowned book *Der Verlust der natürlichen Selbstverständlichkeit* (*The Loss of Natural Self-understandability*), published in 1971. That text presents a theory of schizophrenia that works out the positive character of each individual's world- and self-constitution which, for us, being mentally well, is self-evident but nonetheless means an active achievement, and thus can be lost. Studying psychosis teaches us to look behind such self-evident truths. Closely related to this book are Blankenburg's analysis of "common sense" (Blankenburg 1969). The phenomenon of so-called common sense is in no way naturally given. We need to study its deficits and loss in order to reach its nature, significance, and importance. These studies, inspired by individual clinical cases, are followed by essays that take a more accurate and defined view on psychiatric anthropology. When talking of the essential determinations of existence, it is important for the psychopathologist to find a measurement. Anthropology requires measurements, thought as proportions, and for this purpose initially uses spatial metaphors. Thus one can speak of the height and width of existence, as Binswanger does (Binswanger 1949). But Blankenburg stresses, leaving Binswanger behind, that phenomenological anthropology must go beyond the narrow focus on spatiality alone, reaching emotionality and temporality (Blankenburg 1974).

In close connection with these considerations is the theme of corporality. An exemplary text on the role of the body in psychiatry (Blankenburg 1982a) demonstrates the bodily dimension of human existence as being fundamental and inescapable. In addition to the physical presence given in the term body (*Körper*), the bodily or corporal dimension (*Leib*) contains the personal experience of a human being in terms of his existence, the way he feels and experiences, but also how he realizes his subjectivity in his lived world. Blankenburg lines up closely with phenomenological philosophy, and especially takes Husserl as a starting point of his considerations. As a result, for a variety of psychopathological symptoms, he discusses the proper bodily structure in which they are realized, and argues that without an analysis of these structures, references to symptoms remain abstract. In other texts, Blankenburg takes corporality or embodiment as the starting point for discussing the mind–body problem in general as it arises in psychiatry (1989a, 1996). For psychiatric theory this remains a necessary layer. Thinking corporality, informed, for example, by Merleau-Ponty, is part of the basic science of psychiatry, as much as referring to the spiritual aspects of existence. Both poles are mutually inseparable and dialectically mediated.

PSYCHIATRIC PRACTICE AND PSYCHOTHERAPY

Blankenburg stands between anthropological and Daseinsanalytical psychopathology on the one side, and dialectical philosophy on the other, the latter forming the basis of social psychiatric reforms in the 1970s. With this opening of the theoretical framework, he gave psychiatric anthropology a new opportunity at a time when it was neither fashionable nor regarded as scientifically important.

The practical orientation leads to a modified concept of psychopathology. In his text on basic problems of psychopathology (Blankenburg 1978), he explicates a modified object of psychopathology. First, he notes that psychopathology was caught in a fundamental crisis after the historical developments of both anthropological and social psychiatry. Blankenburg considers it necessary to redefine the object of psychopathology. In contrast to the traditional medical model of disease, which understands symptoms as evidence of objective disease processes and independent of human daily life and habits, a new psychopathology is formed by developing in terms of functioning and behavior. But this new approach is as reductive as objectivist medicine. Against this reference to behavior only, Blankenburg formulates a counter-thesis: The subject of psychopathology should not be deviant behavior but a variety of impairments of abilities to behave or of conduct. This, he claims, is something quite different. Abilities of conduct cannot altogether be subsumed under behavior. It is not about whether someone behaves one way or another, or about behavior as a finished product, but about degrees of freedom to produce whatever behavior. The psychopathological problem is not whether a person behaves in a derogative or unjustified manner, but whether he is able to behave in conformity to norms. The question is if there are abilities or not: "The psychopathologist must look behind the behavior itself to the underlying abilities of conduct and their limitations" (1978: 142). But even the reference to the abilities of conduct is not sufficient. It must be supplemented by the dimension of abilities to experience. Indeed, all experience will be mediated through behavior. Nevertheless, this does not deprive it of its independence. A general subsumption of experience cannot be justified and would lead to a considerable lessening of psychopathological knowledge. Taken together, the disturbances of the abilities to experience and to behave therefore constitute psychopathological findings.

Decisive for the psychopathologists are ultimately impairments of degrees of freedom which by no means must always adequately be reflected in a subject's feeling. These impairments could be understood methodologically most likely in the realm of a psychopathology of freedom, as has already been suggested by the French psychiatrist Ey who defined psychiatry as "la pathologie du sujet et de sa liberté [the pathology of the subject and of its freedom]" (Ey 1973: 1437). Freedom, for psychopathology, serves as an indispensable reference point. Should psychopathology give up this reference point it risks abandoning itself. The phenomenal range of degrees of freedom is nothing abstract, but corresponds to the everyday experience of psychiatrists: "What for theoretical reasoning is accessible at the best through speculation, for practical reasoning—which gains its right from everyday contact to patients—it is a quite differentiable fact modifying the contact itself" (1982b: 37).

Psychopathology is a science that describes limitations of abilities of patients in their concrete biographical situations. It plays out in the tension between autonomy and heteronomy. The restrictions of patients' freedom will be experienced as suffering. This suffering, in the first place, entitles psychotherapists to execute therapy in order to achieve modifications. Thus, the ethics of psychiatry and psychotherapy presupposes some idea of human freedom that is damaged in some particular case and then requires treatment. The notion of suffering with its practical relevance opens up psychiatric theory for sociology and social pathology. Blankenburg distinguishes primary and secondary psychological strain, in analogy to primary and secondary morbid gain (the latter arises only from the effects of a disorder and not by the disorder itself) and presents their appearances in the various psychiatric syndromes. The suffering of a patient must also be understood positively in terms of a call for modification. In psychotherapy, new options of existence have to be found in the face of suffering.

Techniques may be found, for example, from a compound of psychodynamic and existential perspectives, as Benedetti illustrated for the psychotherapy of schizophrenic patients (Benedetti 1983).

The Temporality and Creativity
of Human Beings

A third basic idea is specific to Blankenburg's view on psychopathology: psychopathology is not fixed, it is always developing. The interest of psychotherapists should not be exhausted only in reconstructing the genesis of a symptom. Rather, it is aimed at influencing the current living situation of the patient and his possibilities in the future. Blankenburg discusses temporality as being constitutive for therapy in his late text on the future-II-perspective in its importance for the development of the life-history of the patient (1989b). The grammatical form of future-II leads to a jump forward in which we perceive the open opportunities in the current situation. "Rather, we have to find a way from the imagined future back to the present and into the past" (1989b: 76). The genesis of the self from the future is at least equivalent to one from the past. This demands a change of theoretical perspective (against, e.g. psychoanalysis): "The human ego unfolds no less from the future" (1989b: 79). With such openness for future development, confidence is given back to the patient, which had been shaken by the psychopathological symptoms, and can be regained only in the perspectives of future possibilities.

The therapeutic work between patient and therapist is about enhancing degrees of freedom in the pursuit of life of the patient: "A main desideratum of current psychotherapy is—complementary to the analytical examination of the past—to develop therapies that increase not only 'freedom of' but 'freedom for'. An opening for the future as well as the issue of the maturation of existence [*Zeitigung des Daseins*] in different life situations is among the indispensable tasks of an anthropologically oriented psychotherapy" (1989b: 82). Human beings are characterized by that fact that they are developing from what will come to them in the future, whereas other natural processes can be attributed to what was previous. On a practical level, this results in an altered relationship between patient and therapist. A new layout of the world of the patient who was disturbed in his natural outlining of the world will be recognized as a positive achievement from which something new can develop. Psychotherapy takes the character of a permanent communicative contact and interaction; it is at the same time repetition and creating something new. The therapist is ready for constant interaction because he respects the particular existence of the patient as an opening up of something new, something to be created jointly.

The therapeutic action is understandable only if human existence is looked at from its temporality. A philosophical anthropology as the basic science for psychotherapy, and not only for psychopathology, has to be aware of temporality as an essential category. Blankenburg found this in philosophy, especially in the writings of Husserl and Bergson. With these, and later with Heidegger, temporality is not only one but the essential feature of human existence. This thinking was received from classical writings, especially those of Binswanger and Minkowski. The alterations of time-experience are discussed as the most significant psychopathological phenomena of endogenous depression and schizophrenic psychosis, and from there the general temporality of human existence is deduced.

For Blankenburg, in his later scientific oeuvre, the maturation of existence from a psychiatric point of view is the central theme. The difference between an objective, measurable time and the subjective quality of the maturation of existence is fundamental for the way a human being lives time. This way is often distorted in mental illness and is painfully perceived when the future is closed up or appears as a frozen eternity, lacking everything lively, as in depression; or, when time loses the character of opening up the realm of growing, as in schizophrenic psychosis. Suffering from a mental illness as such has an existential dimension that distinguishes it from suffering from physical illnesses. Psychotherapy has to relate to this fact and becomes the "recovery of the historicity of one's own life story" (1992: 144). Blankenburg always assigns concrete psychotherapeutic techniques to the often abstract appearance of psychopathological constructs with the aim that a patient may be free in terms of his future development and may regain authorship of his life's story.

With this demand concerning the therapeutic attitude Blankenburg completes his enhancements of psychiatric anthropology. Using phenomenology as his main starting point and lasting ideal, he gave phenomenological psychopathology a broader base, even merging in thoughts from competing schools of philosophy as, for example, dialectical philosophy. Thus he contributes to phenomenological psychopathology both as a protagonist and as a critic.

BIBLIOGRAPHY

Benedetti G. (1983). *Todeslandschaften der Seele. Psychopathologie, Psychodynamik und Psychotherapie der Schizophrenie.* Göttingen: Vandenhoeck & Ruprecht.

Binswanger L. (1949). *Henrik Ibsen und das Problem der Selbstrealisation in der Kunst.* Heidelberg: Schneider.

Blankenburg W. (1965a). "Die Verselbständigung eines Themas zum Wahn." *Jahrbuch für Psychologie, Psychotherapie und medizinische Anthropologie* 13: 137–164.

Blankenburg W. (1965b). "Zur Differentialphänomenologie der Wahnwahrnehmung." *Nervenarzt* 36: 285–298.

Blankenburg W. (1967). "Die anthropologische und daseinsanalytische Sicht des Wahns." *Studium Generale* 20: 639–650.

Blankenburg W. (1969). "Psychopathologie des "'Common Sense.'" *Confinia Psychiatrica* 12: 144–163.

Blankenburg W. (1971). *Der Verlust der natürlichen Selbstverständlichkeit. Ein Beitrag zur Psychopathologie der schizophrenen Alienation.* Freiburg, Stuttgart: Enke. New edn. (2012). Berlin: Parodos.

Blankenburg W. (1974). "Grundsätzliches zur Konzeption einer 'anthropologischen Proportion.'" *Zeitschrift für Klinische Psychologie und Psychotherapie* 22: 322–333.

Blankenburg W. (1978). "Grundlagenprobleme der Psychopathologie." *Nervenarzt* 42: 140–146.

Blankenburg W. (1981). "Wie weit reicht die dialektische Betrachtungsweise in der Psychiatrie?" *Zeitschrift für Klinische Psychologie und Psychotherapie* 29: 45–66.

Blankenburg W. (1982a). "Körper und Leib in der Psychiatrie." *Schweizerisches Archiv für Neurologie, Neurochirurgie und Psychiatrie* 131: 13–39.

Blankenburg W. (1982b). "Psychopathologie und psychiatrische Praxis." In W. Janzarik (ed.), *Psychopathologische Konzepte der Gegenwart*, pp. 33–46. Stuttgart: Enke.

Blankenburg W. (1989a). "Phänomenologie der Leiblichkeit als Grundlage für ein Verständnis der Leiberfahrung psychisch Kranker." *Daseinsanalyse* 6: 161–193.

Blankenburg W. (1989b). "Die Futur-II-Perspektive in ihrer Bedeutung für die Psychotherapie." In W. Blankenburg (ed.), *Biographie und Krankheit*, pp. 76–84. Stuttgart: Thieme.

Blankenburg W. (1992). "Zeitigung des Daseins in psychiatrischer Sicht." In E. Angehrn, H. Fink-Eitel, and G. Lohmann (eds.), *Dialektischer Negativismus. Michael Theunisssen zum 60. Geburtstag*, pp. 130–155. Frankfurt am Main: Suhrkamp.

Blankenburg W. (1993). "Die Psychiatrie und das Leib-Seele-Problem." In G. Danzer and S. Priebe (eds.), *Forschen und Denken—Wege in der Psychiatrie*, pp. 67–82. Würzburg: Königshausen & Neumann.

Blankenburg W. (1996). „Überlegungen zum „Selbst"-Bezug aus phänomenologisch-anthropologischer Sicht." In M. Heinze, C. Kupke, S. V. Pflanz, and K. Vogeley (eds.), *Psyche im Streit der Theorien*, pp. 95–122. Würzburg: Königshausen und Neumann.

Blankenburg W. (2007). "Selected Essays." In M. Heinze (ed.), *Psychopathologie des Unscheinbaren*, vol. I. Berlin: Parodos (including Blankenburg 1965a, 1969, 1974, 1981, 1982a, 1989b, and 1992, as quoted above).

Ey H. (1973). *Traité des hallucinations*. Paris: Masson et Cie.

Fuchs T. and Micali, S. (eds.) (2014). *Wolfgang Blankenburg—Psychiatrie und Phänomenologie*. Freiburg: Alber.

Wiggins O. P. (2001). "Husserlian Comments on Blankenburg's "'Psychopathology of Common Sense." *Philosophy, Psychiatry, and Psychology* 8: 327–329.

CHAPTER 22

....

FRANCO BASAGLIA

....

JOHN FOOT

INTRODUCTION

....

THE psychiatrist Franco Basaglia's theoretical ideas have been studied in some depth, while his work inside psychiatric hospitals has also attracted attention.[1] His ideas were derived from a series of phenomenological writers—Sartre, Husserl, Binswanger, Minkowski—and sociologists working on asylums and their history—in particular Erving Goffman (1961). He read Foucault but was more interested in his historical analysis than his theoretical approach. It was also clear that Basaglia was deeply affected in both his practice and theory by the work of Primo Levi on the concentration camp system (Bucciantini 2011). Basaglia traveled widely and studied psychiatric practice inside many asylums in France, Germany, the United Kingdom, and elsewhere. He also adapted his ideas and practice to the situations he found himself in after entering the asylum system in the early 1960s. In this chapter I will argue that it is Basaglia's practice (and its legacy) rather than his theory (although the two often worked together) that marks him out in terms of psychiatric history. In order to do this, I will first refer to Basaglia's life-story, before looking at his theoretical approach to psychiatry. I will then underline how these ideas were put into practice in the period between 1961 and Basaglia's death in 1980.

BIOGRAPHY

....

Franco Basaglia was born in 1924 in Venice. He opposed the ideas and policies of the fascist regime and as a teenager took part in anti-fascist activities. In November 1944, he was arrested and sent to Venice's prison with no sentence. The prison was a forbidding place,

....

[1] For Basaglia's theory, see Colucci and Di Vittorio (2001) and Tarabochia (2013). For his life and practical work, see Foot (2014a, 2014b, 2014c, 2015a, 2015b). Basaglia's writings (often written with his wife Franco Ongaro) were collected in two volumes after his death (Basaglia 1981, 1982).

with daily deportations and an area reserved for Jewish prisoners. It was run by the Nazis and Italian fascists.

Venice was liberated from fascism in April 1945. But Basaglia did not take up a career in politics after the war. He wanted to be an academic and saw himself as an intellectual. For eighteen years he studied medicine and psychiatry in Padua. He was, by all accounts, a brilliant student. He was also unorthodox, becoming interested in new forms of philosophical thought. It was at university and also through a seminar group organized by Pier Francesco Galli in Milan that Basaglia first came into contact with phenomenology—he read Sartre, Binswanger, Husserl, and Minkowski in this period and published academic papers. He also met like-minded younger psychiatrists in Milan and Venice.

Disenchanted with the career prospects offered by the university system, Basaglia became Director of the Psychiatric Hospital in a city called Gorizia in 1961. Gorizia was a Cold War town of just 40,000 people and with numerous soldiers, barracks, and check points. The iron curtain was just yards away. It was also right-wing, with a powerful Christian Democratic Party, a strong neo-fascist presence and a tiny left. Not, perhaps, the obvious place to start a revolution. In November 1961 Basaglia took charge of the asylum, with its 500 patients.

Gorizia's asylum was like many others in Italy—and in the world—at that time. It had the architecture and paraphernalia of containment that had been built up over years—cages for unruly patients, straitjackets, portable electro-shock machines, storerooms for personal belongings which were destined, in many cases, never to be collected. Like many asylums, the buildings were right on the edge of town.

Italy's asylums were regulated by two pre-fascist laws—from 1904 and 1908—which used the phrase "a danger to themselves and to others, or a public scandal" and the fascist criminal code of 1930, which gave patients a criminal record, despite the fact that they had committed no crime and been subject to no trial. There were treatments carried out inside Gorizia's asylum, but it would be difficult to describe them as therapeutic. Inmates were subject (without any choice) to electro-shock and insulin therapy, lobotomies as well as straightforward forms of torture.

Many settled down after a time into what Goffman called in 1961 the "career" of the "perfect patient"—passive, bowed down, accepting of the system, no longer in control of their bodily functions. Their days went by without any real sign of change. Time went on, but they had no sentence to serve. Forms of what would later be called *institutionalization* could be seen everywhere, amongst patients and nurses. Doctors came and went as they pleased, carrying out what R. D. Laing would call the "ceremonial of control" of the ward round before dedicating themselves to their private practices.[2]

Basaglia's first reaction to this place was one of disgust. It also reminded him of his own past and his time in prison (Foot 2015a: 5). Basaglia's mind was made up from the start. He would not accept the way this institution worked. It disgusted him. From the very beginning

---

[2] Basaglia also read Laing in the 1960s, and he was instrumental in the translation of Laing's work into Italian, as he was with Goffman. *The Divided Self* appeared as *L'Io diviso* in 1969 with Einaudi and a preface by Letizia Comba who was part of the Gorizia équipe. Franco Ongaro translated *Asylums*, which also appeared with Einaudi, in 1969, with an introduction by Franco and Franca Basaglia.

he believed that the institution was similar to a concentration camp. He saw it as a place of death, and later defined it as a dumping ground for the poor and the "deviant."[3]

But how could such a place be changed? There was no clear plan at the beginning, apart from a desire to change things. Basaglia's first act as Director was one of resistance. According to a colleague, "On his first day as director in Gorizia, when the head nurse passed him the list of people who had been tied up that night, he said, 'I'm not signing.'" (Foot 2015a: 18).

Basaglia's wide reading of phenomenological texts before arriving in the asylum provided him with a set of ideas and approaches which he then put into practice as Director of an institution. Other texts and experiences were added to the Basaglian "canon" during the 1960s and 1970s. I will now look at this theoretical and philosophical approach in more detail.

BASAGLIA'S THEORETICAL APPROACH

As a student and researcher in the 1950s, Basaglia had become interested in the way that Ludwig Binswanger applied phenomenological ideas to psychiatry. Like Binswanger (and later Laing) Basaglia argued that mental illness could be *understood*. "The condition of the schizophrenic," as Colucci and Di Vittorio put it, "as with that of a sane person, is a way of being in the world. It cannot be excluded from the world of reason as something that is incomprehensible. What is needed is an understanding of *its* reasons and a search for the keys to that understanding" (Colucci and Di Vittorio 2001: 30).

In his day-to-day dealings with patients Basaglia argued that all medical diagnosis should be "placed in brackets" (borrowing from his reading of Husserl) (Colucci and Di Vittorio 2001: 27–29; Sforza Tarabochia 2013: 106–111). This allowed Basaglia and his colleagues to free themselves of preconceived (medical and specialized) ideas and stereotypes about the people they were supposedly "treating." The doctor was no longer a doctor, and the patient was no longer a patient. A series of factors thus came into play beyond a fixed diagnosis—society, the institution itself, as well as personal histories.

Thus, following Husserl, for Basaglia it was important to build up a *relationship* with the people inside the asylum, to listen to their stories. Once again, this was not just a set of ideas—but very much part of daily practice in the Basaglian hospital. For this reason, as well, Basaglia demanded that his équipe were constantly present in the hospital, sometimes for days on end. The Basaglian revolution was about listening, talking, debating, and understanding. In doing so, the barriers created by technical education, white coats, and hierarchies were discarded or broken down. Intersubjective relationships were created (or attempted).

In one case, Basaglia and his first collaborator inside Gorizia, Antonio Slavich, spent four days and nights listening to the traumatic life-story of a patient called Mario Furlan, who had tried to commit suicide on various occasions. Furlan would go on to become one of the patient leaders of the movement inside the hospital. Basaglia did not just removes fences, gates, and barriers—as well as locks on doors—he encouraged the patients to take power.

---

[3] See his accounts in Basaglia 1968, 2000, and Basaglia and Ongaro 1971. Very little of Basaglia's work has been translated into English, although the best collection of his writings is available in English (Scheper-Hughes and Lovell 1987).

Fences were pulled down by the patients themselves. "We put the key in the door," Basaglia later said, "but they (the patients) needed to turn it" (Foot 2015a: 156). In 1965, hospital-wide patient meetings were introduced. Votes were taken and discussions ranged around a variety of issues, from the mundane to the profound.

BASAGLIA'S APPROACH IN PRACTICE

In the hospital itself, fighting against the logic of the institution, Basaglia needed allies. The vast majority of the nursing staff was against change, and the other medics were largely (and often violently) conservative. He decided to recruit like-minded friends and colleagues to create a group—or an "équipe" as it became known. Bit by bit, the balance of power in the hospital began to change. Soon, walls were knocked down and fences removed, the tying up of patients was discouraged and then phased out altogether, and some were even discharged as far as was possible under the 1904 legislation. Electro-shock therapy was reduced (although not phased out entirely). A patient newspaper was set up. A bar was opened in the grounds, as was a hairdresser. Patients got back their clothes, and their dignity. Men and women were allowed to mix together. Many were encouraged to find work, for which they were paid.

These *assemblee* would become the precursors of 1968. Hyper-democracy had been introduced in the heart of one of the most anti-democratic institutions imaginable. This was the overturning, the *negation*, the cultural revolution that Basaglia desired. By this time, he was also influenced by Maoist thought—and his reading of the cultural revolution in China. His aim was to destroy, as he wrote in 1964, the *whole* psychiatric hospital system. Such a radical change was, he argued, necessary and obvious.[4]

Basaglia's initial approach based on his readings of Binswanger and Husserl, amongst others, was continually modified and adapted to cope with the reality of the "total institution." Moreover, other radical texts began to circulate in Italy—and these were read by psychiatrists close to Basaglia. Michel Foucault's *History of Madness* provided, for Basaglia, a critique of reformist approaches to madness and historical context. R. D. Laing's *The Divided Self* (1960) (which saw what was called schizophrenia as understandable and even a rational reaction to the pressures of modernity) was a central text for Basaglia and his équipe (and the movement as a whole). It applied many of Basaglia's own ideas to psychiatric practice and the understanding of mental illness.

But Basaglia was also greatly influenced by sociological texts, above all Erving Goffmans's *Asylums*. Goffman's work—which was translated into Italian by Basaglia's wife and political ally, Franca Ongaro, and recommended for publication by the Basaglias to the Einaudi publishing house in Turin, was central to the movement's analysis of the asylum. Goffman, a Canadian sociologist who had spent two years on the Shetland island of Unst in the 1950s, had immersed himself within the reality of a huge psychiatric hospital in Washington DC for more than a year. His analysis of the reality of the asylums was cold, detached, and devastating. Asylums were "total institutions," which controlled every aspect of the lives of their

---

[4] For the idea of the "therapeutic community" and Basaglia's critique of it see (Foot 2015a: chapter 7).

inmates. The career of the asylum patient ended with complete submission to the system (Goffman 1961; Foucault 1965).[5]

Into this mix of texts and ideas should be added Primo Levi's *If this is a man* (1947). Basaglia had read this book as a young man and it had deeply influenced him. He saw the dehumanization described by Levi in Auschwitz as present in the asylum system, and he made constant comparisons between concentration camps and psychiatric hospitals. This was both an effective propaganda tool (the phrase Asylum = Concentration Camp was a powerful slogan during the 1960s and 1970s in Italy) and a reaction to the physical and moral state of many institutionalized patients within the asylum system. Levi provided Basaglia with a moral critique of the institution of which he was Director. His opposition to the asylum was never just technical, or philosophical—it was also moral and political.

Finally, Basaglia visited asylums that were undergoing change or had already introduced reforms, and applied some of these practices back in Italy. Sometimes, this was a simple matter of practice (as with the meetings he witnessed in the open hospital of Dingleton in Scotland in the 1960s). But there were also theoretical refinements that Basaglia added to his canon of texts, quotations, and baggage of ideas and methods. For example, he was highly critical of some aspects of the Dingleton hospital, arguing that there was a danger of creating a "nice" hospital—a reformist "golden cage"—which would be functional to the system's survival. Basaglia, instead, wanted to destroy the entire system.

By 1968 Gorizia was beginning to have national impact. Gorizia fed into and fed off the movements that exploded across Italy and the world in that year. This transformed asylum was a perfect fit for the ideas of that movement, especially in the early period of change. Italy's institutions were in dire need of serious reform—schools, the army, the Church, prisons, the universities. Doctors, soldiers, prisoners, priests, lecturers, and students all began to "overturn" their own institutions, and called for reform and real change. Gorizia represented the reality of somewhere that had already been transformed by a small, dedicated group of men and women. It became a model.

The Gorizian message reached the general public through the cultural industries. In March 1968, in another moment of perfect timing, a collective book was brought out by the prestigious Einaudi publishing house in Turin. The book was an account of what Basaglia called "the reality of an institution in transformation"—Gorizia. It contained the voices of patients as well as high theory and detailed accounts of debates. Its form, as well as its content, were deeply intertwined with 1968 and its aims.

The Negated Institution: Report from a Psychiatric Hospital was a publishing sensation. It flew off the shelves, and onto the shelves of every budding '68er. It was translated into French, German, Spanish, and Portuguese (but not into English).[6] Students turned up to see Gorizia in droves—and were followed by journalists, photographers, and politicians. Italy's health minister—the Socialist Luigi Mariotti—passed a reform in 1968 that softened the repressive nature of the asylum system. He was scathing about the hospitals he had seen and compared them to "German concentration camps, Dantesque chambers of hell" (Foot 2015a: 75). By 1968 Gorizia was influencing national law and policy.

---

[5] A different version of this Foucault text was published in Italy in 1963 (Foucault 1963).

[6] For this book and its history, see Foot (2015a: chapters 11 and 12).

In 1972, the Gorizia revolution came to an abrupt end. The doctors resigned en masse, claiming at the same time that all but fifty-one of the patients in the hospital were "better." They wrote an open letter, citing Frantz Fanon, to the Provincial Council. The psychiatrists claimed that: "Our presence in the psychiatric hospital, as well as being useless, is damaging for those patients . . . for whom we continue to represent, as psychiatrists, the justification of their internment." The radical doctors left, and normality returned to Gorizia's asylum. Basaglia's revolution moved on.

From Gorizia, the "Basaglians" spread out across Italy—taking over hospitals and psychiatric services in Arezzo, Venice, Ferrara, Pordenone, Udine, and elsewhere. Parallel movements were already in charge in places like Perugia and near Naples. In some places Basaglia was out-flanked on the left by Italian anti-psychiatrists who denied the very existence of mental illness, but still found work high up in the world of psychiatric hospitals. Many asylums remained entirely unreformed.

In the early 1970s Basaglia moved to a bigger city and a larger asylum, in Trieste—close to Gorizia—another Cold War town. When he got there he found another almost unchanged asylum—with familiar features such as cages, bars, and locked wards. Basaglia moved quickly, and he had, this time, full political support. Everything was easier now, and Trieste's asylum opened up to the city, just as the city moved toward the asylum.

In the 1970s, the Trieste asylum would become a magnet for radical psychiatrists. It was in Trieste that new mental health services were first created, beyond the asylum. Basaglia's liberation strategy was increasingly flamboyant. For example, on one occasion, patients were taken up in a chartered plane and flown over Venice—something that was denied to them by law.

The asylum in Trieste soon became a place of pilgrimage for psychiatrists and volunteers. In 1977 Basaglia held a press conference where he announced that the asylum in Trieste was, for all intents and purposes, no longer working as a psychiatric hospital. Across Italy, reformers and politicians began to push for change to the outdated laws governing mental health.

In 1978 the struggle that had started in Gorizia seventeen years earlier finally reached the parliamentary sphere—in Rome. A combination of circumstances had created a legislative vacuum, and in twenty days (without even going to a parliamentary vote) the so-called *Basaglia law* was passed. It is also known—more correctly—as Law 180. Everyone was in favor—apart from the small neo-fascist party. The law called for the closure of all psychiatric hospitals. In addition, no new asylums could be built. The asylum system was over. Psychiatric patients were given back their human and civil rights (within limits). They were patients like the other patients with "normal" illnesses in general hospitals, not a special breed.

The law was a compromise—something of which Basaglia was well aware. It was a victory, but only a partial one. It was a *beginning*, not an end. The next twenty years would see alternative services created right across Italy—day care centers, emergency wards, halfway houses, cooperatives. The vast majority of those 100,000 patients re-entered normal life. Some, quite simply, could not exist outside the asylum. This group was given a technical name—they were called "residuals." The strategy with regard to them was never explicitly spelled out but, in reality, the only thing to do was to wait for them to die.

This process of closure (and of opening up to society) was contradictory. There were suicides and murders. Families often had to take up the slack after hospitals were closed.

Regional differences were huge and the funding and quality of new services varied greatly across the country. Trieste, however, is still a model for psychiatric services post-asylum.

Franco Basaglia died in 1980, from a brain tumor. He was just fifty-six years old. He never had the chance to implement the law that took his name. Italy today has no asylums. It is no paradise, but that system is gone, and it was abolished not for reasons of cost, but for moral and political reasons. The "great internment" described by Foucault gave way, in the 1970s, to a "great liberation." Society absorbed most of the 100,000 inmates who had been kept inside these places. This process was forced on the system from a movement that acted from inside the institutions themselves, in a way that was unique in the Western world. Italy's asylums were closed down by the people who worked inside them. In doing so, these people abolished their own jobs. Today, Basaglia remains a household name in Italy (and not just there). He is still a hugely controversial figure who divides opinion. His legacy is also felt in many other countries, from the United Kingdom to Brazil to the Netherlands to Germany and his theory and practice are studied and discussed within many psychiatric contexts. There are ongoing debates about the effect of the reforms which took his name, and the history of the asylum system he helped to abolish.

BIBLIOGRAPHY

Basaglia F. (ed.). (1968). *L'istituzione negata: Rapporto da un ospedale psichiatrico*. Torino: Einaudi.

Basaglia F. (1981). *Scritti. I. 1953–1968. Dalla psichiatria fenomenologica all'esperienza di Gorizia*, ed. F. Ongaro Basaglia. Torino: Einaudi.

Basaglia F. (1982). *Scritti. II. 1968–1980. Dall'apertura del manicomio alla nuova legge sull'assistenza psichiatrica*, ed. F. Ongaro Basaglia. Torino: Einaudi.

Basaglia F. (2000). *Le conferenze brasiliane*. Milano: Raffaello Cortina Editore.

Basaglia F. and Basaglia Ongaro F. (1971). *La maggioranza deviante. L'ideologia del controllo sociale totale*. Torino: Einaudi.

Bucciantini M. (2011). *Esperimento Auschwitz*. Torino: Einaudi.

Colucci M. and Di Vittorio P. (2001). *Franco Basaglia*. Milano: Bruno Mondadori.

Foot J. (2014a). *La repubblica dei matti. Franco Basaglia e la psichiatria radicale in Italia*. Milan: Feltrinelli.

Foot J. (2014b). "Franco Basaglia and the Radical Psychiatry Movement in Italy, 1961–78." *Critical and Radical Social Work* 2: 235–249.

Foot J. (2014c). "Television Documentary, History and Memory. An Analysis of Sergio Zavoli's *The Gardens of Abel* (1969)." *Journal of Modern Italian Studies* 19: 603–624.

Foot J. (2014d). "Gli esperimenti di Kingsley Hall e Villa 21 a Londra negli anni Sessanta. Mito, memoria e storia." *Memoria e Storia* 47: 65–82.

Foot J. (2015a). *The Man Who Closed the Asylums. Franco Basaglia and the Revolution in Mental Health Care*. London: Verso.

Foot J. (2015b). "Photography and Radical Psychiatry in Italy in the 1960s: The Case of the Photobook *Morire di Classe* (1969)." *History of Psychiatry* 26: 19–35.

Foucault M. (1963). *Storia della follia nell'età classica*. Milano: Rizzoli.

Foucault M. (1965). *Madness and Civilization: A History of Insanity in the Age of Reason*. New York: Pantheon.

Goffman E. (1961). *Asylums. Essays on the Social Situations of Mental Patients and Other Inmates*. New York: Anchor Books.

Goffman E. (1969). *Asylums: le istituzioni totali: la condizione sociale dei malati di mente e di altri internati*, trans. F. Ongaro. Turin: Einaudi.

Laing R. D. (1960). *The Divided Self. An Existential Study in Sanity and Madness*. Harmondsworth: Penguin.

Levi P. (1947). *Se questo è un uomo*. Torino: De Silva.

Scheper-Hughes N. and Lovell A. (eds.) (1987). *Psychiatry Inside Out. Selected Writings of Franco Basaglia*. New York: Columbia University Press.

Tarabochia A. S. (2013). *Psychiatry, Subjectivity, Community. Franco Basaglia and Biopolitics*. Oxford: Peter Lang.

CHAPTER 23

···

FRANTZ FANON

···

LEWIS R. GORDON

INTRODUCTION: PHILOSOPHER, PHYSICIAN, AND MORE

···

FRANTZ Fanon (1925–1961) was a revolutionary philosopher, psychiatrist, playwright, poet, and essayist. This chapter will focus on two of these elements with the others borne in mind.

Although he was an extraordinary psychiatrist, today Fanon is remembered primarily for his work as a philosopher. Physicians who are also remembered as philosophers are not unusual in the history of philosophy. Several noteworthy examples are Imhotep (c. 2667–2600 BCE), Lady Presehet (c. 2500 BCE–?), Aristotle (384 BCE–322 BCE), Ge Hong (283–343 or 363), Tao Hongjing (456–536), John Locke (1632–1704), Anton Wilhelm Africanus Amo (c. 1703–c. 1759), Zhang Xichun (1860–1933), William James (1842–1910), and Karl Jaspers (1883–1969).

Born on the French Caribbean colony (now department) of Martinique, Fanon was affectionately called "Bergson" in his youth. Henri Bergson was the great philosopher and Nobel Laureate who in his time stood for philosophy as Einstein did for physics. A determined humanist dedicated to fighting against degradation and injustice, Fanon was a teenage volunteer in the French resistance against the Nazis in the Second World War and did the same throughout his thirties against the French in the Algerian War of Independence. His training as a soldier, forensic and clinical psychiatrist, and as a philosopher who studied at the University of Lyon with the great phenomenologist Maurice Merleau-Ponty made him a formidable freedom fighter and revolutionary thinker who inspired many fighting for liberation across the then Third World. He died on December 6, 1961 in Bethesda, Maryland, USA, while seeking treatment for leukemia.

Studies and use of Fanon's thought are plentiful across the humanities and social sciences, and, as Nigel Gibson and Roberto Beneduce's *Frantz Fanon, Psychiatry, and Politics* attests, the life sciences (Gibson and Beneduce 2017; see also Desai 2014). Additionally, there is no short supply of biographies of this extraordinarily charismatic thinker (e.g. Bulhan 1985; Cherki 2000; Ehlen 2000; Gordon 2015).

Fanon's contributions to philosophy are many. He was a philosopher who transcended "disciplinary decadence," where intellectuals attempt to reduce reality to their disciplines often through fetishizing their methods. Going beyond that requires a "teleological sus-pension of disciplinarity," where one is willing to suspend one's methods for the sake of de-veloping a sober relationship with reality (Gordon 2006). Fanon saw clearly the struggle of human beings to know and to understand, and he was sensitive to the dangers of forgetting the cultivation of human relationships in practices of social transformation and running institutions.

THEORIZING ANTI-DEHUMANIZATION
UNDER COLONIAL CONDITIONS

The pressing problem at hand, which for Fanon was *dehumanization*, brought him in con-versation with a variety of revolutionary humanist traditions. As he put it, colonialism and the Euromodern world committed a crime against humanity. He thus addressed in his writings, clinical practice, and political work, fundamentally, (1) what it means to be human, (2) challenges of dignity and freedom, and (3) the critical problem of reason—the *sine qua non* of philosophy—being deployed in the interests of human degradation.

The first, germane to the phenomenological study of psychopathology, contributes to phil-osophical anthropology and the constellation of disciplines known as the human sciences. The second speaks to philosophy of liberation, revolutionary social change, and concerns of normative life. The third, however, brings Fanon into debates in much of Euromodern phi-losophy since the thought of the eighteenth-century German philosopher Immanuel Kant and the forms of transcendental argumentation that flowed from his monumental philo-sophical writings.

Transcendental idealism, which Kant also called critical philosophy in his *Prolegomena to Any Future Metaphysics* (1783), explores the conditions of possibility for any idea, any thought, by which reality could be made intelligible. Many proponents and critics of Kant are indebted to this turn. The former set attempts to expand what those conditions are. For instance, whole areas of philosophy have emerged from the idea that one cannot think, the-orize, or philosophize outside of consciousness, language, systems of signs and symbols, or culture (Cassirer 1944; Cornell and Panfillio 2010; Gordon and Gordon 2009). Critics of this view often offer examples of moments of unthinkable breakdowns of the same set of conditions, and they often raise either existential examples of rejecting these or, more nihilistically, the futility of doing so under the weight of powerful, colonizing forces. Critics of the latter often insist that these forces *are* transcendental conditions for such breakdowns (for discussion of both, see Gordon 2018; Rocchi 2018; Thomas 2018). The debates, in short, continue.

Fanon, however, stood both in, and outside of, those conflicts. He brought to them a cen-tral question: What is the impact of colonialism and racism on the conditions of possibility celebrated or rejected on either side of these approaches?

The question was already there, in his heart, from his youth when he realized his reluc-tance to separate people from their embodied existence. Even a cadaver, about which he wrote in *Peau noire, masques blancs* (*Black Skin, White Masks*), was for him deserving of dignity and respect (Fanon 1952). His accepted doctoral thesis (available in Fanon 2016) and several of his essays on psychiatric care are devoted to the importance of always addressing the Other, even when incapacitated by an illness such as Friedreich's ataxia, for the most part socially dead, or physically deceased, as a human being.

Whatever reality may be, the human being, for Fanon, is a relationship of introducing to it a constellation of valuable norms such as dignity, freedom, and truth. He was a critic of capitalism, which he understood as an effort to eliminate any vestige of human relationships in markets. "The market," after all, is an abstraction imposed on the creative ways in which human beings actually exchange or trade in the cultivation of what human beings produce. This is an argument throughout the course of Fanon's career, which he shared with his postdoctoral mentor François Tosquelles, founder of the school of institutional therapy at Saint Alban: it is central to place ourselves in a human and humane relationship with human institutions (Tosquelles 2012).

So let us begin with Fanon's philosophical anthropology and his contribution to philosophy of human science through which his thought on psychopathology emerges.

FACING PSYCHOPATHOLOGY THROUGH INTERROGATING FAILURE

In *Black Skin, White Masks*, a phenomenological dimension of his thought comes to the fore when he methodically demonstrates the failures emerging from any human science or social system attempting to universalize itself under colonial conditions. In philosophical language, such disciplines and societies attempt to be "ontological," absolute, or, simply, what must be. If they were so, they should, then, "work," so to speak, when applied to the study, therapeutic treatment, and governing of people that Euromodern society attempted to dehumanize. In each chapter, Fanon shows layers of failure as the naïve black or colonized protagonist—in phenomenological language, the black steeped in the natural attitude—invests in a system designed for his or her proverbial slaughter.

In his analysis, Fanon joins thinkers such as the Haitian anthropologist, jurist, and philosopher Anténor Firmin and the African-American historian, philosopher, and sociologist W. E. B. Du Bois on the insight of human agency struggling under conditions of double consciousness. The latter refers to black people's experience of how anti-black societies see them as less-than and at times not human. He conjoins such thought with those of Karl Jaspers, Merleau-Ponty, and many other thinkers who share his conviction of the importance of examining what emerges between ontogenetic and phylogenetic explanations—namely, socially produced and experientially lived or meaningful reality.

Announcing at the outset that method must also be held suspect, because colonization achieves its hegemony also at methodological levels, Fanon frees his inquiry of the natural colonized attitude through disarming its legitimacy and ontological status. This act is one of suspension or bracketing, so to speak, without the presupposition of having to do so. Had he announced it as such a methodological move, he would not also have placed phenomenology under critique. This is an ironic movement despite its existential and decolonizing impetus, since, as is well known among students of Husserlian phenomenology, it is a similar impetus that led to transcendental phenomenology as an interrogation of conditions of intelligibility.

Fanon also inaugurated his inquiry through a series of ironic movements. He already places himself in an unusual circumstance since his naïve subject is one who is often talked *about* instead of, in a word, asked. That he is conducting the study raises the question of his status, as well, of investigator. Here, at least methodologically, there is irony. The forensic psychiatrist is, after all, also an investigator. He is in effect conducting an autopsy of a living phenomenon. The inquiry, however, includes forensic psychiatry, in addition to clinical psychiatry, as human science, which means the legitimacy of the forensic stance must also be questioned. The *relationship* to the inquiry is thus directed or, in phenomenological language, *intentional*. This creates an unusual relationship to the naïve subject of the inquiry and the investigator, as they are ultimately one. They diverge, however, at the level of purpose. One is invested in the possibility of the system. The other cannot presume its legitimacy. Let's turn to the first.

The diminutive "black," Fanon shows, blocks paths to public recognition, private affirmations of intimacy, and psychic value. That black is a melancholic being. This is because the black attempts to fit into a system whose legitimacy depends on black absence. It is akin to an insight Fanon realized from some of his "clients" who sought treatment for his or her mental maledictions. Fanon was careful to differentiate "patients" from "clients." A patient is ill; a client is not necessarily so. Some people seek his help because they are having difficulty adjusting to the world in which they are attempting to live. To declare such people "patients" demands a commitment to alleviate their misery. To fix such patients, when they are colonized and racialized peoples, requires making them "happy" living under colonialism, racism, and other forms of degradation. Being at home in such a world is, for Fanon, destructive and obscene.

Fanon showed his clients that their maladjustment to such systems, their anger or consternation, meant they were in fact mentally healthy. This stimulated in many of them a critical reflection: They are not "the problem"; their society, and its concomitant disciplinary practices of rationalization that make it supposedly "normal" to dehumanize them, is the problem. This realization transforms such "blacks," Fanon ultimately argued, into "Blacks."

The Black is an agent of history. Whereas the black cannot imagine a legitimate future with blacks in it, the Black questions any conception of the future premised on her or his disappearance. Such an agent is able to act, to be what Fanon calls "actional." Fanon approaches the naïve black through resources of indirection. He demonstrates failures of language, where even the mastery of the colonial language constitutes an assault on it. As language is quintessentially public, his naïve black flees to the bosom of love only to discover that the price of evasive love is affirmation of self-degradation, since the demand is for, through love, black erasure. Such love is an expression of anti-black racism. Fleeing further into the life of dreams, the free reign of the symbolic collapses into the literal. Like the reputed legendary remark about Freud's cigar, the guns in the dreams of conquered subjects *are guns*. Leaping out as opposition, another possibility is the embrace of the irrational: Become the opposite of all things white. The problem there, however, is that of reaction. Whiteness, which signified death in Fanon's plays and letters, set the conditions to which the black responds. Closed in, lost of action, he is frozen and, in Fanon's words at the conclusion of the fifth chapter of *Black Skin, White Masks*, "without responsibility, straddling Nothingness and Infinity, I began *to weep*" (1952: 114; my translation and emphasis).

The indirect path to this moment of catharsis paves the way for what the naïve black couldn't face at the beginning. The system offers no coherent notion of black normality. The black *is* pathological and lives in the realm of psychopathology in relation to the white—here understood as the human sciences as offered under colonial hegemony—world. To be "well adjusted" is to accept the first-stage double-conscious formulations of the black self. It is to be what that world wants blacks to be, which is, when examined from the standpoint of what it means to be a human being with respect and dignity, abnormal. That black becomes, under stereotypic notions of black "authenticity," the investment of all negative social forces. The black who transcends all that is called "an exception," and, as everyone knows, the exception is not the norm. Even worse, that black is sometimes dubbed an honorary white, an *almost white*, as Fanon concluded at the end of the first chapter of *Black Skin, White Masks*. Or, more to the point, that black, in not manifesting social pathologies or imitating whites, is simply unnatural. In either direction, then, abnormality lurks.

INSIGHTS ON MEANING, REASON, AND DIALECTICS

Fanon showed that so long as one ignores the intervening forces of the social world affected by colonialism and racism, one would be living a lie of false universality. This observation leads to several important philosophical insights.

The first is phenomenological, which addresses the constellation of meanings emerging from our relationships with lived reality—that is, consciousness *of* whatever can be experienced or known. This addresses a concern of philosophy of social science: namely, the problem of "objective social meaning."

No social science is possible without being able to offer what is "normal" and "typical." Fanon showed how the logic of how women and men should behave according to expected norms of the social sciences collapsed whenever race and racism were at work. Proponents of the universality of these sciences would argue that proves something is wrong with race. Fanon argued, however, that, second, such conclusions ignore reality through not asking whether there were flaws in the presumed completeness or scope of such sciences. Couldn't it be that race does not work because, as he argued throughout *Black Skin, White Masks*, there is something in it for which those sciences lack an account? (See also Gordon 2015.)

In one sweep, Fanon puts the issue at center through his poetic formulation of, third, reason walking out whenever the black or the Black walks into the room: "I became disillusioned. That victory played cat and mouse; it mocked me. . . . When I was there, it [reason] was not; when it was there, I was no longer" (1952: 96; my translation). The problem emerges from what we could call "unreasonable reason." How does a philosopher address any form of reason that takes flight when the lover of wisdom's embodiment is black? To force such reason into submission would be a form of "violence." Fanon, thus, raised the problem of having to reason with unreasonable reason *reasonably*.

This problem of "unreasonable reason," which every group nearly crushed beneath the heels of Euromodern colonialism has experienced, raises, fourth, radical problems of justification. If reason is jeopardized, what hope is there for practices of justification? Is justification, in a word, "justified"?

Fanon's radical critique pertains to all forms of reasoning. His position on many proponents of dialectical thinking in his day, for instance, was that they often failed to be dialectical. For example, he pointed out Sartre's enthusiasm for Negritude, which Sartre formulated as a creative black "anti-racist racism," would galvanize blacks for incorporation into the universal working-class struggle. Such absorption, Fanon pointed out, was reclamation of white universality. It was also, and more philosophically rich, a form of anti-dialectical avowed dialectics:

> For once, that born Hegelian had forgotten that consciousness has to lose itself in the night of the absolute, the only condition to attain to consciousness of the self. In opposition to rationalism, he summoned the negative side, but he forgot that this negativity draws its worth from an almost substantive absoluteness. A consciousness committed to experience is ignorant, has to be ignorant, of the essences and the determinations of its being. (1952: 108; my translation)

The problem with many avowed dialectical forms of thought is that they are formulaic: thesis, antithesis, synthesis. That's just not, Fanon objected, how the world works. Failure to understand led, and continues to lead, to the misunderstanding of what was going on beneath many naïve efforts at theory throughout Euromodernity.

A properly dialectical argument first identifies the imposition of contraries, which are both simultaneously universal. If only whites are human, then no other kinds of people are human. Both are universal claims. Euromodern colonialism and its accompanying philosophical anthropology of racism attempted to build, in its many efforts at apartheid or separation, the notion of people who are contraries. If there are human beings who are not whites, then the claim, "Only whites are human," must be false. One could also point to some whites not being human. For example, designated white at birth but kept away from the human world, a feral white child could become a feral, biologically mature creature but not properly a human being.

The error of some dialecticians is that they think that pointing to a contradiction would automatically lead to a linear movement. Fanon, however, showed, not only in *Black Skin, White Masks* but also in his other books (Fanon 1975, 1979), especially *Les Damnés de la terre* (1961) (*The Damned of the Earth*) (available in English translation as *The Wretched of the Earth*), that demonstrating as particular what was previously thought to be universal opens the door to many possibilities (Fanon 1991). Dialectical thinking is *open*.

The openness of thought is relational, which means Fanon, fifth, brings together his phenomenological, forensic, and poetic critical resources with dialectical thinking. The political theorist Jane Anna Gordon calls this "creolizing theory" (Gordon 2014), which is appropriate not only given how Fanon learned to live and think in the Caribbean but also because of what disavowed thinkers have had to do throughout Euromodernity. Never being accepted as "pure" exemplars of any kind of thought—because of the reason that walks out when they walked into the room—many African Diasporic philosophers and physicians had to point out the fallacy of a world premised on racial groups as contraries. It is impossible *to interact*, however, without generating contradictions. Even light is unintelligible without interaction with darkness to bring distinction to appearance.

Fanon the decolonizing thinker thus brings to metacritical levels the philosophical evaluation of thinking. In doing so, he also raises, as we have seen, the problem of the colonization of knowledge and thought and the task of their decolonization—in short, the decolonization of science and philosophy. Nelson Maldonado-Torres calls this Fanon's "decolonial reduction" (Maldonado-Torres 2008). I prefer to call it "Fanonian phenomenology" through which, as his discussion of failure attests, "Fanonian psychoanalysis" also comes to the fore. This movement brings him in conversations with the supposed "greats," since its connection to those ancient philosopher physicians of Kmt (pre-Greco, Latin, and Arabic Egypt), as well as the Athenian gadfly Socrates, is evident. For they, too, were concerned with whether thought and wisdom were in fact dominated by idols.

CONCLUDING OTHER OBSERVATIONS

There are many concrete philosophical observations from Fanon's thought. The first is that if human phenomena are dialectical, existential, and phenomenological, that means their possibilities are open. This means that institutions such as states and ideas such as "sovereignty" and "citizenship" and relationships such as "power" and "community" need not be locked into what their critics have lamented throughout their history. Against anti-statists, Fanon argued that states are and will be what people make them. Similar to the Swiss philosopher, musical composer, and novelist Jean-Jacques Rousseau, who saw sovereignty in a "general will," Fanon saw it as the manifestation of agency and the creative potential of people, which in *The Damned of the Earth* (1961) he called "national consciousness."

Fanon also raised important challenges for the study of ethics, which, in phenomenological psychopathological terms, requires a healthy relationship with others. Colonialism and racism attempt to foreclose such, as we have seen, because of the logic of contraries (*all* versus *none*), against others who are not, for example, white. Thus whites supposedly live in a world of ethics and morals among each other. If they regard blacks and other groups of color as neither selves nor others, and the institutions of power are used to preserve that separation, the result would be people in a "zone of non-being" or a non-place in which ethical and moral relations do not apply. Under such conditions, there isn't accountability for harm done to people in such netherworlds, for "harm" properly happens against those to whom one is accountable.

Those living in such zones do, however, experience selfhood and otherness in relation to each other. They also look at those who dominate them as "others" in such asymmetrical societies. Now the problem unfolds.

To break through the vertical asymmetry and "appear" to those "above" would be a violation of what is presumed justified place of exclusion. As with reason taking flight, so, too, does ethics. Such systems make it unethical and immoral for racially subordinated people to appear. They are governed by a condition of presumed legitimate invisibility. Such societies thus have systems of justice that, from the perspective of those below, depend on injustice. As with unreasonable reason, there is unjust justice. Put concretely, the struggle against a contrarian practice such as racism is not a fight against otherness. An "other" is at least an ethical subject. It is a fight to break vertical barriers.

Colonialism and racism also created the colonization of normative life, which affects psychological wellbeing. Presumed just, changing such systems become acts of injustice and, tragically, violence. This is what Fanon meant when, in the first chapter of *The Damned of the Earth*, he declared that decolonization is always violent. Fanon, however, detested violence. He faced, then, a conundrum. To do nothing in such societies would require maintaining violence and injustice as the embodiments of justice. He thus argued, for the sake of anti-violence, accepting the responsibility for appearances of violence in unjust societies locked in false universalities of their intrinsic justice. The tragedy of this dilemma is brought to the fore in Fanon's case studies of anti-colonial violence and its mental disorders. The agents of violence on whom he focused are colonized subjects fighting for their liberation. In each instance, he studies the after-life of acts of violence, the trauma they bear. Trapped in such, Fanon argues, such subjects would haunt the future with the psychopathology of national trauma.

There is much more to be said about the nuance of Fanon's phenomenological reflections on psychopathology and its relation to concerns of social change, but I would like to conclude with an observation from this question of placing human institutions into human relationships instead of remaining in the grip of dehumanizing norms. At the end of *The Damned of the Earth*, Fanon prescribed setting afoot a "new humanity," which is my preferred term instead of the "new man" familiar to many of his readers. Fanon creatively transformed a powerful insight from the German philosopher and classical philologist Friedrich Nietzsche, who argued against what he called "the last man" and advocated human flourishing in the form of his proscribed "overman"—man, that is, who has gotten over instead of being full of himself.

Fanon creatively extended this observation to the societal level, where the last man's analogue is "the last nation" or "last country" or "last state." Such a nation, country, or state is invested in negative dynamics of power and values such as colonialism, class exploitation, racism, and xenophobia. This list is far from exhaustive. Such societies regard a world in which they don't dominate others to be the equivalent of *the end of the world*. We could call such societal psychopathology immaturity. A mature society, however, regards itself as living among others and thus achieves the "over nation," "over country," or "over state"—that is, institutions that have gotten over themselves. Fanon in effect transforms concerns of global social justice into those also of global social health and the creative possibilities of ideas and ways of living yet to come.

BIBLIOGRAPHY

Bulhan H. A. (1985). *Frantz Fanon and the Psychology of Oppression*. New York: Plenum.

Cassirer E. (1944). *An Essay on Man*. New Haven: Yale University Press.

Cherki A. (2000). *Frantz Fanon: Portrait*. Paris: Éditions du Seuil.

Cornell D. and Panfillio K. (2010). *Symbolic Forms for a New Humanity: Cultural and Racial Configurations of Critical Theory*. New York: Fordham University Press.

Desai M. (2014). "Psychology, the Psychological, and Critical Praxis: A Phenomenologist Reads Frantz Fanon." *Theory and Psychology* 24: 62–63.

Ehlen P. (2000). *Frantz Fanon: A Spiritual Biography*. New York: Crossroads.

Fanon F. (1952). *Peau noire, masques blancs*. Paris: Éditions du Seuil.

Fanon F. (1975). *Sociologie d'une révolution: l'an V de la révolution algérienne*, 2nd edn. [1959]. Paris: François Maspero.

Fanon F. (1979). *Pour la revolution africaine: écrits politiques*. Paris: François Maspero.

Fanon F. (1991). *Les Damnés de la terre* [1961]. Préface de Jean-Paul Sartre. Paris: François Maspero éditeur S.A.R.L./Paris: Éditions Gallimard.

Fanon F. (2016). *Frantz Fanon: Écrits sur l'aliénation et la liberté*, eds. Jean Khalfa and Robert Young. Paris: Éditions la découverte.

Gibson N. C. and Beneduce R. (2017). *Frantz Fanon, Psychiatry, and Politics*. London: Rowman & Littlefield International.

Gordon J. A. (2014). *Creolizing Political Theory: Reading Rousseau through Fanon*. New York: Fordham University Press.

Gordon J. A. and Gordon L. R. (2009). *Of Divine Warning: Reading Disaster in the Modern Age*. New York: Routledge.

Gordon L. R. (2006). *Disciplinary Decadence: Living Thought in Trying Times*. London: Routledge.

Gordon L. R. (2015). *What Fanon Said: A Philosophical Introduction to His Life and Thought*. New York: Fordham University Press.

Gordon L. R. (2018). "Thoughts on Afropessimism." *Contemporary Political Theory* 17: 105–112.

Kant I. (1783). *Prolegomena zu einer jeden künftigen Metaphysik, die als Wissenschaft wird auftreten können. Erstdruck: Riga* (Hartknoch).

Maldonado-Torres N. (2008). *Against War!: Views from the Underside of Modernity*. Durham: Duke University Press.

Rocchi J.-P. (2018). *The Desiring Modes of Being Black*. London: Rowman & Littlefield International.

Thomas G. (2018). "Afro-Blue Notes: The Death of Afro-pessimism (2.0)?" *Theory & Event* 21: 282–317.

Tosquelles F. (2012). "Frantz Fanon à Saint-Alban." In La Fondation Frantz-Fanon (ed.), *Frantz Fanon: Par les textes de l'époque*, pp. 75–89. Paris: Les Petit Matins.

CHAPTER 24

R. D. LAING

ALLAN BEVERIDGE

INTRODUCTION

THE Scottish psychiatrist, Ronald David Laing (1927–89) enjoyed international fame in the 1960s and became a counter-culture icon as a result of his radical pronouncements about psychiatry and the nature of madness. His subsequent fall from grace has tended to obscure the serious intention of his work, particularly his early work in which he drew on existential philosophy and phenomenology to depict disturbed mental states (Beveridge 2011). His first and arguably best book *The Divided Self* attempted to explain schizoid states and schizophrenia (Laing 1960a). At the time it was one of the most accessible books in English on the subject of phenomenology. Many of the classic European texts had not been translated and those that had been, for example, the selections in *Existence: A New Dimension in Psychiatry and Psychology* were often turgid and incomprehensible (May, Angel, and Ellenberger 1958). Laing had read many of the original texts in German and French. He met émigré doctors and analysts fleeing to Scotland from Nazi Europe, several of whom were well-versed in existential philosophy and knew the major contemporary philosophers personally. For example, Laing's mentor, the neurosurgeon, Joe Schorstein was acquainted with Martin Buber, Martin Heidegger, and Karl Jaspers. In addition, Glasgow University was a leading center for European existential philosophy and phenomenology at the time Laing was a medical student. John MacQuarrie, a lecturer in the theology department, co-translated Heidegger's *Being and Time* and also produced an excellent book-length guide to existentialism (MacQuarrie 1973). As a junior doctor in Glasgow, Laing was part of the circle of thinkers who met regularly to discuss continental philosophy. During this period he was producing early drafts of *The Divided Self*, which he read to the group. Given this background, then, Laing was ideally equipped to write on the subject of existential philosophy, phenomenology, and psychiatry.

This chapter will focus on *The Divided Self*. In this book Laing drew on his wide reading in philosophy and literature, but also on his clinical experiences in Glasgow hospitals and in the Army. He also drew on psychoanalytic thinking, particularly object relations theory.

LAING AND THE STANDARD
PSYCHIATRIC INTERVIEW

In a famous set-piece in *The Divided Self*, Laing contrasts the standard psychiatric interview technique as exemplified by Emil Kraepelin with what he calls the "existential-phenomenological construction." He quotes Kraepelin's account of his interview with a patient in front of a class of students. Kraepelin begins:

> The patient I will show you today has almost to be carried into the room, as he walks in a straddling fashion on the outside of his feet. On coming in, he throws off his slippers, sings a hymn loudly, and then cries twice (in English), "My father, my real father!" ... The patient sits with his eyes shut, and pays no attention to his surroundings. He does not look up even when he is spoken to, but he answers in a low voice, and gradually screaming louder and louder. When asked where he is, he says, "You want to know that too? I tell you who is being measured and is measured and shall be measured ..." When asked his name, he screams, "What is your name?" ...
>
> (Laing 1960a: 29–30)

Kraepelin considers that the patient is "inaccessible." He concludes that the patient had not provided a single piece of useful information and that his talk bears no relation to the context of the interview. Laing objects to this construction of the exchange and maintains that the patient is making a meaningful comment on his situation, albeit in a coded manner. Laing suggests that the patient is actually protesting about being paraded in front of students and that he is parodying the inquisitorial style of Kraepelin with his need for "measurement." Laing contends that the patient's behavior can be seen in two opposing ways: either as "signs" of disease, or as "expressive of his existence."

If we see the patient's behavior as signs of disease, then is he is the passive victim of a pathological process. On the other hand, if we see him from Laing's existential perspective, then he is fully autonomous: he possesses agency of his actions. This is a key concept in Laing's existentialist approach. Individuals are held to be fully responsible for their behavior and for their mode of being-in-the-world. When this existential principle is applied to mental illness, individuals are considered to make choices as to how they behave and talk. While Laing grants the patient full control over their self, the price is that there can be no mitigating factors, such as biology or heredity, to absolve the patient of responsibility.

From Laing's point of view, Kraepelin makes no attempt to understand the patient as an individual with his own unique perspective on the situation. Where Kraepelin sees only nonsense in the patient's utterances and behavior, Laing seeks to find meaning. Again, from an existential perspective, it is held that all the actions of human beings are potentially meaningful. Laing's imaginative "construction" of what is happening in the interview has a degree of plausibility. He has certainly alerted us to the fact the patient has a point of view and that he cannot be dismissed as *merely* a collection of symptoms and signs.

The origins of existential psychiatry grew out of the engagement of a number of European clinicians with the philosophical movements known as existentialism and phenomenology.

Existentialism

The period from the mid-1940s to the 1960s was the popular heyday of existentialism (Bakewell 2016). Although its philosophical origins were considerably earlier, the popular preoccupation with existentialism grew out of the carnage of the Second World War and the horrors of the Holocaust. There was a questioning of authority and a need to find meaning in an apparently meaningless world. Victor Frankl, a psychiatrist who survived the concentration camps, wrote *Man's Search for Meaning*, in which he put forward his thesis that the most pressing question for human beings was finding a purpose to their life. For many people, existential ideas about the importance of the individual, the absurdity of existence, and the striving for "authenticity" struck a chord.

Existentialist Philosophy

Existentialism is a philosophy that takes as its starting point the individual's existence (Earnshaw 2006; Dreyfus and Wrathall 2009). It begins with the "individual" rather than the "universal," and does not aim to arrive at general truths. It holds that self and existence can have no fixed definition: each individual is unique and thus escapes categorization. Kierkegaard introduced the idea of "authenticity" and contended that there was public pressure to conform to society, which led to "inauthenticity." Anxiety in the face of death is considered to reveal the banality and absurdity of life, but it can also reveal that the true nature of our lives is based on the choices we make. Warnock emphasizes that existentialists are primarily interested in human freedom (Warnock 1970). Humans have unique power to choose their course of action. What their freedom of choice amounts to and how it is to be described are central concerns of existentialists. Accepting responsibility for the exercise of freedom is the path to authenticity. Existentialists tend to share an opposition to rationalism and empiricism (Dreyfus and Wrathall 2009). Unlike most other philosophies, existential ideas are often expressed through novels and plays, as in the work of Sartre, Camus, and Beauvoir, while Nietzsche and Kierkegaard had a literary rather than a dry technical style of writing. Writers such as Dostoyevsky, Kafka, and Beckett are considered to be part of the existential tradition.

Laing and Existential Analysis

In a paper delivered to the Royal Medical Psychological Association in December 1960, Laing gives his clearest and most comprehensive account of what he means by existential analysis (Laing 1960b). The paper reflects Laing's views on the leading practitioners of existential therapy. He begins by stating that, in the nineteenth century, there were two major trends of philosophical thought: the speculative; and that based on the natural sciences. The existential thinker emerged as a reaction to these two philosophies. To the speculative philosopher he says, and here Laing quotes Feuerbach: "Do not wish to be a philosopher in contrast to being a man . . . do not think as a thinker . . . think as a living, real being . . ." (Laing 1960b: 3). To the natural scientist, he says, "Do not wish to be a scientist in contrast to being a man" (Laing 1960b: 3).

According to Laing, the existential thinker is not irrational. His intention is to articulate the "existence" that each person "is." This is done in opposition to the impersonal abstractions of certain types of philosophy and to technology that turns a man into a thing.

Laing concedes that the language of existential thought can be difficult to understand. He tells his London audience: "It requires an extra effort of goodwill, on the part of older educated Englishman, because many of the propositions of existential thought are not verifiable by the criteria that some influential English philosophers have recently taught" (Laing 1960b: 4).

Here Laing is alluding to Analytic philosophers and their critique of Continental philosophy. Laing goes on to consider what it is to be a human being: It involves taking responsibility for whatever one chooses to do in whatever situation one is in. One is in the world, but one knows that one was not always in the world and that one will not always be in the world. As a result of these considerations a person has to decide how to live their life.

Laing next draws on Heidegger and Sartre: "*My existence* is my way of being-in-the-world." If another person relates to my existence rather than regarding me as an object, then this is, according to Laing, an *existential* relation. Existential psychiatry aims to relate to the patient's way of being-in-the-world.

Laing outlines what he called the basic phenomenological step:

> Existential psychiatry should not be regarded as an *application* of preconceived philosophical speculations to empirical data. Its use of philosophy is to discard preconceptions, or at any rate to make one aware of what they are. One of its basic intentions is to discard any preoccupations which prevent one seeing the individual patient in the light of his own existence. That is, it attempts to understand the patient's complaints in his terms, as well as in our terms.
>
> (Laing 1960b: 6; emphasis in the original)

Laing states that in medicine, one's own experience is the crucible of all clinical judgment. In existential psychiatry, the clinician goes one step beyond this, so that he takes into account not only his experience of the patient but the patient's experience of him. Laing claims that existential analysis is more than just our everyday "common sense" understanding of others. It involves an attempt to understand the patient's being-in-the-world systematically and not simply by flashes of intuition. Furthermore, it is an attempt to do so in a critical way which tests the validity of its propositions. It is a "scientific discipline"—it is existential science, not natural science.

However, the process is hazardous as Laing explains:

> Obviously, the psychiatrist may not step into the patient's experience, he may simply step through the looking-glass into his own projected fantasy, and if he does, there are few signposts to bring him to his senses. It is hazardous also because he lacks at present the security and assurance of well worked out criteria of variability comparable to those that natural science has been able to develop in its relatively long history.
>
> (Laing 1960b: 7)

The core difficulty, then, for the existential analyst is that there is no accepted technique for trying to understand another person's being-in-his-world. It is no use looking to the natural sciences for the answer because they are not directly concerned with human experience and do not possess the appropriate techniques.

THE EXISTENTIAL–PHENOMENOLOGICAL FOUNDATIONS FOR A SCIENCE OF PERSONS

In *The Divided Self*, Laing set out to develop a technique of understanding another person's being-in-his-world. He writes: "Existential phenomenology attempts to characterize the nature of a person's experience of the world and himself. It is not so much an attempt to describe particular objects of his experience as to set all particular experiences within the context of his whole being-in-the-world" (Laing 1960a: 15).

Laing felt that the very language that psychiatrists used to talk about their patients immediately put them at a remove from them. The technical language of psychiatry or psychoanalysis split human beings up verbally. Such language placed man in isolation from his being-in-the-world and from his relation to others. It also broke him up into bits, such as "ego," "superego," and "id." The enterprise to elicit "psychopathology" was flawed from the outset, because it made certain assumptions which served to objectify the person. As a result, Laing argued, it was unable to understand that a person's disorganization represented a failure to achieve a "specifically personal form of unity." Psychopathological terms were abstract and ignored the interpersonal.

He insisted that the proper focus of study was human *existence*, our *being-in-the-world*. Laing writes:

> Unless we begin with the concept of man in relation to other men and from the beginning "in" a world, and unless we realize that man does not exist without "his" world nor can his world exist without him, we are condemned to start our study of schizoid and schizophrenic people with a verbal and conceptual splitting that matches the split up of the totality of the schizoid being-in-the-world.
>
> (Laing 1960a: 18)

Laing contended that "man's being" could be seen from different points of view, for example, as a person or as an organism. How one saw man determined how one related to him and how one conceived of him. Laing maintained it was a common illusion that we somehow increased our understanding of a person if we could translate a personal understanding of him into the impersonal terminology used to describe organisms, and here he referred to the Scottish philosopher, John Macmurray's concept of the "biological analogy." In a celebrated passage Laing writes: "[P]eople who experience themselves as automata, as robots, as bits of machinery, or even as animals . . . are rightly regarded as crazy. Yet why do we not regard a theory that seeks to transmute persons into automata or animals as equally crazy?" (Laing 1960a: 22).

For Laing, existential phenomenology attempted to reconstruct the patient's way of being himself in his world, and this might be done by focusing on the patient's way of being with the therapist. When the patient came to see the psychiatrist, he brought to the meeting "his existence, his whole being-in-his-world." One had to grasp how the patient experienced *his* world. The therapist must try to transpose himself into another strange and alien-world. Only by doing so could he hope to understand the patient's "existential position."

THE EXISTENTIAL–PHENOMENOLOGICAL FOUNDATIONS FOR THE UNDERSTANDING OF PSYCHOSIS

Based on his existential–phenomenological approach, Laing attempted to explain how an individual could develop psychosis. He maintained that the basic premise of *The Divided Self* rested on the concept of what he called "ontological security," the feeling of being at home in the world and with oneself and one's body. According to Laing, most people experienced themselves as real, alive, and more or less worthwhile. They possessed ontological security which they took for granted. They were comfortable with their being-in-the-world. However there were those whose basic ontological position was one of insecurity. Such individuals could not take their realness and aliveness for granted. They were preoccupied with finding ways of "trying to be real" in order to preserve their identity and to prevent the loss of their self.

Laing considered the nature of the relation that ontologically insecure people had with themselves. He contended that they primarily saw themselves as split into mind and body. Further, they most closely identified with the "mind." If this split became extreme, the individual was at risk of developing psychosis. In this context, Laing referred to Rudolf Bultmann and his description of Gnosticism, which conceived of the body as a prison from which the soul needed to escape (Laing 1960a: 69). Miller has argued that the work of Bultmann strongly influenced Laing in *The Divided Self*, especially his depiction of the schizoid condition (Miller 2009).

Laing stated that ontologically insecure individuals tended to have a sense of self which was disembodied, rather than embodied. This self was felt to be their "true" self, and it was often cherished as upholding the ideals of inner freedom, honesty, omnipotence, and creativity. However, because this true self was disembodied, it had no direct contact with real people or real things. In order to communicate with the outside world, the person constructed a "false self," which was identified with the body. However this way of operating in the world was doomed, because it was impossible to maintain. The true self, which was shut away and isolated, was not enriched by outer experience, and, as a consequence, the person's inner world became impoverished. It became unreal, empty, dead, and split. It lost its anchor in reality. The divorce of the true self from the body occurred as a means of defense against the anxieties of participating in the outside world. The estrangement of the true self from the body had the potential to lead to psychosis. Laing thus sought to outline the stages by which the ontologically insecure person could become psychotic.

CONCLUSION

The Divided Self offered an imaginative and, for many, a compelling account of disturbed mental states. Laing's engaging prose style and his references to literature helped to win him a wide readership and to expose complex ideas to a lay audience. However, some commentators felt there were theoretical problems. Laing's attempt to reconcile existentialism with object-relations theory was seen as a doomed project as the two disciplines, philosophy and psychology, are essentially different (Heaton 1991). Laing's discussion of the self seemed to lead to the reification of what some would argue is only a theoretical construct (Berrios and Markova 2003). Nevertheless, Laing's *The Divided Self* was a bold and erudite attempt to synthesize many strands of philosophical and psychoanalytic thought in order to shed light on the mystery of madness.

ACKNOWLEDGMENTS

I would like to thank the R. D. Laing Estate for permission to use R. D. Laing materials. These materials are held at Glasgow University Library Special Collections and include the extensive M. S. Laing archive and Laing's Library.

BIBLIOGRAPHY

Bakewell S. (2016). *At the Existential Café. Freedom, Being and Apricot Cocktails.* London: Chatto & Windus.

Berrios G. E. and Markova I. (2003). "The Self and Psychiatry: A Conceptual History." In T. Kircher and A. David (eds.), *The Self in Neuroscience and Psychiatry*, pp. 9–39. Cambridge: Cambridge University Press.

Beveridge A. (2011). *Portrait of the Psychiatrist as a Young Man. The Early Work and Writings of RD Laing, 1927–1960.* Oxford: Oxford University Press.

Dreyfus H. L. and Wrathall M. A. (eds.) (2009). *A Companion to Phenomenology and Existentialism.* Oxford: Wiley-Blackwell.

Earnshaw S. (2006). *Existentialism.* London: Continuum.

Heaton J. (1991). "The Divided Self: Kierkegaard or Winnicott?" *Journal of the Society for Existential Analysis* 2: 30–37.

Laing R. D. (1960a). *The Divided Self.* London: Tavistock.

Laing R. D. (1960b). MS Laing A116-7. "The Development of Existential Analysis. A Paper given to RMPA, December 1960."

MacQuarrie J. (1973). *Existentialism.* London: Pelican Books.

May R., Angel E., and Ellenberger H. F. (eds.) (1958). *Existence. A New Dimension in Psychiatry and Psychology.* New York: Basic Books.

Miller G. (2009). "R.D. Laing and Theology: The Influence of Christian Existentialism on *The Divided Self.*" *History of the Human Sciences* 22: 1–21.

Warnock M. (1970). *Existentialism.* Oxford: Oxford University Press.

FOUNDATIONS AND METHODS

SECTION EDITORS: ANTHONY VINCENT FERNANDEZ AND RENÉ ROSFORT

CHAPTER 25

....

ON THE SUBJECT MATTER OF PHENOMENOLOGICAL PSYCHOPATHOLOGY

....

ANTHONY VINCENT FERNANDEZ AND ALLAN KØSTER

INTRODUCTION

....

PHENOMENOLOGY is typically characterized as the study of human experience. But, in its philosophical sense, it's more than the study of "what it's like" or "what it feels like" to have experiences. It's not equivalent to a qualitative study or a narrative self-report—although it might draw on evidence from such studies and reports. What, then, is phenomenology in its philosophical sense? Philosophical phenomenology is often characterized as a study of the "structure" of human consciousness, experience, or existence (e.g. Luft and Overgaard 2011; Smith 2018; Zahavi 2012). However, in much of the contemporary phenomenological literature, this key notion of "structure" is left undefined. And, when it is defined, it's typically given only a vague or cursory characterization: "structure" refers to the form or shape, rather than the content, of experience. This gets us a bit closer to what phenomenologists mean by "structure," but contemporary applied phenomenologists deserve something more definite. They deserve a well-articulated framework for conducting their phenomenological investigations.

Psychopathology is, by contrast, an interdisciplinary research program that aims to understand and explain the nature of mental disorders (Jaspers 1997). Today, psychopathology is largely concerned with providing *explanations* of mental disorders—identifying, for example, the genetic, neurobiological, and social factors that contribute to psychopathological conditions. However, psychopathology also requires that we *understand*, not just explain, the conditions in question. Phenomenology, as a descriptive study of lived experience, is one of the major methodological approaches for achieving this kind of understanding (Jaspers 1968).

But when we turn to the phenomenological study of psychopathology, the question of phenomenology's subject matter becomes even more complex. To properly comprehend the psychopathological condition in question, the phenomenologist must articulate the experiential or existential structure of this condition—not just of experience or existence in general. And this requires that the phenomenologist specify how the general structure has been altered or disturbed in this particular case. Ludwig Binswanger, one of the first psychiatrists to apply phenomenology to the study of psychopathology, says, "in the mental diseases we face modifications of the fundamental or essential structure and of the structural links of being-in-the-world as transcendence. It is one of the tasks of psychiatry to investigate and establish these variations in a scientifically exact way" (Binswanger 1958: 194). If, however, we lack a clear account of what we mean by "structure," then the difficulty of doing applied phenomenology is only compounded in its application to psychopathology. As with contemporary phenomenologists in general, phenomenological psychopathologists have not adequately defined this key term. They also use it as a synonym for "form," "shape," and so on (see e.g. Parnas and Zahavi 2002).

In light of this shortcoming in the phenomenological literature, we here provide a detailed account of the phenomenological notion of "structure." We argue that there are at least two distinct kinds or layers of structure that are not properly disambiguated in the literature—what we call "existentials" and "modes." Once we properly distinguish them, we'll have a clearer sense of what it means to articulate both the structure of human experience in general and how experience can be altered or disturbed in particular cases. In the first section, we articulate this distinction with definitions and examples. [1] In the second section, we demonstrate how the distinction between existentials and modes can guide the study of psychopathological and psychologically distressing conditions. Our intention is to provide a means of framing phenomenological investigations and clearly communicating the results of phenomenological studies, which will, in turn, facilitate critical and complementary dialogue—ultimately driving the field of phenomenological psychopathology forward.[2]

The Layers of Phenomenological Research

In this section, we outline the two layers of phenomenological research: existentials and modes. This distinction has foundations in the classical phenomenological texts and is implicit in much of the contemporary phenomenological literature—not only in the study of psychopathology, but also in studies of race, gender, culture, and so on. In this respect, we don't mean to impose an external framework on the field of applied phenomenology. Rather, we provide an explicit articulation of a framework that stands in the background of many contemporary phenomenological studies.

---

[1] The framework that we provide here is based on work that both authors developed separately (in some cases with other co-authors). See e.g. Fernandez (2017); Fernandez and Stanghellini (forthcoming); Fernandez and Wieten (2015); Køster (2017a, 2017b); Køster and Winther-Lindqvist (2018).

[2] While we offer an account of the subject matter of phenomenological psychopathology, we do not intend this to be an account of the subject matter of phenomenological psychiatry more broadly. We take psychopathology to be one component of the broader field of psychiatry, which also includes psychotherapy, psychopharmacology, and so on. In light of this, we acknowledge that there are other phenomenological approaches to psychiatry, such as phenomenological approaches to psychotherapy, that may exceed the boundaries of the framework that we provide here.

The first layer of phenomenological research is "existentials." This term is a Heideggerian coinage, but it can be applied across a variety of phenomenological approaches. As we use it, the term is a rough synonym for what other phenomenologists call "essential" or "ontological" structures of experience.[3]

In *Being and Time*, Heidegger analyzes the structures that are constitutive of human experience and existence. In this respect, he articulates "not just any accidental structures, but essential ones which, in every kind of Being that factical Dasein may possess, persist as determinative for the character of its Being" (Heidegger 1962: 38). By "factical Dasein," he simply refers to a concrete, particular human existence. He aims, therefore, to articulate those structural features that hold for human existence in general, applying across all particular cases. These structural features are what we call "existentials."

But what are existentials? A simple way to conceptualize existentials is to think of them as categories.[4] They are not, however, categories of objects within the world, such as the categories "tree," "bicycle," or "nation." As Heidegger says, "*Existentials* and categories are the two basic possibilities for characters of Being. The entities which correspond to them require different kinds of primary interrogation respectively: any entity is either a '*who*' (existence) or a '*what*' (presence-at-hand in the broadest sense)" (Heidegger 1962: 71; translation modified). When we turn our attention toward the experiencing subject, we no longer concern ourselves with categories of objects within the world. Instead, we concern ourselves with the categorial structures of human experience and existence, such as intentionality, temporality, understanding, selfhood, and affective situatedness, among others. All instances of human existence include these basic structural features. That is, all experience is intentional (i.e. directed toward some object or state of affairs), has a temporal flow, is affectively situated, and so on.

Existentials, like categories, fundamentally differ from the particular phenomena that they encompass. There are, for instance, a variety of ways in which one might be intentionally oriented toward one's environment, various styles of temporal flow, and diverse affective states. When we study the existentials themselves, we don't concern ourselves with the particular ways in which these existentials manifest. We concern ourselves with the existential, or categorial structure, itself. We aim, for instance, to articulate the basic, defining features that hold for any instance of intentionality, temporality, affectivity, and so on. In this respect, the study of existentials is ontological—it's concerned with what it means to *be* this or that kind of being. As phenomenologists, we sometimes ask the big questions, such as "What does it mean to be human?" But we also ask more specific questions, such as "What is intentionality?" or "What is temporality?" When we answer these kinds of ontological questions, we typically do so by articulating a category. To properly understand the being of some

---

[3] We prefer the term "existentials" because it does not require the use of the term "structure." Since much of the ambiguity and vagueness in contemporary phenomenological research stems from an overuse of the term "structure," we prefer to use a label that does not employ this term.

[4] This characterization of existentials is, admittedly, contentious. When Heidegger introduces his notion of existentials in *Being and Time*, he famously says that they "are to be sharply distinguished from what we call '*categories*'—characteristics of Being for entities whose character is not that of Dasein" (Heidegger 1962: 70). However, he here refers to "categories" in a narrow metaphysical sense (e.g. Aristotle's metaphysical categories). Throughout his early lectures, Heidegger used the term "categorial" [*kategorial*] to characterize the very structures that he later rebranded as "existentials" in *Being and Time* (see e.g. Heidegger 2008).

phenomenon, that is, to clarify what it *is*, we have to properly categorize it. We can clarify this approach with the everyday categories noted above. If I ask, for instance, "What is a bicycle?" I'm not asking you to tell me anything specific about *this* bicycle. I'm asking you to articulate the category "bicycle"—that is, the defining features that make something a bicycle. Once I have a sense of these defining features, then I'm in a position to distinguish among those entities that do, or do not, fall into the category "bicycle."

If the study of an existential is like the study of a category, then what does this kind of study look like in practice? We can illustrate the study of an existential with a more detailed analysis of affective situatedness [*Befindlichkeit*].[5] We rely on this as our primary example of an existential for three reasons: First, Heidegger describes the existential of affective situatedness in considerable detail. Second, he clearly distinguishes affective situatedness (i.e. the existential) from particular moods (i.e. the modes of this existential), which will help us clarify the general relationship between existentials and modes. Third, affective situatedness is a central topic in phenomenological psychopathology—especially in the study of affective disorders—which will allow us to easily link this initial sketch of existentials with our discussion of how existentials are studied in phenomenological psychopathology.

As an existential, affective situatedness refers to the fact that we always find ourselves in the world through a particular affective attunement—what Heidegger calls a "mood." Even our everyday "pallid, evenly balanced lack of mood" is still a mood—it's a way of finding ourselves affectively attuned to and situated in the world (Heidegger 1962: 173). And affective situatedness, like all existentials, has "essential characteristics"—that is, a set of defining features that hold for any of the phenomena that belong to this ontological category. Heidegger argues that there are three essential characteristics of affective situatedness: It (1) discloses our thrownness, (2) discloses being-in-the-world as a whole, and (3) lets us encounter the world as meaningful.

(1) By thrownness, Heidegger refers to the experience of what he calls "*the naked that it is and has to be.*" That is, the precarious experience that we don't choose our existence, but always already find ourselves delivered over to and having to exist in a pre-structured historical world. In this sense, Heidegger argues, existence is disclosed to us through affective situatedness as a burden that we have to carry, and this burdensomeness is made apparent by our mood.

(2) When Heidegger says that moods disclose being-in-the-world as a whole, he means that moods aren't internal mental states that simply color an objective world. Rather, as Heidegger says, "[a] mood assails us. It comes neither from 'outside' nor from 'inside'. . ." (Heidegger 1962: 176). Our moods disclose the world, others, and ourselves simultaneously.

(3) When Heidegger says that moods allow us to encounter the world as meaningful, he means that in order to find anything meaningful at all, it must have some kind

---

[5] Heidegger's neologism, *Befindlichkeit*, is remarkably difficult to translate. No English term is an exact correlate. In the Macquarrie and Robinson translation, it is translated as "state of mind," but this translation is rarely used in the English-language scholarship. Alternative translations include "affectedness," "disposedness," "sofindingness," "attunement," and "situatedness," among others. In this chapter, we typically use the term "affective situatedness," but also refer to "attunement" when this captures the distinctive aspect of *Befindlichkeit* that we're trying to express.

of affective pull on us. Which kind of affective pull something has will depend on the mood we happen to find ourselves in. But things can have an affective pull only because we're attuned through some mood or other. As Heidegger says, we must be attuned to the world through a mood to "be 'touched' by anything or 'have a sense for' something" (Heidegger 1962: 177).

In addition to having essential characteristics, each existential can be analyzed by focusing on "general structures." In affective situatedness, Heidegger illustrates this through the example of a concrete mood: fear.[6] He says that the three structural elements of fear are "(1) that in the face of which we fear, (2) fearing, and (3) that about which we fear" (Heidegger 1962: 179). Consider, for example, the experience of coming across a large bear while hiking in the woods. In this case, (1) I am fearful in the face of the bear (i.e. the bear is fearsome); (2) I experience the qualitative feeling of fear; and (3) I am fearful about my own life or the possibility of coming to bodily harm. In like manner, I might be joyful upon receiving a letter of acceptance to my top choice university. In this case, (1) I am joyful in the face of my acceptance; (2) I experience the qualitative feeling of joy; and (3) I am joyful about my future life as a university student or the future prospects for my career. These three elements are not a sequence of events, but a simultaneous structural whole. They constitute the general structure of this existential—and, thus, the general structure of any mood or mode of affective attunement. As Heidegger says, "These possible ways of looking at fear are not accidental; they belong together. With them the general structure of affective situatedness comes to the fore" (Heidegger 1962: 179).

It is, however, important to clarify that, on Heidegger's account, what it means for a mood to be experienced "in the face of" something is a rather permissive criterion. Our mood need not be experienced in the face of an object within the world. As Heidegger clarifies in both *Being and Time* and *The Fundamental Concepts of Metaphysics* (2001), a mood may also be experienced in the face of an event (e.g. being bored at a dinner party) or even in the face of the world as a whole. Moods that take this last form are what Heidegger calls "ground moods" [*Grundstimmungen*]. These are pervasive background feelings that determine the kind of sense and meaning that we are capable of experiencing. Heidegger's concept of ground moods largely overlaps with Matthew Ratcliffe's concept of "existential feelings" (Ratcliffe 2008). In the following section, we'll demonstrate how one might analyze ground moods, or existential feelings, by providing a brief analysis of grief.

To summarize, in much the same way that we distinguish between categories of things—such as "trees," "bicycles," or "nations"—and the particular things that belong to these categories, we can distinguish between the existential itself and the modes that belong to the

---

[6] It may seem strange to refer to fear as a mood rather than an emotion. Moods are often characterized as pervasive background states without a clear object. Emotions, on the other hand, are affective states that are directed toward, or are about, an object. Fear would therefore fall into the category of emotion rather than mood. However, Heidegger's use of the term *Stimmung*, which is translated as "mood," doesn't distinguish between affective states that have, or do not have, an object. While we follow Heidegger's broad use of the term here, his failure to clearly draw a distinction between intentional and non-intentional affective states is one of the motivations behind our move toward Ratcliffe's concept of existential feelings.

existential. The modes of situatedness are moods, or concrete affective attunements, but we can also speak of modes of selfhood, temporality, spatiality, and so on.

APPLICATION IN PHENOMENOLOGICAL PSYCHOPATHOLOGY

Before we demonstrate how to investigate existentials and modes in contemporary applied phenomenology, it will be helpful to distinguish two ways that phenomenologists study modes. First, phenomenologists may study a mode with the aim of understanding it with respect to its generality—that is, with the aim of articulating the essential characteristics or the general structure of the existential that this mode belongs to. Second, phenomenologists may study a mode with respect to its particularity—that is, with the aim of understanding the character of this specific mode. The former investigation is ontological (i.e. a study of the being or essence of a kind of phenomenon); the latter investigation is ontic (i.e. a study of a particular, concrete phenomenon).[7] Heidegger's project is, first and foremost, ontological—it is concerned with the basic structures of human existence in general. By contrast, most studies in applied phenomenology—including phenomenological psychopathology—are ontic insofar as they're concerned with describing particular modes, or ways, of being-in-the-world. However, we argue that these studies can also feed back into the ontological project, helping us delineate and define the existentials themselves. In the following two subsections, we briefly demonstrate how contemporary applied studies can feed back into and clarify our ontological account of the structure of human existence—then, using the example of grief, we provide a more detailed example of the kind of analysis phenomenologists can produce through ontic studies of particular modes.

Refining Our Ontological Accounts of Existentials

If we take existentials as the necessary, invariant structures of human existence and modes as their contingent, variable manifestations, then how should phenomenological psychopathologists investigate existentials? One answer is that the study of existentials simply isn't the business of those doing phenomenological psychopathology—or any form of applied phenomenology, for that matter. Existentials are investigated by the more philosophically minded, pure phenomenologists, who concern themselves with the structure of human existence in general. This position stems from the view that phenomenological psychopathology and other fields of applied phenomenology are *merely* applied. That is, applied phenomenology is merely the ontic study of particular forms of human existence and, therefore, has nothing to say about the structure of existence in general—it simply assumes

---

[7] The distinction between the ontological and the ontic is Heideggerian. However, it's roughly synonymous with the distinction between the transcendental and the empirical, or mundane, which we find in the work of Edmund Husserl and Maurice Merleau-Ponty, among others.

this general structure, which has already been identified and articulated by the classical phenomenologists.

We, however, take a more collaborative, mutually informative view of the relationship between applied phenomenology and what may be called "pure phenomenology" (by Husserl) or "fundamental ontology" (by Heidegger). The latter labels refer to the study of the structure of human experience and existence in general—not its particular manifestations across the human population.[8] If, however, we examine how the classical phenomenologists arrived at their accounts of the essential characteristics and general structure of existentials, we find that they do so by investigating a particular, ontic mode of the existential in question. This approach is similar to Husserl's method of variation, in which you vary a particular phenomenon (real or imagined) to identify the invariant features of this *kind* of phenomenon. Heidegger does not take over this explicit method, but there's a similar approach in the background of his study of existentials.

Regardless of the particularities of the method, it's clear that we don't have immediate insight into the essential characteristics and general structures of existentials. We discover the characteristics and structure through the study of particular modes. And, as with any empirically informed study, we may misidentify the characteristics and structure of the category that the phenomenon belongs to. If our sample of phenomena is too small, we're simply not in a good position to know what these general features are.

The same kind of issue may occur when defining a category of objects within the world. If I tried to identify the defining features of, say, teacups, I might determine that having a handle is one of these defining features. But what if I'm introduced to tea-drinking traditions in East Asia, where it's common for teacups to lack a handle? Once I'm presented with this case, I seem to have two options: I may decide to remove handles as a defining feature of teacups, thus broadening my category; or, alternatively, I may decide that the teacup-like object used in East Asia just doesn't count as a teacup—it's some other kind of object.

There are at least two lessons to be learned from this example: First, if our initial sample of phenomena is too small, we have a greater risk of misidentifying the defining features of the category in question. Second, whether we decide to modify our current category or establish a new one is often a pragmatic issue. If we consider the teacup example, there aren't any a priori criteria that we can use to decide one way or the other in this case. Similar issues arise in the phenomenological study of existentials. We shouldn't assume that the classical phenomenologists got everything right. But we also shouldn't assume that there's only one right way to carve up and characterize the various existentials. Sometimes we have good reason to delimit the domain of experiential phenomena in a new way—and this doesn't necessarily imply that the previous delimitation was wrong.

For an example of this kind of redescription of ontological structures in phenomenological psychopathology, we can turn to Matthew Ratcliffe's work on existential feelings (Ratcliffe 2008).[9] Ratcliffe explicitly adapts his concept of existential feelings from

---

[8] In this chapter, our account of the subject matter of phenomenological psychopathology assumes an invariant existential structure, or set of existentials, exhibited by all human subjects. However, we think that the invariance of existentials is an open question deserving of further discussion and debate. For an account of the possibility of existential or ontological contingency, see Fernandez (2015, 2018).

[9] We here provide only a brief account of Ratcliffe's concept of existential feelings. For further reading, see Ratcliffe (2009, 2013).

Heidegger's notion of affective situatedness, modifying the concept in light of his own aims. One of Heidegger's significant contributions was to outline the very world-opening function of affectivity. However, he doesn't provide a robust taxonomy of affective phenomena. Heidegger's notion of affective situatedness does not, for instance, adequately distinguish between intentional and non-intentional affective phenomena—that is, those that have an object and those that do not. As we noted above, when Heidegger says that moods are experienced in the face of something, he means this in a broad sense. Some moods may have an intentional object within the world, but others are experienced in the face of an event or in the face of the world as a whole.

Ratcliffe, by contrast, more clearly delimits his concept of existential feelings as a separate phenomenological category, or what we call an existential. Existential feelings refer specifically to background feelings that are pre-intentional—that is, feelings that do not have an object, but provide an affective background within which we have other intentional experiences, such as emotions or beliefs. Moreover, Ratcliffe stresses the bodily aspect of existential feelings, which is almost entirely missing from Heidegger's philosophy (see e.g. Aho 2010). Existential feelings are specifically bodily feelings that determine "ways of finding ourselves in the world, existential backgrounds that shape all our experiences" (Ratcliffe 2008: 41). They are simultaneously feelings of ourselves and the world, and include a broad range of affective phenomena, such as feelings of familiarity, alienation, of being or not being at home in the world, of estrangement, and so on. By delimiting the existential in this way, Ratcliffe is able to zero in on a more clearly defined aspect of experience, drawing fine-grained distinctions across its diverse experiential manifestations (Ratcliffe 2008: 53). In the following subsection, we follow Ratcliffe's refinement of Heidegger's notion of affective situatedness, turning to a study of the more clearly delimited phenomena of existential feelings.

Examples of Modal Alterations

What kind of phenomenological insights might be generated when focusing specifically on modal variations in particular experiential states? In the following, we briefly illustrate this by providing excerpts taken from retrospective, phenomenological interviews conducted with persons who have suffered early parental bereavement. The research design included a total of twenty informants who lost a parent between the age of 5–18. They were systematically selected with a current age dispersion between 20–50 years old to more accurately identify potential lasting alterations. Each informant was interviewed for a total of six hours. The interviews were phenomenological in the respect that they were (1) pre-structured by phenomenological insights, specifically with attention to the existential-mode distinction; (2) carried out through a phenomenological-hermeneutic attitude; and (3) subsequently analyzed with the extensive use of phenomenological concepts. Much more could be said about the details of this process, but for the current purpose it will have to suffice to add that although the interviews were conducted through an open and hermeneutic attitude, the specific lines of questioning were guided by pre-established phenomenological insights on various experiential structures, or existentials. For example, part of a two-hour interview devoted to mapping the affective dimension of early parental bereavement was specifically structured to solicit descriptions of potential alterations in existential feelings. This style of questioning not only assumes such an aspect of experience, but is also sensitive to the difficulty of verbalizing or narrating this aspect of experience.[10] To solicit rich descriptions of existential feelings, the interviewer needs to allow for, and perhaps even encourage, the extensive use of metaphors and fuzzy concepts that require greater levels of time, patience, and assistance to adequately articulate. This is, moreover, a standard element of qualitative interview techniques.

Our aim here is not to provide an exhaustive analysis of the effects of bereavement. It is, rather, to demonstrate the utility of the distinction between existentials and modes when applied to specific research contexts. We therefore confine ourselves to a few interview excerpts that are demonstrative of modal alterations in affective attunement. Hence, these should not be read as an attempt to give an exhaustive account of the heterogeneous affective dimension of grief.[11]

It should also be noted that, although it has long been accepted in psychology and psychiatry that grief can become pathological, it is not until recently that systematic discussions and research have been aimed at defining some grief responses as pathological in their own right—that is, as a nosologically distinct category.[12] However, since the specific diagnostic criteria are still debated, we do not confine our phenomenological analysis to modal alterations of *pathological* grief—since the distinctly pathological form of grief has not been clearly identified (Prigerson et al. 2009; Maciejewski et al. 2016). However, this also provides us with an opportunity to demonstrate how phenomenology can contribute to the literature on pathological grief and the process of identifying and characterizing pathological conditions. As we show, phenomenology is an especially powerful tool for distinguishing between subtle experiential alterations and disturbances. Such distinctions can provide psychiatrists with a map of the terrain, which they can use to better distinguishing among those conditions they want to class as pathological, non-pathological, or subthreshold.

The three excerpts exhibited below all display aspects of a particular tendency in the modal alterations of affective attunement that we might characterize as *world-distancing*, which is a particular way in which the world is affectively disclosed. This tendency was consistent across most informants. However, informants exhibited significant scalar differentiations in intensity and frequency. Most informants considered these alterations a new experiential disposition, in the sense that it was not there before bereavement, but has become a recurring experience after bereavement. In multiple cases, it was even considered an experiential constant, that is, as an aspect of experience that was more or less always there.[13]

Let's start with a passage from a 49-year-old man who lost his mother at the age of 12. He describes the emergence of a world-distancing affective attunement in the following way:

[10] For a detailed account on the relation between embodied experiences and narrative see Køster (2017c).

[11] A systematic phenomenological analysis of the modal alteration in affective situatedness following early parental bereavement can be found in Køster (forthcoming).

[12] Prolonged grief disorder is expected to be included in the fortcomming ICD-11.

[13] This, of course, would have to be validated on a much larger sample, which calls for quantitative research methodologies. Migrating the phenomenological insights into operational scales for measuring this on a larger scale is currently being developed by Allan Køster in collaboration with quantitatively orientated grief researchers.

To me this feeling of distancing is similar to a train running. It's my life, and I am on the plat-form watching the train run by. You know, the best metaphor is perhaps looking at a party and, just for a few seconds, having stepped out into the garden and watching the party from afar. You know there are a lot of people, and I have a relation to all of them. Everybody is having fun, but I have stepped outside. I observe it all. And it is perhaps really that observing stance from the outside that best describes the changed feeling, it's a kind of bubbling up. It's a dif-ferent feeling of being in a blur, like things are a bit out of focus because I experience it from afar. When thinking of this state all I can think of is calmness. There is no noise. Perhaps I can describe it by saying there is no sound. And this kind of displacement was not only an initial feeling. It is a recurring feeling, one that has become a property of my way of being . . . In this sense the world has become much more two-dimensional. It has no depth, the world is no longer as nuanced, I think. There are not as many layers, I think, or that's what I am left with when I say that it's soft and calm. You know, when you observe from a distance, you don't get all the details, some of the senses don't exists, as for instance the sense of smell, because you are watching things from afar.

As already noted, a key element in Heidegger's notion of *affective situatedness* and Ratcliffe's *existential feelings* is that they shape how we find ourselves affectively present and situated in the world—that is, our affective attunements open, or disclose, the world in a particular way. How is this aspect of experience altered in this excerpt? First, it's important that the informant himself refers to distancing as a *feeling*. It is a feeling of "*bubbling up*," of "*being in a blur*," a feeling that alters the way the world manifests in the sense that it is now "*more two-dimensional*," without color and lacking in sensory qualities, partially because it is observed from afar. Importantly, this altered state of being-in-the-world should not be seen as a simple deprivation. It also provides a sense of calmness. Elsewhere, the informant refers to what we've called the affective attunement of world-distancing as "*a protective airbag*." The attunement certainly has distressing and debilitating features, but the informant himself experiences his attunement as a kind of defensive stance, protecting him from the harsh re-ality of his loss.

The contours of this description are echoed by a 33-year-old woman who lost her father at the age of 16. However, she adds an important temporal modality to this modal change in affective attunement:

I consider it, this feeling of distancing, as almost a metaphysical feeling. I am in my body but the world is cloudy. I am confined to my own shell, and time has stopped; everybody else is continuing their lives, but I am stuck in stillness. It's a kind a vacuum, where time feels ab-stract. It's a feeling of being fundamentally alone in the world . . . One might perhaps also say that I feel like I am continuously caught behind a glass plate and watching the world and other people through this screen.

Again, she explicitly refers to the sense of distancing as a feeling, in this case a "*metaphys-ical feeling*," that describes a particular way of finding oneself in the world. As emphasized, however, she adds a clear temporal dimension to this experience: distancing is a feeling of being "*stuck in stillness*" because "*time has stopped*," separated from the temporal flow of the world.[14]

---

[14] Thomas Fuchs has argued that depressive disorders often involve temporal and intersubjective desynchronization (Fuchs 2001, 2013). Since we find a similar phenomenon in cases of grief, it may

A 28-year-old woman who lost her mother at age 10 complements these descriptions by elaborating on the social implications of world-distancing as a particular mode of attunement:

> I think it is a bit like being in a bubble; well, it's a feeling of being in a bubble and when somebody is talking to you it just becomes this myriad of words, this stream of fuzzy talk, because it is difficult to localize it, because you are caught in your own bubble. One keeps thinking that this is what is happening, and then that only makes it worse. Often I feel, though, that I am able to tune-in on the conversation, but it is really hard to remain present. I hear the words, but I can't be fully present, so I end up just saying hmmm, and platitudes like "I know that". Sometimes I feel like shaking my head a bit, to see if it disappears, but it's really difficult. It's a bit like having the hiccups and trying to think it away—it does not work. I start thinking that they notice that, they can tell you are not listening. It's really unpleasant. I get this feeling very often, almost daily, since my mum passed. At least it feels like that.

In this passage, she emphasizes how the feeling of distance impacts the capacity to follow the rhythm and resonance of social interaction. She feels cut off from the interaction as a result of the preceding affective state of distance.

Taken together, these excerpts draw out basic contours of modal alterations of affective attunement and affective situatedness that are characteristic of suffering early parental bereavement—even years or decades after the loss. Our focus here has been on world-distancing as an existential feeling, or mode of affective situatedness. The informants report a peculiar way of finding themselves affectively attuned to the world in which the world seems difficult to reach, as if reality is somehow separate from them, on the other side of a barrier. They report feeling alone, regardless of the concrete social situation they currently find themselves in. Moreover, some informants suggest that this disclosure of the world as distant or hard to reach also comes with a sense of softness or calmness. The feeling of being alone and distant makes it difficult to connect with others, but it also protects one from the harsh realities of everyday life.

The specific analyses we've offered here are brief, since our aim is not to provide a detailed analysis of grief, but to provide an illustration of how to conduct a phenomenological study. We can, however, provide a more detailed account of how further analyses of these kinds of interviews might proceed. The essential characteristics and general structure of affective situatedness, or existential feelings, helps us initially identify this specific kind of phenomenon in the informants' reports. But we should also return to these characteristics and structure when performing our analyses. Heidegger, for example, says that an essential characteristic of affective situatedness is that it shapes the meaningfulness of the world, or the kind of sense and meaning that we can find within the world. And Ratcliffe points out that existential feelings determine our sense of reality. In light of these characteristics, we might analyze the informants' reports with the explicit aim of articulating not only which mode of attunement they find themselves in, but also how, exactly, this attunement shapes the meaningfulness of their world and their sense of reality. By describing these characteristics in more detail, we're able to articulate what's distinctive, or perhaps even unique, about the affective dimension of grief.

be worth conducting a comparative study of grief and depression to determine whether there are key differences in the kind of desynchronization experienced by persons in the two groups.

However, it's also important to clarify that despite the consistency of the affective dimension of grief illustrated in these excerpts, we are not suggesting that these alterations constitute a strict invariant structure of the affective dimension of grief and bereavement. What first-person descriptions, such as these, may produce are rather illustrations of modal variations in affective attunement. These variations express *tendencies*, in the sense that they are *typical* or *characteristic* of early parental bereavement, but may not manifest in all cases. This points to a significant difference in the type of knowledge phenomenological analysis can be expected to provide when moving from the ontological focus of philosophical phenomenology to the level of specific empirical cases. As any researcher with experience in empirical case-studies will be able to recognize, real life cases are always ontogenetically specific and context-dependent. Therefore, we should not expect to identify something like an *essence* of grief, or even an essence of the affective dimension of grief. At the ontological level, we might identify an essence of affective situatedness, an essence of temporality, and so on. But, in our ontic, modal investigations, we may be able to identify only what is typical or characteristic of the experience in question. Modal alterations manifest in subtly different ways, which are often difficult to clearly distinguish. The boundaries of modal phenomena, including affective attunements, may often be blurry and ambiguous—not just because we haven't described them in enough detail, but because they are, by their very nature, blurry and ambiguous. In this case, at least, we take ourselves to have articulated certain generalities or tendencies that are typical of, but not necessarily essential to, the experience of early parental bereavement.

CONCLUSION

In this chapter, we've outlined the subject matter of phenomenological psychopathology with the aim of providing a clear, easily applicable framework for conducting studies and reporting the results of one's research. To illustrate this framework, we relied on Heidegger's notion of affective situatedness and Ratcliffe's notion of existential feelings. However, the framework that we've provided is meant to be applicable across the full range of existentials. In addition to affective situatedness, we might study modes of temporality, spatiality, selfhood, intentionality, and so on. To perform a concrete phenomenological study of these modes, one should begin by providing a clear account of the essential characteristics and general structure of the existential in question. Once this has been adequately articulated, then one can investigate the specific modal alterations of this existential, analyzing the various ways in which its characteristics and structure manifest.

For example, to perform a similar phenomenological study of potential modal alternations in temporality following early parental bereavement, we would first need to provide a clear account of temporality's essential characteristics and general structure. Temporality has, for instance, a retentional–protentional structure: We retain what has just been experienced *as* just past and anticipate what is about to come, forming what may be called the specious present or extended now. Moreover, temporality includes the characteristic of conation, or striving, toward some future possibilities. And these possibilities are projected in light of who we already take ourselves to be. In light of this outline of the essential characteristics and general structure of temporality, one could develop a specific interview guide focusing on these aspects of temporality. Once the interviews have been conducted, they should be analyzed utilizing phenomenological concepts to uncover and clearly articulate tendencies and typical modal alterations.

By framing one's study in this way, one can easily compare the results of the study with other studies of modal alterations in the same existential, but across different kinds of conditions. One might, for instance, compare modal alterations in the temporality of grief with modal alterations in the temporality of depression to determine whether these experiences differ and, if so, how. This approach also allows researchers to investigate how modal alterations in one existential may complement modal alterations in another existential that occur in the same condition. One might, for instance, attempt to integrate studies of modal alterations in grief as they occur across the existentials of affectivity, temporality, and selfhood. Such an integration can provide a more complete, holistic account of the experience of grief.

Because many phenomenologists have developed their own distinctive set of concepts and style of phenomenological description, it is often difficult to compare the results of phenomenological studies. This hinders our ability to engage in critical and complementary dialogue, which is key to the continued success of phenomenological psychopathology. We hope that our proposed framework will provide a more effective foundation for such dialogue, ultimately driving the discipline forward.

BIBLIOGRAPHY

Aho K. A. (2010). *Heidegger's Neglect of the Body*. Albany: SUNY Press.

Binswanger L. (1958). "The Existential Analysis School of Thought." In R. May, E. Angel, and H. F. Ellenberger (eds.), *Existence: A New Dimension in Psychology and Psychiatry*, pp. 191–213. New York: Basic Books.

Fernandez A. V. (2015). "Contaminating the Transcendental: Toward a Phenomenological Naturalism." *Journal of Speculative Philosophy* 29(3): 291–301.

Fernandez A. V. (2017). "The Subject Matter of Phenomenological Research: Existentials, Modes, and Prejudices." *Synthese* 194(9): 3543–3562.

Fernandez A. V. (2018). "Beyond the Ontological Difference: Heidegger, Binswanger, and the Future of Existential Analysis." In K. Aho (ed.), *Existential Medicine: Essays on Health and Illness*, pp. 27–42. Lanham: Rowman & Littlefield International.

Fernandez A. V. and Wieten S. (2015). "Values-based Practice and Phenomenological Psychopathology: Implications of Existential Changes in Depression." *Journal of Evaluation in Clinical Practice* 21(3): 508–513.

Fernandez A. V. and Stanghellini G. (forthcoming). "Comprehending the Whole Person: On Expanding Jaspers' Notion of Empathy." In A. L. Mishara, P. Corlett, P. Fletcher, A. Kranjec, and M. A. Schwartz (eds.), *Phenomenological Neuropsychiatry: How Patient Experience Bridges Clinic with Clinical Neuroscience*. New York: Springer.

Fuchs T. (2001). "Melancholia as a Desynchronization: Towards a Psychopathology of Interpersonal Time." *Psychopathology* 34(4): 179–186.

Fuchs T. (2013). "Depression, Intercorporeality, and Interaffectivity." *Journal of Consciousness Studies* 20(7–8): 219–238.

Heidegger M. (1962). *Being and Time*, trans. J. Macquarrie and E. Robinson. New York: Harper Perennial Modern Classics.

Heidegger M. (2001). *The Fundamental Concepts of Metaphysics: World, Finitude, Solitude*, trans. W. McNeill and N. Walker. Bloomington: Indiana University Press.

Heidegger M. (2008). *Phenomenological Interpretations of Aristotle: Initiation into Phenomenological Research*, trans. R. Rojcewicz. Bloomington: Indiana University Press.

Jaspers K. (1968). "The Phenomenological Approach in Psychopathology," trans. J. N. Curran. *British Journal of Psychiatry* 114: 1313–1323.

Jaspers K. (1997). *General Psychopathology*, trans. J. Hoenig and M. W. Hamilton. Baltimore: Johns Hopkins University Press.

Køster A. (2017a). "Embodiment, Knowledge-Generation and Disciplinary Identity." *Constructivist Foundations* 13(1): 70–71.

Køster A. (2017b). "Personal History, Beyond Narrative: An Embodied Perspective." *Journal of Phenomenological Psychology* 48(2): 163–187.

Køster A. (2017c). "Narrative and Embodiment—A Scalar Approach." *Phenomenology and the Cognitive Sciences* 16(5): 893–908.

Køster A. (forthcoming). "Lidelsen i Tabet: Fænomenologiske Betragtninger Over Tabserfaringens Affektive Dybde." *Psyke & Logos*.

Køster A. and Winther-Lindqvist D. A. (2018). "Personal History and Historical Selfhood: A Phenomenological Perspective." In A. Rosa and J. Valsiner (eds.), *Cambridge Handbook of Socio-cultural Psychology*, 538–555. Cambridge: Cambridge University Press.

Luft S. and Overgaard S. (2011). "Introduction." In S. Luft and S. Overgaard (eds.), *The Routledge Companion to Phenomenology*, pp. 1–14. Hoboken: Routledge.

Maciejewski P. K., Maercker, A., Boelen P. A. and Prigerson H. G. (2016). "'Prolonged grief disorder' and 'persistent complex bereavement disorder', but not 'complicated grief', are one and the same diagnostic entity: an analysis of data from the Yale Bereavement Study." *World Psychiatry* 15: 266–275.

Parnas J. and Zahavi D. (2002). "The Role of Phenomenology in Psychiatric Diagnosis and Classification." In M. Maj, W. Gaebel, J. J. López-Ibor, and N. Sartorius (eds.), *Psychiatric Diagnosis and Classification*, pp. 137–162. New York: John Wiley & Sons.

Prigerson H. G., Horowitz M. J., Jacobs S. C., Parkes C. M., Aslan M., et al. (2009). "Prolonged Grief Disorder: Psychometric Validation of Criteria Proposed for DSM-V and ICD-11." *PLOS Medicine* 6(8): e1000121.

Ratcliffe M. (2008). *Feelings of Being: Phenomenology, Psychiatry and the Sense of Reality*. Oxford: Oxford University Press.

Ratcliffe M. (2009). "Existential Feeling and Psychopathology." *Philosophy, Psychiatry, & Psychology* 16(2): 179–194.

Ratcliffe M. (2013). "Why Mood Matters." In M. Wrathall (ed.), *The Cambridge Companion to Heidegger's Being and Time*, pp. 157–176. New York: Cambridge University Press.

Smith D. W. (2018). "Phenomenology." In E. N. Zalta (ed.), *The Stanford Encyclopedia of Philosophy*, (Summer 2018 Edition), https://plato.stanford.edu/archives/sum2018/entries/phenomenology/

Zahavi D. (2012). "Introduction." In D. Zahavi (ed.), *The Oxford Handbook of Contemporary Phenomenology*, pp. 1–4. Oxford: Oxford University Press.

CHAPTER 26

THE PHENOMENOLOGICAL APPROACH

DERMOT MORAN

INTRODUCTION: PHENOMENOLOGY AS THE SCIENCE OF SUBJECTIVITY

PHENOMENOLOGY, broadly speaking, involves the careful, unprejudiced *description* of conscious, lived experiences (Husserl's *Erlebnisse*), precisely according to the manner that they are experienced, without the imposition of external explanatory frameworks, whether these be drawn from the natural or social sciences, from religion, or even from common sense or ordinary language use. In this sense, phenomenology seeks to remain true to what conscious experience—understood in the widest possible sense—reveals to the disciplined observer. Phenomenology, then, must be loyal to the way our experiences are actually given to us (we shall come back to the problem of the right kind of language for describing experiences). Phenomenology aims to recuperate our responses to experience and, in particular, to resist reductionist, scientistic efforts to displace the richness of experience with a narrower, usually more naturalistic account of experience.

The enduring appeal of phenomenology is that it respects the importance and centrality of the first-person point of view. Phenomenology is, as Husserl put it, a science of subjectivity, but it is also a science of subjectivity embodied, embedded, and involved in the intersubjective constitution of objectivity. Phenomenology continues to attract interest because of its strong defence of the ineliminability of subjectivity and its detailed analyses of the structures of conscious life and of the "life-world," the ordinary, everyday, pre-scientific world that we inhabit. Phenomenologists can begin from their own experience, but they are open to understanding other people's experiences, as they are experienced (examples can be found in real life, in literature, or, simply, through the process of imaginative variation, a procedure that Husserl himself practiced). In other words, close attention must be paid to the subject's own account of their experiences, emotions, and how they form their general sense of matters that affect them.

THE PHENOMENOLOGICAL APPROACH: "BACK TO THE THINGS THEMSELVES"

Phenomenology as a movement is usually said to have begun with Husserl's *Logical Investigations* (Husserl 2001), although it has an earlier inauguration in the descriptive psychology of Franz Brentano (Brentano 1995), who was Husserl's mentor for a period in Vienna. Through Husserl's students and followers, it developed into a major philosophical movement in Europe (especially Germany and France) and subsequently in the United States and internationally. The main figures (Husserl, Scheler, Heidegger, Schutz, Sartre, Merleau-Ponty) developed phenomenology in different directions and did not necessarily agree on the central tenets of the approach (Moran 2000). Phenomenology, then, should be understood as a general *approach* rather than a strict *method*. Different phenomenologists, of course, have developed different approaches. Nevertheless, there are certain commonalities which can be observed as broadly characterizing the phenomenological approach. It is best to think of phenomenology not as a set of specific philosophical commitments but rather a disciplined approach that wishes to remain open to the role of subjectivity in the constitution of various forms of objectivity.

Husserl's original slogan was: "Back to the Things Themselves [*Zu den Sachen selbst*]" (Husserl 2001: 168). And this phrase soon became the catch-cry of the phenomenological movement. Husserl means that phenomenology should avoid metaphysical speculation or other forms of theorizing, and, making use of description rather than causal explanation, attempt to gain insight into the *essences* of all kinds of phenomena. Husserl's Freiburg colleague and former assistant, Martin Heidegger, in *Being and Time*, emphasized the specifically *methodological* dimension of phenomenology:

> The expression "phenomenology" signifies primarily a *methodological conception*. This expression does not characterize the what of the objects of philosophical research as subject-matter, but rather the *how* of that research.
>
> (Heidegger 1962: 50)

Heidegger wants to develop phenomenology as a way of making phenomena manifest. In *Being and Time*, Heidegger defines phenomenology as "to let that which shows itself be seen from itself in the very way in which it shows itself from itself" (Heidegger 1962: 58). This formulation is close to that found in Husserl's *Crisis of European Sciences*: "to take the conscious life, completely without prejudice, just as what it quite immediately gives itself, as itself, to be" (Husserl 1970: 233). In both Husserl and Heidegger, then, phenomenology aims at manifestation. At the same time, there is a strong injunction not to tamper with this disclosure or revelation but rather to allow it to manifest itself in its own peculiar way. Human subjects are, as Robert Sokolowski puts it, agents of disclosure, "agents of truth" (Sokolowski 2008).

There is an essential double-sidedness—often called "correlation" to phenomenological intuition. There is, on the one hand, *the object meant* or intended and, on the other hand, the *act of meaning* or *intending* it. Traditional philosophy has tended to emphasize one or the other side of this correlation (i.e. objectivist or subjectivist) and has rarely sought to give credit to the essential subject–object relation and the manner in which experience vacillates backwards and forwards between an object-focus and a subject-focus. Phenomenology argues that the objective view—what Merleau-Ponty calls, in his 1945 *Phenomenology of Perception*, "the view from nowhere [*la vue de nulle part*]" (Merleau-Ponty 2012)—is achieved only by abstracting from the original first-person stance with which humans engage with the world.

Phenomenology, then, offers an important corrective, analyzing and describing the structure of consciousness, intentionality, and embodied being-in-the-world in a way which does not lose sight of the *first-person* perspective, that is, subjectivity both singular and plural (Husserl speaks of the "we-world [*Wir-Welt*]"). For phenomenology, human beings are embodied, intentional meaning-makers, acting and suffering in a surrounding world (the "life-world"), and their subjective slant on matters is not just an annoying inconvenience for the objectivist sciences. Rather, it has to be acknowledged as the very medium of human existence and as the necessary condition for objectivity to be possible. This means phenomenology essentially involves understanding intentionality, the fact that all our lived experiences are about something, have some kind of significance, which is linked to a whole nexus or web of motivations and other intentional implications.

PHENOMENOLOGY AS INTENTIONAL DESCRIPTION OF MEANINGFUL EXISTENCE

Phenomenology essentially *is* intentional description, that is, it aims to describe all kinds of objects in terms of their correlation with subjectivity. Furthermore, phenomenology maintains that intentionality is all-pervasive; all aspects of life involve a coming together of subjective attitude and objective meaning. Besides the intentionality of cognitive states (such as believing, knowing), the intentional structures of perceptions, feelings, moods and emotions, acts of willing and deciding, as well as all kinds of habitual practices, are primary topics of exploration for phenomenologists.

Phenomenology may be characterized initially, very broadly, as a practice of attending to matters that manifest themselves to us ("phenomena" in the widest sense of the word). For Husserl, this meant understanding precisely the essential nature of perception, memory, imagination, temporal consciousness, and other forms of "calling to mind [*Vergegenwärtigung*]," and how these different conscious modalities interweave seamlessly in the stream of consciousness. What is the nature of perception? How are objects experienced in perception? What is their "mode of givenness"? How does perception become altered into a memory or a fantasy? These are typical phenomenological questions. Traditionally, phenomenologists have attempted to describe the essential features of conscious cognitive life, with specific studies of perception (Merleau-Ponty 2012), memory, imagination (Sartre 1962), willing (Pfänder 1967), valuing (Scheler 1973), and judging, but phenomenologists have also sought to describe affective life, feelings, emotions (Sartre 1971; Vendrell Ferran 2015), moods, existential concerns, and various dimensions of lived embodiment (Husserl 1989), and, more generally, "being-in-the-world" (Heidegger's *In-der-Welt-Sein*, Heidegger 1962; and Merleau-Ponty's *être-au-monde*, Merleau-Ponty 2012).

Phenomenological insights (which Husserl called "intuitions [*Anschauungen*]") are understood to be insights into the essential natures of matters (what Husserl called "essential seeing [*Wesensschau*]") that can be read off the phenomena by the trained observer. This intuitionist emphasis has been dismissed as a form of unreliable introspection by its critics (Searle 2000, 2005), but phenomenologists insist that the universal structural features of the experience can be uncovered by remaining attentive to the experience as it unfolds or as it is captured in unprejudiced reflection.

Phenomenology is a discipline, therefore, that tries to be extremely sensitive to the varieties of ways in which *meaning* presents itself to us as living, conscious, embodied subjects embedded in a shared environment, or "life-world [*Lebenswelt*]" (Husserl 1970). For phenomenology, this meaning is not necessarily tied to language and for this reason phenomenologists emphasize the intrinsic meaning involved in pre-linguistic embodied action and perception, in emotional states, moods, and in one's overall embodiment (right down to one's posture, see Straus 1966) and intersubjective relations with others, mediated through empathy (Husserl 1960).

Husserl insisted that phenomenology had to be "presuppositionless": one should not pre-suppose the results of the sciences or even the judgments of common sense. A large part of Husserl's concern is to emphasize the complexity of even simple acts of seeing. There is always, for instance, a combination of present and absent moments, to see the front side is at the same time to have an empty intending apprehension of the rear side of an object in the form of a determinable indeterminacy. It is important not to think that visual perception first and foremost involves "visual sensations," "stimuli," and so on (standard ways of describing experience found in philosophy and psychology since Locke). These descriptions are *not* faithful descriptions of experience, but rather they involve reference to putative theoretical entities ("sense data," "qualia," "stimuli," and so on). First and foremost, one sees physical, spatial entities in the world already endowed with sense, a *flowering apple tree* in the garden (Husserl 2014: 180); one certainly does not *see* sense data, mere patches of green, or some other kind of postulated intermediate entity. Furthermore, as Heidegger emphasizes, what one sees is constrained by one's background assumptions and by the overall context of the "environment [*Umwelt*]" and "life-world [*Lebenswelt*]"). A craftsperson can identify the appropriate tools for a particular task and immediately sees what needs to be done. The gardener identifies some plants as *flowers* and others as *weeds*, not based on botanical classification but based on their usefulness and appropriateness in the context of gardening (itself a cultural and historically inflected practice). This is what Heidegger means when he says we first encounter objects in a practical way as "ready-to-hand [*zuhanden*]" rather than merely as "present-at-hand [*vorhanden*]," objects merely theoretically apprehended, shorn of their context of usefulness (Heidegger 1962; Dreyfus 1991).

Martin Heidegger's *Being and Time* is regarded as one of the most creative and original works of philosophy of the twentieth century. Central to Heidegger's achievement in this work is his radical way of approaching human existence, which both makes the nature of human existence unfamiliar and startling (described in entirely novel terms) and at the same time recognizes the human being's inescapable hunger for familiarity, its anchoring in the routines of the everyday, its self-recognition in terms of the quotidian. Part of Heidegger's originality lies in the way that he emphasizes the "historicality" of human existence. It is not just that all humans live in history and have a history but that their orientation to existence is such as to be intrinsically historical. Being historical is an a priori condition of being human. Human existence then has to be understood in terms of its overall temporal dimensions

THE PHENOMENOLOGICAL REDUCTION: BREAKING WITH THE NATURAL ATTITUDE

Many phenomenologists follow Husserl in insisting that phenomenological description can only be practiced within the performance of the phenomenological reduction. Following the straightforward descriptive psychology of the *Logical Investigations*, around 1905, Husserl realized that he needed to apply a methodological break (which he called *epoché*, borrowing from the Greek Skeptics) with the pre-philosophical "natural" attitude in order to contemplate how meanings and significance are constituted and come to assume the "natural" character that they present to us in ordinary experience. In his *Ideas I*, for instance, Husserl speaks of *epoché* as rigorous "exclusion [*Ausschaltung*]" and an "abstention [*Enthaltung*]" from employing the methods or propositions of the philosophical tradition (Husserl 2014: 52). The *epoché* and the associated "phenomenological reductions" are meant to allow the nature of the experiences to become manifest without distortion and *to lead back* (Latin: *reducere*) to the apprehension of the essential ("eidetic") structures, contents, and objects and how they interconnect with other forms of consciousness. To filter out distortions produced by our everyday, straightforward assumptions and presuppositions (which need not be scientific assumptions, but could include religious beliefs, cultural values, and so on), Husserl proposes a process of suspension or bracketing (*epoché*) and a set of phenomenological and transcendental "reductions" as essential to the phenomenological method.

Heidegger, however, does not make explicit use of Husserl's phenomenological reduction, whereas Husserl thought it as essential to the point of claiming that anyone who misunderstood the importance of the reduction could not be doing phenomenology. Merleau-Ponty accepted a modified version of the phenomenological reduction. He famously said that the lesson of Husserl's reduction was that it could not be carried out to completion because it ran up against the indissoluble life-world—this "rupture can teach us nothing but the unmotivated springing forth of the world" (Merleau-Ponty 2012: lxxvii).

THE NATURAL AND THE TRANSCENDENTAL ATTITUDES

One of phenomenology's greatest and most useful discoveries is that of "the natural attitude [*die natürliche Einstellung*]"—a term Husserl uses from at least as early as 1906–07 but which emerges in print in *Ideas I* (Husserl 2014: 48). Because phenomenology focuses on the manner of experiencing, it necessarily involves interrupting natural, straightforward experiencing (as carried out in what Husserl calls "the natural attitude"). According to Husserl, in our everyday practices and routines, we are in a certain attitude ("the natural attitude") toward things and toward the world, and somehow this is a state of self-forgetfulness. The world presents itself as simply there, given, available to us.

In his mature works, Husserl articulates in some detail the meaning of mundane life in the "natural attitude," which involves all aspects of human engagement with others and with the world as a whole (Landgrebe 1940), the very experience of "being-in-the-world" that Heidegger later explicitly thematizes in *Being and Time*. Disrupting the natural attitude and undermining its hold on us will be central to Husserl's practice of the phenomenological method. By applying a deliberate "exclusion," "suspension," or "bracketing" (*epoché*) of our straightforward commitments, phenomenology hopes to uncover the necessary structures that govern the essence of experiences as such, including the particular character they have in the natural mode of experiencing. This led Husserl in particular to adopt a transcendental stance, which sees consciousness as somehow antecedent to the world, and strongly to oppose all forms of naturalism.

Subjectivity as Embodied, Embedded, and Enworlded

As Husserl's phenomenology developed, he increasingly emphasized that we are *incarnate*, that is to say, embodied, *situated, finite* human beings, already in the world and for whom the world has a given, taken-for-granted, "natural" status. Husserl himself speaks of the "phenomenology of embodiment [*Phänomenologie der Leiblichkeit*]." Similarly, he attended to the enworlded nature of our experience. Much of Husserl's puzzlement came from trying to figure out how it is that the lived world comes to have this *taken-for-grantedness, self-givenness*, and *obviousness* in the natural attitude. Of course, this situatedness and locatedness went on to become the theme of "*In-der-Welt-sein*" in Heidegger or "*être-au-monde*" in Merleau-Ponty.

Phenomenology puts special focus on identifying the a priori frameworks involved in the stream of a coherent, unified conscious life (not just spatiality and temporality, as in the Kantian tradition, but also the a priori structures of human, embodied, social being-in-the-world). Initially phenomenologists, moreover, concentrated primarily on *individual* conscious life, but they (Husserl, Scheler, Stein) soon explored the apprehension of others (in empathy, Scheler 2008), and the constitution of communal, social, and cultural life, indeed the historical dimension of human existence. Classic phenomenology—primarily the work of Husserl, Heidegger, Max Scheler, Edith Stein, Alfred Schutz, Jean-Paul Sartre, and Maurice Merleau-Ponty—proposed a very broad program of research that included essential analyses of all the central aspects of human existence: intentionality, consciousness, perception, embodiment, the "horizontal" nature of experiences, the dimensions of lived temporality, the experience of one's self, the experience of others in "empathy [*Einfühlung*]" (Stein 1989), the experience of alterity, more generally, and intercorporeality, as well as in the understanding of social relations (Stein 2000), intersubjectivity, historicity, sociality, and the whole vague but real experience of "worldhood" (i.e. belonging to an open-ended "life-world" as the ultimate horizon of all experience). Indeed, the classical phenomenological tradition is still a rich source of analyses of phenomena such as imagination, memory, emotions, moods, liminal experiences, the complex character of embodiment or incarnation (with its essential finitude), the experience of lived temporality and historicality, as well as humans' experience of tools, artworks, and the transformation of life in the modern technological world (Heidegger 1977). More recently, phenomenologists have also attended to issues of gender following the explorations of Simone de Beauvoir and Maurice Merleau-Ponty (Young 2005; Butler 2007) and to the construction of social identity (including the sense of belonging to a "group" or larger collective whole).

Husserl, for instance, claims (and here he strongly influenced Merleau-Ponty) that perception is a multimodal achievement, an intertwining of various sense modalities (sight, touch) and of bodily proprioceptive movements (called "kinaestheses" in the psychological terminology of the time) such as eye movements, hand movements, movements of the body (to get nearer, get a better grip, look more closely), involving looking over the object, pointing, grasping, moving around the object, and so on. The body is in the world as the "heart is in the organism," Merleau-Ponty declares (Merleau-Ponty 2012: 209). It is our embodied perception that brings the visible and tangible world alive and Merleau-Ponty in particular shows the entanglement or "chiasme" that is constantly at work between the separate senses (e.g. touch and sight), as well as between body and world (Merleau-Ponty 1968). Moreover, disorders of the embodied relation to the world involve a significant modification of the way the world appears. There is a very fine attunement between lived body and world and it is upset in pathological cases, like the case of the brain-damaged former soldier, Schneider, discussed by Merleau-Ponty (Merleau-Ponty 2012: 105–140). Merleau-Ponty's discussions have inspired a whole phenomenology of embodiment that recognizes the complex manner in which humans are inserted through their "lived," animate bodies into the environing world.

PHENOMENOLOGY AS INTERPRETIVE AND HERMENEUTICAL

Martin Heidegger, especially in *Being and Time* (Heidegger 1962), radicalized Husserl's intentionality to offer a description of human existence (*Dasein*) as essentially *transcending itself* toward the world and developed the conception that human beings can live rather anonymously and "inauthentically" as "the one [*das Man*]," simply following the crowd and doing as others do. But humans can also, through the deep, highly individualizing, existential experience of anxiety (*Angst*), face up to their own intrinsic finitude and mortality and can come face to face with their authentic singularity and freedom to project themselves into a future that they deliberately choose.

Heidegger's introduction of *hermeneutics* (i.e. the theory of interpretation) into phenomenology was a way of neutralizing or at least exposing the operation of prejudice in our understanding. Prejudices for him cannot be eliminated, but at least they can be made transparent, acknowledged, and our corresponding insights put in correlation with these pre-judgments so that our understanding progressed in a "circular" manner (the hermeneutic circle), going backwards and forwards between what is understood and the manner in which it is understood. Heidegger—inspired by Wilhelm Dilthey—combined hermeneutics, the art of interpretative understanding, with phenomenology. Heidegger argued—against Husserl—that pure, unprejudiced description is impossible, since all understanding takes place with the horizon of presuppositions that are essential for the understanding to take place. At best, unrecognized presuppositions or "pre-judgments [*Vorurteilen*]" can be made manifest but they can never be entirely dispensed with. Furthermore, language is essential to understanding and communication, and language always has a particular slant or leaning. Both Heidegger and his student Hans-Georg Gadamer emphasize the centrality of the human capacity for "linguisticality [*Sprachlichkeit*]." As Gadamer asserts in his 1960 *Truth and Method*, "language is the medium of the hermeneutic experience," that is, language is the medium in which understanding is realized (Gadamer 1989: 384). Heidegger's hermeneutical phenomenology focuses more on uncovering the essential "*existentiale*" framework governing what is pre-given and assumed in human existence's (*Dasein's*) practical engagement with the world of interests and "in-order-to's." For Heidegger, humans are already embedded ("*immer schon da*") in a pre-formed, and largely intuitively apprehended, historical and cultural world. Moreover, they are oriented primarily to the future, and the past is always implicitly interpreted in terms of this future project.

Gadamer's own hermeneutics is heavily indebted to phenomenology. He sees his hermeneutics as making manifest or displaying "the matters themselves [*die Sachen selbst*]," shedding light on the essence of these matters in what he calls an "illumination of essence [*Wesenserhellung*]." In fact, hermeneutics, for Gadamer, is the project of self-understanding and understanding others, and as such it can be said to develop a *phenomenology* of the very process of understanding (*Verstehen*).

EXISTENTIAL PHENOMENOLOGY

Phenomenology came to France in the 1930s, primarily through Emmanuel Levinas, Jean-Paul Sartre (especially *Being and Nothingness*, Sartre 1995), and Maurice Merleau-Ponty. Phenomenology now takes on an existential dimension and issues concerning human existence, the experience of freedom, of anxiety, of alienation, the expectation of one's own death, and one's concernful dealings with others, now come to the fore. Sartre and Merleau-Ponty emphasized human embodiment, facticity, being in a situation, the experience of freedom and the experience of being forced to choose in the absence of any objective norms governing the choice. Thus, for example, Sartre, in his 1938 novel *Nausea* (Sartre 1965) describes the experience of vertigo (e.g. standing on a cliff ledge) as precisely the sense of anxiety that overcomes one when one realizes that one's freedom is entirely in one's own hands. The vertigo is not the recognition of the possibility of falling but of the experienced freedom of taking responsibility for the decision *not to jump*.

Merleau-Ponty considered Husserl's emphasis on the *epoché* and phenomenological reduction to be both crucial but problematic. As we saw earlier, Merleau-Ponty denies the possibility of a complete reduction. One can never completely detach oneself from the life-world in which we are embodied and embedded. For Merleau-Ponty, the practice of phenomenological seeing is meant to disrupt the everyday. In his *Phenomenology of Perception*, he writes: "true philosophy entails learning to see the world anew" (Merleau-Ponty 2012: lxxxv). Philosophy will shed light on the "birth of being" for us. Phenomenology aims at "disclosure of the world [*révélation du monde*]" (Merleau-Ponty 2012: lxxvii); its task is to reveal the mystery of the world.

Phenomenological description and taking seriously the obvious experiential evidence that people's emotions, feelings, and moods are intentional (i.e. are about something and are obviously meaningful in some manner) was a very important insight for psychologists and psychiatrists especially in the 1920s. The early phenomenologists, especially Max Scheler and Edith Stein, discussed feelings and emotions. Right at the heart of this approach is that people's moods and traumas are modalities of being-in-the-world. These experiences are lived deeply in the body, in a person's self-experience and in their experience with others. In this regard, Heidegger has made significant contributions with his analyses of "fundamental moods [*Grundstimmungen*]," "disposition/state of mind/attunement [*Befindlichkeit*]," and the experience of "thrownness [*Geworfenheit*]," finding oneself always thrown into a situation. Heidegger is famous for locating authentic self-understanding in a deep anxiety which comes over each human existence at some point. Anxiety is not like fear, a relationship to something in particular, but has as its object one's whole being-in-the-world. One's whole being is experienced as groundless and unsupported. Sartre develops this with his account of vertigo—where one experiences one's own absolute freedom. Vertigo is not so much the fear of falling as the fear of jumping. One's inner freedom is limitless and in this sense truly terrifying, opening up before one like a yawning chasm.

THE APPLICATION OF PHENOMENOLOGY

It is not difficult to see the benefits of phenomenological description for medical diagnoses, for example, the correct recognition of symptoms, and so on. One can also see that literature is a vast repository of such proto-phenomenological description and disambiguation, for example, consider the explorations of jealousy, possessiveness, envy, and so on, in Shakespeare. Of course, the ability to make fine discriminations (as in the case of the professional wine-taster) has to be matched with an equal ability to translate these discriminations into appropriately fine-grained linguistic communication. Literary description has the phenomenological character of being a description from the subjective point of view but of course it has not been methodologically refined and distilled through the techniques of disengagement and bracketing that phenomenology brings to bear. Presumably, literary descriptions do aim at a universality and hence have the claim to eidetic character that phenomenology also seeks. Husserl himself recognized this problem but did not address it centrally, at least until some of his later writings, for instance his essay "On the Origin of Geometry" (Husserl 1970) where he accords to written language an enormously important role in fixing the meanings of ideal objectivities such as occur in mathematics so that they can be accessed as the same over and over again. For Heidegger, however, the issue of language became inescapable and marked a major turning in his conception of phenomenology and its possibilities. Subsequent phenomenology has had to grapple with the complexity of the relationship between language and experience in ways that have frequently challenged many of Husserl's assumptions. This is the case with Jacques Derrida, for instance, insofar as his work is motivated by phenomenology and continues to work within the phenomenological *epoché*, as he himself has attested (Derrida 2011).

Initially, when it originally emerged in Husserl and Scheler, interest in phenomenology was more or less confined to academic philosophy. But it was soon taken up and adapted by other disciplines in the social and human sciences, for example, psychology, psychiatry, psychoanalysis, sociology, literary theory, art criticism, cultural studies, religious studies, and more recently, film theory, gender and identity studies, and studies concerned with human embodiment and intersubjectivity. Both as a strict method and, more generally, as a theoretical approach, phenomenology is now well established not only within theoretical philosophy, but also in various forms of sociology (Schutz 1967; Schutz and Luckmann 1973, 1983), psychology (Gurwitsch 1964), psychiatry and psychotherapy (Binswanger 1963; Straus 1964, 1966; Giorgi 1970, 2009; Gendlin 1981; Heidegger 2001), and, more recently, as a method of qualitative analysis in the social and health sciences (Smith, Flowers, and Larkin 2009). Phenomenology continues to provide a rich resource of procedures and perspectives for illuminating human experiences.

Bibliography

Binswanger L. (1963). *Being-in-the-world: Selected Papers of Ludwig Binswanger*, trans. J. Needleman. New York: Basic Books.

Brentano F. (1995). *Psychology from an Empirical Standpoint*, trans. A. C. Rancurello, D. B. Terrell, and L. McAlister. With a new Introduction by P. Simons. London: Routledge.

Butler J. (2007). *Gender Trouble: Feminism and the Subversion of Identity*. London: Routledge.

Derrida J. (2011). *Voice and Phenomenon. Introduction to the Problem of the Sign in Husserl's Phenomenology*, trans. L. Lawlor. Evanston: Northwestern University Press.

Dreyfus H. L. (1991). *Being-In-the-World. A Commentary on Heidegger's Being and Time, Division I*. Cambridge, MA: MIT Press.

Gadamer H.-G. (1989). *Truth and Method*, trans. J. Weinsheimer and D. G. Marshall. 2nd rev edn. London: Sheed & Ward.

Gendlin E. (1981). *Focusing*. 2nd rev edn. New York: Bantam Books.

Giorgi A. (1970). *Psychology as a Human Science: A Phenomenologically Based Approach*. New York: Harper & Row.

Giorgi A. (2009). *The Descriptive Phenomenological Method in Psychology: A Modified Husserlian Approach*. Pittsburgh: Duquesne University Press.

Gurwitsch A. (1964). *The Field of Consciousness*. Pittsburgh: Duquesne University Press.

Husserl E. (1960). *Cartesian Meditations*, trans. D. Cairns. The Hague: Martinus Nijhoff.

Heidegger M. (1962). *Being and Time*, trans. J. Macquarrie and E. Robinson. New York: Harper and Row.

Heidegger M. (1977). *The Question Concerning Technology and Other essays*, trans. W. Lovitt. New York: Garland Publishing.

Heidegger M. (2001). *Zollikon Seminars: Protocols–Conversations–Letters*, ed. Medard Boss, trans. F. Mayr and R. Askay. Evanston: Northwestern University Press.

Husserl E. (1970). *The Crisis of European Sciences and Transcendental Phenomenology. An Introduction to Phenomenological Philosophy*, trans. D. Carr. Evanston: Northwestern University Press.

Husserl E. (1989). *Ideas Pertaining to a Pure Phenomenology and to a Phenomenological Philosophy, Second Book*, trans. R. Rojcewicz and A. Schuwer. Collected Works III. Dordrecht: Kluwer.

Husserl E. (2001). *Logical Investigations*, 2 vols, trans. J. N. Findlay. Edited with a New Introduction by Dermot Moran and New Preface by Michael Dummett. London and New York: Routledge.

Husserl E. (2014). *Ideas for a Pure Phenomenology and Phenomenological Philosophy. First Book*. General Introduction to Pure Phenomenology, trans. D. O. Dahlstrom. Indianapolis: Hackett.

Landgrebe L. (1940). "The World as a Phenomenological Problem." *Philosophy and Phenomenological Research* 1: 38–58.

Merleau-Ponty M. (1968). *The Visible and the Invisible*, trans. A. Lingis. Evanston: Northwestern University Press.

Merleau-Ponty M. (2012). *The Phenomenology of Perception*, trans. D. A. Landes. London: Routledge.

Moran D. (2000). *Introduction to Phenomenology*. London and New York: Routledge.

Pfänder A. (1967). *Phenomenology of Willing and Other Phaenomenologica*, trans. H. Spiegelberg. Evanston: Northwestern University Press.

Sartre J.-P. (1962). *Imagination. A Psychological Critique*, trans. F. Williams. Ann Arbor: University of Michigan Press.

Sartre J.-P. (1965). *Nausea*, trans. R. Baldick. Harmondsworth: Penguin.

Sartre J.-P. (1971). *Sketch for a Theory of the Emotions*, trans. P. Mairet. London: Methuen.

Sartre J.-P. (1995). *Being and Nothingness. An Essay on Phenomenological Ontology*, trans. H. Barnes. London: Routledge.

Scheler M. (1973). *Formalism in Ethics and Non-Formal Ethics of Values. A New Attempt Toward a Foundation of an Ethical Personalism*, trans. M. S. Frings and R. L. Funk. Evanston: Northwestern University Press.

Scheler M. (2008). *The Nature of Sympathy*, trans. P. Heath. Rev edn with New Introduction by G. McAleer. New Brunswick: Transaction Publishers.

Schutz A. (1967). *The Phenomenology of the Social World*, trans. G. Walsh and F. Lehnert. Evanston: Northwestern University Press.

Schutz A. and Luckmann T. (1973). *The Structures of the Life-World. Vol. 1*, trans. R. M. Zaner, and H. T. Engelhardt Jr. Evanston: Northwestern University Press.

Schutz A. and Luckmann T. (1983). *The Structures of the Life-World. Vol. 2*, trans. R. M. Zaner and D. J. Parent. Evanston: Northwestern University Press.

Searle J. R. (2000). "The Limits of Phenomenology." In Mark A. Wrathall and Jeff Malpas (eds.), *Heidegger, Coping, and Cognitive Science: Essays in Honor of Hubert L. Dreyfus, Vol. 2*, pp. 71–92. Cambridge, MA: MIT Press.

Searle J. R. (2005). "The Phenomenological Illusion." In M. E. Reicher and J. C. Marek (eds.), *Experience and Analysis. Erfahrung und Analyse*, 317–336. Vienna: ÖBV&HPT Verlag, 2005.

Smith J. A., Flowers, P., and Larkin, M. (2009). *Interpretative Phenomenological Analysis: Theory Method and Research*. London: Sage.

Sokolowski R. (2008). *Phenomenology of the Human Person*. New York: Cambridge University Press.

Stein E. (1989). *On the Problem of Empathy*, trans. W. Stein. Collected Works of Edith Stein Vol. 3. Washington, DC: ICS Publications.

Stein E. (2000). *Philosophy of Psychology and the Humanities*. Washington, DC: ICS Publications.

Straus E. W. (ed.) (1964). *Phenomenology: Pure and Applied*. Pittsburgh: Duquesne University Press.

Straus E. W. (1966). *Phenomenological Psychology*, trans. E. Eng. New York: Basic Books.

Vendrell Ferran I. (2015). "The Emotions in Early Phenomenology." *Studia Phaenomenolgica* 15: 349–374.

Young I. M. (2005). *On Female Body Experience: "Throwing Like a Girl" and Other Essays*. Oxford: Oxford University Press.

....

CHAPTER 27

CLINICAL PHENOMENOLOGY: *DESCRIPTIVE, STRUCTURAL, AND TRANSCENDENTAL PHENOMENOLOGY*

....

DOROTHÉE LEGRAND

PHILOSOPHY BECOMING CLINICAL
....

CLINICAL phenomenologists[1] tirelessly hold a reflective stance on their practice, aiming to determine its foundations and delimit its scope. In itself, the reiteration of this effort suggests a resistance of clinical practice to comply with a given philosophical system, and a resistance of philosophy to blend into a given clinical practice. Phenomenology confronts philosophy and clinical practice with a process aiming at a uniformity that constantly fails and thus calls for ceaselessly rethinking their articulation as a never achieved process. Prioritizing *philosophical loyalty* assumes that phenomenology, even if clinical, can in no way give up its philosophical exigency, and cannot accept any compromise that would use the excuse of clinical practice to offload heavy philosophical constraints (Boss 1980: 98). In this case, clinical practice *is* philosophical. However, strictly speaking, clinical practice is *not* philosophical if the clinician, not the philosopher, aims at turning the knowledge of the condition of Being-Human into the acknowledgment of a human being singularly. If it is thus recognized that "the direction of questioning" (Blankenburg 2012: 30)[2] orients differently the investigation depending on whether it is philosophical or clinical,[3] then the guide favored by the clinician will be *clinical fecundity*; the ethics of clinical practice is to be first and always guided

---

[1] Here, under the name "clinical phenomenology," we will speak about different practices of phenomenology in different clinical fields, including psychiatry, psychopathology, clinical psychology, psychoanalysis.

[2] Unfortunately, a lot of the material used in this chapter is not available in English. All quotes from texts that are not available in English have been translated by the author.

[3] Heidegger himself deals with this issue, in concrete terms. *Being and Time* states: "Da-sein is that being whose being itself is at issue. You are concerned with me, and I with you. Thereby, are you doing the analytic of Da-sein? No. But you see me, and I am present to you, within the horizon of the determinations of Da-sein as given by the analytic of Da-sein. We stated that the analytic of Da-sein

by the clinical encounter, by the hospitality given to the other, even at the cost of being un-faithful to the philosophical foundation of this practice. But wouldn't such infidelity call for a philosophical revision? Do we not then enter a dialectical movement between a philo-sophical moment of one's practice and a clinical one? And after such a circulation, wouldn't it be the case that the philosophical and clinical directions of questioning would lose their specificities by merging into one undifferentiated practice?

Here, we will not try to determine whether a clinical practice *is* or *is not* philosophical—as if a definitive criterion could be set; instead we will insist on the *ongoing dynamics* that tie together philosophy and clinical practice, and propose that philosophy *becomes* clinical when, "certainly *without denying* the essential ideas that probably first show themselves *away from the real*, there would be a *necessity* to come closer to the facts where these ideas are, at first, *unrecognizable*, but where they are clarified and *justified* by all the concreteness of human suffering" (Levinas 1984: 408; italics modified). This sentence alone, as it weaves, *without confusing them*, philo-sophical and clinical orientations, allows us to glimpse the *dynamics* of their *unstable* articula-tion. Moreover, it appears here that no choice needs to be made between one's commitment to philosophy and one's engagement into clinical practice: *philosophical fidelity* is *justified* by *clin-ical fecundity*. Conceived of as such, the most fruitful philosophico-clinical joints do not neces-sarily allow or compel us to decide between the fiercest philosophical oppositions. In particular, phenomenology is inherently heterogeneous, and it is by avoiding the exclusion of a given phil-osophical orientation, that is, it is "in virtue of" the articulation of *different* orientations that a "concept is set in motion," and may become clinical (Blankenburg 2012: 33, 171).

BRAIDING PHENOMENOLOGICAL ANALYSIS

Given the complexity of a practice at once philosophical and clinical, the efforts made to determine a field proper to clinical phenomenology have been unceasing. Notably, a divi-sion of labor haunts this domain, according to whether it aims at describing experiential *contents*, the *structure* of these experiences, and/or the *transcendental* constitution of these experiences. This methodological division is supported by the distinction between, on the one hand, that which *would* be directly accessible as immediate data of consciousness and, on the other hand, that which would not be so accessible, and would thus require an analysis.

Emphasizing such division of labor, Karl Jaspers inaugurated the introduction of phenom-enology in clinical practice by stating that "[i]n phenomenology we scrutinize a number of qualities or states and the understanding that accompanies this has a *static* quality" (Jaspers 1997: 27; emphasis in the original). Thus, phenomenology leaves to others to understand and explain "the emergence of one psychic phenomenon from another" (Jaspers 1997: 25). Against such a restriction of the phenomenological scope, it will be assumed here that it is the different descriptive, structural, and transcendental threads that, together, weave

---

interprets the being of this being. And if you now speak to me without doing the analytic of Da-sein, then this is not speaking in an ontological sense. But you are directed toward me as the one who exists in an ontic sense. Dasein analysis is ontic. The analytic of Dasein is ontologic . . . The decisive point is that the particular phenomena, arising in the relationship between the analysand and the analyst, and belonging to the respective, concrete patient, be broached in their own phenomenological content and not simply be classified globally under existentialia" (Heidegger 2001a: 124).

clinical phenomenology. Triple in such a way, phenomenology is nonetheless not omnipotent since, rigorously, one cannot presuppose the possibility of a total clarification of the phenomenon under investigation, even via the descriptions of finely detailed contents of consciousness, complex experiential structures, and universally powerful transcendental processes. Jaspers himself argues that our direct access to psychic states is only superficial, as if we would thereby only touch "the foam on the sea's surface" (Jaspers 1997: 10). To explain psychic depths themselves would require relying upon "extra-conscious mechanisms, unconscious events" which are "never actually experienced" and thus remain inaccessible even to the most advanced description (Jaspers 1997: 10–11). For Jaspers, this is where phenomenology ends; however, this is where it begins for Heidegger.

Phenomenology, Heidegger writes, is a method that, as such, is "directly opposed to the *naïveté* of a haphazard, 'immediate', and unreflective 'beholding'"; phenomenological analysis aims at "something that proximally and for the most part does not show itself at all . . . something that lies *hidden*" (Heidegger 2001: 61; emphasis in the original). As phenomenological, *analysis* is conceived of variously, depending on theoretical positions that otherwise tear apart members of the phenomenological corpus. Nonetheless, practically, it carries at least one consensus: we could not practice clinical phenomenology if we were not making ourselves capable "of welcoming and accepting impartially, without restriction and without being deformed by our own theoretical and intellectual prejudices or by personal and emotional censures, what we always and invariably obtain from our analysands by listening to them and observing them" (Boss 1980: 152). Under the motto "phenomenology," one here aspires to "a description as freed from theory as possible" (Blankenburg 2012: 22). Already, this descriptive approach requires to "return to the thing itself": one must "return" below one's "sedimented attainment," and have the "rigor," the "scientific courage" to renounce them (Maldiney 1986: 11).

Armed with such method, phenomenological clinical practice does not restrict its scope to pathology.[4] Rather, it occurs before any attribution of normality or abnormality, to target what constitutes both.[5] Although this can be taken neither as its birth certificate, nor as its specificity, clinical phenomenology positions itself against any clinical practice that would be "in default of the human dimension": the clinical phenomenologist recognizes that if "the human being is capable of madness," mental suffering is a "properly human dimension" (Maldiney 1986: 9–10; de Waelhens 1972). Accordingly, what clinical phenomenology aims at is the analysis of what it means to "be a human being."

Structural Analysis

In its anthropological vein, the phenomenological analysis of being-human is, notably, an investigation of a singular person's history: listening to the patient as an individual subject aims at a reconstitution of lived experiences and a thoughtful reconstruction of the inner history of life (Binswanger 1994b). This history is the "unique, unrepeatable relation" of

---

[4]   This contrasts with Jaspers 1997: 4, 45–46.
[5]   See e.g. Blankenburg 2012: 27; Binswanger 1971: 149; Binswanger 1994a: 207.

experiential contents, as lived by the individual person. By identifying this history, one is led to "what is most individual in the individual," to the "origin or center of [his] lived experiences" (Binswanger 1994b: 76, 85, 81).[6]

The introduction of such phenomenological anthropology in clinical practice has participated in the evolution from "an objectifying science to a subjectifying science" (Binswanger 1994c: 65). Certainly, "phenomenology is not a purely subjective method" (ibid.) but its clinical practice has been constructed against a conception of the relationship between a clinician and a patient reduced to the treatment of a disease by a therapy. What phenomenology reminds the clinician of is that an encounter essentially consists in "that you never see an isolated phenomenon but the phenomenon always takes place on the background of a self" (Binswanger 1994c: 58).[7] Once this foundation of clinical practice is recognized, research can and must investigate the mode of encounter by which we specifically relate to others as subjects.

Phenomenologically, this primarily means a "return" to the "basic phenomenon" (Binswanger 1994c: 65), that is, the person. No further step is needed with Husserl's phenomenology to recognize that this person, the so-called *subject*, is structurally directed toward something other than himself, the so-called *object*. Such is *intentionality*. Following this structural analysis of consciousness, on the one hand, intentionality, rather than a cut, is a "unitary relation between transcendental subjectivity and transcendental objectivity" (Binswanger 1975a: 207);[8] and on the other hand, intentionality is a transcendence: with the notion of intentionality, "the phenomenologist does not say: there is an object contained in perception" (Binswanger 1994c: 47); rather, he seeks to understand how the subject is structured by "the surpassing towards the world or transcendence" (Binswanger 1965: 17).

However, if "a subject can never be represented in its subjectivity otherwise than as a primary immanence," if, thinking in terms of subjectivity, "one has from the start necessarily attributed to everything else the character of objectivity," if one has "immediately and radically separated the human being from what comes to him" (Boss 1980: 91) then, to grasp the human being in its uniqueness and unity, phenomenological research must "return" from intentionality to a pre-subjective and pre-objective mode of being-in-the-world.[9]

With *this* phenomenology, the clinician defends that being-human never consists in "surpassing oneself subjectively towards things or let them objectively enter into oneself" (Boss 1980: 93, see also 63); rather, one is in contact with the moment where "the union of the subjective and the objective is felt as still un-split" (Blankenburg 1986: 137). Here, with Heidegger, the notion of transcendence changes meaning: being-human is being-in-the-world, that is, it is neither transcending oneself nor being transcended: it is being transcendence. Thus, if clinical phenomenology follows the notion of transcendence as its methodological Ariadne's thread, here it is because it aims at "the description of the modalities of the unity of self and world" (Binswanger 1955b: 228).

Clinical phenomenology here departs from the structural analysis of consciousness in terms of subject–object intentional correlations; resisting any "subjectivation of transcendence" (Boss 1980: 97), its *anthropological* investigation of the meaning of being-*human* becomes an *ontological* investigation of *being*-human. And if the clinician cannot bracket the ontological

---

[6] See also Binswanger 1994a: 214, 1947: 98, 1955a: 235.
[7] See also Binswanger 1994c: 54, 1994a: 205–206.   [8] See also Blankenburg 2012: 23.
[9] See e.g. Binswanger 1947: 101–102; Blankenburg 2012: 12.

dimension of being-human, it is because the question of who the human being is cannot be tackled without referring to the question of the meaning of being (Heidegger 2001: 119–120, see also 122) because "the human being can only be human by understanding being": being-human is "standing in the openness of being" (Heidegger 2001: 121). This definition of the human being, ontological rather than anthropological, is prolonged clinically by the view that human existence is "trans-subjective": it ought to be conceived of as the unity of oneself with "something universal, 'objective,' and impersonal" (Binswanger 1975b: 234). For phenomenology, the challenge of this analysis is nothing minor: from there, it cannot retreat from the exigency to work with what lurks below the conscious subject.

TRANSCENDENTAL ANALYSIS

Always reaching further down, clinical phenomenology then offers not only a *structural* analysis of being-human as being-in-the-world, but also a *transcendental* analysis of being-human as "coming-to-the-world" (Blankenburg 2012: 146). What clinical phenomenology here aims at is not the static description of experiential contents, but the genesis of human existence, its transcendental constitution.[10] Here, clinical phenomenology operates a "return to Husserl"— without unconditionally presupposing subject–object intentionality (Blankenburg 2012: 32).[11]

To account for "the construction, the *constitution*, or the *genesis*" of experience, "we must go down to the first 'beginnings' of conscious experience" (Binswanger 1965: 35; emphasis in the original).[12] Clinical phenomenology is here looking for the constitutive foundation of being-human, and its failure as a "fundamental disorder" (Blankenburg 2012: 15–21). It is the *basis* that is aimed at: whether the transcendental frame continues to support the human being as the very ground of his existence, whether the human being has a relation to himself and to the world that allows him to be transcendentally carried (Blankenburg 1991: 230). Phenomenologically, the return to the base does not operate or does not operate only through a transcendental reduction by which "all given (including the particular empirical subject) is simply described as constituted in the transcendental ego" (Blankenburg 2012: 31); the "source of all constitution" is not only conceptualized as the "pure ego" that would fulfill the function of constituting an experience of "this is me (*Ich bin es*)" (Binswanger 1960: 117). Below such a subjectivist approach,[13] clinical phenomenology is deployed further, by continuously renewing the fruitful infidelities that it operates by each of its motions from Husserl to Heidegger to Husserl. The transcendental "base" is an "evidence," a *selbstverständlichkeit*, namely, that which is self-understood (Blankenburg 2012: 99). A syllabic reading of this single word, *selbstverständlichkeit*, suggests "a relation to the pre-intentional world which is not yet polarized on a human 'I'. What dominates here is an understanding that includes an a-personal, infinitive character. Human consciousness is only the anonymous stage on

---

[10] See also Binswanger 1960: 16–17.   [11] See also Mishara 1986: 181, 186, 191.
[12] See also Binswanger 1960: 13.
[13] "In contrast to Husserl and his phenomenology, . . . being human is fundamentally stated as Dasein. This is done explicitly, as opposed to the characterizations of the human being as subjectivity and as transcendental Ego-consciousness" (Heidegger 2001: 120).

which this is played and we do little more than participating, almost by accident, to this self-understanding of things" (Blankenburg 2012: 99).[14] At its base, far from "our own work," experience appears primarily as the work of a passive synthesis—and here transcendental phenomenology is linked with genetic analysis (Husserl 2001).

Clinical phenomenology is here confronted with "an anonymous transcendental constitution which has always already occurred" (Blankenburg 2012: 106). It does not abandon the subject—it couldn't do so without losing itself as a phenomenological clinical practice—but reveals a subjectivity ordered to "a fundamental receptivity" (Blankenburg 2012: 73); the subject is a "product of coagulation" that emerges from an a-subjective "originary source," from the "anonymous sea of everything that happens 'by itself,'" while one's individual consciousness, "continually forgetful of its origin," erects the "I" as its transcendental source. Being-human here is conceived dialectically as a possibility to "let oneself be as taking foundation and giving foundation," a "mutual relationship between being-summoned-to-respond and being-able-to-respond" (Blankenburg 2012: 124–128, 110).

This characterization of being-human imposes its requirements to the conception and practice of analysis within clinical phenomenology. As a transcendental foundation, the "base" is always presupposed; it not only "does not require clarification," but also it is "largely unfit to clarification" (Blankenburg 2012: 101). Transcendental evidence is "inaccessible," "silenced," subjected to a "constant omission," "fallen into oblivion and ignorance" (Blankenburg 1986: 138).

To lift "the mask of the banal" and reveal the "basal," it is necessary for clinical phenomenologists to practice a transcendental analysis, in order to touch what, by definition, "does not let itself be apprehended in the frame of cognition, which itself remains engaged within the natural evidence." This work thus requires the clinician to take a few steps "in the direction of a self-alienation, a certain detachment from one's anchor in the soil of the healthy habituality of everyday consciousness." This is exactly the *epoché* for clinical phenomenology: a "radical detachment—methodically directed . . . detachment from the evidences of everyday existence" (Blankenburg 2012: 83, 108–109).

The *epoché* is not only the suspension of theoretical knowledge and related judgments; it is not only a methodological prescription to limit the scope of phenomenology to the description of "what is immanent to consciousness" (Binswanger 1994c: 46); rather, the *epoché* is a "technical device of any phenomenological endeavor" and as such it is a "bracketing" of factual reality, a suspension of the banalization of the transcendental base (Blankenburg 2012: 87, 27).[15]

It should be clear that such phenomenological suspension is *not* the pathological loss of natural evidence; the *epoché* is not madness. The patient must make "desperate efforts to maintain a minimum of evidences necessary for survival," and he must fight against the "terror about the lack of ground of his own existence"; conversely, the phenomenologist fights against the "inclination of life" that opposes "considerable resistance against the realization of a *epoché*"; what is "experienced as a singular 'agony'" by one "must be arduously conquered" by the other (Blankenburg 2012: 97, 133, 93, 90). Therefore, the clinician should never neglect the difference between, on the one hand, the phenomenological alienation from his habitual self, which he exercises by practicing the *epoché*, and on the other hand,

---

[14] Heidegger 2001: 122.   [15] See also Binswanger 1960: 16–17.

the pathological alienation from the ground of his existence which the patient is subjected to in an immeasurable *lack of being*. This difference is every time reaffirmed by the "sense of foreignness" which may grab the clinician facing a patient who *irremediably* resists being captured by descriptions and analyses (Blankenburg 2012: 35, see also 81 and 84–85).

Here we will not go into the details of how the transcendental "presupposition" or "trust" could be broken by psychopathology (Binswanger 1960: 16);[16] we will not explore either the different modes of "suppletion" which may occur when the ground collapses and when the "I" must assume itself the task of the transcendental, with the aim to give himself some foundation (Blankenburg 2012: 129–131, 106, 109, 172, 108, 127). Rather, by way of conclusion, we will consider how the phenomenological analysis of being-human informs the clinical encounter.

ENCOUNTERING

As a physician, the clinician may want to intervene in order to "modify the disorders and fill in the lacks"; thereby he would put himself in a position to "master what is 'occurring'" and may try to "understand what is occurring as something a priori defined and modifiable, and thus heteronomous." However, as a phenomenologist, the clinician prefers "to make the 'occurring' emerge" (Blankenburg 1986: 135). But what is "the occurring"?

By letting himself be "engaged-by-the-occurring," the clinician aims at giving a place not only to the disease, but also to the "person of the other human being" who presents himself (Blankenburg 1986: 144). Here, the "occurring" is the other, "uncapturable" (Khun and Maldiney 1986: 24). To allow the encounter with the other, one must suspend the frontier between normality and pathology, and work with the structure and constitution which is common to every human being—which is thus common to both the clinician and the patient. This anthropological orientation of phenomenology argues that the clinical encounter must mobilize the empathy of the clinician (Binswanger 1994c: 55–56),[17] in order to deploy a "relationship of two human beings 'with-each-other and apart-from-each-other' [*miteinander auseinander*]" (Binswanger 1994a: 206).[18]

Yet, there is another reading of the human being's mode of being-with others, a reading which is not only anthropological but ontological, and which "allows us to get rid of the concept of 'psychic empathy', a particularly obscure problem [oppressing] psychology and psychopathology" (Boss 1980: 126). Here, it is argued that the "partnership" between humans is not an empathic projection from one individual to another, but "the carrying of a load distributed upon both the physician and the patient" (Binswanger 1971: 154). As the "originary understanding of being" is a "fundamental feature carrying all of man," each singular human being "participates with others in the opening and clearing of the world" (Boss 1980: 126). Here we must understand that if "phenomenology . . . methodically takes the encounter as the object of its experience" (Blankenburg 1986: 145), such encounter is less

---

[16] See also Blankenburg 2012: 111, 128–129.   [17] See also Binswanger 1960: 70.
[18] See also Boss 1980: 132; Blankenburg 1986: 137; Binswanger 1994c: 36–37, 66; Blankenburg 2012: 88–89.

a relationship between two autonomous and heterogeneous singularities than a relation of the human-being to the "foundation of all that is," to the "originary understanding of Being" (Boss 1980: 87).

Our question reoccurs: What is the "occurring" by which the clinician lets himself be engaged? Is it *Being* for the phenomenologist, whereas it is the *other* for the psychoanalyst? To keep this question open, let us go back to the patient's speech. As reported by Blankenburg, it demonstrates a fundamental lack that tortures patients: "they speak, always anew, of the fact that they need a 'support'" (Blankenburg 2012: 121, see also 19). But who or what could provide such support? Is it *Being* as "anonymous natural evidence"? Is such support provided by *others*, those who can make themselves be "intermediaries of this natural evidence which [the patient] aspires to" (Blankenburg 2012: 122), those through whom there "radiates a force that is formative of the world" (Blankenburg 2012: 138)? Is existential support incarnated by *another singular human being* who not only "gives support but *is* himself this support" (Blankenburg 2012: 120)? We will not close these questions here by giving an answer that would abusively reduce to one the plurality of grounds which could give transcendental support. "All these possibilities constantly impose themselves" on the patient, and the "only thing that is clear" to the phenomenologist who is listening to the patients' voices, is that the human being cannot be for himself his own support (Blankenburg 2012: 122); the man suffers unbearably and intolerably when he "must build his own personal world" (Binswanger 1975b: 235); the world darkens when the human being shines for himself as his own sun.[19]

Let us conclude here by rephrasing this view. Whether one favors one or another approach to clinical phenomenology, the "only thing that is clear" is that, descriptively, structurally and transcendentally, the human being cannot bear isolation—from himself, others, the world, Being. The human being can—and must—be separated—from himself, others, the world, Being—to be a singular subject, but this separation cannot be a rupture. This "cannot" may be diversely interpreted as a vital, existential, anthropological, ontological impossibility. The roots, scope, and consequences of such conceptions of human impossibility are fundamentally different from each other, but for the sake of characterizing clinical phenomenology here, what matters first and foremost is not to construct them as philosophical antinomies but as clinical necessities. Only by setting concepts in motion within such plurality of meanings, can one respect the singularities of others.

Bibliography

Binswanger L. (1947). "Heraklits Auffassung des Menschen." [1935]. In L. Binswanger, *Ausgewählte Vorträge und Aufsätze*, vol. I, pp. 98–131. Bern: Francke Verlag.

Binswanger L. (1955a). "Vom anthropologischen Sinn der Verstiegenheit." [1949]. In L. Binswanger, *Ausgewählte Vorträge und Aufsätze*, vol. II, pp. 235–242. Bern: Francke Verlag.

Binswanger L. (1955b). "Bemerkungen zu zwei wenig beachteten 'Gedanken' Pascals über Symmetrie." [1947]. In L. Binswanger, *Ausgewählte Vorträge und Aufsätze*, vol. II, pp. 226–234. Bern: Francke Verlag.

Binswanger L. (1960). *Melancholie und Manie*. Pfullingen: Günther Neske.

[19] Binswanger, quoting Jeremias Gotthelf: "Think how dark the world would become if man sought to be his own sun" (Binswanger 1975b: 235).

Binswanger L. (1965). *Wahn*. Pfullingen: Günther Neske.

Binswanger L. (1971). "Analyse existentielle et psychothérapie (II)." [1958]. In L. Binswanger, *Introduction à l'analyse existentielle*, trans. J. Verdeaux and R. Khun, pp. 149–157. Paris: Editions de Minuit.

Binswanger L. (1975a). "Heidegger's Analytic of Existence and Its Meaning for Psychiatry." [1958]. In L. Binswanger, *Being-in-the-World, Selected Papers*, trans. J. Needleman, pp. 206–221. London: Souvenir Press.

Binswanger L. (1975b). "Dream and Existence." [1930]. In L. Binswanger, *Being-in-the-World, Selected Papers*, trans. J. Needleman, pp. 222–248. London: Souvenir Press.

Binswanger L. (1994a). "Über Psychotherapie." [1935]. In L. Binswanger, *Ausgewählte Werke, Band 3. Vorträge und Aufsätze*, ed. M. Herzog, pp. 205–230. Heidelberg: Asanger Verlag.

Binswanger L. (1994b). "Lebensfunktion und innere Lebensgeschichte." [1924]. In L. Binswanger, *Ausgewählte Werke, Band 3. Vorträge und Aufsätze*, ed. M. Herzog, pp. 71–94. Heidelberg: Asanger Verlag.

Binswanger L. (1994c). "Über Phänomenologie." [1922]. In L. Binswanger, *Ausgewählte Werke, Band 3. Vorträge und Aufsätze*, ed. M. Herzog, pp. 35–69. Heidelberg: Asanger Verlag.

Blankenburg W. (1986). "Sur le rapport entre pratique psychiatrique et phénoménologique." [1982]. In P. Fédida (ed.) *Phénoménologie, psychiatrie, psychanalyse*, pp. 133–140. Paris: G.R.E.U.P.P.

Blankenburg W. (1991). "Postface." In W. Blankenburg, *La perte de l'évidence naturelle*, trans. J. M. Azorin and Y. Totoyan, pp. 229–233. Paris: Presses Universitaires France.

Blankenburg W. (2012). *Der Verlust der natürlichen Selbstverständlichkeit. Ein Beitrag zur Psychopathologie symptomarmer Schizophrenien* [1971]. Berlin: Parodos Verlag.

Boss M. (1980). *Psychoanalyse und Daseinsanalytik*. Berlin: Kindler Verlag.

De Waelhens A. (1972). *La psychose, Essai d'interprétation analytique et existentiale* Louvain: Editions Nauwelaerts.

Heidegger M. (2001a). *Being and Time*, trans. J. Macquarie and E. Robinson. Oxford: Blackwell.

Heidegger M. (2001b). *Zollikon Seminars. Protocols—Conversations—Letters*, ed. M. Boss, trans. F. Mayr and R. Askay. Evanston: Northwestern University Press.

Husserl E (2001). *Analyses Concerning Passive and Active Synthesis: Lectures on Transcendental Logic*, trans. A. J. Steinbock. Dordrecht: Kluwer Academic Publishers.

Jaspers K. (1997). *General Psychopathology* [1959, 4th edn.], trans. J. Hoenig and M. W. Hamilton. Baltimore: Johns Hopkins Univeristy Press.

Khun R. and Maldiney H. (1986). "Préface." In L. Binswanger, *Introduction à l'analyse existentielle*, trans. J. Verdeaux and R. Khun, pp. 7–24. Paris: Editions de Minuit.

Levinas E. (1984). "In memoriam Alphonse de Waelhens." *Tijdschrift voor Filosofie* 46(3): 405–408.

Maldiney H. (1986). "Daseinanalyse: phénoménologie de l'existant?" In P. Fédida (ed.), *Phénoménologie, psychiatrie, psychanalyse*, pp. 9–28. Paris: G.R.E.U.P.P.

Mishara A. (1986). "L'inconscient chez L. Binswanger." In P. Fédida (ed.), *Phénoménologie, psychiatrie, psychanalyse*, pp. 181–186. (Paris: G.R.E.U.P.P).

CHAPTER 28

GENETIC PHENOMENOLOGY

ANTHONY STEINBOCK

INTRODUCTION

PHENOMENOLOGY is a reflective attentiveness not only to "what" is given in experience, but to "how" those matters are given. Rather than taking our everyday acceptances of reality for granted, it wants "to bracket" them (what is known as the epoché) and trace these acceptances to their origins of sense, namely, to their sense-giving processes (what is known as the reduction). These sense-giving features can be as narrow as a single act of consciousness, or more dynamically, lived-bodily kinaestheses, or again, subjectivity, intersubjectivity, the world-horizon, the earth-ground, or the interrelation of home-worlds and alien-worlds (Steinbock 1995). As such, phenomenology as a whole enquires after modes of meaning givenness (constitution), the structures of those meanings (material or formal essences), the powers and limits of the meaning-giving, and in some instances, the very process of carrying out phenomenology itself.

Accordingly, just what "matters" can be given in phenomenological description depends in part upon how the phenomenologist approaches them. The way of approach we call a "method." Phenomenological method is a style of openness that in turn allows one to be struck by the phenomena, no matter how strangely that experience may seem at first blush.

There are many methodological procedures that characterize the overall project of phenomenology, too many to detail here. However, there are three basic ones that can be recognized as static, genetic, and generative. A static phenomenology can describe both what something is in terms of its essential structures, and how it is given in a slice of time—"now," for example. A genetic phenomenology covers the unfolding of sense (its "genesis"), and its span can be as broad as the life of an individual as described in the process of self-temporalization. A generative phenomenology can be understood in two ways. On the one hand, it deals with the geo-historical, social, normative generation of meaning in home-worlds and alien-worlds as that meaning is generated over the generations; on the other hand, it concerns the whole of phenomenology itself as the very movement of meaning givenness and the generation of structures, spanning more particular static, genetic, and generative dimensions. I will focus on the scope and field of *genetic* phenomenology (Steinbock 1995: chapter 12).

STATIC AND GENETIC METHOD

It was in 1921 that Edmund Husserl, the so-called father of phenomenology, found himself already pushing the bounds of his own previous conception of phenomenological method. It was also at this time that he was led to formulate explicitly the difference between static and genetic phenomenological methods (Husserl 2001: section 4).

Husserl's writings on static and genetic methods not only mark his explicit effort to formulate a difference internal to phenomenological method in terms of static and genetic phenomena; they also show the distinctive traits of each method and how the methods are to be organized in terms of the motivational descriptor of "leading clue." Since the process of questioning back is a questioning after founding relations of validity (accordingly, "the questioning back after genesis"), the question of genesis can operate in tandem with a "regressive" phenomenological approach that questions back archeologically, as it were, into founding layers of experience.

Husserl was not the first to distinguish between static and genetic elements of experience. Husserl himself acknowledges this by referring to the difference between static and genetic method in the same terms Wilhelm Dilthey used for psychology, namely, as "descriptive" [*beschreibende*] and "explanatory" [*erklärende*] (Dilthey 1957). Whereas Dilthey takes description as interpretive description and explanation as something the natural sciences do, Husserl takes descriptive phenomenology in a narrower, "static" sense in order to contrast it with a genetic phenomenological research perspective that takes up an interpretative position with respect to the teleological genesis of sense (Scharff 1976). Lurking in the background of Husserl's formation is not only Dilthey, but also Brentano and his distinction between descriptive psychology and genetic and physiological psychology (Brentano 1924).

The originality of Husserl's distinctions between static and genetic phenomenology consists in the fact that Husserl was led to formulate the difference between methods and matters from motivations internal to the development of phenomenology itself. Because Husserl had described genetic matters that exceeded the scope of static constitution, including phenomena like apperception, normality and abnormality, kinaesthesis, association, etc.—phenomena that came under the general title of "primordial constitution"—Husserl was provoked by the very matters themselves to catch up reflectively with his own descriptions. This means that Husserl had undertaken genetic analyses implicitly without phenomenology having been explicitly cognizant of itself having this genetic methodological dimension (Holenstein 1972; Sakakibara 1997; Donahoe 2004). Moreover, at least on Husserl's own account, his distinction between static and genetic matters pre-dates even this. For example, in June 1918, Husserl writes to Paul Natorp that ". . . already, for more than a decade, I have overcome the level of static Platonism and have situated the idea of transcendental genesis in phenomenology as its main theme" (Husserl 1994: 137).

Looking back from our privileged perspective, with the distinction between static and genetic method and matters already in hand, we can say that Husserl's initial preoccupation was with static phenomena and an approach that was "static." Two aspects are captured under the rubric of static phenomenology. First, there is a constitutive approach that is concerned with *how* something is given or *modes* of givenness, and second, there is a concern with *essential structures*. In Husserl's terminology, a static method can address both "phenomenological" (i.e. constitutive) as well as "ontological" (i.e. essential) dimensions of experience. Thus, a static approach can interrogate the interplay of intention and fulfillment, the meant features of an object, the noetic qualities of an act, etc., as well as the structural or essential possibilities of the particular object or act within the intentional correlation. Here one would examine the structures and the being of these structures (e.g. formal and material essences, regions, and so forth).

By genesis Husserl understands three variations of experience: (1) genesis within the purely active sphere of experience where the ego functions in rational acts; (2) genesis between the active and passive spheres of experience, where we trace the origins of activity in passivity (or between the judicative in the perceptual spheres of experience); and finally, (3) "primordial constitution" as a phenomenology of passive experience or passive genesis of sense, including apperception, motivation, affection and association, kinaesthesis, etc. Ultimately these three dimensions of genesis are bound to the analysis of the genesis of the factical subject or what he calls a "monad."

GENETIC PHENOMENOLOGICAL METHOD

The genuine benefit of a genetic analysis is the fact that it can treat the integrity of the becoming of the individual person in a way that a static or even a generative method might miss. For example, the life of the individual or the synchronic community is something that is treated within the scope of a genetic phenomenology, and the person can be regarded as "absolute" within this dimension. The individual person in this sense has an irreducible sense within genetic self-temporalization, as an individual and not only by having a place within historical "Generativity." The danger with a genetic method alone, however, would be the temptation to understand the individual person as fully self-sufficient or as self-grounding (Steinbock 2014: chapters 1 and 7). If we understand the individual in his or her own way as absolute, this absoluteness is nonetheless grounded in the Generative movement of meaning, and in this way is not self-grounding.

Nevertheless, there are indeed deeper temporal considerations that bear on the subject that are not just momentary conscious intendings. For example, when a reproductive act of remembering is motivated (e.g. by something prominent in the present linking up with a retended past), "I" am awakened to it in a remembering, and a deeper, broader temporal life emerges co-relative to the emergence of an object as such. Remembering is an identifying activity that can repeatedly come back to the same presentation beyond the present, also conferring a density on the object as such over time. Through iterative remembering, we arrive at an identical unending time in the mode of unending past such that the whole of subjectivity, in terms of my genesis of time, cannot have a starting point "in" the past, thus cannot be born, and in this respect "is" "eternal" (Husserl 2001: 468–469).

Accordingly, a genetic phenomenology accounts for how the subject can be given to itself in the process of constituting time; insofar as it is self-temporalizing it constitutes the very sense of past, present, and future, and therefore cannot be "before" or "after" itself. Accordingly, gaps in consciousness like sleep, fainting spells, or any disruption of sense are integrated into a higher arching concordance of temporal continuity such that there are no decisive gaps in such self-temporalization. In this respect, I am given to myself *constitutively* as not arising, not ending, but in the eternal process of self-genesis (Husserl 2001: 467, 469, 471).

Phenomenology of genesis therefore accounts for how I am not temporalized from the outside (i.e. locatable in objective time) since I am the source of that time. To attempt to locate the self-temporalizing process in time would be to presuppose object-time as the already constituted standard, and then to apply it to myself as the measure of temporality, becoming forgetful of myself as self-temporalizing in this very process (Steinbock 2017). Certainly, there are beginnings and endings within temporal genesis. But within the genesis of self-temporalization, I am not before my own birth and I am not after my death, since the very senses of before and after are constituted within temporal genesis.

Husserl thought that the best way to handle more complex matters in phenomenology (like the problem of self-temporalization, or later the problem of cultural communities and historicity, in short, "generativity") was to prepare the groundwork with static investigations. Following such "preparatory" work, it would be suitable to proceed to higher constitutive levels of analysis. Initially, he was led to genetic matters of experience that demanded a formulation of a genetic phenomenological method.

NORMALITY AND ABNORMALITY AS KEY GENETIC MATTERS

What are these genetic matters and clues that motivate a genetic phenomenology? There are several matters that are evoked and described in a genetic phenomenology. They include, but are not limited to, a "phenomenology of the so-called unconscious," the laws of genesis in passive synthesis or laws of association, the intentionality of drive and instinct, the constitution of habit, self-temporalization, and many other themes (Husserl 2001: 201, 214). One main set of themes that arises explicitly when Husserl moves to a genetic method is the complex of "normality" and "abnormality."

Husserl's genetic phenomenology of normality and abnormality gives us clues, but only clues, concerning how we can tell if, for example, a perceptual object is not "real," but merely hallucinatory. This is a complex issue because of the lived process of "normalization" in the dynamic sense of becoming normal (and abnormal) and the constitution of norms within experience.

On the one hand, we would have to ask if the object responds to our efforts to vary it or if it gives itself correlative to kinaesthetic motivations in what he calls a "constitutive duet." If that dynamic tension that qualifies the relation is lost; if the thing is reduced to the subject or the subject to the thing in experience, it could be given as a hallucinatory object. In essence, for Merleau-Ponty, this means that the hallucinatory object lacks the structure of "depth" (Steinbock 1987).

On the other hand, what constitutes the real as such is precisely what is able to count as "objective" in experience. For example, within a *static* dimension of experience, what is given now is "normal," and "real." The system of norms and indexes to experience are given in their complexity, in one stroke, "now." But he asks, what good is this if it is merely given now; it has no temporal density (Husserl 2001: section 24).

When we broaden our analyses to a *genetic* phenomenology, we can account for the enduring appearance of the object as it unfolds concordantly over time and can be identified as such in temporal iterations. The same holds on the side of the lived body in the mode of experiencing. However, even this is incomplete because it might be valid only *for me* in my lifetime.

This motivates the movement to the designation of the real as what is intersubjectively valid, such that objectivity is given in the intersubjectivity of perspectives. This, however, still falls short because of the generative differences of "normal" and "abnormal" life-worlds or "home-worlds" and "alien-worlds." Thus, to give a rich account of the real or the "object" as such, he has to turn to a phenomenological analysis of the normal and the abnormal, and this unfolds in genetic and generative analyses, and to questions of concordance/discordance, optimality/non-optimality, typicality/atypicality, and familiarity/unfamiliarity.

Accordingly, the phenomenology of psychopathology would have to be adduced on both genetic and generative levels. What might be diagnosed as "pathological" in a communal or historical context might be optimal and hypernormal on an individual level. In addition, the optimal individual might throw into relief the historical context as "abnormal" in relation to the new norms that are instituted through the optimal style of the individual. Discordance on one level might be (but is not necessarily) optimal on another.

With these terms—normal and abnormal—he does not mean a statistical, static, medicinal, natural, or innate sense of them. Rather, normal designates the way in which a meaningful world takes shape. The first set of genetic concepts of normal and abnormal are "concordance" and "discordance," respectively. Concordance is the way in which appearances link up and harmonize to form an ongoing, unfolding development of meaning, like when I touch a smooth surface and each smooth aspect harmoniously implicates and confirms the next appearance. A discordance constitutes an anomaly of appearances that ruptures the concordance, and which may continue for an indefinite period of time (instituting an abnormality). However, there is an overarching concordance, and thus an overarching normality when the rupture (anomaly or abnormality) is integrated into the overall flow, or again, when the later harmony of sense matches and reaches back to, while continuing the previous concordance.

THE NORMAL AS THE OPTIMAL

But Husserl adds something more and contributes to his understanding of the "real." Complementing the account of normality as concordance is a deeper analysis of how the lived body is involved with the world *from* a certain perspective. If the lived body is intermeshed in a network of phenomena, as Husserl's analyses point out, then there will be a perspective or a situation that will be preferred as better or best for experiencing. As Husserl maintains, lived-corporeality is a system of good and bad presentations; and to this system, in turn, belongs the idea of optimal modes of *givenness* (Husserl 1973a: 121). These qualitative senses of normality and abnormality that also reach into dimensions of optimality are strikingly similar to some of Georges Canguilhem's early work on the normal and the pathological (Canguilhem 1966), and anticipatory of Maurice Merleau-Ponty's genetic phenomenology of the constitution of the thing (Merleau-Ponty 1946).

First, a system of appearances is optimal insofar as it presents the *most* of the same thing with the greatest richness and differentiation. This is one way in which Husserl understands the "real" thing, namely, as "optimal," and it is the genetic expression of the "objective sense." Here, the optimal is the greatest unity with greatest differentiation, and not just differences. In this instance, one does not understand experience as concordant or discordant; rather, one speaks now of normal experiences being "better," "richer," and abnormal ones as "diminished" or "worse."

To say that we "prefer" such a situation means that "normally" we tend toward the "maximum" of richness or maximum of focus in which the object is both sharp and differentiated, and not when we are aesthetically uncomfortable or unbalanced (for instance, when the light or distance is excessive or deficient). Thus, to see something up close or in bright light does not necessarily mean that we see it optimally. (The same could be said of hearing notes sharply or crisply, on the one hand, and hearing things too loudly, on the other.) Similarly, an optimal (normal) lived body is often considered by Husserl as an integrated, synaesthetic one.

The normal as optimal is what enriches experiences: The abnormal is one that not only gives the perceived object *unusually*, but *worse*, with less abundance of differences so that the experience itself is impoverished. The optimal is not a norm imposed from outside of human experience or, within a genetic framework, stemming from another as given to me. The optimal as norm is itself generated within experience and given as something experienced and experienceable by me. Optima are instituted within experience by the very fact that we take a perspective on things and are embedded in our surroundings, and that as perspectives on the world, we can be more open to the givenness of objects or more closed to them.

For example, I may never have had a pair of glasses, and still have a concordant view of the world. It is "normal" for me on this level of experience as concordant (without comparing them to others). In fact, depending upon the set of experiences, these concordances would be optimal by the mere fact that so far there would be a best among them. All this takes place "pre-reflectively," "passively" without necessarily paying any egoic attention to them. Now, if I try on a friend's pair of glasses, I may become totally disoriented; everything might be too blurry to function. This would constitute an anomaly or abnormality in my experience, constitutively speaking.

But let's suppose that I find a pair of glasses lying around and I put them on, and suddenly the trees have leaves clearly defined, people have spaces between their teeth, I can see street signs now in sharp relief as I go sailing past them in a car. The fact that the glasses interrupted my concordant (normal) view of the world would constitute an abnormality as a discordance. But in terms of optimality, it would constitute a new normality, and a new index to experience!

Norm Transcendence

Particularly striking and clearly original in Husserl's work on normality and abnormality is not only the fact that he attempts to account for the internal development and institution of norms in experience; more provocatively, he accounts for the possibility of *transcending* those norms and instituting new ones, *despite the presence of a norm that already functions teleologically* for anomalies. This is to say both that experience is normal in transcending norms when it is optimalizing or creating new norms, and that anomaly can function innovatively in the *institution of new norms*. It is not given in advance that the anomalies will be simply incorporated into a "higher," overarching teleological or concordant unity.

Even though a new vision can be understood as discordant in relation to the previous one (like in the example of optical surgery where the lived body itself is modified), an optimal vision can supplant the *earlier* one in a kind of re-valuation: The new one *becomes* normal and the old one now refers to the new optimal as *its* norm. Thus, it is possible for new optima to be formed, and it remains a question, observes Husserl, to what extent it is necessary for an originally instituted normal system to maintain perpetually its teleological system of reference.[1]

Since a normal system is not guaranteed in advance and for all time, then what was seen previously only as a discordance, as a deviance, or as a modification can also function creatively as instituting new norms. It can be normalizing in this genetic dynamic sense, and it can only do this by transcending the previous norms. In order to transcend the norm, the fact that the deviation refers back to the norm teleologically cannot be decisive. Such new optima and new norms are constituted, Husserl asserts, "*in spite of the reference back to the earlier norm.*"[2]

Such a conflict of orders is open to what might be called a "transvaluation" of the normal and abnormal. We have seen that from a perspective in which the present norms are lived, a new perception or a new sense could be counted as abnormal. If, however, this discordant perspective were more than simply "new," but also "a 'finer' organization of sense"; if the so-called disruptive, "unusual" or exceptional features of vision or touch were modes of "increased accomplishments," they would not simply be anomalous or abnormal. The new optimal "would not be abnormal, *but more normal than ever, increased normality*, and what was previously called normal [is now called] abnormal."[3] Husserl's statement then implies a two-fold transvaluation. On the one hand, he accounts for the possibility that what is considered anomalous or abnormal on the axis of concordance may issue in a new normality as optimal, and on the other, what was at one time instituted as a norm can be disclosed as "not as normal" or even as abnormal on the axis of optimality (Steinbock 2017).

If we were to advance to the intersubjective sphere of normality on the basis of what has been discussed, we would see similar implications. The greatest number of cases, the majority of instances, the average could not make up a normal society because it may not be optimal in its context; indeed, the average could be abnormal if the average were not optimal or concordant. On the other hand, the view of optimality is not elitist because the

---

[1] Husserl, Ms. D 13 I, 233a: "Ein normales System muß sich also ursprünglich konstituieren. Die Frage is nur, ob es notwendig ist, daß ein solches System immer als Bezugssystem verbleiben muß."

[2] Husserl, Ms. D 13 I, 175a: "(Doch ist denkbar, daß die leibliche Änderung auch 'bessere' Erscheinungen ergibt.) Wer ein pathologisches Sinnesorgan *ursprünglich* hatte, wer seine erste Konstitution mit Erscheinungen geleistet hat, die normal sind,—aber bei nachträglicher Gesundung des Organs wird eine *neue optimale* Erscheinungsgruppe derselben Dinge konstituiert, und die bestimmt nun *trotz der Rückbeziehung auf die frühere Norm*, die für die Durchhaltung desselben notwendig ist, im weiteren Leben (was das Ding selbst ist)." My emphasis.

[3] Husserl, Ms. D 13 XVII, 14: "Dann wäre eine 'feinere' Sinnesorganisation, mit gestigerten Sehleistungen etc., nicht anomal, *sondern erst recht normal, gesteigert normal*, und, was vorhin normal hieß, anomal." My emphasis.

overwhelming majority could express the optimal mode of life for that world. The optimal is not associated with the "few" any more than the abnormal is expressive of so-called "deviant behavior" because it is the richness of the experience that constitutes the optimal, not the number of people who have the experience.

Suffice it to mention that there are two additional conceptual sets of normality and abnormality that pertain to a generative phenomenology (not to be confused with a genetic phenomenology). These other two are typicality and a-typicality, and familiarity and unfamiliarity. Within a generative phenomenology, taking all these meaning-constituting senses of normal and abnormal, the "normal" life-world is constituted as the home-world; the "abnormal" life-world as the alien-world (Steinbock 1995: chapters 11–14).

GENESIS AND STASIS

Conceptually speaking, both genesis and stasis arise co-originally for phenomenology. Yet it was only after explicitly tackling the problems of genesis and more complex features of experience that Husserl *retroactively* understood the problem of genesis not to be more complex than that of stasis, but rather, more concrete and more fundamental. Likewise, static matters were no longer seen to be "simple," but now more *abstract*. This inversion was only discerned after having arrived explicitly at genesis through the leading clue of stasis, even though one could in no way derive genesis from stasis. Husserl came to see genesis as more fundamental than stasis, though pedagogically stasis guided us to the problem of genesis without the latter being reducible to the former (Husserl 1973a: 614–617). In this way, static phenomenology is not to be taken as a final stance for phenomenology, but as a leading clue to constitutive ones, and further, to matters of genesis (and eventually to the problem of generativity) (Steinbock 1995: section 4).

Although it deals with time, Husserl's work on time-consciousness from his *On the Phenomenology of the Consciousness of Internal Time* (Husserl 1991) is not really a full-fledged genetic analysis because it remains too formal: "Mere form is admittedly an abstraction, and thus from the very beginning the analysis of the intentionality of time-consciousness and its accomplishment is an analysis that works on [the level of] abstractions" (Husserl 2001: 173–174). Remaining solely on the level of time-constituting consciousness (in terms of temporal modes of givenness such as impression, retention, protention), is still too formal. This is due to the fact that an inquiry into the question of constitution (which can be static) is not necessarily an inquiry into the problem of genesis. "Another constitutive phenomenology" that is not static, one named "phenomenology of genesis" or "genetic phenomenology," is required for this. It is not until we get to the habitual lived body, the problems of association, affection, concordance of a life, and individuation that the problem of genesis minimally comes into play in a more decisive manner.

Phenomenology of genesis then is the phenomenology of primordial becoming in time, of the genesis of one shape of consciousness emerging from another, acquiring a temporal opacity through the processes of motivation, apperception, affection, association, etc. In short, it is a phenomenology of what Husserl calls at this time, "facticity." Within a static register now, one moves regressively to constitutive phenomenology.

Once Husserl has discussed the problem of genetic method and its matters in relation to static method and its matters, and has done this as a relation of leading clue, a peculiar re-assessment takes shape. I have already noted that the "higher," more complex phenomena of genesis are now seen as more fundamental; in relation to them, static phenomena are grasped *as* "finished," as abstractions from temporality. But to recognize this is to reverse the direction of "leading clue." For now it is no longer static phenomenology as a leading clue to genetic matters, but genesis that orders the investigation into static constitution and into structure. Now one must enquire into the essential relations on the basis of phenomena that are disclosed genetically, which may entail, as it did for Husserl, that one revise the previous results of static analyses from the perspective of genesis—but which nevertheless had served formerly as a leading clue to genesis (see Husserl 2001: 664). This is the reason one can move from a genetic constitutive analysis back to an eidetic analysis, back to examining invariant structures in the natural attitude, back to empirical sciences, etc. It is also now that we are able to grapple with both the genesis of structure (i.e. the structure of individuation) as well as the very structure of genesis.

The formulation of static and genetic methods would not be the ultimate story told for phenomenology—if indeed one could give an exhaustive narrative of the generation of phenomenology and its possibilities. This is because the problem of generativity is a distinctive matter for phenomenology and the most encompassing dimension of phenomenology. It concerns the geo-historical, social, normative dimension of experience. Genetic phenomenology however does provide an opening for novel, dynamic themes concerning our being-in-the-world.

BIBLIOGRAPHY

Canguilhem G. (1966). *Le normal e le pathologique*. Paris: Presses Universitaires de France.

Brentano F. (1924). *Psychologie vom empirischen Standpunkt*, 2nd edn. Leipzig: Meiner.

Dilthey W. (1957). "Ideen über eine beschreibende und zergliedernde Psychologie." In *Gesammelte Schriften: Band 5. Die Geistige Welt*, ed. G. Misch, pp. 139–240. Göttigen: Vandenhoeck & Ruprecht.

Donahoe J. (2004). *Husserl on Ethics and Intersubjectivity: From Static to Genetic Phenomenology*. New York: Humanity Books.

Holenstein E. (1972). *Phänomenologie der Assoziation: Zu Struktur und Funktion eines Grundprinzips der passiven Genesis bei E. Husserl*. The Hague: Martinus Nijhoff.

Husserl E. (1973a). *Zur Phänomenologie der Intersubjektivität: Texte aus dem Nachlaß: Zweiter Teil: 1921–1928*. Husserliana XIV, ed. I. Kern. The Hague: Martinus Nijhoff.

Husserl E. (1973b). *Zur Phänomenologie der Intersubjektivität. Texte aus dem Nachlaß. Dritter Teil: 1929–1935*, Husserliana XV, 614–741, ed. I. Kern. The Hague: Martinus Nijhoff.

Husserl E. (1991). *On the Phenomenology of the Consciousness of Internal Time (1893–1917)*, trans. J. B. Brough. Dortrecht: Kluwer.

Husserl E. (1994). *Briefwechsel. Band V: Die Neukantianer*, ed. K. Schuhmann. Boston: Kluwer.

Husserl E. (2001). *Analyses Concerning Passive and Active Synthesis: Lectures on Transcendental Logic*, trans. A. J. Steinbock. Dordrecht: Kluwer.

Merleau-Ponty M. (1946). *Phénoménologie de la perception*. Paris: Gallimard.

Sakakibara T. (1997). "Das Problem des Ich und der Ursprung der genetischen Phänomenologie bei Husserl." *Husserl Studies* 14: 21–39.

Scharff R. (1976). "Non-Analytic, Unspeculative Philosophy of History: The Legacy of Wilhelm Dilthey." *Cultural Hermeneutics* 3: 295–331.

Steinbock A. J. (1987). "Merleau-Ponty's Concept of Depth." *Philosophy Today* 31: 336–351.

Steinbock A. J. (1995). *Home and Beyond: Generativity Phenomenology after Husserl* Evanston: Northwestern University Press.

Steinbock A. J. (2014). *Moral Emotions: Reclaiming the Evidence of the Heart.* Evanston: Northwestern University Press.

Steinbock A. J. (2017). *Limit-Phenomena and Phenomenology after Husserl.* London: Rowman & Littlefield International.

CHAPTER 29

PHENOMENOLOGY AND HERMENEUTICS

RENÉ ROSFORT

INTRODUCTION

THE relationship between phenomenology and hermeneutics is complicated. They represent two major philosophical traditions that came to fruition in the twentieth century, although both have deep roots in the history of philosophy. The complexity of the relationship is visible in the historical development of the two traditions. Hermeneutics as the systematic study of interpretation goes back to antiquity beginning with the exegesis of the Homeric poems in the sixth century BCE and working its way up through Western intellectual history in myriad forms of interpretation of religious, philosophical, juridical, and literary texts (Grondin 1995; Ferraris 1996; Ramberg and Gjesdal 2014). Phenomenology as a philosophical discipline is much younger, going back only a couple of centuries to G. W. F. Hegel—or even younger still, as some argue, finding its proper beginning with Edmund Husserl at the turn of the twentieth century (Schuhmann 2011; Spiegelberg 1994). Despite its long intellectual history, hermeneutics as a philosophical discipline grows out of phenomenology, and most of the major hermeneutical philosophers of the twentieth century have a background in phenomenology and use phenomenological methods to develop their hermeneutical theories. On the other hand, phenomenology as an interpretation of experience is rooted in the hermeneutical tradition and draws heavily upon examinations of various themes and concepts developed throughout the long history of interpretation of texts (e.g. intention, clarification, understanding, meaning, significance, imagination).

The historical entanglement of phenomenology and hermeneutics is connected with the convoluted conceptual and theoretical relation between the two traditions. On the surface, the distinction between the two philosophical approaches seems uncomplicated: phenomenology is the study of phenomena and hermeneutics is the interpretation of texts. That is to say, phenomenology deals with that which appears or is immediately given, whereas hermeneutics engages with that which has been written down or mediated through language. The aim of phenomenology is therefore to clarify, describe, and make sense of the structures and dynamics of pre-reflective human experience, whereas hermeneutics works with the reflective character of human experience as it manifests in language and other forms of creative signs. On closer inspection, though, the two philosophical approaches overlap with respect to methodology, themes, and philosophical aims, and the development of both approaches in the twentieth century has often taken the form of theoretical exchange and mutual critique. This interplay has led to both a separation of the two approaches into two distinct philosophical disciplines and to a combination in the form of a hermeneutical phenomenology (Greisch 2000).

In what follows, I will focus on the latter attempt to combine phenomenology and hermeneutics into a hermeneutical phenomenology with particular regard to the interrelated issues of interpretation, selfhood, and personal identity. These issues are at the center of the encounter of phenomenology and hermeneutics, and all three play a central role in phenomenological psychopathology.

THE FRAGILE SELF

One of the basic claims of a hermeneutical approach to selfhood is that to be a self is to constantly make sense of and appropriate oneself through interpretations of the multifarious aspects of human identity—concerning, amongst others, experience, biology, culture, history, and ethics. The human self is, therefore, fragile. It is both made and unmade through a hermeneutic, interpretive process.

Human beings are, as Charles Taylor famously argued, self-interpreting animals. We are interested in that which we experience, and with experience comes a need to articulate our experience "to make clearer the imports things have for us" (Taylor 1985: 65). This means, Taylor goes on to argue, that "interpretation is not an optional extra, but an essential part of our existence" (Taylor 1985: 65). To interpret the *what* and the *why* of our experience, however, we need to pay careful attention to *how* we experience that which we experience. This interplay of the interpretative and experiential aspects of human experience is at the core of the relationship of phenomenology and hermeneutics. Human experience is a product of interpretation. Characterizing human experience as interpretation is not to denigrate the importance of experience or to categorize experiential subjectivity as somehow "lower" than scientific objectivity. The interpretative aspect of experience is tied to the peculiar individuality of experience, which means that two human beings never experience the same fact or occurrence in exactly the same way. One of the primary characteristics of human experience is that to experience something is not simply a passive reception of stimuli, but an active engagement with the world.

This is not to say that we can experience what we want to experience or that we somehow create the world that we experience. One of the most important contributions of phenomenology to twentieth-century philosophy is the distinction between subjectivity and subjectivism. Phenomenology is not concerned with describing idiosyncratic experiences, but rather with providing us with methodological tools to describe and makes sense of the impersonal experiential structures and dynamics that constitute human subjectivity (Gallagher and Zahavi 2012: 21–31). The individuality of human experience is bound to and conditioned by those experiential structures, and the sense of being an individual self is experienced through these invariant perceptual and temporal structures.

Still, there is more to the human self than the structures that make up human subjectivity. Hermeneutical phenomenology in the twentieth century developed as an attempt to complement the phenomenological analysis of the experiential structures of subjectivity with an account of the reflective character (e.g. affective, cultural, historical, ethical) selfhood. This is not to say that phenomenology is not interested in selfhood or has not produced influential accounts of selfhood. Rather, it is merely to point out that phenomenological accounts of selfhood are typically interested in minimal accounts of the self that bring out the pre-reflective structures of self-awareness (Zahavi 2005: 99–145; Zahavi 2018; Gallagher 2017), hermeneutical accounts of selfhood are, by contrast, are more fleshed-out, in that they take into account self-reflection, culture, and history. One of the main arguments that led to this hermeneutical development of phenomenology is that to be a self is to do something with what we experience. The hermeneutics of selfhood is produced by the tension between the pre-reflective certainty of being a self and the reflective doubt about how to be the self that one is. That is to say, the field of hermeneutics is grounded in two fundamental experiences, namely the experience of knowing *that* I am and the experience of not being certain of *who* I am. As Paul Ricoeur writes:

> The hermeneutics of the *I am* can alone include both the apodictic certainty of the Cartesian *I think* and the uncertainties, even the lies and the illusions, of the self, of immediate consciousness. It alone can yoke, side by side, the serene affirmation *I am* and the poignant doubt *Who am I?* (2004: 259; translation slightly modified)[1]

Our sense of selfhood is troubled by a sense of otherness. To be the self that I am I have to appropriate myself through a constant interpretation of the otherness that may not feature explicitly in my self-awareness, that I perhaps do not experience clearly or that I may not acknowledge fully, but which nevertheless makes itself known as an inescapable aspect of my identity. The term "otherness" tries to capture the heteronomous aspects of human self-hood that are not explicit in my experience of being a self. This otherness comprises, but is not restricted to, my biological makeup, cultural heritage, and social norms that orient my existence. To take just one example: the complexity of the fact that I am a biological organism on a par with other biological organisms in nature is not explicitly manifest in my experience of being a self. Phenomenology provides methodological tools to deal with my bodily experience, my so-called lived body (*Leib*), but is not able to account for my biological body (*Körper*), that is, the biological workings of, say, my kidney or the effects of my serotonin levels (Olson 1997: 147–148). I need to turn to biology and medicine to understand the

---

[1] The English version translates "l'affirmation sereine: *je suis*" with "the serene assertion *I am.*" I have chosen to maintain the noun "affirmation" because, in Ricoeur's philosophy, this specific noun functions as a technical concept with a fundamental ontological significance. The concept of "affirmation" or "originating affirmation" is meant to capture the basic affirmative character of human existence. Inspired by Spinoza's concept of conatus that designates a general will-to-live, Ricoeur argues that to exist is to want to exist: "Under the pressure of the negative, of negative experiences, we must re-achieve a notion of being which is *act* rather than *form*, living affirmation, the power of existing and of making exist" (2007b: 328; see also Stanghellini and Rosfort 2013: 61, 192–198). In this sense, the notion of affirmation functions as one aspect of the basic dialectical structure of the human being, where the other is the inescapable negation that comes with existing as a finite being (e.g. sickness, grief, fatigue, frustration, depression): "I do not think man directly, but I think him through composition, as the "mixture" of originating affirmation and existential negation. Man is the Joy of Yes in the sadness of the finite" (Ricoeur 1987: 140).

workings of my biological organism, and—perhaps more importantly—to make sense of the effects that these aspects of my body have on my self-awareness and experience of the world. The biological workings of human experience may not be not part of my implicit sense of selfhood, but they are part of the otherness that constitutes my identity. A malfunctioning kidney and critically low levels of serotonin do have a significant effect on my experience (e.g. tiredness, headache, depletion, sadness, irritation), and consequently on my sense of selfhood. A hermeneutical account can integrate the biological explanations of these "phenomenologically blind" aspects of my identity in an account of human selfhood by making them explicit in the interpretative appropriation of selfhood.

Thus, one of the primary differences between phenomenology and hermeneutics is that hermeneutics insists on this interpretative character of selfhood, whereas most contemporary phenomenologists argue for a foundational notion of self as a constitutive feature of experience. The interpretative approach brings out the fragility of our self-awareness by articulating the ambiguous character of human selfhood. Our sense of being a self is the product of an ongoing dialectics of pre-reflective experience and reflective interpretation. This interplay of passivity and activity in the forms of experiential givenness and reflective interpretation, alienation and intimacy, distance and appropriation constitute the philosophical core shared by the major philosophers who worked out the hermeneutical development of phenomenology in the twentieth century.

The Hermeneutical Development of Phenomenology

Martin Heidegger was the first phenomenologist who turned to hermeneutics. His pioneering work was the primary source of inspiration for hermeneutical philosophers in the twentieth century, and continues to heavily influence the development of philosophical hermeneutics in the twenty-first century. It is the hermeneutical core of the existential analysis in his most famous work from 1927, *Being and Time*, that initiated the hermeneutical turn in phenomenology. During the years of the First World War, Heidegger worked intensely with Husserl's newly developed phenomenology, but he grew increasingly critical of Husserl's conception of phenomenology as a "rigorous science." Heidegger's work can be read as a reaction to Husserl's attempt to produce a phenomenology purified of cultural, historical, and existential concerns—focusing on pre-reflective experience in terms of, for example, the temporal structure of perception or the object-directedness of intentionality. Heidegger sets out to deconstruct this scientific ideal of purity by delving into the humdrum of everyday life. In other words, whereas Husserl—or at least the early Husserl—is primarily interested in producing a scientifically rigorous account of the subjective structures of experience, Heidegger—or at least the early Heidegger—is interested in making sense of the existential concerns of a concrete self-in-the-world. As he writes in a series of lectures on phenomenology that he held in the year in which *Being and Time* was published: "The genuine, actual, though inauthentic understanding of the self takes place in such a way that this self, the self of our thoughtlessly random, common, everyday existence 'reflects' itself to itself out of that to which it has given itself over" (Heidegger 1988: 161). Heidegger's hermeneutical transformation of Husserlian phenomenology is a turn from an interest in knowledge to an interest in existence. Or as he puts it in another lecture four years earlier: "What hermeneutics is really meant to achieve is not merely taking cognizance of something and having knowledge about it, but rather an existential knowing, i.e., a *being [ein Sein]*. It speaks *from out of* interpretation and for the sake of it" (Heidegger 1999: 14). Our knowledge is the product of interpretation. As such, interpretation is not a choice or an add-on to the phenomenological description of experience. Experience is configured through interpretation because we are engaged with that which we experience, and we are engaged with experience because experience matters to us.

In fact, for Heidegger one of the primary problems with Husserlian phenomenology is that it does not pay enough attention to the affective aspect of experience. It is the affective aspect that reveals interpretation as an inescapable part of experience. We want to make sense of experience because we are affected by what we experience. Experience is structured normatively, and interpretation is our attempt to make sense the world, other people, and ourselves through the norms and values that orient our existence. As seen in the quote above, Heidegger approaches human selfhood in terms of the normative distinction between inauthentic and authentic existence. Most people, according to Heidegger, live their lives through mindless small-talk and ossified habits, and their engagement with the world and other people is severely limited by hearsay, asinine curiosity, and paralyzing ambiguity (Heidegger 2010: 161–173). The task for a human being is to disentangle herself from the web of idle talk and the empty humdrum of everyday life and to strive for an authentic life by trying to make sense of what she actually cares about. We find ourselves thrown into a world that we have not chosen, and we live a life that we have only partial control over. Heidegger analyzes this existential condition with the concept of *Befindlichkeit*. The concept is translated into English as "attunement"[2] to capture the fact that we experience ourselves as affectively attuned to our existence before our reflective attempt to make sense of ourselves. Heidegger's use of the original German word, however, brings out a more complex understanding of human self-experience. *Befindlichkeit*, in Heidegger's existential analysis, has a twofold significance comprising both the physical and the mental aspect of being-in-the world; or rather, it shows that we cannot separate those two aspects. Our being-in-the-world, our existence, is saturated with affective states. We experience ourselves as situated in a particular time and place, while at the same time experiencing ourselves affected by this particular situation through feelings, emotions, and moods (Heidegger 2010: 130–136).

Heidegger's *Being and Time* introduces an existential hermeneutics that brings out the interpretative character of experience with a particular emphasis on the temporal aspect of human existence. Not long after this seminal work, Heidegger shifted his hermeneutical focus from existential analysis to what he considered to be more fundamental ontological investigations of being in general, and selfhood and subjectivity subsided into the background of the latter part of his authorship. In fact, Heidegger's hermeneutical

---

[2] "*Befindlichkeit*" is notoriously difficult to translate into English. There are a variety of translations in use today (e.g. "affectedness," "disposedness," "sofindingness"). The initial translation was "state-of-mind" (Heidegger 1962). This translation is unfortunate, though, because it seems to work with a distinction between internal, psychological experiences and external experiences of the world that Heidegger's works actually aims to undermine. The most common translation today is "attunement" (Heidegger 2010).

phenomenology does not provide a positive account of what it is to be a human self. The primary strength of Heidegger's work is not the production of positive accounts of specific things, concrete aspects of the world, or solutions to human problems, but rather the deconstructive criticism of various—scientific, philosophical, and religious—existential ideals of what it means to be a human (Gadamer 2004: 253–254). However, as Heidegger's most influential student, Gadamer, writes: "What man needs is not just the persistent posing of ultimate questions, but the sense of what is feasible, what is possible, what is correct, here and now. The philosopher, of all people, must, I think, be aware of the tension between what he claims to achieve and the reality in which he finds himself" (Gadamer 2004: xxxiv).

Gadamer takes it upon himself to develop Heidegger's deconstructive phenomenological hermeneutics into a hermeneutical philosophy more in line with traditional hermeneutics, that is, a hermeneutics aimed at clarifying how the humanities can produce viable solutions to contemporary problems that are not—or cannot be—addressed by the natural sciences. As such, Gadamer's hermeneutical philosophy is not meant to be a contribution to phenomenology, but it has deep phenomenological roots and provides a philosophical articulation of themes that have become central in contemporary phenomenology (Figal 2012: 532). History and language are two of the most important themes that Gadamer deals with in his major work from 1960, *Truth and Method*. The human being exists in and through language, and it is situated in a specific historical tradition. Gadamer's focus is not subjectivity or selfhood, but the historical and linguistic conditions of human interpretation: "The focus of subjectivity is a distorting mirror. The self-awareness of the individual is only a flickering in the closed circuits of historical life. That is why the prejudices of the individual, far more than his judgments, constitute the historical reality of his being" (Gadamer 2004: 278). We think and talk in languages that we have not chosen, whose words carry a historical significance that influence us in ways that are experientially opaque. Moreover, we ourselves change over time, and our understanding of the world, other people, and ourselves is therefore never stable. We are constantly faced with the instability of what we understand, and we have to reappropriate our understanding through interpretation. The task of hermeneutics is to overcome this fundamental alienation that we live with as historical language users.

Gadamer's work is more explicitly hermeneutical than phenomenological in character, meaning that he is more concerned with the textual than experiential conditions of interpretation. Nonetheless, his hermeneutic analysis of the historical and linguistic character of human experience, and his argument for the inescapable interpretative character of this experience, has had an immense impact on the subsequent development of hermeneutical phenomenology.

Hermeneutical Phenomenology

It is in the work of the French philosopher Paul Ricoeur that we find the most elaborate attempt to combine phenomenology and hermeneutics into a proper hermeneutical phenomenology. While Gadamer took Heidegger's deconstructive hermeneutical phenomenology in a more constructive hermeneutical direction with texts and historical traditions as the analytical core, Ricoeur retains Heidegger's existential concern with subjectivity and selfhood in *Being and Time*. Like Gadamer, though, he tries to develop Heidegger's hermeneutical deconstruction into a constructive philosophy aimed at solving concrete existential and societal problems (Ricoeur 2004: 9–10). One of the primary objectives of Ricoeur's philosophy is to provide an account of personal identity, and it is in working out this account that he combines phenomenology and hermeneutics. Ricoeur's basic argument is that the two traditions are entangled to the extent that a separation of the two into distinct disciplines will always result in distorting accounts of human experience and personal identity. Or, as he puts it in an article dedicated to the interplay of the two philosophical traditions: "On the one hand, hermeneutics is erected on the basis of phenomenology and thus preserves something of the philosophy from which it nevertheless differs: *phenomenology remains the unsurpassable presupposition of hermeneutics*. On the other hand, phenomenology cannot constitute itself without a *hermeneutical presupposition*" (Ricoeur 2008: 23–24; emphasis in the original). For Ricoeur, phenomenology is not so much a homogeneous theory as a method, and—as it has become obvious throughout the twentieth century—there are many possible theoretical developments of Husserlian phenomenology. Husserl's insistence on pre-reflective experience and immediate self-awareness neglects, Ricoeur argues following Heidegger, the existential aspects of human experience such as the affective dimension of experience, the question of the will, and the constitutive presence of the other person in human self-awareness (Ricoeur 2007). It is, as we have seen, this existential dimension that is one of the main differences between Husserlian phenomenology and hermeneutics. Contrary to the Husserlian argument that subjectivity functions as the constitutive foundation of experience, hermeneutics, Ricoeur argues, "proposes to make subjectivity the final, and not the first, category of a theory of understanding. Subjectivity must be lost as radical origin if it is to be recovered in a more modest role" (Ricoeur 2008: 34).

The self is not a stable foundation upon which a person can construct a life, but a restless and fragile sense of being someone and wanting to become someone. The self is therefore an existential problem rather than transcendental or constitutive fact, and this existential challenge affects the subjective structures of experience. The pre-reflective structures of experience are not immune to the existential concerns of the experiencing subject nor is the immediate givenness of the world isolated from the personal, historical, or social context in which it is experienced. This is not to say that one cannot or should not investigate the pre-reflective structures of experience or the immediate givenness of the world. On the contrary, as is obvious from both Husserl's work and the work of contemporary phenomenologists, such investigations help us clarify and make sense of fundamental aspects of human experience. And as we shall see, these aspects play a vital role in Ricoeur's hermeneutical phenomenology. What the hermeneutical perspective makes evident is the interpretative foundation of Husserlian phenomenology, namely, that the focus on the pre-reflective structures of experience and the immediate givenness of the world is merely one interpretation or use of phenomenology, and this interpretation needs to be complemented with an existential interpretation in order to provide a satisfactory account of human experience (Ricoeur 2007: 212). As we have seen with Heidegger, this existential interpretation complements the descriptive focus on experiential features of subjectivity in Husserlian phenomenology with an ontological concern that brings out the problems of existing as a self. One way to put it is that while phenomenology concentrates on the *how* of human experience, hermeneutics is concerned with *what* I experience and *why* I experience it in the way that I do. Ricoeur's hermeneutical phenomenology is an attempt to bring into play all three dimensions in the analysis of human experience. The insistence on the existential grounding of experience means that the problem of personal identity is of particular interest to Ricoeur's combination of phenomenology and hermeneutics.

Identity is a problem that the self struggles with throughout her life. Human experience involves an immediate sense of self, that is, a pre-reflective sense of mineness, ownership, and agency. Or as a prominent contemporary phenomenologist argues, selfhood is a constitutive part of experience in the sense "that there is necessarily something it is like for the subject to have or live through the experiences" (Zahavi 2014: 8). Ricoeur's hermeneutical phenomenology uses this sense of self as the experiential foundation of being human. Different from most phenomenological accounts of selfhood, though, Ricoeur argues that we cannot provide a satisfactory account of human selfhood without taking into account the problem of identity. The existential foundation provided by the immediate sense of self is inherently fragile because with the experience of being a self comes also the experience of *wanting to be* a (particular kind of) person. The hermeneutical development of phenomenology is an attempt to explicate and make sense of this conative aspect of experience in terms of what he calls our "effort to exist," "will to exist," or "originating affirmation" (Ricoeur 1977: 46; Ricoeur 1987: 137). This means that, for Ricoeur, we cannot understand what it is to be a self without taking into account the desire or effort to be a particular person. Selfhood, in other words, is entangled with personhood, and our experience of the world, other people, and ourselves is structured and constantly informed by our care about who we *are*, who we *were*, and who we *will be*.

There are no stable or readily identifiable answers to the question of who we are. We can only hope to make sense of our identity through a long detour of interpretations. Interpretation is here understood not exclusively as interpretation of texts, traditions, or cultural artefacts, but also phenomenological and biological interpretations of my body, and ethical interpretations of my relationship with the other person (to mention some of the primary themes of Ricoeur's philosophy). As Ricoeur puts it succinctly: "hermeneutics proves to be a philosophy of detours" (Ricoeur 1992: 17). Inspired by Gadamer's work with textual hermeneutics, Ricoeur goes on to argue that we can indeed use texts and literature as an exercise in self-understanding and as a model for making sense of personal identity. To read a text is to be exposed to a world that is not of our own making, and as such to be confronted with heteronomous perspectives on our conception of the world. In this way, we become distanced from ourselves through reading, and yet we also come to know ourselves through the text: "What would we know of love and hate, of moral feelings, and, in general, of all that we call the *self* if these had not been brought to language and articulated by literature?" (Ricoeur 2008: 84). At work in reading is a dialectics of distance and appropriation that, according to Ricoeur, articulates and clarifies the hermeneutical insistence on the fictional character of selfhood:

> [J]ust as the world of the text is real only insofar as it is imaginary, so too it must be said that the subjectivity of the reader comes to itself only insofar as it is placed in suspense, unrealized, potentialized. In other words, if fiction is a fundamental dimension of the reference of the text, it is no less a fundamental dimension of the subjectivity of the reader. As a reader I find myself only by losing myself. Reading introduces me into imaginative variations of the ego. The metamorphosis of the world in play is also the playful metamorphosis of the ego.
>
> (Ricoeur 2008: 84–85)

This playful or fictional character of the self that is articulated through reading discloses the fragile foundation of human identity. We are not simply what we are in terms of biology, culture, memories, or even in terms of our self-understanding. We need to appropriate our identity through a constant interpretative effort. This is the primary argument of the hermeneutical perspective on personal identity.

This hermeneutical perspective is, however, combined with important phenomenological arguments. Ricoeur's insistence on the long hermeneutical detour over the *what* and the *why* of the identity of a person, that is, the interpretative *explanation* of a person's identity, is accompanied by his argument that if we want to produce a satisfactory account of personal identity we also need to take into account the *how* of a person's identity, that is, the *experience* of being this particular person. Our interpretations need to be rooted in and acknowledge the explanatory importance of experience. This means that we have to take seriously the intentionality of experience and the pre-reflective meaning of experience if we want to make sense of what it means to be a particular person. Language is, as we have seen, fundamental to our interpretation of experience. Nevertheless, Ricoeur's hermeneutical phenomenology shares with Husserlian phenomenology the conviction that language is subordinated to experience, and that linguistic meaning therefore has a derivative character (Ricoeur 2008: 38–40). The point is that identity is not merely a reflective task, but a problem that the person is constantly confronted with in her pre-reflective *experience* of the world, other people, and herself. We are the product of our past and of the culture in which we live, but our identity as persons depends on more than merely the conglomeration of biological development, cultural norms, habit, or memories. In the same way, although our ambitions, our goals, and our ideas about and hopes for the future shape who we are, our identity is also influenced by how we feel, think, and act in the concrete present. Moreover, our identity is deeply affected by how other people see and understand us, and our self-understanding is entangled with interpreting other people's understanding of us. And yet, we are more than what we are in the eyes of other people. The point is that a hermeneutical account of personal identity must take seriously the experience of being the person that I am.

By way of conclusion, I will argue that this interplay of immediate experiential givenness and reflective appropriation makes hermeneutical phenomenology an important tool for phenomenological psychopathology.

HERMENEUTICAL PHENOMENOLOGY AND PHENOMENOLOGICAL PSYCHOPATHOLOGY

Mental suffering comes in innumerable shapes and forms, and to describe and explain mental pain is challenging because of the indeterminate character of human self-experience. The cause of a person's suffering may be evident (e.g. the loss of a loved one), but the experiential character of that suffering indeterminate. And, vice versa, the experience of suffering can be excruciatingly clear while the cause remains obscure. To make sense of suffering we need to examine both the experiential and explanatory aspect of suffering—that is, we have to deal with the *how*, the *why*, and the *what* of the experience of suffering. A person who goes through a prolonged episode of suffering is concerned with how she feels, what she feels, and why she feels the way she does. The questions that accompany severe mental suffering often provoke a sense of losing or having lost oneself. The lack of an obvious cause of suffering or the indeterminate character of that suffering foregrounds a person's sense of identity. Not being able to point to an explicit cause or not being able to make sense of the meaning of one's feelings brings out the fragility of a person's sense of self. Why do I feel the way I do? Is my reaction normal? Am I to blame for what is happening to me? Is it because of something that I have done or because I am actually not who I think I am? These questions do not arise with the same existential urgency when it comes to a broken leg or kidney disease (although one's sense of identity is of course also always affected by a somatic illness; see Wyller 2005). The person's identity is more radically at stake in mental illness due to the lack of determinate experiential givenness or an explicit cause (e.g. the pain of hitting one's toe or the feeling of sadness because of a disparaging remark).

There is important work in phenomenological psychopathology on the role of selfhood in mental illness among which the self-disorder hypothesis of schizophrenia is arguably the most influential (Parnas and Sass 2003; Parnas 2012; Henriksen and Nordgaard 2016). Phenomenological psychopathology primarily focuses on disturbances of the pre-reflective structures of self-awareness such as temporality, embodiment, sense of ownership, and agency. Hermeneutical phenomenology builds on and develops this phenomenological work with a clarification of the reflective aspects of these disturbances of our implicit sense of self. The argument is that we cannot hope to provide a satisfactory account of the disturbed sense of self without an account of personhood (Stanghellini and Rosfort 2013). I am a self who is also a person, and to be a person is to be an embodied, social, and rational being who has to make sense of these aspects of her identity. In this sense, the notion of personhood is broader than the notion of selfhood as it is typically used in phenomenological psychopathology, involving the biological, social, and ethical aspects of human suffering. Moreover, the notion brings out the conative aspects of human identity, that is, the fact that we are not merely the self that we experience ourselves to be. We want to be a particular kind of self, and we have ambitions, dreams, and hopes for the future that affect our experience of suffering.

The experience of being a self involves, as we have seen, a need to make sense of experience, and in particular to make sense of who we are, what we are, and why we feel, think, and behave the way we do. These questions concern not merely the experiential aspects of personal identity, but also the biological, social, and ethical aspects of what it means to be a person, and as such they go beyond the scope of a strictly phenomenological account of selfhood. To make sense of a person's suffering it is not sufficient to clarify the experiential structures and dynamics of self-awareness. We also need to take into account the biological and sociocultural factors that shape—and in some cases are part of the cause of—my suffering, and the ethical considerations that inform and orient my thinking about how to live with my suffering. A person is not merely who she experiences herself to be, and her mental illness is more complex than her experience of it. This is of course a trivial observation. What is not trivial, though, is how to make sense of this complexity of mental illness. Phenomenological psychopathology provides us with an explanation of the experience of suffering, but we need other approaches to clarify and make sense of the "phenomenologically blind" aspects of a mental illness. Hermeneutical phenomenology provides an account that allows us to integrate a phenomenological approach with other approaches such as biological, sociological, and ethical approaches to mental illness. This account provides the philosophical foundation for a dialectical model of mental illness that understands the patient as an autonomous person who is constantly trying to make sense her own suffering (Jaspers 1997: 414–424; Stanghellini and Rosfort 2015a, 2015b). This model is person-centered in the sense that understands personal identity as a critical part of mental illness. To fully understand a person's experience of and life with a mental illness, we need to acknowledge that her sense of identity is involved in her mental suffering. As we saw in the first section, hermeneutics works with a fragile concept of selfhood. The experience of being a self is always accompanied by an experience of not being who I am, that is, an experience of otherness. This otherness constantly disturbs my sense of identity, and to live with this fragile sense of self I need to acknowledge that I am more than my sense of self. I am also the otherness that constitutes my identity as the person I am (my body, the world, and other people). To exist as a person is to constantly interpret and appropriate this otherness as part of the person that I am.

The strength of hermeneutical phenomenology lies in providing methods (most influentially, but not exclusively, narrative theories) to articulate these various aspects of personal identity through a phenomenological approach. The argument is that we cannot make sense of personal identity without articulating and interpreting the complexity of our experience of identity. This complexity grows out of experience, so to speak, in the form of the questions that we ask about who we are, what we are, what we have done, and what we should do. Hermeneutics allows us to deal with this complexity rather than being paralyzed by it. The contribution of hermeneutical phenomenology to phenomenological psychopathology is to be found precisely here. The dialectical model of mental illness understands that the biological, cultural, and ethical aspects of mental illness are not merely "add-ons" to a primary or foundational phenomenological account of selfhood, but are critical for our approach to and understanding of the suffering person. The person is both a patient and an agent in her experience of her mental illness. That is to say, that her suffering is her individual suffering because she always does something with her suffering, and yet she suffers from the otherness of her suffering in the sense that there are biological, social, and ethical aspects of her suffering that are out of her control. This dialectics of selfhood and otherness is at the heart of the hermeneutical approach to the patient as autonomous person who tries to make sense of herself in her experience of a mental illness. One of the major strengths of this account is that it allows us to see that a phenomenological approach to psychopathology is not necessarily in conflict with a biological, social, or ethical account. A hermeneutical development of phenomenological psychopathology is, in this sense, a theoretical foundation for a constructive interdisciplinary dialogue with other approaches to mental illness.

Bibliography

Ferraris M. (1996). *The History of Hermeneutics*, trans. L. Somigli. Atlantic Highlands: Humanities Press.

Figal G. (2012). "Hermeneutical Phenomenology." In D. Zahavi (ed.) *The Oxford Companion to Contemporary Phenomenology*, pp. 525–542. Oxford: Oxford University Press.

Gadamer H.-G. (2004). *Truth and Method* [1960], trans. J. Weinsheimer and D. G. Marshall. London: Continuum.

Gallagher S. (2017). "Self-defense: Deflecting Deflationary and Eliminativist Critiques of the Sense of Ownership." *Frontiers in Psychology* 8: 1–16.

Gallagher S. and Zahavi D. (2012). *The Phenomenological Mind*, 2nd edn. London: Routledge.

Greisch J. (2000). *Le cogito herméneutique. L'hermeneutique philosophique et l'héritage cartésien*. Paris: Vrin.

Grondin J. (1995). *Sources of Hermeneutics*. New York: State University of New York Press.

Heidegger M. (1962). *Being and Time* [1927], trans. J. Macquarrie and E. Robinson. Oxford: Blackwell.

Heidegger M. (1988). *The Basic Problems of Phenomenology* [1975], trans. A. Hofstadter. Bloomington: Indiana University Press.

Heidegger M. (1999). *Ontology—The Hermeneutics of Facticity* [1988], trans. J. van Burren. Bloomington: Indiana University Press.

Heidegger M. (2010) *Being and Time* [1927], trans. J. Stambaugh and D. J. Schmidt. Albany: State University of New York Press.

Henriksen M. G., Nordgaard J. (2016). "Self-disorders in Schizophrenia." In G. Stanghellini and M. Aragona (eds.), *An Experiential Approach to Psychopathology: What is It like to Suffer from Mental Disorders?* pp. 265–280. Berlin: Springer.

Jaspers K. (1997). *General Psychopathology*, trans. J. Hoenig and M. W. Hamilton. Baltimore: The Johns Hopkins University Press.

Olson E. T. (1997). *The Human Animal: Personal Identity Without Psychology*. Oxford: Oxford University Press.

Parnas J. (2012). "The Core Gestalt of Schizophrenia." *World Psychiatry* 11: 67–69.

Ramberg B. and Gjesdal K. (2014). "Hermeneutics." *The Stanford Encyclopedia of Philosophy* (Winter 2014 edn.) Edward N. Zalta (ed.), https://plato.stanford.edu/archives/win2014/entries/hermeneutics/

Ricoeur P. (1977). *Freud and Philosophy: Essay on Interpretation* [1965], trans. D. Savage. New Haven, CT: Yale University Press.

Ricoeur P. (1987). *Fallible Man* [1960], trans. C. A. Kelbley. New York: Fordham University Press.

Ricoeur P. (1992). *Oneself as Another* [1990], trans. K. Blamey. Chicago: University of Chicago Press.

Ricoeur P. (2004). *The Conflict of Interpretations: Essays in Hermeneutics* [1969], ed. D. Ihde. London: Continuum

Ricoeur P. (2007a). *Husserl. An Analysis of His Phenomenology* [1967], trans. E. G. Ballard and L. E. Embree. Evanston: Northwestern University Press.

Ricoeur P. (2007b). *History and Truth* [1965], trans. C. A. Kelbley. Evanston: Northwestern University Press

Ricoeur P. (2008). *From Text to Action. Essays in Hermeneutics, II* [1986], trans. K. Blamey and J. B. Thompson. London: Continuum.

Sass L. A. and Parnas J. (2003). "Schizophrenia, Consciousness, and the Self" *Schizophrenia Bulletin* 29: 427–444.

Schuhmann K. (2011). ""Phenomenology": A Reflection on the History of the Term." In S. Luft and S. Overgaard (eds.), *The Routledge Companion to Phenomenology*, pp. 657–688. Abingdon: Routledge.

Spiegelberg H. (1994). *The Phenomenological Movement: A Historical Introduction*, 3rd edn. Berlin: Springer.

Stanghellini G. and Rosfort R. (2013). *Emotions and Personhood: Exploring Fragility—Making Sense of Vulnerability*. Oxford: Oxford University Press.

Stanghellini G. and Rosfort R. (2015a). "Disordered Selves or Persons with Schizophrenia." *Current Opinion in Psychiatry* 28: 256–263.

Stanghellini G. and Rosfort R. (2015b). "The Patient as an Autonomous Person: Hermeneutical Phenomenology as a Resource for an Ethics for Psychiatrists." In John Z. Sadler, K. W. M. Fulford, and Werdie van Staden (eds.), *The Oxford Handbook of Psychiatric Ethics*, pp. 319–335. Oxford: Oxford University Press.

Taylor C. (1985). "Self-interpreting Animals." In C. Taylor, *Human Agency and Language: Philosophical Papers 1*, pp. 45–76. Cambridge: Cambridge University Press.

Wyller T. (2005). "The Place of Pain in Life." *Philosophy* 80: 385–393.

Zahavi D. (2005). *Subjectivity and Selfhood: Investigating the First-Person Perspective.* Cambridge: The MIT Press.

Zahavi D. (2014). *Self and Other: Exploring Subjectivity, Empathy, and Shame.* Oxford: Oxford University Press.

Zahavi D. (2018). "Consciousness, Self-Consciousness, Selfhood: A Reply to some Critics." *Review of Philosophy and Psychology*. Online first: doi: 10.1007/s13164-018-0403-6

CHAPTER 30

INTROSPECTION, PHENOMENOLOGY, AND PSYCHOPATHOLOGY

LOUIS SASS AND ADAM FISHMAN

INTRODUCTION

"INTROSPECTION" and "phenomenology" refer to the two most prominent scientific or philosophical programs or traditions—or sets of programs or traditions—to study subjectivity: to describe, from within, the "what-it-is-like" of human consciousness or experience. The relationship between the approaches falling under these rubrics is exceptionally difficult to define, however. Outsiders, especially hostile ones, but also some insiders, tend to treat them as equivalent—with phenomenological method sometimes simply assumed to be a form of "introspection," and "introspection" just understood to mean a focusing on the "phenomenology" or subjective character of mental life. The approaches do share some common ancestry, stretching back at least to Descartes and Kant and including more recent thinkers about consciousness or subjectivity such as Brentano, Bergson, and William James.[1]

The views of insiders to the two sets of programs or traditions are extremely divergent, however. They range from the claim that the relevant methods can be complementary or even overlapping to the point of equivalence, to the insistence, by Edmund Husserl and some of his followers, that to describe phenomenology as a form of introspection is "preposterous" (Zahavi 2011: 16). There is, in fact, a strong tradition *within* phenomenology (summarized later) of *criticizing* introspection or introspectionism, and seeking to define phenomenology in a way that would sharply dissociate it from the supposed weaknesses or errors of introspection. The phenomenological arguments against "introspection" can sound pertinent and powerful, yet may also seem, at other moments, somewhat overdrawn or even inaccurate. The reasons for these wavering reactions make some sense once one recognizes the

---

[1] We thank Matthew Ratcliffe, Dan Zahavi, Jeffery Geller, and Anthony Fernandez for helpful suggestions. Much of the research for this chapter was done by A. F., the analysis and writing primarily by the senior author, L. S.

ambiguities inherent in both notions; for, in fact, there are *several* ways of understanding each of these key terms. It seems that "introspection"—perhaps "phenomenology" as well—is a kind of "floating signifier," and that any adequate comparison of the two must take these ambiguities into account.

A thorough treatment of this complex topic would require a great many pages. Our strategy in this chapter will be to focus on criticisms of introspection by members of the phenomenological tradition. We will be interested in the nature and validity of these criticisms, but also in the extent to which they really do differentiate between the two programs or traditions. We will concentrate on three examples of "introspection": the Cornell school of E. B. Titchener and the German Würzburg School, both from the early twentieth century, as well as a contemporary group of French researchers who seek the "explicitation" of consciousness or subjectivity. Some differences between the perspectives of Husserl, phenomenology's founder, and those of Heidegger and Merleau-Ponty will be considered. We will end by considering phenomenological psychopathology in light of these issues. As we shall see, the reasons for criticizing "introspection," and distinguishing it from true "phenomenology," may seem less cogent or apt when one considers certain versions of "introspection," and when one includes phenomenological psychopathology under the rubric of "phenomenology."

PHENOMENOLOGICAL CRITICISMS
OF INTROSPECTION

The phenomenological attack on "introspection" can be traced back to Husserl himself, who clearly associated it with the dreaded "psychologism" that he himself had espoused in his earliest writings, but rejected vigorously after some decisive criticism from the philosopher Frege (Kusch 1995; Vermersch 2011).[2] Husserl's arguments have been echoed by Merleau-Ponty (1945), Gurwitsch (1966), and some contemporary Husserlians (e.g. Zahavi 2007).

Epoché

Phenomenologists have argued that introspection suffers from a failure to carry out the "bracketing" or *epoché* that is the first, largely negative, move in any phenomenological investigation. *Epoché* is an act of "abstention" or putting into parentheses (neither believing nor denying, nor even doubting) of all common-sense assumptions (of the "natural attitude") as well as of theoretical claims *about* experience, mind, or the world, in order to make way for a presuppositionless and unprejudiced investigation of what actually appears in our conscious experience (Merleau-Ponty 1945: 86). Introspectionists are criticized for relying

---

[2] The very intensity of Husserl's repudiation of introspection and naturalism, together with his inconsistent recognition/denial of their possible "interpenetration" (see Merleau-Ponty 1964), suggests he might have been, in some sense, intellectually *traumatized* by this experience (Vermersch 2011). This, obviously, is itself a psychologistic suggestion—though interesting nonetheless.

on "predetermined categories," categories decided upon before the investigation and therefore imposed *upon* experience rather than elicited *from* it (Overgaard et al. 2008: 110).

Intentionality

A second key criticism is the claim that introspectionists fail to transcend a misleading sub-
ject/object distinction that contradicts the object- or world-directed nature of actual subjective life. The very term "introspection," it is said, implies a deplorable "Cartesianism": the
assumption that subjectivity is some sort of inward or inner object or quasi-object
("intro . . .") that could be inspected (". . . spection") at a kind of remove (Zahavi 2011).[3] It is
noted that Husserl, by contrast, followed Brentano in considering consciousness to be fundamentally "intentional" or object-directed. This means that the subjectivity to which one
returns in phenomenological reduction (the Latin "*reducere*" means to withdraw or lead
back to) must *not* be conceived as a "mysterious inner world" or "state of consciousness"
to be grasped through "a very peculiar kind of act—'inner perception' or introspection"
(Merleau-Ponty 1945: 58). Rather, it is a veritable streaming-*outward* that we simply *are*, and
that is simply inconceivable (and indescribable) apart from the objects *toward which* it aims.

Transcendental

A third phenomenological criticism is the claim that introspectionists adopt a "naturalism"
regarding consciousness, thereby failing to recognize the *transcendental* or, we might say,
truly *constituting* nature of subjectivity (Zahavi 2011: 16f.). Consciousness is not a mere
"sector of being" that happens to involve "inner events" (Merleau-Ponty 1964: 59–61) yet can
be studied like the objects of physics, chemistry, or biology. Consciousness, writes Merleau-
Ponty, needs to be understood as "a totality with no equivalent at all among the things of
nature" (1945: 58) since it is the very domain *within which* both meaning and the world itself actually *come into being*. "Acts of consciousness" therefore require *transcendental* clarification; they constitute a "privileged realm" and need to be considered "with regard to
their . . . presentational function"—as that "*through*" which "objects, processes, events, and
occurrences . . . display themselves" (Merleau-Ponty 1945: 90; Gurwitsch 1966: 90).

Merleau-Ponty brings the intentionality and transcendental insights together in these
lapidary lines on subjectivity: "The interior and the exterior are inseparable. The world is
entirely on the inside, and I am entirely outside of myself" (1945: 469). This is more or less
what Husserl meant when he spoke, in his *Cartesian Meditations*, of "transcendence [a going
beyond] *within* immanence" (Moran and Cohen 2012: 162). Phenomenology, he might have
said, is not a matter of looking at the *within*; rather, it is a matter of looking *at* the world *from*
within—but, of course, with a heightened awareness of precisely this *from-ness*.

---

[3] There may be something literal-minded about taking the term "introspection" too seriously,
especially if one recognizes, as did both Heidegger and the later Husserl (together with his student Eugen
Fink 1995: 88ff.), that language, whose origins lie mainly in concrete experience of the physical world
(*within* the natural attitude), is *inevitably* misleading when applied to experience or human existence
as such.

Eidetic Intuition

A fourth way of distinguishing introspection from phenomenology is to note that introspection fails to seek "eidetic intuition" (*Wesenschau*) through "eidetic reduction," which is meant to be the key source of generalization in Husserlian phenomenology. Unlike more standard forms of generalization or abstraction, this phenomenological "intuition of essences" is not supposed to be reliant on fallible empirical observation, for example, on a gathering of subjective reports. Indeed it is "not concerned with matters of fact or existence, but [with] the necessary and essential . . . [with] essences of a universal character" (Moran and Cohen 2012: 92): "Prior to knowledge of the factical world," wrote Husserl, "there is universal knowledge of those essential possibilities without which no world whatever, and this includes the factical world as well, can be thought of as existing" (Husserl 1997: 487).

The eidetic reduction is supposedly grounded in something whose universality and truth can be recognized with an intuitive (viz. immediately perceived) certitude somewhat akin to the truth of logic and mathematics (Moran and Cohen 2012). It involves "regaining" the sense of things or events that, though "not thematized," were always present "in our spontaneous, unreflective experience" (Merleau-Ponty 1964: 55). It depends on a kind of imaginative variation whereby one discovers, with clarity and confidence, something one had already known in some more obscure, perhaps pre-reflective way.

An example of eidetic intuition is the controlled process whereby phenomenological reflection discerns the essence of a particular mode or element of experience through acts of controlled imaginative variation—so that, for example, by pure reflection on, and imaginative variation of, one's own experiences (or memories thereof), one identifies the invariants that make a perception a perception, rather than an act of remembering, imagining, or dreaming. Many Husserlians (but not all phenomenologists, as we shall see later (Merleau-Ponty 1964)) consider the eidetic reduction (speaking of essences) an *essential* feature of any investigation of subjectivity that is truly "phenomenological."

Resumé

We have described four criticisms, each linked to a core notion definitive of phenomenology, at least in its Husserlian form. Two of these criticisms—intentionality and the transcendental dimension—pertain to how *subjectivity itself* is conceived. The other two—bracketing and the eidetic reduction—concern the appropriate *method for studying* subjectivity.

PHENOMENOLOGICAL CRITICISMS APPLIED TO CLASSICAL INTROSPECTIONISTS

Titchener

Both the absence of bracketing and the neglect of "intentionality" seem readily apparent in the introspection advocated by the early twentieth-century Cornell psychologist E. B.

Titchener—a British transplant and former pupil of Wilhelm Wundt who is often treated as the quintessential example of an introspectionist. Titchener's naturalism is apparent in his invoking of chemistry and physics as models for the study of subjective experience (Beenfeldt 2013: 34; Boring 1953: 173) and in lines such as these: "... the introspective methods thus do us the same service in psychologising that 'observation and experiment' do in natural science"; its limitations are "of the same sort as the 'limitations' of a microscope or a camera" (Titchener 1912: 508, 498). As we shall see, rather than bracketing all presuppositions, Titchener seems to have accepted the assumption—typical of the empiricist and associationist traditions, and of sense-data theorists—that "consciousness is a mosaic of sensory data and images derived from these data," as in Hume's account of "impressions" and "ideas" (Gurwitsch 1966: 159).

Central to Titchener's approach was the attempt to avoid what he termed the "stimulus error" or the "meaning error." These refer to reports of experience that describe the actual worldly *object*, naively perceived, or else the experienced *meaning*, naively registered, rather than truly describing the associated and underlying "impression," "sensation," "mental process," or "mental material itself" (Boring 1921). Titchener followed Wundt in distinguishing between "mediate" and "immediate" experience. He believed that psychology, through "hard introspective labor," should focus on the latter, which he equated with "experience dependent on an experiencing person [or] organism" (Heidbreder 1933: 123, 126, 129).

In his vision of *perception*, Titchener resembled a sense-data theorist who believes that what one truly sees, in visual perception, is not the *external stimulus*—say, a table or a tomato on a plate—but the *sensation* or "immediate experience [of] color and brightness and spatial pattern" (Heidbreder 1933: 129): for example, a "red patch of a round and somewhat bulgy shape, standing out from a background of other color-patches [in a] field of color [that is] directly present to my consciousness" (Price 1932: 3, quoted in Pepper 1942: 26). This conflicts with the emphasis on intentionality put forward in the phenomenological tradition: "To say that I am . . . oriented toward sensations is all just pure theory," wrote Martin Heidegger (1982: 63). "Perception is directed toward the extant being itself..."

Regarding the experience of meaning in *thinking* and *understanding*, Titchener stressed the role of specific *imagery*—which itself is quasi-sensory, and ultimately *derived* from sensations.

It might seem natural to assume that one's experience of the meaning of an abstract concept would itself occur in some kind of highly abstract medium. But according to Titchener, introspection, properly conducted, shows that the experience of the meaning even of highly abstract concepts or notions is *always* actually mediated by concrete, sensory, even quasi-physicalistic images. "All the [introspectionist] reports," he wrote, "show the same features: visual images, pictorial or symbolic; internal speech; kinaesthetic images; organic sensations. Nowhere a sign of the imageless component!" (Titchener 1910: 516). A clear example comes from one trained introspector who investigated his own experience of the meaning of "meaning" itself (obviously a highly abstract concept), and "discovered" this notion to be associated, at least in *his* consciousness, with something very concrete: namely, the image of "the blue-grey tip of a kind of scoop, which has a bit of yellow above it (presumably a part of the handle), and which is just digging into a dark mass of what appears to be plastic material" (Titchener 1910: 519, discussed in Sass 1994: 90).

According to one historian of psychology, Titchener's method of so-called "introspection" actually consisted of "a Byzantine and heavily theory-laden procedure of 'psychological analysis' or regimented 'analytic attention' designed to generate data confirming a set of assumptions regarding mental ontology taken over from British associationism [which is closely allied with empiricism and sense-data theory], while at the same time shielding those assumptions from disconfirming evidence" (Beenfeldt 2013: 67).

Instances such as the above (e.g. the "blue-grey tip") also seem to illustrate the potentially misleading effect that the act or attitude of intense self-observation can have, as noted by various general critics of introspection who warn of a misleading potential in what may amount to a kind of alienating and reifying stare (Sass 2017: chapter 7). It is noteworthy that reports by such psychological investigators as Titchener, or by contemporary subjects asked to adopt his version of introspective technique (Hunt and Chefurka 1976), can display close parallels with the experiences of psychiatric patients who manifest intense and dysfunctional forms of self-consciousness—of alienating "hyperreflexivity." In accord with this orientation or stance, some patients with schizophrenia or depersonalization disorder may come to lose the sense of being grounded in an active and coherent subject position, while generating subjective phenomena (neither fully perceptual nor fully imaginary) with a quality aptly characterized as "phantom concreteness" (Laing 1965; Sass et al. 2013; Sass 2017: chapter 7).

The Würzburg School

The phenomenological criticisms seem to apply less clearly, however, to the introspectors of the Würzburg School—who included Oswald Külpe, Karl Bühler, and Narziss Kaspar Ach. In the early twentieth century, the famous "imageless-thought controversy" pitted the Würzburgers against the Titchenerian introspectionists. The controversy turned on the Würzburger claim that unbiased introspection actually revealed elements and acts of consciousness, including "dispositions of consciousness" and "determining tendencies" that did not, in fact, contain any of the sensory or image-like qualities that the Titchenerian sensationists seemed to find (or to project?) wherever they observed.

At a certain point the Würzburg investigators, who were influenced by Brentano's "act psychology" approach, had begun to look not for the "abstract sensory elements to which experience was to be reduced" but for "the subjective acts which make experience of various kinds possible" (Danziger 1980: 255). The Würzburgers may well have continued to view these acts of consciousness themselves in overly object-like ways, tending to treat them as additional items in the inventory of an inner life conceived as being a "little tag end of the world" (Husserl 1960: 24)—as some phenomenologists might wish to claim. However, the Wurzbürger attitude toward the nature of these "acts" does seem to have been more open, and their bracketing more thorough, than that of the Titchenerians. Further, these latter points should be considered in light of two (closely related) facts: 1) that the truly transcendental nature of consciousness is difficult and perhaps impossible to capture fully in human language or thought (Fink 1995), and 2) that bracketing or reduction can, in any case, *never* be absolute or complete: indeed, "The most important lesson of the reduction is the impossibility of a complete reduction," as Merleau-Ponty put it in a famous line from his *Phenomenology of Perception* (1945: lxxvii).

It may well be that the Würzburgers did not sufficiently appreciate the truly *constituting* nature of consciousness—its status as that which brings the experiential universe itself into manifestation. But as we have seen, they did shift the focus from object-like *contents* of awareness (understood almost as inner "things," subsisting *within* the container of consciousness) by emphasizing the *psychological acts* that make awareness possible. And they did define mental processes in terms of their actual lived objects or meanings. All this suggests some implicit—if not, perhaps, sufficiently theorized or emphasized—appreciation of the need for bracketing, and also of the intentional and perhaps even the transcendental nature of consciousness or mind.

PHENOMENOLOGICAL CRITICISMS APPLIED TO CONTEMPORARY INTROSPECTIONISTS

Contemporary "Introspectionists"

If we turn to contemporary schools, the distinction between "phenomenology" and "introspection" becomes still harder to draw.

One common feature of *contemporary* introspectionists is a commitment to avoiding any imposition of theoretical as well as everyday prejudices onto lived experience—which, of course, is equivalent to advocating bracketing or *epoché*. They all instruct subjects "not to employ implicit or explicit theories about consciousness prior to the experiment" (Overgaard et al. 2008: 116). This is true of Hurlburt's (2011) Direct Experience Sampling method, of the so-called "New Introspectionists" (Overgaard et al. 2008), and of a third, largely French group of investigators on whom we will now focus. These latter offer a particularly sophisticated meditation on a possible methodology for introspection. Since they term their method "explicitation," we refer to them as the "explicitationists."

"Psycho-Phenomenological Introspection"

Though strongly influenced by the biologist and student of Buddhism, Francisco Varela, who dubbed his own approach "neurophenomenology," Pierre Vermersch, Michel Bitbol, and Claire Petitmengin often use the word "introspection" to describe their own approach. In a phrase that throws their intellectual hybridity into relief, Vermersch refers to their method as "psycho-phenomenological introspection" (2009: 25). None of the explicitationists is entirely satisfied with the term "introspection," however—some are even tempted to reject it (Petitmengin and Bitbol 2009: 379). But as Vermersch (2011) points out, virtually all the possible semantic alternatives—including "reflection," "immanent view," and "inner viewing" (all of which have been used by Husserl himself, e.g. 1977: 19–20)—*also* rely on metaphors, often similar ones, that can be equally misleading.

As the phrase "psycho-phenomenological introspection" suggests, explicitation incorporates phenomenological insights and was expressly designed to avoid the criticisms directed at classical introspectionism (Bitbol and Petitmengin 2013: 273). The proposed method includes the three moves sometimes identified as crucial in a phenomenological study: *epoché*, focused description, and intersubjective corroboration (Gallagher and Zahavi 2012).

The explicitation interview attempts to bring the interviewee into more direct contact with their experience—not only by resisting the infiltration of prejudices but also (more originally) by encouraging a re-inhabiting of the original experience at issue by adopting an "evocation position," a state of trance-like receptivity (cf. Maurel 2009: 64). This is achieved by having the interviewee describe a specified moment of experience in concrete terms, by focusing the interviewee initially on the sensorial surround of the episode in question (Maurel 2009), and sometimes by having the interviewee re-enact physical gestures performed during the moment described. The interviewer may mirror the interviewee's gestures and repeat their phrases in order to guide and deepen their attention to the particulars of the experience. The goal is to move attention "from the narrow *content* to the complete *act* of consciousness," which, according to Bitbol and Petitmengin (2013: 273), is "tantamount to performing the phenomenological reduction."

The explicitationists thus speak of seeking "descent to close contact with the very flesh of [one's] experience (and away from abstraction)". Only after this "descent" is the experimenter meant to undertake what they describe as "an ascent towards general concepts and structures" (Bitbol and Petitmengin 2013: 273). And this ascent, in turn, is done while attempting to bracket theoretical and common-sense assumptions as much as possible, thereby adopting a "bottom-up" approach that is designed to ensure "high fidelity" to concrete experience.

The explicitationists have been criticized by a Husserlian phenomenologist for adopting the term "introspection," since this term seems to endorse, at least tacitly, "the idea that consciousness is inside the head and the world outside" (Zahavi 2011: 17)—an idea that would supposedly neglect the fundamental *intentionality* of conscious existence. But the explicitationists deny that they are "diverting" attention from external objects "toward an inner world." Actually, they claim, their methods of evocation and exploration tend to *weaken* rather than reinforce the distinction between "internal" and "external," bringing the introspecting individual more in touch with the "permeable" nature of the "separation" sometimes "perceived between an inner and an outer world" (Petitmengin and Bitbol 2009: 379).

It has been suggested, as well, that the explicitationists risk treating consciousness as a "mere sector of being," and thereby neglecting, presumably, its *transcendental* status as the condition for the appearance of the world (Zahavi 2011: 17). It is difficult, however, to see just how this criticism would have any *special* application to the explicitationist approach—as opposed to being taken to apply, perhaps on principle, to just about *any* attempt to describe the actual lived experiences of particular individuals (and this would include phenomenological psychopathology; see later).[4] Such a criticism would, in any case, need to be considered in light of Merleau-Ponty's claim that "the transcendental attitude is already implied in

---

[4] On this issue, consider Husserl's comment on "phenomenological psychology" in his 1928 Amsterdam lectures: "Even as an eidetic phenomenologist, the psychologist is transcendentally naïve. However much he or she may try to put everything psychophysical out of play in directing his/her interest toward the purely mental, these are still actual or possible 'minds,' minds thought of completely in the relative sense of this word as always the minds of bodies out there, that is to say, mind of concrete human beings in a spatial world" (1997: 242). But for skepticism about the cogency of Husserl's transcendental-phenomenology-vs-phenomenological-psychology distinction, see Welton (2000: 67, 114f., 267–269).

the psychologist's descriptions, so long as they are faithful descriptions" (1945: 60)—for this suggests that proper consideration of actual subjective life (an, in part, empirical project) will, when *properly* conducted, naturally lead one to acknowledge the intentional and constituting dimensions of consciousness.

The knottiness of the introspection/phenomenology relationship becomes even more apparent if we consider, in concluding, two forms of diversity *within* phenomenology: 1) differing views regarding the phenomenological project itself, especially its methodology; and 2) the distinction between more purely philosophical versus more applied (psychological or psychopathological) forms of phenomenological inquiry.

Varieties of Phenomenology

So far, we have presented Merleau-Ponty and Heidegger as essentially consistent with Husserlian tradition. There are, however, important differences to be considered. These pertain less to the vision of subjectivity itself (to its intentional and transcendental nature) than to methodological issues.[5]

Epoché

It is well known that Heidegger advocated a *hermeneutic* approach to phenomenology. This meant questioning the possibility of pristine intuition and pure description, within a more or less straightforward *epoché*, in favor of accepting the *necessary* role of presuppositions in the self-critical, endless, and always somewhat obscure, back-and-forth processes inherent in acts of interpretation and understanding. On this account of the famous "hermeneutic circle," pre-judgments are more difficult to remove but also more valuable to retain than Husserl seems to have recognized.

Adopting this sort of hermeneutic vision might, in fact, introduce some doubt about the degree of emphasis, found in Husserl as well as in virtually all contemporary schools of introspection, on attempting to eschew presuppositions. Such attempts are not without some heuristic value, of course; for even if incapable of being fully achieved, they surely *do* constitute an important moment in the overall interpretive phenomenological procedure. Emphasis on bracketing or faithful explicitation should not, however, be allowed to obscure the potential contribution of interpretive or hermeneutic dialogue in which the experimenter (first as interviewer, later as analyst) might play a more active role in suggesting and weighing possible interpretations, albeit in an appropriately skeptical, flexible, and self-critical fashion (more on this later).

---

[5] Ideally we would also consider the variation *within Husserl himself*, not only his development over time, but also possible internal inconsistencies: e.g. on the importance of the "life-world," the value of "induction" (see Merleau-Ponty 1964), and the unavoidability of error in any attempt to describe the "transcendental" (see Fink 1995).

Eidetic Reduction

A second issue concerns the sharpness of the distinction between what might be considered eidetic or transcendental versus empirical or factual aspects of, and approaches to, human experience. This distinction is examined in Merleau-Ponty's essay, "Phenomenology and the Sciences of Man" (1964), which offers a subtle discussion and ambivalent critique of Husserl's presentation of eidetic intuition (*Wesenschau*).

There Merleau-Ponty argues that Husserl *did* acknowledge, at least implicitly, a similarity between phenomenological *Wesenschau* and more standard, "inductive" forms of investigation. But Merleau-Ponty also argues that Husserl failed to acknowledge this true "homogeneity" in a full or explicit manner; and failed as well to appreciate the value and necessity not only of a dialectic between empirical observation and abstract essences, but also of the "interpenetration of psychology and phenomenology" that Merleau-Ponty (1964: 73) views as a key source of phenomenological insight. Philosophy, writes Merleau-Ponty (1964: 92), "must begin by understanding the lived experiences." He echoes Heidegger (perhaps also the explicitationists): "Finally this essence is accessible only in and through the individual situation in which it appears. When pushed to the limit, eidetic psychology becomes analytic-existential" (Merleau-Ponty 1964: 95).

Merleau-Ponty here clearly tilts toward a hermeneutic rather than a foundationalist or logic-inspired vision of phenomenological inquiry. Indeed his views erode any too-sharp differentiation between a supposedly essence-oriented, transcendental condition of true "phenomenology" versus a "merely" empirical approach supposedly exemplified by "introspection," phenomenological psychology, or phenomenological psychopathology. The phenomenologist, writes Merleau-Ponty, must in fact "find a way of knowing which is neither deductive nor purely empirical," thereby avoiding both the Scylla of psychologism and the Charybdis of logicism (1964: 55). "It is essential," in any case, "that this abstract phenomenology [with its interest in essences] should come into contact with the facts . . ." (Merleau-Ponty 1964: 91).

To illustrate what "contact with the facts" can mean, Merleau-Ponty (1964) describes Husserl's encounter, in the mid-1930s, with French philosopher and anthropologist Lucien Lévy-Bruhl's writings on the experience of time and myth in the tribal or "primitive" mind. "Before this," writes Merleau-Ponty, "Husserl had maintained that a mere imaginative variation of the facts would enable us to conceive of every possible experience we might have" (1964: 90). Pure eidetic intuition is supposed to yield "a body of apriori knowledge that is not in any way a matter of empirical fact but of universal principles" (Palmer in Husserl 1997: 210)—namely, what Husserl (1997: 487) termed a "philosophical knowledge of the given world [that] allows us to grasp *the invariant essential form, the pure ratio of the world,* including all of its regional spheres of being." Husserl's encounter with Lévy-Bruhl's compelling account of people described as living in a "flowing present," devoid of "historical time," shook his belief in such a capacity (1964: 90–91). The encounter forced Husserl to recognize that "the imagination, left to itself, is unable to represent the possibilities of existence which are realized in different cultures" (Merleau-Ponty 1964: 90).

To this latter point we might add: "which are realized in different psychopathological conditions."

Many of the points discussed in this chapter can, in fact, be illuminated by brief consideration of phenomenological psychopathology. Phenomenological psychopathology might well seem vulnerable to some of the same criticisms that Husserl had directed at introspection—for it too is largely an empirical enterprise, and one that can hardly be grounded in a purely eidetic form of intuition.

PHENOMENOLOGICAL PSYCHOPATHOLOGY

It seems clear that phenomenological psychopathologists—students of abnormal subjectivity—attempt to adopt both the intentional and transcendental standpoints. Appreciation of the world-directed as well as subjective/constituting nature of their object of study (that is, of abnormal subjectivity) is illustrated by phenomenological descriptions of, for example, typically schizophrenic, manic, or psychotically depressed ways of experiencing time and space, or the overall "atmospheric" qualities of their lived world or experiential universe (for a review, see Sass and Pienkos 2013). It is difficult, however, to see how either the eidetic reduction (*Wesenschau*) or the *epoché* could be appropriate in phenomenological psychopathology—at least in anything like a pure form.

How, after all, could a phenomenological psychiatrist or psychologist (unless, of course, she has *herself* been psychotic) rely primarily on her own, taken-for-granted understanding of human experience as a way of discovering—via some kind of a priori eidetic reduction—the essential features of, say, the "delusional mood" in prodromal schizophrenia? Phenomenological psychopathology obviously involves a sort of second-person or third-person phenomenology. Here the need for a careful gathering and sifting of subjective reports from patients or other sufferers is perfectly obvious—yet this is the very sort of empirical enterprise that seems to be excluded in Husserl's vision of *Wesenschau* or eidetic intuition (at least prior to his encounter with Lévy-Bruhl).

A second point pertains to the issue of bracketing or *epoché*, and to the need for a more hermeneutic approach.

That phenomenological psychopathology involves empirical examination does not imply that its investigations should be purely *empiricist* in nature—in the sense of being grounded in experiences devoid of interpretation or conceptual understanding. One could, after all, hardly hope to imagine, or intellectually to grasp, the altered time-experience in schizophrenia, depression, or mania if one lacked all theoretical understanding of the nature of temporality in normal persons—including, for example, such notions as William James's "specious present" or Husserl's "duration block" of "retention/primal-impression/protention" (Fuchs 2013).

To explore a patient's abnormal experience of self, time, space, or atmosphere, for example, it is necessary to pose some quite specific but open-ended questions (typically a "semistructured interview") that, at the very least, identify these domains and ask about some possible ways in which they might in fact be altered (Nordgaard et al. 2013). This suggests the need for something closer to a hermeneutic dialogue than to the pristine bracketing of assumptions on which both Husserl and recent introspectionists place so much emphasis.

Consideration of the source of these guiding concepts, so crucial for effective interviewing as well as subsequent analysis, does suggest, however, that something like an eidetic orientation—even if not in a purist, quasi-logicist form—cannot be entirely dismissed. For as Husserl noted, to grasp such concepts as "percept" or "image," "perception" or the "imaginary," also of time, space, or selfhood—all necessary for inquiry into subjective dimensions of psychopathology—does require some consulting of one's own experience, without which they would remain empty words. This is the contribution of Husserl's *eidetic psychology*, which Merleau-Ponty (1964: 58) describes as "a reflective effort by which we clarify the fundamental notions which psychology [and, we would add, psychopathology] uses constantly, through a contact with our own experience."

This does not mean, however, that empirical consideration of actual experiences, including abnormal ones, does not *also* have the potential to contribute to our *refinement* of the basic concepts. With psychotic disorders, the "refinement" in question may even turn out to be revolutionary, in the sense that the researcher must strive to conceive what may not, at least at first, seem to be imaginable, thereby coming to construct concepts that might not otherwise have existed. The study of basic-self or ipseity disturbances in schizophrenia might, for instance, inspire phenomenologists and other philosophers to question the necessary universality of what is sometimes called the *cogito*, while also suggesting, to some, the need to distinguish between different aspects of basic self-experience (namely, "possession" versus "agency") that had not previously been appreciated (Zahavi 2005).[6]

All this shows, according to Merleau-Ponty, "that knowledge of essences is altogether experiential, that it does not involve any kind of supersensible faculty," but *also* "that any knowledge of facts always involves an a priori understanding of essence" (1964: 72). As Merleau-Ponty (1964: 58) suggests, it is too simple to say that whereas "knowledge of facts belongs to psychology," the "definition of the notions which will enable us to understand these facts belongs to phenomenology." "Empirical psychology" is *not*, in fact, always and only "preceded by an eidetic psychology" (Merleau-Ponty 1964: 58), as Husserl sometimes claimed, since it sometimes has an impact on eidetic psychology itself. It is difficult to imagine a more compelling illustration of the hermeneutic vision of truth-seeking as a constant tacking back and forth—between theory and evidence, between essence and existence.

CONCLUSION

The relationship between introspection and phenomenology is far from straightforward, and must be understood in light of the heterogeneous nature of the various projects and approaches that have adopted these labels. Depending on how one understands each term, "introspection" and "phenomenology" can seem either mutually congruent or radically at odds.

---

 [6] Another possible example is "phantom concreteness," a phenomenon that might suggest the possibility of a mode of experience that merges aspects of perception and imagination in unanticipated ways.

BIBLIOGRAPHY

Beenfeldt C. (2013). *The Philosophical Background and Scientific Legacy of E.B. Titchener's Psychology*. Cham: Springer.

Bitbol M. and Petitmengin C. (2013). "A Defense of Introspection from Within." *Constructivist Foundations* 8: 269–279.

Boring E. G. (1921). "The Stimulus Error." *American Journal of Psychology* 32: 449–471.

Boring E. G. (1953). "A History of Introspection." *Psychological Bulletin* 50: 169–189.

Danziger K. (1980). "The History of Introspection Reconsidered." *Journal of the History of the Behavioral Sciences* 16: 241–262.

Fink E. (1995). *Sixth Cartesian Meditation*, trans. R. Bruzina. Bloomington: Indiana University Press.

Fuchs T. (2013). "Temporality and Psychopathology." *Phenomenology and the Cognitive Sciences* 12: 75–104.

Gallagher S. and Zahavi D. (2012). *The Phenomenological Mind*, 2nd edn. London: Routledge.

Gurwitsch A. (1966). "The Phenomenological and the Psychological Approach to Consciousness." In A. Gurwitsch (ed.), *Studies in Phenomenology and Psychology*, pp. 89–106. Evanston: Northwestern University Press.

Heidbreder E. (1933). *Seven Psychologies*. Englewood Cliffs: Prentice Hall.

Heidegger M. (1982). *The Basic Problems of Phenomenology*. trans. A. Hofstadter. Bloomington: Indiana University Press.

Hunt H. T. and Chefurka C. M. (1976). "A Test of the Psychedelic Model of Altered States of Consciousness." *Archives of General Psychiatry* 33: 867–876.

Hurlburt R. (2011). *Investigating Pristine Inner Experience*. Cambridge: Cambridge University Press.

Husserl E. (1960). *Cartesian Meditations*, trans. D. Cairns. Dordrecht: Springer.

Husserl E. (1977). *Phenomenological Psychology: Lectures, Summer Semester, 1925*, trans. J. Scanlon. The Hague: Martinus Nijhoff.

Husserl E. (1997). *Psychological and Transcendental Phenomenology*, trans. T. Sheehan and R. E. Palmer. Dordrecht: Kluwer.

Kusch M. (1995). *Psychologism*. London: Routledge.

Laing R. D. (1965). *The Divided Self*. Harmondsworth: Penguin.

Maurel M. (2009). "The Explicitation Interview: Examples and Applications." *Journal of Consciousness Studies* 10–12: 58–89.

Merleau-Ponty M. (1945). *The Phenomenology of Perception*, trans. D. A. Landes, 2012. London: Routledge (*note*: marginal French pagination cited here).

Merleau-Ponty M. (1964). "Phenomenology and the Sciences of Man." In J. Edie (ed.), *The Primacy of Perception*, pp. 43–95, trans. J. Wild. Chicago: Northwestern University Press.

Moran D. and Cohen J. (2012). *The Husserl Dictionary*. London: Continuum.

Nordgaard J., Sass L., and Parnas J. (2013). "The Psychiatric Interview: Validity, Structure, and Subjectivity." *European Archives of Psychiatry and Clinical Neuroscience* 263: 353–364.

Overgaard M., Gallagher S., and Ramsøy T. (2008). "An Integration of First-person Methodologies in Cognitive Science." *Journal of Consciousness Studies* 15: 100–120.

Pepper S. (1942). *World Hypotheses*. Berkeley: University of California Press.

Petitmengin C. and Bitbol M. (2009). "The Validity of First-person Descriptions as Authenticity and Coherence." *Journal of Consciousness Studies* 16: 363–404.

Price H. H. (1932). *Perception*. London: Methuen.

Sass L. (1994). *The Paradoxes of Delusion*. Ithaca: Cornell University Press.

Sass L. (2017). *Madness and Modernism, Insanity in the Light of Modern Art, Literature, and Thought, Revised Edition*. Oxford UK: Oxford University Press. (orig: New York: Basic Books, 1992)

Sass L. and Pienkos E. (2013). "Space, Time, and Atmosphere: A Comparative Phenomenology of Melancholia, Mania, and Schizophrenia, Part II." *Journal of Consciousness Studies* 20: 131–152.

Sass L., Pienkos E., and Nelson B. (2013). "Introspection and Schizophrenia: A Comparative Investigation of Anomalous Self Experiences." *Consciousness and Cognition* 22: 853–867.

Titchener E. B. (1910). *A Textbook of Psychology*. New York: Macmillan.

Titchener E. B. (1912). "The Schema of Introspection." *The American Journal of Psychology* 23: 485–508.

Vermersch P. (2009). "Describing the Practice of Introspection." *Journal of Consciousness Studies* 16: 20–57.

Vermersch P. (2011). "Husserl the Great Unrecognized Psychologist! A Reply to Zahavi." *Journal of Consciousness Studies* 18: 20–23.

Welton D. (2000). *The Other Husserl*. Bloomington: Indiana University Press.

Zahavi D. (2005). *Subjectivity and Selfhood*. Cambridge, MA: MIT Press.

Zahavi D. (2007). "Killing the Straw Man: Dennett and Phenomenology." *Phenomenology and the Cognitive Sciences* 6: 21–43.

Zahavi D. (2011). "Varieties of Reflection." *Journal of Consciousness Studies* 18: 9–19.

CHAPTER 31

....

PHENOMENOLOGY AND THE COGNITIVE SCIENCES

....

SHAUN GALLAGHER

INTRODUCTION

....

PHENOMENOLOGICAL approaches to experience are traditionally understood to rely on first-person reflection. In settings that involve clinical psychopathology, however, phenomenology has relied on second-person methods, such as interviews and the reports and vignettes that result from them. For the phenomenological psychiatrist, what is important, at least as a starting point, is understanding the lived experience of the patient, and not just the objective symptoms that can be checked off on a diagnostic list (see Parnas and Gallagher 2015). In contrast to phenomenology, cognitive science offers third-person explanations, often posed at the subpersonal level and with special attention paid to neural processes. Cognitive science is sometimes viewed as supporting a medicalized approach to psychopathology, and in some sense opposed to a phenomenological approach. Phenomenology taken in a strict sense, following the work of Husserl, brackets the kind of naturalistic explanations found in cognitive science and offers a transcendental analysis of experience. For these reasons phenomenology and cognitive science have been understood to be mutually exclusive approaches.

Over the past two decades, however, there have been various efforts to naturalize phenomenology (e.g. Petitot et al. 1999; Zahavi 2010). Rather than taking phenomenology and cognitive science as mutually exclusive, they have been framed as mutually constraining (Varela 1996), or mutually enlightening (Gallagher 1997). On the one hand, these attempts have been controversial, encountering resistance from both cognitive scientists (e.g. Dennett 2002; Metzinger 1995) and phenomenologists (e.g. Lawlor 2009). Cognitive scientists, however, often misconstrue phenomenology as psychological introspection; and phenomenologists usually consider the idea of mutual constraints as contradictory. On the other hand, one can find some support for the idea that phenomenology and cognitive science are not necessarily opposed. Thus Husserl himself maintains that "every analysis or theory of transcendental phenomenology—including . . . the theory of the transcendental constitution of an objective world—can be developed in the natural realm, by giving up the transcendental attitude"

(Husserl 1970: 159). Husserl was not anti-science, even if he was anti-scientistic. Others in the phenomenological tradition have made significant advancements toward establishing a mutually enlightening relationship with empirical science. Thus, Gurwitsch, Sartre, and Merleau-Ponty pursued what could be generally called phenomenological psychology. Gurwitsch appealed to gestalt psychology, animal studies, and developmental psychology to support his phenomenological accounts (Gurwitsch 2009: 246). Sartre played off of empirical psychology in his analysis of the imagination, making references to experimental research (e.g. Sartre 2004: 107ff.). Merleau-Ponty (Merleau-Ponty 2012) is well known for his integration of phenomenology, psychology, and neurology. He made extensive use of the experimental literature and case studies, and in his lectures he discussed a "convergence" of phenomenology and psychology, explicating various misunderstandings on both sides of this relationship (Merleau-Ponty 1964; Merleau-Ponty 2010: 317).

Most of the theoretical debates about naturalizing phenomenology have taken place outside discussions of psychopathology. Such debates have more to do with philosophy of mind, cognitive neuroscience, and studies of consciousness. In some sense, however, similar but more pragmatic debates emerge in psychiatric and clinical studies. Phenomenological psychiatrists have insisted, since the time of Jaspers (Jaspers 1963), on the importance of first-person lived experience for understanding disorders such as depression, schizophrenia, and anxiety disorders, and in many instances they have questioned whether third-person explanations in terms of neuroscience can tell us anything useful for actually treating such disorders (e.g. Sass 2004; Sass and Parnas 2007). Cognitive neuroscience, in contrast, has focused on working out explanations in terms of brain mechanisms and their failures (e.g. Frith 1992), with little attention paid to first-person reports.

Working toward a mutual enlightenment approach, in this chapter I discuss two questions that may throw some light on the relationship between phenomenology and cognitive science in the context of understanding psychopathology.

(1)   To what extent should we trust patients' first-person reports?
(2)   How can phenomenology contribute to cognitive explanations of psychopathology?

INTERPRETING FIRST-PERSON REPORTS

Even if, in contrast to cognitive science, which sometimes reduces first-person phenomenological reports to third-person data (e.g. Dennett 1991) or dismisses them as irrelevant (e.g. Spaulding 2010), phenomenology takes first-person reports seriously, there is still a question: What does it mean to take such reports seriously? On one view, it could mean that we take them strictly at face value. On another view it may mean that we balance our interpretation of them by drawing on larger explanatory contexts that may include cognitive science.

Billon and Kriegel (2015) argue in favor of taking first-person reports at face value. They consider psychopathological counterexamples to what they call "subjectivity theories of consciousness" which posit a constitutive connection between phenomenal experience and what phenomenologists call the "mineness" of experience (see e.g. Gallagher and Zahavi 2015; Zahavi 2005). They cite Jaspers as a proponent of such a theory.

> Self-awareness is present in every psychic event . . . Every psychic manifestation, whether per-
> ception, bodily sensation, memory, idea, thought or feeling carries *this particular aspect of*
> *"being mine,"* of having an "I"-quality, of "personally belonging," of it being one's own doing.
> We have termed this *"personalization."*
>
> (Jaspers 1963: 121; italics original)

In defending such theories, they insist on the idea that we need to interpret patients' reports
at face value. Here I want to set aside the status of subjectivity theories of consciousness and
focus on the issue of taking patients' reports at face value.

Billon and Kriegel note that schizophrenic patients with symptoms of thought insertion or delusions of control often expressly disown some of their mental states (thoughts or
intentions). They cite one of Jaspers's patients:

> I have never read nor heard them; they [inserted thoughts] come unasked; I do not dare to
> think I am the source but I am happy to know of them without thinking them. They come at
> any moment like a gift and I do not dare to impart them as if they were my own.
>
> (Jaspers 1963: 123)

In the case of thought insertion patients describe thoughts that appear to happen "in them,"
but that are not their own thoughts. These appear to be reports of phenomenal or conscious
experience that lack subjectivity or the character of mineness.

> Importantly, patients suffering from thought insertion and alien control seem to mean what
> they say: they reject watered-down or metaphorical interpretations . . . Jaspers was thus
> confronted with the following dilemma: either (a) we can make sense of the patients' reports,
> but subjectivity theories should be rejected, or (b) subjectivity theories need not be rejected,
> but the patients' reports must be deemed unintelligible or incomprehensible.
>
> (Billon and Kriegel 2015: 32)

Jaspers categorized such experiences as cases of depersonalization (Jaspers 1963: 121), although he claims that such experiences are incomprehensible since "we are not able to
have any clear sight of a psychic event without our self-awareness being involved" (Jaspers
1963: 578). If that is the case, Jaspers concluded, only a neuroscientific explanation can make
sense of such unintelligible delusions and in this case phenomenological psychopathology is
of limited value.

If we take the patient's report at face value, however, and try to make sense of it, then it
suggests that there are conscious experiences that do not have the character of mineness.
This is especially so if we treat the patients as generally rational. As Billon and Kriegel point
out, one finds similar reports in cases of somatoparaphrenia, depersonalization, and other
cases of non-delusional alienation symptoms, where patients manifest rational behavior
outside of these symptoms.

In response to this problem of understanding a first-person experience that lacks a sense
of mineness, one view seemingly denies the face value of the patient's report. For example, a
number of theorists claim that when the patient describing thought insertion says that the
thought is not his own, he really means that he is not the agent of that thought (Campbell
1999; Gallagher 2000; Stephens and Graham 2000). This view depends on a distinction between sense of self-agency (SA) and sense of mineness or ownership (SO). Although the
patient seems to be saying that he is not the owner of the thought, he is in fact complaining
that the thought is something he experiences, or that it appears in his own stream of

consciousness, which seems to suggest that there is SO for the thought. What the patient means, on this view, is that the thought seems to be generated by some other agent—thus, he has no SA for the thought. This interpretation, however, according to Billon and Kriegel, is "uncharitable to the patients" since we are not taking their first-person reports at face value. Moreover, they argue, explanations in terms of SA do not explain the fact that the thought feels alien.

An alternative proposal is that there is a failure to reflectively endorse the thought as one's own. The patient judges the thought not to fit with her own theory or narrative about herself and for that reason either denies that she is the agent (Stephens and Graham 2000), or denies that she is the owner of the thought (Bortolotti and Broome 2009). This judgment, however, is a matter of mental state attribution or a reflective process rather than a matter of first-order experience. A related proposal is suggested and developed by Billon (2013). He argues that the subject does not have phenomenal experience of the thought that he labels as inserted. Rather, the phenomenology of inserted thoughts is purely a second-order (reflective) phenomenology. Specifically, the inserted thought lacks phenomenality and therefore subjectivity (a quality of ownership the subject can attribute to himself).[1] Billon and Kriegel (2015), however, argue that this does not explain the alien feeling of the thought since a person may experience unbidden thoughts he does not endorse, but, in contrast to thought insertion, he does not fail to judge them as his own thoughts.

More positively, Billon and Kriegel argue that rather than taking the alien character of the experience as a case of something (agency or endorsement) going missing, we should consider that the alien character is something added to the thought (also Zahavi and Kriegel 2015). Moreover, this interpretation is more faithful to the face value of the patient's reports since they complain of something alien being inserted into their experience, not of something missing.

Such interpretations rely on taking the first-person report of the patient seriously. If the subject says "This is not my thought," he is, in effect, denying SO for that thought (Billon 2013: 299). Does taking the subject's first-person report seriously mean that one needs to take it literally, in this case as a statement about SO? Surely we should not assume that the schizophrenic subject is adopting the philosophic-scientific conceptual distinction between SO and SA and is using it to express his complaint. Indeed, as Billon and Kriegel suggest, "we cannot reasonably expect [patients] to spontaneously master some conceptual distinctions that philosophers have just started to draw rigorously" (Billon and Kriegel 2015: 45). Only if we knew that the subject adopted such a specialized vocabulary would we be required to follow what Billon defines as the "Phenomenological principle: If the patient says that an occurrent thought is not his, then it is not subjective [i.e. owned]" (Billon 2013: 299). Indeed, the paradoxical nature of the report of thought insertion is that when the subject says "This is not my thought," the subject is not complaining that the thought is not part of his experience—indeed, his complaint is precisely that the alien thought is part of his experience, and he might better say: "This thought does not feel like mine, although it is mine insofar as it is something that I experience."

---

[1] I will not try to adjudicate among these interpretations in this chapter. I have done so elsewhere and have argued that both Billon and Bortolotti and Broome's interpretations ultimately lead back to problems with SA (see Gallagher 2015, 2017a, 2017b).

Phenomenology is not just a method of describing or taking things at face value. It is a form of inquiry into first-person lived experience, and this sometimes involves interpretations that may be informed by other types of investigations (Gallagher and Zahavi 2012). On this view, the proper phenomenological principle is actually a hermeneutical principle, namely, through interview and careful interpretation we discern the patient's lived experience. That interpretation should be informed and/or confirmed by what we know via other methods. It is important to get the phenomenology right, but this does not mean that one ought to accept the first-person report at face value. One's interpretation should be balanced by other evidence. If, for example, evidence from cognitive science suggests that brain processes that correlate with the sense of agency are disrupted in patients who experience thought insertion or delusions of control (e.g. Daprati et al. 1997; Haggard et al. 2003; Jeannerod 2009) this may count as indicative of how we should understand a patient's report. In fact, however, it can go the other way as well; a patient's phenomenological report, and its interpretation, can motivate empirical experiments that seek to identify processes that might contribute to explaining the anomalous or alien experience. To the extent that the communication between phenomenology and empirical science goes both ways on this kind of issue, this would count as a form of mutual enlightenment.

Phenomenological Interventions in Cognitive Explanations of Psychopathology

Phenomenology and Empirical Studies

Empirical sciences that study proper and pathological functioning are not interpretation-free, of course. There may be general agreement about the fact that neuronal processes in the inferior parietal cortex are activated under certain experimental conditions, or in some pathological cases. The interesting question then is what such activation means. I will first look at two examples of how phenomenology can inform the interpretation of experimental results.

In the first example, Farrer et al. (2003) found activation in the inferior parietal cortex associated with a disruption in the sense of agency. They explain this as follows:

> We have proposed the activity seen in inferior parietal cortex relates to the feeling of loss of agency associated with the discrepancy between intended actions and sensory feedback. However, from the experiment discussed so far it is possible that the activity in this region relates solely to the sensory discordance. The feeling of agency might relate to activity in other regions. We think this is unlikely on the basis of various pathological cases in which the primary disorder concerns the feeling of agency rather than sensory discordance.
>
> (Farrer et al. 2003: 329)

Yet they also note that lesions of the inferior parietal cortex may be associated with somatoparaphrenia—where a patient may experience her limb as an alien object and believe that it belongs to another person (Farrer et al. 2003: 329). Somatoparaphrenia, however, is usually interpreted to be about a failure of the sense of ownership (or a disownership), rather than the sense of agency. What would allow us to say clearly whether it is SO or SA that is disrupted?

Likewise, in a second example experiment, Farrer and Frith (2002) associate activation of the anterior insula with a positive experience of agency. They explain this as follows:

> One aspect of the experience of agency that we feel when we move our bodies through space is the close correspondence between many different sensory signals. In particular there will be a correspondence between three kinds of signal: somatosensory signals directly consequent upon our movements, visual and auditory signals that may result indirectly from our movements, and last, the corollary discharge [efferent signal] associated with motor commands that generated the movements. A close correspondence between all these signals helps to give us a sense of agency.
>
> (Farrer and Frith 2002: 601–602)

Yet the integration of somatosensory signals with visual and auditory signals is often interpreted to be the basis for the sense of ownership for one's body and one's actions. For example, Tsakiris and Haggard (2005) associate SO with sensory integration, and they note that activity in the insula is found in the absence of movement, which implies that this area may in fact reflect body-ownership rather than agency. The question is once again, what would allow us to say clearly whether it is SO or SA that is disrupted?

In Farrer et al. (2003), subjects were not asked to describe their experience. They were simply asked, after they moved a joystick ostensibly controlling movement on a computer screen, whether the movement of a hand on the computer screen represented "their own movement, their own movement distorted, or the movement of another agent" (Farrer et al. 2003: 325). Is a question about one's "own" movement in contrast to another's movement a question about ownership or agency?

Farrer and Frith (2002) elicited no reports from their subjects. Rather, the subjects were informed whether they were actually controlling the movement on the computer screen or not. The experimenters were looking for neural correlations that discriminated between when the subject knew she was in control versus when she was told that she was not in control of the movement (although in each case she was moving the joystick). There is much more to be said about these experiments (see Gallagher 2017), but the question here is what the experimenters took as the basis for their interpretation concerning SA and SO.

Both studies started by assuming a phenomenological distinction between SA and SO (Gallagher 2000), with the intent of trying to identify the neural correlates of SA. Yet it was never clear what the subjects were actually experiencing. In this case, there was no clear attempt to confirm the interpretation of the experimental results by consulting the subjects' phenomenology. This is a good example of how phenomenology did contribute to these experiments (by "frontloading" phenomenological distinctions between SA and SO; see Gallagher 2003), but could have played a further confirmatory role with respect to interpreting the results.

Phenomenology and Cognitive Theory

Outside of experimental situations, when one is attempting to develop a cognitive theory that would explain psychopathological symptoms, such as delusions of control or thought insertion in schizophrenia, phenomenology may also be relevant. Frith (1992), for example, developed an influential explanation of exactly such symptoms based on cognitive neuroscience. His explanation relied on an important insight about motor control processes that help to explain differentiations between self-generated movement and movement that is not self-generated. He relied on the notion of a comparator (or forward model) mechanism responsible for self-monitoring, and proposed that this self-monitoring process was disrupted in cases of delusions of control and thought insertion. Whether comparator models provide an adequate account of delusions of control is still a controversial question (see e.g. Friston 2012; Grünbaum 2015; Langland-Hassan 2008; Synofzik, Vosgerau, and Newen 2007), although there is some empirical evidence and reasonable intuitions to support it. The explanation involves the idea that a copy of the efferent signal or motor command (efference copy) somehow is not properly delivered to the forward comparator, although reafferent signals or sensory feedback registering the actual movement is properly delivered. Because of the failure of efference copy or the forward comparator, the agent's intention is not registered and there is a mismatch between intended movement and actual movement. This is interpreted as a disruption in the sense of agency for that movement, thus seeming alien to the subject. This explanation correlates nicely with phenomenological reports concerning the disruption in SA in delusions of control (see previous section).

The problem, however, is that when this explanation is applied to thought insertion, it does not seem phenomenologically accurate. Frith's model assumes that, as in the case of a motor action, in the case of thinking we experience an effortful intention. The intention to think, according to Frith, is the element that bestows a sense of agency for the thought. Likewise, just as in the case of motor control, an efference copy corresponding to the generation of thought is sent to a comparator, which also registers the occurrence of the actual thought, normally matching up intention and thought. If something goes wrong with the efference copy or the comparator, thought occurs which seems not to be generated by the subject, and it appears to be an alien or inserted thought. From the perspective of phenomenology, however, the idea that there is an intention to think in most cases of thinking is questionable. In this respect, however, one might object that phenomenology cannot tell us anything about subpersonal processes. Yet it is not always clear that Frith takes the notion of intention to think to be only a subpersonal event since the missing intention seemingly reaches consciousness under the description of a loss of SA—"I did not intend to think this thought." Even if phenomenology cannot say anything directly about subpersonal processes, however, phenomenology can offer some helpful clues about what must be happening at that level if there is some correlating conscious experience (e.g. thinking) that the subpersonal processes are meant to explain. Phenomenologically, an intention to think would itself be a form of thinking, and if it were necessary to have an intention to think for every thought that one thinks, one would have an infinite regress (Gallagher 2004).[2] Would this same logic apply to an intention to think even if the intention were subpersonal? And what precisely is a subpersonal intention if it is not simply a process that corresponds to a personal-level phenomenon? Answers to these questions are not clear since the Frithian model does not define the notion of an intention to think in a precise way.

---

[2] Akins and Dennett (1986: 517) also suggest that the idea of having an intention to think leads to a "never-beginning regress of intentions to form thoughts."

This is not the only problem with Frith's model. It is not clear how this explanation would discriminate between unbidden thoughts that, as Frankfurt puts it, "strike us unexpectedly out of the blue . . . thoughts that run willy-nilly through our heads" (Frankfurt 1976: 240), and inserted thoughts. It is also not clear why one would need subpersonal efference copy or comparator mechanisms for motor control correction (that typically allow us to keep our actions on track) when we have the capability to keep our thoughts on track at the personal, experiential level. John Campbell interprets Frith's notion of a lack of metarepresentational self-monitoring as a lack of introspective monitoring: "it is the match between the thought detected by introspection, and the content of the efferent copy picked up by the comparator, that is responsible for the sense of ownership of the thought" (Campbell 1999: 617). Not only does this again run into the infinite regress problem if one needs an intention to introspectively monitor, in addition if the failure of self-monitoring in schizophrenia involves a lack of introspection, this runs counter to clinical reports where schizophrenic subjects report hyperreflectivity that in some cases means an excess of introspection rather than a lack of introspection (Sass and Parnas 2003).

My point here is not to defeat Frith's explanation but to suggest that systematic phenomenology (as well as clinical phenomenological reports) can contribute something important to theory development even when the theory is framed as a neurocognitive theory.

Conclusion

I have argued that even in its central business of trying to understand a subject's lived experience, and especially in cases of clinical psychopathology, phenomenology is not about taking patients' reports at face value. Rather, phenomenology can best understand the patient by tempering interpretations with evidence and best explanations from empirical scientific approaches, including cognitive neuroscience. I have also argued, however, that we should not simply accept at face value what is on offer in such cognitive approaches to psychopathology. In this respect, phenomenology can play a critical but productive role making both experimental interpretation and theory formation more precise.

Let me add a large qualification to the previous discussion, however. If outside of studies of psychopathology there has been some productive interaction between phenomenology and the cognitive sciences, this has been primarily by way of phenomenology pushing cognitive science toward a more embodied and situated perspective following, for example, the inspiration of Merleau-Ponty (see e.g. Varela, Thompson, and Rosch 1991; Gallagher 2005).[3] A more embodied and situated approach to psychopathology is still to be developed (see, however, Fuchs and Schlimme 2009; Röhricht et al. 2014). As things continue to move in that direction, the idea of a mutual enlightenment between phenomenology and embodied cognitive science can only benefit our understanding of psychopathology.

---

[3] By "situated" I mean especially analyses that make reference to the social situation and the patient's intersubjective relations. In this respect, e.g. the concept of sense of agency is not treated as merely the result of internal brain processes but may also be modulated by social context (see e.g. Gallagher 2017).

ACKNOWLEDGMENTS

The author thanks the Humboldt Foundation's Anneliese Maier Research Award for supporting this research.

BIBLIOGRAPHY

Akins K. A. and Dennett D. (1986). "Who May I Say is Calling?" *Behavioral and Brain Sciences* 9: 517–518.

Billon A. (2013). "Does Consciousness Entail Subjectivity? The Puzzle of Thought Insertion." *Philosophical Psychology* 26: 291–314.

Billon A. and Kriegel U. (2015). "Jaspers' Dilemma: The Psychopathological Challenge to Subjectivity Theories of Consciousness." In R. Gennaro (ed.), *Disturbed Consciousness: New Essays on Psychopathology and Theories of Consciousness*, pp. 29–54. Cambridge: MIT Press.

Bortolotti L. and Broome M. (2009). "A Role for Ownership and Authorship in the Analysis of Thought Insertion." *Phenomenology and the Cognitive Sciences* 8: 205–224.

Campbell J. (1999). "Schizophrenia, the Space of Reasons and Thinking as a Motor Process." *The Monist* 82: 609–625.

Dennett D. C. (1991). *Consciousness Explained*. Boston: Little and Brown.

Dennett D. C. (2002). "The Fantasy of First-person Science." http://ase.tufts.edu/cogstud/papers/chalmersdeb3dft.htm

Daprati E., Franck N., Georgieff N., Proust J., Pacherie E., Dalery J., and Jeannerod M. (1997). "Looking for the Agent: An Investigation into Consciousness of Action and Self-consciousness in Schizophrenic Patients." *Cognition* 65: 71–86.

Farrer C. and Frith C. D. (2002). "Experiencing Oneself vs. Another Person as being the Cause of an Action: The Neural Correlates of the Experience of Agency." *Neuroimage* 15: 596–603.

Farrer C., Franck N., Georgieff N., Frith C. D., Decety J., and Jeannerod M. (2003). "Modulating the Experience of Agency: A Positron Emission Tomography Study." *Neuroimage* 18: 324–333.

Frankfurt H. (1976). "Identification and Externality." In A. O. Rorty (ed.), *The Identities of Persons*, pp. 239–251. Berkeley: University of California Press.

Friston K. (2012). "Prediction, Perception and Agency." *International Journal of Psychophysiology* 83: 248–252.

Frith C. D. (1992). *The Cognitive Neuropsychology of Schizophrenia*. Hillsdale: Erlbaum.

Fuchs T. and Schlimme J. E. (2009). "Embodiment and Psychopathology: A Phenomenological Perspective." *Current Opinion in Psychiatry* 22: 570–575.

Gallagher S. (1997). "Mutual Enlightenment: Recent Phenomenology in Cognitive Science." *Journal of Consciousness Studies* 4: 195–214.

Gallagher S. (2000). "Philosophical Conceptions of the Self: Implications for Cognitive Science." *Trends in Cognitive Sciences* 4: 14–21.

Gallagher S. (2003). "Phenomenology and Experimental Design." *Journal of Consciousness Studies* 10: 85–99.

Gallagher S. (2004). "Neurocognitive Models of Schizophrenia: A Neurophenomenological Critique." *Psychopathology* 37: 8–19.

Gallagher S. (2005). *How the Body Shapes the Mind*. Oxford: Oxford University Press.

Gallagher S. (2015). "Relations between Agency and Ownership in the Case of Schizophrenic Thought Insertion." *Review of Philosophy and Psychology* 6: 865–879.

Gallagher S. (2017). "Multiple Aspects in the Sense of Agency." *New Ideas in Psychology* 30: 15–31.

Gallagher S. (2017a). "Deflationary Accounts of the Sense of Ownership." In F. de Vignemont and A. Alsmith (eds.), *The Subject's Matter*, pp. 145–162. Cambridge, MA: MIT Press.

Gallagher S. (2017b). "Self-defense: Deflecting the Deflationary and Eliminativist Critiques of the Sense of Ownership." *Frontiers in Psychology* 8: 1612. doi.org/10.3389/fpsyg.2017.01612

Gallagher S. and Zahavi D. (2012). *The Phenomenological Mind*. London: Routledge.

Gallagher S. and Zahavi D. (2015). "Phenomenological Approaches to Self-consciousness." In E. N. Zalta. *The Stanford Encyclopedia of Philosophy*. http://plato.stanford.edu/archives/spr2015/entries/self-consciousness-phenomenological/

Grünbaum T. (2015). "The Feeling of Agency Hypothesis: A Critique." *Synthese* 192: 3313–3337.

Gurwitsch A. (2009). *The Collected Works of Aron Gurwitsch (1901–1973). Vol. 1: Constitutive Phenomenology in Historical Perspective*, trans. and ed. J. García-Gómez. Dordrecht: Springer.

Haggard P., Martin F., Taylor-Clarke M., Jeannerod M., and Franck N. (2003). "Awareness of Action in Schizophrenia." *Neuroreport* 14: 1081–1085.

Husserl E. (1970). *Cartesian Meditations*, trans. D. Cairns. The Hague: Martinus Nijhoff.

Jaspers K. [1913] (1963). *General Psychopathology*, trans. J. Hoenig and M. W. Hamilton. Manchester: Manchester University Press.

Jeannerod M. (2009). "The Sense of Agency and its Disturbances in Schizophrenia: A Reappraisal." *Experimental Brain Research* 192: 527–532.

Langland-Hassan P. (2008). "Fractured Phenomenologies: Thought Insertion, Inner Speech, and the Puzzle of Extraneity." *Mind & Language* 23: 369–401.

Lawlor L. (2009). "Becoming an Auto-affection (Part II): Who Are We? Invited Lecture, ICNAP, 2009. Available at: http://www.icnap.org/meetings.htm

Merleau-Ponty M. (1964). "Phenomenology and the Sciences of Man." In M. Merleau-Ponty (ed.), *The Primacy of Perception*, trans. J. Wild, pp. 43–95. Evanston: Northwestern University Press.

Merleau-Ponty M. (2010). *Child Psychology and Pedagogy: The Sorbonne Lectures 1949–1952*, trans. T. Welsh. Evanston: Northwestern University Press.

Merleau-Ponty M. (2012). *Phenomenology of Perception*, trans. R. Landes. London: Routledge.

Metzinger T. (1995). "Introduction: The Problem of Consciousness." In T. Metzinger (ed.), *Conscious Experience*, pp. 3–37. Exeter: Imprint Academic.

Parnas J. and Gallagher S. (2015). "Phenomenology and the Interpretation of Psychopathological Experience." In L. Kirmayer, R. Lemelson, and C. Cummings (eds.), *Revisioning Psychiatry Integrating Biological, Clinical and Cultural Perspectives*, pp. 65–80. Cambridge: Cambridge University Press.

Parnas J. and Zahavi D. (2002). "The Role of Phenomenology in Psychiatric Diagnosis and Classification." In M. Maj, W. Gaebel, J. J. López-Ibor, and N. Sartorius (eds.), *Psychiatric Diagnosis and Classification*, pp. 137–162. West Sussex: Wiley.

Petitot J., Varela F. J., Pachoud B., and Roy J.-M. (eds). (1999). *Naturalizing Phenomenology: Issues in Contemporary Phenomenology and Cognitive Science*. Stanford: Stanford University Press.

Röhricht F., Gallagher S., Geuter U., and Hutto D. (2014). "Embodied Cognition and Body Psychotherapy: The Construction of New Therapeutic Environments." *Sensoria: A Journal of Mind, Brain & Culture* 56: 11–20.

Sartre J.-P. (2004). *The Imaginary: A Phenomenological Psychology of the Imagination*, trans. J. Webber. London: Routledge.

Sass L. A. (2004). "Some Reflections on the (Analytic) Philosophical Approach to Delusion." *Philosophy, Psychiatry, & Psychology* 11: 71–80.

Sass L. A. and Parnas J. (2003). "Schizophrenia, Consciousness, and the Self." *Schizophrenia Bulletin* 29: 427–444.

Sass L. A. and Parnas J. (2007). "Explaining Schizophrenia: The Relevance of Phenomenology." In M. C. Chung, K. W. M. Fulford, and G. Graham (eds.), *Reconceiving Schizophrenia*, pp. 63–96. New York: Oxford University Press.

Spaulding S. (2010). "Embodied Cognition and Mindreading." *Mind and Language* 25: 119–140.

Stephens G. L. and Graham G. (2000). *When Self-Consciousness Breaks: Alien Voices and Inserted Thoughts*. Cambridge, MA: MIT Press.

Synofzik M., Vosgerau G., and Newen A. (2007). "Beyond the Comparator Model: A Multifactorial Two-step Account of Agency." *Consciousness and Cognition* 17: 219–239.

Tsakiris M. and Haggard P. (2005). "Experimenting with the Acting Self." *Cognitive Neuropsychology* 22: 387–407.

Varela F. J. (1996). "Neurophenomenology: A Methodological Remedy for the Hard Problem." *Journal of Consciousness Studies* 3: 330–349.

Varela F., Thompson E., and Rosch E. (1991). *The Embodied Mind*. Cambridge, MA: MIT Press.

Zahavi D. (2005). *Subjectivity and Selfhood: Investigating the First-person Perspective*. Cambridge, MA: MIT Press.

Zahavi D. (2010). "Naturalized Phenomenology." In S. Gallagher and D. Schmicking (eds.), *Handbook of Phenomenology and Cognitive Science*, pp. 3–20. Dordrecht: Springer.

Zahavi D. and Kriegel U. (2015). "For-me-ness: What it is and what it is Not." In D. Dahlstrom, A. Elpidorou, and W. Hopp (eds.), *Philosophy of Mind and Phenomenology*, pp. 36–53. London: Routledge.

....

CHAPTER 32

PHENOMENOLOGY, NATURALISM, AND THE NEUROSCIENCES

....

MASSIMILIANO ARAGONA

THE LANDSCAPE

....

WORDS may have different meanings depending on the context of use. Consequently, the relationship between phenomenology, naturalism, and the neurosciences may vary depending on the semantic interpretation of these terms.

Phenomenology

It is a general approach but also a more specific philosophical research program. As a general approach, phenomenology is the study of phenomena as they appear. If we use the term in this general sense, phenomenology is compatible with different philosophical perspectives and also with various scientific approaches. However, used as a synonym for "description of the phenomenon," phenomenology loses any specificity and can be used even for the individuation of the explanandum in neoempiricist explanations, for example, the influential theory developed by Carl G. Hempel and Paul Oppenheim (Hempel and Oppenheim 1948). As a philosophical research program, phenomenology is a typical example of continental philosophy, encompassing topics like ontology, epistemology, hermeneutics, and ethics. There is "no unique and definitive definition of phenomenology" because a "unique and final definition of phenomenology is dangerous and perhaps even paradoxical as it lacks a thematic focus" (Farina 2014: 50). However, we can start from its recognized father, Edmund Husserl, and use his ideas as a core prototype. He founded phenomenology as a philosophical method whose motto was to go back to the "things themselves" (Husserl 2001: 168). There is some support for an ontological interpretation of this claim but here it is more important to explore the epistemological import of Husserl's ideas. In his view, rigorous knowledge is based on a thorough analysis of the way things are given to our consciousness; that is, whatever we know, we know it from the vantage point of our own experience, and there is no access to reality independent of our experience. Objects of knowledge are not independent, objective facts; they are the result of an intentional act of knowing, that is, they exist as objects of knowledge only in relation to a subjective pole that knows them. Husserl calls *epoché* the methodical act of bracketing, of suspending our obvious trust in naturalistic beliefs regarding both the certainty of science and the objectivity of the common-sense world. By focusing on our act of knowing and on things as they present themselves in our conscious field, we can realize that common objects are the product of a complex process of synthesis grounded on manifold partial perspectives. Husserl calls *imaginative variation* the act of imagining what things would be like if we progressively add or subtract their qualities. By consistently applying this method we discover that the object maintains its identity even without some qualities (e.g. of a chair we can progressively change the color, the material of which it is made, etc., and we still have a chair), but finally we arrive at one point when if we subtract a last feature the object is no more itself. This quality that cannot be removed without the elimination of the object is its essential characteristic, its *eidos*, in Husserl's words.

Starting from this core view, the history of phenomenology undertook different developments that in some cases significantly diverged from Husserl's original ideas. There is no space here to follow these developments, but at least we shall stress that French scholars mainly developed the existential import of these views, in close connection with psychopathological and psychoanalytic reflections and also with influences from linguistics, anthropology, and Hegel's philosophy. In Germany, one of the closest collaborators of Husserl, Martin Heidegger, progressively diverged from the transcendental philosophy of his teacher to highlight ontological themes and transformed phenomenology into a philosophical hermeneutics. In his inquiry into Being, Heidegger begins his analysis from the existing being (*Seiende*) that concretely poses the question of Being (*Sein*) and for whom the answer is relevant. That being is the human being (*Dasein*), "and this is why his philosophy can also be read as an anthropology whose key concepts are relevant for psychopathology" (Stanghellini and Aragona 2016: 7). These concepts, presented in *Being and Time* (Heidegger 1927), are general categories indicating fundamental ways of being-in-the-world. They include being-in (*In-sein*), being immersed in (*Sein-bei*), being-with (*Mit-Dasein*), temporality (*Zeitlichkeit*), spatiality (*Räumlichkeit*), understanding (*Verstehen*), and thrownness (*Geworfenheit*), and have been considered the "guidelines for reconstructing the life-world a person lives in" (Stanghellini 2013: 344). According to Alfred Kraus, Heidegger's existential categories must be understood ontologically as characteristics of the *Dasein*, in preparation for an inquiry into the fundamental question of Being. In contrast, their use in psychopathology has an ontic orientation, that is, they are concerned with factual phenomena of a concrete person (Kraus 2010).

To summarize, phenomenology is a term used in different contexts with important differences in meaning but with a shared family resemblance. In general, we may consider an investigation "phenomenological" if it is grounded on philosophical phenomenology, existential thinking, or hermeneutics.

Naturalism

In general, naturalism is the view that only natural laws and forces operate in the world and that supernatural or spiritual forces do not really exist. It is also defined as "a sympathy with the view that ultimately nothing resists explanation by the methods characteristics of the natural sciences" (Blackburn 2005: 246). However, we can distinguish the strong idea of naturalism that arises from these definitions from a weaker version. The strong version has an ontological part: what *really* exists in the world is *only* matter, that is, reality has no place for "supernatural" or "mental" entities. It also has a methodological claim: everything should be explained by science with its proper methods and this is the only way to acquire real knowledge. The weaker version has also two corresponding parts. The ontological claim is that reality is larger than nature and that some non-natural, ideal entities somehow exist. Accordingly, this weaker version of ontological naturalism would accept that mental and social phenomena (e.g. numbers, moral duties, social organizations) are somehow real but would say that they do not belong to the natural order. At this point, there are two methodological possibilities. One is to say that only natural entities can be studied scientifically, hence ideal entities must remain outside the domain of scientific inquiry. But this approach would have difficulty justifying the scientific status of mathematics. To save mathematics as a science, the other possibility is to make a further distinction between empirical and non-empirical sciences, which is the classic distinction between synthetic and analytic sciences. Indeed, neopositivism and logical empiricism were based on these assumptions and were able to trace a clear distinction between scientific knowledge and non-scientific discourses based on their criterion of significance. When these perspectives collapsed and W. V. O. Quine dismissed the analytic/synthetic distinction as a dogma, the consequence was the proposal of a naturalized epistemology based on experimental psychology and hence on natural science. In other words, this discipline should study natural phenomena[1] in experimental conditions in which controlled inputs elicit registrable outputs (Quine 1969). What is the consequence of these philosophical positions for the sciences of mind?

On the strong version of naturalism, cognitive neuroscientists should embrace a form of naturalism that is physicalist, reductionist, and eliminativist. Physicalist in the sense that only mass, energy, and the other physical and chemical properties accepted by the scientific community are allowed in a scientific view of the world. Reductionist, meaning that all scientific phenomena should be ideally reduced to the microlevel of physical laws. Eliminativist because it is claimed that mental phenomena should be reformulated in scientific terms while the corresponding "mental" terms should be eliminated from the scientific terminology. On the weak version, it may be accepted that mental phenomena are somehow real. There is, however, a dilemma here: either mental phenomena are reducible to scientific procedures and thus naturalized, or they remain as sociocultural constructions or ineffable subjective experiences. In this case, they may be still accepted as real (this is the difference with the stronger version), but not as part of the natural order, hence they are left outside the field of inquiry pertaining to science.

In the end, whatever form of naturalism we choose in our approach to mental phenomena and psychopathological syndromes, the result does not change much: in order to treat them scientifically we should remove their subjective qualities and reduce the phenomenon to its underlying neurobiological processes. As epiphenomenal qualities, mental experiences might be aesthetically interesting but would have no scientific value (as if we were contemplating the beauty of light emission while studying the rules governing the emergence of an optic phenomenon).

---

[1] This phenomenalism is, of course, quite different from phenomenology in the specific sense described above.

The Neurosciences

Contemporary neurocognitive sciences are the product of extraordinary technological developments that gave researchers the possibility a) to directly study brain functioning in vivo while performing neuropsychological tasks, with an unprecedented spatial and/or temporal resolution,[2] and b) to interfere or modulate brain functioning while the experimental subject is performing the requested task. This technological possibility fueled research programs based on *embodiment* theories, here intended as the philosophical/methodological stance arguing that the mind does not operate in a vacuum but is strictly intertwined with the body and its environmental interactions (*situatedness*). In cognitive sciences, this is promoting a shift from functionalism to embodiment, and from explicit to implicit cognition. Functionalism refers to the classic cognitive idea that what characterizes the mind is not its material constitution but its functional organization, so we may reproduce mental activity in a computer or other devices. On the contrary, the view of the embodied mind claims that because the mind arises from biological constitution, we should not study functional organization in general but its concrete emergence from brain functioning. Explicit cognition refers to classical "theory-theory" models in cognitive sciences, in which the language of mind (*mentalese*) makes logical inferences and predictions from available data, while in the cognitive model of implicit cognition there is a pre-reflective automatic activation of brain areas or neurons directly stimulated by salient stimuli.

There is little doubt that the development of neuroimaging and neurophysiological technologies has resulted in a better knowledge of brain structure and function. As a consequence, the distance between effective activity in brain networks and the proxies representing them (e.g. brain images or records of electrical activity) is significantly reduced. There are still some problems "internal" to this domain. These are technical problems (i.e. spatial or temporal resolutions) as well as epistemological ones: for example, the subtraction techniques used in fMRI research rely on the assumption that the subtracted images acquired during the rest condition are somehow neutral while we know that there is brain activity also in this state (on methodological limitations, see Uttal 2003). However, despite these limitations the progress is evident and substantiates the trust in further advancements.

Even more promising are the possibilities opened by technological instruments that stimulate brain activity or that may interfere selectively with brain activity while the subject is performing a task. At the moment the temporal and spatial limitations of these instruments are significant, yet technological advancements promise to improve the situation, and their potentiality in neuropsychological research is high.

In general, current neuroscientific developments are clearly part of a naturalistic scientific enterprise, and their successes in the study of brain functioning are evident. Nevertheless, this has also raised epistemological challenges. To what extent can we extend technologies developed to study the brain to phenomena that go beyond neurology? Today the common view among neuroscientists, psychiatrists, and some philosophers is that the neurosciences can study not only the neurobiological bases of mental disorders

---

[2] This does not mean that it is optimal. Some instruments have very good temporal resolution but lower spatial resolution; in some instances it is the opposite; some are in the middle. However, every year new technological advancements improve the situation and promise to overcome current limitations.

and psychopathological symptoms, but also normal processes like empathy or ethical decisions (e.g. Bernhardt and Singer 2012; Aishwarya and Malik Ali 2017). In fact, in the last two decades new disciplines have been formed such as neurophenomenology, neuroethics, neuroeconomy, and neuropolitics, to name just a few. In the next section, we will focus on the neurophenomenological program as an example of naturalization of a philosophical perspective driven by the advancement of cognitive neuroscience.

NEUROPHENOMENOLOGY: IS A NATURALIZED PHENOMENOLOGY POSSIBLE?

The most famous integration of phenomenology and naturalistic research programs in the neurosciences is called "Neurophenomenology." We will concentrate on Francisco Varela's influential model, which aims to find "meaningful bridges between two irreducible phenomenal domains" (Varela 1996: 340), that is, phenomena that are present in first-person experience at one side, and third-person phenomena established by the cognitive sciences and neuroscientific technologies at the other. The basic claim is that instead of being subjective "noise," first-person accounts should be taken "seriously as [a] valid domain of phenomena" (Varela 1996: 346) that enriches the experimental setting. First-hand experience can be explored and analyzed by a proper method "inspired from the style of inquiry of *phenomenology*" (Varela 1996: 347). This method is clearly indebted to Husserl's phenomenology (including the terms employed, such as phenomenological reduction, intentionality, etc.). However, phenomenology is used in a wider sense, including several elements taken from other traditions like Asian contemplative meditation. This account of phenomenology deserves a critical discussion but for reasons of space this will not be done here. Instead we will focus on the other basic claim of Varela's neurophenomenology, namely that first-person experiences provide valid data that can be correlated with third-person data collected in the cognitive neurosciences. On his view, both domains of phenomena have equal status and are not reducible to one another. The working hypothesis is that "[p]henomenological accounts of the structure of experience and their counterparts in cognitive science relate to each other through reciprocal constraints" (Varela 1996: 343). Neurophenomenology explores the bridge between them with a "stereoscopic perspective" (Varela 1996: 344) in which neuroscientific questions can be guided by first-person phenomenological evidence, and third-person neuroscientific evidence can suggest new articulations of the phenomenological descriptions. According to Varela, "[s]cience and experience constrain and modify each other as in a dance" (Varela 1996: 347). Varela did not provide his account with concrete examples of how all this should work, but confined himself to a general outline. Hence, years later the challenge of the "explanatory gap" in the relationship between first-person subjective experience and third-person neuroscience still had "to be adequately bridged" (Lutz and Thompson 2003: 32). Antoine Lutz and Evan Thompson have presented a suggestive experiment where in a perceptive task the basic and variable electroencephalographic (EEG) activity unrelated to the task itself was not considered as "noise," as is usually the case. Instead, the activity was related to different experiential states of the subject (some subjects were focused on the task, others were distracted, and so on). What is relevant here is that since its early formulation, neurophenomenologists following Varela have progressively added complexity to the model. On the phenomenological side, the methodology to produce and record subjective reports was integrated with so-called second-person methods in order to improve its reliability (Olivares et al. 2015). At the neuroscientific side, it is claimed that the study of single neural processes or structures is not of much use because the neural processes relevant in neurophenomenological studies are those involving "the transient selection of a distributed neural population that is both highly integrated and differentiated, and connected by reciprocal, transient, dynamical links. A prelude to understanding the neural processes crucial for consciousness is thus to identify the mechanisms for large-scale brain processes, and to understand the causal laws and intrinsic properties that govern their global dynamical behaviours" (Lutz and Thompson 2003: 40). Finally, to reduce the explanatory gap between the two poles of the correlation, that is, phenomenological and neuroscientific evidence, a third domain was introduced: "Formal models and analytical tools from dynamical systems theory, grounded on an embodied-enactive approach to cognition" (Lutz and Thompson 2003: 34).

Up until now, we have looked at Varela's neurophenomenology and its development in Varela's followers. Varela is also one of the editors of an influential book explicitly aimed at naturalizing phenomenology (Petitot et al. 1999) that suggests there are different ways the project might proceed. In the foreword the editors assert that "Husserlian phenomenology cannot become instrumental in developing cognitive science without undergoing a substantial transformation" (Petitot et al. 1999: xiii). One of the editors of the book, Jean Petitot, was particularly active in suggesting this *instrumental* transformation of phenomenology, so we turn to his proposal. In an early paper, Petitot (1995) argues that through the eidetic method, phenomenology studies the qualitative and macroscopic (morphological) structure of the world of things. He then goes on to introduce a bifurcation. If phenomenology joins these morphological concepts to descriptive ones, then we have a descriptive phenomenology. On the contrary, if these morphological phenomena are joined to geometrical concepts, then we have a naturalized phenomenology aimed at mathematically explaining the emergence of the vague morphological essences on physicalist bases. This requires a change in the language used by phenomenologists to describe phenomena, which should be dErivable from the formalisms of physical objectivity. Indeed, there should be a shift from a pre-physical descriptive phenomenology to a post-physical objectivation in which a concept is understood only when it can be transformed in a mathematical system to construct the phenomena themselves. This conclusion is in line with the following sentence co-authored by Varela: "it is not enough that such a phenomenology be descriptive and analytical; it should also be explanatory" (Roy et al. 1999: 19). However, despite this early overlapping, there is a significant conceptual difference between Petitot's mathematical and explanatory reformulation of phenomenology, and Varela's proposal concerning distinct domains in reciprocal constraints.

To sum up, in current programs of naturalized phenomenology there is some heterogeneity at various levels. For the purpose of this chapter, it is noteworthy that there are differences in both the way the term phenomenology is used and the kind of cognitive and/or neuroscientific data to be correlated to such a phenomenology. In general, it is clear that Husserl would have strongly rejected these programs, his conception of phenomenology being anti-naturalistic. In fact, despite many differences in their respective views, a naturalized phenomenology would be a paradox or nonsensical not only for Husserl but also for Heidegger, Gadamer, and many classical as well as contemporary phenomenologists.[3] Thus, in order to produce a naturalized phenomenology the first thing to do is to reject the way Continental philosophy intends phenomenology and to radically change its meaning and role.[4] Accordingly, if we remain within the original spirit of phenomenology we must reply negatively to our question: a naturalized phenomenology is an oxymoron.

However, knowledge often progresses when recognized authorities are challenged and their ideas are critically reviewed. Thus we can argue that we are free to use the term phenomenology in a variety of ways, depending on our aims. If I understand Petitot's proposal, his mathematized phenomenology would be very different not only from traditional philosophical phenomenology but also from Varela's usage, and maybe more akin to Noam Chomsky's generative grammar (Chomsky 1956). Another possibility is to use phenomenology as a synonym for detailed phenomenal description of first-person experiences. They could be derived (as Varela suggests) from the application at the descriptive level of Husserl's analyses and conceptual distinctions (e.g. his fine-grained description of temporality),[5] as well as other phenomenological distinctions traced by other authors (e.g. Heidegger's existential structures). Moreover, these descriptions could be further enriched by using introspective methods of various kinds, resources from meditation techniques, intersubjective (second-person) co-constructions and validations, and so on. Although it uses concepts elaborated in the second part of the twentieth century, the epistemological structure of such an approach is akin to the approach explored by Karl Jaspers more than a century ago (the first edition of his *General Psychopathology* appeared in 1913). Jaspers used the term phenomenology quite freely as a synonym of detailed description of lived experiences, and also added that every phenomenon, even the most complex one (like the change of the entire personality structure at the onset of some pathological conditions), could be reduced to the effect of an underlying genetic or neurobiological causal alteration: "Every concept in phenomenology and the psychology of meaningful phenomena becomes drawn into the domain of causal thinking to serve as an element of causal explanation. The units of phenomenology (e.g. hallucinations, modes of perception, etc.) are explained by bodily events. Complex meaningful connections in their turn are considered as units (e.g. a manic syndrome plus all its contents can be regarded as the effect of a cerebral process . . .)" (Jaspers

---

[3] e.g. De Preester states that a "naturalized phenomenology is no longer phenomenology" (De Preester 2002: 645), and Zahavi adds that "Husserl was a staunch anti-naturalist. . . . And to suggest that the phenomenological account could be absorbed, or reduced, or replaced by a naturalistic account was for Husserl sheer nonsense" (Zahavi 2013: 30). As we will see below, both authors look for another way to introduce a phenomenological stance in scientific research.

[4] Petitot's attempt to quote a sentence of Husserl to support the idea that his proposal is not in contradiction to Husserl's ideas is unconvincing (Petitot 1995).

[5] As argued by Helena De Preester: "In spite of differences in method and object, it may be possible to preserve the descriptive results of Husserl's phenomenology. In other words, it might be possible to implement Husserl's descriptive results in the natural realm" (De Preester 2002: 642). Zahavi makes a distinction between the original transcendental philosophy characterizing Husserl's phenomenology (whose naturalization is a nonsense) and a phenomenological psychology as "a form of descriptive, eidetic, and intentional psychology which takes the first-person perspective seriously, but which . . . remains within a pre-philosophical attitude" (Zahavi 2013: 38).

1963: 305).[6] Now, following this model we explain the phenomenon if we discover the causal connection linking the emerging symptom to the underlying brain dysfunction. As a case in point, an epileptic first-person phenomenon like déjà vu can be explained as output of a depolarization in some brain areas (Illman et al. 2012).

This neurophenomenological approach provides new perspectives on phenomenology and, as argued by Morten Overgaard, "[p]henomenology, especially phenomenological psychology, could potentially enrich cognitive neuroscience by adding to it a more precise description of its object of research" (Overgaard 2004: 369). However, Jaspers was well aware that although it was always possible to use this method, in practice many phenomena of psychopathological interest were not explainable in this way. Accordingly, he proposed to develop an alternative method to understand the motivational chain giving meaningfulness to human experiences and actions (Rosini et al. 2013). On the contrary, Varela proposed this method as anti-reductionist and as a way to solve the hard problem of consciousness, being apparently unaware of its reductionist implications. In sum, phenomenology in this naturalized sense is a way to improve phenomenal descriptions of subjective experiences in order to make them reliable and suitable to be correlated to neurocognitive evidences. However, this deeply changes the phenomenological program: "naturalization is an epistemological reversal which alters the status of consciousness from primal region (source) to region in the world" (De Preester 2002: 645). In other words, it transforms phenomenology into the servant of a reductionist research program, that is, a new version for the twenty-first century of the Kraepelinian and neo-Kraepelinian ideal of using refined psychopathological descriptions as starting points for the explanatory reduction to neurobiological dysfunctions.

Finally, another possibility is to use phenomenology as "phenomenological psychology" in a different and longer project in which "a naturalization of phenomenology might not only entail a modification . . . of transcendental philosophy, but also a rethinking of the concept of nature—a rethinking that might ultimately lead to a transformation of natural science itself. . . . it should, however, be obvious that the task is daunting and that there is still a long way to go" (Zahavi 2013: 41). Skepticism about the possibility of phenomenology to change the way scientists operate is mandatory. Nevertheless, in Zahavi's paper there is a less demanding proposal that is feasible: to let phenomenology and natural sciences enter into a dialogue in which each influences the other's approach. Phenomenological analyses might suggest to the experimenter possible variations to the experimental design, in order to consider some phenomenal issues or details of which he was unaware. Conversely, the phenomenologist could be solicited by some experimental findings to reconsider his phenomenological analysis to see if the phenomenon addressed could be more complex than previously thought (Zahavi 2013: 41). If I understand correctly, this proposal differs from Varela's in a key point: there would be no mutual constraints but a free choice to be influenced from what is emerging in the other field.[7]

---

[6] This does not mean that Jaspers is a reductionist but only that he does not see the search of a causal explanation of mental phenomena as an incoherent or impossible stance. However, he stresses that, to be coherent, those working with this explanatory perspective should avoid psychological reflections because they are outside their disciplinary field. In his psychopathology Jaspers proposes a methodological pluralism with several disciplines cooperating, everyone from its perspective, to the never-ending task of understanding human beings.

[7] I sympathize with this view, although I would not call it a naturalized phenomenology but a model of possible dialogue between disciplines.

CONCLUSION

This debate about phenomenology, naturalism, and the neurosciences solicits a reflection about the role of philosophy in the dialogue with current cognitive neurosciences. The latter are naturalistic research programs whose aim is scientific explanation of observed phenomena. Applied to psychopathology, mental phenomena are outputs of underlying cognitive information processing that, in turn, is grounded on brain activity. We may discuss if the cognitive level is just a provisional step along the way to the "real" explanation in neurobiological terms, but this does not change too much for our ends. We may also discuss if, to be suitable for explanatory research, mental phenomena must be objectively measurable, and consequently if we should exclude from our list of explananda subjective complaints. It seems that neurophenomenology has its place here, its fundamental claim being that first-person experiences cannot be dismissed because they are fundamental elements for a complete scientific explanation. Consequently, neurocognitive sciences should include them in their research programs. Along this way, phenomenology provides a method for eliciting and describing subjective experiences in order to make them suitable for explanatory research. However, in Varela's neurophenomenological program this is not fundamental because other methods can be used as well for the same purposes. Hence, in neurophenomenology the role of phenomenology is secondary, and the research program remains shaped by the naturalistic approach of cognitive neurosciences looking for explanatory correlations between phenomena and underlying cognitive and brain activities.

The problem is therefore not only that neurophenomenology betrays Husserl's orthodoxy. In fact, every phenomenologically oriented psychopathologist did the same using phenomenology and hermeneutics rather freely for his own purposes, largely unconcerned with philosophical orthodoxy. The main problem is that neurophenomenology neglects the fundamental contribution of phenomenological psychopathology, which shows that naturalistic explanation is just one of the available methods, and that other methods are more appropriate to study the essential meaning of mental phenomena, to be understood within the broader context of the way a person is in his/her social and cultural world. In other words, the point is not just to include subjective experiences in the field of interest of neuroscientists. This is important but it is not enough. A key issue is to become aware that mental phenomena are not items that we find ready-made in nature and that we can simply observe and describe. Instead, they are the complex result of a hermeneutic construction in which brain activity, lived experience, capability of self-interpretation of proper experiences,[8] and dialogical negotiation with surrounding environment,[9] strictly interact (Berrios 2013; Aragona and Marková 2015). On this, Continental philosophy as hermeneutics has much more to say than simply aiding neurocognitive scientists in the description of mental explananda. To conclude, instead of reducing phenomenology to a methodological tool, we should improve the dialogue between phenomenological psychology and psychopathology at one side, and experimental studies on the other side. Reciprocal constraints

---

[8] Based on personal, social, and cultural abilities, available idioms of distress, etc.
[9] Including familial and social environment as well as, in the case of mental symptoms, the clinician cooperating with the patient in the understanding of his/her problems.

and bridge laws implicitly introduce a reductionist naturalization, while we need mutual respect of the different domains involved, and a free decision to be open to the knowledge emerging in the other field.

BIBLIOGRAPHY

Aishwarya S. and Malik Ali K. (2017). "Neuromarketing and Neuroethics—An Emerging Trend on Evaluation of Emotional Responses of Consumers to Marketing Stimuli." *International Journal of Innovative Research in Management Studies* 1: 27–30.

Aragona M. and Marková I. (2015). "The Hermeneutics of Mental Symptoms in the Cambridge School." *Revista Latinoamericana de Psicopatologia Fundamental* 18: 599–618.

Bernhardt B. C. and Singer T. (2012). "The Neural Basis of Empathy." *Annual Review of Neuroscience* 35: 1–23.

Berrios G. E. (2013). "Formation and Meaning of Mental Symptoms: History and Epistemology." *Dialogues in Philosophy, Mental and Neuro Sciences* 6: 39–48.

Blackburn S. (2005). *The Oxford Dictionary of Philosophy*. Oxford: Oxford University Press.

Chomsky N. (1956). "Three Models for the Description of Language." *IEEE Transactions on Information Theory* 2: 113–124.

De Preester H. (2002). "Naturalizing Husserlian Phenomenology: An Introduction." *Psychoanalytische Perspectieven* 20: 633–647.

Farina G. (2014). "Some Reflections on the Phenomenological Method." *Dialogues in Philosophy, Mental and Neuro Sciences* 7: 50–62.

Heidegger M. (1927). *Sein und Zeit*. Halle: Max Niemeyer.

Hempel C. G. and Oppenheim, P. (1948). "Studies in the Logic of Explanation." *Philosophy of Science* XV: 135–175.

Husserl E. (2001). *Logical Investigations, Vol. 1 (1900)*. Abingdon and New York: Routledge.

Illman N. A, Butler C. R., Souchay C., and Moulin C. J. A. (2012). "Déjà Experiences in Temporal Lobe Epilepsy." *Epilepsy Research and Treatment* Article ID 539567.

Jaspers K. (1963). *General Psychopathology*, 4th German edn. [1946]. Manchester: Manchester University Press.

Kraus A. (2010). "Existential A Prioris and the Phenomenology of Schizophrenia." *Dialogues in Philosophy, Mental and Neuro Sciences* 3: 1–7.

Lutz A. and Thompson E. (2003). "Neurophenomenology." *Journal of Consciousness Studies* 10: 31–52.

Olivares F. A., Vargas E., Fuentes C., and Martínez-Pernía D., and Canales-Johnson A. (2015). "Neurophenomenology Revisited: Second-person Methods for the Study of Human Consciousness." *Frontiers in Psychology* 6: 673.

Overgaard M. (2004). "On the Naturalising of Phenomenology." *Phenomenology and the Cognitive Sciences* 3: 365–379.

Petitot J. (1995). "La réorientation naturaliste de la phénoménologie." *Archives de Philosophie* 58: 631–658.

Petitot J., Varela F. J., Parchoud B., and Roy J. M. (eds.) (1999). *Naturalizing Phenomenology*. Stanford: Stanford University Press.

Quine W. V. (1969). *Ontological Relativity and Other Essays*. New York: Columbia University Press.

Rosini E., Di Fabio F., and Aragona M. (2013). "1913–2013: One Hundred Years of General Psychopathology." *Dialogues in Philosophy, Mental and Neuro Sciences* 6: 57–66.

Roy J.-M., Petitot J., Pachoud B., and Varela F. (1999). "Beyond the Gap: An Introduction to Naturalizing Phenomenology." In J. Petitot, F. J. Varela, B. Parchoud, and J. M. Roy (eds.), *Naturalizing Phenomenology*, pp. 1–83. Stanford: Stanford University Press.

Stanghellini G. (2013). "Philosophical Resources for the Psychiatric Interview." In K. W. M. Fulford (ed.), *The Oxford Handbook of Philosophy and Psychiatry*, pp. 320–355. Oxford: Oxford University Press.

Stanghellini G. and Aragona M. (2016). "Phenomenological Psychopathology: Toward a Person-centered Hermeneutic Approach in the Clinical Encounter." In G. Stanghellini and M. Aragona (eds.), *An Experiential Approach to Psychopathology*, pp. 1–43. Berlin: Springer.

Uttal W. R. (2003). *The New Phrenology: The Limits of Localizing Cognitive Processes in the Brain*. Cambridge, MA: MIT Press.

Varela F. J. (1996). "Neurophenomenology. A Methodological Remedy for the Hard Problem." *Journal of Consciousness Studies* 3: 330–349.

Zahavi D. (2013). "Naturalized Phenomenology: A Desideratum or a Category Mistake?" *Royal Institute of Philosophy Supplement* 72: 23–42.

CHAPTER 33

....

NORMALITY

....

SARA HEINÄMAA AND JOONA TAIPALE

INTRODUCTION

....

PHENOMENOLOGY offers two kinds of resources for the study of mental disorders. On the one hand, we find a set of analytical concepts developed for the illumination of the conditions and the limits of experiencing. These include the concepts of concordance and optimality that explicate two different senses of normality operative in human experiencing. On the other hand, phenomenology also offers systematic investigations of several different types of psychic and psychophysical disorders, ranging from depression and eating disorders to psychosis and schizophrenia.

In concrete phenomenological inquiries, these two types of resources—analytical-conceptual and thematic—often intermingle. This is due to the fundamental philosophical tasks that phenomenology sets itself. Because it aims at disclosing the conditions of the possibility of all experiencing it does not limit itself to ordinary experiences or to the statistically most common or most dominant forms of experiencing. Rather, it studies experience in its greatest possible variety and plurality. Individual experiences merely serve as examples that allow us to notice, highlight, and scrutinize general forms of experiencing. Thus, empirically unusual and statistically exceptional types of experiences are as important as ordinary experiences and may sometimes be more illuminative for the task at hand. Husserl even argues that the phenomenologist may profit more from the arts, poetry, and history than from the empirical sciences of the psyche (e.g. Husserl 1963: 184), since phenomenology is not an inquiry into actual or real experiences but is a science of possibilities. The aim is to maximize variance, not similarities.

For reasons of accessibility, our exposition will discuss the analytical-conceptual and thematic resources of phenomenology in parallel. We will articulate the main conceptual tools that Husserl offers for the analysis of the normality and abnormality of experiencing and also look into the types of phenomena that Husserl himself analyzed while developing these concepts. At the same time, we will discuss some of the main contributions of classical and contemporary phenomenologists in the study of psychiatric disorders. Here our aim is to clarify the theoretical character of these contributions and to draw attention to the methods and the types of results that phenomenologists provide for the study of the human psyche.

Preparatory Remarks: On the Character of Phenomenological Inquiries

Before getting deeper into the Husserlian concepts on normality and abnormality, it is necessary to make a few preparatory remarks about Husserl's investigations. Three methodological factors must be emphasized in particular since they separate phenomenology from empirical studies of human behavior and psyche, on the one hand, and from alternative philosophical studies of the mind and consciousness, on the other hand.

Philosophical Analysis of Constitution

The first thing to notice is that Husserl's concepts of normality and abnormality are transcendental-philosophical concepts and not empirical ones. They are devised for the purpose of studying pure experiences and experienced phenomena and of analyzing the processes of sense-constitution essential to all possible experiencing. So, in this context, "normal" does not refer to what is empirically general or average, nor to what is quantitatively common or statistically noteworthy. Nor is it about the standards of the social behavior of human beings as described and interpreted by anthropology and the human and social sciences. In the context of Husserlian phenomenology, normal is what contributes to sense-constitution, and abnormal is whatever disrupts the lattices of sense. "[N]ormality is a mode pertaining to constitution," Husserl writes in his manuscripts (Husserl 1973b: 68, cf. 1973b: 123, 154, 1973c: 35; Steinbock 1995, 2003; Taipale 2012, Heinämaa 2013; Taipale 2014: 123–124).

A simple example helps to illuminate how the concepts of normality figure in phenomenological inquiries into sense-constitution. When I enter bright daylight from a movie theatre, the light temporarily blinds my vision. The situation is anomalous or abnormal in phenomenological terms, not in respect to the quantity of light or in respect to the relative rareness of the situation, but because the appearances that now are formed in my stream of consciousness deviate from the system of appearances established in the darkness of the theatre (cf. Lobo 2013). What has been appearing and what now appears do not cohere, and thus for a moment I fail to make sense of the seen environment. A passing condition such as this can be said to be phenomenologically anomalous or abnormal.

A recurrent example from Husserl's own works brings to the fore another idea of abnormality central to phenomenological inquiries into sense-constitution: When I try on new eyeglasses and scan my surroundings with them, then the appearances that I have of things systematically diverge from the ones that I have had, and thus they break the established harmony and coherence of appearing. The new appearances with the spectacles are abnormal in the same sense as the new appearances in the case of bright sun light. However, Husserl points out that since my eyesight with new spectacles gives the environment to me more fully and in more detail and specification than my vision without glasses, it *normalizes* my vision in an important sense despite its discordance with my earlier experiences. To be sure, my new vision with spectacles deviates from my earlier visions and interrupts their coherent progression, but at the same time it promotes distinction and articulation in the appearing field, brings a new clarity in respect to visible objects, and allows me to make sense of the perceptual field.

A situation such as this can be said to be phenomenologically normal but in a different sense from the example above: whereas normality there meant coherence between experiences, it here means added clearness and determinacy in respect to the experienced objectivity. Both ideas of normality concern sense-constitution: the first highlights the mutual coherence between appearances and the second highlights the correlation between appearances and the objects intended.

Intentionality and the Subject–Object Correlation

Another basic thing to notice is that since phenomenology studies sense-constitution in terms of intentionality, that is, in terms of the correlation between the subject-related intentions and the objects intended, it is bound to illuminate both the subjective and the objective side of constitutional normality.

A familiar example of this duality of correlative analyses is provided by the everyday experience of spatiality. While the environing world usually gives itself to us with the sense of stability or steadiness, we may occasionally encounter the world without any fixed directions or clear spatial structure or order. This happens, for example, in the transitional states of falling into sleep and awaking from sleep. Marcel Proust's *Remembrance of the Things Past* involves an illuminative description of the situation:

> [W]hen I awoke like this [rabidly], and my mind struggled in an unsuccessful attempt to discover where I was, everything revolved around me through the darkness: things, places, years. My body, still too heavy with sleep to move, would make an effort to construe the form which its tiredness took as an orientation of its various members, so as to induce from that where the wall lay and the furniture stood, to piece together and to give a name to the house in which it must be living.
>
> (Proust 1981: 10)[1]

Here it is not only the attended objects and the environing space that lack stable structures but also the bodily subject of experiencing. In the semi-awakened state between sleep and wakefulness, my own sensing-moving, perceiving, and governing body operates in a non-unitary, irregular manner. The perceiving self, as well as the perceived environment, falters and flickers in search for coherence and stability. So, in this case, there is a rupture both on the subjective and on the objective side of experiencing (cf. Reyes Melero 2013: 105–107).

A different experiential alteration, almost contrary, can be identified in depressive conditions: instead of dispersing or fluctuating, one's own body is experientially solidified and hardened and the limits and structures of the environing space are rigidified and closed. Thomas Fuchs describes such changes as follows:

---

[1] Merleau-Ponty, *Phenomenology of Perception*, includes a phenomenological analysis and interpretation of the form of experience described by Proust (1995: 74–75, 145–146, cf. 163–164). See also Merleau-Ponty's extensive discussion of sleep in his lectures on *Institution and Passivity* (2010).

Thus, melancholia may be described as a reification or *corporealization* of the lived body … The melancholic patient experiences a local or general oppression, anxiety and rigidity (e.g., a feeling of an armor vest or tire around the chest, lump in the throat, or pressure in the head). Sense perception and movement are weakened and finally walled in by this rigidity, which is visible [for others] in the patient's gaze, face, or gestures. To act, patients have to overcome their psychomotor inhibition and to push themselves to even minor tasks, compensating by an effort of will what the body does not have by itself any more. With growing inhibition, their sensorimotor space is restricted to the nearest environment, culminating in depressive stupor.

(Fuchs 2005: 98–99, cf. Fuchs 2002; Micali 2013)

Some mental illnesses manifest even more profound changes on the subjective side of experiencing and in the core structures of subjectivity itself. Rather than just affecting the patient's experiences of her own body, schizophrenia seems to damage the articulation of selfhood and mineness which are traditionally taken to be a priori forms of all experiencing or of all human experiencing. On the basis of this insight, phenomenologists have argued that such conditions involve, not just abnormal changes in the contents of conscious states, but also profound changes in the *intensity of self-awareness* (Parnas and Sass 2001; Parnas and Handest 2003; Parnas, Sass, and Zahavi 2013).

Phenomenologists have also clarified the experiential dimensions of chronic depression and manic-depressive alteration. These studies show that pathological states may effect profound changes in the *temporal* structures of subjectivity. In experiences of depression, the past weighs heavy and seems to haunt the subject and contaminate each present moment. Extreme depressive states undermine the temporal flow comprehensively and disrupt its rhythmic progress: the future may seem completely blocked or endlessly delayed or postponed. In the manic phases of the bipolar condition, in contrast, the future seems to condense into the present, and its endless possibilities seem to be available all at once (Schwartz and Wiggins 2017). Thus, the patient may be severely estranged from social relations by the experiential fact that for her future possibilities are all given at once and with equal intensities whereas for others such possibilities present themselves in a serial fashion and in diverse temporal distances. Depressive experiences, broadly put, are conceptualized in contemporary phenomenology not as lacks or deficiencies but as modifications of experiential duration and subjective time and as concomitant modifications in affective intersubjectivity.

All in all, inquiries into the experiential dimensions of mental disorders suggest that the structures of subjectivity are not static forms but are dynamically developing, and potentially also deteriorating. This insight motivates one of Merleau-Ponty's main arguments in *Phenomenology of Perception*: If consciousness were a universal power of signification or a continuum of pure acts of thinking (*cogito*), he contends, then illness would not be able to attack consciousness and conscious subjects at all. The term "mental illness" would merely be an oxymoron or else display a conceptual confusion (Merleau-Ponty 1995: 110).

Model of Perception

The third methodological point to emphasize is that the concepts of normality were developed by Husserl originally for the purpose of illuminating the intentional structures of *perceptual* experience and thing-constitution. When introducing these concepts, Husserl did not study the emotive and axiological forms of experiencing (i.e. emotions, desires, and feelings), or on the structures of our communicative or goal-directed practical lives. The primary model for inquiries into normality and abnormality in Husserlian phenomenology is the normality of perception (cf. Breyer 2010; Wehrle 2010; Doyon and Breyer 2015; Doyon 2018).

However, Husserl soon started to apply the concepts of normality in the analysis of other forms of experiencing. On the one hand, he carried the concepts of normality and abnormality over from the analysis of perception to the study of memory and imagination and the so-called "higher mental capacities," most importantly, intelligence, reason, and linguistic communication. Thus, we find in his extensive manuscripts, reflections concerning dementia, insanity, infancy, and animality (Husserl 1973a–c, cf. Husserl 1988: 187; Taipale 2012: 147–155; Heinämaa 2014a; Fernandez 2016).

On the other hand, Husserl also transferred the concepts of normality from the analysis of subjectivity to the analysis of intersubjectivity. This became topical when he proceeded from the study of the doxic experiences of perception and cognition to practical and axiological experiences and the forms of objectivity constituted in such experiences, that is, values and goals.

When analyzing the structures of intersubjectivity, Husserl made a distinction between abnormal worlds and the normal environing world (*Umwelt*). He called the abnormal worlds *alien-worlds* (*Fremdenwelt*) and the normal world *home-world* (*Heimwelt*) (Husserl 1973c: 176 n. 1, 214, 2008: 336–337; Steinbock 1995; 2003; Taipale 2010; Staiti 2011; cf. Waldenfels 2004). The basis of this distinction is in the concept of *practice* and the related concept of *membership* in a practical community (Heinämaa 2013). This means that ultimately the distinction between the home-world and alien-worlds is drawn on the basis of familiar and unfamiliar practices. Our home-world is the practical world in which we participate and are members, and the alien-world is any world of foreign practices, that is, practices in which we do not or cannot participate, due to varying differences in our practical orientation, skills, capacities, interests, and callings.

The simple example of participating in a scientific conference illuminates these distinctions. The elements of such conferences are normal to us due to our familiarity with the academic practices of research and debate that contribute to the constitution of the culture of scientific knowledge. In Germany and Austria, however, the scholarly audience may applaud after presentations by knocking instead of clapping. Despite the unfamiliarity of the gesture to Anglophone researchers, we can immediately make sense of it as an appraisal on the basis of the shared practical setting of the situation. The home-world of the scholarly practice of arguing and reasoning may thus prevail over national home-worlds.

On the other hand, if the guiding aims of the people attending an event differ radically and comprehensively, then the constitution of a common world may be impossible and we find ourselves at the border between the normal and the abnormal, home-world and alien-world. An illuminating example is offered by Jane Champion's movie *The Piano*: A small European frontier-community organizes a Christmas pageant and invites their Māori neighbors to the event. The play that the Europeans perform happens to be a comic version of *Bluebeard*, involving a scene in which the main character beheads his next female victim. When the performance proceeds to this dramatic scene, the Māori audience, unfamiliar with the theatrical traditions of the Europeans and their performance customs, storms the stage and tries to hinder the event from happening.

It is crucial to emphasize that the concepts of normal world and abnormal world, or home-world and alien-world, are subject-relative, that is, always given to an individual or collective subject. Thus, no world is home-world as such, and no world is alien-world as such, but only in relation to some subject, individual, or collective (e.g. Husserl 1973c: 233; cf. Steinbock 1995, 2003; Waldenfels 2004).

With these three methodological remarks in mind, we can turn to Husserl's concepts of normality and distinguish between two main meanings crucial to phenomenological studies of experiencing.

ANALYTICAL CONCEPTS OF CONCORDANCE AND OPTIMALITY

Husserl operates primarily with two concepts of normality. On the one hand, he defines normality by concordance (*Einstimmigkeit*) and, on the other hand, he defines normality by optimality (*Optimalität*). An experience is said to be normal in the sense of concordance if it coheres with other experiences while maintaining the identity of the experienced object (Husserl 1973a: 364–366, 1973c: 165, 1980: 490, 1986: 83); and an experience is said to be normal in the sense of optimality if it contributes to the richness and differentiation of the experience in respect to the intended object (Husserl 1973a: 379, 2005: 53, 55). Both concepts characterize experiences with intentional objects and with horizons of co-intendings, but whereas concordance is determined in respect to *other experiences*, optimality is determined in respect to *the intended object*. Thus understood, concordance is about consistency or harmony between experiences, while optimality is about the clearness, richness, and fullness of experiencing.

The example discussed in the first section of the chapter helps to illuminate these two senses: When I put on new eyeglasses with high-definition lenses, I see better than I did without the glasses. The new appearances are optimality-normal in respect to the richness or sharpness of the seen objectivities and the visual field as a whole. At the same time, the very same appearances are concordance-abnormal in respect to my earlier visions; they deviate from the established harmony between my experiences (e.g. Husserl Ms. D 13, I, 175a). The optician may even warn me that I first need to move cautiously with the new spectacles, especially when standing up, since my visual and kinesthetic systems (the brain) only gradually adjust to the new type of visual information provided by the glasses.

Both sets of concepts, those of concordance and those of optimality, can be used in the analysis of the structures of subjective modes of experiencing as well as those of intersubjective modes of experiencing. An experience can, for example, be concordant in respect to the earlier experiences of the subject and her individual history of experiencing, and at the very same time be discordant in respect to the experiences of other subjects and a community of subjects (cf. Taipale 2014: 130–133).

For example, a person who is blind from birth is statistically deviant and anomalous in comparison to the majority of the population. However, her experiences, like those of the sighted, proceed in a concordant manner forming a harmonious whole in which local deviations and temporary interruptions are possible. Thus, we can say that her present perceptions, here and now, are concordance-normal in respect to her earlier experiences and her general way of experiencing.

Moreover, a person blind from birth is also concordance-normal in respect to the *community* of the blind (cf. Reyes Melero 2013: 110–111). It is not only that she can enter into relations of mutual communication and understanding with all members of this community (cf. Heinämaa 2013), but also that she can take part in the distinctive practices of this community, including practices of writing and reading (the Braille notation), practices of training and handling animals (e.g. seeing-eye dogs), and special practices of tool-use (e.g. item identification instruments, talking products, canes). Moreover, these practices can be learned and they have their intersubjective histories and traditions in which they are transmitted to new generations. To the sighted they are unfamiliar and unknown, and thus we can say that the sighted person is concordance-abnormal in respect to the historical community of the blind.

Alternative appearance systems cannot be put in an order of preference by the concepts of concordance. When a rupture or a series of ruptures has first disrupted the old order and finally replaced it with a new concordant order, there is no way of comparing the two orders, the old one and the new one, in terms of concordance-normality. In terms of concordance, the two systems are symmetrical: both are abnormal from the point of view of the other. For the blind the world of the sighted is unfamiliar and remains so, and for the sighted the world of the blind is equally alien. Thus, other concepts are needed to capture the *normative* sense of normality implicit in both common sense and scientific discourses. The concept of optimality serves some of these purposes.

Let us illuminate the relations between the concepts of concordance and optimality by developing the example of the eyeglasses: I put on the spectacles, and everything gives itself to me in clear contours; I take off the spectacles, and everything in fuzzy.[2] However, nothing in the orderly relations between the "fuzzy" things in the "fuzzy" world tells me that they should be clearer. The idea of fuzziness is as if borrowed from the world ordered by the spectacles. It is of course possible, and probable, that without the eyeglasses I will not grasp all the things that would be given to me if I were to examine the environment with the eyeglasses. For example, I may not notice that a bus to my work place is approaching since I do not identify the route number marked on its front. But lacking these distinctions is not an internal defect of the world that I grasp with my bare eyes. It is a defect only in relation to the clearer and sharper world given by the eyeglasses (and my interest in identifying the route number). This must not be misunderstood as implying that the world without the eyeglasses would not have any ruptures. It has its own internal ruptures. For example, when tears fill my eyes or when the driving lights of the approaching bus suddenly blind me, I momentarily see nothing—all established distinctions are lost and the world is torn apart for some time.

The transition toward optimality may be quite challenging. For example, a person who is blind from birth and gains eyesight by an organic transplant proceeds from abnormality to normality in terms of optimality. Her condition is new, conflicting with her earlier

---

[2] Notice that the terms "distinct" and "fuzzy" already depend on the concept of optimality to be explained. We use them here, however, to avoid introducing additional technical terminology.

experiences, and may elicit many different kinds of emotive responses. Similarly, a person who has been deaf from birth and gains hearing by a transplant inserted in her skull, usually reacts either with joy or with terror. In both cases, the perceptual field is enriched by new unfamiliar types of elements and relations. The integration of these and the establishment of a new coherence demands reorganization of the whole perceptual field and its different modalities: visual, auditory, tactile, and kinesthetic (cf. Heinämaa 2014b, 2014c; Slatman 2014). It also requires that the person develops new skills and dispositions and learns new ways of acting. If these can be gained, the person ends up with an environing world with more distinction and richness in respect to many objectivities.

Husserl argues that the optimal trumps the concordant in a similar manner also on the level of intersubjective experience as long as social acts of communication are available and operative. He explicates this idea by discussing the example of color blindness. The argument is that if a community of color blind people came into communicative contact with a community of people who are not color blind, then the color blind community would immediately, without any further ado, "recognize that their world is not the optimal" (Husserl 1973b: 33). At the same time, Husserl also argues that in their full senses, the terms "the world" and "the thing" refer to objectivities that are accessible to all experiencing subjects independently of differences in their apparatuses of sensibility: "[I]t belongs to the actually existing thing to be capable of being experienced as the *same* for 'everyone', with everyone's sensibility, which can be 'normal' or 'abnormal'" (Husserl 1992: 363–364; Staiti 2011; Carr 2014; cf. Tani 2004).

PHENOMENOLOGY OF PSYCHOPATHOLOGY—AN OVERVIEW

Since its onset, the phenomenological tradition has had a considerable interest in questions of psychopathology. The concrete analyses and descriptions that phenomenologists have offered have served two kinds of purposes. On the one hand, scholars have used clinical examples of experiential aberrations in order to highlight, *ex negativo*, the conditions of normal experiencing as well as the essential structures of all experiencing. On the other hand, the other strong tendency in the tradition has been the attempt to describe the phenomenological structure of various pathological phenomena in their own terms. These two lines of research often complement one another. Of the classical phenomenologists, Merleau-Ponty has been recognized as one of the most influential proponents of the former approach, but at the same time he has positively contributed to our understanding of various pathological experiential conditions and dysfunctions per se (see e.g. Merleau-Ponty 1995: 138).

One of the general tenets of the phenomenological approach to psychopathological phenomena lies in its capacity to complement psychological and psychiatric, and more generally all third-person analyses and explanations. With its first-person methods of variation, dismantling, construction, interpretation, and hermeneutic clarification, phenomenology offers crucial information about the ways in which people suffering from mental illnesses experience the world and about the structures of their experiences—information that remains unreachable from a third-person standpoint. By such studies, phenomenology significantly contributes both to our understanding of the meanings and the experiential genesis of mental disorders and to our understanding of "what it is like" to suffer from mental illnesses and to be a patient (e.g. Fisher 2014; Svenaeus 2018).

In the tradition of phenomenological psychopathology, particular weight has been given to analyses of schizophrenia and depression. Karl Jaspers, Ludwig Binswanger, Eugène Minkowski, Wolfgang Blankenburg, and Kimura Bin are the main pioneers in this field. Their contributions to the understanding of psychic disorders have mainly concerned the ways in which patients' experiences of themselves, other persons and the intersubjective environment alternate and transform during sickness. The result of the analyses show that mental disorders affect the fundamental structures of temporality, embodiment, and selfhood, and thus in a comprehensive and global way impair the patients' possibilities of relating to the others and to the world as a whole (e.g. Jaspers 1919; Binswanger 1960; Minkowski 1970; Blankenburg 1971; Bingswanger 1975 [1949]; Kimura 1992; Bingswanger 1993 [1930]; Jaspers 1997 [1913]; cf. Sass 2001).

During the last few decades, these traditional lines of research in phenomenological psychopathology have been carried over and developed further by many new phenomenologists and clinical researchers, including Thomas Fuchs, Louis Sass, Josef Parnas, Dan Zahavi, Osborne Wiggins, Giovanni Stanghellini, and Matthew Ratcliffe. These scholars, and many others, have significantly reinforced and increased the conceptual, descriptive, and methodological tools of phenomenology for the theorization of psychopathology, thus remarkably furthering also the clinical lines of research.

At the same time, phenomenologists have expanded their inquiries to cover various new types of psychic and psychophysical disorders, including different forms of autism and eating disorders (e.g. Legrand 2013; Svenaeus 2014; Fuchs 2015; Legrand and Briend 2015). In autism research, phenomenologists have challenged accounts that analyze the disorder dominantly by the negative terms of lack or deprivation. In this line, it has been argued that the core of autism is not owing to diminished social awareness but rather must be understood in terms of *heightened* social awareness (e.g. Fuchs 2005: 101, cf. Fuchs 2015). To this end, Louis Sass, Josef Parnas, and Dan Zahavi have introduced the idea of *hyperreflexivity* (Sass, Parnas, and Zahavi 2011). Adopting the term from Merleau-Ponty, they underline that psychophysical disorders may be owing not only or mainly to deficits, shortages or lacks, but also to the unusual intensification of various experiential functions or structures.

A culmination of this new research activity, is the establishment of the so-called *EASE* scale in the early 2000s. The abbreviation stands for "Examination of Anomalous Self-Experience." As characterized by its developers, the EASE is "a symptom checklist for semi-structured, phenomenological exploration of *experiential* or *subjective* anomalies that may be considered as disorders of basic or 'minimal' self-awareness" (Parnas et al. 2005). This descriptive scale has been devised in collaboration between phenomenologists, psychiatrists, and clinical psychologists on the basis of self-descriptions obtained from schizophrenic patients, and it has a strong diagnostic and differential-diagnostic relevance. Its theoretical and practical usages demonstrate the power of the first- and second-person methods of phenomenology.

Conclusion

On the basis of our explications of the Husserlian concepts of normality and abnormality, we can now draw three general conclusions.

First, the phenomena of normality and abnormality cannot be adequately analyzed by mere quantitative concepts. Normality and abnormality are not merely statistical or stochastic measures but involve deep *experiential* structures and *constitutional* dimensions. The phenomenological methodology allows us to disclose these dimensions. Instead of being analyzed from the third-person perspective, clinical disorders and behavioral disruptions are studied in this framework from the perspectives of the persons who undergo them and suffer from them (cf. Merleau-Ponty 1995: 120).

Georges Canguilhem emphasizes the social and existential implications of this methodological factor in *The Normal and the Pathological*. He famously points out that many conditions that are rendered pathological by common standards of measurement may be both experienced and understood as normal by the persons experiencing them. Moreover, Canguilhem also argues that experiential life is not merely receptive of and submissive to external norms but is also norm-instituting or normalizing (Canguilhem 1991: e.g. 338–339; cf. von Wright 1963). Thus, the pathological is not simply abnormal in the sense of lacking the norm or diverting from common norms or working against them; it also establishes its own normality.

Second, the phenomenological concepts of normality are not defined by any ideas of *naturalness or nativity*, and correspondingly abnormality is not identified with unnaturalness or artificiality. What is experientially normal may well be artificial, human-made, or culturally mediated; and, on the other hand, many natural and innate processes and situations may be experientially abnormal.

Third, since sense-constitution is a dynamic process and not a static principle or a creative act performed once and for all, the phenomenological concepts of normality and abnormality are *dynamic* concepts. Experiences that are deviant in the framework of the already constituted senses are able to institute new sense and thus establish new systems of normality. What is normal in one experiential context may turn out to be abnormal in another, and what has been abnormal for many generative communities for several centuries may become normal for new persons in new situations and with new experiential horizons.

Bibliography

Binswanger L. (1960). *Melancholie und Manie: Phänomenologische Studien*. Pfullingen: Neske.

Binswanger L. (1975). "Heidegger's Analytic of Existent and Its Meaning for Psychiatry" [1949], trans. J. Needleman. In J. Needleman (ed.), *Being-in-the-World: Selected Papers of Ludwig Binswanger*, pp. 206–221. London: Condor Books.

Binswanger L. (1993). "Dream and Existence" [1930], trans. J. Needelman. In K. Hoeller (ed.), *Dream and Existence: Studies in Existential Psychology and Psychiatry*, pp. 81–105. Atlantic Highlands: Humanities Press International.

Blankenburg, W. (1971). *Der Verlust der natürlichen Selbstverständlichkeit. Ein Beitrag zur Psychopathologie symptomarmer Schizophrenien*. Stuttgart: Enke.

Breyer T. (2010). "Unsichtbare Grenzen: Zur Phänomenologie der Normalität, Liminalität und Anomalität." In P. Merz, A. Staiti, and F. Steffen (eds.), *Geist—Person—Gemeinschaft: Freiburger Beiträge zur Aktualität Husserls*, pp. 109–128. Würzburg: Ergon.

Canguilhem G. (1991). *The Normal and the Pathological* [1943], trans. C. R. Fawcett and R. S. Cohen. New York: Zone Books.

Carr D. (2014). "The Emergence and Transformation of Husserl's Concept of World." In S. Heinämaa, M. Hartimo, and T. Miettinen (eds.), *Phenomenology and the Transcendental*, pp. 175–189. London: Routledge.

Doyon M. (2018). "Husserl and Perceptual Optimality." *Husserl Studies*. doi.org/10.1007/s10743-018-9224-9

Doyon M. and T. Breyer (eds.) (2015). *Normativity in Perception*. Basingstoke: Palgrave, MacMillan.

Fernandez A. V. (2016). "Phenomenology, Mental Illness, and the Intersubjective Constitution of the Lifeworld." In S. W. Gurley and G. Pfeifer (eds.), *Phenomenology and the Political*, pp. 199–214. Lanham: Rowman & Littlefield International.

Fisher L. (2014). "The Illness Experience: A Feminist Phenomenological Perspective." In L. Käll (Ed), *Feminist Phenomenology and Medicine*, pp. 27–46. New York: SUNY Press.

Fuchs T. (2002). "The Phenomenology of Shame, Guilt and the Body in Body Dysmorphic Disorder and Depression." *Journal of Phenomenological Psychology* 33: 223–243.

Fuchs T. (2005). "Corporealized and Disembodied Minds: A Phenomenological View of the Body in Melancholia and Schizophrenia." *Philosophy, Psychiatry & Psychology* 12: 95–107.

Fuchs T. (2015). "Pathologies of Intersubjectivity in Autism and Schizophrenia." *Journal of Consciousness Studies* 22: 191–214.

Heinämaa S. (2013). "Transcendental Intersubjectivity and Normality: Constitution by Mortals." In D. Moran and R. T. Jensen (eds.), *The Phenomenology of Embodied Subjectivity*, pp. 83–103. Dordrecht: Springer.

Heinämaa S. (2014a). "The Animal and the Infant: From Embodiment and Empathy to Generativity." In S. Heinämaa, M. Hartimo, and T. Miettinen (eds.), *Phenomenology and the Transcendental*, pp. 129–146. London: Routledge.

Heinämaa S. (2014b). " 'An Equivocal Couple Overwhelmed With Life': A Phenomenological Analysis of Pregnancy." *philoSOPHIA* 4: 12–49.

Heinämaa S. (2014c). "Transformations of Old Age: Selfhood, Normativity, and Time." In S. Stoller (ed.), *Simone de Beauvoir's Philosophy of Old Age*, pp.167–187. Würzburg: Walter de Guyter.

Husserl E. (1963). *Ideas: General Introduction to Pure Phenomenology* [1913], trans. W. R. Boyce Gibson (Husserliana 3, ed. W. Biemel). New York, London: Collier.

Husserl E. (1973a): *Zur Phänomenologie der Intersubjektivität: Texte aus dem Nachlass, Erster Teil, 1905–1912*. Husserliana 13, ed. I. Kern. The Hague: Martinus Nijhoff.

Husserl E. (1973b): *Zur Phänomenologie der Intersubjektivität: Texte aus dem Nachlass, Zweiter Teil, 1921–1928*. Husserliana 14, ed. I. Kern. The Hague: Martinus Nijhoff).

Husserl E. (1973c), *Zur Phänomenologie der Intersubjektivität: Texte aus dem Nachlass, Dritter Teil, 1929–1935*. Husserliana 15, ed. I. Kern. The Hague: Martinus Nijhoff.

Husserl E. (1980). *Phäntasie, Bildbewusstsein, Erinnerung: Zur Phänomenologie der anschaulichen Vergegenwartigungen. Texte aus dem Nachlass (1898–1925)*. Husserliana 23, ed. E. Marbach. The Hague, Netherlands: Martinus Nijhoff.

Husserl E. (1986). *Aufsätze und* Vorträge *1911–1921, Mit ergänzenden Texten.* Husserliana 25, eds. T. Nenon and H. R. Sepp. The Hague, Netherlands: Martinus Nijhoff.

Husserl E. (1988). *The Crisis of European Sciences and Transcendental Philosophy: An Introduction to Phenomenology* [1954], trans. D. Carr (Husserliana 6, ed. W. Biemel). Evanston: Northwestern University.

Husserl E. (1992). *Experience and Judgment: Investigations in a Genealogy of Logic* [1939], trans. J. S. Churchill and K. Ameriks. Evaston: Northwestern University Press.

Husserl E. (2005). *Wahrnehmung und Aufmerksamkeit, Texte aus dem Nachlass (1893–1912).* Husserliana 38, eds. T. Vongehr and R. Giuliani. New York: Springer.

Husserl E. (2008). *Die Lebenswelt: Auslegungen der vorgegebenen Welt und ihrer Konstitution, Texte aus dem Nachlass (1916–1937).* Husserliana 39, ed. R. Sowa. New York: Springer.

Jaspers K. (1919). *Psychologie der Weltanschauungen.* Berlin: Springer.

Jaspers K. (1997). *General Psychopathology I–II* [1913], trans. J. Hoenig and M. W. Hamilton. Baltimore: Johns Hopkins University Press.

Kimura B. (1992). "Réflexion et soi chez le schizophrène," trans. Joël Bouderlique. In Y. Pélicier (ed.), *Écrits de Psychopathologie Phénoménologique*, pp. 117–127. Paris: Presses Universitaires de France.

Legrand D. (2013). "Inter-subjectively Meaningful Symptoms in Anorexia." In R. T. Jensen and D. Moran (eds.), *The Phenomenology of Embodied Subjectivity*, pp. 185–201. Dordrecht: Springer.

Legrand D. and F. Briend (2015). "Anorexia and Bodily Intersubjectivity." *European Psychologist* 20: 52–61.

Lobo C. (2013). "Self-variation and Self-modification or the Different Ways of Being Other." In R. T. Jensen and D. Moran (eds.), *The Phenomenology of Embodied Subjectivity*, pp. 263–283. Dordrecht: Springer.

Merleau-Ponty M. (1995). *Phenomenology of Perception* [1945], trans. C. Smith. London: Routledge.

Merleau-Ponty M. (2010). *Institution and Passivity: Course Notes from Collège de France (1954–1955)* [2003], trans. L. Lawlor and H. Massey. Evanston: Northwestern University Press.

Micali S. (2013). "The Alteration of Embodiment in Melancholia." In R. T. Jensen and D. Moran (eds.), *The Phenomenology of Embodied Subjectivity*, pp. 203–219. Dordrecht: Springer.

Minkowski E. (1970). *Lived Time: Phenomenological and Psychological Studies* [1933], trans. N. Metzel. Evanston: Northwestern University Press.

Parnas, J. and L. A. Sass (2001). "Self, Solipsism, and the Schizophrenic Delusions." *Philosophy, Psychiatry, & Psychology* 8: 101–120.

Parnas J. and P. Handest (2003). "Phenomenology of Anomalous Self-experience in Early Schizophrenia." *Comprehensive Psychiatry* 44: 121–134.

Parnas J., P. Møller, T. Kircher, J. Thalbitzer, L. Jansson, P. Handest, and D. Zahavi (2005). "EASE: Examination of Anomalous Self-experience." *Psychopathology* 38: 236–258.

Parnas J., L. A. Sass, and D. Zahavi (2013). "Rediscovering Psychopathology: The Epistemology and Phenomenology of the Psychiatric Object." *Schizophrenia Bulletin* 39: 270–277.

Proust M. (1981). *Remembrance of Things Past: Volume I: Swann's Way* [1871], trans. L. Davis. London: Penguin Books.

Reyes Melero I. de los (2013). "The Body as a System of Concordance and the Perceptual World." In R. T. Jensen and D. Moran (eds.), *The Phenomenology of Embodied Subjectivity*, pp. 105–120. Dordrecht: Springer.

Sass L. (2001). "Self and World in Schizophrenia: Three Classic Approaches." *Philosophy, Psychiatry, & Psychology* 8: 251–270.

Sass L., J. Parnas, and D. Zahavi (2011). "Phenomenological Psychopathology and Schizophrenia: Contemporary Approaches and Misunderstandings." *Philosophy, Psychiatry, & Psychology* 18: 1–23.

Schwartz M. and O. Wiggins (2017). "What Phenomenology has to Offer Psychiatry? Aberrant Temporality Is a Core Phenomenon of Diverse Mental Disorders." Key note paper presented at *Issues in Contemporary Phenomenology*. University of Warsaw, Polish Academy of Sciences, Polish Phenomenological Association, Warsaw, March 23–26, 2017.

Slatman J. (2014). *Our Strange Body: Philosophical Reflections on Identity and Medical Interventions*. Amsterdam: Amsterdam University Press.

Staiti A. (2011). "Different Worlds and Tendency to Concordance: Towards a New Perspective on Husserl's Phenomenology of Culture." *The New Yearbook for Phenomenology and Phenomenological Philosophy* 10: 127–143.

Steinbock A. (1995). *Home and Beyond: Generative Phenomenology After Husserl*. Evanston: Northwestern University Press.

Steinbock A. (2003). "Generativity and the Scope of Generative Phenomenology." In D. Welton (ed.), *The New Husserl: A Critical Reader*, pp. 289–325. Indianapolis: Indiana University Press.

Svenaeus F. (2014). "The Body Uncanny: Alienation, Illness, and Anorexia Nervosa." In L. Käll (ed.), *Feminist Phenomenology and Medicine*, pp. 201–222. New York: SUNY Press.

Svenaeus F. (2018). *Phenomenological Bioethics: Medical Technologies, Human Suffering, and the Meaning of Being Alive*. London: Routledge.

Taipale J. (2010). "Normalität." In H-H. Gander (ed.), *Husserl-Lexikon*, pp. 212–214. Darmstadt: Wissenschaftliche Buchgesellschaft.

Taipale J. (2012). "Twofold Normality: Husserl and the Normative Relevance of Primordial Constitution." *Husserl Studies* 28: 49–60.

Taipale J. (2014). *Phenomenology and Embodiment: Husserl and the Constitution of Subjectivity*. Evanston: Northwestern University Press.

Tani T. (2004). "Life and the Life-World." In D. Moran and L. Embree (eds.), *Phenomenology: Critical Concepts in Philosophy IV: Expanding Horizons of Phenomenology*, pp. 399–417. London and New York: Routledge/Taylor & Francis

Waldenfels B. (2004). "Homeworld and Alienworld." In D. Moran and L. Embree (eds.), *Phenomenology: Critical Concepts in Philosophy IV: Expanding Horizons of Phenomenology*, pp. 280–291. London and New York: Routledge/Taylor & Francis.

Wehrle M. (2010). "Die Normativität der Erfahrung." *Husserl Studies* 26: 167–187.

von Wright G. (1963). *The Varieties of Goodness*. London: Routledge & Kegan Paul.

SECTION THREE

KEY CONCEPTS

SECTION EDITORS: MATTHEW R. BROOME
AND GIOVANNI STANGHELLINI

CHAPTER 34

....

SELF

....

DAN ZAHAVI

INTRODUCTION

....

WHY an entry on the self in a handbook on phenomenological psychopathology? The answer is obvious. Many of the central figures in classical psychiatry considered disorders of the self to play a prominent role in a variety of psychopathological phenomena. Consider, for instance, Jaspers who back in 1913 employed the notion of *Ichstörungen* (self-disorders) in his account of schizophrenia or Minkowski who decades later wrote: "The madness . . . does not originate in the disorders of judgment, perception or will, but in a disturbance of the innermost structure of the self" (Minkowski 1997: 114). In contemporary phenomenological psychopathology, Josef Parnas and Louis Sass have developed such ideas further by arguing that schizophrenia involves transformations and alterations of the very basic sense of self and that such self-disorders may be ascribed a generating, pathogenic role. They antecede, underlie, and shape the emergence of later and psychotic pathology and may thus unify what, from a purely descriptive psychiatric standpoint, may seem to be unrelated or even antithetical syndromes and symptoms (Sass and Parnas 2003).

Both Sass and Parnas explicitly affirm their commitment to a phenomenological understanding of selfhood (cf. Sass 2000; Parnas 2003). The self has been discussed extensively in phenomenological philosophy, however. Indeed, even a quick survey will reveal a plethora of partially overlapping, complementary and at times conflicting notions and definitions of the self in the works of such authors as Husserl, Scheler, Heidegger, Gurwitsch, Stein, Sartre, Merleau-Ponty, Henry, etc. In the following short overview, a selection is consequently required. My aim will be to highlight some of those aspects and ideas that have been taken up by and been of inspiration to psychiatrists (for a more extensive treatment cf. Zahavi 1999, 2003, 2005, 2014).

PRE-REFLECTIVE FOR-ME-NESS

....

One way to pinpoint some of the central phenomenological insights concerning selfhood is to proceed *via negativa*. What conception of self do the phenomenologists typically reject? Two different ideas come to mind: 1) According to one classical conception, the self must be considered a transcendental principle of unity. It is a necessary precondition for synchronically and diachronically ordered experiences, but it is not itself a datum of experience. We can infer that it must exists, but it is not itself experientially present. Were it given, it would be given for someone, that is, it would be an object and therefore no longer a self (cf. Natorp 1912). 2) According to another currently popular approach, there is nothing primitive or fundamental about selves, rather they are the outcome of complicated processes of social constructions, being more a matter of politics and culture, than of science and nature.

In contrast to both of these proposals, most phenomenologists would defend the experiential presence of the self; it is a fundamental and pre-reflective feature or character or dimension of experience rather than some high-level social construct or hidden non-experiential transcendental precondition.

Let me provide a few examples from the corpus of phenomenological writings to substantiate this claim. In the lecture course *Grundprobleme der Phänomenologie* from 1919/20, for instance, Heidegger argues that any worldly experiencing involves a certain component of self-acquaintance and self-familiarity, any experiencing is characterized by the fact that "I am always somehow acquainted with myself" (Heidegger 1993: 251). This self-acquaintance is not occurring outside of or independently of my worldly engagement, rather the self-acquaintance is only to be found in intentional life, that is, self-acquaintance is always the self-acquaintance of a world-immersed self. When looking at concrete life experience we will consequently come across a co-givenness of self and world. Or as Heidegger writes in a later lecture course, the "co-disclosure of the self belongs to intentionality" as such (Heidegger 1988: 158).

Another recurrent idea in the phenomenological literature is that the primary manifestation of self is pre-reflective rather than reflective or introspective. This is also an idea we find in Heidegger:

> Dasein, as existing, is there for itself, even when the ego does not expressly direct itself to itself in the manner of its own peculiar turning around and turning back, which in phenomenology is called inner perception as contrasted with outer. The self is there for the Dasein itself without reflection and without inner perception, *before* all reflection. Reflection, in the sense of a turning back, is only a mode of self-*apprehension*, but not the mode of primary self-disclosure.
>
> (Heidegger 1988: 159)

We find a related conception in Merleau-Ponty, who writes that we at the root of all our experiences and all our reflections find a being who immediately knows itself, not by observation, not by inference, but through direct contact with its own existence (Merleau-Ponty 2012: 390). But as he then also goes on to say, "there is no 'inner man,' man is in and toward the world, and it is in the world that he knows himself" (Merleau-Ponty 2012: lxxiv).

Similar ideas can also be found in Husserl and Sartre. For both of them, consciousness is fundamentally characterized by intentionality. It is this intentional life that is at one and the same time self-involving and world-disclosing. This involvement already occurs pre-reflectively and must be considered an essential and constitutive feature of experience. As Sartre writes:

> It is not reflection which reveals the consciousness reflected-on to itself. Quite the contrary, it is the non-reflective consciousness which renders the reflection possible; there is a pre-reflective cogito which is the condition of the Cartesian cogito.
>
> (Sartre 2003: 9)

> This self-consciousness we ought to consider not as a new consciousness, but as *the only mode of existence which is possible for a consciousness of something.*
>
> (Sartre 2003: 10)

> [P]re-reflective consciousness is self-consciousness. It is this same notion of *self* which must be studied, for it defines the very being of consciousness.
>
> (Sartre 2003: 100)

As for Husserl, he often argues that the stream of consciousness is characterized by a "Für-sich-selbst-erscheinens," that is, by a self-appearance or self-manifestation (Husserl 1959: 189, 412, 2001: 44, 46). Husserl also speaks of an "inner consciousness" which is a non-thematic and non-objectifying form of self-awareness that precedes reflection (Husserl 1952: 118), and insists that conscious life has the general structure *ego-cogito-cogitatum* (Husserl 1950: §14, 1954: §50). When being intentionally directed at an object, we are never conscious of it *simpliciter*, but always of the object as appearing in a certain way, say, as judged, seen, hoped, feared, remembered, smelled, anticipated, tasted, etc. The same object, with the exact same worldly properties, can present itself in a variety of manners. It can be given as perceived, imagined, or recollected, etc. But when articulating the character of our experiential life, it is not sufficient merely to consider the intentional object and the intentional act. Experiences are not simply states that happen to occur anonymously; they are all characterized by their irreducible first-person character; they are like something *for me*. Experiences are in short Janus-faced: they are of something other than the subject and they are like something for the subject. There is always a genitive and dative of manifestation.

As should be clear by now, when the phenomenologists are discussing selfhood, they are typically not preoccupied with a question that has dominated much of the discussion of personal identity in analytic philosophy, namely the question concerning diachronic persistency: What kind of features (if any) allows P_2 at t_2 to be identical with P_1 at t_1? Rather their basic interest concerns the relation between consciousness, self-consciousness, and selfhood. Consider Gurwitsch's classical distinction between an egological and a non-egological theory of (self)consciousness (Gurwitsch 1941). Whereas an *egological* theory would claim that when I watch a movie by Hitchcock, I am not only intentionally directed at the *movie*, nor merely aware of the movie being *watched*, I am also aware that it is being watched by *me*, a *non-egological* theory would omit the reference to a subject of experience and simply say that there is an awareness of the watching of the movie. Or as Lichtenberg phrased it in his classical objection to Descartes: we only know of the existence of our sensations, ideas, and thoughts. Experiences simply take place, and that is all. To say cogito and to affirm the existence of an I is already to say too much (Lichtenberg 2000: 190).

What eventually dawned on a number of phenomenologists was that one might deny that each and every experience contains an explicit reference to an ego, understood as an inhabitant in or possessor of consciousness, without opting for the view that our experiential life is anonymous. Rather than being impersonal, consciousness remains characterized by a basic dimension of selfhood precisely because of its ubiquitous self-consciousness. To quote the central passage from Sartre once again: "pre-reflective consciousness is self-consciousness. It is this same notion of self which must be studied, for it defines the very being of consciousness" (Sartre 2003: 100). Or as Michel Henry would put it, the most basic form of selfhood is the one constituted by the very self-manifestation of experience (Henry 1963: 581, 1965: 53). Thus, rather than defining self-consciousness on the basis of a preconceived notion of the self, the notion of self is derived from a correct understanding of self-consciousness. Pre-reflective self-consciousness does not amount to a consciousness of a separate and distinct self. But pre-reflective self-consciousness is ineliminable first person, and that is all that is needed in order to warrant the notion of an experiential self (cf. Zahavi 2009, 2014). To use vocabulary from analytic philosophy of mind, one might say that experience necessarily involves what-it-is-likeness, and experiential what-it-is-likeness is necessarily what-it-is-like-*for-me*-ness (Zahavi and Kriegel 2016).

Even Husserl, who famously opted for and operated with a variety of different notions of ego, would not have disagreed. Husserl's notion of *pure ego* is, as he writes, not something secret or mysterious, but simply a name for the subject of experience (Husserl 1952: 97). The stream of consciousness is not a mere bundle of experiences, rather all experiencing is the experiencing of a subject that does not stream like its experiences (Husserl 1952: 103, 277). But although the pure ego must be distinguished from the experiences in which it lives and functions, it cannot in any way exist independently of or be thought in separation from them (and vice versa) (Husserl 1952: 98–99, 1976: 123–124).

One can see the phenomenological proposal as occupying a middle position between two opposing views. According to the first view, the self is some kind of unchanging soul substance that is distinct from and ontologically independent of the worldly objects and conscious episodes it is directed at and the subject of. According to the second view, there is nothing to consciousness apart from a manifold or bundle of changing experiences. There are experiences and perceptions, but no experiencer or perceiver. A third option is available, however, the moment one realizes that an understanding of what it means to be a self calls for an examination of the structure of experience, and vice versa. Thus, *the experiential self* is not a separately existing entity, it is not something that exists independently of, in separation from or in opposition to the stream of consciousness, but neither is it simply reducible to a specific experience or (sub-)set of experiences; nor is it for that matter a mere social construct that evolves through time. Rather, and to repeat, the (minimal or experiential) self can be identified with the ubiquitous first-person character of the experiential phenomena (Zahavi 2014). The experiential self is consequently, and very importantly, not some experiential object. It is not as if there is a self-object in addition to all the other objects in one's experiential field. Rather the claim is that all of these objects, when experienced, are given in a distinctly first-person way. In short, if we want to "locate" the experiential self, we shouldn't look at *what* is being experienced, but at *how* it is being experienced.

The account just given only constitutes the starting point of a phenomenological exploration of self, however, and it has been further developed in various directions by different phenomenologists. Whereas the link between intentionality and selfhood has been emphasized, it is, for instance, natural also to inquire into the relationship between selfhood and embodiment or selfhood and temporality. With a few noticeable exceptions (Michel Henry comes to mind), most phenomenologist have also emphasized the embodied and temporal character of the self. The short argument being that if experience is essentially embodied and temporal, so is selfhood. In addition, few of the phenomenologists have thought that this rather thin notion of self—as Stein remarks at one point, "the pure 'I' has no depth" (Stein 2008: 110)—could stand alone and have tried to complement it with richer notions of self, that to a larger extent incorporates features such as historicity, sociality, and normativity. Sartre has, for instance, discussed how my encounter with others furnishes me with a new ontological dimension (Sartre 2003: 245), and Husserl has argued that the personal ego has a different type of historicity and individuality than the pure ego. The former is constituted through the commitment to specific normative standards, through the establishment of enduring habits, and through the appropriation of others' attitudes toward oneself. Indeed to exist as a person is for Husserl to exist socialized in a communal horizon (Husserl 1952: 204–205, 265–270). I am, in short, not merely a pure and formal subject of experience, but also a person with abilities, dispositions, habits, interests, character traits, and convictions, and to focus exclusively on the former is to engage in an abstraction (Husserl 1962: 210).

PATHOLOGY OF SELF

Let me in conclusion return to pathology. Even if self and consciousness ordinarily go together, might pathology (for instance, cases of thought insertion) present us with relevant exceptions, that is, with cases where experiences are anonymous and unowned in that they lack for-me-ness altogether? This is a view that has been defended by some (cf. Metzinger 2003; Lane 2012). But even though inserted thoughts are felt as intrusive and strange, it is not obvious that they lack ownership altogether, since the afflicted subject remains aware that it is he himself rather than somebody else who is experiencing these alien thoughts. Claiming that the experiences of a patient suffering from thought insertion do not entirely lack first-person character and that such phenomena do not involve a complete effacement of for-me-ness is not, however, to deny that the clinician should recognize that schizophrenia does, in fact, involve a fragile and unstable first-person perspective. But there is an important difference between claiming that thought insertion exemplifies a state-of-mind with no for-me-ness, and saying that the for-me-ness that is retained is frail (cf. Parnas and Sass 2011: 532). Frail in what sense? In the sense that the patient no longer simply takes the for-me-ness for granted, it has lost some of its normal obviousness, familiarity, and unquestionability, and doesn't effortlessly lead to or permit reflective self-ascription (Sass and Parnas 2003: 430). In other words, we are clearly dealing with a kind of self-alienation or alienated self-consciousness, but as these phrasings also make clear, some dimension of self and self-consciousness remains preserved.

One lesson to learn is that we might have to distinguish more carefully between two different phenomenological claims: a minimalist one and a more robust one (cf. Zahavi 2014). On the minimalist reading, the for-me-ness of experience simply refers to the subjectivity of experience, to the fact that the experiences are pre-reflectively self-conscious and thereby present in a distinctly subjective manner, a manner that is not available to anybody else. This feature is arguably retained in the pathological cases. On a slightly more robust reading, the for-me-ness of experience can refer to a sense of endorsement and self-familiarity; to the quality of "warmth and intimacy," that James claimed characterizes our own present thoughts (James 1890: 239). This feature can be disturbed and perhaps even be completely absent in certain forms of pathology.

BIBLIOGRAPHY

Gurwitsch A. (1941). "A Non-Egological Conception of Consciousness." *Philosophy and Phenomenological Research* 1(3): 325–338.

Heidegger M. (1988). *The Basic Problems of Phenomenology*, trans. A. Hofstadter. Bloomington & Indianapolis: Indiana University Press.

Heidegger M. (1993). *Grundprobleme der Phänomenologie (1919/1920)*. Gesamtausgabe Band 58. Frankfurt am Main: Vittorio Klostermann.

Henry M. (1963). *L'essence de la manifestation*. Paris: Presses Universitaires de France.

Henry M. (1965). *Philosophie et phénoménologie du corps*. Paris: Presses Universitaires de France.

Husserl E. (1950). *Cartesianische Meditationen und Pariser Vorträge*. Husserliana I. Den Haag: Martinus Nijhoff.

Husserl E. (1952). *Ideen zu einer reinen Phänomenologie und phänomenologischen Philosophie. Zweites Buch. Phänomenologische Untersuchungen zur Konstitution*. Husserliana 4. Den Haag: Martinus Nijhoff.

Husserl E. (1954). *Die Krisis der europäischen Wissenschaften und die transzendentale Phänomenologie. Eine Einleitung in die phänomenologische Philosophie*. Husserliana 6. Den Haag: Martinus Nijhoff.

Husserl E. (1959). *Erste Philosophie (1923/24). Zweiter Teil. Theorie der phänomenologischen Reduktion*. Husserliana 8. Den Haag: Martinus Nijhoff.

Husserl E. (1962). *Phänomenologische Psychologie. Vorlesungen Sommersemester 1925*. Husserliana 9. Den Haag: Martinus Nijhoff.

Husserl E. (1976). *Ideen zu einer reinen Phänomenologie und phänomenologischen Philosophie. Erstes Buch. Allgemeine Einführung in die reine Phänomenologie*. Husserliana 3. Den Haag: Martinus Nijhoff.

Husserl E. (2001). *Die "Bernauer Manuskripte" über das Zeitbewußtsein (1917/18)*. Husserliana 33. Dordrecht: Kluwer Academic Publishers.

James W. (1890). *The Principles of Psychology*. London: Macmillan and Co.

Jaspers K. (1913). *Allgemeine Psychopathologie*. Berlin: Springer.

Lane T. (2012). "Toward an Explanatory Framework for Mental Ownership." *Phenomenology and the Cognitive Sciences* 11(2): 251–286.

Lichtenberg G. C. (2000). *The Waste Books*, trans. R. J. Hollingdale. New York: The New York Review of Books.

Merleau-Ponty M. (2012). *Phenomenology of Perception*, trans. D. A. Landes. London: Routledge.

Metzinger T. (2003). *Being No One*. Cambridge, MA: MIT Press

Minkowski E. (1997). "Du symptome au trouble générateur." In *Au-delà du rationalisme morbide*, pp. 93–124. Paris: Éditions l'Harmattan.

Natorp P. (1912). *Allgemeine Psychologie*. Tübingen: J.C.B. Mohr.

Parnas J. (2003). "Self and Schizophrenia: A Phenomenological Perspective." In T. Kircher and A. David (eds.), *The Self in Neuroscience and Psychiatry*, pp. 217–241. Cambridge: Cambridge University Press.

Parnas J. and Sass L. A. (2011). "The Structure of Self-Consciousness in Schizophrenia." In S. Gallagher (ed.), *The Oxford Handbook of the Self*, pp. 521–546. Oxford: Oxford University Press.

Sartre J.-P. (2003). *Being and Nothingness: An Essay in Phenomenological Ontology*, trans. H. E. Barnes. London and New York: Routledge.

Sass L. (2000). "Schizophrenia, Self-experience, and the So-called 'Negative Symptoms.'" In D. Zahavi (ed.), *Exploring the Self*, pp.149–182. Amsterdam: John Benjamins.

Sass L. A. and Parnas J. (2003). "Schizophrenia, Consciousness, and the Self." *Schizophrenia Bulletin* 29(3): 427–444.

Stein E. (2008). *Zum Problem der Einfühlung.* Freiburg: Herder.

Zahavi D. (1999). *Self-Awareness and Alterity: A Phenomenological Investigation.* Evanston: Northwestern University Press.

Zahavi D. (2003). "Phenomenology of Self." In T. Kircher and A. David (eds.), *The Self in Neuroscience and Psychiatry*, pp. 56–75. Cambridge: Cambridge University Press.

Zahavi D. (2005). *Subjectivity and Selfhood: Investigating the First-Person Perspective.* Cambridge, MA: The MIT Press.

Zahavi D. (2009). "Is the Self a Social Construct?" *Inquiry* 52(6): 551–573.

Zahavi D. (2014). *Self and Other: Exploring Subjectivity, Empathy, and Shame.* Oxford: Oxford University Press.

Zahavi D. and Kriegel U. (2016). "For-Me-Ness: What It Is and What It Is Not." In D. O. Dahlstrom, A. Elpidorou, and W. Hopp (eds.), *Philosophy of Mind and Phenomenology: Conceptual and Empirical Approaches*, pp. 36–53. London: Routledge.

CHAPTER 35

···

EMOTION

···

RENÉ ROSFORT

INTRODUCTION

UNDERSTANDING the role of emotions in mental illness is challenging due to the multifarious character of human emotions. Emotions are mental phenomena, and as such they are informed and shaped by the particularly human cognitive makeup involving consciousness, language, and rationality. Emotions are also thoroughly embodied phenomena produced by biological functions that do not require cognition, rationality, or language. Adopting either the biological or the cognitive perspective on emotions has a significant bearing on how one interprets human emotional life, and emotion research in the past century and a half has been dominated by the debate between these two perspectives (de Sousa 2010; Plamper 2012).

Advocates of the biological approach, often neuroscientists and evolutionary psychologists, argue that human emotions are feelings or perceptions of bodily functions. On this approach, our experience of emotions is the result of cross-species biological "affect programs," meaning that humans share several of their so-called "basic" emotional reactions such as fear, surprise, anger, joy, and sadness with other non-human primates. An emotion is a complex conglomeration of chemical and neural responses to the environment that most of the time take place without conscious knowledge. Our experience or feeling of fear, joy, or sadness is a (secondary) function of physiological changes, and the principal to this argument of this approach is that to understand this experience we must examine the biological properties and dynamics at play in this organism-environment relation (e.g. Panksepp 1998; Damasio 2003; Ekman 2003; Prinz 2004). Philosophers, on the other hand, often adopt a conceptual approach arguing that human emotions are to be explained in terms of their rational or cognitive aspects. Although most philosophers, of course, acknowledge that emotions are embodied, biological phenomena, they argue that human emotions are characterized by cognitive or intentional structures that require a conceptual approach focusing on beliefs, representations, and rational evaluations. Understanding why we are afraid or why we feel proud, we need to examine the cognitive structures or propositional content of our fear and pride (e.g. Gordon 1987; Nussbaum 2001; Solomon 2007; Morton 2013).

This debate is of particular interest to psychopathology, since it plays into the debate be-tween biologically oriented psychiatry and more cognitive (e.g. psychological, anthropolog-ical, social) approaches to mental illness (Borch-Jacobsen 2009: 185–196; Zachar 2014; Maj 2016;). Conceiving emotions as either basically biological or primarily cognitive phenomena determines the ensuing psychopathological interpretation of mental disturbances in the sense that one explains these disturbances as the result of either biological dysfunctions or cognitive problems. Phenomenology provides an alternative perspective on emotions that brackets the question of biological or cognitive priority in order to make explanatory room for investigations of the experience of emotion. This, in turn, allows phenomenological psy-chopathology to use the lived experience of mental disturbances as the starting point for the examination and treatment of mental suffering.

THE EXISTENTIAL SIGNIFICANCE OF HOW WE FEEL

The phenomenological approach to emotions found its conceptual beginning, as is the case with many phenomenological topics, in Heidegger's methodological reworking of Husserl's phenomenology. While Husserl's phenomenology focused on complex analyses of experi-ence trying to uncover the experiential structures and dynamics responsible for the consti-tution of world, self, and intersubjectivity, Heidegger criticized this account for ignoring the affective aspect involved in our concrete or factual experience of the world. We do not merely experience the world. We are engaged in the world, and our experience is qualified by our affective being-in-the-world. This means that we cannot clarify, let alone make sense of, our experience by disregarding of our felt encounter with the world or to suspending the affective resonance of our experiences. We need to substitute, Heidegger argues, the strict phenomenological approach with an existential analysis that takes seriously the affective dimension of human experience (e.g. Heidegger 1988: 227; Heidegger 1999: 16; Heidegger 2001: 84–87).[1]

The affective dimension is important for Heidegger because of the existential significance of how we feel. Two interconnected notions, *mood* and *attunement*, are fundamental for Heidegger's analysis (Heidegger 2010: 134–142). Our experience of and thinking about the world are not neutral but always characterized by a certain mood (*Stimmung*) and a partic-ular way of being attuned to the world and to ourselves (*Befindlichkeit*). In fact, it is the affec-tive character of our experience and thinking that make experience and thinking matter to us. We *exist* in the world, and our existence in the world is constitutionally characterized by our care about *how* we are in the world. The German word *Befindlichkeit* captures two basic aspects of the existential character of our being-in-the-world. We find ourselves *situated* in the world (*sich befinden*), that is, *exposed to* and *engaged with* the world. This being situated in the world, in turn, elicits certain affective experiences revealing how we feel about our

---

[1] The references to Heidegger's works are to the English translation, but the page numbers refer to the authoritative German edition of his complete works (*Martin Heidegger. Gesamtsausgabe*. Frankfurth am Main: Vittorio Klosterman 1975–). The page numbers of the German edition are reproduced at the top of the page in the English translations.

situation (*befinden sich*) by way of certain moods which make "manifest 'how one is and is coming along'" (Heidegger 2010: 134).

Heidegger's analysis of the affective dimension of our experience is shaped by his particular—and one could argue idiosyncratic—interpretation of our being-in-the-world, and, as Herbert Spiegelberg has noted, this hermeneutical foundation can make his analysis of the psychological character of emotional experience "limited and slanted," and "it must not be mistaken for an all-embracing one" (Spiegelberg 1972: 20). The strength of Heidegger's phenomenology of affectivity lies not in his specific analysis of various emotional experiences, which does not go beyond sketchy outlines, but rather in the methodological insistence on the existential significance of how we feel. Heidegger argues convincingly that emotional experience tells us something significant not only about our experience, but more importantly about our life, and in this way his "phenomenological hermeneutics provides the horizon against which man's psyche stands out in depth" (Spiegelberg 1972: 21).

Heidegger's insistence on the existential significance of emotional experience echoes Max Scheler's earlier phenomenological exploration of human emotional life. Scheler's theory revolves around the idea that the various aspects of emotional experience "correspond to the structure of our entire human existence," and "[a]ll 'feelings' possess an experienced related-ness to the I (or the person)" (Scheler 1973: 332; translation slightly modified). But while Scheler makes emotional experience the heart of a philosophical anthropology, Heidegger rejects the idea of a philosophical anthropology. There are several reasons for this rejection, but it is probably connected with two basic aspects of Heidegger's philosophy: on the one hand, his general refusal of diluting or contaminating the purity of philosophical inquiry with empirical disciplines such as biology and psychology and, on the other, his reluctance to reduce the onto-logical exploration of philosophy to an anthropomorphic enterprise (Heidegger 1997: 207–213).

Subsequent phenomenological generations inherited Heidegger's (and Husserl's) skepticism of empirical investigations, but most contemporary phenomenologists acknowledge that the existential meaning of our emotional life cannot be explored without taking into consideration what Scheler calls the place of the human being in cosmos (Scheler 2009). This means that while Heidegger early on left the existential analysis to deal with questions about fundamental ontology or being in general, the succeeding phenomenological tradition has used his methodology rather unorthodoxly to investigate central aspects of philosophical anthropology such as, among other things, the body, imagination, habits, values, and sociocultural norms (e.g. Sartre 1994; Bollnow 1941; Strasser 1977; Ricoeur 1987; Schmitz 1989; Fuchs 2000; Ratcliffe 2008; Stanghellini and Rosfort 2013). The reason for this seems obvious. As Heidegger himself argued, the affective dimension of experience reveals that our experiences matter to us. Emotions are existential phenomena characterized by the way they touch or affect us (Latin *afficere*) and how they move us (Latin *emovere*) to feel, think, or act in a particular way. They express our care about the world, ourselves, and other people, and it is thus difficult, if not impossible, to investigate emotional experience without interpreting how we feel our emotions.

DESCRIBING AND INTERPRETING

Fundamental to the phenomenological approach to emotion is the argument that the interpretation of the existential significance of our feelings, that is, *why* we feel the way we do, has to begin with a systematic description of *how* we feel. The methodological awareness of the task of working out the dialectics between interpreting and describing a feeling (our own or that of another person) is part of what distinguishes the phenomenological approach from the cognitive and biological approaches to emotions. The distinction between these two aspects of our understanding of emotions is based on the acknowledgment that description is interpretation. The phenomenological description is not simply a description of phenomena, but a theoretical constructed description aimed at articulating significant features of immediate or pre-reflective experience. Phenomenology does not purport to present a completely accurate or comprehensive description of the immediate feeling of an emotional experience. As Stephan Strasser argues, the epistemological problem of emotions is that at the core of emotional experience are affective impressions that are not easily rationalized or conceptually grasped. These affective impressions present "a not-fully-rationalizable form of apprehending reality [*Wirklichkeiterfassung*]," and "the echo of feeling [*Gefühlswiderhall*] which an object produces thus immediately predispose us before any knowledge of facts has intervened as complement and as mediation" (Strasser 1977: 132–133; translation slightly modified). On the other hand, we cannot describe emotional experiences without pre-established knowledge, concepts, and words. The acknowledgment of this dialectics explains why we need to suspend our conceptions or preconceived interpretation of reality in order to describe the experience of reality. Although we cannot descriptively capture the feeling of an emotion, our descriptive endeavors can be more or less distorting, and the methodological distinction between description and interpretation provides us, so the phenomenological argument goes, with a more accurate picture of a person's emotional experience. This methodological distinction is also the reason why phenomenological accounts of emotions normally start with the broad and amorphous concept of affectivity rather than the concepts of emotion, feeling, passion, sentiment, sensation, and moods. To categorize our affective as emotions, sensations, passions, moods, or sentiments is a matter of interpretation. Our emotional vocabulary has undergone significant changes over the last century, and our emotional concepts are constantly shaped by the dominant sociocultural norms (Dixon 2003). The phenomenological destabilization of established emotional vocabulary is thus part of the suspension of preconceived interpretations in order to describe the pre-reflective experience of emotions.

In other words, if our interpretation of a person's emotions is not anchored in a systematic description of how the particular person actually feels, we risk interpreting that person's feelings through our own preconceptions and ideas about what those feelings mean rather than allowing the person's experience to shape and guide our interpretation.

EMOTIONS, SENSATIONS, AND MOODS

Phenomenological accounts of emotions share a basic distinction between intentional and non-intentional feeling. This is not surprising given the central role that the concept of intentionality plays in phenomenology. Experience is not disembodied registration of indifferent phenomena, but permeated by structured and embodied relations to phenomena embedded in a context that procures significance to experience. Experiencing is to experience something, and the concept of intentionality allows us to investigate this pre-reflective rela-tion between our experience and the phenomena that we experience. Intentionality, in other words, discloses the constitutional interdependence of world and mind, and examining the intentional structures and dynamics of experience provides a methodological means to es-cape preconceived distinctions between mind and world, the internal and the external, sub-ject and object, that characterize other philosophical approaches to the human mind.

Human emotional life is not an amorphous conglomeration of feelings, but experi-enced as a structured engagement with the world. We do not merely feel. Our feelings are constitutive of how we perceive, move, think, and act in the world. The distinction between intentional and non-intentional emotional experiences is based upon the ex-periential fact that many of our feelings are experienced as structured phenomena that relate us to something other than ourselves. These structured affective phenomena are what we typically understand as emotions, for example, love, surprise, hate, jealousy, pride, shame, and ambition. What characterizes these structured affective phenomena or emotions is that they are directed at objects and express our personal engagement in and with the world. As Paul Ricoeur argues, "[F]eeling [*sentiment*] interiorizes reason and shows me that reason is my reason, for through it I appropriate reason for myself . . . In short, feeling reveals the identity of existence and reason: it personalizes reason" (Ricoeur 1987: 102). My feelings of gratitude, love, or anger are directed at someone or something, and this intentional structure provides the framework for a systematic analysis of our emotions in terms of temporality (how long do the feelings last?), embodiment (how do they make me feel?), relation (at who or what are they directed?), and context (in which situation do they occur?). This intentional analysis allows us to explore and interpret how emotions disclose our being-in-the-world, and although we are affected by these feelings pre-reflectively, they move our thinking, are a constitutional part of our understanding, and motivate our actions.

Not all of our feelings are experienced as intentionally structured phenomena, however. There is more at work in our emotional life than the structured emotions that we have names for. The intentional analysis also reveals affective phenomena that are non-intentional, that is, unstructured feelings without a relation to an explicit object or tied to a specific situa-tion. We experience transient bodily sensations and periods of peculiar moods that do not disclose a specific relation to an object or tell us something particular about the situation in which we find ourselves. And yet, they still affect the way we experience the world, other people, and ourselves. These non-intentional feelings can be described in terms of their tem-poral character (e.g. momentary or long-lasting) and the way they affect our experience (e.g. disturbing or encompassing).

Bodily sensations such as pain, discomfort, or pleasure come and go, often undetected, and we become aware of these inchoate sensations because of their disturbing—painful, annoying, or wearisome as well as pleasurable, exciting, or stimulating—effect on our ex-perience. Bodily sensations are non-intentional in the sense that they are closely tied to a complex physiological web of homeostatic regulation or bodily functions that most of the time take place without conscious appraisal. This does not mean, however, that non-intentional sensations are without a significant relation to our conscious emotional life. Stephan Strasser, who provides a careful phenomenological analysis of bodily sensations, understands them as the result of "the pre-intentional functioning of the human being," and he argues that this biological aspect of our emotional life "ought not to be compared with a concealed, buried geological layer. It reaches into the sphere of experience, it intersects with the intentions, it colors itself with its feelings [*Gefühlen*]" (Strasser 1977: 218). Bodily sensations affect *the way* we experience, and although we are often unaware of these sensations or able to disregard them, they are not without existential significance. As Strasser argues: "The pre-intentional life is, on the one hand, more primitive than the intentional one . . . but, on the other hand, it rests upon the forms of function which likewise show themselves receptive to higher contents. Precisely for this reason it is not absurd to think that there are pre-intentional modes of behavior which belongs to the specific possibilities of human existence" (Strasser 1977: 218–219; see also Ricoeur 1966: 85–134; Jaspers 1997: 108–118; Fuchs 2000: 87–150; Stanghellini and Rosfort 2014).

While bodily sensations are normally experienced as transient, circumscribed, and disturbing the attentional foreground of experience, moods, on the other hand, last longer, possess an encompassing character, and are part of the background of experience. Another difference between moods and sensations regards the bodily aspects of these feelings. Like all emotional experiences moods are deeply embodied phenomena, but whereas bodily sensations often make us aware of particular aspects or parts of our body, a mood typically affect our bodily engagement with the world, that is, the way our body as an organ for our interaction with the world. When my arm itches or my head hurts my attention is directed to these parts of my body. In anxiety, joy, boredom, or sadness, on the other hand, it is my bodily engagement with the world that is changed. A mood affects my experience of the world to the extent that the experiential distinctions between world, body, self, and other vanish or at least become blurred. It can thus be difficult, if not impossible, to locate the origin or cause of a mood. The feelings involved in a mood expose the merging of inner and outer, my feeling and the atmosphere in which I am situated.

Jaspers describes how this disturbance or collapse of my intentional engagement with the world takes on a dramatic character in delusions: "Everything gets a *new meaning* [*eine neue Bedeutsamkeit*]. The environment is somehow different—not to a gross degree—perception is unaltered in itself but there is some change which envelops everything with a subtle, pervasive and strangely uncertain light. A living-room which was formerly felt as neutral or friendly now becomes dominated by some indefinable mood [*Stimmung*]" (Jaspers 1997: 98 [82]; translation slightly modified). Klaus Conrad points to the experiential feature of mood in the prodromal stages of schizophrenia in his seminal analysis of the so-called *Trema*:

> The very background from which palpable things arise has lost its neutrality. What makes us tremble are not the trees and the bushes that we see, neither is it the whisper in the treetops nor the ululation of the owl that we hear, rather all that constitutes the background, all the surrounding space [*Umraum*] from which trees and bushes, whisper and ululation arise: they are precisely *the very obscurity and background*
>
> (Conrad 1958: 41; my translation)

As these descriptions of Jaspers and Conrad show, changes in our mood have a global transformative effect on our experience, and this global character entails that disturbances of our mood can have a dramatic effect on our understanding of the fundamental significance of experience of reality (Heidegger 2010: 186). It is, in other words, reality, and our place in reality, that is at stake in moods.

Making Sense of Emotional Experience

This phenomenological typology of three basic types of emotional experiences—emotion, sensations, and moods—is, of course, not an exhaustive description of human emotional life. It is an example of how a phenomenological approach to emotions attempts to start with a structured description of emotional experience. This descriptive attempt is, as mentioned, an interpretation. It is an interpretation, however, aimed at articulating how we feel emotions, that is, how emotions affect our experience of ourselves, other people, and the world. This descriptive articulation of *how* we feel provides a foundation for our more explicit interpretive endeavors to understand *what* emotions are and *why* we feel the way we do. Articulating our emotional experience in terms of intentional emotions and non-intentional bodily sensations and moods discloses a basic interplay of autonomy and heteronomy, or self and otherness, at work in human emotional life. We shape our emotional life in the sense that we use our feelings to orient and inform our engagement with the world. In this sense, we are, as the cognitive approach argues, responsible for our emotions, or at least for how we think about and act on our emotions. On the other hand, though, there are, as the biological approach argues, aspects of our emotional life over which we really do seem to have no control. Bodily sensations are experienced as something that happen to me, an anonymous or otherness beyond my control, while self and otherness are obscurely entangled in moods. A stomach pain or a throbbing headache can disturb our thinking to the extent that we lose control of our actions. A persistent anxiety or protracted sadness can have such a disorienting effect on our thinking that the meaning of our existence collapses. The question of responsibility is always at stake in our emotional life, but it becomes particularly blurred in these non-intentional aspects of our emotional life. The phenomenological description provides us with an articulation of this interplay of autonomous and heteronomous forces at work in our experience of emotions. This descriptive articulation allows the phenomenological approach to investigate how an experience feels before explaining that experience in terms of either cognitive or biological processes.

This phenomenological foundation has the psychopathological advantage over other approaches to emotions—for example, the cognitive or the biological—that it gives explanatory priority to the person's lived experience of emotions. The articulation of *how* a person feels provides the material for the psychopathological interpretation of *why* the person feels the way she does. This priority of the person's experience at the core of phenomenological psychopathology has both diagnostic and therapeutic gains. Diagnostically it allows for a more comprehensive understanding of the emotional aspect of mental disturbances. The complexity of the affective disturbances involved in the mental disturbance is approached with both a nuanced articulation of the feelings themselves and attention to the more comprehensive existential significance of those feelings. This investigation of the interplay of feeling and significance gives both experiential nuance and contextual depth to the interpretation of symptoms. Therapeutically it enables the patient to work with the disturbances of her emotional life through a better understanding of the autonomous and heteronomous aspects of her feelings. An understanding acceptance of the passivity at work in our emotions allows the patient to actively appropriate this otherness that is out of her control and incorporate it into her existence. As Wolfgang Blankenburg argues in relation to anxiety disorders, this understanding of the ambiguity of passivity and activity in anxiety teaches the patient "not to turn his back to anxiety, but instead of running from it have the 'courage to be anxious' or summon up the *why* of anxiety. This free repetition out of one's own intention, that is, a free confrontation with anxiety, can bring out *that which causes anxiety*, and in turn lead to a new 'self-appropriation' [*Sich-selbst-Ergreifen*]" (Blankenburg 1993: 327–328; author's trans.).

The diagnostic and therapeutic advantage of a phenomenological account of emotion stems from the dialectics of description and interpretation of the existential significance of our emotional experience. This does not mean, however, that phenomenological psychopathology can be practiced in isolation form the cognitive and biological investigations of emotions. Emotions disclose what we care about, and structure or disturb our engagement with the world, our relation to ourselves, and interaction with other people. To make sense of this existential significance of our emotions we cannot but combine our phenomenological work with an explicit hermeneutical endeavor (Strasser 1977: 124; Ricoeur 2008). This hermeneutical aspect of phenomenology is primarily aimed at interpreting the existential significance of emotions, but existential significance of our emotional experience cannot be explained merely by our experience of emotions. Emotions are deeply embodied mental phenomena that go beyond our experience of them, and we therefore need both cognitive (philosophical, anthropological, sociological) and biological investigations to make sense of the existential significance of emotions (Stanghellini and Rosfort 2013). The principal phenomenological argument, though, is that these interpretative endeavors must begin with how a person experiences her emotions.

Bibliography

Blankenburg W. (1993). "Affektivität und Personsein aus psychiatrischer Sicht. Am Beispiel von Angst und Hoffung im menschlichen Dasein." In H. Fink-Eitel and G. Lohmann (eds.), *Zur Philosophie der Gefühle*, pp. 307–333. Frankfurt am Main: Suhrkamp.

Bollnow O. F. (1941). *Das Wesen der Stimmungen*. Frankfurt: Klostermann.

Borch-Jacobsen M. (2009). *Making Minds and Madness: From Hysteria to Depression*. Cambridge: Cambridge University Press.

Conrad K. (1958). *Die beginnende Schizophrenie: Versuch einer Gestaltanalyse des Wahns*. Stuttgart: Georg Thieme Verlag.

Damasio A. R. (2003). *Looking for Spinoza. Joy, Sorrow, and the Feeling Brain*. London: Heinemann.

de Sousa R. (2010). "The Mind's Bermuda Triangle: Philosophy of Emotions and Empirical Science." In P. Goldie (ed.), *The Oxford Handbook of Philosophy of Emotions*, pp. 93–117. Oxford: Oxford University Press.

Dixon T. (2003). *From Passions to Emotions: The Creation of a Secular Psychological Category*. Cambridge: Cambridge University Press.

Ekman P. (2003). *Emotions Revealed: Understanding Faces and Feelings*. London: Weidenfeld & Nicolson.

Fuchs T. (2000). *Leib, Raum, Person. Entwurf einer phänomenologischen Anthropologie*. Stuttgart: Klett-Cotta.

Gordon R. M. (1987). *The Structure of Emotions: Investigations in Cognitive Philosophy.* Cambridge: Cambridge University Press.

Heidegger M. (1988). *The Basic Problems of Phenomenology*, trans. A. Hofstadter. Bloomington: Indiana University Press.

Heidegger M. (1997). *Kant and the Problem of Metaphysics*, trans. R. Taft. Bloomington: Indiana University Press.

Heidegger, M. (1999). *Ontology—The Hermeneutics of Facticity*, trans. J. van Burren. Bloomington: Indiana University Press.

Heidegger M. (2001). *Phenomenological Interpretations of Aristoteles: Initiations into Phenomenological Research*, trans. R. Rojcewicz. Bloomington: Indiana University Press.

Heidegger M. (2010). *Being and Time*, trans. J. Stambaugh and revised by D. J. Schmidt. New York: State University of New York Press.

Jaspers K. (1997). *General Psychopathology*, trans. J. Hoenig and M. W. Hamilton. Baltimore: John Hopkins University Press.

Maj M. (2016). "The Need for a Conceptual Framework in Psychiatry Acknowledging Complexity While Avoiding Defeatism" (Editorial). *World Psychiatry* 15: 1–2.

Morton A. (2013). *Emotion and Imagination.* Cambridge: Polity.

Nussbaum M. C. (2001). *Upheavals of Thought: The Intelligence of Emotions.* Cambridge: Cambridge University Press; Evanston: Northwestern University Press.

Panksepp J. (1998). *Affective Neuroscience: The Foundations of Human and Animal Emotions.* Oxford: Oxford University Press.

Plamper Jan (2012). *Geschichte und Gefühl: Grundlagen der Emotionsgeschichte.* München: Siedler Verlag.

Prinz J. J. (2004). *Gut Reactions: A Perceptual Theory of Emotion.* New York: Oxford University Press.

Ratcliffe M. (2008). *Feelings of Being: Phenomenology, Psychiatry and the Sense of Reality.* Oxford: Oxford University Press.

Ricoeur P. (1966). *Freedom and Nature: The Voluntary and the Involuntary*, trans. E. V. Kohák. Evanston: Northwestern University Press.

Ricoeur P. (1987). *Fallible Man*, trans. C. A. Kelbley. New York: Fordham University Press.

Ricoeur P. (2008). "Phenomenology and Hermeneutics." In P. Ricoeur, *From Text to Action: Essays in Hermeneutics II*, trans. K. Blamey and J. B. Thompson, pp. 23–50. London: Continuum.

Sartre J.-P. (1994). *Sketch for a Theory of the Emotions*, trans. P. Mairet. London: Routledge.

Scheler M. (1973). *Formalism in Ethics and Non-Formal Ethics of Value: A New Attempt toward the Foundation of an Ethical Personalism*, trans. M. S. Frings and R. L. Funk. Evanston: Northwestern University Press.

Scheler M. (2009). *The Human Place in Cosmos*, trans. M. S. Frings. Evanston: Northwestern University Press.

Schmitz H. (1989). *Leib und Gefühl. Materialien zur einer philosophichen Therapeutik.* Paderborn: Junfermann.

Solomon R. C. (2007). *True To Our Feelings: What our Emotions Are Really Telling Us.* Oxford: Oxford University Press.

Spiegelberg H. (1972). *Phenomenology in Psychology and Psychiatry: A Historical Introduction.* Evanston: Northwestern University Press.

Stanghellini G. and Rosfort R. (2013). *Emotions and Personhood: Exploring Fragility—Making Sense of Vulnerability.* Oxford: Oxford University Press.

Stanghellini G. and Rosfort R. (2014). "Jaspers on Feelings and Affective States." In T. Fuchs, T. Breyer, and C. Mundt (eds.), *Karl Jaspers' Philosophy and Psychopathology*, pp. 149–168. Dordrecht: Springer.

Strasser S. (1977). *Phenomenology of Feeling: An Essay on the Phenomena of the Heart*, trans. R. E. Wood. Pittsburgh: Duquesne University Press.

Zachar P. (2014). *A Metaphysics of Psychopathology*. Cambridge, MA: The MIT Press.

CHAPTER 36

THE UNCONSCIOUS IN PHENOMENOLOGY

ROBERTA LANFREDINI

PHENOMENOLOGY AND THE OBJECTIFYING ATTITUDE

THE word "phenomenology" is linked to the metaphor of light. Almost all its notions imply a shedding of light onto something: phenomenon, manifestation, evidence, clarity, distinction, perspective, part, datum, essence. In phenomenology we also speak of interior gaze, of intentional putting into focus, of attentional ray, of intuitive replenishment. Seeing is always seeing something. And seeing something means enclosing, limiting in relation to a background. Viewing also has the task of abstracting: abstraction isolates and, hence, illuminates certain properties, putting others into the shade. In Husserl's phenomenology, the concept which expresses better than any other this "irradiating" of consciousness is intentionality (Husserl 1900–1). Any phenomenon is always related to a state of consciousness; no objects exist that are not in the cone of light of an intentional *Erlebnis*. So Husserl proposes an objectifying attitude, "the Ego is, in an eminent sense, directed toward the objectively given, is abandoned to what is objective" (Husserl 1912–1929: 12). This thesis, which indicates an undiscussed priority of the theoretical attitude, is moderated by the acknowledgment of the fact, fundamental for introducing a possible phenomenology of the unconscious, that the objectifying attitude is founded on a terrain of passivity, pre-categoriality, pre-givenness, a terrain which Husserl does not hesitate to call "confused."

Every spontaneous act, after being performed, necessarily passes over into a confused state; the spontaneity, or if you will, the activity, to speak of it more properly, passes into a passivity, although of such a kind that (. . .) it refers back to the originally spontaneous and articulated performance. This reference back is characterized as such by the I-can or the faculty, which evidently belongs to it, to "reactivate" this state (Husserl 1912–1929: 13–14).

And yet, for Husserl, there exists the possibility of "reactivating" the "non-objectifying" (implicit, tacit, passive) dimension, that same dimension which will later become central in the Heideggerian notion of Dasein, rendering it objectifying (explicit, manifest, active), thanks to a modification of the attitude which renders possible the continuous interpenetration of the two spheres. This means interpreting non-objectifying acts as potentially convertible into objectifying acts. Thus, the theoretical object "reveals" its passivity and, on the other hand, the stratum of passivity (confused, indeterminate) always has the possibility of passing over into its active double. Something similar occurs in the distinction, fundamental in phenomenology, between *actuality* and *inactuality* [*Inaktualität*] or, if we wish, between object and background. In this case, too, as in that of the distinction between passivity and activity, the possibility is revealed of one dimension pouring into the other.

It is the essence of a waking Ego's stream of mental processes that the continuously unbroken chain of cogitations is continually surrounded by a medium of non-actionality which is always ready to change into the mode of actionality just as, conversely, actionality is always ready to change into non-actionality (Husserl 1912–1929: 72–73).

The distinction between passivity and activity on the one hand and between actuality and inactuality on the other offers us two types of consideration. The first is that consciousness never consists solely in activity or solely in actuality.

It is likewise obviously true of all such mental processes that the actional ones are surrounded by a "halo" of non-actional mental processes (Husserl 1912–1929: 72).

The second consideration is that every state of passive or inactual consciousness can always, as an essential law, re-emerge into activity or actuality; and hence can re-enter the grasp of the "awakened Ego." Passivity, or inactuality, as *modifications* of activity and actuality, are derived from and subordinate to the latter pair. The priority of attention, putting into focus, the Ego's grasp on the tacit horizon, once again confirms the priority of light over darkness.

THE DARK DIMENSION OF SUBJECTIVITY: THE PHENOMENON OF RETENTION

The general question which must be addressed is whether phenomenology is capable of conceiving and making functional a more substantial and incompatible darkness. Because this happens it is necessary for the phenomenological description to allow for the possibility of being free from the "grasp" of an "awakened," vigilant, present "I." That is, an "I" for whom the world opens up as his or her *own* world, and for whom what is hidden, or vague, or inaccessible becomes such in that it is located on the horizon of what the gaze actually "seizes." The word horizon is significant because it implies the centrality of the notion of *representation* at the expense of the notion of *immersion*. Speaking of requires addressing the problem by using a register that is no longer static and spatial (passivity as pre-categorical; inactuality as background, or halo) but dynamic and temporal. Immersion in fact implies a continuous slippage of the present into the just-been and, for this reason, a continuous difficulty of perceptual "grasp." From this point of view, the continually interpenetrating and mediating relationship between impression and retention renders ungraspable the "now-point" of consciousness. Thus, the lapse of time renders consciousness opaque, posing the problem of a possible unconscious dimension in the very heart of phenomenology (i.e. the temporal flow of consciousness). In fact, within consciousness itself, the lapse of time shows a point of opacity in the intersection between impression and retention, a threshold in which the impression fades, making itself available for the acceptance of un-conscious or, rather, "anonymous" contents. However, the fact remains that, for Husserl, the pre-reflective dimension can only be spoken of in reference to consciousness; which means presupposing once again the centrality and solidity of the intentional structure and the "awakened I." (Husserl 1912–1929, 1913). If, from the phenomenological point of view, consciousness is *everything*, and if it is true that nothing escapes consciousness (nothing of the world and nothing of oneself, temporal form constitutes the display of consciousness itself. The problem is that in this *everything* which unfolds temporally (according to a struc-ture with a retentional perspective, a primary impression and a protentional perspective) a dimension is introduced which is not "present" to consciousness, and which therefore in some way escapes it. In open contrast, it would seem, with the thesis many times reiterated by Husserl, that "everything which we call *object*, of which we speak, which we confront as actuality which we hold as possible or probable, no matter how indeterminately we think it, is precisely therefore already an object of consciousness" (Husserl 1912–1929: 322). The dimension which flees the "radiation" of consciousness is that of affection. This, connected to the *retentional* element, refers to "the entire realm of associations and habits" (Husserl 1912–1929: 233). This realm includes "sensibility, what imposes itself, the pre-given, the driven in the sphere of passivity. What is specific therein is motivated in the obscure back-ground" (Husserl 1912–1929: 234).[1]

What Husserl calls "the case of zero degree affection" (Fuchs 2000; Heller-Roazen 2007) presents implicit motivations, associations, and habits proper to sensibility and impulse, not immediately susceptible to a rational grasp or to irradiation by the awakened con-sciousness. Nevertheless, in *Analysen zur passiven Synthesis* (Husserl 1920–1926; Lohmar 1998), Husserl explicitly declares the possibility of an "intentional capture" even of this silent dimension, by means of the phenomenon of so-called *reawakening*, from which the attempt to realize a "phenomenology of the unconscious" (Bernet 1996, 2003; Depraz 2013; Lohmar and Brudzińska 2012). Freud's thesis, according to which unconscious dream formations do not acknowledge the rules of logic and temporal coherence, and hence constitute a dimension wholly independent of consciousness, is completely denied by Husserl, for whom the unconscious is always mediated by intentional consciousness. The phenomenological deformation of the Freudian notion therefore resides in the in-evitability of a reflexive grasp even of those experiences which, on first consideration, seem to be marked by immersion in a complete passivity. The primacy of the passive syn-thetic constitutions "fills" the space of an "unconscious of consciousness" which forms part of the temporal structure of consciousness: that is, the place in which consciousness becomes opaque and resides in the impression of retention being diminished, in its be-coming obscure and plunging into indistinctness. This "diminution" of the impression of retention is also a matter of consciousness. The "lived unconscious" is always mediated by reflection, and the passive, anonymous consciousness is always susceptible of being explicated by the awakened I. Retentions, considered in themselves, are not intentional.

---

[1] The reference to psychoanalysis is explicit here: "The 'motives'" are often deeply buried but can be brought to light by 'psychoanalysis.' A thought 'reminds' me of other thoughts and calls back into memory a past lived experience, etc. In some cases it can be perceived. In most cases, however, the motivation is indeed actually present in consciousness, but it does not stand out; it is unnoticed or unnoticeable ('unconscious')" (Husserl 1912–1929: 234).

In fact, in restraining the perceptual present, making it slip into the "just-been" before sinking into the more distant horizon of consciousness, they do not offer a genuine "past." The only act capable of offering the past in its true sense is remembering, which, by means of the phenomenon of associative reawakening, permits the retentions sunk in the past to "reawaken," making them emerge intentionally. Therefore, the retentions, becoming ever more distant, continue to subsist as a passive stratum of consciousness, and in a certain sense independently of conscious "grasp"; though the fact remains that this grasp is always free to reactivate the sunken retentions by means of association, making them emerge as "past" through the phenomenon of reawakening. The reactivation of the retentional flow brings the now "past" object back to the actuality of consciousness, giving it back its "sense": an object as an object (*ein Gegestand als Gegenstand*) gives itself uniquely for use by an active consciousness, and the passive contents must, if they are not to vanish in the unity of consciousness, avoid the retentional sinking into an unconscious that is, so to speak, absolute. In this sense, affection will never be pure passivity, but always passivity energized by some activity, and the reawakening through memory takes on the appearance of a reflexive revolution with respect to a pre-constituted whole, one therefore predisposed to emerge from the darkness of passivity into the light of activity. Through the phenomenon of reawakening, the unconscious thus becomes, to all intents and purposes, a lived experience of my own. Therefore, it is not only the activity of consciousness which is rooted in passivity, but passivity is already in turn predisposed to activity: that is, to rationality. Husserl's phenomenology of the unconscious brings it back into the domain of the analytic of consciousness. In this schema, everything is directly to the emergence of givenness and to the transparency of consciousness. The unconscious, for all that it is *sunken*, is the "thing" of consciousness.

The conception of the unconscious as strictly anchored to the priority of the impression and to the primary consciousness of the now-point is noted by Michel Henry as one of the most critical points in Husserl's phenomenology. The process in which the now-point, and the impression given in it, change constantly into the past in an uninterrupted slippage, "this continual sinking of being into the abys of a nothingness that continually opens up below it is what gives Husserlian description its fascinating, even hallucinatory character, as well as its incoherence and absurdity" (1990: 30). This incoherence and absurdity resides in reading the continuum of consciousness as an incoherent passage between being and nothing, which has the task of guaranteeing the return to being and its continuous outpouring into an always new now-point that is destined to fall constantly into an ever deeper past. Now, this movement leaves phenomenological description "stumbling like a drunken man," since "one who stands on the crest of the now not only has one foot on the ground and the other in the void but is also continually falling from the ground and into the void" (Henry 1990: 30), thereby rendering this very continuum of consciousness broken and constantly interrupted. The predominance of the primary consciousness of the now thus deprives impression of its function as a *donation*. In fact, affectivity is not the keystone, but the result, the hinge. And it is not the slipping and sinking of the now-point that is grasped by retention, but that "longitudinal intentionality" (Henry 1990: 28) which runs along the whole flow, giving it continuity. Restoring the experience of the past, the just-been, to a primary consciousness entails a considerable shift in the standpoint of phenomenology toward the unconscious. The unconscious is no longer the present incessantly sinking into the past, but the past which incessantly maintains the present.

IT IS FELT IN US: THE IMPERSONAL IN THE FLESH

In Husserl's phenomenology, essentially tied to the present of consciousness, the concept of the unconscious is assimilated into the non-conscious: that is, into what is simply no longer present. Husserl's first preoccupation is to guarantee the "offered-ness" of the perceptual present. Retention itself displays a present in the form of the just-been and not a genuine past. The past to which Husserl refers is always relative to the capacity of the awakened consciousness to illuminate parts of the world and of consciousness itself, mediating that "activity of overview," that attitude to reflective distance which Merleau-Ponty sees as the essential hallmark of Husserlian phenomenology (Merleau-Ponty 1945; Behnke 2002). This is a conception which foregrounds cognitive activities at the expense of ontological ones, representation at the expense of being. According to Merleau-Ponty, the re-designation of the past as such, is revealed in the ontological dimension of phenomenology. It is, in fact, in the notion of incarnation and of *en-être* that Merleau-Ponty discovers the deep reasons of Freudianism. From its very beginnings, phenomenology has been founded on a paradox: on the one hand the subject is *in the world* but not only *of the world*; on the other hand, it is conscious of the world while at the same playing a part in it. All this is translated into the concept of *en-être*; not disembodied consciousness, but organic matter, flesh, *res viva*. In contradiction to Husserl, the visible is not "in front of" the subject, but is "an encompassing, lateral investment, *flesh*" (Merleau-Ponty 1964: 217). Being surrounds, absorbs, passes through the subject. Flesh, as "interiorly worked-over mass" (Merleau-Ponty 1964: 147), thus becomes the ontological characterization of Being and of its many-layered, multifaceted nature, of which the body is one variant. The subject is neither consciousness nor mere intentionality, but "the massive unity of Being . . ., it is the wild, non-refined, vertical Being" (Merleau-Ponty 1964: 202–203), which renders me visible and the things seen: "since vision is a palpation with the look, it must also be inscribed in the order of being that it discloses to us; he who looks must not himself be foreign to the world that he looks at" (Merleau-Ponty 1964: 134). In this sense, being is *reversibility*, that same reversibility which we experience in the example of the two hands touching each other; which is never coincidence because there is always a gap that is irremediably hidden from me: that is, the *between* of my flesh and the flesh of the world. The subject is enveloped by the world; the world passes through the subject. The visible is always previously structured by the invisible, identity by difference. The invisible is not that which excluded by the visible, but is that which is intrinsic to the visible: every visible is also invisible. The invisible is the *Urpräsentation* of the *Nichturpräsentierbar* (originating presentation of the unpresentable); it is a *cavity* of the visible, one of its *folds*, its *reverse side*; "it is pure transcendence without an ontic mask" (Merleau-Ponty 1964: 229).

In this powerful reprise of the ontological theme, which constitutes an unmasking of gnoseological conceptions taken for granted, the fleshly subject is the correlative of a pre-egological subject; the subject, as a synthesis of visible and invisible, is "a Self-presence that is not an *absence from oneself*, a contact with Self *through* the divergence (*écart*) with regard to Self" (Merleau-Ponty 1964: 192), an opening to the world before it is a representation of the world. Psychoanalysis and ontology are united in thinking about the incarnation and initiation of the subject: in Merleau-Ponty, as in Freud, "with the first vision, the first contact, the first pleasure, there is initiation, that is, not the positing of a content, but the opening of a dimension that can never again be closed, the establishment of a level in terms of which every other experience will henceforth be situated" (Merleau-Ponty 1964: 151). In this pre-objective and pre-egological dimension, composed of non-representational acts (since they do not give objects, and are *fungierende*) (Merleau-Ponty 1964: 238), "inside Being," the unconscious is located. In this sense, phenomenology can loosen the conceptual crystallizations of psychoanalysis: the unconscious, exceeding any naturalistic configuration, its rootedness in the world and openness to the world. To a psychological psychoanalysis which considers the Ego as an autonomous function and presents an objectifying conception of reality, Merleau-Ponty, by reclaiming Lacan, counterpoises an ontological re-reading of Freud. What Lacan criticizes is in fact the illusion of the datum of perception as such and the definition of the subject as the site of the unity of experience. The subject is in fact, before all else, *acted*; not activity but, first of all, passivity. Thinking about "an ontological psychoanalysis" (Merleau-Ponty 1964: 270) means going beyond a naturalistic and causal conception of psychic life, but also avoids flattening it onto a "humanistic" and "existential" dimension. In the dimension of concrete ontology, psychoanalysis takes on the role of deconstructing the head-to-head contraposition between subject and object in favor of the auscultation of that atemporal and indestructible dimension in us that is the unconscious; an unconscious which is not here reduced to a psychology of events and of unconscious psychic realities, but read as the reversible, the reverse side of consciousness; that primary experience of absence which only a phenomenology that descends "into its own subsoil" can glimpse, and which Lacan has called our "mooring to being." For Merleau-Ponty, therefore, the unconscious is not a totality of primary instincts which burst into consciousness, nor a place in which repressed representations dwell, but the "censored chapter" of the subject's history, the truth of which is written elsewhere: in the body, in impenetrable memories, in distortions, and so on. The unconscious is the invisible which gives our history and our experience the visible form that it has; that which organizes our experience without positively giving itself. The relationship between consciousness and unconscious is not therefore a relationship between two realities, but a relation between the presence and absence of the same reality; an absence which, for this very reason, is not a nothingness.

The constant use of the impersonal form ("is thought in me," "is perceived in me," etc.) indicates a new openness of phenomenology to an ontology of the transindividual or of the intercorporeal; indeed, sensation's "origin is anterior to myself, it arises from *sensibility* which has preceded it and will outlive it, just as my birth and death belong to a natality and a mortality which are anonymous" (Merleau-Ponty 1964: 250–251). The subject, as Lacan says, *is spoken*. Our whole experience is inserted, therefore, into a general flux which flows inside me without my being the cause of it. Conceiving of perception not as a personal act but as an impersonal fabric in which other beings are no more than "variations of ourselves," radically changes the phenomenological perspective. From being personal, this perspective makes itself impersonal, from solipsistic it becomes relational: all beings are reciprocally constituted out of a common flesh, out of matter which is *in itself* expressive. This once again underlines the rooting in the world, situated existence, *être au monde*.

ARCHAEOLOGY OF THE SELF

According to Ricoeur (1965, 1990), the great merit of psychoanalysis consists in the attempt to insert identity into the crack between conscious and psychic. Beyond the intentional and voluntary dimension, there is a primary experience which includes the "I" that I desire, the "I" that I live, and existence in general as body. Freud suggested calling latent acts pre-conscious, provisionally unconscious but disposed to becoming conscious. It is the repressed processes which are properly unconscious and cannot become conscious unless mediated: that is, by means of representations which stand in for them. For Freud, we can therefore speak of an unconscious only if we encounter a repression which does not suppress or negate a drive, but prevents its becoming conscious. For Ricoeur, the unconscious in Husserl is in reality identifiable with the pre-conscious of psychoanalysis.

An authentic phenomenology of the unconscious cannot dispense with the question of memory. To the enigmatic question *whose is the memory?* Ricoeur offers an equally enigmatic reply: *memory is of the past.* We can speak about the past in two ways: in the sense of *Vergangenheit*: that is, as that which is no longer, or which has disappeared because of the corrupting and destructive power of time; but also in the sense of the *Gewesen*, as *having-been*. In this second sense, the past indicates the anteriority of being in a positive form, an absence not guaranteed by memory but nonetheless susceptible to being evoked by it. We say that the past *is no longer there*; but we also say that *the past has been*: with the first expression we underline its disappearance, its absence in respect of our possibility of acting upon it; with the second we instead underline its full anteriority with respect to any forgotten or remembered event. According to Ricoeur, it is a grammatical error to make the past into a noun, treating it as a place, or as a storehouse in which lived experiences would be deposited after they have passed. In this sense, the metaphor of the imprint of a seal on wax, often used in speaking of memory, reinforces the idea of a recollection as localized, as if it could be gathered and stored somewhere, in a place which might preserve it and from where can be extracted so as to evoke it, recalling it to memory. In fact, there exists a deep and unrememberable *having-been past*, a *Gewesenheit* which Ricoeur compares to the Freudian Unconscious, something so forgotten that it can never be conscious.

Time, as a desire to be and an effort to exist, as a vital fact in which the "patchiness" of the psyche or of consciousness plays a part, enables the conversion of traditional science into hermeneutic science, as indeed psychoanalysis is configured to be, through which the subject's psyche-soma withdraws from any attempt at deterministic description. For Ricoeur, the truest essence of the psychic resides in the concept of incommunicable otherness, in which it is *becoming conscious* that reproduces the meaning of consciousness itself. In this sense, Ricoeur attributes to Freud the great theoretical responsibility for an overturned *epoché*, which has the purpose of treating as a whole that which is other in relation to consciousness itself: beyond intentionality there exists an unconscious thought, a lacuna, an anteriority of the drive over volition. The dimension of beyondness and otherness which characterizes consciousness, which in Kant resides in the limit, which cannot be crossed, of the noumen, is now located in the very heart of the subject as its own most intimate self.

This is the basis on which is founded the distinction, present in both Husserl and Freud, between representation [*Vorstellung*] and psychic representing [*Vorstellungrepräsentanz*]. The latter, concerning the receptive side of the Ego, its constitutive passivity, tells us that responsibility for meaning goes far beyond conscious intentionality, since it is rooted in the drive-work of the unconscious in the recognition of that energetic thrust rooted in the subject and at the same time other than it. Freud claims that the instinct per se is unknowable, and enters the psychic field by means of indices of representation. So, the point at which meaning and force coincide must be identified not in conscious representations but in representations of the instinct; that is, what Ricoeur calls a quasi-language. The notion of representation emphasizes the fact that responsibility for meaning also belongs to the instinctual work of the unconscious, to its primeval energetic thrust.

Consciousness, far from being the first and absolute source, receives and produces its meanings from the starting point of an energetic and vital dimension which is largely endured. One of the great outcomes of psychoanalysis is that the Ego is not the instinct's *origin*, but its *goal*, and that consciousness is not so much that which posits something as a becoming conscious of something, starting from a "dark depth"; that same dark depth which phenomenology itself takes as its starting point.

Freud and Ricoeur are moved by the same impulse: that of bringing the activity of the Ego back to its root in the drive and in the body, a root in which the conflict between the components of the psyche is primary and can never be definitively resolved. But with a substantial difference. For Ricoeur, the unconscious cannot be substantivized: reduced, that is, to a mere cause of which consciousness would simply constitute the effect. If that were the way things are, the relationship between consciousness and the unconscious would inevitably be lost and, with it, the therapeutic relationship. What interests Ricoeur is the path back to the negative character of the unconscious. In fact, for him, a decisive factor in treatment is an extension of the field of consciousness by means of the continuous integration of the unconscious resources which as a consequence releases the affects from their contracted state.

Thanks to this "unrememberable" we draw on the mythic depth, that same background which gives memory the resource with which to combat oblivion. From this dark and subterranean spring emerge both the oblivion of erasure and the energy that is made available for the work of memory. We can in fact think of memory as an active, living force. But to do this, we need to acknowledge that memory is not only concerned with the past, but also with the present and the future. The future reverberates in the past, and the past, moving into the present, gives the future its direction. This perspective, dispensing with the retrospective illusion of fatality, is capable of modifying the weight of the past by passing beyond the irreversible having-been of events. Thus, guilt, the precondition not maintained, the evil perpetrated or suffered, are not mere boulders which the past loads onto the shoulders of the present and the future. Forgiveness, the fulfillment of responsibilities, the remedy for an evil, in fact offer the possibility of "reopening" the past and of changing its meaning, thereby re-clarifying the future. Furthermore, the future, once blocked, retroactively modifies the past, understood as a compulsion to repeat, unreflective habit, action motivated by painful, repressed memories. This renewal of the past is what permits cure.

BIBLIOGRAPHY

Behnke E. A. (2002). "Merleau-Ponty's Ontological Reading of Constitution." In T. Toadvine and L. Embree (eds.), *Phénoménologie de la perception in Merleau-Ponty's reading of Husserl*, vol. 45, pp. 31–50. Netherlands: Kluwer Academic Publishers.

Bernet R. (1996). "The Unconscious between Representation and Drive: Freud, Husserl and Schopenhauer." In J. Drummond and J. G. Hart (eds.), *The Truthful and the Good. Essays in Honor of Robert Sokolowski*, pp. 81–96. Cham/Heidelberg/New York/Dordrecht/London: Springer.

Bernet R. (2003). "Unconscious Consciousness in Husserl and Freud." In D. Welton (ed.) *The New Husserl. A Critical Reader*, pp. 199–219. Indianapolis: Indiana University Press.

Depraz N. (2013). "Consciousness and First-Person Phenomenology: First Steps Towards an Experiential Phenomenological Writing and Reading." In S. Menon, A. Sinha, and B. V. Sreekantan (eds.), *Interdisciplinary Perspectives on Consciousness and the Self*, pp. 127–149. India: Springer.

Fuchs T. (2000). *Leib, Raum, Person. Entwurf einer phänomenologischen Anthropologie.* Stuttgart: Klett-Cotta.

Henry, M. (1990). *Phénoménologie matérielle*; Eng. trans. *Material Phenomenology*. New York: Fordham University Press, 2008.

Heller-Roazen D. (2007). *The Inner Touch: Archaeology of a Sensation*. New York: Zone Books.

Husserl E. (1900–1901). *Logische Untersuchungen*; Eng. trans. *Logical Investigations*, Vol. II, London and New York: Routledge, 2001.

Husserl E. (1912–1929). "Ideen zu einer reinen Phänomenologie und einer phänomenologischen Philosophie, Zweites Buch, Phänomenologischen Untersuchungen zur Konstitution"; Eng.trans. *"Ideas Pertaining a pure Phenomenology and to a Phenomenological Philosophy, Second Book."* In *Studies in the Phenomenology of Constitution*. Dordrecht, Boston, London: Kluwer, 1989.

Husserl E. (1913). "Ideen zu einer reinen Phänomenologie und einer phänomenologischen Philosophie: Allgemeine Einführung in die reine Phänomenologie"; Eng.trans. "Ideas Pertaining to a pure Phenomenology and to a Phenomenological Philosophy, First Book." In *General Introduction to a Pure Phenomenology*. The Hague, Boston, Lancaster: Martinus Nijoff, 1983.

Husserl E. (1920–1926). *Analysen zur passiven Synthesis*; Eng. trans. *Analyses Concerning Passive and Active Synthesis: Lectures on Transcendental Logic.* Dordrecht, Boston, London: Kluwer, 2001.

Lohmar, D. (1998). *Erfahrung und kategoriales Denken*. Hume, Kant und Husserl über vorprädikative Erfahrung und prädikative Erkenntnis. Dordrecht-Boston: Kluwer Academic Publishers.

Lohmar, D. (2009). Die Entwicklung des Husserlschen Konstitutionsmodells von Auffassung und Inhalt, in "Studia Universitatis Babeş—Bolyai," LI V, 2.

Lohmar, D. and Brudzińska, J. (eds.) (2012). *Founding Psychoanalysis Phenomenologically: Phenomenological Theory of Subjectivity and the Psychoanalytic Experience*. Dordrecht-Heidelberg-London-New York: Springer.

Merleau-Ponty M. (1945). *Phénoménologie de la perception*; Eng. trans. *Phenomenology of Perception*. London: Routledge, 1962.

Merleau-Ponty M. (1964). *Le visible et l'invisible*; Eng. trans. *The Visible and the Invisible*. Evanston: Northwestern University Press, 1968.

Ricoeur P. (1965). *De l'interprétation: Essai sur Freud*; Eng. trans. *Freud and Philosophy: an Essay on Interpretation*. New Haven: Yale University Press, 1970.

Ricoeur P. (1990). *Soi-même comme un autre*; Eng. trans. *Oneself as Another*. Chicago: University of Chicago Press, 1992.

CHAPTER 37

....

INTENTIONALITY

....

JOEL KRUEGER

INTRODUCTION

....

RIGHT now, you're probably conscious of many things: for example, the words on the page—or rather the meaning of the words on the page as your eyes skim across them. But you're probably conscious of other things, too: the slight twinge in your back from sitting too long, the faint aroma of coffee in the mug on your desk, or the nagging feeling that you've forgotten to do something. These different things are *objects* of your consciousness.

This feature of consciousness—its ability to be about things—is what philosophers call "intentionality." The term comes from the Latin verb *intendo*, which means to aim, hold out, or stretch. In this technical sense, intentionality refers to the way consciousness can stretch out or be directed toward objects internal (images, memories, etc.) and external (things, relations, and events in the world). Conscious mental states are never empty but always *of* or *about* something.

Phenomenologists argue that intentionality is a central feature of consciousness. Edmund Husserl, the founder of phenomenology, appropriated the notion from his teacher Franz Brentano, who rejuvenated discussions of intentionality found in medieval philosophers like Thomas Aquinas, John Duns Scotus, and William of Ockham. And these thinkers appropriated discussions going back to Greek philosophers like Aristotle and Empedocles. We also find sophisticated discussions of intentionality in non-Western traditions—for example, sixth- and seventh-century Indian Buddhist thinkers like Dignāga and Dharmakīrti (Coseru 2012).

I focus here on phenomenological approaches to intentionality since they're particularly relevant to psychopathology. Not only have phenomenologists spent more time considering intentionality than other philosophical traditions. They've also broadened discussions to consider intentionality's embodied and affective dimensions—themes helpful for understanding the character of some psychopathological conditions. Phenomenologists are concerned not simply with the formal or logical properties of intentionality (cf. Searle 1983) but rather with how intentionality is integral to *subjectivity*. This qualitative orientation can help illuminate the lived experience of psychopathological conditions, some of which appear to involve subtle disturbances of intentionality.

BRENTANO ON INTENTIONALITY

Phenomenologists take their characterization of intentionality from Brentano, who looked to construct a "descriptive psychology" (or what he sometimes calls "phenomenology"): a descriptive analysis of experience from the inside (Brentano 1995a). Brentano insists that intentionality must be at the center of this project. Intentionality, he tells us, "is characteristic exclusively of mental phenomena. No physical phenomenon exhibits anything like it. We can, therefore, define mental phenomena by saying that they are those phenomena which contain an object intentionally within themselves" (Brentano 1995b: 68). For Brentano, intentionality not only distinguishes mental from physical phenomena. It also gives individual mental states their distinctive character: "Every mental phenomenon includes something as an object within itself, although they do not all do so in the same way. In presentation something is presented, in judgment something is affirmed or denied, in love loved, in hate hated, in desire desired, and so on" (Brentano 1995b: 68).

Several points are important. First, Brentano argues that each type of conscious act is constituted as the kind of act it is only via its relation to its intentional object. An act of perception is only such in relation a perceptual object; likewise, other conscious mental states like beliefs, desires, memories, and emotions. Accordingly, to understand the ontology of consciousness, we must investigate the different relations that connect conscious acts with their respective intentional objects. As later phenomenologists will insist, this feature of intentionality illustrates that consciousness is a *relational* phenomenon. We are "through and through compounded of relationships with the world" (Merleau-Ponty 2002: xiv).

Second, looking at how conscious acts relate to their intentional objects allows us to individuate different acts. The same intentional object—a bottle of Belgian beer, say—can be the intentional object of multiple conscious acts. I can *believe* the beer is in my refrigerator, *desire* the beer, and upon opening my refrigerator, visually *perceive* the beer. In each case, the bottle of beer stands in a distinct relation to the act within which it is present *as* intentional object. And this is significant, phenomenologists insist, because these different relations enable us to distinguish the character and structure of different conscious acts within the inventory of all possible mental activity. Intentionality is the tool that enables these taxonomic considerations.

Finally, this way of thinking about intentionality is different from other ways of characterizing mind–world relations as primarily involving *causality*. Intentional relations need not be causal relations; minds can intend non-existent objects like unicorns and Sherlock Holmes—or existent objects beyond our perceptual reach (e.g. distant planets), or even objects that once existed but no longer do (e.g. my deceased grandmother). To be clear, the intentional relation *itself* is, in these cases, very real. I can feel strongly about a fictional literary character, say, or be moved by the memory of my beloved dead grandmother. But neither the literary character nor my beloved grandmother exist as objects in the world. The form of my conscious relation to them will, accordingly, be different than mind–world relations characterized exclusively by appealing to causal descriptions involving existent entities. This is particularly useful in the context of phenomenological psychopathology, which may involve investigating how individuals experientially relate to non-existent individuals, objects, and events.

Beyond Brentano: Mental, Bodily, and Affective Dimensions of Intentionality

Although nearly all major phenomenologists quibble with different parts of Brentano's analysis—especially his idea that intentional objects are "in" consciousness as mental intermediaries between mind and world—they nevertheless agree that investigations of consciousness must begin with intentionality. But phenomenologists also move beyond Brentano in a number of important ways.

To see how this is so, we can note first that phenomenologists insist that minds are irreducibly *embodied* (Gallagher and Zahavi 2008: chapter 7). The things we think and experience—and the way we think and experience them—reflect aspects of the physical structure of our body as well as the things our body can do. So, intentionality for phenomenologists is rooted in our bodies and agency. This motor dimension has to be part of a full picture of intentionality.

Additionally, phenomenologists argue that we don't just think thoughts or perceive things. We *feel feelings*. And these feelings—affective phenomena like emotions, moods, and bodily states—play an important role in shaping how the world and other people show up for us, experientially (Colombetti 2014). Feelings are an essential part of the way we are intentionally open and responsive to our world.

Phenomenologists thus move beyond Brentano by developing a multidimensional approach to intentionality that respects not only its mental character but also its embodied and affective dimensions. Next, I will consider these three dimensions of intentionality—*mental intentionality, motor intentionality*, and *affective intentionality*—in turn.[1] To be clear: from a phenomenological perspective, these dimensions are interrelated. Intentionality is an integrative achievement not of minds, brains, or bodies but of *persons*—subjects open and responsive to physical and social environments. So, while we can make a conceptual distinction between these different dimensions to clarify intentionality's overall structure—as well as differentiate various ways intentionality that becomes disturbed in psychopathology—we should remain mindful that these dimensions are interwoven within the practice of intentionality conceived of as an embodied and situated activity of the whole person.

Mental Intentionality

For Husserl, the structure of intentionality can be analyzed into two components: the object as intended by consciousness (*noema*), and the conscious act that intends the object (*noesis*). In other words, *noema* picks out the object-side of the intentional relation (i.e. *what* is given to consciousness) whereas *noesis* picks out the subject-side (i.e. *how* the "what" is given to consciousness). For example, if I remember the front door of my grandmother's house, the

[1] Phenomenologists like Husserl and Merleau-Ponty speak of *act* vs. *operative* intentionality to mark a difference between thinking of intentionality as a feature of conscious acts vs. embodied actions. For simplicity, I adopt more straightforward terminology.

noema is the door-as-remembered; it is *what* is made present to consciousness. The *noesis* is the act of remembering; it is *how* the door is made present to consciousness. However, if I visit my grandmother's home, the intentional object will remain the same—her front door—but now the noetic structure through which I intend the front door will be different. It will now be a perceptual act—and the *noesis–noema* structure of that act will vary accordingly. Husserl argues that *all* conscious acts have this noetic structure. It is the basic framework for our intentional engagement with the world.[2]

In addition to its noetic structure, Husserl describes another important feature of mental intentionality. He says intentionality "wants to go to the object itself . . . that is, to an intuition that gives the object itself, to an intuition that is in itself the consciousness of having the object itself" (Husserl 2001: 126). He continues: "This directedness is . . . a striving, it is from the very beginning 'driving at' a satisfaction" (Husserl 2001: 126). There are several points here worthy of consideration.

Perhaps most important is that, for Husserl, intentionality is not a passive state in which the external world presses itself onto a yielding observer but instead a dynamic, temporally extended *activity* (i.e. a kind of "striving" or "driving at satisfaction"). This claim aligns Husserl with contemporary enactive approaches to perception stressing the interdependence of perception and action (e.g. Bower and Gallagher 2013; Hurley 1998; Noë 2004; Thompson 2005).

Consider seeing a red ball. When we see the ball, we don't actually see the whole thing. We only see the part or "aspect" facing us. Nevertheless, Husserl insists we *experience* the ball as a complete three-dimensional object with density, spatial extension, and unseen parts potentially capable of being seen. These unseen parts are part of the content of our experience, co-given alongside the visible parts: "Of necessity a physical thing can be given only 'one-sidedly' . . . A physical thing is necessarily given in mere 'modes of appearance' in which necessarily a *core of 'what is actually presented'* is apprehended as being surrounded by a horizon of *'co-givenness,' which is not givenness proper*, and of more or less vague *indeterminateness*" (Husserl 1998: 94).

For Husserl, this feature of our experience can be understood by looking at the intentional structure of perception's "striving" character. The reason unseen parts of the ball are co-given is because we experience the ball as offering possibilities for engagement— what James Gibson terms "affordances" (1966, 1979)—that provide increasingly determinate specifications of the ball's nature. Put otherwise, the ball affords various interactions (touching, handling, picking up, throwing, etc.) specified both by (1) our possession of kinaesthetic capacities (e.g. the ability to turn our torso, tilt our head, reach for the ball and grasp it) as well as (2) our implicit practical knowledge of how *exercising* these capacities will reliably alter our experience by bringing hidden sides into view. These affordances are part of the noematic content of perception.

Additionally, since intentionality is embodied and situated, Husserl argues that this striving isn't just going on in our head. It's a *relational* process through which we stretch outside of ourselves and interact with the world. And the objects partially constitutive of these relations present qualities—again, given as noematic content—affording different kinds of

---

[2] How we ought to understand the ontological status of the *noema* continues to be a matter of debate in the literature. See Gallagher 2012: 69–71.

interaction; they establish an object's *meaning*. Taking seriously the striving character of intentionality thus illuminates how perception involves a "constitutive duet" between subject and object (Husserl 2001: 52).

MOTOR INTENTIONALITY

As we've seen, Husserl is sensitive to the role embodiment plays in shaping the character and content of intentionality. But Merleau-Ponty takes this idea further. He argues that we are fundamentally animate bodies open and responsive to a meaningful environment; this bodily openness is constitutive of our being-in-the-world. And this openness means that our embodied being is intentional *all the way down*—including prenoetic levels of worldly engagement (Gallagher 2005). For Merleau-Ponty, this is a "deeper" intentionality "beneath the intentionality of representation" (2002: 140 n. 54).

Merleau-Ponty observes that, within the ebb and flow of everyday life, we routinely act—in an organized and purposive way—without conscious reflection, planning, or even full awareness. "Motor intentionality" refers to the integrated suite of skills, capacities, and habits—not all of which are available to consciousness—that enable this unreflective action (Rietveld 2008). It picks out a way of being directed toward the world different than we find within the noetic structure of mental intentionality (Dreyfus 2005; Kelly 2002).

Consider reaching for a coffee mug while reading the newspaper. We don't first locate the mug—along with different parts of our body—and then think about various movements and postural adjustments needed to carry out our reach. Instead, we simply reach for the mug spontaneously—and crucially, our grasp calibrates itself accordingly. Body and world together organize a coherent and meaningful experience. As Merleau-Ponty puts it, "From the outset the grasping movement is magically at its completion; it can begin only by anticipating its end" (2002: 119).

Once again, this dimension of intentionality is rooted in our embodiment. This is because we don't merely inhabit our bodies as *objects*, as physical things with properties similar to other objects in the world. We also *live through* our bodies onto the world; we experience them from the inside, as *subjects* (Carman 1999). Accordingly, we can unthinkingly grasp the mug because have an immediate proprioceptive and kinaesthetic sense of where our limbs are in space and what sort of skilful actions are possible *within* that space. This is a tacit pre-reflective bodily awareness operative without deliberate reflection (Legrand 2007). Moreover—and to return to an earlier point—we immediately perceive the mug as *meaningful*: as an artefact affording a range of different interactions determined by the structure of the cup, the context in which we encounter it, and our preeflective awareness of our body as an intentional vehicle.

For Merleau-Ponty, motor intentionality is pervasive throughout everyday life: changing gears while driving, brushing our teeth, tying our shoes, typing on our laptop, stroking our child's cheek while singing a lullaby, playing tennis, practicing guitar scales, lunging for the bottle of wine about to fall off the table, and many other contexts of spontaneous action. In these cases, there is a particular form of bodily understanding of objects and environments—as well as our situatedness within these environments—that allows us to be immediately open and responsive to the things happening around us. For Merleau-Ponty, "[t]hese elucidations enable us clearly to understand motility as basic intentionality. Consciousness is in the first place not a matter of 'I think that' but of 'I can'" (2002: 159).

AFFECTIVE INTENTIONALITY

For phenomenologists, affective states are not internal states hidden away inside brains and bodies. They are embodied and enactive processes that connect us to a shared world and guide our dealings with it (Colombetti and Krueger 2015; Krueger 2014; Krueger and Szanto 2016). Importantly, they also have a revelatory character that shapes how the world shows up for us in our experience (Slaby and Stephan 2008).[3]

Heidegger, for example, argues that moods aren't simply add-ons providing color to other mental phenomena. Moods are examples of affective phenomena that disclose the world *as being* a certain way. A mood, he says, "has always already disclosed, in every case, Being-in-the-world as a whole, and makes it possible first of all to direct oneself toward something" (Heidegger 1962: 176). For Heidegger, moods set up our encounter with the world by constituting our sense of belonging to it. They reveal the world as a space of practical purposes, values, goals, and activities—a space of *meaning*—and in this sense they are *primordial* phenomena presupposed by the intelligibility of our thoughts, experiences, and actions (Ratcliffe 2008: 48).

Sartre offers a vivid example of the revelatory character of affectivity. After reading a text late into the night, we find it increasingly difficult to focus on the words or their meaning. For Sartre, our eyestrain is first "indicated by objects of the world; that is, by the book which I read. It is with more difficulty that the words are detached from the undifferentiated ground which they constitute; they may tremble, quiver; their meaning can be derived only with effort . . ." (1989: 332). In this case, as focusing on the words becomes more difficult, we shift our attention from the words (experienced as blurry, unstable, or lacking meaning) to the affective quality of the pain around our eyes and temples. For Sartre, this case highlights the Janus-faced intentional structure of affectivity: affective states convey information about self *and* non-self.

This revelatory role of affectivity is supported by different streams of empirical work. Several studies indicate that subjects estimate the grade of an incline to be steeper when wearing a heavy backpack as opposed to not wearing one, or when they feel fatigued as opposed to refreshed (Proffitt et al. 1995; Proffitt et al. 2001). Even the presence of a supportive friend—actually present or merely imagined—leads subjects to perceive the incline as less steep than when alone (Schnall et al. 2008). The affective support we receive from others shapes how we perceive the world and its affordances. A similar dynamic appears to be at work in the social world. There is evidence, for example, that shared affect is a crucial component of empathy. It allows individuals to pick up on the ways others are responsive to environmental affordances, and in so doing, to share and understand their perspective on the world (Kiverstein 2015).

---

[3] For a detailed look at the role of emotions in mental illness, see Stanghellini and Rosfort 2013.

Without this orienting function of shared affect, however—such as in autistic spectrum disorder (ASD)—individuals struggle to get grip on what others find important in a given situation and have difficulty relating to them. This absence of "affective framing" (Maiese 2015) is one of the reasons people with ASD struggle to comfortably inhabit the common space of the social world.

DISRUPTIONS OF INTENTIONALITY

Phenomenologically informed psychopathologists argue that the generative disorder of schizophrenia is a disturbance of the first-person perspective (Sass and Parnas 2003; see also Henriksen and Nordgaard 2014; Krueger and Henriksen 2016). According to this so-called ipseity-disturbance model (IDM), this disturbance can include a diminished sense of existing as a bodily subject, a weakened sense of ownership of one's thoughts and experience, a gradual fragmentation or loss of coherence of the field of awareness, and disturbed self–world, self–other boundaries (Parnas et al. 2005).

These phenomenological descriptions can be enriched by highlighting how various forms of *intentional* disruptions co-occur with or exacerbate disruptions of *ipseity*. For example, Fuchs (2007) draws on Husserl's (1991) analysis of "inner time-consciousness" to relate schizophrenic disorders to the temporal structure of consciousness. For Husserl, the temporal microstructure of consciousness—as intentional—consists of a dynamic self-organizing process comprised of both a *retention* of what I have just seen, heard, or thought, as well as an anticipatory *protention* of what I expect to continue seeing, hearing, or thinking. This temporal synthesis is a tacit background process organizing our experiences into sequences of coherent units.

In schizophrenia, this temporal microstructure of intentional consciousness can become fragmented (Fuchs 2007: 233). Consequently, patients' capacity to make sense of situations, experiences, and the behavior of others is impaired. In the early stages of psychosis, for instance, experiences such as the loss of one's train of thought, difficulty following conversations, or difficulty maintaining narrative coherence are common (see also Gallagher 2007). One patient reports: "I'm a good listener but often I'm not really taking it in. I nod my head and smile but it's just a lot of jumbled up words to me" (McGhie and Chapman 1961: 106).

This temporal disruption also destabilizes the dynamics of *motor* intentionality. One patient says:

> I found recently that I was thinking of myself doing things before I would do them. If I am going to sit down, for example, I have got to think of myself and almost see myself sitting down before I do it. It's the same with other things like washing, eating, and even dressing . . .
>
> (McGhie and Chapman 1961: 107)

In these cases, patients take up normally spontaneous, unreflective actions in a deliberate and thoughtful way; each movement is considered in isolation from the others, leading to a "disautomation" compromising their ability to negotiate physical and social environments (Fuchs 2007: 233). Maiese highlights how this disautomation also involves a disruption of *affective* intentionality—a disturbance of what she terms "affective framing"—in that "the body is no longer 'feelingly' integrated into its lived environment" (Maiese 2015: 180). This loss of bodily-affective responsivity results in a diminished sense of ownership, agency, and control. Disturbances of motor and affective intentionality also characterize some of the disruptions of embodiment, spatial cognition, and perception of social and environmental affordances characteristic of conditions like depression and Moebius Syndrome (de Haan et al. 2013; Slaby et al. 2013; Krueger and Taylor Aiken 2016). In sum, focusing on disruptions of intentionality—along with approaches like IDM—can in this way deepen and enrich our understanding of core disturbances involved in different psychopathologies.

BIBLIOGRAPHY

Bower M. and Gallagher S. (2013). "Bodily Affects as Prenoetic Elements in Enactive Perception." *Phenomenology and Mind* 4: 109–131.

Brentano F. (1995a). *Descriptive Psychology*, trans. B. Müller. London: Routledge.

Brentano F. (1995b). *Psychology from an Empirical Standpoint*, trans. A. C. Rancurello, D. B. Terrell, and L. L. McAlister. London and New York: Routledge.

Carman T. (1999). "The Body in Husserl and Merleau-Ponty." *Philosophical Topics* 27(2): 205–226.

Colombetti G. (2014). *The Feeling Body: Affective Science Meets the Enactive Mind*. Cambridge, MA: MIT Press.

Colombetti G. and Krueger, J. (2015). "Scaffoldings of the Affective Mind." *Philosophical Psychology* 28(8): 1157–1176.

Coseru C. (2012). *Perceiving Reality: Consciousness, Intentionality, and Cognition in Buddhist Philosophy*. New York: Oxford University Press.

de Haan S., Rietveld E., Stokhof M., and Denys D. (2013). "The Phenomenology of Deep Brain Stimulation-Induced Changes in OCD: An Enactive Affordance-Based Model." *Frontiers in Human Neuroscience* 7: 1–14.

Dreyfus H. L. (2005). "Merleau-Ponty and Recent Cognitive Science." In T. Carman and M. Hansen (eds.), *The Cambridge Companion to Merleau-Ponty*. Cambridge: Cambridge University Press.

Fuchs T. (2007). "The Temporal Structure of Intentionality and Its Disturbance in Schizophrenia." *Psychopathology* 40(4): 229–235.

Gallagher S. (2005). *How the Body Shapes the Mind*. Oxford, New York: Oxford University Press.

Gallagher S. (2007). "Pathologies in Narrative Structures." *Royal Institute of Philosophy Supplements* 60: 203–224.

Gallagher S. (2012). *Phenomenology*. New York: Palgrave Macmillan.

Gallagher S. and Zahavi D. (2008). *The Phenomenological Mind: An Introduction to Philosophy of Mind and Cognitive Science*. New York: Routledge.

Gibson J. J. (1966). *The Senses Considered as Perceptual Systems*. Boston: Houghton Mifflin.

Gibson J. J. (1979). *The Ecological Approach to Visual Perception*. Hillsdale: Lawrence Erlbaum Associates.

Heidegger M. (1962). *Being and Time*, trans. J. Macquarrie and E. Robinson. New York: Harper and Row Publishers.

Henriksen M. G. and Nordgaard, J. (2014). "Schizophrenia as a Disorder of the Self." *Journal of Psychopathology* 20: 435–441.

Hurley S. (1998). *Consciousness in Action*. Cambridge, MA: Harvard University Press.

Husserl E. (1991). *On the Phenomenology of the Consciousness of Internal Time*, trans. J. B. Brough. (1991 edition). Dordrecht, Boston: Springer.

Husserl E. (1998). *Ideas Pertaining to a Pure Phenomenology and to a Phenomenological Philosophy—First Book: General Introduction to a Pure Phenomenology*, trans. F. Kersten. Dordrecht: Kluwer Academic Publishers.

Husserl E. (2001). *Analyses Concerning Passive and Active Synthesis: Lectures on Transcendental Logic*, trans. A. J. Steinbock. Dordrecht: Kluwer Academic Publishers.

Kelly S. D. (2002). "Merleau–Ponty on the Body." *Ratio* 15(4): 376–391.

Kiverstein J. (2015). "Empathy and the Responsiveness to Social Affordances." *Consciousness and Cognition* 36: 532–542.

Krueger J. (2014). "Varieties of Extended Emotions." *Phenomenology and the Cognitive Sciences* 13(4): 533–555.

Krueger J. and Henriksen M. G. (2016). "Embodiment and Affectivity in Moebius Syndrome and Schizophrenia: A Phenomenological Analysis." In J. E. Hackett and J. A. Simmons (eds.), *Phenomenology for the 21st Century*, pp. 249–267. Basingstoke: Palgrave Macmillan.

Krueger J. and Szanto T. (2016). "Extended Emotions." *Philosophy Compass* 11: 863–878.

Krueger J. and Taylor-Aiken A. (2016). "Losing Social Space: Phenomenological Disruptions of Spatiality and Embodiment in Moebius Syndrome and Schizophrenia." In J. Reynolds and R. Sebold (eds.), *Phenomenology and Science*, pp. 121–139. Basingstoke: Palgrave Macmillan.

Legrand D. (2007). "Pre-reflective Self-as-Subject from Experiential and Empirical Perspectives." *Consciousness and Cognition* 16(3): 583–599.

Maiese M. (2015). *Embodied Selves and Divided Minds*. New York: Oxford University Press.

McGhie A. and Chapman J. (1961). "Disorders of Attention and Perception in Early Schizophrenia." *British Journal of Medical Psychology* 34(2): 103–116.

Merleau-Ponty M. (2002). *Phenomenology of Perception*, trans. C. Smith. New York: Routledge.

Noë A. (2004). *Action in Perception*. Cambridge, MA: MIT Press.

Parnas J., Moller P., Kircher T., Thalbitzer J., Jansson L., Handest P., and Zahavi D. (2005). "EASE: Examination of Anomalous Self-experience." *Psychopathology* 38(5): 236–258.

Proffitt D. R., Bhalla M., Gossweiler R., and Midgett J. (1995). "Perceiving Geographical Slant." *Psychonomic Bulletin & Review* 2(4): 409–428.

Proffitt D. R., Creem S. H., and Zosh W. D. (2001). "Seeing mountains in Mole Hills: Geographical-slant Perception." *Psychological Science* 12(5): 418–423.

Ratcliffe M. (2008). *Feelings of Being: Phenomenology, Psychiatry and the Sense of Reality*, 1st edn. New York: Oxford University Press.

Rietveld E. (2008). "Situated Normativity: The Normative Aspect of Embodied Cognition in Unreflective Action." *Mind* 117(468): 973–1001.

Sartre J.-P. (1989). *Being and Nothingness*, trans. H. E. Barnes. London: Routledge.

Sass L. A. and Parnas, J. (2003). "Schizophrenia, Consciousness, and the Self." *Schizophrenia Bulletin* 29(3): 427–444.

Schnall S., Harber K. D., Stefanucci J. K., and Proffitt D. R. (2008). "Social Support and the Perception of Geographical Slant." *Journal of Experimental Social Psychology* 44(5): 1246–1255.

Searle J. R. (1983). *Intentionality: An Essay in the Philosophy of Mind*. Cambridge: Cambridge University Press.

Slaby J. and Stephan, A. (2008). "Affective Intentionality and Self-consciousness." *Consciousness and Cognition* 17(2): 506–513.

Slaby J., Paskaleva A., and Stephan A. (2013). "Enactive Emotion and Impaired Agency in Depression." *Journal of Consciousness Studies* 20(7–8): 33–55.

Stanghellini G. and Rosfort R. (2013). *Emotions and Personhood: Exploring Fragility, Making Sense of Vulnerability*. Oxford: Oxford University Press.

Thompson E. (2005). "Sensorimotor Subjectivity and the Enactive Approach to Experience." *Phenomenology and the Cognitive Sciences* 4(4): 407–427.

CHAPTER 38

PERSONHOOD

RENÉ ROSFORT

INTRODUCTION

THE notion of personhood plays a fundamental, but challenging role in contemporary mental health care. One of the principal reasons for the complicated status of personhood is that it functions as both a descriptive and normative notion. What it means to understand and treat the patient as a person has been an open question in psychiatry, at least since the humanitarian reforms pioneered by, among others, Philippe Pinel and Vincenzo Chiarugi around the turn of the nineteenth century (Weiner 2008; Scull 2015: 202–223). The notion of personhood has a long history, drawing upon both philosophy and theology (Strawson 1959; Sturma 1997: 44–57; Taylor 1989: 127–142), but the modern understanding of being a person is a child of the Enlightenment's—and in particular Immanuel Kant's—call for autonomy and responsibility that in mental health care brought about a new way of seeing the patient. The patient is no longer to be understood merely as a passive object of her or his illness, but as an autonomous person whose thoughts, actions, and self-understanding are a constitutive part of the illness itself. This recognition of the patient as an autonomous person was the first major step toward the consolidation of psychopathology as an indispensable aspect of psychiatry. To understand mental suffering we need to understand how the person experiences, thinks about, and deals with her or his suffering. The notion of personhood is challenging, however, due to the fact that personhood is an idea that we need to acknowledge in order to see it. Personhood is a normative notion, meaning that the act of recognition—that is, the norm that we should acknowledge a human being as a person—is a prerequisite for actually seeing a person (Kant 1996a: 79–81). Personhood is not a feature of a human being that we can describe, measure, or examine on a par with, for example, a kidney or the amygdala. As philosopher Robert Spaemann argues: "There is no characteristic that can be called 'being a person'. Rather, we say that certain beings are persons due to specific characteristics that we have already identified" (Spaemann 1996: 14; author's trans.). In other words, to understand a human being—oneself as well as another—as a person is a way of seeing. We have to want to see a human being as more than just a lump of meat. This means that seeing every human being as a person is a choice or—as some would argue—an ethical demand.

The notion of personhood has not been a central notion in the phenomenological tradition as, for example, the notions of subjectivity, intentionality, or life-world. One reason for this is the interplay of descriptive and normative features at work in the notion. On the one hand, personhood engages with the individual psychological make-up of the subject that goes counter to phenomenology's transcendental ambition to arrive at an impersonal account of subjective experience (e.g. Husserl 2001: 40–55; Gallagher and Zahavi 2012: 19–21). Understanding what it means to be a person entails an insistence on the individual character of experience. One human being cannot experience the experience of another human being. While the biological functions and the subjective structures of experience can be investigated from an impersonal third- or first-person perspective, the texture or flesh of an actual human experience is uniquely personal. This is to say that to make sense of a particular person's experience, we need to take into account the innumerable—and more or less articulate—aspects that make up a particular personality, that is, physical appearance, nationality, language, upbringing, education, tastes, dislikes, concerns, ambitions, ideals, dreams, and so on. This inordinate descriptive particularity is part of what makes personal experience phenomenologically suspect. Another thing that makes the notion of person sit uneasily with the phenomenological tradition is the aforementioned normative character of the notion. Most phenomenologists understand their work as primarily, or exclusively, concerned with a descriptive clarification of subjectivity, experience, and selfhood. As we have seen, we cannot describe a person without first acknowledging the norm of personhood. This means that the notion of personhood cannot be logically or descriptively distilled from our examinations of human biology or human experience. It is a normative perspective on what it means to be human. And as such it is something that we choose to adopt in our approach to human beings, and this choice entails several questions: Why should we consider human beings as persons? What, if anything, distinguishes a person from a thing or a nonhuman animal? And, perhaps most importantly, beside the historical fact that in psychiatry it has become an ethical obligation to treat patients as persons is there any psychopathological advantage to be gained from examining human beings as persons in addition to, say, biological organisms or experiencing selves?

In what follows, I will address these questions by looking at the interplay of descriptive and normative aspects of personhood, arguing that the notion is of vital importance to phenomenological psychopathology. In fact, despite the modest life of the notion in the phenomenological tradition, several major phenomenologists, both in philosophy and psychopathology, have contributed with careful investigations of what it means to be a person. Here I will primarily draw upon the work by the French philosopher Paul Ricoeur who, arguably, has worked out the most detailed phenomenological account of personhood.

SUBJECTIVITY, SELF, AND PERSON

Human experience is subjective in the sense that a human being's experience of the world involves an experience of experiencing the world. We are self-aware of our experience, though most of the time this self-awareness plays a tacit role in the background of everyday experience. But when something disturbs our experience of the world—for example, when we make mistakes, when facing mental or physical difficulties, when we find ourselves at the center of attention, or in philosophical moments—we become aware that our experience is *our* experience. We are not merely experiencing something. We are involved in our experience and that experience *matters* to us. Phenomenology offers methodological tools to explore the basic structures of our experience and to engage with the relation between self-awareness and experience. This exploration provides us with both a clarification of the various aspects of subjectivity and an account of selfhood. While the former is primarily concerned with investigating the experiential features of self-awareness such as intentionality, temporality, spatiality, embodiment, intersubjectivity, the latter, examines our sense of being self that is, what it means to be a self that is aware of itself in experiencing the world, other people, and itself. These two aspects of the phenomenological exploration of experience are obviously interconnected, but exactly how the two aspects are connected remains an open question. Most contemporary phenomenologists argue that subjectivity involves some sense of selfhood, but there is significant disagreement over whether selfhood can be reduced to a minimal pre-reflective sense of agency and ownership (Legrand 2011; Gallagher 2012b; Zahavi 2014) or requires a more reflective sense of identity (Grøn 2004; Figal and Espinet 2012; Tengelyi 2012).

This disagreement stems from the tectonic shift in the foundation of the phenomenological landscape sat in motion in the late 1920s by Heidegger's critique of Husserl's transcendental conception of subjectivity, and by Heidegger's subsequent hermeneutical approach to the question of being a self. While Husserl's phenomenology is preoccupied with a meticulously detailed examination of the pre-reflective, transcendental structures of experience, subjectivity, and self-awareness, Heidegger's phenomenological work engages with a so-called hermeneutics of facticity that while still having transcendental ambitions is primarily concerned with making sense of the feelings, cares, and concerns of the self (Heidegger 1999, 2010). One of the main differences between the two phenomenological projects concerns the notion of selfhood. Husserl's notion of selfhood is a thin one derived from his scientifically careful descriptive analysis of the experiential structures of subjectivity and remains a minimal, pre-reflective sense of agency and ownership working in the background of experience. Heidegger's notion of selfhood, on the other hand, goes way beyond the descriptive analysis of the experiential features of subjectivity. It is a thick notion informed by his existential interpretation of anxiety, boredom, fear, care, and depicts a self-struggling with the challenges of human identity.

Heidegger soon lost interest in questions of subjectivity and selfhood and turned his attention to being in general, but his hermeneutical phenomenology found fertile soil among the first generation of French phenomenologists. In this generation Emmanuel Levinas and Paul Ricoeur are the ones who spent most time and intellectual energy on trying to make sense of what it means to be a person. Both authors use Heidegger's ontological explorations of selfhood as the template of their own work, but they do so in significantly different ways. Levinas criticizes Heidegger (and most of thinkers in the Western philosophical tradition) for privileging ontology over ethics being more interested in sophisticated speculations about the nature of the world than trying to make sense of our responsibility to the human being standing in front of us. Levinas sees it as his task to revert this understanding of philosophy arguing that ethics should the primary aim of our reflective efforts. His lifework is therefore dedicated to a meticulous and careful examination of the explicit ethical demand involved in our meeting with the other human being (Levinas 1969, 1981). While Levinas throughout his career remains skeptical of the ontological implications in the notion of personhood and therefore avoids dealing systematically with the notion (Ferretti 2003), the interplay of ethical and ontological aspects of personhood is a key issue in Ricoeur's philosophy. In fact, Ricoeur criticizes Levinas for producing an asymmetrical account of selfhood that dismisses the ontological aspects of being a self for sake of the ethical concern for our responsibility to the other (Ricoeur 1992: 335–341). Ricoeur's argument is that, however, we cannot hope to understand ethics without ontology—and vice versa. That is to say, that we cannot come to understand *how* to behave if we do not examine *what* it is to be human, and we cannot understand what it is to be human without understanding our responsibility to the other person. And the core of Ricoeur's argument is exactly that the notion of personhood helps us to brings out and examine this this interplay of ethics and ontology, that is, the normative and descriptive factors that make human beings human.

For more than half a century, Ricoeur patiently developed Heidegger's phenomenological hermeneutics of selfhood into a complex account of personhood. This account is grounded in what Ricoeur takes to be a basic experiential tension in human self-awareness between selfhood and otherness, involving, the tension between the voluntary and the involuntary, the active and the receptive, the autonomous and the heteronomous aspects of subjectivity (Ricoeur 1966). Ricoeur uses this tension to develop Heidegger's existential analysis of human feelings and care into a full-fledged hermeneutical phenomenology of the biological, cultural, and ethical factors involved in being a person. Personhood, for Ricoeur, is a necessary notion in our exploration of what it means to be human, since the notion of selfhood is not sufficient to make sense of the peculiar fragility of human identity. The notion of personhood allows us to explore the tension between selfhood and otherness, that is, the innumerable ways that our experience of being a self is troubled by an otherness that challenges our understanding of what and who we are. The notion is thus more comprehensive than the notion of selfhood in that it investigates the ways otherness disturbs and challenges our experience of identity. Personhood, in other words, helps us to make sense of the fact that we are biological organisms whose identity cannot be reduced to a biological constancy, but is dependent upon how we experience and think about ourselves, and upon how other people see us. As Ricoeur argues, the fragility of human identity is rooted in the various ways in which our biology challenges our experience of being an autonomous self:

> It is always the moment of nature, the otherness of life, that, in the proper sense of the word, fosters and nourishes the oppositions of each consciousness to the other than itself . . . And the very term "self"—*Selbst*—proclaims that self-identity continues to be carried by this self-difference by this ever-recurring otherness residing in life. It is life that becomes the other, in and through which the self ceaselessly achieves itself.
>
> (Ricoeur 1970: 472)

This insistence on the biological roots of the fragility of human identity marks a significant break with the phenomenological approach of Husserl and Heidegger, both of whom were dismissive of a biological intrusion into phenomenology (Zahavi 2010; Gallagher 2012a). For Ricoeur, however, to make sense of what it means to be a person phenomenology cannot but take into account the biological aspects of human identity (e.g. height, skin color, metabolism, kidney function). In fact, the biological character of our identity is one of the major sources of otherness that a person needs to deal with throughout her life. Our body constantly challenges our experience of ourselves. We can never fully understand or appropriate our own body, and part of what it means to be a person is to acknowledge that the biological otherness of our embodiment is an integral part of our identity (Ricoeur 1966: 409–443). The fact that our experience of who we are is disturbed by that which we cannot understand or appropriate means that human identity is intrinsically fragile. Our self-understanding cannot but be at odds with what we are. This means that even though we in a sense are what we are with all our concrete particularities, in another sense we are not what (we think) we are (Ricoeur 1992: 317–319). To exist as a person over and through time is to experience one-self as different from how one understands oneself to be and from the person one wants to be. In fact, the identity of a person is fragile because it cannot be grounded in an impersonal otherness (biological, social, or cultural) or in an intimate sense of selfhood (pre-reflective or reflective). Rather, to be a person is the task of becoming the concrete person that one is through the encounter with the otherness that is an inescapable part of one's identity.

SEEING A PERSON

The notion of personhood thus serves to make sense of the problem that our identity is a fact that is also a task. One could say that our identity is a normative fact. We are the bi-ological organism that we are, but our experience of continuity is nevertheless a fact that is constantly disturbed. When we try to understand ourselves and to make sense of what we say and do, we are confronted with multifarious experiences of otherness that turn our identity into a question (Grøn 2017: 16–20). These experiences that disturb our sense of identity stem, as mentioned, from the opaque biology of our bodies, but also, and often more manifestly, from our own—more or less articulate—idea(l)s about the person that we would like to be, and from the way other people see us. My identity is a question not only about what I am and who I feel or think myself to be, it also depends upon my ideas about how—and sometimes even who—I would like to be and upon the way other people see me. This combination of descriptive and normative features makes personhood "a projected synthesis that seizes itself in the representation of a task, of an ideal of what the person should be" (Ricoeur 1986: 86). In being the person that we are, we are confronted with the task of holding together, trying to make sense of, and living with *what* we are, *who* we want to be, and *how* other people see us. The notion of personhood involves the normative demand that we recognize and respect every human being as a person (Kant 1996b: 210–211). In this sense, all human beings are to be seen as persons. And yet, to be a person is also to be a certain kind of person—both in our own eyes and in the eyes of other people. Persons are individuals, and as such they come in as many forms and shades as there are human beings. Persons are considerate, mean, passionate, dull, kind, reserved, good, melancholic, ambitious, shy, bad, obnoxious, outgoing, prying, invidious, cool, sin-cere, joyful, anxious, reticent, and so on. It is this interplay of normative universality and descriptive individuality that makes seeing a person—ourselves as well as other people—a challenging task.

To see a person is to see an individual, concrete person who is more than what can be seen or explained. The notion of personhood serves, as mentioned, to make sense of the fragile character of human identity as a restless interplay of selfhood and otherness. This means that to see a human being as a person is, on the one hand, to respect this human being's experience of being an autonomous self and, on the other, to acknowledge the limits of that autonomy. A person is responsible for the person that he or she is, and yet due to the constitutive otherness (e.g. body, world, other people) involved in the identity of a person this responsibility is not a simple fact. In fact, trying to make sense of and appropriate the person that we have become is a task that plays a major role in the person that we are, and the person that we will be.

Seeing a human being (ourselves as well as another) as a person is to see that human being as an autonomous and responsible person who is more than merely a product of (mental, social, biological) causal factors. A person is autonomous in the sense that her sense of self is a fundamental part of her identity. And yet, to be a person is more than our sense of self. The way other people see us is constitutive of the person that I am. I am not entirely in control of how other people see me, and my identity as a person depends on their recognition and respect. My identity is in this sense out of my hands, as it is with respect to the biological factors that make up who I am, and it is this interplay of autonomy and heteronomy that makes personal identity a question of appropriation. Being the person that I am requires that I appropriate my identity. This appropriation is difficult because it involves appropriating both my own sense of who I am and the way that other people see me. Ricoeur argues that this appropriation always takes place through narratives, that is, through the stories that we tell about ourselves because "the vicissitudes of life . . . remain in search of narrative configuration" (Ricoeur 2005: 103). Narratives help us to see the unique person that every human being is by articulating (some of) "the vicissitude of life" that we cannot see. Personal narratives give voice to an autonomy that is repeated at risk of being forgotten, and it helps us to make sense of heteronomous aspects of a human identity that the person is not responsible for. In this sense, narratives bring awareness to the interplay of normative universality (every human being is a person) and descriptive individuality (every person is a certain kind of person) constitutive of being a person.

The normative demand involved in the notion of personhood is meant to secure a person's autonomy. The demand to see a human being as an autonomous person is not only directed at our relation to other people. It also concerns the way we relate to ourselves. Being a person requires that I appropriate and take responsibility for the person that I am even though my identity is not entirely of my own making. To be a person is therefore a task that weighs heavily upon me, and which can become unbearable. Narratives can make us aware of the burden of identity and help us to make sense of the concrete problems that a person faces in her struggle for becoming the person that she, feels, understands, and wants herself to be.

Personal Suffering

It is this articulation of the problems of identity that makes the notion of personhood vital to phenomenological psychopathology. The notion is particularly useful when it comes to making sense of and dealing with the alienating aspect of mental illnesses. The disturbance of self-awareness involved in mental illness often entails a sense of alienation and unbearable passivity. As Wolfgang Blankenburg argues, "[t]he dynamic of anonymized processes of disease overtakes the subject's biography, and a human destiny becomes a 'destiny of drives and impulses'" (Blankenburg 1986: 98). Our identity is at stake in suffering. Our experience of being a self is troubled, and in severe cases it is so dramatically disturbed that we lose our sense of agency and ownership of our experiences and actions. And yet, "suffering is one of the most vivid forms of self-consciousness" (Ricoeur 1966: 450).

This ambiguity of suffering is constitutive of human identity. It is in and through suffering that we become the person that we are. In fact, the fragility of our identity is that which makes us that individual person that each and every one of us is. We are persons simply by being human, but we become the persons that we are through the challenges of suffering. Pain is not something that we simply feel. We are not mere passive victims of pain. Of course pain can be so excruciating that the experience is completely drained of thought and reflection. But in the afterglow of pain, thought re-emerges. We do something with what we feel. We relate ourselves to our feelings, or as Karl Jaspers argues, we always position ourselves to our suffering (Jaspers 1997: 414–427). In this sense, human suffering is always personal suffering. The notion of personhood can be of help when trying to make sense of how and why we suffer the way we do. In our attempts to describe and make sense of a person's suffering, it allows us to maintain both the irreproducible descriptive particularity of that person's suffering and the normative demand involved in personal suffering, namely, that in suffering we are dealing with a struggle of and for autonomy. This struggle is about appropriating and making sense of the unbearable passivity involved in suffering. And although the ethical demand to be (and to recognize the other person as) an autonomous person who takes responsibility for one's actions have a universal aim, the particularity of suffering tells a story about the irreplaceable individual in front of us who suffers. As Eugène Minkowski notes, "[t]he human person forms herself in the crucible of suffering. Through suffering the person affirms herself; she looks beyond, she sees beyond" (Minkowski 1999: 812; my translation). Understanding suffering as personal suffering is not simple. It involves a recognition of the interplay of selfhood and otherness in our self-awareness, the intimate alienation at the core of human identity that makes the person that we are a never-ending task. Minkowski argues that it is this ambiguity of suffering, a paralyzing passivity and active engagement, that makes our suffering personal:

> Suffering is an integral part of the human existence. Actually, it is more than a part; it marks existence and situates it. Suffering produces pain, and this is not a simple tautology. It hurts, and how! But it is a hurting that we do not know how to compare with any other. It takes place within the human "pathos," and through this the human being recognizes her human aspect . . . We find our person profoundly engaged in suffering. Suffering is in us, and in suffering we get in touch with ourselves and with existence. It is not human misery, but human suffering.
>
> (Minkowski 1999: 801; my translation)

Distinguishing suffering and misery is fundamental to phenomenological psychopathology because it allows both the patients and the mental health-care professional to recognize the patients as an autonomous person (Stanghellini and Rosfort 2015). While misery emphasizes the passivity of pain, suffering underscores the interplay of activity and passivity that makes human pain personal suffering. We engage with our suffering and with the world through suffering, as Minkowski argues, and in this engagement we are searching for the meaning(s) of our suffering. Suffering can be so unbearable that the patient is no longer able to see himself as a person. His sense of self can become so dramatically disturbed that his identity is submerged in anonymous and alienating processes of painful otherness.

A narrative reconfiguration of his suffering structured around the notion of personhood can help the mental health professional recognize the patient as a person, and the patient to appropriate his pain and make the otherness part of who he is. Suffering in this sense lets us see the individual person that we are through personal challenges that all human beings share.

BIBLIOGRAPHY

Blankenburg W. (1986). "Biographie und Krankheit." In K.-E. Bühler (ed.), *Zeitlichkeit als psychologisches Prinzip. Grundfragen der Biographie-Forschung*, pp. 85–13. Köln: Janus Presse.

Ferretti G. (2003). "Variazioni nel concetto di persona e paradossi dell'identità." In G. Ferretti, *Il bene al-di-là dell'essere: Temi e problemi levinassiani*, pp. 21–92. Napoli: Edizioni Scientifiche Italiani.

Figal G. and Espinet D. (2012). "Hermeneutics." In S. Luft and S. Overgaard (eds.), *The Routledge Companion to Phenomenology*, pp. 496–507. London: Routledge.

Gallagher S. (2012a). "On the Possibility of Naturalizing Phenomenology." In D. Zahavi (ed.), *The Oxford Handbook of Contemporary Phenomenology*, pp. 70–93. Oxford: Oxford University Press.

Gallagher S. (2012b). "Multiple Aspects in the Sense of Agency." *New Ideas in Psychology* 30: 15–31.

Gallagher S. and Zahavi D. (2012). *The Phenomenological Mind*, 2nd edn. London: Routledge.

Grøn A. (2004). "Self and Identity." In D. Zahavi, T. Grünbaum, and J. Parnas (eds.), *Structure and Development of Self-Consciousness: Interdisciplinary Perspectives*, pp. 123–156. Philadelphia: John Benjamins Publishing Company.

Grøn A. (2017). "Eindruck—Ausdruck." In S. Frohoff, T. Fuchs, and S. Micali (eds.), *Fremde Spiegelungen. Interdisciplinäre Zugange zur Sammlung Prinzhorn*, pp. 11–20. Paderborn: Wilhelm Fink.

Heidegger M. (1999). *Ontology—The Hermeneutics of Facticity* [1923], trans. J. van Bureen. Bloomington: Indiana University Press.

Heidegger M. (2010). *Being and Time* [1927], trans. J. Stambaugh, revised by D. J. Schmidt. Albany: State University of New York Press.

Husserl E. (2001). *Logical Investigations, vol. 1* [1900], trans. J. N. Findlay. London: Routledge.

Jaspers K. (1997). *General Psychopathology* [1959], trans. J. Hoenig and M. W. Hamilton. Baltimore: Johns Hopkins University Press.

Kant I. (1996a). "Groundwork of the Metaphysics of Morals" [1785], trans. M. J. Gregor. In I. Kant, *Practical Philosophy*, pp. 37–108. Cambridge: Cambridge University Press.

Kant I. (1996b). "Critique of Practical Reason" [1788], trans. M. J. Gregor. In I. Kant, *Practical Philosophy*, pp. 135–276. Cambridge: Cambridge University Press.

Legrand D. (2011). "Phenomenological Dimensions of Bodily Self-Consciousness." In S. Gallagher (ed.), *The Oxford Handbook of the Self*, pp. 204–227. Oxford: Oxford University Press.

Levinas E. (1969). *Totality and Infinity: An Essay on Exteriority* [1961], trans. A. Lingis. Pittsburgh: Duquesne University Press.

Levinas E. (1981). *Otherwise than Being or Beyond Essence* [1974], trans. A. Lingis. Pittsburgh: Duquesne University Press.

Minkowski E. (1999). *Traité de psychopathologie* [1966]. Le Plessis-Robinson: Institut Synthélabo pour le progress de la connaissance.

Ricoeur P. (1966). *Freedom and Nature: The Voluntary and the Involuntary* [1950], trans. E. Kohak. Evanston: Northwestern University Press.

Ricoeur P. (1970). *Freud and Philosophy: An Essay on Interpretation* [1965], trans. D. Savage. New Haven: Yale University Press.

Ricoeur P. (1986). *Fallible Man* [1960], trans. C. A. Kelbley. New York: Fordham University Press.

Ricoeur P. (1992). *Oneself as Another* [1990], trans. K. Blamey. Chicago: University of Chicago.

Ricoeur P. (2005). *The Course of Recognition* [2004], trans. D. Pellauer. Cambridge, MA: Harvard University Press.

Scull A. (2015). *Madness in Civilization: A Cultural History of Insanity, from the Bible to Freud, from the Madhouse to Modern Medicine.* London: Thames & Hudson.

Spaemann R. (1996). *Personen. Versuch über den Unterschied zwischen "etwas" und "jemand."* Stuttgart: Klett-Cotta.

Stanghellini G. and Rosfort R. (2015). "The Patient as an Autonomous Person: Hermeneutical Phenomenology as a Resource for an Ethics for Psychiatrists." In J. Z. Sadler, K. W. M. Fulford, and W. van Staden (eds.), *The Oxford Handbook of Psychiatric Ethics*, pp. 319–335. Oxford: Oxford University Press.

Strawson P. (1959). *Individuals: An Essay in Descriptive Metaphysics.* London: Methuen & Co Ltd.

Sturma D. (1997). *Philosophie der Person: Die Selbstverhältnisse von Subjektivität und Moralität.* Paderborn: Ferdinand Schöningh.

Taylor C. (1989). *Sources of the Self. The Making of Modern Identity.* Cambridge: Cambridge University Press.

Tengelyi L. (2012). "Action and Selfhood: A Narrative Interpretation." In D. Zahavi (ed.), *The Oxford Handbook of Contemporary Phenomenology*, pp. 265–286. Oxford: Oxford University Press.

Weiner D. B. (2008). "The Madman in the Light of Reason. Enlightenment Psychiatry. Parts One and Two." In E. R. Wallace and J. Gash (eds.), *History of Psychiatry and Medical Psychology*, pp. 255–303. New York: Springer.

Zahavi D. (2010). "Naturalized Phenomenology." In D. Schmicking and S. Gallagher (eds.), *Handbook of Phenomenology and Cognitive Science*, pp. 3–19. Dordrecht: Springer.

Zahavi D. (2014). *Self and Other: Exploring Subjectivity, Empathy, and Shame.* Oxford: Oxford University Press.

CHAPTER 39

BEFINDLICHKEIT
Disposition

FRANCESCA BRENCIO

INTRODUCTION

THIS chapter is dedicated to *Befindlichkeit*, a key concept expressed in Martin Heidegger's work *Being and Time* (1962). *Befindlichkeit* means "disposition," both in terms of being-in-situation and being situated. In order to explain why disposition is of interest to mental health clinicians, I will show the link between disposition and situatedness through three steps: the meaning of the "there" of "being-there" (following the English translation of the German word *Dasein*); the meaning of situatedness; and the meaning of moods in situatedness. Finally, I will show why disposition is related to psychopathology and clinical practice.

Being and Time represents Martin Heidegger's magnum opus. Published in 1927, it rapidly became one of the most significant and controversial philosophical texts of the twentieth century and it brought Heidegger international acclaim and notoriety, also confirming his distance from Husserl's phenomenology.[1] The genesis of *Being and Time* is well known:[2] *Sein und Zeit* is left interrupted due to "a matter of language," since the metaphysical language is

---

[1] On this topic, see Husserl E. (1968). *Letters to Roman Ingarden*. The Hague, Martinus Nijhoff; Husserl E. (1994). "Randbemerkungen Husserls zu Heideggers Sein und Zeit und Kant und das Problem der Metaphisik." *Husserl Studies* 11, pp. 3–63; Husserl E. (1997). *Psychological and Transcendental Phenomenology and the Confrontation with Heidegger (1927–1931)*. Dordrecht: Kluwer Academic Publishers. Due to the abundance of critical literature on this issue, I refer the reader to Boedeker E. C. (2005). "Phenomenology." In Hubert L. Dreyfus and Mark A. Wrathall (eds.), A Companion to Heidegger, pp. 156–172. Oxford: Blackwell Publishing; Crowell S. G. (2001). *Husserl, Heidegger, and the Space of Meaning: Paths Toward Transcendental, Phenomenology*. Evanston: Northwestern University Press; Crowell S. G. (2005). "Heidegger and Husserl: The Matter and Method of Philosophy." In Hubert L. Dreyfus and Mark A. Wrathall (eds.), A Companion to Heidegger, pp. 49–64. Oxford: Blackwell Publishing; Stapleton T. (1983). *Husserl and Heidegger: The Question of a Phenomenological Beginning*. Albany: State University of New York Press.

[2] See Kiesel T. (1993). The Genesis of Heidegger's Being and Time. Berkley: University of California Press.

not able to name what Being is.[3] With *Being and Time* emerges the only question that will engage Heidegger's thoughts for the rest of his life: the question of Being (*Sein*), in German *Seinsfrage*. The ontological question—what is the Being?—will cross the philosopher's meditation as Ariadne's thread and with his 1927 book Heidegger tries to answer this question with an analysis of the only being able to pose this question, the human being. However, it would be a mistake to consider *Being and Time* as an anthropological or psychological work on human being, since Heidegger's intention is to provide an analysis of the ontological constitution of being using a phenomenological approach. This is why Heidegger will use the word *Dasein*—in English, being-there—to pursue his goals.

What does *Dasein* mean? It is not simply the German expression for "existence," not equivalent to *anthropos*, not *homo sapiens*, not man in general, not human being and not even the transcendental *consciousness*; similarly, *Dasein* is not the "I" or the *ego*. Rather *Dasein* means the *way* through which human being *has to be*. For Heidegger being-there (*Dasein*) is not to be understood in terms of everyday human existence or embodied agency but—from his earliest Freiburg lectures onward—as an unfolding historical horizon or space of meaning that is already "there" (*Da*), prior to the emergence of the human body and its various capacities: "The *Da* in *Being and Time* does not mean a statement of place for a being, but rather it should designate the openness where beings can be present for the human being, and the human being also for himself."[4] Heidegger insists that *Dasein* is not to be interpreted as a concrete subject, such as *être-la*,[5] "here" in a determinate place. *Dasein* is "there" prior to the practical involvements of the subject: "The 'essence' (*Wesen*) of this entity lies in its 'to be' [*Zu-sein*]. Its Being-what-it-is [*Was-sein*] (*essentia*) must . . . be conceived in terms of its Being (*existentia*)."[6] The first feature of *Dasein* is to *have to be* (*zu-sein*) and its essence lies in its existence: "*Dasein* brings its 'there' along with it. If it lacks its 'there', it is not factically the entity which is essentially *Dasein*."[7]

For Heidegger the fundamental state of *Dasein* is its being-in-the-world: being-there and world are not separated but must be grasped together, avoiding the Cartesian dualism between subject and object and overcoming the subjectivism on which all Western philosophy is based. Being-in-the-world is a unitary phenomenon that characterizes every relationship; it is not a kind of "property" of human being, but rather the fundamental assumption of our existence: " 'Being-in' is thus the formal existential expression for the Being of *Dasein*, which has Being-in-the-world as its essential state."[8] Human being's primordial being-in-the-world is not an abstraction but always a concrete occurrence. Its being-in-the-world occurs and fulfils itself only in and as the manifold particular modes of human behavior; this kind of being presupposes a unique openness of man's existence. It has to be an openness into which

[3] Cf. M. Heidegger, *Letter on Humanism*, in *Pathmarks*, edited by W. McNeill, Cambridge University Press, 1998, pp. 249–250 [*Brief über den Humanismus*, in *Wegmarken*, Hrsg. von F.-W. von Herrmann, Klostermann Verlag, Frankfurt am Main 2004, *Gesamtausgabe* 9].

[4] M. Heidegger, *Zollikon Seminars*, trans. F. Mayr and R. Askay, Evanston: Northwestern University Press, 2001, p. 120 [*Zollikoner Seminare*, Hrsg. von M. Boss, Klostermann Verlag, Frankfurt am Main 1994, *Gesamtausgabe* 89].

[5] Cf. M. Heidegger, *Zollikon Seminars*, p. 120.

[6] M. Heidegger, *Being and Time*, trans. J. Macquarrie and E. Robinson, (New York: Harper & Row, 1962), [*Sein und Zeit*, Hrsg. von F.-W. von Herrmann, Klostermann Verlag, Frankfurt am Main 1977, *Gesamtausgabe* 2]. p. 67.

[7] M. Heidegger, *Being and Time*, p. 133.   [8] M. Heidegger, *Being and Time*, pp. 78–79.

the particular beings which man encounters can disclose themselves as the beings they are, phenomenologically, with all the context of their meaningful references.

The basic state of *Dasein* is its *being situated*, or in other words, its relationship with spatiality: being-in-the-world stresses the topological feature of *Dasein*, its being in a place and to be situated. The situatedness is a constant feature of *Dasein* and "the primacy of such situatedness is to be found . . . in the question of the nature of such situatedness, our own existence is itself brought into question."[9] Finding ourselves already into situatedness, means find ourselves gathered to a "there" (being-*there*[10]). The way in which our situatedness arises is most clearly evident in the German word *Dasein*, being-there: "By focusing on existence as 'Dasein', Heidegger is able to draw attention to the way in which existence is indeed a matter of situatedness—to exist, to be 'in the world', is to have a concrete 'there'."[11] As Heidegger says, "by its very nature, *Dasein* brings its 'there' along with it. If it lacks its 'there', it is not factically the entity which is essentially *Dasein*; indeed, it is not this entity at all. *Dasein is its disclosedness,* . . . *'Dasein is* its 'there'."[12]

Disposition: The situatedness is strictly related to the existence's facticity and it becomes manifest to us through our own moods and affectivity, through the way we "find ourselves," what Heidegger calls *Befindlichkeit*, in English "disposition."[13] We find the notion of *Befindlichkeit* in the §29 of chapter 5 (I section) of *Being and Time*. *Befindlichkeit* first appears in Heidegger's work as a translation of the Aristotelian notion of διάθεσις (disposition). It is in the years 1924–1927 that Heidegger develops a concept of disposition that constitutes a radicalization of the Husserlian phenomenological approach, in order to provide a concrete account of a phenomenological "beginning" (*Anfang*) and to offer a description of human being in terms of "living life" (*das Lebende*).[14] *Befindlichkeit* is not a

---

[9] J. Malpass, *Heidegger's Topology. Being, Place, World*, The MIT Press, Cambridge Massachusetts 2006, p. 41.

[10] "To translate 'Dasein' as 'being-there', while it does mean that the sense of 'here' that can be involved with '*Da*' is lost, nevertheless makes clear the way in which *Dasein* is indeed a mode of being that is characterized by its 'there'—it is its *there*—although how this 'there' is to be understood remains itself in question," J. Malpass, *Heidegger's Topology. Being, Place, World*, p. 50.

[11] J. Malpass, *Heidegger's Topology. Being, Place, World*, p. 47.

[12] M. Heidegger, *Being and Time*, p. 171.

[13] The word *Befindlichkeit* is one of the most difficult to translate in English. In the essay entitled "Affectivity in Heidegger I: Moods and Emotions in Being and Time," Andreas Elpidorou and Lauren Freeman provide a broad account of how *Befindlichkeit* has been translated into English by various scholars, such as "state of mind," "findingness," "affectivity," "disposition," "attunement," and many others. For a detailed reconstruction of the different translations, cf. A. Elpidorou and L. Freeman, "Affectivity in Heidegger I: Moods and Emotions in Being and Time," *Philosophy Compass*, vol. 10, issue 10, 2015, pp. 661–671. My choice to translate *Befindlichkeit* with "disposition" is due to the use of the German reflexive verb *sich befinden*, which literally means "finding oneself." In the ordinary way of speaking, the colloquial sentence "Wie befinden Sie sich?" means "how is it going?" or "how do you feel?" etc. In everyday language this expression refers to the situation in which someone finds him/herself situated. It is starting from this situated experience that the world and some entities in the world are disclosed to *Dasein*: the "disposition" is both this being into a situatedness, as ontological and constitutive dimension, and being open to the world. "Disposition" is the key to transcendence and to openness, as we will see later in the chapter.

[14] Cf. Beaufret J. (1974) Husserl et Heidegger. In Dialogue avec Heidegger III. Paris: Les Editions de Minuit; Bernet R. (1988). "Transcendance et intentionalité: Heidegger et Husserl sur les prolégomènes d'une ontologie phénoménologique." In F. Volpi et al. (eds.), Heidegger et l'Idée de la phenomenology, pp. 195–215. Dordrecht: Kluwer Academic Publishers; Hopkins B. (1993). Intentionality in Husserl and Heidegger: The Problem of the Original Method and Phenomenon of Phenomenology. Dordrecht: Kluwer Academic Publishers; Keller P. (1999). *Husserl and Heidegger on Human Experience.*

starting point in the context of Heidegger's understanding of fundamental structures of *Dasein*, rather it is a point of arrival in his pathway toward phenomenology and its roots, precisely, into Heidegger's relationship with Aristotle, a central point of his philosophical education.[15] According to Heidegger, Aristotle is the first philosopher to have investigated affects or passions (the πάθη) and to have stressed how human being is constitutively a *being-in*, because of this being is always determined by affects. *Being-in* indicates again a kind of situatedness, our being into an emotional state: "It is, above all, decisive that we lose composure, as in the case of fearing without encountering something in the environing world that could be the direct occasion of fear. In this being-a-matter-of-concern of the πάθη, corporeality is co-encountered in some mode or another."[16]

In the summer 1924 lectures on Aristotle's *Rhetoric*, Heidegger shows how philosophical logos and propositional judgment of philosophical discourse are both grounded in everyday speech, originating from factical existence, in which situation, affects, and moods disclose the determination of *Dasein*. Affect is thus a constitutive phenomenon of discursive disclosure and logos is a fundamental characteristic of the *Dasein* whose capacity for meaningful disclosure is grounded in affect. In the discourse we find the disposition (διάθεσις) of the hearer and the importance of affects (πάθη). The affects play a fundamental role in the determination of being-in-the-world, of being-with-and-toward-others: "These πάθη, 'affects,' . . . are concerned with a disposition of living things in their world, in the mode of being positioned toward something, allowing a matter to matter to it."[17] In these years (1919–1924)[18] Heidegger is working on the issue of living being: this is why we find the language typical of philosophy of life (*Lebensphilosophie*) such as in the lecture courses of 1918, *The Idea of Philosophy and the Problem of Worldview* and *Phenomenology and Transcendental Philosophy Value*, where Heidegger insists on the supremacy of life, understood as pre-theoretical, on the theoretical dimension: "This primacy of the theoretical must be broken, but not in order to proclaim the primacy of the practical, and not in order to

Cambridge: Cambridge University Press; Richardson W. J. (1963). *Heidegger. Through Phenomenology to Thought*. Dordrecht: Springer; Taminiaux J. (1994). "The Husserlian Heritage in Heidegger's Notion of the Self." In T. Kisiel and J. van Buren (eds.), *Reading Heidegger from the Start: Essays in his Earliest Thought*. Albany: State University of New York Press; von Hermann F.-W. (1988). *Der Begriff der Phänomenologie bei Heidegger und Husserl*. Frankfurt am Main: Klostermann Verlag.

[15] The lecture *Phänomenologische Interpretationen zu Aristoteles: Einführung in die Phänomenologische Forschung* (winter semester 1921–1922), the course entitled *Grundbegriffe der aristotelischen Philosophie* (summer semester 1924), and the lecture *Platon: Sophistes* (winter semester 1924–1925) are important pathways of Heidegger's understanding of the Aristotelian concepts πάθη (affects) and διάθεσις (disposition). On this topic cf. C. Hadjioannou, "*Befindlichkeit as Retrieval of Aristotelian διάθεσις: Heidegger Reading Aristotle in the Marburg Years*," in T. Keiling (ed.), *Heideggers Marburger Zeit: Themen, Argumente, Konstellationen*, Klostermann Verlag, Frankfurt am Main 2013, pp. 223–236; F. Volpi, *Heidegger e Aristotele*, Padova: Daphne Editrice, 1984; W. Walter Brogan, *Heidegger and Aristotle: The Twofoldness of Being*, New York: SUNY, 2005.

[16] M. Heidegger, *Basic Concepts of Aristotelian Philosophy*, translated by R. D. Metcalf and M. B. Tanzer, Bloomington: Indiana University Press, 2009, pp. 139–140 [*Grundbegriffe der aristotelischen Philosophie*, Hrsg. Von M. Michalski, Klostermann Verlag, Frakfurt am Main 2002, *Gesamtausgabe* 18].

[17] M. Heidegger, *Basic Concepts of Aristotelian Philosophy*, p. 83. Cf. P. L. Coriando, *Affektenlehre und Phänomenologie der Stimmungen: Wege einer Ontologie und Ethik des Emotionalen*, Klostermann Verlag, Frankfurt am Main 2002, pp. 91–116.

[18] See Van Buren J. (1994). *The Young Heidegger*. Bloomington: Indiana University Press.

introduce something that shows the problems from a new side, but because the theoretical itself and as such refers back to something pre-theoretical."[19]

The philosophy of living being grounds Heidegger's own understanding of *Befindlichkeit*, as an a priori constitutive part of *Dasein's* facticity, together with moods (*Stimmungen*). According to Heidegger, it is through moods that we can know the world in general and the possibility of "truth." Whereas modern philosophy holds that "truth" is a function of propositional logic, Heidegger argues that it is pre-predicative mood that "founds all predicative truth."[20] Disposition expresses the fact that human beings are always situated into a mood and always opened to the world. For these reasons, Heidegger argues that *Befindlichkeit*, as an ontological structure, discloses the ontic experience of the world through moods. *Befindlichkeit* is a "fundamental *existentiale*,"[21] namely it is a basic existential way in which *Dasein* is its "there." Heidegger writes: "In having a mood, *Dasein* is always disclosed mood wise as that entity to which it has been delivered over in its Being; and in this way it has been delivered over to the Being which, in existing, it has to be. 'To be disclosed' does not mean 'to be known as this sort of thing.'"[22] According to Heidegger, moods are not a kind of psychological state that we experience within a given world. Mood is a "background through which it is possible to encounter things in the ways that we do, as 'there', 'not there', 'mattering', 'not mattering', 'for this' or 'for that.'"[23] Heideggerian moods have neither an "internal" nor an "external" phenomenology: "A mood assails us. It comes neither from 'outside' nor from 'inside', but arises out of Being-in-the-world, as a way of such Being. . . . The mood has already disclosed, in every case, Being-in-the-world as a whole and makes it possible first of all to direct oneself towards something."[24] A mood is a "background to all specifically directed intentional states. It is part of the structure of intentionality and is presupposed by the possibility of encountering anything in experience or thought."[25] Even though moods are considered to be psychological phenomena, Heidegger insists on the fact that psychology is not able to grasp the ontological importance of mood under the light of an ontological perspective. He writes: "Having a mood is not related to the psychical in the first instance, and is not itself an inner condition . . . . It is in this that the *second* essential characteristic of states-of-mind shows itself. We have seen that the world, *Dasein*-with, and existence are *equiprimordially*

[19] M. Heidegger, *Towards the Definition of Philosophy*, translated by T. Sadler, London, Continuum, 2002, p. 47 [*Zur Bestimmung der Philosophie*, Hrsg. von B. Heimbüchel, Klostermann Verlag, Frankfurt am Main 1999, *Gesamtausgabe* 56/57].

[20] Cf. K. Held, "Fundamental Moods and Heidegger's Critique of Contemporary Culture," in J. Sallis (ed.) *Reading Heidegger: Commemorations*, Indianapolis: Indiana University Press, 1993, pp. 28–30.

[21] Cf. M. Heidegger, *Being and Time*, p. 173.   [22] M. Heidegger, *Being and Time*, p. 173.

[23] M. Ratcliffe, "The Phenomenology and Neurobiology of Moods and Emotions," in D. Schmicking and S. Gallagher (eds.), *Handbook of Phenomenology and Cognitive Sciences*, Springer 2010, p. 128.

[24] M. Heidegger, *Being and Time*, p. 176

[25] M. Ratcliffe, *The Phenomenology and Neurobiology of Moods and Emotions*, p. 128. On this topic I refer the reader also to Ratcliffe M. (2009). "Existential Feeling and Psychopathology." Philosophy, Psychiatry, & Psychology 16(2): 179–194; Ratcliffe M. (2009). "The Phenomenology of Moods and the Meaning of Life." In Peter Goldie (ed.), The Oxford Handbook of Philosophy of Emotion, pp. 349–371. Oxford: Oxford University Press; Ratcliffe M. (2013). "Why Moods Matter." In Mark A. Wrathall (ed.), The Cambridge Companion to Heidegger's Being and Time. Cambridge: Cambridge University Press.

disclosed; and state-of-mind is a basic existential species of their disclosedness, because this disclosedness itself is essentially Being-in-the-world."[26]

Befindlichkeit works on two levels: on one hand, it shows how *Dasein* is essentially always *disclosed* to the world, to others and to entities; on the other hand, it shows how *Dasein* is always orientated toward both a horizontal and a vertical axis. Every mood and all consequential feelings activate this double axis and illuminate *Dasein*'s ability to understand of itself, its existence, its being-with the others (*Mit-sein*), and its way of behaving.[27] Heidegger identifies three ontological features of *Befindlichkeit*: the first is that it discloses to *Dasein* its thrownness; the second is that moods disclose being-in-the-world as a whole, and third is that *Befindlichkeit* implies a disclosive submission to the world, out of which we can encounter something that matters to us.

Fear, anxiety and psychopathology: In §30 of chapter 5 of *Being and Time*, Heidegger analyzes the phenomenon of fear (*Furcht*)[28] and in §40 the phenomenon of anxiety (*Angst*), as modes of *Befindlichkeit*. Fear has always an object and according to Heidegger it is always characterized by three elements: (1) what in the face of which we fear, (2) fearing, and (3) what about which we fear. On the contrary, anxiety is characterized by the absence of a definite object. Anxiety blocks any possibility to be open to others and to situations. Anxiety breaks the transparency of self-constitution and the human being loses its capacity to recognize itself in relation to others: "Anxiety thus takes away from *Dasein* the possibility of understanding itself, as it falls in terms of the 'world'."[29] In anxiety, "one has an 'uncanny' feeling. Here the peculiar indefiniteness of that which *Dasein* finds itself involved with anxiety initially finds expression: the nothing and nowhere. But uncanniness means at the same time not-being-at-home."[30] In anxiety *Dasein* faces with its own "uncanniness," the mode of not-being-at-home (*Unheimlich*) and this can be experienced as a kind of disconnection from reality. Anxiety is the collapse of the meaning of life and it is interpreted as a pulling away from nothingness, as Heidegger writes in *What is Metaphysics?* (1929): "Anxiety does not let such confusion arise. Much to the contrary, a peculiar calm pervades it. . . . The indeterminateness of that in the face of which and for which we become anxious is no mere lack of determination but rather the essential impossibility of determining it. . . . In anxiety, we say, 'one feels ill at ease.' . . . All things and we ourselves sink into indifference. This, however, not in the sense of mere disappearance. Rather in this very receding, things turn toward us. . . . Anxiety reveals the nothing."[31] However, anxiety also has a positive meaning, since it discloses *Dasein* as being-possible. It means that anxiety makes manifest in *Dasein* its "*being towards* its own most potentiality-for-Being-that is, its *being-free for* the freedom of choosing itself and taking hold of itself."[32] Anxiety brings *Dasein* face to face with its *being free for* the authenticity of its being, and for this authenticity as a possibility which it always is. *Befindlichkeit* also illuminates the relationship with the others (human beings, entities,

---

[26] M. Heidegger, *Being and Time*, p. 176.

[27] Cf. P. L. Coriando, *Affektenlehre und Phänomenologie der Stimmungen: Wege einer Ontologie und Ethik des Emotionalen*, pp. 1–10, 117–153; F.-W. von Herrmann, *Hermeneutische Phänomenologie des Daseins. Eine Erläuterung von "Sein und Zeit"*, vol. 3, pp. 28–45.

[28] Cf. M. Heidegger, *Being and Time*, pp. 179–182.   [29] M. Heidegger, *Being and Time*, p. 231.

[30] M. Heidegger, *Being and Time*, p. 188.

[31] M. Heidegger, *"What is Metaphysics?"* in *Pathmarks*, p. 88.

[32] M. Heidegger, *Being and Time*, p. 232.

word, nature, etc.): working on the ontological disclosure of *Dasein*,[33] it increases our ability to feel empathy (*Einfühlung*) as consequence of the constitutive being-with the others (*Mitsein*) of *Dasein*.

Why is disposition related to psychopathology and clinical practice and why is it of interest to mental health clinicians? At first sight we may think we are faced only with a theoretical construction that has nothing to do with mental health or psychopathology: with some little exception for the Zollikon seminars, Heidegger is usually considered a philosopher who is not so interested in issues connected to mental health. However, this is a prejudice that needs to be broken, going directly to his works. With the notion of *Befindlichkeit* we are faced with four important issues that are connected with psychopathology and with phenomenological psychopathology: first, we are faced with the constitutive situation (or ontological, using Heidegger's word) of being into situation and being situated, typical of every human being. These features stress how our existence and also our health are never disembodied from the situation in which we find ourselves: the situatedness is the prominent peculiarity of our life and it shows the kind of relationship we have with ourselves and with the world around us.

In second place, *Befindlichkeit* shows that situatedness is always aimed to openness: being open toward others, toward events, also toward illness allows human being to search for meanings and possibilities of understanding, to face delusions and to break the wall of sufferance that can paralyze people affected by mental disorders or who have experienced a trauma. For example, in the frame of emotional trauma, such as grief, the unity of temporality is devastatingly disturbed: people are frozen in an eternal present in which they remain forever trapped, or to which they are condemned to be perpetually returned.[34] Faced with loss, a sense of a foreshortened future pervades human being and doesn't allow us to distinguish the experience of time itself from the experience of temporal properties.[35] A traumatic event or situation creates psychological trauma when it overwhelms the individual's ability to cope, and leaves that person fearing death, annihilation, mutilation, or psychosis. The individual may feel emotionally, cognitively, and physically overwhelmed. Trauma comes in many forms, and there are vast differences among people who experience trauma. Both in trauma and in psychopathological phenomena (i.e. depression, anxiety) the sense of life is altered; this alteration is not only related to the content of what has happened, but is also a formal alteration insofar as the experience of being determined by the past and of how it is resolved undergoes a profound change, which has a bearing on everything in the past, consolidating memory falsifications and fabrications. Traumatic events usually elicit a closure of human being not more able to recognize its constitutive openness and breaking trust in interpersonal relationships.

In the third place, Heidegger's interpretation of anxiety, in the frame of modes of *Befindlichkeit*, approaches the human being and its suffering from a phenomenological

---

[33] F. Brencio, "Heidegger and Binswanger: Just a Misunderstanding?" *The Humanistic Psychologist*, vol. 43, issue 3, 2015, pp. 278–296.

[34] Cf. R. Stolorow, *Trauma and Existence*, New York: Francis and Taylor 2007.

[35] Cf. M. Ratcliffe, M. Ruddell, and B. Smith, "What is a "Sense of Foreshortened Future?" A Phenomenological Study of Trauma, Trust, and Time," *Frontiers in Psychology*, vol. 5, 2014, pp. 1–11.

point of view. By anxiety Heidegger does not mean common anxiousness which is ultimately reducible to fearfulness, but rather the fundamental characteristic that shows us who we really are, what our lives are really about, and our possibility to choose what is really important in our existence. In anxiety we lose the experience of our ordinary identity, we are frozen and we cannot feel "at home" in the world. Anxiety seems to mean a breakdown of all ordinary understanding and activity in the space of a moment. The alienation that comes from this hiatus—being-in-the-world and yet feeling one is not-being-at-home in the world—shows us that the world, in this particular moment, has nothing to offer us. The possibility of the future loses its meaning and the world suddenly falls away. Anxiety shows the horizon of being in which *Dasein* manifests itself as the possibility in which man encounters what is most essential in itself.

Finally, in the fourth place, disposition illuminates the understanding of moods (*Stimmungen*) and the relationship between feelings (*Gefühle*) and emotions (*Emotionen*). Moods and feelings are the grounds of our experience of reality and more generally of the world. According to Heidegger it is the mood that attunes one to the world and gives meaning—this is why in anxiety, as noted earlier, the world collapses completely. Heidegger's conception of moods and their phenomenology provide some support in psychopathology: for example, Sass (1994) suggests that schizophrenia involves a general diminution of bodily feelings, accompanied by exaggeration of specific affective responses;[36] Stanghellini (2004) stresses the role played by changes in feelings and observes that distortions of feeling, in the sense of disembodiment, are a source of altered experience—the feeling of being disconnected to oneself.[37]

Under this light, Heidegger's notion of disposition can help psychopathology in providing a new paradigm for understanding both the human being and the pathologies of existence: "Paramount in Heidegger's contribution was his insistence on the structural unity of *Dasein*, which has introduced into phenomenological clinical psychology a framework for interpreting psychopathological phenomena within the context of the person's being-in-the-world as a whole, a scope scarcely approached in academic psychology. In other words, phenomenological psychologists now use philosophical resources to move beyond the description of more or less isolated mental states to the gestalt "existence".[38] Heidegger seeks interpretively to restore the unity of our being, split asunder in Cartesian dualism. His analysis of the human being is the reconstitution of a whole: the point is not to reconstitute the ontic process of a causal series of events but to see the ontological unit of an articulated multiplicity.[39]

[36] Cf. L. Sass, *The Paradoxes of Delusion: Wittgenstein, Schreber and the Schizophrenic Mind*, Ithaca, Cornell University Press 1994.

[37] Cf. G. Stanghellini, *Disembodied Spirits and Deanimated Bodies: The Psychopathology of Common Sense*, Oxford, Oxford University Press 2004.

[38] F. J. Wertz, "Phenomenological Currents in Twentieth-Century Psychology," in H. L. Dreyfus and M. A. Wrathall (eds.), *A Companion to Phenomenology and Existentialism*, Oxford: Blackwell Publishing 2006, pp. 401–402.

[39] F. Brencio, "World, Time and Anxiety. Heidegger's Existential Analytic and Psychiatry," *Folia Medica*, vol. 56, issue 4, pp. 297–304.

BIBLIOGRAPHY

Beaufret J. (1974). *Husserl et Heidegger*. In Dialogue avec Heidegger III. Paris: Les Editions de Minuit.

Bernet R. (1988). "Transcendance et intentionalité: Heidegger et Husserl sur les prolégomènes d'une ontologie phénoménologique." In F. Volpi, et al. (eds.), *Heidegger et l'Idée de la phenomenology*, pp. 195-215. Dordrecht: Kluwer Academic Publishers.

Blattner W. (2006). *Heidegger's Being and Time*. New York: Continuum.

Boedeker E. C. (2005). "Phenomenology." In Hubert L. Dreyfus and Mark A. Wrathall (eds.), *A Companion to Heidegger*, pp. 156-172. Oxford: Blackwell Publishing.

Brencio F. (2015). "Heidegger and Binswanger: Just a Misunderstanding?" *The Humanistic Psychologist* 43 (3): 278-296.

Brencio F. (2015). "World, Time and Anxiety. Heidegger's Existential Analytic and Psychiatry." *Folia Medica* 56(4): 297-304.

Brogan W. W. (2005). *Heidegger and Aristotle: The Twofoldness of Being*. New York: SUNY.

Coriando P. L. (2002). *Affektenlehre und Phänomenologie der Stimmungen: Wege einer Ontologie und Ethik des Emotionalen*. Frankfurt am Main: Klostermann Verlag.

Crowell S. G. (2001). *Husserl, Heidegger, and the Space of Meaning: Paths Toward Transcendental, Phenomenology*. Evanston: Northwestern University Press.

Crowell S. G. (2005). "Heidegger and Husserl: The Matter and Method of Philosophy." In Hubert L. Dreyfus and Mark A. Wrathall (eds.), *A Companion to Heidegger*, pp. 49-64. Oxford: Blackwell Publishing.

Elpidorou A. and Freeman L. (2015). "Affectivity in Heidegger I: Moods and Emotions in Being and Time." *Philosophy Compass* 10(2): 661-671.

Hadjioannou C. (2013). "Befindlichkeit as Retrieval of Aristotelian διάθεσις: Heidegger Reading Aristotle in the Marburg Years." In T. Keiling (ed.), *Heidegger's Marburger Zeit: Themen, Argumente, Konstellationen*, pp. 223-236. Frankfurt am Main: Klostermann Verlag.

Heidegger M. (1962). *Being and Time*, trans. J. Macquarrie and E. Robinson. New York: Harper & Row [*Sein und Zeit*, Hrsg. von F.-W. von Herrmann, Klostermann Verlag, Frankfurt am Main 1977, *Gesamtausgabe* 2].

Heidegger M. (1998). "Letter on Humanism." In *Pathmarks*, pp. 239-276, edited by W. McNeill. Cambridge: Cambridge University Press [*Brief über den Humanismus*, in *Wegmarken*, Hrsg. Von F.-W. von Herrmann, Klostermann Verlag, Frankfurt am Main 2004, *Gesamtausgabe* 9].

Heidegger M. (2001). *Zollikon Seminars*, trans. F. Mayr and R. Askay. Evanston: Northwestern University Press [*Zollikoner Seminare*, Hrsg. von M. Boss, Klostermann Verlag, Frankfurt am Main 1994, *Gesamtausgabe* 89].

Heidegger M. (2002). *Towards the Definition of Philosophy*, trans. T. Sadler. London: Continuum, 2002 [*Zur Bestimmung der Philosophie*, Hrsg. von B. Heimbüchel, Klostermann Verlag, Frankfurt am Main 1999, *Gesamtausgabe* 56/57].

Heidegger M. (2009). *Basic Concepts of Aristotelian Philosophy*, trans. R. D. Metcalf and M. B. Tanzer. Bloomington: Indiana University Press [*Grundbegriffe der aristotelischen Philosophie*, Hrsg. Von M. Michalski, Klostermann Verlag, Frakfurt am Main 2002, *Gesamtausgabe* 18].

Held K. (1993). "Fundamental Moods and Heidegger's Critique of Contemporary Culture." In J. Sallis (ed.), *Reading Heidegger: Commemorations*, pp. 286-303. Indianapolis: Indiana University Press.

Hopkins B. (1993). *Intentionality in Husserl and Heidegger: The Problem of the Original Method and Phenomenon of Phenomenology.* Dordrecht: Kluwer Academic Publishers.

Husserl E. (1968). *Letters to Roman Ingarden.* The Hague, Martinus Nijhoff.

Husserl E. (1994). "Randbemerkungen Husserls zu Heideggers Sein und Zeit und Kant und das Problem der Metaphisik." *Husserl Studies* 11: 3–63.

Husserl E. (1997). *Psychological and Transcendental Phenomenology and the Confrontation with Heidegger (1927–1931).* Dordrecht: Kluwer Academic Publishers.

Keller P. (1999). *Husserl and Heidegger on Human Experience.* Cambridge: Cambridge University Press.

Kiesel T. (1993). *The Genesis of Heidegger's Being and Time.* Berkley: University of California Press.

Malpass J. (2006). *Heidegger's Topology.* Being, Place, World. Cambridge, MA: The MIT.

Ratcliffe M. (2009). "Existential Feeling and Psychopathology." *Philosophy, Psychiatry, & Psychology* 16(2): 179–194.

Ratcliffe M. (2009). "The Phenomenology of Moods and the Meaning of Life." In Peter Goldie (ed.), *The Oxford Handbook of Philosophy of Emotion,* pp. 349–371. Oxford: Oxford University Press.

Ratcliffe M. (2010). "The Phenomenology and Neurobiology of Moods and Emotions." In D. Schmicking and S. Gallagher (eds.), *Handbook of Phenomenology and Cognitive Sciences,* pp. 123–140. Berlin: Springer.

Ratcliffe M. (2013). "Why Moods Matter." In Mark A. Wrathall (ed.), *The Cambridge Companion to Heidegger's Being and Time,* pp. 157–176. Cambridge: Cambridge University Press.

Ratcliffe M., Ruddell M., and Smith B. (2014). "What is a 'Sense of Foreshortened Future?' A Phenomenological Study of Trauma, Trust, and Time." *Frontiers in Psychology* 5: 1–11.

Richardson W. J. (1963). *Heidegger. Through Phenomenology to Thought.* Dordrecht: Springer.

Sass L. (1994). *The Paradoxes of Delusion: Wittgenstein, Schreber and the Schizophrenic Mind.* Ithaca: Cornell University Press.

Stanghellini G. (2004). *Disembodied Spirits and Deanimated Bodies: The Psychopathology of Common Sense.* Oxford: Oxford University Press.

Stapleton T. (1983). *Husserl and Heidegger: The Question of a Phenomenological Beginning.* Albany: State University of New York Press.

Stolorow R. (2007). *Trauma and Existence.* New York: Francis and Taylor.

Taminiaux J. (1994). "The Husserlian Heritage in Heidegger's Notion of the Self." In T. Kisiel and J. van Buren (eds.), *Reading Heidegger from the Start: Essays in his Earliest Thought,* pp. 269–290. Albany: State University of New York Press.

Van Buren J. (1994). *The Young Heidegger.* Bloomington: Indiana University Press.

Volpi F. (1984). *Heidegger e Aristotele.* Padova: Daphne Editrice.

von Hermann F.-W. (1988). *Der Begriff der Phänomenologie bei Heidegger und Husserl.* Frankfurt am Main: Klostermann Verlag.

von Herrmann F.-W. (2008). *Hermeneutische Phänomenologie des Daseins. Eine Erläuterung von "Sein und Zeit."* Frankfurt am Main: Klostermann Verlag. (3 volumes).

....

CHAPTER 40

VALUES AND VALUES-BASED PRACTICE

....

K. W. M. (BILL) FULFORD AND
GIOVANNI STANGHELLINI

INTRODUCTION

"VALUES" is one of those terms that, although familiar in everyday discourse, has no settled meaning. Values are "what matters" or that which "is important." But what matters or is important covers a diversity of concepts (such as needs, wishes, preferences, strengths, limitations, and virtues) the meanings of which are both individually complex (reflecting as they do the variety of personal, cultural, and historical values) and collectively conflicting (what we need and what we want, e.g. are often in conflict).

The diverse meanings of "values" are reflected in a corresponding diversity of philosophical and phenomenological accounts. It would take a much longer chapter than this even to list the variety of these accounts let alone do justice to the many insights they offer. Rather than attempting anything in the way of a comprehensive review, therefore, we focus on the challenges presented by values in psychopathology and the resources of values-based practice in responding to them. We describe two case studies, respectively of delusion and of anorexia, and then consider the extent to which these are capable of wider generalization drawing on the resources of phenomenological psychopathology and the phenomenology of values.

FIRST CASE STUDY: SIMON'S STORY

Simon (40) was a black, American lawyer threatened by legal action from a group of colleagues. Although he had long since given up his religious faith, he responded to this crisis by praying at a small altar that he set up in his front room. After an emotional evening's "outpouring", he discovered that the candle wax had run down marking certain words and phrases of his bible. The marked passages meant nothing to Simon's peers but he interpreted them as a direct communication from God signifying that "I am the living son of David . . ."

Simon's experiences are consistent with "delusional perception" as defined in psychiatric diagnostic schedules such as the PSE (Present State Examination) (Wing, Cooper, and Sartorius 1974). Delusional perception in DSM (Diagnostic and Statistical Manual) (American Psychiatric Association (APA) 2013) is among the Criterion A symptoms for schizophrenia. Yet in Simon's case his experiences turned out to be empowering rather than disabling. Guided by the marked passages in his bible from this and subsequent similar episodes Simon won his case, his reputation soared, and he went on to establish a research trust for the study of religious experience.

THE CHALLENGE OF VALUES IN SIMON'S STORY

How the positive outcome of Simon's story should be understood takes us straight to the challenge of values in psychiatric diagnosis. Why? Because the difference between a diagnosis of psychotic disorder and religious experience in Simon's case lies not in his experiences as such but in how their effects on his life are evaluated. In DSM a diagnosis of schizophrenia requires that in addition to one or more Criterion A symptoms (such as delusional perception) the person concerned should also satisfy a criterion of clinical significance, Criterion B. To satisfy Criterion B the person concerned must show a 'level of functioning in one or more major areas, such as work, interpersonal relations, or self-care, (that) is markedly below the level achieved prior to the onset (APA 2013: 99). Simon, therefore, although satisfying Criterion A, does not on the information available satisfy Criterion B, for although he was indeed functioning differently as a result of his experiences, his functioning (as a lawyer) was above rather than (as required by Criterion B) below the level achieved prior to the onset.

But this is where values come in. For DSM's Criterion B is a *value* criterion: it requires not just a change in Simon's functioning but one or more value judgments about whether any change is *above* the level previously achieved (i.e. a change for the *better* = *not* ill) or *below* that level (i.e. a change for the *worse* = *ill*). It may be of course that with further information the diagnostic picture will become less clear-cut. His interpersonal functioning, for example, might have taken a turn for the worse. But this reinforces the evaluative nature of Criterion B. For this mixed picture then requires evaluations not merely of Simon's level of functioning within any one area (work functioning in this instance) but between other areas as well (enhanced work functioning versus deterioration in interpersonal relations).

Simon's story is the tip of a values iceberg; values are critical too in other areas of psychopathology such as depression (Fulford et al. forthcoming); and values of various kinds occur throughout both DSM (Sadler 2005) and ICD (Fulford 1994). But values are challenging. They are challenging for theory: they raise questions about the very status of mental disorder that in turn beg deep underlying questions about the relationship between evaluative and descriptive meaning (Fulford 1989). Values are challenging too for empirical research (Stanghellini and Ballerini 2007; Fulford et al. 2014). And they are challenging above all clinically in the balanced (diagnostic as well as therapeutic) judgments they entail. Getting the balance wrong is an important factor driving abuses of psychiatry (as in the former USSR, Fulford et al. 1993). Getting the balance right on the other hand is a key factor in contemporary person-centered approaches to psychiatric care based on co-production and recovery of individual quality of life (Allott et al. 2005). So how do we go about getting the balance of values right?

RESPONDING TO THE CHALLENGE: ANALYTIC PROCESS

Getting the balance right starts with taking the significance of values in psychiatric diagnosis seriously. For some, like Thomas Szasz (1960), for example, psychiatric diagnostic values show psychiatry to be outwith medical science. For others, such as R. E. Kendell (1975) and Christopher Boorse (1975, 1976), they show that psychiatric science is at a primitive stage of development. Neither approach amounts to a basis for taking the values in question seriously (other than by way of elimination). Work in analytic philosophy of values by contrast takes these same values fully seriously in showing them to be a reflection of the diversity of human values and as such fully consistent with the science of medicine.

The work in question is derived from the mid-twentieth-century "Oxford School" of ordinary language philosophy exemplified by J. L. Austin (1956–1957), R. M. Hare (1952), and others. Work in this tradition, applied to medicine (Fulford 1989), shows that values are implicit in all medical diagnostic concepts but become visible only in areas like psychiatry where the values in question are diverse and hence tend to come into conflict. In other words values are in this respect like the air we breathe—everywhere and everywhere important but noticed only when (as when the air is in short supply) we have difficulty breathing. So understood therefore the visibility of values in psychiatric diagnosis is a mark neither of psychiatry being outwith medical science (as Szasz thought) nor of some supposed deficiency in psychiatric science (as Kendell, Boorse, and others argued) but rather of the diversity of human values in the areas of human experience and behavior (such as belief, desire, volition, motivation, identity, sexuality, and so forth) with which psychiatry is characteristically concerned (Fulford 1989).

The practical counterpart of this analytically derived way of understanding psychiatric diagnostic values is a skills-based approach to balanced clinical decision-making called values-based practice (Fulford 2004). Far from being anti-scientific, values-based practice so derived is a partner to evidence-based practice. Values-based practice, as Figure 40.1 indicates, relies on learnable clinical skills and other process elements that, together with evidence-based practice, support balanced decision-making in individual cases within frameworks of shared values. (See generally, Fulford, Peile, and Carroll 2012.)

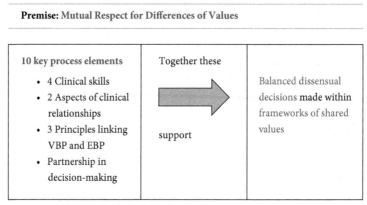

FIGURE 40.1 A summary of values-based practice.

There are many other resources for working with values in medicine: ethics, health economics, decision analysis, and so forth. The role of values-based practice among these other resources remains controversial (Loughlin 2014) but it is nonetheless currently being successfully applied in a number of areas particularly of bodily medicine such as surgery (Handa et al. 2016). Progress in mental health, however, despite a number of well-supported initiatives, has been slower. There are various reasons for this (Fulford et al. 2015). What these come down to is that the particular diversity of values in mental health makes them in various respects more challenging than their counterparts in bodily medicine. Our second case study illustrates one particular aspect of the more challenging nature of values in mental health and how phenomenology extends the resources of analytically derived values-based practice in responding to them.

SECOND CASE STUDY: ANNA'S STORY

Anna is a young woman whose clinical picture satisfies DSM criteria for anorexia nervosa (APA 2013). She shows: a) significantly low body weight for her age due to "restriction of energy intake"; b) "Intense fear of gaining weight or of becoming fat"; and c) "Disturbance in the way (she experiences her) body weight or shape, undue influence of body weight or shape on self-evaluation, or persistent lack of recognition of the seriousness of (her) current low body weight." Anna also shows a number of associated features: her "self-esteem . . . (is) highly dependent on (her) perceptions of body weight and shape." Also, "weight loss (is) . . . viewed (by her) as an impressive achievement and a sign of extraordinary self-discipline, whereas weight gain (was) perceived as an unacceptable failure of self-control." Like many others she "lacks insight" into her condition and was brought to "professional attention by family members." Next to these symptoms, Anna says she has a troubled experience of her body from a first-person perspective: "I don't feel my body. It changes in shape and consistency according to situations." She compares her body to a "wobbling liquid whose shape changes when I'm in the presence of other people." She feels shame and disgust for her body. Yet, surprisingly she seeks identity through the others' gaze that "makes me sense my body from without myself." Also, she seeks a sense of herself through starvation aimed at salvation in thinness.

THE CHALLENGE OF VALUES IN ANNA'S STORY

Anna's story may seem at first glance diagnostically value-free. The "weight loss," "energy intake restriction," and "intense fears" respectively of Criteria a) and b), although requiring judgments (e.g. *significantly* low body weight, *intense* fear of gaining weight), are in principle straightforwardly descriptive. Unlike Simon, furthermore, there are no functional criteria of clinical significance required for a DSM diagnosis of anorexia. Functional consequences of anorexia are noted by DSM (343) but are not diagnostic.

Closer inspection shows however that in addition to these descriptive features, values are integral not only to diagnosis in Anna's story but also, as we will see, to treatment. As to diagnosis, the descriptive elements of Criterion a) (such as weight loss) are not in themselves diagnostic since they are features equally of non-pathological states of fasting (as in hunger strikers). Nor is intense fear of weight gain (Criterion b)) as such diagnostic: such fears may be normal in some groups (such as fashion models) and, anyway, according to DSM (342), they are not always present in anorexia. Something more than or additional to these descriptive criteria is thus needed to differentiate anorexia as a mental disorder from non-pathological fasting.

In Simon's story the equivalent "something more," required to mark out pathological delusional experiences from non-pathological counterparts such as spiritual experiences, was provided by the evaluative diagnostic elements in DSM's Criterion b). In Anna's story the relevant evaluative elements are to be found in DSM's Criterion c) for anorexia. With the relevant evaluative elements italicized, Criterion c) reads "*disturbance* in the way (she experiences her) body weight or shape, *undue* influence of body weight or shape on self-evaluation, or persistent lack of recognition of the *seriousness* of (her) current low body weight."

The evaluative elements of Criterion c) for anorexia, like their counterparts in Criterion b) for schizophrenia, are explicit and as such accessible to the balancing processes of values-based practice. Again, the required balancing may seem straightforward in Anna's case. Anna will of course balance the requisite values very differently from her family and the medical professionals involved. This is of the essence of her story. But from everyone else's perspective it seems straightforwardly the case that in terms of the values expressed in Criterion c), that the way Anna experiences her body weight or shape is not just different but *disturbed*; that her perceived body weight or shape is not merely influencing but having an *undue* influence on her self-evaluation; and that while she recognizes that her body weight is low she does indeed show a persistent lack of recognition of the *seriousness* of her condition. Anna then unlike Simon is ill and, correspondingly, in need of medical treatment. It is with treatment, however, that phenomenology comes into play.

RESPONDING TO THE CHALLENGE: A PHENOMENOLOGICAL DEPTH DIMENSION

The phenomenological tradition offers a rich resource of work on values. We return to this resource in the next section. Of particular relevance to Anna's story however is Sartre's phenomenology of the body. As developed in *Being and Nothingness* (1986), Sartre's phenomenology of the body gives a depth dimension to our understanding of the values in Anna's story providing both a deeper understanding and approach to treatment.

The insight comes from Sartre's conceptualization of the "lived body for others." Phenomenology distinguishes two dimensions of corporeality, the body-subject and body-object. The body-subject is the body experienced from within, my own direct experience of my body, my direct awareness of myself as a spatiotemporal embodied agent in the world. The body-subject is thus a first-person perspective. The body-object by contrast is a third-person perspective. The body-object is the body thematically investigated from without, as by natural sciences such as anatomy and physiology, for example. In his phenomenology of the body Sartre added a third dimension of corporeality that he called the "lived-body-for-others." This third dimension of corporeality reflects the apprehension of one's own body from the vantage point of someone else. It is a reflection of one's own body as looked at by another person. When I become aware that someone is looking at me, I realize that my body can be an object for that other person. "With the appearance of the Other's look," writes Sartre (1986), "I experience the revelation of my being-as-object." The upshot of this is a feeling of "having my being outside . . . [the feeling] of being an object." Thus, one's identity becomes reified by the gaze of the Other and reduced to the external appearance of one's own body.

Sartre's lived-body-for-others gives a precise way of characterizing Anna's experience. Anna's presenting concerns are about fasting aimed at reducing her body size. But behind these presenting concerns, as one of us has reported in detail elsewhere (Stanghellini and Mancini 2017), is Anna's awareness of her own body. Anna experiences her body first and foremost as an object being looked at by another (as Sartre's lived-body-for-others) rather than from a first-person perspective (as a body-subject). Since she cannot have an experience of her body from within, she apprehends her body from without through the gaze of the Other. Her body is to her as she described it a "wobbling liquid" that may change when she is in the presence of other people. Her body, so to say, takes the shape that the Others' gaze imposes upon it. This is the source of her exaggerated concern to take responsibility for the way she appears to others. The Others' gaze makes her feel shame or disgust for her body. Lacking a stable first-person experience as a body-subject she seeks identity through starvation aimed at salvation in thinness.

In Anna's case therefore (and by extension in other similar cases, see next section), the negative values defining her presenting problems (starvation aimed at thinness) are underpinned by and reflect a deeper underlying set of values concerned with her negative experience of her lived body as a lived-body-for-others. In terms of DSM's Criterion c), the "*disturbance* in the way (Anna experiences her) body weight or shape," the "*undue* influence of body weight or shape on (Anna's) self-evaluation," and Anna's "persistent lack of recognition of the *seriousness* of (her) current low body weight," all stem from this core psychopathological change in body image. This is the insight on Anna's values (fasting, thinness, and shaping up, importance of the way she appears to others) suggested by Sartre's phenomenology of the body. But given this insight it is small wonder that when it comes to treatment, tackling Anna's presenting symptoms head-on will prove ineffective. Treatment may of course involve a range of measures including, where appropriate, medical interventions. But so far as the presenting problems in her behavior (fasting) and her motivating values (thinness and shaping up) are concerned any chance of effective intervention depends on therapy engaging with the underlying disturbances in the way she experiences her body.

Again, we do not have space here to follow through in detail the implications for therapy of this Sartrean way of understanding anorexia. But one way of achieving such engagement is with a phenomenologically informed therapeutic values-based interview (Stanghellini and Mancini 2017). This approach starts from a recognition that the values by which the presenting symptoms of people like Anna are (in part) defined (values of fasting and thinness) *are driven by a deeper set of values concerned with their disturbed lived-body-for-others.* There will thus be no way of convincing them that their values of thinness and fasting are wrong, since, given the reality (for them) of their need to experience their own body as an object being looked at by others, they are right. Instead of tackling their presenting symptoms head-on therefore the aim of therapy is to help them make sense of their drive for thinness and starvation by putting them in touch with the *core psychopathological anomaly from which these stem*—namely, their difficulties in feeling their own body in the first-person perspective and in sustaining a stable and continuous sense of themselves as embodied agents.

The psychopathological core of the life-world of persons like Anna is not feeling oneself in the first-person perspective, and in particular feeling extraneous from one's body and emotions. This entails a fleeting feeling of selfhood and an evanescent sense of identity. This vulnerable awareness of oneself is disturbing and generates the need to appraise oneself in alternative ways. One of the coping strategies or alternative means of self-recognition in these persons is feeling their body through the gaze of Others. Obviously, this coping strategy is not voluntarily adopted. A second way to regain a sense of themselves is identifying oneself through one's passion for thinness as passions representing a rupture in the fleeting character of their emotional and bodily life. The ossification of this passion and of the related value is the expression of the need to compensate for the disturbing, shameful, and anxiogenic fleeting sense of selfhood and identity.

If we want to understand what it is like to live with anorexia and bulimia it's a mistake to see Anna's values as merely imperfect cognition or as a kind of irrational or delusional belief about one's body or nutrition. Anna's values are a kind of *religion* that goes beyond the rationality/irrationality divide. It is about the worth of life and the way to make one's life meaningful. Food has a moral value: it is a sin and a temptation. Fatness has a moral value too as indicative of laziness, lack of self-care, and self-control. Thinness is more valuable than anything else including health. Strict rules are needed not to do wrong and to be led astray. Starvation is the unique salvation practice.

The values-based therapeutic interview thus aims to put people like Anna in touch with their underlying values as a step toward developing more effective and less destructive coping strategies. The depth dimension of understanding added by phenomenology to values-based practice is thus essential to meeting the values challenges presented by Anna's story. Sartre's phenomenology of the body explains the origins of the values driving Anna's presenting anorexic symptoms and behaviors. This in turn informs treatment. Phenomenology however does not thereby remove the need for analytically derived values-based practice. To the contrary it shows the need at least in cases like Anna's for a double engagement with it. Values-based practice is required for engagement first with the values challenges of her presenting symptoms. In this respect the engagement is similar to that required with Simon. But with Anna values-based practice is also required for engagement with the further values challenges arising from the origins of her presenting symptoms in underlying areas of psychopathology. What is required then in mental health, at least in cases of the kind exemplified by Anna's story, is a combined values-based practice drawing equally on the process elements of analytically derived values-based practice and the depth dimension of understanding provided by phenomenology. In the next section we look at the extent to which this combined values-based practice may be generalized to other areas of psychopathology.

GENERALIZING FROM OUR CASE STUDIES

To a first level of generalization we have noted already the clinical and empirical evidence showing that the values evident in Simon's story are, as we put it, but the tip of an evaluative iceberg. There are similar indications in Anna's case. Pro-Ana websites (as they are called) provide ample evidence of the extent to which people with anorexia may share Anna's values. Empirical studies of anorexia furthermore point to underlying body image disturbances consistent with the above Sartrean analysis of Anna's experiences (Tan et al. 2006; Hope et al. 2011). Further evidence of such disturbances has been provided by a questionnaire developed by one of us (Stanghellini et al. 2012) called IDEA (IDentity and EAting disorders). Used with large samples both of patients and of the general population the IDEA questionnaire has shown that people affected by or prone to feeding and eating disorders tend to have a reduced first-person apprehension of their body, experiencing it rather through the gaze of the Other (Stanghellini et al. 2012; Castellini et al. 2015; Stanghellini et al. 2015).

In this final section we indicate the further scope for generalization from our case studies afforded by the rich resources available respectively from phenomenological psychopathology and from the phenomenology of values.

PHENOMENOLOGICAL PSYCHOPATHOLOGY

The long tradition of phenomenological studies of schizophrenia has particular potential as the basis for future work in this area. Descriptions of what are in effect values in persons with schizophrenia can be found in Kretschmer (1921), Berze and Gruhle (1929), Minkowski (1927), Binswanger (1956), and Blankenburg (1969, 1971). The experiences of a person with schizophrenia are said to reflect a "crisis in common sense" resulting in "antagonomia" (literally, striving against rules) and "idionomia" (a belief in the radical uniqueness and exceptionality of one's own as against other people's view of how things are) (Stanghellini and Ballerini 2007). Such accounts are presented descriptively. Yet their impact on the life of the person concerned depends on their evaluative content. Antagonomia, for example, reflects the evaluative element in a form of more basic socialization abnormality characteristic of schizophrenia called "heteronomic vulnerability" (Stanghellini and Ballerini 2007).

So understood, antagonomia (the value shaping the schizophrenic persons' worldview and driving their actions), distancing oneself from others, instead of being a merely descriptively defined symptom of a mental disorder, becomes understandable as a natural consequence of one's feeling vulnerable to the destructive "force" emanating from the Other ("heteronomic vulnerability"), jeopardizing one's own self-integrity and bodily boundaries. Also, antagonomia is seen as a way to preserve (the value of) one's own exceptionality ("idionomia") driving (as the corresponding action) the need to take an eccentric stand in the face of commonly shared assumptions and the here and now of the Other.

In being presented descriptively such accounts of the phenomenological psychopathology of schizophrenia mirror the failure to recognize values for what they are in empirically derived diagnostic criteria (such as those of DSM). There is a similar failure of recognition in Sartre's phenomenology of the body. Notwithstanding the ethical roots of existentialism, Sartre positioned his phenomenology of the body essentially as an ontological rather than ethical study. This is why generalizing from our two case studies to other areas of psychopathology requires, in addition to the depth dimension of understanding available from phenomenological psychopathology, the insights also of analytic philosophy of values. In

Simon's case it was analytic philosophy of values that provided the key insight into the nature of psychiatric diagnostic values as a reflection of the diversity of human values rather than of some (supposed) deficiency in psychiatric science. It was from this key insight that practical ways of working with such diversity in the form of values-based practice were derived. Anna's case, similarly, illuminated as it was by the depth dimension of understanding provided by the phenomenology of the body, far from eliminating the need for analytically derived values-based practice, required, as we put it, a double engagement with it. It is to the further resources for this double engagement available from the phenomenology of values that we turn next.

THE PHENOMENOLOGY OF VALUES

Again, we do not have space here to cover the phenomenology of values in detail but will focus instead on its potential contribution to the combined phenomenological/analytic, values-based practice needed to meet the particular challenges of values in mental health. To anticipate, analytically derived values-based practice in the form summarized above is cast mainly in cognitive terms. This, as we have seen, is important heuristically. It is also important practically in the relative perspicuity of the process elements derived from it (summarized in Figure 40.1). The phenomenology of values adds to the cognitive aspects of values by which analytic values-based practice is constituted corresponding affective and conative aspects. These aspects of values are represented also in analytic moral philosophy: emotivist theories, for example, make central the affective aspects of values (Stevenson 1937); and Austin, among others, worked on the nature of agency (Austin 1956–1957). But phenomenological value theory is distinctive in offering a holistic approach, an approach that connects the cognitive, affective, and conative aspects of values one with another and with other aspects of the life-world of the individual concerned including their identity.

The theories in question were not developed with the challenges of psychopathology in mind. But their potential in this respect is well-illustrated by the work of three classical figures in phenomenology, Edmund Husserl, Max Scheler, and Paul Ricouer. Husserl's value theory (1908–14) makes the phenomenological three-way understanding of values explicit by setting his value theory within his wider account of mental phenomena as comprising cognitive, affective, and conative elements. Husserl argued that although what is valued is framed cognitively (it is perceived, remembered, imagined, etc.), actually attaching value (valuing something as good, or bad, or with indifference) always involves affect. Thus, the act of valuing in an affective act that is related to the cognitive apprehension of an object, that is, the very same object is apprehended cognitively (e.g. perceptually) and affectively (i.e. emotionally intuited). It is the latter that leads to conative or volitional (i.e. choosing) mental processes.

Scheler takes us further toward a holistic understanding of values by linking values with persons (Scheler 1927). Along with most other phenomenologists, Scheler took the affective faculty to be essential at least for moral values. But people, Scheler recognized, experience themselves simultaneously at different levels, caught "in between" the possibilities of good and evil, of spirit and flesh, of animal life and the divine. Our values, Scheler argued, are thus necessarily "stratified": there are values of the Holy and Unholy (the Divine), psychic values (the Beautiful and the Ugly, Right and Wrong, Truth and Falsehood), vital values (Noble and Vulgar), sensual values (the Agreeable and Disagreeable), and values of utility (Economics, Government). Scheler's account of shame and repentance (Scheler 1927) illustrates the "in-between" in action. The basic condition for feeling shame, he argued, is an imbalance between the claims of spiritual personhood and embodied needs. In shame what Scheler characterizes as "spirit" and "flesh," eternity and time, essence and existence, come together in tension. To be a human being is precisely to experience simultaneously these two orders of being such that one is unable to sever either without losing one's very humanity. Yet it is in this tension too that the possibility of repentance arises. To be a person means to be able to acknowledge and consequently extinguish in repenting one's having-been-bad while simultaneously becoming good. Scheler's account of repentance thus highlights in a way that goes beyond the resources of a merely cognitive values-based practice the dynamic and temporal nature of personhood and its links with personal values.

Like Scheler, Ricouer (1950) shows, in this case through his concept of motivations, how values come into conflict one with another. Ricouer goes further however in giving us an account of how we resolve value conflicts through the exercise of feelings and imagination.

Values, Ricouer argued, are based on motivations, ranging from bodily motivations to motivations of pure reason. Bodily motivations are involuntary and bound to our basic needs such as thirst and hunger. Rational motivations are voluntary and include the capacity to transcend our bodily needs. Feelings, understood as spontaneous beliefs about what is good or bad, highlight motives and it is the relative strengths of our feelings that produces actions. For instance, I decide not to follow the bodily motive of hunger where this is outweighed by the rational motive of shaping up. Imagination in Ricouer's phenomenology is what enables a person to break with the immediate satisfaction of a bodily motive. It is through imaginative comparison that we are able to compare one motive with another and to balance their respective satisfactions. The way we balance motivations over a period of time amounts to what Ricouer called a "quest for legitimacy" through which we establish our unique identity.

CONCLUSION

An indication of the potential of phenomenological value theory for a combined values-based practice is the extent to which each of the theories just outlined illuminates one or another component of the process of analytically-derived values-based practices. An important point of congruence, for example, in Husserl's phenomenology, is between his comparative affects (affects that value something as better or worse than something else) and the outputs of analytic values-based practice in balanced decision-making between values. The importance of tensions between "stratified values" in Scheler's theory is congruent similarly with (and in this respect gives substance to) the complex and conflicting values with which the process of values-based practice is concerned. Ricouer's theory has much to say that is relevant to the outcomes and process of values-based practice but in addition speaks to its premise of mutual respect. In analytic values-based practice this premise is derived semantically (i.e. from the meanings of value terms; Fulford 2014). But mutual respect is a consequence also of Ricouer's quest for legitimacy. For the quest is mutual, it is a quest for the recognition of our values by others. Our own values, therefore, to the extent that they embody our identity as unique individuals, are rooted in and depend critically on the mutual respect of others.

As we have indicated the connections between the phenomenology of values and values-based practice remain potential. Our point for now is that there is no barrier of principle to such connections being made. The complementarities just outlined suggest that, in the context at least of phenomenological psychopathology, making such connections would be both heuristically productive and practically rewarding.

ACKNOWLEDGMENTS

Simon's story is based on one of a number of cases collected by Mike Jackson as part of his doctoral work and published in Jackson M. and Fulford K. W. M. (1997) "Spiritual Experience and Psychopathology." *Philosophy, Psychiatry, & Psychology* 4(1): 41–66.

BIBLIOGRAPHY

Allott P., Fulford K. W. M., Fleming B., Williamson T., and Woodbridge K. (2005). "Recovery, Values and e-Learning." *The Mental Health Review* 10(4): 34–38.

American Psychiatric Association. (2013). *DSM-5.* Washingston, London: American Psychiatric Publishing.

Austin J. L. (1956–57). "A Plea for Excuses." In J. L. Austin, *Proceedings of the Aristotelian Society*, 57: 1–30. Reprinted in White A. R. (ed.) (1968) *The Philosophy of Action*, pp. 19–42. Oxford: Oxford University Press.

Berze J. and Gruhle H. W. (1929). *Psychologie der Schizophrenie.* Berlin: Springer.

Binswanger L. (1956). *Drei Formen Missgluckten Daseins.* Tubingen: Max Niemeyer Verlag.

Blankenburg W. (1969). "Ansaetze zu einer Psychopathologie des 'common sense.'" *Confinia Psychiatrica* 12: 144–163.

Blankenburg W. (1971). *Der Verlust der Naturalichen Selbverstandlichkeit.* Stuttgart: Enke.

Boorse C. (1975). "On the Distinction between Disease and Illness." *Philosophy and Public Affairs* 5: 49–68.

Boorse C. (1976). "What a Theory of Mental Health Should Be." *Journal for the Theory of Social Behaviour* 6: 61–84.

Castellini G., Stanghellini G., Godini L., Lucchese M., Trisolini F., and Ricca V. (2015). "Abnormal Bodily Experiences Mediate the Relationship between Impulsivity and Binge Eating in Overweight Subjects Seeking Bariatric Surgery." *Psychotherapy and Psychosomatics* 84: 124–126.

Fulford K. W. M. (1989, reprinted 1995 and 1999). *Moral Theory and Medical Practice.* Cambridge: Cambridge University Press.

Fulford K. W. M. (1994). "Closet Logics: Hidden Conceptual Elements in the DSM and ICD Classifications of Mental Disorders." In J. Z. Sadler, O. P. Wiggins, and M. A. Schwartz (eds.), *Philosophical Perspectives on Psychiatric Diagnostic Classification*, pp. 211–232. Baltimore: Johns Hopkins University Press.

Fulford K. W. M. (2004). "Facts/Values. Ten Principles of Values-Based Medicine." In J. Radden (ed.), *The Philosophy of Psychiatry: A Companion.* pp. 205–234. New York: Oxford University Press.

Fulford K. W. M. (2014). "Living with Uncertainty: a First-Person-Plural Response to Eleven Commentaries on Values-based Practice." In M. Loughlin (ed.), *Debates in Values-based Practice: Arguments For and Against*, chapter 13. Cambridge: Cambridge University Press.

Fulford K. W. M., Smirnov A. Y. U., and Snow E. (1993). "Concepts of Disease and the Abuse of Psychiatry in the USSR." *British Journal of Psychiatry* 162: 801–810.

Fulford K. W. M., Peile E., and Carroll, H. (2012). *Essential Values-based Practice: Clinical Stories Linking Science with People*. Cambridge: Cambridge University Press.

Fulford K. W. M., Bortolotti L., and Broome M. (2014). "Taking the Long View: An Emerging Framework for Translational Psychiatric Science." Special Article for *World Psychiatry* 13(2): 108–117.

Fulford K. W. M., Dewey S., and King M. (2015). "Values-based Involuntary Seclusion and Treatment: Value Pluralism and the UK's Mental Health Act 2007." In J. Z. Sadler, W. van Staden, and K. W. M. Fulford (eds.), *The Oxford Handbook of Psychiatric Ethics*, chapter 60, pp. 839–860. Oxford: Oxford University Press.

Fulford K. W. M., Crepaz-Keay D., and Stanghellini G. (forthcoming). "Depressions Plural: Pathology and the Challenge of Values." In C. Foster and J. Herring (eds.), *Depression and the Law*. Oxford: Oxford University Press.

Handa I. A., Fulford-Smith L., Barber Z. E., Dobbs T. D., Fulford K. W. M., and Peile E. (2016). "The Importance of Seeing Things from Someone Else's Point of View." BMJ Careers onlinejournal. http://careers.bmj.com/careers/advice/The_importance_of_seeing_things_from_someone_else's_point_of_view

Hare R. M. (1952). *The Language of Morals*. Oxford: Oxford University Press.

Hope T., Tan J., Stewart A., and Fitzpatrick R. (2011). "Anorexia Nervosa and the Language of Authenticity." *Hastings Center Report* 41(6): 19–29.

Husserl E. [1908–1914] (1998). *Vorlesungen ueber Ethik und Wertlehere*. In Husserliana 28. Published in English Dordrecht, Boston (MA), London: Kluwer, LLIX-523.

Kendell R. E. (1975). "The Concept of Disease and its Implications for Psychiatry." *British Journal of Psychiatry* 127: 305–315.

Kretschmer E. (1921). *Korperbau und Charakter*. Berlin: Springer. Published in English (1925). *Physique and Character*. New York, Brace & Company.

Loughlin M. (ed.) (2014). *Debates in Values-based Practice: Arguments For and Against*. Cambridge: Cambridge University Press.

Minkowski E. (1927). *La Schizophrenie. Psychopatologie des schizoides et des Schizophrenes*. Paris: Payot.

Ricouer P. (1950). *Le volontaire et l'involontaire*. Paris: Aubier. Published in English (1996). *Freedom and Nature*. Evanston: Northwestern University Press.

Sadler J. Z. (2005). *Values and Psychiatric Diagnosis*. Oxford: Oxford University Press.

Sartre J. P. (1986). *Being and Nothingness*, trans. H. E. Barnes. London: Routledge.

Scheler M. (1927). Der Formalismus in der Ethik und die materiale Wertethik: Neuer Versuch der Grundlegung eines ethischen Personalismus, Gesammelte Werke, vol. 2. Bern, Munich: Francke, 1954. Published in English (1973). Formalism in Ethics and Non-Formal Ethics of Values: A New Attempt Toward a Foundation of An Ethical Personalism, trans. M. S. Frings and R. L. Funk. Evanston: Northwestern University Press.

Stanghellini G. (2016). *Lost in Dialogue. Anthropology, Psychopathology, and Care*. Oxford, Oxford University Press.

Stanghellini G. and Ballerini M. (2007). "Values in Persons with Schizophrenia." *Schizophrenia Bulletin* 33(1): 131–141.

Stanghellini G., Castellini G., Brogna P., Faravelli C., and Ricca V. (2012). "Identity and Eating Disorders (IDEA): A Questionnaire Evaluating Identity and Embodiment in Eating Disorder Patients." *Psychopathology* 45: 147–158.

Stanghellini G., Trisolini F., Castellini G., Ambrosini A., Faravelli C., and Ricca V. (2015). "Is Feeling Extraneous from One's Own Body a Core Vulnerability Feature in Eating Disorders?" *Psychopathology* 48(1): 18–24.

Stanghellini G. and Mancini M. (2017). *The Therapeutic Interview. Emotions, Values and the Life-world*. Cambridge: Cambridge University Press.

Stevenson C. L. (1937). "The Emotive Meaning of Value Terms." *Mind* 46: 14–31.

Szasz T. S. (1960). "The Myth of Mental Illness." *American Psychologist* 15n: 113–118.

Tan J. O. A., Hope T., Stewart A., and Fitzpatrick R. (2006). "Competence to Make Treatment Decisions in Anorexia Nervosa: Thinking Processes and Values." *Philosophy, Psychiatry, & Psychology* 13(4): 267–282.

Wing J. K., Cooper J. E, and Sartorius N. (1974). *Present State Examination (PSE). Measurement and Classification of Psychiatric Symptoms; An Instruction for PSE and CATEGO Program*. London: Cambridge University Press.

CHAPTER 41

....

EMBODIMENT

....

ERIC MATTHEWS

THE EMBODIED SUBJECT

....

To understand the concept of embodiment (or the embodied subject), as it has figured in recent discussions among philosophers, psychiatrists, neuroscientists, and cognitive scientists, it is important to see it in the context of the perennial debate about the nature of mental life (including mental disorder). In the last few centuries, it has been widely assumed that our choice on this question is limited to only two positions, which are seen as diametrically opposed: namely, "substantial dualism" and "materialism." The concept of human beings as embodied subjects has been proposed as a third option, which escapes the perceived shortcomings of both dualism and materialism. We can therefore understand this third option better by first briefly outlining each of the traditional views, and the problems in them which the concept of embodiment seeks to resolve.

The most fully elaborated form of dualism was developed by the French philosopher, René Descartes (1595–1650), and hence is often called "Cartesian dualism." Descartes argued that the human mind must be regarded as something quite different in character from anything physical (including the human brain). The mind, for him, was a "thinking thing," without physical properties: it was invisible, intangible, and occupied no space, and so was not subject to physical laws. As he expressed it, it was an "immaterial substance." By calling it a "substance," he meant that it was capable of existing independently—in particular, its existence was independent of that of anything physical, including even the human body. The body, including the brain, was a part of "material substance," that is, of the physical world. As such, like all other physical objects, it was visible and tangible, it occupied space, and functioned in accordance with the laws of physics (which, for Descartes, essentially meant mechanics). Although the mind had, strictly speaking, no location, it was thought of as metaphorically "inside" the human being, the site of her "inner life," in the sense that it was accessible only to the person whose mind it was, by "introspection." The body, on the other hand, was accessible, like all other physical objects, to anyone equipped with the relevant senses. A human being, in short, was a compound of two quite distinct parts—hence the view's designation as "dualism."

Even in Descartes's own time, a number of thinkers saw problems in dualism. Most obviously, there was the question of how "mind" and "body" could interact. Such interactions are a familiar part of everyday life, and the growth of greater scientific knowledge of the brain has revealed more of them: for instance, some kinds of brain damage have been seen to lead to loss of memory, and even personality change. In psychiatry, in particular, we need to account for the obvious role which brain dysfunctions seem to play in various forms of mental disorder. The dualist conception of "mind" and "body" as distinct "substances," each operating according to different laws, has been seen as making it impossible to account for such interactions between them, and so has been rejected by many as unscientific.

Most of those who reject dualism on these grounds have concluded that we must accept instead that the mind is not a separate substance from anything physical, but is part of the material world. In particular, they have identified what we customarily call "mind" with the brain. This is understandable, since the brain is the part of the material world which is most centrally concerned with our "mental" functioning—with thoughts, emotions, desires, moods, and so on. "Materialism" thus usually means the identification of "mind" with "brain," or (perhaps better) the identification of thoughts, emotions, desires, moods, and other elements in our mental life with processes going on in the brain, or states of the brain. It is then assumed that our thoughts, emotions, etc. can be fully explained as caused by other brain processes and states. This appears to avoid the dualist problem of accounting for "mind–brain interaction," since mind and brain are one and the same.

PHENOMENOLOGY AND EMBODIMENT

There are problems in both dualism and materialism. One central problem with dualism is that it situates our "minds" outside the world that we think about. Our relation to the things and people around us, and even to our own bodies, thus becomes that of a detached observer, rather than of someone who participates in, or experiences, the world. Materialists do not have that problem: but their identification of our minds with our brains, seen as one kind of mechanical system, makes us just one kind of object in the world. As such, we are causally (that is, passively) affected by other objects, but do not actively engage with the world in the way required for genuine experience.

The problems in both views can be seen as a consequence of the assumption, typical of most traditional Western philosophy, that our primary relation to the world was cognitive—that of ourselves, as knowers ("knowing subjects"), to a reality which is "objective," in the sense that it is as it is independently of how we "subjectively" experience it. Then the task of both philosophy and science is to strive for objective knowledge in that sense. Developments in philosophy in the twentieth century led to a questioning of this assumption. The work of the later Wittgenstein was one of these developments: but more important from the present perspective were elements in the "phenomenological" tradition initiated by Edmund Husserl (1859–1938). The formulation of the concept of human beings as embodied subjects, however, is mainly due to the work of certain critics, within the phenomenological tradition, of aspects of Husserl's original presentation of his philosophy. Most notable among these critics were Martin Heidegger (1889–1976), Jean-Paul Sartre (1905–1980), and, above all, Maurice Merleau-Ponty (1908–1961).

At the heart of phenomenology, as these critics saw it, is the insight that any account that we can give of the world, ourselves, and our relation to the world, must ultimately get its meaning for us from our own experience of living in the world. The idea of an "objective" account of the world, in the sense of one totally independent of how we experience things, must thus be devoid of content. Without human experience, Merleau-Ponty argues, "scientific symbols would be meaningless" (Merleau-Ponty 2012: lxxii). Theoretical science cannot give us the most fundamental account of reality, since it is itself dependent on our pre-theoretical encounters with things and people. Phenomenology aims to "rediscover this naïve contact with the world" (Merleau-Ponty 2012: lxx). It attempts to give an account of ourselves and our world which is not intended to explain them theoretically, but simply to describe our experience of them as it is before we begin to theorize about it, in science or in more traditional philosophy. Such a description should clarify what it is that we are seeking to explain by our scientific theories.

To understand ourselves and our world thus requires us to start by reflecting on what it is like to be ourselves, living in the world in the ways we do. That is, we need to reflect on what Heidegger, Sartre, and Merleau-Ponty all call our "being-in-the-world." If we approach our being-in-the-world without assumptions, we can see that it is primarily a matter of our practical and emotional engagement with things and people, rather than of the detached observation of pure cognition. We move about the world, have purposes related to our situation, use objects to realize these purposes, feel emotions about things and people, and see things and people as meaningful in relation to these purposes and emotions. For example, a hammer has the meaning of a "tool," and our native place has the meaning of "home." Detached cognition enters in, and has value for us, only in its relation to this practical and emotional engagement. As Merleau-Ponty expresses it, our consciousness is primarily not a matter of theoretical thinking about things, but of practical dealings with them—what Merleau-Ponty actually says is "Consciousness is originarily not an 'I think that', but rather an 'I can'" (Merleau-Ponty 2012: 139).

If we are in the world in this active and engaged way, then we are neither, as in dualism, a mind, loosely attached to a body, nor, as in materialism, a purely physical object (a body, and especially a brain) which is passively affected by other objects. Rather, each of us is a living human being, who is both a "subject" and an "object," and whose "subjective," or mental, life is inseparably connected with her "objective," or bodily, life: in short, we are embodied subjects. Our thoughts and feelings about the world, and our desires in relation to it, are not purely "inner events": what thought or feeling we are having can be determined only by its role in our dealings with the world. This rules out both the Cartesian identification of thoughts, etc. with events in the soul, and the materialist identification of them with events in the brain. Indeed, as the contemporary German philosopher and psychiatrist, Thomas Fuchs, argues, materialism in this respect contains relics of dualism. Thoughts, etc., Fuchs says, are "life-performances," which can be attributed only to a "being of flesh and blood and only in connection with his life-situation" (Fuchs 2008: 354, translation by E. M.).

Conversely, a person's body is not just one kind of object for her, like the chair she sits on, or the cars that she sees passing on the road. Her principal experience of her body is, as Merleau-Ponty puts it, as "the vehicle of being-in-the-world" (Merleau-Ponty 2012: 84). Her body provides her individual perspective on the world, the here and now from which she necessarily experiences things. Sartre makes the important point that my body exists, not only for me, but also for others. I am aware of the Other primarily as an object in my world, but a special kind of object, who also views *me* as an object in his or her world. As Sartre says, "I never apprehend the Other as body without at the same time in a non-explicit manner apprehending my own body as the center of reference indicated by the other" (Sartre 1969: 344). Thus, living one's own body is also necessarily living in an *intersubjective* world—a world in which our relations with others, in society and culture, are part of what we are ourselves.

For some purposes, of course, we can regard even our own bodies as one kind of physical object. For instance, a medical student might take her own body as a mere instance when studying how the human body generally functions. This would be different from the way in which she experiences her body in acting in the world—for example, in using her hands in caring for patients. In some of his works, Husserl makes this distinction in terms of two German words for "body," *Körper* and *Leib* (e.g. Husserl 1970: 107). By *Körper* (usually translated as "physical body"), he means the body considered as one more object in the world, to be described and explained in the same terms as any other physical object. By *Leib* (usually translated as "living body"), he means the body as experienced by someone as the vehicle of their life.

Being embodied in the way human beings are is being a member of a particular human society. Being aware of oneself as an individual subject, engaged in the world from a particular point of view, is necessarily being aware too of other subjects with whom one can communicate, by verbal language and other means. An "I" is necessarily part of a "we." The possibility of communication, whether in words or in other ways, depends on culturally shared meanings. For example, what it means to say "I love you" will differ depending on the concept of love which exists in the speaker's and hearer's culture. In this way, the cultural context in which human beings live gives a particular coloring to the emotions, desires, beliefs, purposes, etc. which they have. This is a further reason for not identifying our "mental" life with brain processes or brain-states.

To say that human beings are embodied subjects is to say, in summary, that their existence—their actions, their thoughts, their feelings, and so on—is primarily as a kind of living beings. It is rooted in their nature as a particular biological species, with needs, and with desires and thoughts relating to those needs. Like all complex animals, their dealings with their environment are active and purposeful, not a matter of mechanical responses to stimuli. But they differ from other species in that they are members of a particular society, who communicate with other members through language and meaningful action. This gives a cultural context to their behavior, which they can and do develop by reflection. Merleau-Ponty says, for this reason, that "Man is an historical idea, not a natural species" (Merleau-Ponty 2012: 174). To understand human behavior, therefore, we must take account of this constant interplay between physiology, personal reflection, and cultural context.

RELEVANCE OF EMBODIMENT TO PSYCHIATRY

Embodiment has been described, in the Preface to a recent collection of articles, as "on the way to becoming a major paradigm of psychopathology" (Fuchs et al. 2010). It has been "on the way" for a considerable time. For instance, Heidegger's account of the human mode of being as being-in-the-world was already an influence on the "existential analysis" developed by Ludwig Binswanger (see Binswanger 1963) and on the "phenomenological psychiatry" of Eugene Minkowski (see Minkowski 1970). More recently, Merleau-Ponty's more extensive account of embodiment has influenced such psychiatrists and philosophers as Sass (see e.g. Sass 2001), Stanghellini (see e.g. Stanghellini 2004), and Fuchs (see e.g. Fuchs 2008). In the 1960s, the controversial psychiatrist R. D. Laing, influenced more by Sartre than by Merleau-Ponty, gave a phenomenological account of the experience of schizophrenia as a kind of divorce between the self and its body, so that the self was experienced as a mere "onlooker," with no direct participation in the world around him or her (see Laing 2010, especially chapter 4).

The appeal of the idea of embodiment in this context is that it is seen as providing a more coherent and richer account of mental disorder than dualism or materialism. From a dualist perspective, a "mental" disorder can only mean a disturbance of the functioning of "mental substance." Healthy mental functioning, for Descartes, is rational functioning, so disorder must take the form of *irrational* thoughts, beliefs, feelings, desires, and so on. One of Descartes's own examples is that of those "madmen" who are "so damaged by the persistent vapours of melancholia that they firmly maintain they are kings when they are paupers" (Descartes 1984: 13). This wording seems to imply that Descartes believed that such delusions are the product of what we should call biochemical disturbances in the brain, causing the mind to deviate from rationality—as in such modern hypotheses as that of a dopamine imbalance in schizophrenia. But this would be inconsistent with dualism, which makes it impossible to account for such causal relations between the two substances. On the other hand, if a person arrived at such a delusion as a result of her own (presumably illogical) thinking, then that would be a matter for intellectual criticism, rather than therapy. It might be possible for Cartesian dualists to think of mental disorders as having a "mental" cause if they thought of mental substance as including an "unconscious mind," in which persisting psychological traumas were stored, causing disorders in adult life. But, first, this would be inconsistent with Cartesian dualism: Descartes effectively *defines* mental substance as fully conscious. And secondly, it would still underestimate the role of brain dysfunction, and the corresponding value of physical treatments.

The opposing materialist identification of the mind with the brain, considered as a purely physical system, seems to imply that what we call "mental disorder" is really nothing but the distressing outcome of certain kinds of brain dysfunction. An example might be depression, which is commonly seen as caused by such things as serotonin imbalances. This seems, however, to play down the importance of the particular kind of distress, some of which concerns bodily experience, which people with mental disorders suffer, as expressed in its relation to the patient's own past experience and the distorted relations with other human beings which it produces. For the same reason, it does not give an adequate account of the valuable role played in treatment by "talking therapies." Some materialists might suggest that a talking therapy could cause changes in the nervous system, and so in the mental disorder. But this would be a misunderstanding of the implications of strict materialism. Talking therapies can work only if the patient *understands* the therapist's words, and understanding is not a purely physical process. Strict materialism implies that the only genuine causal relationships are those in which a physical process leads to an equally physical change. On a strict materialist view, such talking therapies would seem to be no more relevant to, say, depression or obsessive-compulsive disorder than to epilepsy or motor neurone disease.

The concept of embodiment, by contrast, allows us to regard mental disorder as a disturbance, not merely of a part of a human being, but of the human being as a whole. This chimes better with the reality of such disorder, as experienced by sufferers. It can be seen as a disturbance of someone's whole being-in-the-world, an unsatisfactory relation to other things and people, resulting from disturbing experiences, and the essential role in those experiences played by brain dysfunction, disorders of brain chemistry, etc. Both brain dysfunctions and traumatic experiences can thus be relevant (in different proportions in different cases) to the explanation and treatment of the disorder.

To sum up, the concept of human beings as embodied subjects implies that we can understand human mental life, including its disorders, only if we take into account *both* the brain processes which make it possible *and* the meaning which is given to our thoughts, emotions, etc. by our relation to the world, especially the "human world" of other people and society. This point can be illustrated by briefly considering three examples, in which writers with considerable clinical experience have used this concept as a framework for understanding some common mental disorders. First, Glas, in discussing pathological anxiety, argues that to understand it might require us to see it *both* as "rooted in a dysbalance of a physiological equilibrium" *and* as "the expression of a frustrated urge for self-realization" (Glas 2003: 222). Both, including their interaction with each other, would need to be taken into account in order to understand this as a problem in the person's being-in-the-world. Secondly, Gillett considers the phenomenon of anorexia in young women. A full understanding of this phenomenon as a human experience, he suggests, may have to include possible disturbances in brain functioning, causing a malfunction suppressing the desire to eat. But this on its own would not explain everything about the disorder: for example, the fact that the young women seem unable to see how desperately thin they are, or their horrified denial that they have in fact gained weight, or their tendency to engage in other self-harming behaviors (Gillett 2003: 150). Finally, Fuchs suggests that we might see schizophrenia as a "circular process," in which neuropsychological and biochemical dysfunction both gives rise to, and is in turn affected by, psychosocial alienation (Fuchs 2009: 230).

BIBLIOGRAPHY

Binswanger L. (1963). *Being-in-the-World*. New York: Basic Books.

Descartes R. (1984). *The Philosophical Writings of Descartes, Volume II*, trans. J. Cottingham, et al. Cambridge: Cambridge University Press.

Fuchs T. (2008). *Leib und Lebenswelt: neue philosophisch-psychiatrische Essays*. Kusterdingen: Die Graue Edition.

Fuchs T. (2009). "Embodied Cognitive Neuropsychiatry and its Consequences for Psychiatry." *Poiesis and Praxis* 6: 219–233.

Fuchs T., et al. (eds.) (2010). *The Embodied Self: Dimensions, Coherence and Disorders*. Stuttgart: Schattauer GmbH.

Gillett G. (2003). "Form and Content: The Role of Discourse in Mental Disorder." In K. W. M. Fulford, et al. (eds.), *Nature and Narrative: An Introduction to the New Philosophy of Psychiatry*, pp. 139–153. Oxford: Oxford University Press.

Glas G. (2003). "Anxiety—Animal Reactions and the Embodiment of Meaning." In K. W. M. Fulford, et al. (eds.), *Nature and Narrative: An Introduction to the New Philosophy of Psychiatry*, pp. 231–249. Oxford, Oxford University Press.

Husserl E. (1970). *The Crisis of European Sciences and Transcendental Phenomenology*, trans. D. Carr. Evanston: Northwestern University Press.

Laing R. D. (2010). *The Divided Self: An Existential Study in Sanity and Madness* (Penguin Classics edition). London: The Penguin Group.

Merleau-Ponty M. (2012). *Phenomenology of Perception*, trans. D. A. Landes. London: Routledge.

Minkowski E. (1970). *Lived Time: Phenomenological and Psychopathological Studies*, trans. N. Metzel. Evanston: Northwestern University Press.

Sartre J.-P. (1969). *Being and Nothingness: An Essay on Phenomenological Ontology*, trans. H. E. Barnes. London and New York: Routledge.

Sass L. (2001). "Self and World in Schizophrenia: Three Classic Approaches in Phenomenological Psychiatry." *PPP: Philosophy, Psychiatry, Psychology* 8: 251–270.

Stanghellini G. (2004). *Disembodied Spirits and Deanimated Bodies: The Psychopathology of Common Sense*. Oxford: Oxford University Press.

CHAPTER 42

....

AUTONOMY

....

KATERINA DELIGIORGI

INTRODUCTION

....

AUTONOMY is a dominant notion in patient care because it expresses the value of respect for the other person; to recognize someone's autonomy is simply to treat them as someone, not as some thing. The way theories of autonomy articulate this basic value, focusing on individual choice and fostering an ideal of self-sufficiency, is deeply at odds with the phenomenological tradition. As we shall see, one of the aims of phenomenology is to correct the "individualistic drift" of modern philosophy and allow for a fresh conception of the relation of self to world and self to others.[1] My task in this article is to examine how such revision can yield a phenomenological understanding of autonomy and how this can be used to modify established clinical practice.

As used in contemporary philosophy, "autonomy" is not a single concept. It stands for a family of concepts that includes agential freedom, will and volition, choice, deliberation, control, and action. What unites these concepts is a concern with individual choice: the self or "autos" in "autonomy." This concern reflects a philosophical and also cultural idea that as mature, rational beings we should not be under tutelary guidance, rather we should be let free to lead our own lives as we see fit and others ought to respect our choice of life.[2]

Varieties of Autonomy

Within the broad family of autonomy, three conceptions stand out in the current discussion: personal, moral, and substantive.

The most familiar is personal autonomy. A key reference remains Gerald Dworkin's paper for the Hastings Center. The paper's defense of personal autonomy serves two immediate

---

[1] See Renault (1997) for a clear statement of this diagnosis, the term "individualistic drift" is his (at 148).

[2] That others may not interfere with one's choice of life is succinctly expressed in John Stuart Mill's "very simple principle" that "the only purpose for which power can be rightfully exercised over any member of a civilized community, against his will, is to prevent harm to others. His own good, either physical or moral, is not sufficient warrant" (Mill 1989: 13).

aims: to respond to philosophical skepticism about free will and to show why it might be wrong to use techniques of manipulation that take the individual out of the decision process. Personal autonomy speaks to the idea that our choices should be free from external interference and that they should be ours. Dworkin encapsulates these ideas in the formula "autonomy equals authenticity + independence" (Dworkin 1976: 26).

The originator of the moral conception is Immanuel Kant. For Kant autonomy is a moral demand on individuals. Morality makes a distinctive claim on us: it enjoins us to do the right thing just because it is the right thing to do.[3] In recognizing the authority of morality, each individual places himself under the moral law, which legislates unconditionally for every rational being. Failure to be autonomous, or more correctly, to act autonomously, amounts to choosing ends without regard for the law.

Although substantive conceptions of autonomy vary a great deal, their common aspiration is good self-management. The typical autonomous agent exhibits a range of epistemic and motivational virtues. For example, she ensures that her ends fit her overall intentions or plans, her means are appropriate, that the likely consequences of the proposed action are taken into account, that any contradictory desires and distracting emotions are controlled.[4] Because she exhibits these virtues, the agent's claim that her way of managing her affairs be respected by others is plausible: she has the authority she has earned by conducting herself autonomously.

Problems can be raised for all three conceptions and, as we shall see, have been raised especially sharply by phenomenologists: fragile and highly dependent agents appear to be excluded by the substantive conception; the formal understanding of the good in the Kantian conception threatens to detach morality from everyday life; finally, the model of self-knowledge used in the personal conception assumes an unexamined mind–world epistemic dualism.[5] In some ways, addressing this last issue is a priority for phenomenology and sets the stage for how autonomy may be rethought within a phenomenological context.

Personal autonomy contains a negative claim addressed to others, roughly "do not meddle in my affairs," and a positive claim expressing the thought that one is in charge of one's affairs, because they make authentic or, in the substantive models, fully thought through choices. What count as mine are mental items, desires, the beliefs that guide those desires, the plans we make on the basis of such beliefs and desires, and the emotions that support or scupper our plans. To adjudicate between these different mental items and decide which ones truly are our own, we need to know them. An autonomous agent must know her mind. On a widespread view, we know our mental states, by looking inwards, by introspection.[6] By contrast, we know things about the world by observing, experimenting, testing. So mind and world are known in radically different ways: only the latter can be the topic of scientific study. It seems then that if we want to study the mind scientifically, the best way is by ridding ourselves of the idea that there is anything "inner" for us to observe, and adopting a reductivist materialist approach to explaining human behavior.

---

[3] For a book-length treatment of Kantian autonomy, see Deligiorgi 2012.

[4] A representative range of views is gathered in Taylor 2005.

[5] For critical engagement, see Anderson and Christman 2005; for specifically phenomenological engagement and focus on the philosophy of mind, see Woodruff Smith and Thomasson 2005.

[6] See Goldman 2006.

PHENOMENOLOGY: THE HISTORICAL CONTEXT

Starting with Franz Brentano in the 1870s and explicitly formulated as a philosophical program of investigation by Edmund Husserl in the 1900s, phenomenology aims to counter both the reductivist and the introspective approaches for the study of mind outlined above. Brentano distinguishes between "genetic psychology" (Brentano 1995), the empirical study of psychology, which employs the methods of the natural sciences to discover causal explanations or correlations, and descriptive psychology or phenomenology. Descriptive psychology, especially as Husserl develops it, is a philosophical discipline that studies the essential characteristics and interrelations of all psychic phenomena. The procedure to elicit these essential characteristics is called "eidetic variation" and it is a highly structured process of abstraction from basic pre-reflective experiences.[7] What matters for our present discussion is not the detail of the phenomenological method but its ambition. Phenomenology breaks new ground because it does not split the world into inner and outer, each requiring a different approach. The starting point of the investigation of all phenomena is recognition that at the basis of all propositions are conscious states, stretches of consciousness of a subject. The importance accorded to the first person perspective has given rise to two different senses of "phenomenology," phenomenology as Husserl practices it, is not concerned with the qualitative character of conscious states, or "what is like . . .?" questions, rather it is concerned with "what is . . .?" questions and aspires to be a rigorous science. There is another sense of "phenomenology," as we shall see shortly, that aims precisely to recover the qualitative aspects of experience. What matters for the moment is Husserl's radical vision of a science that is not reductively materialistic, but which is premised on a rethinking of the mind–world relation.

Where does this radical rethinking leave the aspiration to be autonomous and the claim that one's individual autonomy be respected? Husserl was highly responsive to the philosophical and cultural idea that we should not be under tutelary guidance, but he did not articulate a positive ideal of personal autonomy; he thinks rather that emancipation from external forces puts individual enquirers on the path to objectivity (Husserl 1970: 7–8). With respect to more narrowly moral matters, Husserl is sympathetic to Kant, because Kant's ethics is directed by the idea of an objective good, the moral law, but also critical of the abstract conception of the good (Husserl 1988: 235). The concern to root goods to the world of individual strivings and emphasis of reasoning and willing well brings Husserl's ethics close to contemporary substantive conceptions of autonomy (Husserl 1988: 145).

The conceptual shift toward substantive ideals of agency, which include good reasoning and sound willing, amounts, however, to a move away from the basic intuition that individual choice ought to be respected even if it falls short of the ideal. In the phenomenological tradition, there are two interesting ways of grappling with this issue. One is to radicalize the idea of personal autonomy. Jean-Paul Sartre's conception of freedom as a condition for radical self-creation illustrates this. Sartre conceptualizes individual life as a life of abandonment, without any objective markers to show to how it should be lived. Individuals have to

---

[7] A relatively clear explanation of the process of eidetic variation in relation to perception can be found in Husserl 1969: 70–71.

confront the fact of their freedom, which means that "moral choice is comparable to the construction of a work of art" (Sartre 1946: 45). This very austere picture of individual choice resembles the personal conception of autonomy but it permits no connection to a basic shared value, that of respect for each other, from which personal autonomy still draws its normative force.

An alternative path is to change the conversation and this is what Karl Jaspers (1963) does when he brings together phenomenology and psychopathology in his 1913 work, *General Psychopathology*. Departing from Husserlian orthodoxy, Jaspers has a view of philosophy as a passionate, engaged activity that can deepen our understanding of historical and cultural phenomena, by analyzing how individuals engage with and make sense of their social world. In his early work on psychopathology, but also in his later work on religion and politics, he champions a philosophy that seeks to encompass human life as a whole made of many mutually irreducible parts. These philosophical commitments result in a highly distinctive phenomenology of psychopathology: patient self-description, the account of what an experience is like, has a clear role in the classification of the psychic phenomena, and empathy has a role in understanding the patient's experience. Subjective symptoms, Jaspers writes, "can only become an inner reality for the observer by his participating in the other person's experiences, not by any intellectual effort" (Jaspers [1912]1968: 1313). So here we have an account of an intersubjective relation that requires attending to the other person and thus expresses respect for the other person, but without issuing into a defense of autonomy, because its normative foundation is the recognition of human dependence and fragility.

AUTONOMY AND PHENOMENOLOGICAL PSYCHOPATHOLOGY

Given this complex philosophical inheritance, phenomenologists working in contemporary psychopathology and bioethics respond to demands of clinical practice, which includes a clinical discourse around autonomy, by identifying a set of priorities that cut across intra-disciplinary boundaries:[8]

(a) the first-person perspective is essential to the phenomenological approach, so the experience of the patient should count (Toombs 1992, 2001; Mullen 2007; Giorgi 2009; Fuchs 2010, 2013; Martin and Hicherson 2013; Stanghellini and Rosfort 2013)

(b) human beings are to be treated as wholes not as sets of symptoms and psychological processes; this often means an emphasis on embodiment (Toombs 1992, 2001; Mullen 2007; Giorgi 2009; Martin and Hicherson 2013).

(c) human beings, their decisions, capacities, and symptoms, are to be considered within their social and cultural context (Mullen 2007; Fuchs 2010, 2013; Martin and Hicherson 2013)

---

[8] For the ways in which different traditions of phenomenology contribute to clinical practice, see Toombs 2001 and Broome, Harland, Owen, and Stringaris 2014.

(d)   the aim, or one of the aims, of the medical encounter should be to understand what is going on, make sense of things without aiming at finality; sometimes empathy is key; generally, modesty, provisionality, and open-endedness are to be accepted, indeed valued (Toombs 1992; Mullen 2007; Giorgi 2009; Martin and Hicherson 2013; Stanghellini and Rosfort 2013)

The list is illustrative of the pluralistic landscape of current practice. The question now is how any of these priorities intersect with recognizable conceptions of autonomy.

In many cases, the overarching aim seems to be to encourage practitioners to be more autonomous, in the sense of emancipating themselves from diagnostic formulae and tools (Toombs 1992; Mullen 2007; Martin and Hicherson 2013). For example, having identified shortcomings in current diagnostic tools for schizophrenia, which are both fragmented and too unwieldy, Mullen argues that reliance on these tools may encourage a loss of the capacity to listen properly and attend to the patient's life and state of mind. Martin and Hicherson similarly identify problems with clinical assessments of patient competence when it comes to making decisions about treatment. The gold standard in clinical and legal practice is the MacArthur Competence Assessment Tool, which consists of a short structured interview and a scoring system allowing the quantitative psychological assessment of the patient. By placing high value on individual cognitive performance of the patient, the tool ignores the decision context, the complex temporality experienced by the patient, and the lived experience of judgment by patient and assessor. And similar concerns about the way questionnaires fail to capture the experience of the patient and limit the communication are raised by Toombs (1992: 26–30). But these calls for the practitioner to think for herself are aimed at fostering sensitivity to the particularity of each situation.

Explicit attempts to think of patient autonomy within a phenomenological context tend to assume a substantive conception that comes close to ideas of human flourishing. The most explicit such model is developed in a series of articles by Thomas Fuchs, who argues for the importance both diagnostically and in terms of treatment of having an integrative conception of autonomy (Fuchs 2010, 2013).

The question is to what extent is it useful to think of these approaches as phenomenological reconceptions of autonomy? The basic value expressed by the concept of autonomy is respect for the other person, so invocation of autonomy can function as a reminder that one treats a who not a what (see e.g. Stanghellini and Rosfort 2013). As we saw, commitment to the basic value of respect can take very different forms. Historically, autonomy in the clinical context is aimed at placing limits on paternalistic interference. The phenomenological priorities listed earlier have different set of targets, such as dependence on formulae for diagnosis and treatment, and top-down, piecemeal approaches to patient care. These phenomenological targets can be usefully seen as extensions of the idea of autonomy and as contributions to thinking how a substantive conception in particular can have application in the clinical context.

More challenging for phenomenologists is the way the normative balance is tipped toward being in charge of one's own affairs. Autonomy in all three conceptions we discussed earlier states that one is or is helped to become in charge of one's life, by controlling what is external or alien. This idea fits well the medical model of psychopathology. So we speak of mental illness, disorder, dysfunction, distress, and aim to cure or to alleviate what we diagnose as pathological. By contrast, the phenomenological injunction is to seek meaning in the experience. This is reflected clearly in the acceptance of provisionality and open-endedness in (d). Taking this idea of meaning in the experience a bit further we can look at notable examples in the phenomenological literature about the revelatory value of anxiety and insomnia as states that tell us something important about our standing in the world.[9] While such insight into our condition can be described as an attainment, it is quite different from the achievement of rational self-constitution, which remains the goal of personal, moral, and substantive conceptions of autonomy.

Acknowledgments

Thanks to Lambert Wiesing and to the editors for their helpful comments.

Bibliography

Anderson J. and Christman J. (eds.) (2005). *Autonomy and the Challenges of Liberalism: New Essays.* Cambridge: Cambridge University Press.

Brentano F. (1995). *Descriptive Psychology,* trans. Benito Müller. London: Routledge.

Broome M. R, Harland R., Owen G. S., Stringaris S. (eds.) (2014). *The Maudsley Reader in Phenomenological Psychiatry.* Cambridge: Cambridge University Press.

Deligiorgi K. (2012). *The Scope of Autonomy. Kant and the Morality of Freedom.* Oxford: Oxford University Press.

Dworkin G. (1976). "Autonomy and Behavior Control." *The Hastings Center Report* 6(1): 23–28.

Fuchs T. (2010). "Subjectivity and Intersubjectivity in Psychiatric Diagnosis." *Psychopathology* 43: 268–274.

Fuchs T. (2013). "Existential Vulnerability. Towards a Psychopathology of Limit Situations." *Psychopathology* 46: 301–308.

Giorgi A. (2009). *The Descriptive Phenomenological Method in Psychology: A Modified Husserlian Approach.* Pittsburgh, PA: Duquesne University Press.

Goldman A. (2006). *Simulating Minds.* Oxford: Oxford University Press.

Hand S. (ed.) (1989). *The Levinas Reader: Emmanuel Levinas.* Oxford: Blackwell.

Husserl E. (1969). *Cartesian Meditations. An Introduction to Phenomenology,* trans. D. Cairns. The Hague: Martinus Nijhoff.

Husserl E. (1970). *The Crisis of European Sciences and Transcendental Phenomenology,* trans. D. Carr. Evanston: Northwestern University Press.

Husserl E. (1988). *Vorlesungen über Ethik und Wertlehre 1908–1914,* ed. U. Melle. Dordrecht, Boston, London: Kluwer.

Jaspers K. [1913] (1963). *General Psychopathology,* trans. J. Hoenig and M. W. Hamilton. Chicago: University of Chicago Press.

Jaspers K. [1912] (1968). "The Phenomenological Approach in Psychopathology." *British Journal of Psychiatry* 114: 1313–1323.

Martin W. and Hicherson, R. (2013). "Mental Capacity and the Applied Phenomenology of Judgement." *Phenomenology and the Cognitive Sciences* 12(1): 195–214.

---

[9] See Hand 1989 and Staehler 2009.

Mill J. S. (1989). *On Liberty and Other Writings*. Cambridge: Cambridge University Press.

Mullen P. E. (2007). "A Modest Proposal for Another Phenomenological Approach to Psychopathology." *Schizophrenia Bulletin* 33(1): 113–121.

Renault A. 1997. *Era of the Individual. A Contribution to a History of Subjectivity*. Princeton: Princeton University Press.

Sartre J.-P. (1946). *Existentialism is a Humanism*, trans. Bernard Frechtman. New York: Philosophical Library.

Staehler T. (2009). *Plato and Levinas. The Ambiguous Out-side of Ethics*. New York: Routledge.

Stanghellini G. and Rosfort R. (2013). "Empathy as A Sense of Autonomy." *Psychopathology* 46: 337–344.

Toombs S. K. (1992). *The Meaning of Illness: A Phenomenological Account of the Different Perspectives of Physician and Patient*. Philosophy and Medicine Series, 42. Dordrecht: Kluwer.

Toombs S. K. (ed.) (2001). *The Handbook of Phenomenology and Medicine*, Philosophy and Medicine Series, 68. Dordrecht: Kluwer.

Woodruff Smith D. and Thomasson A. L. (eds.) 2005. *Phenomenology and Philosophy of Mind*. Oxford: Oxford University Press.

CHAPTER 43

....

ALTERITY

....

SØREN OVERGAARD AND MADS GRAM HENRIKSEN

INTRODUCTION

....

ALTERITY—or otherness—is a key notion in phenomenology. In this chapter, we distinguish between a broad and a narrow definition of alterity. We then go on to outline classical and contemporary phenomenological analyses of experiences of alterity in the narrow sense of the term. We consider analyses of normal experiences of alterity that are found in the philosophical literature as well as analyses of pathological experiences described in phenomenological psychopathology.

BROAD AND NARROW DEFINITIONS OF ALTERITY

....

Within phenomenology, one can distinguish between a broad and a narrow definition of the term "alterity." According to the *broad* definition, there are "three fundamentally different types of alterity: alterity in the form of (1) non-self (world), (2) oneself as Other, and (3) Other self" (Zahavi 1999: 195). On this broad understanding, "alterity" refers to anything that eludes or transcends a subject's grasp. Thus, inanimate objects and, more generally, the so-called "external" world transcend our grasp insofar as it is not possible to perceive all aspects of them at once. For example, we always see a cube from a particular vantage point, which means that we never strictly speaking see more than three of its six sides. Yet, in some sense we are perceptually aware of the "unseen" sides as well, that is, we see the cube *as* having sides that are not currently seen, thus "transcending" our current experience of it (Husserl 2001: 40–41). Strange as it may sound, we also transcend ourselves in various ways. For example, as embodied subjects we have external appearances that routinely escape us. Mirrors aside, we generally do not see our own face or back. Finally, as many philosophers have noted, other subjects (or minds) elude us in even more profound ways than we elude ourselves. For, in addition to whatever transcendence pertains to their bodies, the minds of others are *in principle* inaccessible to us, it might be said. While others' bodies are as perceptible as inanimate objects are, it seems there simply is no such thing as perceiving another person's mind or their mental states or episodes. This is the source of the philosophical problem of other minds (see Overgaard 2012).

Although, as we will see, phenomenologists have tended to question the assumption that another's mentality is imperceptible, most classical and contemporary phenomenologists accept that other subjects or minds are radically transcendent in a way inanimate things are not. Husserl thus maintains that the other subject is "the only transcendence really worthy of the name" and that "everything else we call transcendence, such as the objective world, is *based* upon the transcendence of other subjectivities" (Husserl 1959: 495; our translation, italics in original). Similarly, Levinas affirms that "[t]he absolutely other is the Other [*Autrui*]" (Levinas 1969: 39). Such remarks point to a *narrow* definition of "alterity." Narrowly defined, "alterity" refers exclusively to another agent, subjectivity or mind, or what is *experienced* as such.[1] The rationale behind restricting the use of the term "alterity" in this way is that only other subjects present an in-principle limitation to our knowledge or grasp, as we shall see in the next section. In the remainder of the essay, we will focus on the narrow sense of alterity.

HUSSERL AND MERLEAU-PONTY ON EXPERIENCES OF ALTERITY

In this section, we outline core parts of Husserl's and Merleau-Ponty's broadly convergent classical phenomenological analyses of the experience of alterity, and briefly compare these with the proposals of Sartre and Levinas. Husserl's and Merleau-Ponty's analyses take their point of departure in the mentioned idea that, as subjects of experience and action, we experience ourselves as embodied. Briefly, the "transcendence" (or "alterity" in the *broad* sense) of material objects such as tables resides in the fact that such objects are always experienced as containing "more" than what is currently perceived. Seated at a table, one sees only the table top—partly occluded, perhaps, by books, coffee cups, etc.—and perhaps two legs of the table. At the same time, one is tacitly aware of the table as having an underside, of the table as having more legs than are currently in view, and of the table top as continuing uninterrupted beneath the occluding books and cups. According to Husserl and Merleau-Ponty, one is aware of the hidden aspects of things as aspects that *would* come into view if one were to move in particular ways. This highlights the crucial role of the body (*Leib*), which anchors us in our world, enables it to appear experientially, and is the seat of our power of locomotion. For Husserl and Merleau-Ponty, therefore, only an embodied subject can experience "transcendent," material objects (Husserl 2001: 39–53; cf. Merleau-Ponty 2012: 334).

According to Husserl and Merleau-Ponty, we experience our own subjectivity as embodied. Thus, the question is not how we can reach other minds "hidden behind" their bodies (see Merleau-Ponty 1964: 52–53), but rather how their bodies can appear to us as

---

[1] One might also define "alterity" as all that is experienced as "not me" or "other-than-me" (cf. the "non-self" criterion in the broad definition). If alterity is defined in this way, then there is no alterity in our normal experiences of ourselves. But inanimate objects as well as animate creatures would still count as "other."

bodies of the right sort, namely as other embodied *subjects*. Husserl's guiding idea is that we must experience our own body and the body of another as forming a "pair," appearing as two of a kind (Husserl 1995: 112). In brief, if a person touches a table top with her hand, this action is at the same time subjective and bodily; and if she watches her hand as it explores the table top, it visually appears to her as such. If she notices another person's hand moving across the table top, she will immediately see it as a subjective organ exploring the table top, just like her own hand.

Husserl and Merleau-Ponty emphasize that although this experience is a perceptual experience of the other's embodied subjectivity and not the result of an inference (Husserl 1995: 111), this experience is importantly different from the perception of physical objects such as tables and trees (Merleau-Ponty 2012: 190–191). While the table never shows all of its sides at once, it nevertheless has no sides or aspects that cannot be perceived. Even the naked wood under the wood stain can be perceived, if we are willing to damage the surface. Other subjects, by contrast, have aspects that essentially are unperceivable, Husserl thinks. We can see another's joy in her smile, and we can to some degree appreciate what it is like for her to feel this joy. But the precise subjective "feel" of her joy as she experiences it is in principle beyond our perceptual grasp (Husserl 1995: 109; Merleau-Ponty 2012: 372). More generally, although we may understand how the world looks from another's perspective, we can never literally see things through another person's eyes or undergo their experiences as they undergo them. Indeed, according to Husserl and Merleau-Ponty, this must be so. As the former puts it, "if what belongs to the other's own essence were directly accessible, it would be merely a moment of my own essence, and ultimately he himself and I myself would be the same" (Husserl 1995: 109). In the words of Merleau-Ponty, the other's dimension of inaccessibility is the "price" we must pay for there to be others in the world at all (2012: 379).

Husserl and Merleau-Ponty do not believe that we only experience alterity in concrete face-to-face encounters with others. Their point is not merely that our interactions with others may be—and perhaps increasingly are—mediated in various ways, for example, we send text messages, emails, and interact via social media. More important is the fact that we even experience the inanimate objects around us as testifying to the presence of others. In cultural objects, for example, we experience "the near presence of others under a veil of anonymity. *One* uses the pipe for smoking, the spoon for eating" (Merleau-Ponty 2012: 363; cf. Heidegger 2007: 153–154). The very environments in which most of us live are infused with alterity in the shape of roads, fields, parks, and so on. However, inanimate objects are experienced as having a *derived* alterity (in the narrow sense) about them, in contrast to the intrinsic alterity of other people.

Although the Husserlian and Merleau-Pontian perspectives on alterity are endorsed by many contemporary phenomenologists, they are not the only perspectives we find within the phenomenological tradition. Sartre's analysis of alterity, for example, takes its point of departure in what he perceives as a weakness of the Husserlian account. For Husserl, as Sartre reads him, the paradigmatic encounter with another is a situation in which *I* observe and interpret another person. In other words, "*the Other* is still an object *for me*" (Sartre 1989: 255), that is, something I inspect with my gaze, much as I inspect other items in my environment. Sartre acknowledges that other people are very special objects, according to Husserl, given that I am said to experience them as able to sense, feel, and think. But these abilities are ultimately properties that I attribute to a certain type of observed object. By contrast, Sartre claims that the paradigmatic encounter with another subject is the situation in which

I experience *myself* as his or her *observed object*. Importantly, I can experience another's presence as "the *one who looks at me*" (Sartre 1989: 257) in situations in which I precisely do not see any others. Sartre offers the famous example of a Peeping Tom observing some scene through a keyhole. When he takes himself to be alone, the voyeur is pure "looking": fully absorbed by the scene, he is scarcely aware of himself or his actions. But the moment he hears (or believes he hears) footsteps in the corridor behind him, everything changes. Now he experiences himself as the shameful, contemptible voyeur exposed as such by the look of the unseen person behind him (Sartre 1989: 259–260).

Levinas agrees with Sartre that it is problematic to think the paradigmatic experience of alterity is that of observing a special object. But Levinas is skeptical of Sartre's positive account, since it seems merely to reverse the relation of observer and observed. For Levinas, the exemplary experience of alterity does not consist in experiencing oneself to be an object or "theme attended to by the other, but rather in submitting oneself . . . to a morality" (Levinas 1969: 86). In other words, we fundamentally experience others as creatures that have some sort of *moral claim* on us. Levinas realizes that our treatment of others may not always seem to bear this out. But he insists that some vague awareness of a moral demand or obligation is nevertheless part and parcel of normal experiences of others. The slight discomfort we feel—be it ever so slight—as we hurry past a beggar in the street testifies to this, Levinas thinks. After all, we experience nothing comparable when we walk past a tree or a lamppost.[2]

After this brief sketch of some classical phenomenological analyses of "normal" experiences of alterity, we will now consider some rather less normal ways in which alterity may show up in our experiences.

Alterity and Psychopathology

From the very outset, human beings are socially minded creatures. Yet, social relations are not always unproblematic. Even in normal conditions, relating to others can be difficult and, as Sartre (1989) vividly has described, our interpersonal struggles may have high stakes, potentially drawing our freedom or self-understanding into question. Turning to psychopathology, we may observe various disturbed forms of relating to others, of perceiving others, as well as, more broadly, disturbed experiences of the boundary between self and non-self. In the characterological traits and behavioral tendencies, which define personality disorders in ICD-10 (WHO 1992), certain deviating, largely persistent and inflexible patterns of relating to others form important diagnostic criteria. These include unwarranted suspiciousness toward others (paranoid personality disorder) and callous unconcern for others (dissocial personality disorder). The involved personality disorders illustrate disturbed *forms of relating to others* but the involved *perceptions of others* are also not entirely unaffected. For example, the enduring, rigid perception of others as, in these cases, either basically threatening or worthless does not permit others to appear in their full transcendence and freedom. There exist,

---

[2] For a fuller account of Sartre's take on alterity, see Overgaard (2013), on which we have drawn in this section. See Critchley (2002) for a helpful introduction to Levinas's take on the topic.

however, also more profound forms of "disturbed alterity" in psychopathological conditions. In the following, we explore some of these in the case of schizophrenia.

Setting aside psychotic experiences for now, many patients with schizophrenia report persisting difficulties in relating to others (Salice and Henriksen 2015). These difficulties are often present long before the onset of psychosis and may lead to social withdrawal and isolation. Social difficulties were addressed by many classical psychiatrists, especially under the headings of (schizophrenic) "autism" (e.g. Minkowski 1927: 29–30; Bleuler 1950: 63–68; Binswanger 1987: 85) and lack of "common sense" (Blankenburg 2001), and they were considered essential features of the clinical picture of schizophrenia. In brief, autism and problems with common sense are considered indicative of a disturbance of the pre-reflective attunement with others and the world we share, for example, reflected in an inadequate grasp of the tacit rules of social interaction or by an inability to take for granted what others consider obvious.

Problems with common sense are often associated with excessive tendencies to hyper-reflect (in an attempt to decode the meaning of everyday objects or social situations) and a fundamental, yet regularly ineffable feeling of being profoundly different from others (*Anderssein*) or simply "wrong" (Parnas and Henriksen 2014: 253). The root of this unsettling feeling is often a persisting experience of being *ontologically different* from others (Parnas and Henriksen 2014: 253) or, as Saks puts it, "not really human" (Saks 2007: 193). In their ontological solitude, patients may, for example, perceive others as deeply enigmatic, as imbeciles concerned primarily with superficial (material) aspects of existence, as "robot-like" or as "mere extras" in their life (e.g. reflected in certain solipsistic "Truman show"-like experiences).

Many patients also report transitivistic phenomena, that is, transient experiences of permeability or blurring of self–other boundaries. For example, patients may experience being as if "mixed up" with another and being unable to tell which thoughts originate in whom. They may also experience being "transparent" or "radically exposed" (Henriksen et al. 2010) in the sense that it is as if others somehow are able to "see" or "know" their thoughts.[3] In our view, the non-psychotic, anomalous self-experiences ("self-disorders"), of which we have described a few above, constitute important sources of social anxiety, social withdrawal, and of the social difficulties frequently reported by patients (cf. Salice and Henriksen 2015: 167).

In acute psychosis, the experience of alterity may undergo dramatic changes. Among the diagnostically important first-rank symptoms of schizophrenia, initially described by Schneider (1950), we find delusion of thought insertion, withdrawal or broadcasting, and passivity phenomena. These delusions articulate *primary* pathological experiences of someone or something placing alien thoughts in one's mind, extracting or stealing certain thoughts, having access to one's thoughts (e.g. others can hear the thoughts if they stand close by), and controlling one's body, actions, or will, etc.

Other important and frequently reported first-rank symptoms are auditory verbal hallucinations in the form of a running commentary or discussing "voices." Here, parts of the patients' inner speech or dialogue appear to have become automated, morbidly

---

[3] In clinical settings, sustained avoidance of eye contact may be a sign of the patient harboring transitivistic experiences.

objectified, and acquired auditory or quasi-auditory qualities, allowing the patients to "hear" their loud and unfamiliar thoughts as alien voices (Stanghellini and Cutting 2003; Henriksen et al. 2015). Crucially, the "objects" of such delusional and hallucinatory experiences are typically not unproblematically inscribed in the intersubjective world. Rather, they always appear "insufficiently objective" and continue to carry a residual layer of subjectivity (Parnas and Henriksen 2016: 82). In short, primary delusion and auditory verbal hallucination in schizophrenia seem to presuppose and occur in another "modal space," looming up before the patient alone (Sass 1994: 46; Ratcliffe 2012; Parnas and Henriksen 2016)—as Merleau-Ponty puts it with regard to hallucinations, they "play out on a different stage than that of the perceived world" (2012: 355). This observation has been partly corroborated by Aggernæs (1972), who explored the "status of reality" of hallucinatory experiences in schizophrenia and found inter alia that patients typically experience their hallucinatory "voices" as intrinsically "private," that is, the "voices" are *experientially given* to them (i.e. not *inferred* by them) in such a way that they usually do not expect others to be able to hear the "voices" they hear.

According to Schneider, permeability of self–other or self–world boundaries ("'Durchlässigkeit' der 'Ich-Umwelt-Schranke'") and the implied waning sense of self are crucial sources of the first-rank symptoms (1950: 136). In schizophrenia, the tacit sense of self-presence, which usually persists across the flux of time and changing modalities of consciousness, saturating our experiential life with an indefinite, yet vital feeling of "mineness," is unstable or threatened (Parnas and Sass 2011; Parnas and Henriksen 2014: 254–255). Recently, Parnas and Henriksen (2016: 83–85) have argued that this wavering sense of self-presence in schizophrenia may "de-structure" experiential life, affecting the very articulation of the "me-not-me" or "self–other" distinction and thereby enabling a "radical alterity" or "another presence" to emerge in the midst of the patient's own subjectivity (cf. Henriksen and Parnas 2014: 545). This "radical alterity" may take several different forms in the pre-psychotic stage of the illness, for example, a feeling that some of one's thoughts are not really one's own, experiences as if one's body, parts of it, or one's own bodily movements are not truly one's own, permeability of self–other boundaries, and the experience as if something or someone in one's peripersonal space is "drawing near" (*Anwesenheit*). In different illness stages and depending on the patient's "psychotic work" (Ey 1973),[4] this "radical alterity" may materialize into a persecuting, influencing, or hallucinatory other (Parnas and Henriksen 2016: 85). In brief, radical alterity seems to enable a profound sense of self-alienation to grow from within the disturbed subjectivity. Although experiences of radical alterity need not be, and typically will not initially be, experiences of alterity in the narrow sense that we have focused on in this chapter, some of them may eventually develop into an experience of another agent's or pseudo-agent's presence in the midst of one's own subjectivity—for example, someone (or something) listening to, looking at, or touching you (i.e. delusion of being bugged, filmed, or controlled, respectively) or speaking to or about you (i.e. auditory verbal hallucination) (Ey 1973).

---

[4] Ey employs the term "psychotic work" (*le travail psychotique*) to denote the cognitive efforts involved in making sense of one's pathological experiences.

CONCLUSION

We have outlined a broad and a narrow definition of "alterity" within the phenomenological literature. We have also provided examples from classical and contemporary phenomenology of both normal and pathological experiences of alterity. Finally, we have highlighted the idea that "radical alterity" is a central feature of the phenomenology of schizophrenia.

BIBLIOGRAPHY

Aggernæs A. (1972). "The Experienced Reality of Hallucinations and Other Psychological Phenomena: An Empirical Analysis." *Acta Psychiatrica Scandinavica* 48: 220–238.

Binswanger L. (1987). "Extravagance, Perverseness, Manneristic Behaviour and Schizophrenia," trans. J. Cutting. In J. Cutting and M. Shephard (eds.), *The Clinical Roots of the Schizophrenia Concept*, pp. 83–88. Cambridge: Cambridge University Press.

Blankenburg W. (2001). "First Steps Toward a Psychopathology of "Common Sense"," trans. A. L. Mishara. *Philosophy, Psychiatry & Psychology* 8: 303–315.

Bleuler E. (1950). *Dementia Praecox or the Group of Schizophrenias*, trans. J. Zinkin. New York: International University Press.

Critchley S. (2002). "Introduction." In S. Critchley and R. Bernasconi (eds.), *The Cambridge Companion to Levinas*, pp. 1–32. Cambridge: Cambridge University Press.

Ey H. (1973). *Traité des hallucinations, Tome I et II*. Paris: Masson.

Heidegger M. (2007). *Being and Time*, trans. J. Macquarrie and E. Robinson. Oxford: Blackwell.

Henriksen M. G., Škodlar B., Sass L. A., and Parnas J. (2010). "Autism and Perplexity: A Qualitative and Theoretical Study of Basic Subjective Experiences in Schizophrenia. *Psychopathology* 43: 357–368.

Henriksen M. G. and Parnas J. (2014). "Self-disorders and Schizophrenia: A Phenomenological Reappraisal of Poor Insight and Noncompliance." *Schizophrenia Bulletin* 40: 542–547.

Henriksen M. G., Raballo A., and Parnas J. (2015). "The Pathogenesis of Auditory Verbal Hallucinations in Schizophrenia: A Clinical-Phenomenological Account." *Philosophy, Psychiatry, & Psychology* 22(3): 165–181.

Husserl E. (1959). *Erste Philosophie (1923/24). Zweiter Teil*. Husserliana VIII. Ed. R. Boehm. The Hague: Nijhoff.

Husserl E. (1995). *Cartesian Meditations: An Introduction to Phenomenology*, trans. D. Cairns. Dordrecht: Kluwer Academic Publishers.

Husserl E. (2001). *Analyses Concerning Passive and Active Synthesis*, trans. A. J. Steinbock. Dordrecht: Kluwer Academic Publishers.

Levinas E. (1969). *Totality and Infinity: An Essay on Exteriority*, trans. A. Lingis. Pittsburgh: Duquesne University Press.

Merleau-Ponty M. (1964). *Sense and Non-Sense*, trans. H. L. Dreyfus and P. A. Dreyfus. Evanston: Northwestern University Press.

Merleau-Ponty M. (2012). *Phenomenology of Perception*, trans. D. Landes. London: Routledge.

Minkowski E. (1927). *La Schizophrénie. Psychopathologie des Schizoïdes et des Schizophrènes*. Paris: Payot.

Overgaard S. (2012). "Other People." In D. Zahavi (ed.), *The Oxford Handbook of Contemporary Phenomenology*, pp. 460–479. Oxford: Oxford University Press.

Overgaard S. (2013). "The Look." In S. Churchill and J. Reynolds (eds.), *Jean-Paul Sartre: Key Concepts*, pp. 106–117. Durham: Acumen.

Parnas J. and Sass L. A. (2011). "The Structure of Self-consciousness in Schizophrenia." In S. Gallagher (ed.), *The Oxford Handbook of the Self*, pp. 521–546. Oxford: Oxford University Press.

Parnas J. and Henriksen M. G. (2014). "Disordered Self in the Schizophrenia Spectrum: A Clinical and Research Perspective." *Harvard Review of Psychiatry* 22(5): 251–265.

Parnas J. and Henriksen M. G. (2016). "Mysticism and Schizophrenia: A Phenomenological Exploration of the Structure of Consciousness in the Schizophrenia Spectrum Disorders." *Consciousness and Cognition* 43: 75–88.

Ratcliffe M. (2012). "Phenomenology as a Form of Empathy." *Inquiry* 55: 473–495.

Saks E. R. (2007). *The Center Cannot Hold*. New York: Hyperion.

Salice A. and Henriksen M. G. (2015). "The Disrupted 'We': Schizophrenia and Collective Intentionality." *Journal of Consciousness Studies* 22(7–8): 145–171.

Sartre J.-P. (1989). *Being and Nothingness*, trans. H. E. Barnes. London: Routledge.

Sass L. A. (1994). *The Paradoxes of Delusion*. Ithaca: Cornell.

Schneider K. (1950). *Klinische Psychopathologie*. Stuttgart: Georg Thieme Verlag.

Stanghellini G. and Cutting, J. (2003). "Auditory Verbal Hallucinations—Breaking the Silence of Inner Dialogue." *Psychopathology* 36: 120–128.

World Health Organization (WHO) (1992). *The ICD-10. Classification of Mental and Behavioural Disorders: Clinical Description and Diagnostic Guidelines*. Geneva: WHO.

Zahavi D. (1999). *Self-Awareness and Alterity: A Phenomenological Investigation*. Evanston: Northwestern University Press.

CHAPTER 44

....

TIME

....

FEDERICO LEONI

FROM BEING TO TIME

....

THE problem of time plays a central role in modern philosophy; it is not simply a privileged object of inquiry, but also the background of any other inquiry. Philosophical investigations no longer revolve around Being, as it was the case with the ancients and, emblematically, with Aristotle. With Descartes, and later on with Kant, Husserl, and Heidegger, Being is no longer interrogated directly, but only indirectly. It seems that the moderns cannot reach Being anymore, unless through a long detour in the course of which the journey itself becomes the final destination. For the moderns, the subject is the door leading to Being, and the subject has become essentially temporal. As a result, time has become, first, the door leading to Being and, ultimately, Being itself. In his *Discours de la méthode* (1637) and *Meditationes de prima philosophia* (1641), Descartes (1999), with the famous exercise of methodical doubt, has brought us to the threshold of this development. My own experience might play tricks on me, Descartes argues: I might be dreaming what I see; an evil genius might be implanting all sorts of illusions in my mind. However, the fact that I am having an experience and I am thinking is indubitable, and implies that, as I think, I also exist—at least as a thinking being. For Descartes, this tiny but indestructible evidence is the only foundation on which a new and hopefully conclusive form of knowledge can be built.

It is clear that at the core of Descartes's intellectual gesture lies a powerful cultural strategy: this is the Trojan horse of a resolutely anti-traditionalist battle, so to speak, a battle for the necessity of getting rid of what we think we know just because others have claimed or substantiated it. My self, my clear critical consciousness is the only criterion of validity, the only testing ground for a knowledge that aspires to the status of science. However, there is another, more properly philosophical side to Descartes's attitude. The forced passage through the needle eye of the *cogito* implies that it would be naive to speak directly of things, reality or Being, because first of all we must become aware of the fact that the things of which we speak are, in fact, *spoken* things, and, in a broader sense, the things of which we have experience, perception, memory, and so on. In other words, there are never simply "things," but there is always and primarily our experience of things. The subject therefore is not just the criterion of a free rational examination, but has become the epistemological foundation of knowledge in general and the speculative root of a more or less explicit reduction of Being to being-thought. More precisely, it is the presence of the subject to itself that becomes foundational.

On closer inspection, the Cartesian subject is in fact a presence that relates to itself as a presence, a relationship of the subject with itself. "I know that I am thinking, I feel that I am feeling, I experience the fact that I am having this experience": this doubling is fundamental and inescapable. It is a recursive, circular, and autoaffective operation, which creates the space in which every other presence can find its place and meaning precisely as a presence that meaningfully exists for the subject only within such absolute dimension. This way, the question of time—implied or outlined in embryo in these pages—timidly enters the scene, ready to take center stage in modern philosophical debates. Once the pieces of the philosophical game are positioned in this way, the centrality of time becomes necessary and unavoidable. To be sure, the subject's presence to itself remains a profound mystery, which allows for different readings already in Descartes and in the discussions he entertains with his interlocutors. The first possibility is that such self-presence is immediate, instantaneous, and extra-temporal—an intuition enclosed in a sort of eternal instant. Here, time is a motionless instant. The second possibility is that this self-presence is mediated, articulated in a kind of syllogism, so that this experience (which is the key to all other experiences) becomes a construction, a discourse that leads from premises to conclusions. Time itself here becomes speech, journey, chronology, and movement. In one way or another, however, once the subject has taken a foundational role, the foundation of everything in fact coincides with the enigma of the unity of the subject with itself and the mystery of its temporalization or self-temporalization.

Time and Subject

There is a more or less direct line that connects Descartes to Kant in relation to this problem. Kant's famous metaphor of the Copernican revolution, which opens the *Critique of Pure Reason* (1781), almost literally reproduces the Cartesian approach and its method of inquiry. To this date, Kant argues, philosophers have followed a Ptolemaic approach. They addressed the problem of knowledge by placing the object of knowledge at center stage, with the knowing subject rotating around it. This resembles a bit what the ancients did, who—precisely from a Ptolemaic perspective—placed Being at the center (as in Aristotle) and from it directly derived certain characteristics or, if you will, a certain knowledge concerning those characteristics. The earth was at the center of the universe, and it laid down the laws for its inhabitants. Being dictated the rules of the philosophical game and imposed its contents on any form of knowledge about Being, that is, on ontology or metaphysics. However, from now on, says Kant, we must proceed in the opposite direction: a Copernican approach must be adopted. We must put the subject at the center and let the object orbit around it. In other words, it is time to admit that there is no such thing as a direct access to the object, but only an indirect one, mediated by the stained glass of our mind and the transcendental bias of our experience. The object can no longer prescribe its laws to our experience; rather, it is the subject that dictates the law of its experience to an object that is no longer "in itself" but always and only "for us." Essentially, we *are* time, and the law of our experience is nothing but the law of self-temporalization of the subject.

Kant's treatment of the problem of time is extremely complex and profound and can of course only be sketched here. Let us say first of all that the Copernican revolution, in the Kantian sense, still implies that the subject receives a series of impressions "from the outside"—a "rhapsody" of sensible data, as Kant writes in order to emphasize the disorderly nature of this process. However, the very nature of the Copernican revolution suggests that such disorder is then inscribed in a form, in a pattern, or in a grid, which operates "from the inside" of the subject. The nature of this form or pattern or grid is precisely temporal. It works roughly in the following way: first, we must assume that the subject is present to itself or, better, that it has become one with this activity of making itself present to itself. Kant calls this activity "synthetic unity of transcendental apperception." In other words, the subject keeps relating to itself and reuniting with itself, in a kind of dull pulsation or secret litany: "I, who am still myself, who am still myself. . . ." This subject or unitary and continuous activity is the point where a kind of space emerges in which the multiplicity of experience can be accommodated. This manifold experience finds its place in a series of distinct and discontinuous locations created by that pulsation or litany. Kant calls this activity "analytic unity of transcendental apperception." From the encounter between the raw material of sensitivity and the a priori form of the litany, a sort of transcription emerges that is experience itself, a transcription that we could picture as the marks left by the pen of a seismograph which records, in a necessarily linear manner, the motions of the earth on a roll of paper that eternally rotates in a circular manner and, moreover, around a motionless pivot. Here is the second version of this pulsation or litany of experience: "I, who am still myself, have now heard this, and I, who am still myself and therefore can say that before I heard this, I have now heard also that, and then I, who am still myself and heard this and that, perceive now this other thing."

It is easy to realize that, in a nutshell, Kant's treatment of the problem already followed the path later taken by Husserl's and Heidegger's investigations and perhaps even included their solutions to it. In Kantian terms, we could say that the unity of the subject is the matrix of the unity of the object. In other words, the self-temporalization of the subject—its being in relationship with itself or its being *nothing but* a relationship with itself—constitutes the very structure of the object, the locus in which the object can manifest itself in a variety of ways; in short, it represents the meaning of its objectivity understood as a peculiar "thingly" substance or depth.

TIME AND BODY

This is the path later followed by Husserl. His phenomenology is always, on the one side, a phenomenology of perception focusing on the world's self-donation to a subject that records its presence through the senses, and, on the other hand, a phenomenology of time or (as reads the title of a volume collecting his lectures on the topic) of "inner time-consciousness," namely a phenomenology of the way in which the sensible presence of things is recorded through the original, affective, and autoaffective presence of the subject to itself. It is easy to detect the influence of the Kantian model. However, Husserl's analysis, when compared to Kant's, strikes for its exceptional accuracy and descriptive concreteness, and even more for the extraordinary attention devoted to the problem of the subject's self-temporalization as autoaffection. Husserl literally shifts the Kantian temporal synthesis backward and relocates it in the depths of the body, thereby transferring what Kant called the "I think" directly into the *Leib*, to use the language of Husserl's phenomenology. It is a move of enormous consequences, because it means to shift the synthesis from the "I"—which Kant always kept distinct from the disorder and meaninglessness of sensitivity—to the very dimension of sensitivity and passive perception. As a result, sensitivity emerges as a faculty endowed with a form of its own, a capacity to generate order and meaning or to embody all possible meanings, without the need for additional disembodied and multi-layered transcendental foundations.

This overall development is clearly visible if one follows the path that leads from the lectures on the *For the Phenomenology of the Consciousness of Inner Time* (1991; which collect texts of the 1893–1917 period) and from *Ideas for a Pure Phenomenology and a Phenomenological Philosophy* (1913) to the late and extraordinary *Lectures on Passive Synthesis* (1920–26). In brief, one could say that for Husserl, and especially for the late Husserl, time coincides with the subject, but the subject is the body. With its paradoxical overtones, the expression "passive synthesis" is clear evidence of such development—in fact, when read through the lenses of traditional philosophy, it sounds like a true oxymoron. For Kant, the synthesis is an active process performed by the subject or, as I said above, the subject itself as process and activity. Passivity, instead, means receptivity of chaotic and meaningless sensitive data independently of time and the order provided by it. For Husserl, on the contrary, synthesis and temporalization happen *before* any subjective act and process of temporalization.

We could find this bodily comprehension of time operating in some ways already in Husserls's notes *For the Phenomenology of the Consciousness of Inner Time*. Presence, he says, always undergoes two different tensions, two peculiar intentionalities, retention and protension, which form the depth and the sense of presence itself. Retention retains past within presence. Protension opens presence to the future. But retention and protention are not operations of the subject, are not intentionalities enacted by consciousness, are not active and objectivating syntheses. They are forms of immanent, asubjective, passive intentionality, immanent to sensible presence itself. Long before subject, its intentionality, its imaginative syntheses and its semiotic operations, presence itself is "operating" and "anonymous" intentionality, as the late Husserls says. And the form of this immanent intentionality is double. On the one side persistence of the presence and inner modification of presence in past (retention); on the other side anticipation of future and modification of presence itself in future (protension). Time is this continuous yet articulated bodily structure, this immanent yet self-unfolding and self-transcending complexity, this material and sensible passivity yet capable of engendering transcendence and subjectivation. And it is this body-time which is altered, differently articulated, peculiarly accentuated, within the different forms of psychopathological experience.

The example of the two hands touching each other, in Husserl's *Ideas for a Pure Phenomenology*, is perhaps the clearest and most accurate example of the enormous attention devoted to this knot between time and body within phenomenological tradition. By touching the left hand, Husserl writes, the right hand plays a subjectivating function, while the touched left hand is objectified. The two experiences can be reversed at any moment: the touching hand can always become the touched one and vice versa. However, both hands are part of a body that through them touches and recognizes itself, while at the same time evading and alienating itself. What for Kant was a peculiarity of the self, namely a relationship with itself through which the self alienates itself in order to recognize itself as identical with itself, thereby being simultaneously one and many, eternal and temporal, transcendental and empirical—all this is "backdated," so to speak, by Husserl and relocated at the level of the living body. Husserl's example was further expanded by Maurice Merleau-Ponty in one of the most famous chapters of his last and unfinished work, *The Visible and the Invisible* (1968). Merleau-Ponty's notion of "flesh" exemplifies this complex relocation of the transcendental into the body and its unstable pulsation between the anonymity of a desubjectivized flesh and the emergence of a subjectivized body—a body still poised over a desubjectivization that is both menacing and joyous, full of anguish and eroticism.

TIME AND EVENT

In Heidegger also there is no subject, but there is *Dasein*, the "being-there," or "being-here," according to the translation of the German term regularly employed by Heidegger—since his early masterpiece *Being and Time* (1927)—in place of the traditional term for "subject." *Dasein*, however, as Heidegger clarifies, is always and immediately *In-der-Welt-Sein*: "being-in-the-world." For Heidegger "always" or "immediately" do not mean "at a second moment in time," as when subject encounters the world or something in the world is perceived by a subject. On the contrary, what he means is that our being-in-the world is still the world: it is a "fold" of the world and not something different from it. In other words, the being-in-the-world is the world folding on itself and revealing itself as other than itself and, at the same time, as nothing other than itself.

To Heidegger's radically phenomenological gaze, every previous phenomenological study of experience appears built on a prejudice, or at least on a too restricted and unduly generalized factor, that of the cognitive relationship. The cognitive relationship theory presupposes a subject distinct from the world, which only at a second moment in time, and somehow accidentally, encounters the world. Hence stems the primacy accorded to *perception* in the phenomenology of Husserl and Merleau-Ponty, and also the idea that the subject was an insufficient category that needed to be expanded in the direction of the body as a locus of sensitivity. This meant to transfer to the body what Kant had located in a transcendental sphere created in the image and likeness of a self. Heidegger thinks differently. He believes that the act of *doing*, and not simply knowing, provides the raw material for a phenomenology of experience and existence. By definition, this act is not contemplative and does not presuppose an observing subject and an observed object or an essentially perceiving subject waiting for a series of stimuli coming from an object. The object is first encountered in a dimension of use, instrumentality, solidity, resistance, and physical contact. The hand, rather than the eye, is at the center of Heidegger's investigation. Heidegger substitutes the subject for a hand that interacts concretely and immediately with the world. In place of the object, he places a thing, whose concreteness, everyday nature, and materiality are brought to the foreground through his lively descriptions. The profound meaning of Heidegger's view is that experience is not an arrow going from the subject to the object or from the object to the subject, but is rather like an open space stretching between subject and object, a third space of which the subject and the object are the effects, or, worse, the abstractions. There is a world, and there is a being-in-the-world, precisely because there is a dense network of practices, occupations, gestures, and affections in which we are always immersed unknowingly and unintentionally, or at least independently of a previous awareness or decision.

The consequence of this, however, is that time is no longer *in* the subject, as Kant or the early Husserl thought. Nor is it in the body, as the late Husserl believed. Nor is it exactly in the extended, intercorporeal, and even interspecific body, which ultimately coincides with the world itself, as Merleau-Ponty suggested with his notion of flesh. Time is the world folding on itself and unfolding away from itself in every occurring gesture or practice or event, be it great or small, epochal or ordinary. Time, more precisely, is Being folding itself, thereby sending itself to itself, in itself, and away from itself. Time is this triple movement that Being itself undergoes, or more precisely performs, or more simply *is*. Time *is* Being: this is the conclusion Heidegger famously reached—thirty years after the publication of *Being and Time*—in a lecture he entitled, with a significant inversion, *On Time and Being* (1962). The journey begun with Descartes comes to an end and seems to have inverted its course. Our temporality is not the stuff of Being. On the contrary, the temporality of Being is what constitutes us. Such abyssal temporality is the unfolding of Being in its infinite forms, including those of our world and our being-in-the-world.

FROM PHENOMENOLOGY TO PSYCHOPATHOLOGY

Phenomenological psychopathology is profoundly indebted to this long tradition of philosophical discussions on the nature of time and has derived from it the idea that in the psychopathological experience the possibility of temporalization or self-temporalization is impaired, the synthetic activity of what Kant called the self is difficult or impossible, the Husserlian autoaffective dimension of the living body is lacerated, and the event of Being as a modern dimension of temporality in the Heideggerian sense is forcluded. However different, all these forms of experience have something in common: their temporality is "out of joint," to use Shakespeare's expression. As a result, the subject's experience, which revolves around time or takes the form of those deeper processes that we gather under the notion of "time," is in turn out of joint and has become literally delusional.

Of course, this kind of temporal dislocation comes in different forms depending on the patient, and, more generally, varies according to his or her psychopathological condition (melancholy, mania, schizophrenia, paranoia, obsession, and so on). In his most pronounced Husserlian phase, Binswanger (*Melancholy and Mania* (1960)) believed that if Husserl's temporal synthesis required a "moment of living presence"—which included the dimensions of retention and protention—then each major form of psychopathological experience stemmed from the collapse of the inner proportion or balance between those three dimensions. According to this view, a melancholic experience is one in which retention has crushed all other temporal dimensions, turning the past into an unchangeable and impenetrable burden. In the manic experience, instead, the subject's presence has freed itself from retention and protention and has completely abandoned itself to a shimmering, elusive, and insubstantial present. In the schizophrenic experience, finally, protention has prevailed over presence and retention, thereby reorganizing time and experience around a distressing future, which must be constantly deciphered in its catastrophic and essentially unavoidable coming.

According to Kimura Bin's extraordinarily eloquent rendering (*Écrits de psychopathologie phénoménologique* (1992)) of this type of structural phenomenology of psychopathological experience, the melancholic experience takes place essentially *post festum*, the manic experience *intra festum*, and the schizophrenic one *ante festum*. Bin borrows these Latin expressions from the Marxist philosopher György Lukacs, who used them to designate the Revolution as the feast or event par excellence. However, if we understand the event as something that is happening here and now, the melancholic person is, for the Japanese psychiatrist, essentially incapable of participating in it because the structure of his temporality inevitably transforms the present event into a past one; the manic person, on the other hand, can never participate in the event because somehow he coincides with the event itself and with its kaleidoscopic changeability; the schizophrenic person, finally, can never participate in the event because the event is always still to come and is perceived as so unprecedented that it becomes incommensurable with what is already known and ultimately unbearable. Bin's analysis and reinterpretation of psychopathology draws, on the one hand, from Husserl's transcendental approach and, on the other, from Heidegger's deconstruction of transcendental subjectivism and from his event-centered ontology. Quite originally, Kimura Bin has also combined these ideas with themes typical of Japanese philosophy, in particular the notion of *aida* ("in-between"), propounding a new interpretation of schizophrenic experience as a disruption of the accessibility of the space "in between" (*L'Entre. Une approche phénoménologique de la schizophrénie* (2000)).

Similarly, in his extraordinary reinterpretation of phenomenology and phenomenological psychopathology, Henri Maldiney (*Penser l'homme et la folie à la lumière de la Daseinsanalyse* (1991)) has combined two different approaches, one influenced by Husserl and Merleau-Ponty, the other indebted to the extreme consequences of Heidegger's ontology. On the one hand, Maldiney argues, if the temporal synthesis coincides with the bodily synthesis, then the transcendental temporal structural flaw that Binswanger and others have constantly emphasized in psychopathological experience turns out to be, in fact, a transcendental structural flaw of the body itself. More precisely, it turns out to be a structural flaw of one's body as a transcendental entity, as a body able to play its constitutive role with respect to experience. On the other hand, Maldiney goes on, if the temporal synthesis is not the act of a subject or a subjective body, but rather the very event of Being (or Being itself as an event), then the alteration that Binswanger's psychopathology identified in the structures of the transcendental temporal synthesis should be seen—at a more profound level—as a failed relationship with the event or with Being, or as a failed relationship of the event with itself or of Being with itself (at least if one carries to its ultimate consequences Heidegger's elimination of the subject and its translation in terms of an ontology of the event).

Kimura's and Maldiney's models represent some of the most advanced contributions to the phenomenological–psychopathological reflection and outline a still unexplored field of research that promises to be extremely fruitful in terms of conceptual advancement.

BIBLIOGRAPHY

Binswanger L. (1960). *Melancholie und Manie*. Pfullingen: Neske.
Descartes R. [1637/1641] (1999). *Discours on Method, Meditations on First Philosophy*. Indianapolis: Hackett Publishing Company.

Heidegger M. [1927] (2010). *Being and Time*. Albany: SUNY Press.

Heidegger M. [1962] (2002). *On Time and Being*. Chicago: University of Chicago Press.

Husserl E. [1893–1917] (1991). *For the Phenomenology of the Consciousness of Inner Time*. Dordrecht, Boston: Kluwer.

Husserl E. [1920–1926] (2001). *Analysis Concerning Passive and Active Synthesis*. Dordrecht, Boston: Kluwer.

Husserl E. [1913] (2014). *Ideas for a Pure Phenomenology and a Phenomenological Philosophy*, three volumes. Indianapolis: Hackett Publishing Company.

Kant I. [1781] (1999). *Critique of Pure Reason*. Cambridge, New York: Cambridge University Press.

Kimura B. (1992). *Écrits de psychopathologie phénoménologique*. Paris: Presses Universitaires de France.

Kimura B. (2000). *L'Entre. Une approche phénoménologique de la schizophrénie*. Paris: Millon.

Maldiney H. (1991). *Penser l'homme et la folie à la lumière de la Daseinsanalyse*. Grenoble: Millon.

Merleau-Ponty M. [1964] (1968). *The Visible and the Invisible*. Evanston: Northwestern University Press.

CHAPTER 45

···

CONSCIENCE

···

MARCIN MOSKALEWICZ

Every human being has a conscience . . . It follows him like a shadow when he plans to escape

(Kant 1996: 146)

Conscience must apply a measuring stick to the situation one is confronted with, and this situation has to be evaluated in the light of a set of criteria, in the light of a hierarchy of values. These values, however, cannot be espoused and adopted by us on a conscious level—they are something that we are

(Frankl 1992: 146)

Clinical experience teaches us about the great role played by the disquiet of conscience in the pathogenesis of mental disorders

(Kępiński 2001: 123)

What does the conscience call to him to whom it appeals? Taken strictly, nothing. The call asserts nothing, gives no information about world-events, has nothing to tell

(Heidegger 1962: 318)

CONSCIOUSNESS AND CONSCIENCE

···

COULD a lack of conformity to what is considered morally good be related to allegedly undeserved suffering of the mind? Evoking conscience, our inner ethical compass, might seem as a step back to premedical models of illness and those religious conceptions that considered it as a punishment for immoral conduct. The idea, however, is less controversial than it initially appears. Both regular disease and mental illness are ethically based concepts (Fulford 1995). Furthermore, in contemporary psychopathology a clear-cut distinction between morally wrong acts and a disease is not always strictly held. If too scrupulous a conscience of a *typus melancholicus*, his excessively *conscientious* personality, makes him prone to a depressive disorder (Tellenbach 1972), unremitting efforts to preserve a clear conscience may lead to adaptation issues. On the other hand, psychopaths do not feel guilt or remorse because they lack conscience (Hare 1999). Addictions are difficult to convincingly conceptualize without at least some reference to the notions of weakness of will and personal responsibility (Graham and Poland 2011; Radoilska 2013). A more recent idea of a moral injury exemplifies the possibility of a damage done to one's conscience by participating in or committing immoral acts (Litz et al. 2009), where shattering one's deeply held moral beliefs leads to abnormal anxiety, suicidality, and addiction. Some claim that conscience is a neurocerebral function that is a psychosocially configured phylogenetic precondition of mental illness in general (García-Valls 2016). It is, therefore, quite conceivable that too weak or too scrupulous conscience could contribute to the development of mental pathology.

But the difficulty remains, and it partly lies within the definition. The concept of conscience serves as an umbrella term that has been given so many different philosophical exposures that it cannot be immediately clear what it actually denotes. In contemporary English, conscience is the consciousness of one's moral worth. The term is mostly used when there is a conflict between one's own and communal values. It indicates recognition of this conflict with a concomitant need to follow an inner guide. Etymologically, conscience originates in Latin *conscientia* meaning knowledge of something or being aware of something, which goes back to the Greek term συνείδησις (*syneídēsis*). Both concepts are derivatives of verbs denoting acquiring knowledge. In Antiquity, the term meant mostly consciousness. The view of conscience as the consciousness of good and evil systematically grew in the Middle Ages. Starting with Descartes, consciousness has been freed from the moral connotations of conscience and the differentiation of meaning took place in various modern languages (Krokos 2013).

Due to its modern semantic baggage, unlike values and moral responsibility, conscience is seldom talked about in phenomenological psychopathology, but it does not mean it is irrelevant. The principal distinction between any phenomenological view of conscience and the more common sense view, which will be called psychological (as witnessed by the aforementioned examples) is that upon the psychological account conscience is that part of consciousness we are guided by and follow, mostly in the case of a conflict of values, whereas phenomenological conscience is given before any self-conscious theorizing. Psychological conscience is a reflective awareness of one's own acts in terms of right and wrong. It becomes apparent through an evaluative judgment related to personal moral standards that can be also related to supposedly divine or non-transcendent moral laws. Even if psychological conscience refers to what phenomenological conscience gives us directly (and not to abstract values or social *mores*, which to be sure are independent of it), it is argumentative. It is an inner judge that prohibits, inhibits, and exercises control over oneself. When we (rightly) assert that a psychiatric intervention may foster moral growth (Pearce and Pickard 2009), we are usually referring to that reflective level. In a more phenomenological exposition, however, conscience—not unlike the Husserlian account of consciousness in general (Zahavi 2003)—accompanies (at least some, if not all of) our conscious acts as a pre-reflective awareness. It is pre-reflective in the sense that "there are no *considerations* to weight *pro-et-contra*, there is nothing for me to *deliberate* about" (Backström 2007: 323). Is it also pre-reflective because it is silent—when we present a concrete message of conscience in positive terms, we are already psychologically responding to its call. Values given through phenomenological conscience are not what we reflect upon—they are ourselves (Frankl 1992). Phenomenological conscience is more original than a fear-based superego. It is not separated from psychological moral life but makes it possible. Moreover, conscience from this perspective is not so much a conscience of something. Rather, as we shall see, it is objectless. Its object, as paradoxical as it seems, is nothing—a non-existent potentiality of being. This article presents a phenomenological view of conscience in its biological and existential manifestations as derived from the work of Antoni Kępiński (1918–1972) and Martin Heidegger (1889–1976), in relation with Viktor Emil von Gebsattel's (1883–1976) notion of existential neurosis. It is argued that these manifestations are two sides of the same coin of becoming, which points to the most original phenomenon of temporality.

CONSCIENCE AS NATURAL SELF-CONTROL

The notion of conscience features prominently in the work of Antoni Kępiński, one of the major Polish psychiatrists of the twentieth century. A graduate of the Jagiellonian University in Cracow and the University of Edinburgh, Kępiński was an influential advocate of humanist, axiological, and dialogical psychiatry. His work presents a mixture of phenomenology focused upon understanding the phenomenon of life and first-person experience of mental illness, and anti-naturalistic system theory (Kapusta 2007; Maciuszek 2015). Kępiński proposed that we look at mental disorders from a moral point of view, in which values provide a unity to constantly developing personhood.

> If we look in this way at neuroses, antisocial behaviors, psychosomatic illnesses, addictions, etc., they appear, at least to an extent, as consequences of breaching the moral order. People suffering from these conditions experience a living hell for transgressing moral law inherent in nature, for their harsh negative feelings, for their laziness and reluctance to take the effort of living, for their egoism, etc. Obviously, we have no right to deprecate them. Evil, same as death, is intrinsic to the process of life
>
> (Kępiński 2001: 119)

Kępiński usage of the word "moral" is disjoined from a conventional moral or immoral conduct. His theory presents a variation of psychophysical monism, in which the measure of good and evil is life itself. Good is what allows the growth of negative entropy and leads to positive affects, evil is what amplifies the processes of entropy and destruction (Kępiński 2001). There is a dialectics of creation and destruction at play in all life forms, and, because of that, there is an ontological-axiological *conflict* within a human being.

Kępiński argued that all organisms are autonomous, open, self-regulating, and teleological systems in constant metabolism of energy and information with the environment. They are organized by primary values that orient them toward the future and provide order to lived experience (Kępiński 2001, 2016). Inspired by the cybernetic model of feedback loops, Kępiński defined the highest among the systems of self-control in living organisms as conscience. From cellular to conscious and collective levels, all life constantly passes through three temporal phases—planning, realization, and assessment. Conscience helps to perpetuate the exchange of energy and information and prevents the spatiotemporal collapse that would reduce the metabolism. As such, conscience is an innate, embodied, and constitutive element of the self.[1] The role of the basic, constitutional conscience, which is literally a "biological conscience" (Kępiński 2001: 107) is to lead an organism toward its greatest possible development.[2] What might this greatest possible development be?

Unfortunately, we do not have a direct control upon constitutional conscience and are unable to know its actual "aims." Biological conscience manifests itself at a conscious level through "pangs" that are analogous to positive and negative affects understood in terms of a natural system of compensation. In other words, there is a reward for good and punishment for evil in nature itself. This conception begets obvious complications and some scholars rightly suggest that it should be limited to value-based intentional feelings involving the self (guilt, remorse, hatred) and not to organic, bodily feeling, such as tiredness (Maciuszek 2015). Breaking an innate moral order is supposed to lead to human suffering, but this moral order has nothing to do with any rational natural law (Kępiński was not a Thomist). Rather, it is merely focused on the preservation of (individual and species) life. The moral law is apparently the potentiality of being understood in a non-deterministic way—the perpetuation of life through development of new forms of interaction with the environment. In the manner reminiscent of Hans Jonas's phenomenological philosophy of biology (Jonas 2001), in which all organisms care for their own being, Kępiński points toward freedom pervading all life forms.

BEYOND VIRTUE AND VICE

This conception reminds us of the ancient idea of a continuum between vice and illness and a possible identity between moral virtue and mental health. Analogically to the aforementioned moral injury, two notions of evil—evil as sin (committed) and evil as experience (suffered)—appear as intrinsically connected. However, Kępiński's understanding of the continuum is neither reductive—vice is just a disease, nor inflationary—mental illness is really a vice, in the sense that Irwin (2013) proposes. It is because neither wrongdoing nor mental illness is prior in his account—they are simply two facets of the same phenomenon. As von Gebsattel (1964) explains, the question about mental illness that assumes the dualism of somatic and psychological causes is wrongly asked. Analogically, a schism into two types of treatment, the physical and the moral, is a symptom of warped epistemology. Modern decoupling of facts and values—or consciousness and conscience—is itself a part of the trouble.

The examples Kępiński uses in the quote (addiction, antisocial personality) suggest that the inflationary reading is the more appropriate one. On the reductive reading, there is little space for the notion of moral responsibility for one's predicament—and, hence, for autonomy and freedom which Kępiński would have defended. However, the anti-psychiatrist conclusion—that we are dealing with a primarily moral problem (Harcourt 2013)—is far from what Kępiński proposed. Rather, since conscience is essentially a biological

---

[1] We shall skip the question of whether all living organisms indeed have a biological conscience and limit ourselves to human beings.

[2] Kępiński distinguishes three layers of conscience. The constitutional conscience that embodies the natural moral order occupies the bottom. A further layer, which is similar to the Freudian superego, grows during early development. Finally, a psychological conscience operates fully consciously. There is a tension between these three layers as, e.g. the second or the third layer may influence and distort the underlying order. Alternatively, the damage of the constitutional conscience puts the weight of decision-making upon the psychological conscience, which supposedly leads to a permanent anxiety.

phenomenon, vice appears as a sort of natural defect. The natural moral order lies in the very process of temporal becoming. To borrow a phrase from existential philosophy, the essence of nature lies in its existence—and, therefore, the natural moral order, as the article will argue further on, rests on the potentialities of being in an undetermined future.

CONFLICT AND TRANSCENDENCE

From the perspective of biological conscience, life appears as a task that requires self-regulation. It demands a transcendence of oneself (Murawski 1987). Kępiński's absolute morality is nothing more than the natural *telos* of nature, which, upon a closer look, appears as the undetermined potentiality of being. There are no goals in nature beyond the increase of negative entropy. Conscience as self-control extends beyond the present and is inversely proportional to life dynamics. Humans are cursed to live more in the past and future than in the present (Kępiński 2016). An elementary anxiety resulting from impossibility to achieve future projects in the form they were planned pervades the process of the exchange of energy and information with the environment. This anxiety stems neither from the past (unrealized plans) nor from the future (anticipation of failure), but since the two are intertwined, from the temporal movement itself (Kępiński 2001). The anxiety-based ontological-axiological conflict of becoming generates the movement of human life. When unresolved, this conflict contributes to what is conventionally called a mental illness (to be sure, this does not imply that all mental illness is a result of the unresolved conflict). But since the two operate at the same level, (at least some) mental illness *is* this impossibility to cope with the conflict in a constructive way. Meanwhile, the possibility of coping given through a degree of freedom stems from the neurophysiological autonomy of an organism.

We are touching here upon the essence of what von Gebsattel (1964) termed an existential neurosis—a struggle between two elementary forces of becoming, transcendence and nihilism. The nihilistic tendency, much like Kępiński's entropy, preconditions creativity. As the conflict is the origin of mental suffering, this view fits into the psychodynamic tradition. Consciously, the conflict manifests itself as a tension between a given lack of meaning and a search for meaning. The existential neurosis also has an intrinsic social aspect, which von Gebsattel presents in the Heideggerian spirit. Originally, everyone is a part of the collective [*das Man*] and its values, a functionary of the system. This is not a quasi-antipsychiatric claim that the social average is sick—the idea is that the statistically normal occupies merely the surface of the anthropological truth. The system, whatever its actual content, is a universal point of departure for individualized vital becoming. There is no cure for existential neurosis beyond transcending oneself and not succumbing to nihilism. This transcendence reaches toward the future and, when it becomes an ethical action, even toward the "infinite" (Minkowski 1970: 118). Heidegger's notion of conscience will clarify this issue.

THE CALL OF CONSCIENCE

Like Kępiński's, Heidegger's conscience does not refer to any reflective theorizing, least to any transcendent principles or norms of one's own culture. Unlike Kępiński's, it has the character of revelation (Heidegger 1962). It reveals human existence in its naked truth—as finite and permeated by guilt and angst. As far as the practical side of Heidegger's fundamental ontology is concerned, conscience plays an elementary role—it manifests finitude at the level of human experience. Like psychological conscience, it points toward guilt, but not in the ordinary meaning of breaching a moral requirement. Existential conscience reveals original guilt accompanying temporal becoming—being guilty of what has not happened and of what will not be chosen. Only because of it, one can *become* guilty in the common sense of the word.

Heidegger's conscience calls oneself to oneself. What is calling is the potentiality of being that does not yet exist—the unrealized *potential of oneself*. It does not, however, call toward any concrete possibilities of authentic existence as different from the inauthentic one, in which choices have been already made by others. It literally gives one nothing—it merely opens oneself toward the indefinite future. But this nothing is given in a positive sense—as something that one must face. Conscience opens an "abyss of nothingness," to use Hannah Arendt's phrase, which appears "before any deed that cannot be accounted for by a reliable chain of cause and effect and is inexplicable in Aristotelian categories of potentiality and actuality" (Arendt 1978: 207). In other words, it abolishes the sequence of temporal flow and discloses the previously inexistent potentialities of being, different from the future projected and planned in the bygone present. We could say, following Backström, that conscience reminds us of what we don't want to be reminded of. It is "a manifestation of our very openness for each other" (Backström 2007: 330), which is the root of our moral life and is itself situated beyond any explicit moral principles. The psychiatrist, Medard Boss, Heidegger's friend who worked with him closely on the psychopathological application of his philosophy, defined mental health precisely in terms of openness toward the possibilities of being (Boss 1983). This openness toward nothingness—and toward the other, to complement Heidegger's view—is clearly terrifying and one eagerly (and understandably) attempts to cover it up.

> The irremediable insubstantiality of one's own existence cannot be measured by any criterion of some fuller and more successful existence, which is why it can be used as a point of departure of a non-normative approach to psychopathological phenomena. It is this irremediable insubstantiality that is the source of all mental suffering the psychotic and neurotic individuals try to cope with by means of various cover-ups
>
> (Kouba 2014: 123)

Even if anyone may hear the universal message of conscience and choose resolute and authentic existence, it certainly does not imply having a good conscience, which (in some metaphysical way) could defend him from mental illness. Acting in accordance with one's existential conscience does not automatically lead to a betterment of life. But, in certain circumstances, facing nothingness may ease the troubles imposed by psychological conscience so that neurotic guilt and anxiety understood as psychiatric symptoms disappear.[3]

---

[3] Psychological conscience may well internalize the denial of freedom and contribute to an automatic way of being. One example for Kępinski were the Nazis, for whom obedience became the principal rule of conscience and a means to escape from the natural freedom (Kępiński 1983). Such collective "conscience," however, clearly wipes out conscience understood as openness, and it is a product of secondary, reflective mediation between one's own and communal values. Hence, even if someone evokes the concept of conscience when speaking of his moral demands, he may refer to morality in the ordinary sense of *mores* and thus misinterpret conscience.

One of von Gebsattel's anankastic patients was suffering from the pangs of conscience reproaching him for not doing anything well enough (von Gebsattel 1954). It took him hours to accomplish ordinary activities. The patient feared odors that were spread all around him causing pain, shame, and disgust. The underlying threat, von Gebsattel surmised, was coming from the "un-form" or death, and the patient's behavior was a defense mechanism against decay. But his actual disturbance was the impossibility of overcoming nihilism that was blocking his transcendence of himself. His struggle with different forms of decay was really a struggle with his own death—with his nihilistic tendencies. The patient couldn't cope with nothingness. Temporarily speaking, he could not break away from the past and the all-pervading guilt. Certainly, conscience would not solve his predicament of blocked becoming by enabling him to tell right from wrong. However, if the repulsive odors represent death, hearing the call of existential conscience would address the underlying trouble. It could bring trust into the world in all its unpredictability and allow the patient to live with things being otherwise than imagined. It would free his psychological conscience from moral prohibitions, ease the guilt, and reduce the symptoms. Since it is impossible to overcome nihilism without realizing it first, acknowledging nothingness underlying all becoming—nothingness that is the core of human vulnerability—would be the first step to achieve mental health.

Contemporary person-centered understanding of mental illness presents an analogous approach even if without explicitly utilizing the concept of conscience. Giovanni Stanghellini defines mental pathology as an incapacity to risk "the leap to the Other" (Stanghellini 2017: 91). Temporarily speaking, the future is the other (Levinas 1987). Mental pathology understood as an interruption of a dialogue with the alterity of others and oneself is the interruption of the dialogue between the present and the yet-to-come (and not just a predictable future whose seeds are anchored in the present). The latter, as far as it has to do with the indefinite potential of oneself and the world, is nothingness.

Being personally engaged in this dialogue with nothingness, patients play an active role not only in making sense of their experiences and presenting symptoms, but also in the course and outcome of their illness. They are responsible for it in the same way that we are all responsible for our involuntary dispositions. For example, the feeling of ontological eccentricity, a core value of persons with schizophrenia, even if given and not chosen, has a voluntary component (Binswanger 1992). Detachment from the shared world has a value that motivates autistic behavior (Stanghellini and Ballerini 2007). The notion of responsibility without blame, as defined by Hannah Pickard (Pickard 2011) could be well extended beyond personality disorders to people with schizophrenia, who may be held responsible for their preference of eccentricity, even if they are not blameworthy and should not be blamed by their caregivers. Although (at least some) people with schizophrenia are following their psychological conscience, they are not following the call of existential conscience—or their life potential tacitly controlled by what Kępiński meant by constitutive conscience aimed at the greatest possible development—that tells them to open themselves to the possibility of *being different* from what they are. They reject common sense just to dwell in their idiosyncratic worldview.[4] Asking the question whether their values are indeed *theirs* and not a *result*

---

[4] We must be careful in distinguishing schizophrenic praise of eccentricity from Heidegger's highly individualistic account of resoluteness as a response to the call of conscience.

of their disease would move us back to the reductive reading. The choice at stake, the choice of conscience, is not merely psychological but intrinsic to existential becoming.

CONCLUSION

Typically, conscience is related to an evaluative judgment. It has to do with the consciousness of what one has done or is planning to do, for which one is morally responsible. Such a conscience either points back and reproves or points forward and warns. When one does not follow its orders, it adds to one's guilt feelings. And when it is either too weak or too scrupulous, it may contribute to the development of mental illness. In a more phenomenological account, conscience is a silent witness that is pre-reflectively and pre-theoretically *lived through* conscious acts and that preconditions the evaluative judgment. Conscience as a biological–existential phenomenon operates *beyond* concrete moral principles. This claim does not imply that conscience cannot become "erroneous" (to borrow a phrase from the Catholic tradition). Its erring, however, has nothing to do with any single moral laws, but only with the possibilities of one's being in the undetermined future.

The phenomenon of original conscience that facilitates lived becoming (transcendence of oneself) and that can be described in the language of phenomenological biology or existential philosophy is, therefore, substantially different from the evaluative judgment. Original conscience reveals primordial anxiety and guilt as well as other truths of the precarious human existence, of which nothingness is the ultimate ground. Following its call requires certain courage of despair, to use Paul Tillich's term, which allows taking the anxiety of being upon oneself. It is the courage to be oneself in the face of meaninglessness—to confront and not hide away from underlying nothingness, and to take the risk of facing the future despite a threat by non-being. The recognition of nothingness through conscience implies an affirmation and thus overcoming of nihilism—"the acceptance of the power of being, even in the grip of nonbeing" (Tillich 1952: 176). Existential anxiety is not a state to dwell in but a means to remove the anxiety of ordinary conscience. Retreat into obsessive conscientiousness or an antisocial disregard of the moral dimension of life are both a means to avoid true conscience. Controlling oneself or the other covers the underlying nothingness and substitutes an open, undetermined future with a predictable pattern. On the other hand, living in existential truth can facilitate mental health (Yalom 1980). Such an understanding of conscience may help to inspire values-based practice by pointing at an underlying, shared framework of becoming which operates beyond the plurality and variability of psychological values and conditions the very possibility of finding an agreement between conflicting worldviews.

ACKNOWLEDGMENT

The project has received funding from the European Union's Horizon 2020 research and innovation programme under the Marie Sklodowska-Curie grant agreement No 659205.

Bibliography

Arendt H. (1978). *The Life of the Mind. Vol II. Willing.* San Diego, New York, London: Harcourt Brace and & Company.

Backström J. (2007). *The Fear of Openness. Essays on Friendship and the Roots of Morality.* Åbo: Åbo Akademi University Press.

Binswanger L. (1992). "Drei Formen mißglückten Daseins." In M. Herzog (ed.), *Ausgewählte Werke Band 1*, pp. 233–418. Heidelberg: Roland Asanger Verlag.

Boss M. (1983). *Existential Foundations of Medicine and Psychology*, trans. S. Conway and A. Cleaves. New York, London: Jason Aronson.

Frankl V. E. (1992). *Man's Search for Meaning. An Introduction to Logotherapy.* Boston: Beacon Press.

Fulford Bi. (1995). *Moral Theory and Medical Practice.* Cambridge: Cambridge University Press.

García-Valls P. R. (2016). "¿Qué es la conciencia?" In M. I. López-Ibor Alcocer, J. A. Gutiérrez, and J. A. Sacristán (eds.), *Psiquiatría: situación actual y perspectivas de futuro*, pp. 221–250. Madrid: Fundación López-Ibor, Fundación Lilly.

Gebsattel V. E. F. von. (1954). *Prolegomena einer Medizinischen Anthropologie.* Berlin, Göttingen, Heidelberg: Springer Verlag.

Gebsattel, V. E. F. von. (1964). *Imago Hominis.* Beiträge zu einer personalen Anthropologie Schweinfurt: Verlag Neues Forum.

Graham G. and Poland J. (eds.) (2011). *Addiction and Responsibility.* Cambridge, MA and London: MIT Press.

Harcourt E. (2013). "Aristotle, Plato, and the Anti-Psychiatrists: Comment on Irwin." In K. Fulford, M. Davies, R. Gipps, G. Graham, J. Sadler, and G. T. T. Stanghellini (eds.), *The Oxford Handbook of Philosophy and Psychiatry*, pp. 47–52. Oxford: Oxford University Press.

Hare R. D. (1999). *Without Conscience: The Disturbing World of the Psychopaths Among Us.* New York, London: Guilford Press.

Heidegger M. (1962). *Being and Time.* Oxford: Basil Blackwell.

Irwin T. (2013). "Mental Health as Moral Virtue: Some Ancient Arguments." In K. Fulford, et al. (eds.), *The Oxford Handbook of Philosophy and Psychiatry*, pp. 37–46. Oxford: Oxford University Press.

Jonas H. (2001). *The Phenomenon of Life. Toward Philosophical Biology.* Evanston: Northwestern University Press.

Kant I. (1996). *The Metaphysics of Morals*, trans. and ed. M. Gregor. Cambridge: Cambridge University Press.

Kapusta A. (2007). "Life Circle, Time and the Self in Antoni Kępiński's Conception of Information Metabolism." *Filosofija, Sociologija* 18(1): 46–51.

Kępiński A. (1983). *Rytm Życia.* Kraków: Wydawnictwo Literackie.

Kępiński A. (2001). *Lęk.* Kraków: Wydawnictwo Literackie.

Kępiński A. (2016). *Melancholia.* Kraków: Wydawnictwo Literackie.

Kouba P. (2014). *The Phenomenon of Mental Disorder: Perspectives of Heidegger's Thought in Psychopathology.* London: Springer.

Krokos J. (2013). *Conscience as Cognition. Phenomenological Complementing of Aquinas's Theory of Conscience.* Frankfurt am Main: Peter Lang.

Levinas E. (1987). *Time and the Other.* Pittsburgh: Duquesne University Press.

Litz B. T., et al. (2009). "Moral Injury and Moral Repair in War Veterans: A Preliminary Model and Intervention Strategy." *Clinical Psychology Review* 29: 695–706.

Maciuszek J. (2015). *Obraz człowieka w dziele Kępińskiego*. Toruń: Wydawnictwo Naukowe Uniwersytetu Mikolaja Kopernika.

Minkowski E. (1970). *Lived Time. Phenomenological and Psychopathological Studies*. trans. N. Metzel. Evanston: Northwestern University Press.

Murawski K. (1987). *Jaźń i sumienie. Filozoficzne zagadnienia rozwoju duchowego człowieka w pracach Carla Gustawa Junga i Antoniego Kępińskiego*. Wrocław: Zakład Narodowy im. Ossolińskich.

Pearce S. and Pickard H. (2009). "The Moral Content of Psychiatric Treatment." *British Journal of Psychiatry* 195: 281–282.

Pickard H. (2011). "Responsibility Without Blame: Empathy and the Effective Treatment of Personality Disorder." *Philosophy, Psychiatry, & Psychology* 18(3): 209–224.

Radoilska L. (2013). *Addiction and Weakness of Will*. Oxford: Oxford University Press.

Stanghellini G. (2017). *Lost in Dialogue. Anthropology, Psychopathology and Care*. Oxford: Oxford University Press.

Stanghellini G. and Ballerini M. (2007). "Values in Persons with Schizophrenia." *Schizophrenia Bulletin* 33(1): 131–141.

Tellenbach H. (1972). *Melancholy*. Pittsburgh: Duquesne University Press.

Tillich P. (1952). *The Courage to Be*. New Haven and London: Yale University Press.

Yalom I. D. (1980). *Existential Psychotherapy*. New York: Basic Books.

Zahavi D. (2003). *Husserl's Phenomenology*. Stanford: Stanford University Press.

CHAPTER 46

··

UNDERSTANDING AND EXPLAINING

··

CHRISTOPH HOERL

INTRODUCTION

WE have some intuitive idea that psychiatric disorders constitute a distinct sub-group of disorders—a very specific way of being unwell. But what distinguishes this way of being unwell from other ways of being unwell? In this chapter, I want to consider this question in light of a distinction that looms large in Karl Jaspers's *General Psychopathology*, and which has been at the heart of phenomenological psychiatry ever since. This is the distinction between *understanding*, on the one hand, and *explaining*, on the other. I will first outline one way of fleshing out what the distinction between understanding and explaining comes to. Having done so, I will suggest that one possible way of thinking of what is distinctive specifically of psychiatric disorders is that they constitute a particular kind of challenge to understanding: there is a sense in which they both defy and call for understanding at the same time.[1]

THE BASIC DISTINCTION

As characterized by Jaspers, there are a number of different dimensions to the difference between understanding and explaining. For instance, explaining is said to result from repeated observations, whereas understanding is gained directly "*on the occasion* of confronting human personality" (Jaspers 1997: 303) and is in this sense more akin to a form of direct perception (Jaspers 1997: 313). More specifically, understanding is obtained in the course of exercising empathy, or "sink[ing] ourselves into the psychic situation" of the other person (Jaspers 1997: 301), whereas explaining is based on drawing inductive inferences from the observation of regularities. Understanding proceeds "from within" whereas explaining

---

[1] Evnine (1989: 11), too, suggests that we should characterize psychic illness "precisely by the difficulties it presents for understanding."

proceeds "from without" (Jaspers 1997: 27). Other terminological contrasts that Jaspers also uses to illustrate the difference between understanding and explaining are that between the "subjective" and the "objective," and that between the "qualitative" and the "quantitative."

Arguably, however, no precise theoretical framework for capturing the distinction between understanding and explaining emerges from these remarks. For instance, Jaspers provides no detailed account of what he means by "empathy," the cognitive capacity that underpins understanding. He simply seems to take an already existing understanding of the notion for granted. Furthermore, he says that "[e]very concrete event—whether of a physical or psychic nature—is open to causal explanation in principle, and psychic processes too may be subjected to such explanation" (Jaspers 1997: 305). Thus, his remark that understanding proceeds "from within" whereas explaining proceeds "from without" must mean something different from the claim that understanding deals with the "inner" mental life whereas explaining deals only with its outward manifestations.

There is one aspect of Jaspers's characterization of the contrast between explaining and understanding, though, that might seem especially puzzling at first sight: Jaspers describes explaining as the "perception of causal connection" (Jaspers 1997: 27), and generally seems to equate explaining with explaining causally (see e.g. Jaspers 1997: 301). Yet, his descriptions of the object of understanding, too, seem replete with what, on the face of it, are clearly causal terms. Thus, he says, for instance, that understanding is concerned with "psychic *reactions* to experience, . . . the *development* of passion, the *growth* of an error, [or] the *effects* of suggestion" (Jaspers 1997: 302f., my emphases). In each case, he arguably doesn't just have a temporal sequence in mind, but specifically a causal one. But then in what sense is understanding different from the grasp of causal connections involved in explaining?

I think there is a way of resolving this last puzzle that can also help shed light on some of the other characterizations Jaspers gives of the distinction between understanding and explaining. The phrase Jaspers actually uses most frequently when speaking of the distinctive subject matter of understanding is "how one psychic event emerges from another" (Jaspers 1997: 27, repeated e.g. at 301). Again, this seems to indicate a causal connection, but it is also suggestive of the idea that understanding involves causal knowledge of a particular sort. Consider the following passage from Elizabeth Anscombe's article "Causality and Determination":

> [C]ausality consists in the derivativeness of an effect from its causes. This is the core, the common feature, of causality in its various kinds. Effects derive from, arise out of, come of, their causes. [A]nalysis in terms of necessity or universality does not tell us of this derivedness of the effect; rather it forgets about that. For the necessity will be that of laws of nature; through it we shall be able to derive knowledge of the effect from knowledge of the cause, or vice versa, but that does not show us the cause as source of the effect.
>
> (Anscombe 1981: 136)

The question Anscombe is concerned with in this passage concerns the relationship between two types of claims, sometimes referred to as *singular causal claims* and *general causal claims*, respectively. General causal claims state causal laws—"smoking causes heart disease" is a standard example. They are what Anscombe means when she speaks of an analysis of causal connections "in terms of necessity or universality,"[2] and her claim is that such an

---

[2] Whether causal laws should actually be thought of as stating or implying relations of necessity or universal generalizations is a further question, which we can set aside for present purposes.

analysis leaves out what it actually is that causation consists in. Insofar as such causal laws hold, they hold only because of a more fundamental type of causal relation obtaining on the level of particular events, as expressed by singular causal claims such as "Jane's smoking caused her heart disease." What makes such claims true are just facts about that specific individual and what happened to her, independently of whether such facts also form parts of a wider pattern.

In light of these considerations, one way of making sense of what Jaspers means when he says that understanding is concerned with "how one psychic event emerges from another" is in terms of the idea that understanding furnishes us specifically with knowledge of instances of singular causation in the psychic domain—of how, in Anscombe's similar vocabulary, psychic events "derive from, arise out of, come of" each other. It is this kind of causal knowledge that we gain when we are able to "sink ourselves into the psychic situation" of the other. Explaining, by contrast, as Jaspers thinks of it, seems to be concerned with establishing general causal laws—it may be successful in identifying repeated patterns, but, in doing so, it deals with causal connections only "from without" insofar as it delivers no insight into what the relevant causal connection actually consists in. This would also explain why Jaspers thinks that understanding requires "a fresh, personal intuition . . . on every occasion" (Jaspers 1997: 317): certain psychic events may give rise to others in an individual case in a way that is understandable, even though it is not true that they do so generally.[3]

UNDERSTANDING AND THE NATURE OF PSYCHIATRIC DISORDER

Why might it be important, as Jaspers clearly thinks it is, for the psychiatrist to exercise understanding, rather than just seeking to explain? I think one line of thought that can be seen to emerge from *General Psychopathology* is that not achieving at least some level of understanding in the context of dealing with psychiatric patients would constitute a particular kind of epistemic failure—a failure to recognize their illness for the particular type of illness it is.

There are two aspects to this line of thought, which I want to connect to two sets of remarks Jaspers makes. The first of them concerns the relationship between psychic illness and what Jaspers terms "the objective mind":

> The basic phenomenon of mind is that it arises on psychological ground but is not something psychic in itself; it is an objective meaning, a world which others share. The individual acquires a mind solely through sharing in the general mind . . . The general or objective mind is currently present in social habits, ideas and communal norms, in language and in

[3] As the passage from Anscombe I have quoted in the text continues: "If A comes from B, this does not imply that every A-like thing comes from some B-like thing or set-up or that every B-like thing or set-up has an A-like thing coming from it; or that given B, A had to come from it, or that given A, there had to be B for it to come from. Any of these may be true, but if any is, that will be an additional fact, not comprised in A's coming from B. If we take 'coming from' in the sense of travel, this is perfectly evident" (Anscombe 1981: 136).

the achievements of science, poetry and art. . . . This objective mind is substantially valid and cannot fall sick. But the individual can fall sick in the way in which he partakes in it and reproduces it

(Jaspers 1997: 287)

This conception of the "objective mind," with its Hegelian undertones, may seem rather alien from the perspective of contemporary philosophy of mind.[4] However, I think at least part of the basic point Jaspers is trying to get at can be readily understood. At least implicit in this passage seems to be the idea of a certain priority that the understandable has in our grasp of what psychic illness consists in. The idea, more specifically, would be that psychic illness can only be recognized for what it is by recognizing the patient as someone in possession of a capacity to partake in practices that are understandable, and, in this sense, sharing in the general mind. For what psychic illness consists in is precisely a situation in which this capacity malfunctions.[5]

We can perhaps draw a (limited) analogy here with some remarks Brian O'Shaughnessy (2000) has made about the relation between consciousness and other "states of consciousness." Consciousness, in this context, is conceived of as the condition of being in touch with reality, the kind of condition we normally enjoy during our waking hours. As O'Shaughnessy argues, consciousness, thus understood, is not just one amongst a number of possible states of consciousness such as dreaming or being in a trance. It occupies a special position amongst them—"a position of absolute pre-eminence in the mind" (O'Shaughnessy 2000: 78)—for these other states of mind are what they are only because they are "privative derivatives [of it], modes of not being in it" (O'Shaughnessy 2000: 73).

In a similar vein, we can see Jaspers arguing that psychic illness cannot be understood fully unless we recognize it as a state that is a privative derivative of our normal ability to engage in understandable practices. As a result, though, psychiatric disorders both seem to call for understanding at the same time as defying understanding. They call for understanding insofar as they call for treating the patient as one capable of engaging in understandable practices. However, insofar as it is precisely that capacity that goes awry in psychic illness, they also, at the same time, defy understanding: to think that the patient could be understood "without remainder," as it were, would constitute a failure to see psychic illness for what it is.

While this kind of view might seem paradoxical at first sight,[6] I think we might be able to make sense of it by connecting it to some remarks Jaspers makes about the difference between schizophrenic delusions and a phenomenon such as general paralysis, a degenerative mental disorder occurring in late-stage syphilis. He says:

---

[4] Perhaps less so the associated idea that understanding is closely connected to participating in joint activities, which Jaspers elsewhere expresses as follows: "We understand other people, not through considering and analysing their mental life, but by living with them in the context of events, actions and personal destinies" (Jaspers 1968: 1313). A similar view can be found expressed more recently, for instance, in Heal (2005).

[5] See also the following remark: "The essence of being human and of being a sick human shows itself in the way in which the individual appropriates structures of the mind to his own use and modifies them" (Jaspers 1997: 287f.).

[6] On related issues, see also Eilan (2000).

In the one case, it is as if an axe had demolished a piece of clockwork—and crude destructions are of relatively little interest. In the other it is as if the clockwork keeps going wrong, stops and then runs again. In such a case we can look for specific, selective disturbances. But there is more than that; the schizophrenic life is peculiarly productive. In certain cases the very manner of it, its contents and all that it represents can in itself create quite another kind of interest; we find ourselves astounded and shaken in the presence of alien secrets, which in this sense cannot possibly happen when we are faced with the crude destruction, irritations and excitements of General Paralysis.

(Jaspers 1997: 576f.)

One way of interpreting Jaspers's clockwork metaphor, and the idea that "schizophrenic life is peculiarly productive" is that, in psychic illness, the particular way in which reason goes awry is not just a diminution or breakdown of mental powers, as it is in general paralysis, but is itself an instance of the phenomenon of "psychic events emerging from one another" that understanding makes manifest. So the idea would be that there is something in principle understandable, at least to some degree, about the process that leads to the pathology, even though, at the same time, the end product of that process—the pathology itself—constitutes an impairment in normal abilities to partake in practices that are understandable.

What might such an attempt at understanding the emergence of pathological thought look like? A question along these lines has recently been discussed by Kenneth Kendler and John Campbell (2014), who consider it specifically in the context of suggestions about the involvement of dopamine in delusion formation. Considered on its own, the idea that dopamine irregularities cause psychotic syndromes obviously belongs firmly into the category of what Jaspers calls explanation. That is to say, we may perhaps be able to establish a link between the two phenomena by observing a general pattern of correlations between them, but this only gets at the causal connection "from without," it gives us no insight into what the causal connection consists in.[7]

As Kendler and Campbell explain, though, what we know about the role of dopamine might also allow us to frame some more specific hypotheses about individual cases. In this context, they consider specifically the way in which midbrain dopamine (DA) neurons have been implicated in the encoding of motivational salience. In a passage quoted by Kendler and Campbell, Kapur (2003) writes:

Dopamine mediates the conversion of the neural representation of an external stimulus from a neutral and cold bit of information into an attractive or aversive entity. In particular, the mesolimbic dopamine system is seen as a critical component in the "attribution of salience," a process whereby events and thoughts come to grab attention, drive action, and influence goal-directed behavior because of their association with reward or punishment.

(Kapur 2003: 14)

As Kendler and Campbell point out, against the background of this specific role dopamine neurons have in motivation it becomes possible for us to imagine, at least to some extent, what it would be like to live with a dopamine system that has a tendency to fire at inappropriate times. More specifically, they suggest that in imagining this, we might render the

---

[7] A crucial background issue here is that while we seem to have conceptions for "mechanisms" by which one event causes another both for events within the biological domain and for events within the psychological domain, we have no similar such conception of a "mechanism" connecting events across those two domains. On connected issues, see Campbell (2017).

formation of delusions of reference understandable. They consider the example of a patient who is watching the nightly news when his dopamine neurons misfire. As they write:

> He has the sense of some immediate meaning and importance in the commentator's comments. He seeks to "discover the meaning" of the event and realizes that the commentator really is looking at him, and notices that his newscast may contain hidden messages to him. It takes little imagination to realize how easily a delusion of reference might emerge from this primary experience.
>
> (Kendler and Campbell 2014: 3)

Kendler and Campbell's main interest seems to be in the idea that this way of "expanding the domain of the understandable in psychiatric illness," by taking account of findings in neuroscience, might help us account for the *content* of particular delusions, such as delusions of reference. As I said before, though, we need to be wary of thinking that psychiatric patients could be understood "without remainder," for that would arguably constitute a failure to see their illness for what it is. This is a common problem with approaches to delusions Campbell elsewhere describes as "empiricist" because they construe delusional beliefs as "a broadly rational reaction to some very unusual experiences" (Campbell 2001: 91)—arguably, to do so amounts to a failure to acknowledge their delusional nature.

I think it is therefore important also to recognize another dimension to Kendler and Campbell's example. Note that, in the process of imagining what it would be like to live with a misfiring dopamine system, as they describe it, another thing that arguably becomes understandable is how difficult it would be in such a situation to retain a capacity to "think straight"—that is to say, how being assailed by events and thoughts that appear to demand our attention or carry a special significance would undermine one's ability to react to one's experience in a "broadly rational" manner in the first place.

If this thought is along the right lines, understanding can uncover more than just connections between individual mental events—how one might, for example, form beliefs with a certain content in response to certain kinds of experience. It can also uncover some of the preconditions of our very ability to engage in practices that are understandable, and how that ability might itself be impacted upon by particular kinds of experiences. It is in this sense that understanding might be seen, not just as one approach to psychiatric phenomena amongst others, but as something that plays a crucial role in our ability to see psychic illness for the particular type of illness it is.

Conclusion

I have outlined one interpretation of Jaspers's distinction between understanding and explaining, taking as my lead his characterization of understanding as being concerned with "how one psychic event emerges from another" (Jaspers 1997: 27). On this interpretation, understanding furnishes us specifically with knowledge of instances of singular causation in the psychic domain. Moreover, I have suggested that there is a special sense in which psychiatric disorders both call for and defy such understanding, insofar as they involve psychic events giving rise to a situation in which the very ability to partake in understandable practices is impaired.

Why did Jaspers think that understanding was of particular importance in clinical practice? Even if understanding can be interpreted as conveying a type of causal knowledge, it is at least not obvious that he thought it had some privileged instrumental value in the context of therapy. Rather, as I have suggested in this chapter, another reason for thinking that understanding has an essential role to play in psychiatry is that it is essential to a grasp of the very nature of psychic illness—that is, of the particular way of being unwell that having a psychiatric disorder, distinctively, consists in.

ACKNOWLEDGMENT

Parts of this chapter draw on ideas that are further elaborated in C. Hoerl (2013). "Jaspers on Explaining and Understanding in Psychiatry." In G. Stanghellini and T. Fuchs (eds.), *One Century of Karl Jaspers' General Psychopathology*, pp. 107–120. Oxford: Oxford University Press.

BIBLIOGRAPHY

Anscombe G. E. M. (1981). "Causality and Determination." In: *Metaphysics and the Philosophy of Mind: Collected Philosophical Papers Volume II*, pp. 133–147. Oxford: Basil Blackwell.

Campbell J. (2001). "Rationality, Meaning, and the Analysis of Delusion." *Philosophy, Psychiatry, & Psychology* 8(2): 89–100.

Campbell J. (2017). "Validity and the Causal Structure of a Disorder." In K. S. Kendler and J. Parnas (eds.), *Philosophical Issues in Psychiatry IV: Classification of Psychiatric Illness*, pp. 257–273. Oxford: Oxford University Press.

Eilan N. (2000). "On Understanding Schizophrenia." In D. Zahavi (ed.), *Exploring the Self*, pp. 97–113. Amsterdam: John Benjamins.

Evnine S. J. (1989). "Understanding Madness?" *Ratio* 2(1): 1–18.

Heal J. (2005). "Joint Attention and Understanding the Mind." In N. Eilan, C. Hoerl, T. McCormack, and J. Roessler (eds.), *Joint Attention: Communication and Other Minds*, pp. 34–44. Oxford: Oxford University Press.

Jaspers K. (1968). "The Phenomenological Approach in Psychopathology." *The British Journal of Psychiatry* 114(516): 1313–1323.

Jaspers K. (1997). *General Psychopathology*, trans. J. Hoenig and M. W. Hamilton. Baltimore: Johns Hopkins University Press.

Kapur, S. (2003). "Psychosis as a State of Aberrant Salience: A Framework Linking Biology, Phenomenology, and Pharmacology in Schizophrenia." *American Journal of Psychiatry* 160: 13–23.

Kendler K. S. and Campbell J. (2014). "Expanding the Domain of the Understandable in Psychiatric Illness: An Updating of the Jasperian Framework of Explanation and Understanding." *Psychological Medicine* 44(1): 1–7.

O'Shaughnessy B. (2000). *Consciousness and the World*. Oxford: Clarendon Press.

DESCRIPTIVE PSYCHOPATHOLOGY

SECTION EDITORS: MATTHEW R. BROOME
AND ANDREA RABALLO

CHAPTER 47

··

CONSCIOUSNESS AND
ITS DISORDERS

··

FEMI OYEBODE

INTRODUCTION

CONSCIOUSNESS is one of the most challenging contemporary scientific and philosophical problems. In this chapter I shall focus on the subjective state of awareness of the sensible world, which terminates when we go to sleep or are comatose, or dead. However, it is important to emphasize that I am not referring, merely, to the distinction between asleep or awake. To be awake presupposes being conscious. My focus is on the process of being *conscious of* something, a key feature of Husserl's phenomenology termed intentionality, rather than merely being awake. In other words, it is the process of being conscious of something, in the sense in which I am aware that I can see a particular object, hear a particular conversation, recall an episode of my life, or imagine a given situation. To make the point more forcefully, I am not merely writing this sentence but I am intimately aware that it is *me* writing this sentence.

At the outset it is important to distinguish consciousness from attention. Attention refers to the capacity to focus our interest or consciousness on specific aspects of the objective world. This might entail selecting, shifting, and thereby focusing attention, for example, on a passing vehicle rather than on a lamppost. No doubt both processes are related but there is empirical work to show that both processes can operate independently of one another. The global workplace theory, an influential psychological model of consciousness, uses a theater metaphor in which attention resembles choosing a television channel and consciousness is the picture on the screen (Baars and Franklin 2007). The distinction that is being drawn here is that between selecting an experience and being conscious of the selected event. It is a truism that we are only conscious of a fraction of the information processing going on in our brain at any one time. The function of attention seems to be to select some aspects of stimulus input defined by location in space, a given feature such as shape or by an object. Whereas the function of consciousness pertains to summarizing all the information from the environment that we need in order to ensure that it is available for planning, decision-making, language, rational thought, and setting long-term goals (Tononi and Koch

2008). This is what Jaspers refers to as "the immediate experience of the total psychic state" (Jaspers 1997). Finally, there is the question whether consciousness is unitary. A full discussion of this issue is outside the scope of this chapter. Empirical studies conducted by Robert Sperry (1913–1994) (Sperry 1968) and also by Gazzaniga (2000) raised the possibility that in patients who had undergone surgical division of the corpus callosum, each cerebral hemisphere appeared to experience its private and separate sensations and to have independent consciousness. On the other hand, Gazzaniga and colleagues argued from the same empirical findings that there was only a single consciousness, located in the left hemisphere, always seeking to interpret and explain external events. There is a related but distinct issue, which is not whether consciousness is simple or unitary but whether consciousness is global in nature such that all modular brain functions relate equally to a singular consciousness system or rather whether each specialist brain function such as perception or memory has its own consciousness system. In other words, whether in the event of abnormalities in the visual system, for example, there may be impairments in the awareness of visual experience without corresponding impairments in awareness of auditory experience. There is empirical evidence to support this latter view: in Anton's syndrome, in which there is impaired awareness of blindness, there is no corresponding general or global impairment of consciousness awareness in other perceptual modalities. Also in "blindsight," which like Anton's syndrome, results from injury to the primary visual cortex, subjects can respond to visual stimuli that they do not consciously see. These two examples demonstrate that it is too soon to conclude that a full description of consciousness as a psychological system is yet available to us.

It is often stated that any theory of consciousness must attempt to explain certain basic facts about mental life, namely that a) consciousness has a subjective nature that is united by a unique individual inner perspective; b) that conscious awareness appears to have a quality that is recalcitrant to physical or materialist description; and c) that conscious experience is directed toward objects, that is, it is intentional in nature. It is the particularly striking inner subjective aspect of conscious awareness that is of prime concern to psychiatrists and I turn to it in the next section. It is not the purpose of this chapter to examine whether or not consciousness is a phenomenon that resists cognitive neuroscience reduction. Indeed, phenomenological analysis brackets this discussion whilst engaging in exploration of the acts of consciousness and its objects. In this chapter it is accepted that consciousness is always directed toward objects, that it is intentional in nature.

Consciousness has a pivotal role in Husserl's (1859–1938) phenomenology. Phenomenology is the study or description of phenomenon and it involves the description of things as one experiences them (Hammond, Howarth, and Keat 1991). In other words, phenomenology is concerned in part with subjective conscious experience. For Husserl, consciousness is intentional. In *Cartesian Meditations* he wrote:

> Conscious processes are also called *intentional*; but then the word intentionality signifies nothing else than the universal fundamental property of consciousness: to be consciousness *of* something.
>
> (Husserl 1977: 33)

Husserl's conception of consciousness demands that consciousness and its intentional object be inseparable. This point is well made by Hammond et al.:

Acts of consciousness and objects of consciousness are essentially interdependent: the relation between them is an "internal" not an "external" one. That is to say, one cannot first identify the items related and then explore the relations between them; rather one can identify each item in the relation only in reference to the other item to which it is related. Acts of consciousness are directed upon objects such that one cannot investigate the acts independently of their objects; and the objects are always objects for consciousness such that one cannot investigate objects independently of investigating the conscious acts of which they are objects.

(Hammond et al. 1991: 48–49)

In Husserl's terminology, the term "noetic" describes acts of consciousness and "noematic" refers to the objects of consciousness. Acts of consciousness include such possible modes as perception, retention, recollection, expectation, etc. Objects of consciousness include any conceivable object.

To be more exact, Husserl's phenomenology regards consciousness not as "a particular mundane domain among other domains" but acts of consciousness

are considered solely as experiences of objects, in and through which objects appear, present themselves, and are apprehended as what they are. If consciousness is a unique realm of absolute priority, it is because it is the medium of access to whatsoever exists and is valid.

(Gurwitsch 1976: 166)

Aron Gurwitsch's (1901–1973) account re-emphasizes the primacy of consciousness in the phenomenological reduction but acknowledges that in the natural attitude (without the introspection and analysis of phenomenology) psychology, neuroscience, and psychiatry have different concerns that include establishing how acts of consciousness are causally related to physiological or functional processes.

From the accounts above, it is obvious that there are tensions between the manner in which consciousness is envisaged in the natural attitude and the notion of consciousness as revealed in phenomenological reduction. Phenomenological reduction of consciousness poses problems for psychopathology particularly as psychopathology relates to abnormalities of consciousness. First, strictly speaking, all psychopathology is best regarded as abnormality of consciousness. In other words abnormalities of perception, of memory and its various functions, and of the imagination are ultimately abnormalities of acts of consciousness. In this account even behavior is tractable back to consciousness and its contents. Secondly, given that consciousness and its objects are inseparable, it is problematic to deal separately with abnormalities of consciousness as distinct from descriptions of the objects of consciousness. To develop this point, it is problematic to discuss levels of and qualities of consciousness, for example, as distinct from acts of consciousness or objects of consciousness. This issue identifies a particular conflict between a neuroscience approach to the notion of consciousness as opposed to the conceptualization of consciousness drawn from a phenomenological standpoint. Finally, phenomenological analysis requires a description of subjective experience. But, abnormalities of consciousness, as usually construed in psychopathology, concern experiences that are characterized by demonstrable impairments of the capacity to accurately report subjective experiences.

Karl Jaspers's (1883–1969) approach was to eschew the problem posed by inseparability of acts of consciousness and the objects of consciousness by giving an account that treated consciousness as distinct from acts of consciousness. He identified three aspects of consciousness, namely a) actual inner awareness, b) a subject–object dichotomy, and c) knowledge of a conscious self. In this account, Jaspers used the metaphor of a stage, very reminiscent of the metaphor of a theater that has currency today and that of a medium. These metaphors allowed Jaspers to refer to the idea that "the stage can shrink (narrowing of consciousness) or the medium can grow dense (clouding of consciousness)" (Jaspers 1997). For Jaspers, loss of actual inner awareness is synonymous with loss of consciousness. In Jaspers's conception, attention is conceived as either an active or passive turning toward an object and the degree of clarity and distinctness of the content of consciousness is referred to as the field of attention. Finally, Jaspers also comments on the role of attention for "rousing further associations . . . guiding notions, set tasks, target ideas . . .," etc. (1997).

In summary, consciousness is pivotal in Husserl's phenomenology and hence it is equally important in clinical psychopathology. Phenomenological reduction emphasizes the inseparability of acts of consciousness and objects of consciousness. Yet in the natural attitude consciousness is treated as a distinct feature of mental life without any logical dependence on acts of consciousness or objects of consciousness. Even though this tension between the natural attitude to the term consciousness and the understanding that one reaches following radical phenomenological reduction exists, it is a tension that is at its sharpest in discussing abnormalities of consciousness. And, this tension is further accentuated by the fact that abnormalities of consciousness rely on observations of behavior rather than, as is usually the case in psychopathology, on reports of subjective experience.

Finally, empirical experience is contrary to the propounded understandings of consciousness—abnormalities of consciousness are evident in the observed limitations in conscious awareness in patients with various kinds of disturbances that impair consciousness. These limitations in consciousness are independent of abnormalities of acts of consciousness and objects of consciousness even where these two aspects of consciousness are themselves compromised. To emphasize this point, in an individual who is observed not to be alert, it can also be the case that their perceptual experiences are abnormal as are the perceived objects that they report. Yet, the fact of abnormalities in acts of consciousness and reported in the objects of consciousness are distinct from the demonstrable impairments in consciousness per se. This, in my view, confirms that Jaspers's account is more suited to discussing abnormalities of consciousness in psychopathology.

In the next section, I propose to deal with abnormalities of consciousness under the following headings: a) dimensional changes in levels of consciousness; b) qualitative changes of consciousness; c) disorders of attention, and d) disorders of awareness.

DISORDERS OF CONSCIOUSNESS

Dimensional Changes in Levels of Consciousness

Impairment of consciousness can be seen as a continuum from alertness through to drowsiness and ultimately coma and death. Lishman (1998) makes the point that "considerable difficulties can surround the conceptual levels of consciousness of patients with acute organic reactions, partly because of problems inherent in the use of certain terms and partly because of the expectation that impaired consciousness must necessarily be accompanied by decreased responsiveness to stimuli … In most conditions impairment of consciousness is accompanied by diminished arousal and alertness."

Clouding of Consciousness

Clouding of consciousness represents the early stage on the continuum from alertness to coma and is characterized by deterioration in thinking, attention, perception, memory in the context of drowsiness, and diminished awareness of the environment.

Drowsiness

Drowsiness can be conceptualized as a further stage from clouding of consciousness toward coma. It is characterized by slowed actions, slurred speech, sluggish responses, and marked lowering of vigilance and awareness of the immediate environment. There is unimpaired avoidance of painful stimuli. Coughing and swallowing reflexes are present but reduced. Muscle tone is low.

Coma

Coma is the term used to describe an unconscious state in which there are no verbal responses or indeed any responses to painful stimuli. The righting response of posture is lost, reflexes and muscle tone may still be present but reduced, breathing is slow, deep, and rhythmic, and the skin may be flushed. Distinct stages of coma have been identified and described by Teasdale and Jennett (1974).

QUALITATIVE CHANGES OF CONSCIOUSNESS

The dimensional alterations in consciousness as described above rarely presents solely as disturbance of consciousness. There is usually an admixture of alterations in consciousness itself as described above, changes in acts of consciousness such as perception, and also variations in the subjective experience of objects of consciousness. The term "delirium" covers these abnormal experiences.

Delirium

Lipowski (1990) defines delirium as "a transient organic mental syndrome of acute onset, characterized by global impairment of cognitive functions, a reduced level of consciousness, attentional abnormalities, increased or decreased psychomotor activity and a disordered sleep–wake cycle." Subjective accounts of delirium are rare and there is the problem that the experiences during an episode occur in the context of reduced level of conscious awareness and the accounts are retrospective in nature.

Crammer's account (Crammer 2002) stands out primarily because he was a psychiatrist describing his experiences and he understood (in retrospect) the nature and quality of the experiences. He wrote:

> During the period 26–30 November I was, for the most part, completely unconscious, unaware of the passage of time, the presence of visitors, the attention of nurses and doctors or my transfer by trolley or ambulance from ward to ward and hospital to hospital. However, within that period there were several brief fluctuations (perhaps 5 min or so) in degree of awareness, and subsequently I could recall having some human contact and some idea (partly mistaken) about my whereabouts and state of health in these episodes. In the first two episodes I accepted that I was ill in some quite unspecified way and thought that I was to be transferred for operation (unspecified) first to India and then to Australia; in the fourth episode, although much the same in feeling, I thought that I was changing planes on the flight home from Australia.

Crammer describes his subjective experiences and also attempts to explain them in retrospect. He wrote:

> I come half-awake lying on a vague bed in a very vague room with two young women (in white coats?) standing by my side. I identify them as physiotherapists. One is dark-haired (Indian?) and says nothing; the other is fair, does the talking and laughingly tells me that I need an operation and it will be best for me to transfer to India for it, perhaps to a Christian Mission hospital, possibly called Vellore, with which they have a staff exchange programme (clearly the dark-haired girl). I receive this information passively without curiosity: I do not know or care where I am, or what is wrong with me, although I am prepared to believe I have something requiring treatment and am reassured that it will be well done. I fail to be myself, not very aware of surroundings and with no recollection of any injury or hospitalization.

He continued:

> [T]he idea of India may have been prompted by the (Indian?) nurse and perhaps by an unconscious memory of a fall in India 3 years earlier [and the idea of Australia by the fact that on] admission to hospital I had been struck by the Australian accents of some of the nurses (and I had read previously in the local paper that Oxford hospitals had imported numbers of Australians to help), although all this was out of the conscious mind. Perhaps an Australian nurse helped me into the ambulance.

Crammer attempts to make sense of his experience in retrospect. He is fully aware of the vagaries of memory and the likelihood of bias but nonetheless his explanations demand our attention.

> The impairment of understanding—disorientation, misidentification of others, development of false beliefs—which is the central disturbance in the confusional state, developed slowly as consciousness declined and was based in memory failure and inattention. I believed that I was living in Australia, presumably because of an overheard voice, and thereafter held to this belief and denied that I could be or ever had been in the John Radcliffe Hospital (in reality, previously I had been both an out-patient and an in-patient). I thought that I had been at a doctor's social and checking-in for a flight home. A woman in a white coat was a physiotherapist, not a doctor; the doctor who later inspected my monitors was a flight engineer and the nurse was a check-in girl . . . These are not absurd answers to the self-posed questions (who, where, what

is this?) but near-misses based on brief, limited sensory impression with limited associative memory, a sort of guess without any uncertainty or any correction in relation to previous experience or immediately subsequent events, processes that go on all the time in normal life.

Fleminger (2002), in his comments on Crammer's account, made the point that Crammer's experience was akin to dreaming but remembered with more vividness than dreams. He questioned whether the traditional approach of considering delirium as arising from disturbance of consciousness was appropriate and proposed that it might be better to consider delirium as a disturbance of the sleep–wake cycle (arousal) which is why it resembles dreaming so much and why it is more common in individuals with sleep deprivation.

Twilight State

Twilight state is a descriptive term for a condition in which there is a) an abrupt onset and termination; b) variable duration from a few hours to several weeks; and c) the occurrence of unexpected violent acts or emotional outbursts during otherwise normal, quiet behavior (Lishman 1998). Consciousness is often impaired and there may be dream-like states, delusions, or hallucinations. It is associated with epilepsy, alcohol intoxication, brain trauma, and dissociative disorders (fugue).

It is an important condition because of its place in forensic settings where it is often used as a legal defense for violent behavior. In the forensic context it is important to demonstrate prior occurrences of similar episodes with inexplicable behaviors and other objective evidence of physical or psychiatric disorders.

Twilight state is insufficiently differentiated from oneroid state. Meduna (1950) characterized these phenomena as dominated by confusion, apprehension, fear, hallucinations, and the feeling that events were unreal. Meduna thought the condition was comparable to Kahlbaum's catatonia because it was an independent disorder of unreality. Reports suggest that the patient may experience elaborate visual hallucinations in the context of impairment of consciousness, marked emotional change including terror or exaltation in response to the hallucinations. There may be other hallucinations including auditory and tactile ones (Oyebode 2015). A published case by Fink and Taylor reports the essential features of this state (Fink and Taylor 2003).

> [He] talked continuously, night and day. His speech was comprehensible. He was apprehensive, fearful, and hid when people came to the house lest they should kill him. He feared that the police were out to get him. On the fourth, he was mute and catatonic. Progressively he refused food, was negativistic, grimaced and postured, with waxy flexibility and echopraxia. When mutism lifted, his confusional state came to the surface. He thought he had grenades in his pockets, and that his father had lost his legs. He failed to recognize his parents.

Stupor

Stupor is a term that refers to "a symptom complex whose feature is a reduction in, or absence of, relational functions: that is, action and speech" (Berrios 1996). It is distinct from coma in that it does not lie along a continuum from wakefulness to coma. It is principally characterized by mutism and akinesis. The patient is fully awake, alert with eyes that are open even if not focused or engaged in direct gaze. There may be impairment of consciousness but this is rarely clearly evident. How far this condition is similar to or identical with the medical condition akinetic mutism in which lesions in the diencephalon and upper brainstem are present is unclear. Locked-in syndrome is a variety of akinetic mutism.

Stupor reportedly occurs in schizophrenia as part of catatonia, and in mood disorders including both depressive and manic phases. It may be surprising that mania, a condition that is usually conceived of as presenting with elevated mood, increased energy, and marked restlessness can also present in a stupor and in such cases it

> is usually characterized by psychomotor manifestations . . . as the prominent feature: some patients lie [in bed] showing very severe inhibition for a long time. Their limbs are cold; they refuse food, and every attempt to feed them is vain due to their opposition; for months they are mute. Only the facial expression, which shows no trace of depression and often shows a slight smile, reveals that a case is not typical circular [manic-depressive] stupor with depressed mood . . . Considerable retardation in their movements can be observed immediately: the gait is heavy and leaden; they hesitate to shake hands; and their writing is clearly slowed down.
>
> (Salvatore et al. 2002)

In depressive stupor:

> The patient, usually, is confined to bed, is mute, inactive and un-cooperative. His bodily needs require attention in every way; he has to be fed, washed and bathed . . . On the surface it may seem as if there was a total absence of feeling or emotion, but that is more apparent than real, for, after recovery, many patients give a vivid account of the distress which they have experienced. The idea of death is believed by some to be almost universal.
>
> (Henderson, Gillespie, and Batchelor 1962)

DISORDERS OF ATTENTION

To recapitulate, attention is designed to present to the mind, with clarity and vividness, an appropriate selection, only of some of the objects in our environment, where there are several, simultaneous possible objects. It includes the capacity to focus, sustain, disengage, and shift attention. There is a passive and an active element to attention, the former controlled in a bottom-up approach by external stimuli and the latter controlled in a top-down approach by the individual's goals or expectations. There is also an attentional capacity, which is the extent of the inherent or intrinsic processing capacity of the attentional system. A full description of the current cognitive neuroscience model of attention is outside of the scope of this chapter.

There is little doubt that there are attentional problems, demonstrable on formal cognitive neuropsychological testing, associated with psychiatric disorders. Thus, impairments of attention and/or working memory are demonstrable in diverse conditions such as generalized anxiety disorder, depressive disorder, bipolar disorder, schizophrenia, and organic brain disorders such as delirium and dementia. Attentional disturbance is a core aspect of attention deficit hyperactivity disorder.

Subjective accounts of abnormal attention are at their most rich and detailed in the seminal studies of McGhie and Chapman (1961). In Chapman's later paper he gave several examples of problems with attention (Chapman 1966):

> I can't shut things out of my mind and everything closes in on me. It stops me thinking and then the mind goes blank and everything gets switched off. I can't pick things up to memorize because I am so absorbing everything around me and take in too much so that I can't retain for any length of time—only a few seconds, and I can't do simple habits like walking or cleaning my teeth. I have to use all my mind to do these things . . . (case 10).

> At times there is nothing to hold the mind and this is when I go into a trance (case 15).

> It happens when I'm watching the television as well and my concentration drifts away and focuses on any point in the room and I can't pick anything up that is going on. I go into a daze because I can't concentrate long enough to keep up the conversation and something lifts up inside my head and puts me into a trance . . . (case 12).

> Nothing settles in my mind—not even for a second. It just comes in and then it's out. My mind goes away—too many things come into my head at once and I lose control. I get afraid of walking when this happens. My feet just walk away from me and I've no control over myself . . . (case 29).

These subjective descriptions draw attention to a number of cognitive difficulties including problems with focusing attention, of disengaging from environmental cues, of selecting from a range of possible cues in the environment and thereby feeling overwhelmed by information. The difficulties described above have now been incorporated into the notion of Basic Symptoms that are conceived as subtle subclinical disturbances in mental processes that are the most direct expressions of the underlying neurobiological aberrations of psychosis (Schultze-Lutter et al. 2016). These are disparate difficulties and probably reflect distinct neural underpinnings. The most distinct subjective description refers to being overwhelmed by information. This speaks to Broadbent's theory (Broadbent 1966) in which he proposed a sensory buffer which allows only certain sensory data to pass through a filter for later processing and that this filter prevents overloading of the limited capacity mechanism beyond the filter. McGhie and Chapman's own view is expressed as follows:

> Now let us suppose that there is a breakdown in this selective-inhibitory function of attention. Consciousness would be flooded with an undifferentiated mass of incoming sensory data, transmitted from the environment via the sense organs. To this involuntary tide of impressions there would be added the diverse internal images, and their associations, which would no longer be coordinated with incoming information. Perception would revert to the passive and involuntary assimilative process of early childhood and, if the incoming flood were to carry on unchecked, it would gradually sweep away the stable constructs of a former reality.
>
> (McGhie and Chapman 1961)

John Cutting interprets these accounts differently. He made the point that the patients had heightened attention rather than that the proposed sensory buffer was unable to streamline what information was available for processing (Cutting 2011). Furthermore, Cutting used the term "lures" to describe features of the environment that seemed to capture the attention of patients with schizophrenia in such a manner that they were unable to disengage their attention. In cognitive neuroscience terms, this implies an impairment of passive attention as well as problems with disengaging and shifting attention.

In mood disorders, Cutting makes the case that patients are as prone to "lures" as they are in schizophrenia, the difference being that rather than objects, it is people who are the "lures" in mood disorders. The subjective description to support this view is drawn from Minkowski (1970: 329).

> I feel that, when you insist, I ought to submit to your will and do what you demand of me. It irritates me to be someone's fool, but I am incapable of resisting; I feel that you have control of me. I don't dare do anything unless you ask me to. I do everything unconsciously. If you insist that I go out, I will go out. I can't resist anymore. It is atrocious! After dinner, when the others get up from the table, I get up automatically, carried along by their movements. I am the reflection of others. In sum, I vibrate with people, I reflect their movements; it is their vibrations that make me vibrate myself.

Minkowski classifies this as an example of the influence of events, words, and people on patients in depressive states. I am uncertain that this is an example of passive attention, namely of what Cutting terms "lures." Nonetheless, it is incontrovertible that depressed mood is associated with gloomy thoughts, memories of past morbid incidents to such a degree that there is marked impairment of concentration and attention. This suggests that both active and passive attention may be "lured" by negative aspects of the patient's inner world.

Disorders of Awareness

There are a number of neuropsychiatric conditions that illustrate the relationship between disorders of attention and impaired conscious awareness of objects. These conditions are complex and are not completely understood. They include unilateral neglect; anosodiaphoria (lack of concern about hemiparesis); defective appreciation of hemiparesis with rationalization; denial of hemiparesis; and unawareness of hemiparesis (anosognosia).

In their seminal paper, Paterson and Zangwill (1944) described unilateral neglect in a previously healthy male who suffered a penetrating injury of the right parietal occipital region following an explosion in 1943. He lost consciousness for two or three minutes and showed minimal post-traumatic and retrograde amnesia. On recovery his most significant deficit was a strong neglect of the left side of space. He collided with objects on his left and left food on the left side of his dish. It was concluded that the lesion was on the upper borders of the supramarginal and angular gyrus on the right side (Mattingley 1996).

The aim in this section is not to examine in detail the varying hypotheses and findings regarding these disorders of conscious awareness but to draw out the fact that syndromes of unawareness exist and that these syndromes make clear that consciousness involves attentional systems and that these systems require intact brain function in particular hemispheres and regions. These conditions in which individuals demonstrate a degree of unawareness or denial of hemiplegia have been recognized for well over a century by, amongst others, Babinski, Lhermitte, and Critchley.

Stuss and Benson (1986) described a classic case of denial of hemiplegia.

> A 62-year old man suffered a subarachnoid haemorrhage. A right middle cerebral artery was demonstrated and successfully ligated, but the patient awoke with left hemiplegia. At first he

vehemently denied the hemiplegia. At this time he was disoriented and had a retrograde amnesia covering at least 2 years prior to the surgery. When evaluated early one morning about 2 weeks post-operatively, he spontaneously described his paralysis, was oriented to both time and place, but had no memory of his cranial surgery.

In another case they described the extent to which individuals with anosognosia will go to deny their disability.

A 57-year old hypertensive man sustained an acute intracerebral haemorrhage involving the right putamen. On admission to hospital he was stuporous with profound left hemiplegia, left hemisensory loss, and left hemianopsia . . . He was disoriented for time and place, could not remember his doctors' names, and actively denied any physical disability. When asked if he could walk or dance, he would immediately say yes; when asked to raise his arms or legs, he would raise the right limbs and insist that both arms or legs had been raised. When his hemiplegia was demonstrated to him he would accept the obvious fact and repeat the examiner's statement concerning the cause of his disability but within minutes, if asked whether he had any disability, he would adamantly deny disability.

These accounts of unilateral neglect and anosognosia emphasize the fact that consciousness has neural underpinning and that attention to both right and left visual fields, is probably controlled by the right hemisphere whereas the dominant hemisphere (the left hemisphere in right-handed individuals) only oversees the contralateral visual fields. Hence damage to the dominant hemisphere is not followed by unilateral neglect or anosognosia since the right hemisphere continues to monitor sensory information from all fields. Damage to the right hemisphere on the other hand is accompanied by hemineglect and anosognosia for the left visual field. But, these matters also pertain not merely to visual fields to also to how our bodies are experienced. This is made most manifest in a case that presented following embolism of the right cerebral artery reported by Critchley.

[I]t felt as if I was missing one side of my body (the left), but it also felt as if the dummy side was lined with a piece of iron so heavy that I could not move . . . I even fancied my head to be narrow, but the left side from the centre felt heavy, as if filled with bricks.

(Critchley 1950)

The example of blindsight highlights a different understanding of the nature of consciousness. Cortical blindness occurs when the posterior cerebral arteries, which supply the visual cortex are occluded. Bilateral occlusion produces total blindness but several studies since the early reports by Riddoch (1917) have shown that patients with this condition can "see" in their blind visual fields. The intriguing fact is that these patients are not aware of their capacity to "see"; in other words they are not consciously aware of having seen anything. Individuals with blindsight can detect simple patterns, the presence and direction of motion, and can detect and discriminate wavelength. However, the subjects are not aware of having seen anything. From the investigation of these subjects Zeki (1993) concluded that the "integrity of the visual cortex is necessary for the *conscious* experience of vision." Exploration of the neural basis of blindsight forces the conclusion that there are different kinds of awareness. Young, for example, makes the case for phenomenal awareness, access awareness, monitoring, and executive awareness. He argued that:

We might have expected that the existence of a unitary conscious mechanism would predict that all impairments would simultaneously compromise phenomenal awareness, access awareness, and monitoring to equivalent extents. Instead, one has to wonder whether the subjective unity of conscious phenomena is not largely illusory. Even if there were multiple conscious mechanisms, why should they not feel unified in operation? What else could they feel like?

(Young 1994)

Young is arguing that our subjective sense of the unity of conscious experience is not an implacable obstacle to the possibility of different neural mechanisms underlying different forms of conscious awareness. But, more crucially, impairment of consciousness can occur without our explicit knowledge of it, and with other areas of cognitive function being spared. These empirical facts pose serious challenges to how consciousness is construed in radical phenomenological analysis.

CONCLUSIONS

Consciousness is a pivotal aspect of Husserl's phenomenology. Indeed, it could be argued that it is consciousness that reveals to our inquiry all the subjective contents of experience. In this regard it is presupposed in any analysis of the total state of the psyche. Nonetheless, when psychic life takes place in the context of impairment of consciousness it makes the subjective experience inaccessible for phenomenological analysis. It is inevitable that in these situations we come to rely more on observations and analysis of fragments of information that are divulged to us.

There is an obvious dimensional variation in the clarity of conscious awareness ranging from full alertness to coma and there are also significant qualitative changes associated with delirium that consist of more than alteration in conscious awareness but include changes in levels of activity, impairment in acts of consciousness such as perception and memory, and significant changes in the symbolic contents of consciousness. The role of attention in consciousness is complex but important. Attention and its disorders demonstrate that consciousness too is unlikely to be singular in nature but is probably a composite of differing elements that are unified in subjective experience.

BIBLIOGRAPHY

Baars B. J. and Franklin S. (2007). "An Architectural Model of Conscious and Unconscious Brain Functions: Global Workspace Theory and IDA." *Neural Networks: The Official Journal of the International Neural Network Society* 20(9): 955–961. doi:10.1016/j.neunet.2007.09.013

Berrios G. E. (1996). *The History of Mental Symptoms: Descriptive Psychopathology Since the Nineteenth Century*. Cambridge: Cambridge University Press.

Broadbent D. E. (1966). *Perception and Communication*. Oxford: Pergamon. doi:9781483225821

Chapman J. (1966). "The Early Symptoms of Schizophrenia." *The British Journal of Psychiatry: The Journal of Mental Science* 112(484): 225–251.

Crammer J. L. (2002). "Subjective Experience of a Confusional State." *The British Journal of Psychiatry: The Journal of Mental Science* 180: 71–75.

Critchley M. (1950). "The Body-Image on Neurology." *The Lancet* 255(6600): 335–341.

Cutting J. (2011). *A Critique of Psychopathology*. Mill Wood: Forest Publishing Company.

Fink M. and Taylor M. A. (2003). *Catatonia: A Clinician's Guide to Diagnosis and Treatment*. Cambridge, New York: Cambridge University Press.

Fleminger S. (2002). "Remembering Delirium." *British Journal of Psychiatry* 180: 4–5.

Gazzaniga M. S. (2000). "Cerebral Specialization and Interhemispheric Communication." *Brain: A Journal of Neurology* 123(7): 1293–1326.

Gurwitsch A. (1976). *The Field of Consciousness*. Pittsburgh: Duquesne University Press.

Hammond M., Howarth J., and Keat R. (1991). *Understanding Phenomenology*. Oxford, Cambridge MA: Basil Blackwell.

Henderson D. K., Gillespie R. D., and Batchelor I. R. (1962). *Henderson and Gillespie's Textbook of Psychiatry for Students and Practitioners*. Oxford: Oxford University Press.

Husserl E. (1977). *Cartesian Meditations: An Introduction to Phenomenology*. The Hague: M. Nijhoff.

Jaspers K. (1997). *General Psychopathology*. Baltimore: Johns Hopkins University Press.

Lipowski Z. (1990) *Delirium: Acute Confusional States*. New York: Oxford University Press.

Lishman W. A. (1998). *Organic Psychiatry: The Psychological Consequences of Cerebral Disorder*. Oxford, Malden MA: Blackwell Science.

Mattingley J. B. (1996). "Paterson and Zangwill's (1944) Case of Unilateral Neglect: Insights from 50 Years of Experimental Inquiry." In C. Code, C.-W. Wallesch, Y. Joanette, and A. R. Lecours (eds.), *Classic Cases in Neuropsychology*, 243–262. Hove: Psychology Press.

McGhie A. and Chapman J. (1961). "Disorders of Attention and Perception in Early Schizophrenia." *British Journal of Medical Psychology* 34(2): 103–116.

Meduna L. J. (1950). *Oneirophrenia; The Confusional State*. Urbana: University of Illinois Press.

Minkowski E. (1970). *Lived Time: Phenomenological and Psychopathological Studies*. Evanston: Northwestern University Press.

Oyebode F. (2015). *Sims' Symptoms in the Mind: Textbook of Descriptive Psychopathology*. Edinburgh: Saunders Elsevier. doi:9780702055560

Paterson A. and Zangwill O. L. (1944). "Disorders of Visual Space Perception Associated with Lesions of the Right Cerebral Hemisphere." *Brain: A Journal of Neurology* 67(4): 331–358.

Riddoch G. (1917). "Dissociation of Visual Perceptions Due to Occipital Injuries, with Especial Reference to Appreciation of Movement." *Brain: A Journal of Neurology* 40: 15–57.

Salvatore P., Baldessarini R. J., Centorrino F., Egli S., Albert M., Gerhard A., and Maggini C. (2002). "Weygandt's on the Mixed States of Manic-Depressive Insanity: A Translation and Commentary on its Significance in the Evolution of the Concept of Bipolar Disorder." *Harvard Review of Psychiatry* 10(5): 255–275.

Schultze-Lutter F., Debbane M., Thoodoridou A., Wood S. J., Raballo A., Michel C., Schmidt S. J., Kindler J., Ruhrmann S., and Uhlhaas P. J. (2016). "Revisiting the Basic Symptom Concept: Toward Translating Risk Symptoms for Psychosis into Neurobiological Targets." *Frontiers in Psychiatry* 7: 9. doi: 10.3389/fpsyt.2016.00009

Sperry R. W. (1968). "Hemisphere Deconnection and Unity in Conscious Awareness." *The American Psychologist* 23(10): 723–733.

Stuss D. T. and Benson D. F. (1986). *The Frontal Lobes*. New York: Raven Press.

Teasdale G. and Jennett B. (1974). "Assessment of Coma and Impaired Consciousness. A Practical Scale." *Lancet* 2(7872): 81–84.

Tononi G. and Koch C. (2008). "The Neural Correlates of Consciousness: An Update." *Annals of the New York Academy of Sciences* 1124: 239–261. doi:10.1196/annals.1440.004

Young A. (1994). "Neuropsychology of Awareness." In A. Revonsuo and M. Kamppinen (eds.), *Consciousness in Philosophy and Cognitive Neuroscience*, 173–203. Hillsdale, NJ: L. Erlbaum.

Zeki S. (1993). *A Vision of the Brain*. Oxford: Blackwell Scientific Publications.

CHAPTER 48

THE EXPERIENCE OF TIME AND ITS DISORDERS

THOMAS FUCHS

INTRODUCTION

SINCE Minkowski (1933/1970), von Gebsattel (1954), Straus (1966), and Tellenbach (1980), temporality has been a major subject of phenomenological psychiatry. Drawing on philosophical concepts of Bergson, Husserl, and Heidegger, these authors have analyzed psychopathological deviations of time-experience mainly from an individual point of view, for example, as a slowing-down or inhibition of lived time in depression or obsessive-compulsive disorder. Their analyses are still highly valuable today, but may be carried further by introducing concepts such as *embodied* and *intersubjective temporality* into psychopathology. The following overview introduces some conceptual distinctions that are important for analyzing disturbances of temporality in psychopathological conditions (cf. Table 48.1). On this basis, major psychiatric disorders such as schizophrenia, melancholic depression, and obsessive-compulsive disorder will be presented as paradigm cases for a psychopathology of temporality.

IMPLICIT AND EXPLICIT TEMPORALITY

To begin with, I will introduce the distinction between *implicit* and *explicit* temporality, or in other words, between time as pre-reflectively lived and time as consciously or reflectively experienced (see also Table 48.1).

Implicit Time

Implicit or lived time means to experience the movement of life without awareness of the time passing, usually while being absorbed in some activity and oriented toward one's

Table 48.1 Forms and dimensions of temporality

Form	Dimensions and aspects
Implicit temporality	(1) Retention / presentation / protention (2) Conation (drive, striving, affection) Intersubjectivity: bodily resonance, intercorporeality
Bodily temporality	Bodily protentionality or potentiality; "intentional arc" Body memory
Explicit temporality	Past–present–future Temporal emotions: sadness, guilt versus hope, longing, etc. Intersubjectivity: synchronization–desynchronization
Biographical temporality	Autobiographical/narrative self-coherence
Existential temporality	Thrownness–project Awareness of finitude Seeking for meaning

immediate goals. Implicit temporality thus constitutes the always present undercurrent of our experience (Fuchs 2013). This undercurrent requires two conditions:

(1) The first condition relates to the continuity of pre-reflective awareness. Husserl famously argued that this continuity of "inner time-consciousness" is not a sequence of single instants but is based on the transcendental synthesis of three moments: presentation, retention, and protention (Husserl 2012: 44). *Presentation* consists of the "primal impression" as the experience given at each moment. *Retention* means remaining aware of what has just been experienced even as it slips away. *Protention* is the open anticipation of experiences yet to come—the sense of imminence. Speech is a good illustration of this: we hear the currently spoken words (presentation), but are also aware of the words we have just heard (retention) and anticipate certain words to come next (protention). This enables us to listen to and understand the sentence as a whole. Retention and protention may not be confounded with recollection and expectation, for they are an intimate part of the experienced present. Taken together, the three moments can also be referred to as the "width of presence" or the "duration block" (Zahavi 2008: 56).

(2) The second condition for implicit temporality is less related to a cognitive process than to a dynamic and affective dimension of lived time. It can be captured by concepts such as drive, striving, urge, or affection. This second condition thus concerns the affective-conative aspect of temporality, or in short, *conation* (from Latin *conatio* = striving, seeking) (Fuchs 2013). It functions as the root for spontaneity, affective directedness, attention, and the pursuit of goals that are key aspects of psychic life. The importance of the conative momentum for the experience of temporality is clearly demonstrated when changes occur in basic motivational states, for example, in mania and depression: both severely affect the patients' sense of time, on the one hand in the direction of acceleration, on the other as a retardation (see below).

The implicit dimension of temporality may also be related to the *lived body*, for it is essentially opened up by its protentions, potentialities, and capacities. Drawing on Merleau-Ponty's notion of the "intentional arc," as the bodily mediated directedness of our attention and activity toward its goal, we may say that this arc is based on both aspects of implicit temporality: on the *cognitive* component of the temporal synthesis or continuity, and on the *affective-conative* tension necessary to perform an act or pursue a goal. Moreover, it is mainly through our acquired bodily skills and habits that we usually pursue our goals and perform our actions as familiar temporal sequences; lived temporality is thus crucially based on what may be termed *body memory* (Casey 2000; Fuchs 2000a, 2012). In sum, implicit time may be regarded as the manifestation of the continuous, teleological, and intentional processes of life: "Lived time is connected with the experience of the embodied human subject as being driven and directed towards the world in terms of bodily potentiality and capability" (Wyllie 2006: 173).

Explicit Time

We do not only experience temporality pre-reflectively, however. Often we become very explicitly aware of time, for example, when coming too late to a meeting, when awaiting a long wished-for holiday, or when we contemplate the memories of a past loved one. A gap then arises between plan and execution, desire and fulfillment, or presence and loss (Fuchs 2013). If the gap occurs between the present and the past, we experience a segment of time as "no longer," and we feel time moving on relentlessly, while separating us from what we are missing. If we experience the gap between the present and the future, we are awaiting the "not yet" or "yet-to-come." Both in missing a lost object and in awaiting the future, we experience temporality as segmented and partly separated from the present. We are no longer immersed in our activities, and there is a sense in which time even seems to negate implicit or lived time. This becoming-explicit of time may also entail its apprehension as an independent and inexorable power that dominates us (Fuchs 2013: 80).

Explicit time is constituted by the three components of past, present, and future. These are experienced as closely bound up with certain time-specific emotions: the "now" with surprise, astonishment, or shock; the "no longer" with regret, grief, or remorse; the "not yet" with desire, impatience, yearning, or hope. Like retention, presentation, and protention, the dimensions of past, present, and future require some form of synthesis. Here, however, we are no longer dealing with a passive or automatic process on the transcendental level, but with an active synthesis by the subject. It is the personal, extended, or *narrative self* that binds the three parts together, namely through constantly creating and modifying a more or less coherent autobiographical story. The personal self is thus capable both of appropriating its lived life as a narrative entity and of projecting itself into the future, on the basis of what the person has experienced to date.

The personal self may thus be regarded, in Heidegger's terminology, as a dialectic unity of "thrownness" (*Geworfenheit*) and "project" (*Entwurf*), or as a "thrown project" (*geworfener Entwurf*). It fulfils itself in time—indeed, "the living of time and the fulfilment of the self are two aspects of the same process" (Theunissen 1991: 305). By actively living time and *leading* our life, we realize or "temporalize" ourselves. Awareness of one's mortality is a crucial aspect of this existential temporality, for the urge or need to develop overarching projects and to seek for a meaningful coherence of our experiences, deeds, and goals ultimately emerges from the anticipation of death, that means, from the irretrievability and the finiteness of explicit time.

INTERSUBJECTIVE TEMPORALITY

After distinguishing implicit and explicit temporality, we now turn to their intersubjective dimension. For this, we have to conceive of time as *a relational order of processes* which resonate or in other ways interact with one another. On the implicit level, we find that social interactions are basically characterized by intercorporeality, that means, an ongoing attunement of bodily and emotional communication, or an *interbodily resonance* (Froese and Fuchs 2012). From early childhood on, the microdynamics of daily interaction entail an unconscious synchronization of movements, gestures, and expressions that is part of the implicit "social sense" (Bourdieu 1990; Ramseyer and Tschacher 2006; Tschacher, Rees, et al. 2014). This implies a tacit sense of being temporally connected with others, which Minkowski (1933/1970) has called "lived synchronism"; one could also speak of a *basal contemporality*.

As a rule, we are hardly aware of this basal synchronism. On an explicit level, however, intersubjective time manifests in the various forms of social coordination or "timing" where synchronicity tends to be established deliberately and by convention: through daily and weekly routines, calendars, time scheduling, appointments, etc. This temporal coordination with others does not remain constant, however, but repeatedly passes through phases of *desynchronization*, of which we may distinguish two kinds: a state of being "too late" and of being "too early" in relation to external social processes. In other words, we may experience a *synchronicity*, a *retardation*, or an *acceleration* of our own time as against the intersubjective or "world time" (Figure 48.1).

Intersubjective *synchronicity* or the experience of a shared "*now*" is constituted through the presence of the other and through our shared referral to the world, as in joint attention or joint action. Presence in the full sense always means the actual or imagined presence of others (Pokropski 2015). It can also be made explicit by using indexical words such as "here," "now," "today," etc. Thus, the word "today" inserts the pre-reflectively shared situation into an explicit and external order of time: "today" means the world-day shared by all of us, and thus entails an alignment of implicit time with the world time. This is the basis of all explicit forms of temporal coordination.

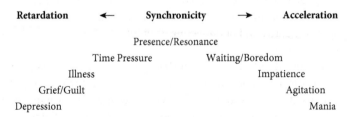

FIGURE 48.1 Synchronization and desynchronization of one's own and world time (Fuchs 2013).

On the other hand, the *"too early"* or the *acceleration* of one's own time with respect to external processes, makes *waiting* necessary, thus imposing on us a slower time structure to which we can respond with patience or impatience. *Boredom* also highlights unpleasantly the discrepancy between one's own drive or interest and the lack of external stimulation or possibilities for action. Restlessness and agitation as a further acceleration of one's own time can develop into *manic excitement* in pathological cases. Here the individual's time gets more or less decoupled from natural and social rhythms.

In contrast, the *"too late"* or the *retardation* of one's own time is usually experienced as more unpleasant. As a counterpart to waiting, there first arises the time pressure, which results from having to catch up on a delay. Other experiences of backlog may be more painful: *illness*, for example, means a deceleration, a loss of ability to act, and thus a partial exclusion from the life of others. *Grief* reflects a break which has been experienced in one's synchronicity with others—the mourner cannot disengage from the shared past, whereas the social time keeps moving on (Fuchs 2018). *Guilt* also has a retarding structure as its sufferer holds fast to omissions of the past. Finally, a more or less marked desynchronization from intersubjective time is characteristic of severe depression.

To summarize: Intersubjective time can be considered a relational arrangement of individual and social processes which are characterized by synchronizations and desynchronizations. While lived or implicit time is basically associated with synchrony, the experience of explicit time arises particularly in desynchronized states: as the "too early" or "too late," and thus as time which "creeps" or "rushes," which "flies" or against which one is fighting. The irreversibility and dominance of time is experienced first and foremost in discrepancies or separations from others to whom our lived time is attuned. Time which faces us from outside in seeming independence is in fact experienced primarily *in relationships* with others—that is, in desynchronizations of intersubjective time.

PSYCHOPATHOLOGY OF TEMPORALITY

On this basis, major psychiatric disorders such as schizophrenia, melancholic depression, and obsessive-compulsive disorder will briefly be presented as paradigm cases for a psychopathology of temporality.

Schizophrenia

In schizophrenia, major symptoms such as thought disorder, thought insertion, or passivity experiences may be explained by a weakening of the synthesis of inner time-consciousness (Gallagher 2000; Fuchs 2000b: 144f., 2013; Mishara 2007; Vogeley and Kupke 2007). The transition from simple disturbances of attention or speech to thought blockages and interferences, and finally to inserted thoughts, cannot be explained as mere concentration deficits at the level of semantic connections (Fuchs 2013). Rather, the disturbance must be localized at the transcendental level where the temporal coherence of consciousness as such is constituted. The disturbance of temporal continuity on this level—certainly correlated to neurophysiological dysfunctions[1] —then leads to a fragmentation of the intentional arc and an intrusion of unfitting thoughts or impulses into awareness. In speaking, for example, the patients may no longer be able to span the intentional arc of a meaningful sentence; speech becomes incoherent, or they have to use single words to explicitly "build up" the sentence. The single elements of thought, perception, or action then become disconnected fragments, which may even appear to the patient as alienated or opaque phenomena (Fuchs 2007).

The fragmentation of inner time-consciousness implies not only a weakening of the intentional arc, but also a failure of the inhibition of inappropriate thoughts or movements. Appearing "out of the blue," so to speak, they can only be experienced in the retentional mode, which means that they will appear to the patient as a surprise or with a "transcendental delay" (Fuchs 2013). As a result, they lose their sense of mineness and are experienced as alien elements intruding into the patient's stream of consciousness, finally appearing as thought insertions, voices or "made" movements (passivity experiences). Thus, the disintegration of the intentional arc and the fragmentation of self-coherence entails an externalization of the remaining fragments, resulting in the typical first-rank symptoms of schizophrenia.

Finally, *delusions* may also be related to the disturbance of temporality. The basic disintegration of inner time-consciousness leads, as we have seen, to fragmented thoughts, sensations, or movements that are not immediately experienced as one's own. These fragments of the broken intentional arc may be in a sense re-temporalized on the explicit level, namely by integrating them in a delusional narrative. The patient now experiences "others" as influencing him, moving his limbs, inserting thoughts into his head. Although these delusional explanations might lessen the burden of the temporal self-disintegration, they come at the price of an increased disconnection from the temporality shared with others. For the deluded patient, there is no open intersubjectivity any longer, because the delusion has always already determined what others could possibly mean or intend. The loss of the patient's ability to shift between different perspectives excludes all other possibilities of interpretation. The frozen, idiosyncratic reality of the delusion thus arrests the course of explicit or biographical time in order to compensate for the fragmentation of lived time (Fuchs 2013, 2015).

In sum, from a phenomenological point of view, key schizophrenic symptoms may be described as disturbances of the transcendental constitution of the "inner time-consciousness" or of lived time. The fragmentation of the normally continuous implicit flow of time is also what Stanghellini et al. (2016) have found in their research on altered time-experience in schizophrenia. This disturbance manifests itself in disorders of thought and attention, a disintegration of intentional acts, a fragmentation of basic self-coherence, and, in acute psychosis, in an externalization of the fragments in the form of first-rank symptoms.[2]

---

[1] There is increasing neuropsychological evidence of these disturbances of temporal integration. e.g. schizophrenia patients exhibit reduced attention spans, disturbances in planning, initiation, sequencing, and synchronization of speech as well as in the performance of other activities (Andreasen et al. 1998; Vogeley and Kupke 2007).

[2] Of course it should be added that basic disturbances of temporality may also affect the level of explicit time. Thus, the fragmented identity of the subject becomes dubious and uncertain, and the patient might wonder whether he still is the same person as he was before.

Affective Disorders

If we compare this analysis with the alterations of temporality in *affective disorders*, we find quite a different picture: Both in depression and mania, the synthesis and continuity of inner time-consciousness always remains intact. What is either lacking or exaggerated instead are the *conative dynamics*, and thus the affective tension that carries the intentional arc forward. In contrast to the fragmentation of lived time in schizophrenia, affective disorders therefore show a *retardation* or an *acceleration* of lived time, subjectively experienced as time "slowing down" or "speeding up" (cf. Fuchs 2013 and chapter XX, this volume).

This difference has also been confirmed in comparative studies by Stanghellini et al. (2016, 2017). Thus, for example, the schizophrenic blockade and incoherence of thought is fundamentally different from the inhibition and retardation of thinking found in severe depression. This illustrates again the difference between the transcendental synthesis and conative dynamics of lived time: The first signifies the temporal sequencing and structuring of the flow of consciousness, whose disturbances are manifested in cognitive symptoms. The second means the affective or vital dynamics of the flow, which may be altered in terms of drive, goal-directedness, and velocity. In experimental tests of time ratings, depressives' experience of time was repeatedly demonstrated to be slowed down, whereas manic patients showed a speeded-up temporality (Bech 1975; Kitamura and Kumar 1982; Münzel et al. 1988; Mundt et al. 1998; Bschor et al. 2004).

The disturbance of temporality in depression is twofold: On the one hand, there is a loss of drive, appetite, libido, interest, and attention, that means, a reduction of the *conative-affective dynamics*, leading to psychomotor inhibition and to a slowing-down of lived time. This is also expressed in an increasing rigidity and reification of the lived body, in bodily heaviness, exhaustion, oppression, and general anxiety (Fuchs 2005; Ratcliffe 2013). On the other hand, this is connected with a *loss of intersubjective synchronicity*: depressive patients lack the bodily resonance of emotions that is necessary for intercorporeality. The resulting lack of expressive communication is felt by others as an irritating failure of attunement. The patients themselves feel the painful incapacity to empathize with other people, to be addressed or affected by them. Hence, the failure of conative-affective dynamics is accompanied by a loss of basal contemporality or a *social desynchronization* (Fuchs 2001).

A more detailed analysis of temporality in affective disorders will be given in chapter XX.

Obsessive-Compulsive Disorder

Obsessive-compulsive disorders (OCD) may be conceived as disturbances of the implicit time of pre-reflective, spontaneous becoming which normally underlies the enactments of life. Implicit time, as we have seen, enables the performance of intentional arcs of perceiving and acting as well as the transition to new arcs of action which need not be deliberately "set in motion" each time. In OCD, however, the flow of intentional arcs is inhibited, and a *pathological explication of the implicit* arises (Fuchs 2011): For example, the morning toilet and dressing consists of an endless sequence of single actions painstakingly registered and set apart from each other; the housework must be worked through in accordance with a detailed item list; the act of closing the door must be repeated several times in a determined way, etc.

The temporality of OCD is thus characterized by an inhibition or hold-up of lived time which instead of continually flowing is made into an explicit sequencing, or rather, a stuttering. The patients are unable to abandon themselves to the stream of becoming and instead try to monitor and control their life in a hyperreflexive manner (Fuchs 2011). Two components of the temporal disturbance may be distinguished:

(1) First, we find in OCD patients an overall attempt to inhibit the passage of time as the *power of change*. For any change is experienced as a potential threat or harm, as a contamination, loss, decay, or obliteration. Thus, hesitation, indecisiveness, procrastination, or hoarding are typical means to arrest the flow of time. Even more, checking, controlling, washing, or cleaning should alleviate the anxious apprehension of the future and the fear of an ever impending harm. The patients are desperately trying to preserve a pristine state of their belongings, their body, or their environment, in order to "freeze time," as it were; for letting go would seem to surrender them to the unfathomable perils of life, and finally to death.

(2) The second component is a characteristic *feeling of incompleteness* or imperfection, a tormenting sense that one's actions or experiences are not "just right" and therefore have to be repeated endlessly, which underlies many symptoms in OCD. First described by Janet as "*sentiment d'incomplétude*," later by Straus (1948/1987) and von Gebsattel (1954: 128ff.), it has recently been investigated in more detail in the context of psychotherapeutic approaches (Summerfeldt 2004; Coles and Ravid 2016). Explanations in terms of a sensory-affective dysfunction with a possible neurophysiological origin have also been proposed (Subirà et al. 2015).

From a phenomenological point of view, however, the sense of completeness may not just be localized merely at the end of a sequence. Rather, it means the fulfillment of an overarching temporal *gestalt*, namely the intentional arc as a whole, which is experienced integrally at the end. If this holistic gestalt is dissolved into single elements, which are only effected externally and bit by bit, then the individual may well monitor his actions meticulously; nevertheless, the unity of action is lost, and a feeling of fulfillment cannot ensue. Since the patient is not really involved in his own actions, they appear at the end as if "not done."

Importantly, the pathological explication or dissolution of lived time in OCD is not the result of a cognitive incoherence as in schizophrenia (in OCD, there are no "gaps" in the stream of consciousness). Rather it arises from an inhibition caused by the patient's vain attempt to avoid the threatening passage of time and to alleviate the anxiety connected with its progress. In order to arrive at a controlled progression and termination of actions nevertheless, patients frequently try to establish *counting rituals*. Numbers divide the qualitative lived time in homogeneous quantitative units that may then be executed or repeated in a seemingly rational manner (brushing one's teeth for twelve minutes, check the light twenty times, etc.). However, the sequence of numbers also means a "bad infinity" (Hegel) which in the long run is not capable of restraining the constant urge for security. Usually, the number of repetitions or the length of an action must continuously be raised. The result is the well-known phenomenon of being desperately stuck in a repetitive present like in a hamster wheel, leaving the patient no exit to an open future.

CONCLUSION

This chapter has introduced some general concepts of temporality which are suitable for analyzing disturbances of temporalization in psychiatric disorders. The distinction of lived and experienced, or implicit and explicit time allows to understand and explain symptoms of major disorders, for example, as a fragmentation or a retardation of lived time, or as a pathological explication of normally implicit components of the stream of consciousness. Moreover, the concepts of synchronization and desynchronization connect the analysis of time with intersubjectivity, that means, with the social origins as well as the social manifestations of mental illness.

Three examples of an application of these concepts were presented: Central symptoms of schizophrenia such as thought disorder, thought insertion, or passivity experiences may be regarded as manifesting a disturbance of inner time-consciousness. Major depression, on the other hand, may be conceived as an inhibition of the conative-affective dynamics of life which leads to a desynchronization from intersubjective time. Finally, in obsessive-compulsive disorder the flow of lived time is inhibited and dissolved into repetitive elements in order to alleviate the anxious apprehension of the future and the tormenting feeling of incompleteness. However, through avoiding the future, the obsessive patient gets stuck in a present that is completely determined by the past, as an "eternal recurrence of the same." These examples should suffice to point out that a comprehensive psychopathology of temporality is both a major desideratum and a promising project for the future.

BIBLIOGRAPHY

Andreasen N. C., Paradiso S., and O'Leary D. S. (1998). "Cognitive Dysmetria" as an Integrative Theory of Schizophrenia: A Dysfunction in Cortical-Subcortical_Cerebellar Circuitry?" *Schizophrenia Bulletin* 24: 203–218.

Bech P. (1975). "Depression: Influence on Time Estimation and Time Experience." *Acta Psychiatrica Scandinavica* 51: 42–50.

Bourdieu P. (1990). *The Logic of Practice.* Stanford: Stanford University Press.

Bschor T., Ising M., Bauer M., Lewitzka U., Skerstupeit M., Müller-Oerlinghausen B., and Baethge C. (2004). "Time Experience and Time Judgment in Major Depression, Mania and Healthy Subjects. A Controlled Study of 93 Subjects." *Acta Psychiatrica Scandinavica* 109: 222–229.

Casey, E. (2000). *Remembering. A Phenomenological Study.* Bloomington: Indiana University Press.

Coles M. E. and Ravid A. (2016). "Clinical Presentation of Not-Just right experiences (NJREs) in Individuals with OCD: Characteristics and Response to Treatment." *Behaviour Research and Therapy* 87: 182–187.

Froese T. and Fuchs T. (2012). "The Extended Body: A Case Study in the Neurophenomenology of Social Interaction." *Phenomenology and the Cognitive Sciences* 11: 205–236.

Fuchs T. (2000a). "Das Gedächtnis des Leibes." *Phänomenologische Forschungen* 5: 71–89.

Fuchs T. (2000b). *Psychopathologie von Leib und Raum. Phänomenologisch-empirische Untersuchungen zu depressiven und paranoiden Erkrankungen.* Steinkopff: Darmstadt.

Fuchs T. (2001). "Melancholia as a Desynchronization. Towards a Psychopathology of Interpersonal Time." *Psychopathology* 34: 179–186.

Fuchs T. (2005). "Corporealized and Disembodied Minds. A Phenomenological View of the Body in Melancholia and Schizophrenia." *Philosophy, Psychiatry & Psychology* 12: 95–107.

Fuchs T. (2007). "The Temporal Structure of Intentionality and its Disturbance in Schizophrenia." *Psychopathology* 40: 229–235.

Fuchs T. (2011). "The Psychopathology of Hyperreflexivity." *Journal of Speculative Philosophy* 24: 239–255.

Fuchs T. (2012). "The Phenomenology of Body Memory." In S. Koch, T. Fuchs, M. Summa, and C. Müller (eds.), *Body Memory, Metaphor and Movement*, pp. 9–22. Amsterdam, Philadelphia: John Benjamins.

Fuchs T. (2013). "Temporality and Psychopathology." *Phenomenology and the Cognitive Sciences* 12: 75–104.

Fuchs T. (2015). "The Intersubjectivity of Delusions." *World Psychiatry* 14: 178–179.

Fuchs, T. (2018). "Presence in Absence. The Ambiguous Phenomenology of Grief." *Phenomenology and the Cognitive Sciences* 17: 43–63.

Gallagher S. (2000). "Self-reference and Schizophrenia: A Cognitive Model of Immunity to Error through Misidentification." In D. Zahavi (ed.), *Exploring the Self: Philosophical and Psychopathological Perspectives on Self-experience*, pp. 203–239. Amsterdam, Philadelphia: John Benjamins.

Gebsattel E. von. (1954). *Prolegomena einer medizinischen Anthropologie*. Berlin, Göttingen, Heidelberg: Springer.

Husserl E. (2012). *Cartesianische Meditationen*. Hamburg: Felix Meiner Verlag.

Kitamura T. and Kumar R. (1982). "Time Passes Slowly for Patients with Depressive State." *Acta Psychiatrica Scandinavica* 65: 415–420.

Minkowski E. (1933). *Le temps vécu. Etudes phénoménologiques et psychopathologiques*. Paris: Press Universitaires de France; Eng. trans. N. Metzel. *Lived Time. Phenomenological and Psychopathological Studies*. Evanston: Northwestern University Press, 1970.

Mishara A. L. (2007). "Missing Links in Phenomenological Clinical Neuroscience: Why We Are Not There Yet." *Current Opinions in Psychiatry* 20: 559–569.

Mundt C., Richter P., van Hees H., and Stumpf T. (1998). "Zeiterleben und Zeitschaetzung depressiver Patienten." *Nervenarzt* 69: 38–45.

Münzel K., Gendner G., Steinberg R., and Raith L. (1988). "Time Estimation of Depressive Patients: The Influence of the Interval Content." *European Archives of Psychiatric and Neurological Sciences* 237: 171–178.

Pokropski M. (2015). "Timing Together, Acting Together. Phenomenology of Intersubjective Temporality and Social Cognition." *Phenomenology and the Cognitive Sciences* 14: 897–909.

Ramseyer F. and Tschacher W. (2006). "Synchrony: A Core Concept for a Constructivist Approach to Psychotherapy." *Constructivism in the Human Sciences* 11: 150–171.

Ratcliffe M. (2013). "A Bad Case of the Flu? The Comparative Phenomenology of Depression and Somatic Illness." *Journal of Consciousness Studies* 20: 198–218.

Stanghellini G., Ballerini M., Presenza S., Mancini M., Raballo A., Blasi S., and Cutting J. (2016). "Psychopathology of Lived Time: Abnormal Time Experience in Persons with Schizophrenia." *Schizophrenia Bulletin* 42: 45–55.

Stanghellini G., Ballerini M., Presenza S., Mancini M., Northoff G., and Cutting J. (2017). "Abnormal Time Experiences in Major Depression: An Empirical Qualitative Study." *Psychopathology* 50: 125–140.

Straus E. (1948/1987). *On Obsession: A Clinical and Methodological Study*. New York: Johnson Reprint Corp.

Straus E. (1966). *Phenomenological Psychology*. New York: Basic Books.

Subirà M., Sato J. R., Alonso P., do Rosário M. C., Segalàs C., Batistuzzo M. C., and Pujol J. (2015). "Brain Structural Correlates of Sensory Phenomena in Patients with Obsessive-Compulsive Disorder." *Journal of Psychiatry and Neuroscience* 40(4): 232.

Summerfeldt L. J. (2004). "Understanding and Treating Incompleteness in Obsessive-Compulsive Disorder." *Journal of Clinical Psychology* 60: 1155–1168.

Tellenbach H. (1980). *Melancholy. History of the Problem, Endogeneity, Typology, Pathogenesis, Clinical Considerations*. Pittsburgh: Duquesne University Press.

Theunissen M. (1991). *Negative Theologie der Zeit*. Frankfurt am Main: Suhrkamp.

Tschacher W., Rees G. M., and Ramseyer F. (2014). "Nonverbal Synchrony and Affect in Dyadic Interactions." *Frontiers in Psychology* 5: 1323.

Vogeley K. and Kupke C. (2007). "Disturbances of Time Consciousness from a Phenomenological and a Neuroscientific Perspective." *Schizophrenia Bulletin* 33: 157–165.

Wyllie M. (2006). "Lived Time and Psychopathology." *Philosophy, Psychiatry, & Psychology* 12:173–185.

Zahavi D. (2008). *Subjectivity and Selfhood. Investigating the First-Person Perspective*. Cambridge, MA: MIT Press.

CHAPTER 49

ATTENTION, CONCENTRATION, MEMORY, AND THEIR DISORDERS

JULIAN C. HUGHES

INTRODUCTION

CONSCIOUS living things attend and remember. Human beings are by nature self-conscious and typically we express our self-conscious awareness and reflection through language. Furthermore, language defines us as human beings. So the importance of attention, concentration, and memory is that these phenomena are closely tied to our sense of being the sort of beings that we are.

In this article I shall, first, define the terms as they have been described in texts of descriptive psychopathology; and, secondly, before some concluding remarks, describe the disorders of attention, concentration, and memory as they occur in a variety of conditions.

WHAT ARE ATTENTION AND CONCENTRATION?

The *Shorter Oxford English Dictionary* defines attention as:

> The action, fact, or state of attending or giving heed; the mental faculty of attending, attentiveness; application of the mind, consideration, thought;

and concentration as:

> The continued focusing of mental powers and faculties on a particular object.

Whilst the definition of "attention" seems in part tautological (attention is attending!), it is also the "application of the *mind*"; and concentration—which is defined elsewhere as "attention sustained for some duration of time" (Sims 1988: 30)—is similarly the continuing focus of "*mental* powers and faculties" (emphasis added).

Attention and concentration can be regarded as the means by which we, as minded individuals, interact with the world. They, like memory, are intentional mental states in the sense that they always imply an object: we attend to or concentrate on *something*. As is well known, it was Franz Brentano (1838–1917) who introduced the notion of "intentionality" back into contemporary thought from its use by scholastic thinkers in the Middle Ages. It was one way to characterize mental from physical phenomena. Mental phenomena take in and contain an object intentionally; but mental phenomena show intentional inexistence, because what is contained in the mental just is not physically present. It is of note that "attention" and "intentional" share the similar Latin root *tendere*, which suggests stretching out, a directedness toward something. This is again to suggest the importance of these mental phenomena for our being-in-the-world. They are the means by which we give heed to the world in order to consider it. If they go wrong, then our grasp of the world is changed, distorted, or lessened.

Karl Jaspers stated simply of attention, "This determines the clarity of our experience" (Jaspers 1997: 140). Earlier he wrote: "Normal people can concentrate on any task which is set them, but with alteration in the total psychic state, this capacity steadily decreases" (Jaspers 1997: 140). When Jaspers referred to the "total psychic state," he was thinking of "a total state of consciousness which makes it possible for individual phenomena to arise" (Jaspers 1997: 137). He went on to say:

> In psychic life, everything is connected with everything else and each element is coloured by the state and context in which it occurs. . . . Each single element, every perception, image or feeling differs according to whether it occurs in a state of clear or clouded consciousness.
>
> (Jaspers 1997: 137)

Andrew Sims makes the same link between attention, concentration, and consciousness:

> Attention is a different function from consciousness, but dependent upon it. Thus, variable degrees of attention are possible with full consciousness, but complete attention and concentration is impossible with diminished consciousness.
>
> (Sims 1988: 30)

A distinction can be made between attention and awareness:

> Attention and awareness are not precisely distinguished, but *attention* refers to the objective observation of another person, object or event, whilst *awareness* is the subjective description of the state in which the percepts may be received.
>
> (Sims 1988: 30)

Thus, there can be a background awareness of something going on, say in the street outside, but my attention is fixed on what is happening in the room, until suddenly the noise outside captures my attention. Sims also picks up Kräupl Taylor's distinction between *vigilance* and *absorption*. One person may be too absorbed by what is happening inside to notice what is going on in the street; another, who is too vigilant, might not be able to concentrate on what is going on inside because of the slightest thing that occurs outside. According to Kräupl Taylor:

> When the reactivity of the mind is high, this is subjectively experienced as full, clear or lucid consciousness. . . . A lucid sensorium [or consciousness] is objectively noticed as a state of alertness, attentiveness, or vigilance.
>
> (Kräupl Taylor 1979: 215)

So attention and concentration are important for how we see and relate to the world, are intimately connected to consciousness, but are fragile to those conditions that might affect consciousness.

WHAT IS MEMORY?

Memory is not one thing. A phenomenological account of memory, therefore, would include many things. John Hodges (2007) has provided a useful overview of the major subdivisions of memory (see Figure 49.1).

The main division is between declarative (explicit) and procedural (implicit) memory. Declarative memory is "available to conscious access and reflection," whereas procedural memory refers to learned responses which are not a matter of conscious reflection (Hodges 2007: 6).

Procedural memory is split into three types. Conditioning and priming are similar: one thing leads to another based on a type of memory. In the classical conditioning experiments of Ivan Pavlov, a stimulus (such as a bell) leads to a response (dogs salivating). In tests of priming, the subject is asked to recall some words and a prompt is then used to elicit the correct answer, even though the original word has been forgotten. In the first case, the dog has remembered at some level that the bell signifies food. In the second case, the subject has forgotten the words at a conscious level, but the prompts are enough to encourage the right answer, so something was remembered. Day-to-day procedural memory is easily understood in terms of motor skills such as driving and playing a musical instrument. These are

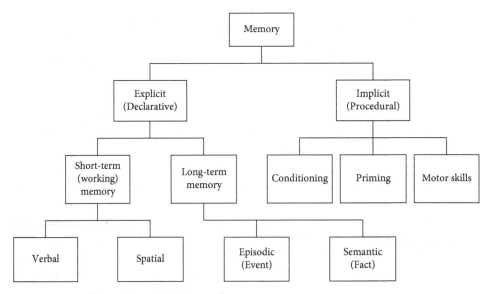

FIGURE 49.1 The major subdivisions of memory.

Adapted from John R. Hodges, *Cognitive Assessment for Clinicians*, 2nd edn., 7, Figure 1.3 © 1994, Oxford University Press. Reproduced by permission of Oxford University Press https://global.oup.com/academic/product/cognitive-assessment-for-clinicians-9780192629760?q= Cognitive%20Assessment%20for%20Clinicians&lang=e n &cc=g b

things we can just do, once we have acquired the necessary skills, without reflection. I can remember how to drive without thinking about how to drive.

Declarative memory is split into short-term (or working) memory and long-term memory. Short-term memory is, strictly speaking, that part of the memory "responsible for the immediate recall of small amounts of verbal . . . or spatial material" (Hodges 2007: 8). It is the sort of memory involved in remembering a telephone number just long enough to use it. The material is then usually forgotten.

Long-term memory is split into episodic and semantic memory. Episodic memory is the memory of personal episodes, which are time- and context-specific: Auntie Bertha being stung by a bee on the beach in Bognor for instance. Semantic memory, on the other hand, does not depend on time or place, but is our store of knowledge. This includes our memory for the meaning of words (such as "bee" and "beach") as well as our recall of factual information.

Another important distinction, which is relevant to clinical practice, is between antero-grade and retrograde memory. Anterograde memory refers to new memories being formed; whilst retrograde memory refers to information learned previously. A person may still be able to recall events and information from years ago, but not remember what has just happened.

So memory is not just one thing. The distinctions can be made even finer. There are differences between recalling and recognizing; and differences between recalling words and recognizing faces and the other way around. Memory is a pervasive feature of our mental lives. As with problems affecting attention and concentration, disturbances of memory are likely to have profound effects on our psychic lives generally.

DISORDERS OF ATTENTION AND CONCENTRATION

Attention and concentration are affected by a great variety of disorders. Sims (1988: 31) lists organic states, such as "head injury; acute toxic confusional states . . . epilepsy; raised intra-cranial pressure; and brain stem lesions" as causing inattention, usually in conjunction with lowering of conscious level. Psychogenic states, such as dissociative amnesia, may also alter attention (Sims 1988: 31). In this section I shall give examples from just a sample of possible disorders.

Mania is characterized, as well as by elation, by *distractibility*, which is an inability to retain attention, so that something external quickly intrudes on the conversation and adds to the impression of flight of ideas. In addition, the person with mania or hypo-mania may well feel that those around are slow in their thoughts. The rapidity of thought, which frequently combines with grandiose thinking, is also a sign of poor attention or contributes to it.

On the other hand, in depression, it can be hard for the person to keep up with others be-cause the thinking of the depressed person feels slow.

> Mrs. Jones believes she is suffering from dementia. She finds it difficult to concentrate on what is going on around her. She has been feeling very low for some time and is unable to maintain her interest in things, which she also feels must reflect her increasing dementia. But people tell her that she is depressed. In a test of her mental functioning, in which she felt she had done

very badly, she was told that her memory was good, even though she forgot some words she was meant to remember and even though, when asked to spell a word backwards, she could not concentrate on the task and felt desperate about it.

The cognitive profile suggested in the case of Mrs. Jones is typical of depression, where tests that require concentration can seem too much for the person, despite other cognitive functions being maintained.

In delirium, an acute confusional state, it becomes difficult for the person to maintain attention or to shift attention in an appropriate manner. In part this links to the perceptual disturbances, such as illusions, and associated delusions which can develop. As in the case of Mr. Stewart, in delirium there can be marked fluctuations in the person's conscious level, which inevitably has an impact on attention and concentration.

> Mr. Stewart was brought into hospital by his daughter. He had been feeling unwell for some time. He is now in a side room. He becomes sure that the doctors are poisoning him with the wrong medication because the clock on the wall keeps looking like a snake. He is also hearing noises which he thinks are the staff lining up outside his room to come in and kill him. When they do come in, they ask him all sorts of questions. But he cannot focus on them for more than a few seconds both because he is fearful about what the doctors intend to do and because he is distracted by the changing appearance of the clock.

Children with hyperkinetic disorders are overactive. But they also have marked inattention, which is regarded as a central feature and has led to the term "attention deficit disorder." The *International Classification of Diseases* (ICD-10) comments:

> Impaired attention is manifested by prematurely breaking off from tasks and leaving activities unfinished. The children change frequently from one activity to another, seemingly losing interest in one task because they become diverted to another . . .
>
> (WHO 1992: 263)

In a variety of conditions, regarded as neurotic and stress-related, such as panic and generalized anxiety, phobic disorders, post-traumatic stress disorder, and obsessive-compulsive disorder, attention and concentration can be affected.

> Since arriving in England, Anas Ahmadi has suffered from flashbacks to his last few months in Syria, when frequent rocket attacks targeted his own and nearby villages. He remains hypervigilant, often feeling tense and on edge, his attention attracted by every loud noise or unusual movement in his vicinity. He sometimes forgets that he is now in a safe country and thinks he is back near Damascus. His concentration on the tasks he should be doing can be impaired.

Disorders of attention and concentration can also appear in schizophrenia and other psychotic states, in part because the person might be distracted by their psychotic experiences. Jaspers describes "thought block" in schizophrenia as an interruption of concentration:

> They suddenly cease to reply, stare in front, and do not seem to understand anything. After a time (minutes or seconds) this ceases, only to recur again a little later.
>
> (Jaspers 1997: 142)

Increasingly, cognitive dysfunction is a recognized aspect of schizophrenia, not solely when it is chronic:

> Impaired attention is considered a primary cognitive deficit in schizophrenia. Individuals who are genetically predisposed to schizophrenia have poor ability to maintain their attention even prior to the first psychotic episode . . . . By the time patients experience their first episode of psychosis, attentional impairments are typically present and of moderate severity . . .
>
> (Bowie and Harvey 2006)

As in a number of disorders, such as obsessive-compulsive disorder, anorexia nervosa, and autism, so too in schizophrenia, lack of cognitive flexibility as shown by difficulties in set- or task-shifting can also be problematic for, and a manifestation of, problems in attention and concentration. Such executive dysfunction has general implications for the ways in which other cognitive functions are managed. We can see, therefore, that attention and concentration can be affected by a number of mental disorders and are manifestations of some of these disorders, with profound implications for the people concerned.

DISORDERS OF MEMORY

Confabulation "is a falsification of memory occurring in clear consciousness in association with an organically derived amnesia" (Sims 1988: 44). This can occur in a variety of conditions, but is frequently associated with the Korsakov syndrome (dense amnesia, lack of insight, and confabulation), which in turn is associated with heavy drinking. It is caused by a lack of Vitamin B1, also known as thiamine. But Korsakov's can be caused by a variety of organic conditions (e.g. tumours or strokes) that might affect the mammillary bodies or other regions of the brain associated with dense amnesia, such as the thalamus; and confabulation can occur in other pathologies as well. For instance, it can occur in dementia, where there is a regrettable tendency to label confabulated beliefs as delusions, whereas they are merely the person's attempt to account for a gap in memory.

> Ms. Harbottle has dementia and lives in a care home. Every morning she puts on her glasses which sit on the bedside table. But increasingly they are not there when she awakens. She starts to think that someone else is coming into her room and moving them. It must be the staff in the home. When she complains, staff inevitably find her glasses elsewhere and give them back to her with the explanation that she must have put them down herself and forgotten. She objects to this, because she never recalls putting them elsewhere. Now she finds other things in unexpected places, as if someone is constantly in her room moving objects. Again the staff tell her that she obviously forgets where she puts things.

Such experiences inevitably lead to paranoia and could be labeled as psychotic rather than as a memory problem, with unfortunate implications for treatment.

Kräupl Taylor described Mr. B., who in 1926 was overcome by carbon monoxide fumes and became unconscious. A week later he showed signs of the Korsakov syndrome:

> He could not remember anything since the accident, was unable to retain new experiences, and had difficulty in orienting himself in space and time.
>
> (Kräupl Taylor 1979: 258–259)

Mr. B was paid a considerable disability pension. Controversy then arose about whether or not his symptoms were veridical. Thirty years later it was confirmed that mostly he had been shamming, even if the original disorder had a true organic basis. Oliver Sacks, too, presents an interesting account of his patient, Jimmie G., who had Korsakov's, where "the memory traces were fugitive in the extreme, and were apt to be effaced within a minute, often less, especially if there were distracting or competing stimuli" (Sacks 1986: 26).

Transient global amnesia occurs in otherwise healthy people who are unable to remember new things for even a short while. After a few hours, things return to normal but the person is left with a dense memory deficit for the time of the attack.

Disturbances in memory also occur in delirium, but this is "largely secondary to diminished attention" (Hodges 2007: 30). People with delirium will show confabulation too. When people recover from a delirium, say after an infection, they will usually have a dense amnesia for the time that they were ill, "although where fluctuation has been marked islands of memory may remain" (Hodges 2007: 30).

Schizophrenia is also associated with poor memory (Rushe et al. 1999). But memory disorders are mostly associated with the dementias (Hughes 2011a) and can vary according to the type of dementia. Alzheimer's disease shows a gradual onset of memory impairment, where this typically affects episodic memory early (whereas in dementia with Lewy bodies memory loss is seen slightly later), but Alzheimer's still affects both semantic and procedural memory.

> Mr. Chaudhry developed memory impairment some years ago. Initially he was seen in a memory clinic and was told that he had mild cognitive impairment. But later he was told that he had dementia. Although at first he would only forget things that had just happened, later it started to affect his use of language. He became disoriented, forgetting the date and where he was living. At about this time, his family had to stop him from driving because he seemed to be losing the necessary skills. He then started to find it difficult to recognize the faces of his friends and family. As the dementia worsened, he lost other skills too, such as his ability to feed himself. In the more advanced stages of his Alzheimer's disease, he forgot how to speak English and reverted to his native tongue. In the end he seemed to live in a small space of time, where he could only recall what had just happened.

Vascular dementias and stroke disease can cause more localized cognitive impairment, perhaps affecting the memory for words and language at an early point, rather than episodic memory. In semantic dementia too, which is one type of frontotemporal degeneration, there is an early and prominent loss of the memory for words (Hodges and Patterson 2007). Memory disorders, therefore, like attention and concentration, suggest a variety of possible pathologies and will cause a variety of subjective difficulties, from the embarrassment of word-finding problems to the tragedy of forgetting a loved one.

CONCLUSION

Problems with attention, concentration, and memory occur in a great variety of conditions. In this sense they contribute to trans-nosography, because several different psychiatric diseases share these common psychopathological dimensions. Not infrequently there is a discrepancy between the person's subjective experience of problems with attention, concentration and memory, and the objective reality. For instance, the person with dementia might not recognize the extent of his deficits on objective testing; whereas the person with depression might ardently believe that she has dementia and is performing very badly on tests when in fact she is doing well. But depression can be prodromal to dementia, so the observed cognitive deficits are both significant to the person and significant clinically as markers of a potentially unifying underlying pathology. And understanding the mismatch between objective symptoms and subjective experience in the person with dementia, who lacks insight into his condition, is important if we are to know how to communicate with and help him to live with dementia. Our ability to attend and to remember is vital to our standing because of our situated nature as beings who act on and interact with the world, which we do primarily as embodied agents (Hughes 2011b).

Attention, concentration, and memory, therefore, are intimately connected to our standing as selves-in-the-world. When I cannot attend or concentrate sufficiently, my grasp on the world diminishes, which may or may not be pathological. When I cannot remember, my reality is circumscribed, which may or may not be a difficulty. The importance of these phenomena is their essential tendency to connect us to the world and to each other as minded individuals.

BIBLIOGRAPHY

Bowie C. R. and Harvey P. D. (2006). "Cognitive Deficits and Functional Outcome in Schizophrenia." *Neuropsychiatric Disease and Treatment* 2(4): 531–536.

Hodges J. R. (2007). *Cognitive Assessment for Clinicians*, 2nd edn. Oxford: Oxford University Press.

Hodges J. R. and Patterson K. (2007). "Semantic Dementia: A Unique Clinicopathological Syndrome." *The Lancet Neurology* 6(11): 1004–1014.

Hughes J. C. (2011a). *Alzheimer's and Other Dementias: The Facts*. Oxford: Oxford University Press.

Hughes J. C. (2011b). *Thinking Through Dementia*. Oxford: Oxford University Press.

Jaspers K. (1997). *General Psychopathology. Volume I*, trans. J. Hoenig and M. W. Hamilton. Baltimore, London: Johns Hopkins University Press. [Originally published (1959). *Allgemeine Psychopathologie* by Berlin, Heidelberg: Springer-Verlag.]

Kräupl Taylor F. (1979). *Psychopathology: Its Causes and Symptoms*. Sunbury-on-Thames: Quartermaine House.

Rushe T. M., Woodruff P. W. R., Murray R. M., and Morris, R. G. (1999). "Episodic Memory and Learning in Patients with Chronic Schizophrenia." *Schizophrenia Research* 35(1): 85–96.

Sacks O. (1986). *The Man Who Mistook His Wife for a Hat*. London: Picador.

Sims A. (1988). *Symptoms in the Mind: An Introduction to Descriptive Psychopathology*. London: Baillière Tindall.

World Health Organization (WHO) (1992). *The ICD-10. Classification of Mental and Behavioural Disorders: Clinical Descriptions and Diagnostic Guidelines*. Geneva: World Health Organization.

CHAPTER 50

THOUGHT, SPEECH, AND LANGUAGE DISORDERS

JOHN CUTTING

INTRODUCTION

DISORDERS of thought, speech, and language are prolific in psychotic and brain-damaged subjects. Understanding of the topic has been blighted by inapt terminology, failure to appreciate that items in psychiatric and neurological lexicons often refer to the same entity, uncertainty about what constitutes thought or speech as opposed to language, and shifting psychological models during the twentieth century as to the nature of the mind. The most insightful contributions have been those of linguists and neuropsychologists. Phenomenological psychopathologists have largely shunned the topic. I shall nevertheless consider what phenomenological philosophy has to offer.

DESCRIPTIVE PSYCHOPATHOLOGY

The plethora of psychiatric and neurological terms are laid out in Table 50.1. Speech disorders are the simplest to categorize. Either there is a reduction (poverty of speech) or absence (anarthria, mutism); excess (logorrhoea, pressure of speech); or repetition (echolalia, if of others' speech; stereotypy, if of one's own speech).

The three generic disorders of language are aphasia, non-aphasic misnaming, and some aspects of formal thought disorder. Aphasia has many subdivisions, but all are essentially breakdowns in the structural elements of language—its phonemes, syntax, and semantics. Non-aphasic misnaming, a term introduced by Weinstein and Kahn (1952), is a disorder of the fourth element of language—its pragmatics, the way it is put to use. Neologisms (non-dictionary words), paraphasias (actual words used wrongly), and stilted or out-of-focus phrases occur. Whereas aphasia results from damage within the Broca-Wernicke axis in the left hemisphere, non-aphasic misnaming accompanies a variety of focal lesions outside this region—frontal, right-hemispheric—as well as generalized dysfunction—delirium, concussion. Some aspects of the umbrella term, formal thought disorder, are also disturbances

Table 50.1 Inventory of thought, speech, and language disorders

Item	Meaning of item
Speech disorder anarthria mutism	absence of speech
poverty of speech	reduced speech
logorrhoea pressure of speech	excess speech
echolalia	repetition of others' speech
stereotypy of speech	repetition of own speech
Language disorder *generic terms:*	
aphasia	phonemic, syntactic, and semantic breakdowns in language
non-aphasic misnaming	pragmatic breakdown in language
formal thought disorder (some aspects)	pragmatic breakdown in language; phonemic, syntactic, and semantic hypervalence
specific entities:	
neologism	non-dictionary word
paraphasia	actual word used wrongly
Thought disorder	
generic terms:	
formal thought disorder (some aspects)	illogical, inconsequential, or impoverished expression of thought
specific entities:	
illogicality	illogical expression of thought
poverty of content of thought	impoverished thinking
flight of ideas	exuberant thinking
derailment (tangentiality, knight's move thinking, loss of goal, incoherence)	inconsequential expression of thought
loss of dreaming	absence of dreams
loss of imagery	absence of imagery

of pragmatic language, and are indistinguishable from the neologisms, paraphasias, and odd turns of phrase evident in non-aphasic misnaming. Others are the opposite of aphasia, and consist of a preoccupation with, elaboration of, the phonemics, grammar, and formal meaning of words.

Genuine thought disorder is apparent in yet other components of formal thought disorder, in the form of seemingly illogical, inconsequential, and impoverished ways of expressing some idea. A number of metaphors have been proposed in an attempt to portray this—tangentiality, derailment, knight's move thinking, loss of goal, and incoherence. Andreasen's (1979) investigation into all this demonstrated that raters were unreliable in distinguishing between these. A quantitative assessment of whether thoughts were impoverished (poverty of content of thought) or exuberant (flight of ideas) was more reliable in Andreasen's study.

Other aspects of thinking—dreaming, imagery—can also be impaired in psychopathological situations.

Nosological Specificity

Despite the problematical nature of some of the supposed entities, there is a surprisingly strong link between some of them and specific diagnostic categories. Formal thought disorder, particularly poverty of content of thought, is highly indicative of schizophrenia (Andreasen 1979). Mutism (Braun et al. 2004), loss of dreaming (Herschmann and Schilder 1919), and loss of imagery (Hurlburt 1990) are characteristic of depressive illness. Flight of ideas and pressure of speech, in combination, are virtually pathognomonic of mania. In delirium non-aphasic misnaming predominates (Weinstein and Kahn 1952). Of all the conditions which commonly present to psychiatrists, dementia is the only one where aphasia appears.

Psychological Accounts

Psychological approaches in the case of formal thought disorder have been of two main sorts. Either an intrinsic disturbance of language and thinking is denied, and the various manifestations attributed to non-specific motivational, emotional, or attentional factors. Or, an intrinsic problem is deemed genuine, but a single overarching explanation is offered for all of them: for example, recrudescence of primitive, illogical thought patterns (Storch 1924), regression to childish ways of thinking (Vygotsky 1934), or loss of abstract attitude (Goldstein 1939).

Each proposal has eventually been rebutted by experimental work. To give some examples: Owen et al. (2007) showed that people with schizophrenia were *more* not less logical than normal controls on syllogisms, refuting two of the theses in one go—their superior performance a blow to any non-specific motivational impairment and questioning the very notion that they were illogical at all. Cameron (1938) found marked differences between six-year-olds and schizophrenics in a reasoning test, undermining Vygotsky's thesis. Shimkunas (1972) found schizophrenics to be *more* not less *abstract*, contra Goldstein.

Linguistic Analysis

The proper analysis of language disorder is linguistics and this has considerably clarified the pot-pourri of abnormalities known as formal thought disorder, in itself and with respect to aphasia and non-aphasic misnaming.

If we start with aphasia, which is the simplest of the three, the new words are composed of substitutions or deletions governed by rules intrinsic to normal language formation itself: phonemic transpositions between similarly articulated phonemes—*pears* becoming *bears* (Blumstein 1995); syntactic changes in the direction of simplification—abandonment of articles, agreement markers, and auxiliary verbs—hence a telegrammatic style (Caplan 1995); semantic anomalies are words with a similar lexical form but not primarily a similar sound or category membership—hence *walk* for walking but not *sneeze* for snooze or *dog* for cat (Rapp and Caramazza 1995).

In formal thought disorder the precise opposite occurs. Chaika (1974) observed:

> an inappropriate noting of phonological features, e.g. "I had a little goldfish too like a clown. Happy Halloween down".

She also pointed out:

> preoccupation with too many of the semantic features of a word, e.g. "My mother's name was Bill and Coo. St. Valentine's Day is the official startin' of the breeding season of the birds. All buzzards can coo".

This is not the sort of speech encountered in aphasia, but rather a hyper-alertness to phonological and semantic cues. Their grammatical deviance too is quite unlike the paring down of syntactical complexity seen in aphasia, but instead a profusion of suffixes and prefixes, as in these neologisms from my subjects: "talkable people" (talked a lot), "deep thoughtedness" (able to think deeply), and "hermatergised" (made into a hermit). Bleuler (1911/1950) had already noticed this: "bemillioned" (received millions), "enchambered by winter" (house-bound). I consider these to be "hyperphoneticism," "hypergrammatism," and "hypersemanticism" (to coin further neologisms, hopefully in the interests of science). To complicate matters, however, this hyperactivity in the first three components of language is coupled with pragmatic deviance.

Non-aphasic misnaming is pure pragmatic language disorder. The features, in Weinstein and Kahn's (1955) account, are: "paraphasic misnaming," for example, wheelchair called *chaise longue*; inappropriate reference to body in the third person, for example, disabled limb described as "He's very limpy"; and "stilted, ornate and pedantic" phrases, for example, when asked why he had gone to the doctor one patient replied, "lack of precision in dealing with my friends."

We can now formulate the three entities as follows: aphasia is a breakdown in phonetics, syntax, and semantics; non-aphasic misnaming is a breakdown in the pragmatics of language; formal thought disorder is the most complex, as it is a combination of phonetic, syntactic, and semantic hyperactivity along with pragmatic language breakdown (and some further genuine anomalies of thinking).

NEUROPSYCHOLOGICAL CONTRIBUTIONS

With an eye to our later phenomenological analysis we can abstract from the neuropsychological literature two general principles about the nature of speech and language.

The first, uncovered by decades of work by Russian linguists and neurologists, and summarized by Glezerman and Balkowski (1999), is that any word plays a dual role in the scheme of things. Its core status in modern humans (in the left hemisphere) is as a category, whose meaning depends on its contrast with other words rather than any faithful portrayal of a life experience—for example, a pond is *not* a river and *not* a lake rather than that collection of water in our home village. Its other role is as a sign for this very last sort of experience, a situation attested to in numerous accounts of primitive languages. Per Cassirer (1944):

> The Bakairi language—an idiom spoken by an Indian tribe in Central Brazil—has an individual name for each species of parrot and palm tree whereas there exists no name to express the genus "parrot" or "palm".

Secondly, this duality between word as category and word as sign for collective experience is so marked that under experimental conditions which isolate each hemisphere's contribution to language in modern humans one can lay bare the two separate roles. Take this experiment carried out by Deglin (1993). Subjects were asked questions in the immediate aftermath of receiving electroconvulsive therapy (ECT) to either the right or left hemisphere for their psychiatric condition, essentially inducing a brief uni-hemispheric mode of being human. Under conditions of left hemisphere suppression (right hemisphere alone viable) they were asked whether some object, for example, brother, was appropriately named or whether another name would do, for example, sister, or even a made-up word. The subjects replied along the lines of this one, who said "Brother, that's someone who's a blood relation and that's why it's a brother. You can't call it anything else!" When their right hemisphere was suppressed (left hemisphere alone viable) they replied that "brother" could easily be called something else. The author concluded:

> The right hemisphere does not know that a verbal sign is arbitrary and conventional. It appears in fact that for the right hemisphere the verbal sign is as firmly attached to the object, indeed part of the object, as its form, colour or smell.

Extant Phenomenological Psychopathology

As mentioned, the greatest psychopathologists of the past—Minkowski, Binswanger, Blankenburg—wrote nothing on our topic. The only psychopathologist of any standing who did was Goldstein, primarily a neurologist but related to and mentored by Cassirer (1874–1945), one of the great philosophers of the twentieth century, who, although not usually regarded as a phenomenological philosopher, was exquisitely aware of the issues.

What Goldstein (Gelb and Goldstein 1925) and Cassirer (1929/1957) appreciated about aphasia was something that no one else had properly grasped, which was that a brain-damaged subject might be unable to utter a particular word in one context, but could do so in another. For example, one patient could not name a watch [*Uhr*] but when asked what time it was readily replied "*ein Uhr*" [one o'clock]. This showed that the very same word "*Uhr*" was unavailable in one situation and available in another, an indictment of all theories which treated aphasia as a static loss of word retrieval. Goldstein went on to formulate schizophrenic language and thought as a loss of the abstract attitude. This was wrong but his insight into the dynamic nature of aphasia chimes with the Russian studies on a word's dual status and informs our general formulation.

PHILOSOPHICAL RESOURCES OF
THESE PSYCHOPATHOLOGICAL ISSUES

Thought, speech, and language disorders at first sight offer a bewildering array of seemingly random entities. As we have shown, a psychological account of these misses the point by either denying the intrinsic linguistic nature of most of them or by proposing a single explanation which is then easily rebutted. Carefully conducted linguistic analyses, however, reveal clear differences between the three generic varieties—aphasia, non-aphasic misnaming, and formal thought disorder—and show that each is predominantly a language disorder but of a different sort from the others. Neuropsychological investigations, and the only extant phenomenological study of the matter, uncover an overriding duality in the way a single word functions in human discourse: 1) as a virtual property of a *thing* experienced; and 2) as an arbitrary name for the *sort of thing* by which experience can be categorized.

What can the chief phenomenological philosophers—Husserl, Heidegger, Merleau-Ponty, Scheler—offer us, such that we can say that there is a viable philosophical phenomenological psychopathology of the matter in question which linguistic and neuropsychological approaches have not exhausted?

Each of these philosophers had a different view of language and there is certainly no consensus as to the phenomenology of language. Husserl (1929) was of the opinion that speech localized and temporalized an ideal meaning. This was a top-down approach, whereby language substantiated itself as speech in the here and now of an individual speaker. Thought was primary, and language and speech a particular mode of this. Heidegger, in two articles in particular in his many writings on language—"Language" (1959/1971a) and "The Nature of Language" (Heidegger 1959/1971b), took the opposite line. For him, language was the primary means whereby human beings could not only think but be human beings at all and, furthermore, have any sense of things around them:

> Where word breaks off no thing may be.
>
> (Heidegger 77)

Merleau-Ponty's (1960/1964) *On the Phenomenology of Language* charts a middle path between these extremes of thought as language and language as thought. Ever alert to the human being's dual status as perceiver being perceived or toucher being touched, and to how this breaches the divide between idealism and realism, he formulates language in a similar way, as a revelation of the *other* by virtue of the meaning I put into my speech:

> When I speak or understand, I experience that presence of others in myself or of myself in others which is the stumbling-block of the theory of intersubjectivity . . . To the extent that what I say has meaning, I am a different 'other' for myself when I am speaking; and to the extent that I understand, I no longer know who is speaking and who is listening.
>
> (Merleau-Ponty 1960/1964: 97)

Scheler (1926/2008), who wrote very little about language, nevertheless foresaw the results of the aforementioned neuropsychological investigations, and had a completely different view on language from the other three philosophers dealt with here:

> Whatever meaning we derive from an object originally belongs to that object, and not to our subsumption or meaning which we put on to it . . . The sequence is object → word, not word → object . . . The original meaning adhering to something actually forms the basis of the qualities.

(Scheler 1926/2008: 396)

With the gradual individualization of the human being, Scheler goes on to say, thinking takes different turns, the result of pondering on one's operations on objects of various sorts, culminating in a matrix of their essences. This allows different levels of sophistication of language but this is always the handmaiden of thought, not the other way round.

Scheler's view conforms better than the others to the neuropsychological and psychopathological facts with which we are confronted. Were speech the temporalization and spatialization of a universal grammar, as Husserl, and later Chomsky, opined, why should the word "*Uhr*" come and go in someone with brain damage or the word "brother" be both a property of an object and an arbitrary name depending on which hemisphere is in play. If language were the "making of man" and "where word breaks off no thing may be" (Heidegger) how is it that severe aphasics such as Broca's (1861) original case "Tan tan," so-called because that was his only word, are apparently no less human and no less aware of things than the rest of us, as evidenced by "Tan tan's" undiminished ability to communicate his needs using this single word. If Merleau-Ponty was right in supposing that language opens up the world of the other to us why was it that one severely aphasic patient (Sacks 1985) was reputedly more adept at identifying which politicians were lying on television than when he had his full language faculties.

Only Scheler's view, or some similar thesis, which acknowledges the primacy of the object and a word's original enmeshment in this but not its genesis, and which envisages further stages in thought development, each with a different sort of linguistic contribution, can do justice to the psychopathology on display in this field. Only some such thesis can explain the multiplicity apparent here—a failure of language as communication (non-aphasic misnaming), a different sort of failure of language as a set of phonemic, syntactic, and semantic disordered rules with preserved communication (aphasia), and a dual failure of language as communication breakdown coupled with idiosyncratic disregard of the rules governing the formation of the core elements of language.

BIBLIOGRAPHY

Andreasen N. C. (1979). "Thought, Language, and Communication Disorders." *Archives of General Psychiatry* 36: 1315–1330.

Bleuler E. (1911/1950). *Dementia Praecox*. New York: International University Press.

Blumstein S. E. (1995). "The Neurobiology of the Sound Structure of Language." In M S. Gazzaniga (ed.), *The Cognitive Neurosciences*, pp. 915–929. Cambridge, MA: MIT Press.

Braun C. M. J, Dumont M., Duval J., and Hamel-Hébert I. (2004). "Speech Rate as a Sticky Switch: A Multiple Lesion Case Analysis of Mutism and Hyperlalia." *Brain and Language* 89: 243–252.

Broca P. (1861). "Remarques sur le siège de la faculté du langage articulé, suivies d'une observation d'aphémie." *Bulletin de la Société Anatomique de Paris* 6: 330–357.

Cameron N. (1938). "Reasoning, Regression and Communication in Schizophrenia." *Psychological Monographs* 50: 1–34.

Caplan D. (1995). "The Cognitive Neuroscience of Syntactic Processing." In M S Gazzaniga (ed.), *The Cognitive Neurosciences*, pp. 871–879. Cambridge, MA: MIT.

Cassirer E. (1929/1957). *The Philosophy of Symbolic Forms Vol 3*. New Haven: Yale University Press.

Cassirer E. (1944). *An Essay on Man*. New haven: Yale University Press.

Chaika E. (1974). "A Linguist Looks at 'Schizophrenic' Language." *Brain and Language* 1: 257–276.

Deglin V. L. (1993). "Die paradoxale Mentalität oder warum Fiktionen die Realität ersetzen." In P. Grzybek (ed.), *Psychosemiotik—Neurosemiotik*, pp. 55–93. Bochum: Universitäts Verlag Dr. Norbert Brockmeyer.

Gelb A. and Goldstein K. (1925). "Psychologische Analysen hirnpathologischer Fälle." *Psychologische Forschung* 6: 127–214.

Glezerman T. B. and Balkowski V. I. (1999). *Language, Thought and the Brain*. New York: Kluwer Academic.

Goldstein K. (1939). "The Significance of Special Mental Tests for Diagnosis and Prognosis in Schizophrenia." *American Journal of Psychiatry* 96: 575–588.

Heidegger M. (1959/1971a). "Language." In *Heidegger's Poetry, Language, Thought*, pp. 189–210. New York: Harper & Row.

Heidegger M. (1959/1971b). "The Nature of Language. In *Heidegger's On the Way to Language*, pp. 57–108. New York: Harper & Row.

Herschmann H. and Schilder P. (1919). "Träume der Melancholiker nebst Bemerkungen zur Psychopathologie der Melancholie." *Zeitschrift für die gesamte Neurologie und Psychiatrie* 53: 130–160.

Hurlburt R. T. (1990). *Sampling Normal and Schizophrenic Inner Experience*. New York: Plenum Press.

Husserl E. (1929). "Formale und transzendentele Logik." *Jahrbuch für Philosophie und phänomenologische Forschung* 10: 1–298.

Merleau-Ponty M. (1960/1964). "On the Phenomenology of Language." In *Merleau-Ponty's Signs*, pp. 84–97. Evanston: Northwestern University Press.

Owen G. S., Cutting J., and David A. S. (2007). "Are People with Schizophrenia More Logical than Healthy Volunteers? *British Journal of Psychiatry* 191: 453–454.

Rapp B. C. and Caramazza A. (1995). "Disorders of Lexical Processing and the Lexicon. In M. S. Gazzaniga (ed.), *The Cognitive Neurosciences*, pp. 901–913. Cambridge, MA: MIT Press.

Sacks O. (1985). *The Man who Mistook his Wife for a Hat*. London: Duckworths.

Scheler M. (1926/2008). *The Constitution of the Human Being*. Milwaukee: Marquette University Press.

Shimkunas A. M. (1972). "Conceptual Deficit in Schizophrenia: A Reappraisal." *British Journal of Medical Psychology* 45: 149–157.

Storch A. (1924). "The Primitive Archaic Forms of Inner Experiences and Thought in Schizophrenia." *Nervous and Mental Diseases Monographs* 36.

Vygotsky L. S. (1934). "Thought in Schizophrenia." *Archives of Neurology and Psychiatry* 31: 1063–1077.

Weinstein E. A. and Kahn R. L. (1952). "Nonaphasic Misnaming in Organic Brain Disease." *Archives of Neurology and Psychiatry* 67: 72–79.

Weinstein E. A. and Kahn R. L. (1955). *Denial of Illness.* Charles C Thomas Springfield 111.

CHAPTER 51

....

AFFECTIVITY AND
ITS DISORDERS

....

KEVIN AHO

INTRODUCTION

....

THE impact of phenomenology on our current understanding of psychopathology is informed, largely, through the ways in which it challenges traditional psychological and be-
haviorist views that regard emotions and moods in terms of subjective mental states that
(1) reside "inside" the minds or brain of the individual; (2) are generally caused by external
stimuli; and (3) generate evidence that can be identified in the "outer" behavior—for example, speech patterns, posture, movements, facial expressions, etc.—of the individual.
Martin Heidegger's phenomenology of "mood" (*Stimmung*) has been especially influential in dismantling this view. By interpreting the human being not as a substance—as an
encapsulated mind or *ego cogito*, for instance, or some combination of physical and mental
substance—but in terms of the unitary activity of "being-in-the-world," Heidegger dissolves
the "inner/outer" distinction by positing how moods disclose the way we are already affectively bound up in the world. Thus, in *Being and Time*, he writes, "A mood assails us. It comes
neither from 'outside' nor from 'inside', but arises out of being-in-the-world . . . Having a
mood is not related to the psychical . . . and is not itself an inner condition which then reaches
forth in an enigmatical way and puts its mark on things and persons" (1927/1962: 137).

On this account, moods are not to be viewed as fleeting or contingent aspects of human
experience. They are, rather, constitutive of what it means "*to be*" human, which means we
are structurally affective or "mooded" (*stimmungsmässigen*) beings. Heidegger refers to this
structure of existence in terms of *Befindlichkeit*, a notoriously difficult word to translate that
is sometimes rendered as "affectedness" but is perhaps best understood as "situatedness"
in the sense that a condition or structure of being human is that we invariably "find"
(*finden*) ourselves bound up in worldly situations where things—for example, people, cultural practices, natural events, equipment, etc.—affectively "matter to" us in specific ways.[1]

....

[1] *Befindlichkeit* is derived from "*befinden*" ("to find oneself in a certain state or situation") as in
the ordinary expression "*Wie befinden Sie sich?*" which means "How are you?" or more literally,
"How do you find (*finden*) yourself?" It has, over the years, been translated in a number of ways as

Understood this way, we cannot help but find ourselves in moods because we are already woven into a normative field or horizon of meaning that makes particular emotions possible, where, for instance, a thunder storm can disclose itself *as frightening*, a long lecture *as boring*, or an impending ski trip *as exciting*.[2] This means "emotions" are distinct from "moods" in the sense that the former are intentionally specific; they have the character of being "about" something insofar as they are directed at particular objects, events, and situations in the world. They also have determinate causes and are relatively intense, focused, and short-lived. Moods, on the other hand, are more enduring, unfocused, and indeterminate; they do not have an intentional correlate and are, consequently not directed at particular objects in the world but to the world *as a whole*. Moods are atmospheric or global feelings-states to the extent that they both affectively color and open up a person's perceptual field or horizon of awareness (Stanghellini and Rosfort 2013). This explains why Heidegger says: "Moods are *not side-effects*, but are something which in advance determines our being with one another. It seems as though moods [are] in each case already there . . . like an atmosphere in which we immerse ourselves in each case and which then attunes us through and through" (1995: 67). When exploring the nature of psychopathology then, it important to take care in distinguishing between different kinds of affective states. There is a profound difference, for instance, between a person who is depressed *about something* or anxious *toward someone* on the one hand, and a person who is globally depressed and anxious. In the latter instance, depression and anxiety constitute an a priori background or horizon on the basis of which a person can affectively experience or perceive anything. Moods are not generalized and diffuse emotions but, rather, serve as the condition for the possibility of emotions, for anything to affectively "matter" to us in the first place (Fuchs 2013). On this account, it is usually a person's moods, not their emotions that are illuminated in psychopathologic states.

When we are healthy and going about our daily lives, this background sense of "mattering" is so close and familiar that it withdraws to the extent that we are unaware of our moods. This poses unique challenges for psychologists and psychiatrists because moods are generally disclosed to us pre-reflectively, that is, "*prior to* all cognition and volition, and *beyond* their range of disclosure" (Heidegger 1927/1962: 136). We cannot get behind our moods and examine them from a perspective of objectivity and detachment because this dispassionate perspective *is itself* a mood. Thus, the best way to gain access to the lived experience and meaning of psychopathology is not by taking an attitude of theoretical detachment but by attending to first-person descriptions of how the affective and orienting structure of *Befindlichkeit* is disrupted or breaks down. The following draws on experiential accounts to illuminate this structural disruption from three different perspectives: embodiment, being-with-others, and temporality.

"state of mind" (Heidegger 1927/1962), "affectedness," (Dreyfus 1991), "disposition" (Wrathall 2001) and "findingness" (Haugeland 2013). I follow Guignon's (1984) translation as "situatedness" because it best captures the sense of being bound up in an affective context or situation (Elpidorou and Freeman 2015).

[2] This is why Heidegger says, "The fact that moods can deteriorate and change over time means simply that in every case Dasein [human existence] always has some mood" (1927/1962: 134).

EMBODIMENT

One way to grasp how *Befindlichkeit* dissolves the "inner/outer" distinction is to see it in terms of what Matthew Ratcliffe calls "existential feeling," that is, both a "feeling of the body" and a "way of finding oneself in the world" (2008: 2). Like moods, existential feelings are not directed at specific objects or situations in the world but serve, rather, as the background orientation or grip that structures our affective experience of objects and situations. When we are healthy this mediating grip remains hidden or concealed from us in the sense that we are not self-consciously aware of it.[3] A signature aspect of the existential feeling of health, then, is our affective connection with the world, a taken-for-granted bond that makes it possible to intentionally move through lived space, to reach out and handle equipment, engage with others, and perform workday tasks. In this state, the body is not a conspicuous "physical object" (*Körper*) that I am contingently connected to. It is, rather, a "lived body" (*Leib*), the living medium through which I engage the world and affectively experience things, and it disappears in the spontaneous performance and flow of these tasks (e.g. Aho and Aho 2008; Gadamer 1996; Leder 1990; Sveneaus 2000).

Psychopathological states tend to disrupt the mediating activity of existential feeling, resulting in ordinary tasks presenting themselves as difficult if not impossible. First-person accounts often refer to feelings of being "immobilized," "frozen," "stiffened," and "paralyzed" (Fuchs 2005; Karp 1996). Pulled out of its seamless bond with the world, our body reveals itself as an obstacle or burden, as a clumsy, lethargic, and heavy object. In this state, the sufferer becomes acutely aware of bodily phenomena that were previously concealed in the flow of everydayness such as constriction in the chest when breathing, nausea in the stomach, pain in the joints, or pressure and a dull ache in the head (Ratcliffe 2015). In severe cases the body is described in a depersonalized way as not even belonging to oneself, showing up as "unreal," "alien," or even "dead" as can be the case in Cotard's syndrome, where a sufferer may no longer feel their own body or the sensations of taste, smell, and touch (Fuchs 2005, 2013). When we experience our corporeality in this way, lived space invariably begins to close up or shrink as perception, sensory motor function, and bodily movement become increasingly inhibited and constrained resulting in slowed speech patterns and postural changes such as a bowed head, lowered shoulders, and a sluggish gait (Fuchs 2005).

BEING-WITH-OTHERS

As a way of finding oneself in a world, existential feelings also disclose the unique ways in which this world is shared or inter-affective. On this view, I am not an isolated and self-enclosed subject of experience but a situated or public way of being, and I understand who

---

[3] Hans Georg-Gadamer (1996) describes the inconspicuousness of health in the following way: "Health is not a condition that one instrospectively feels *in oneself*. Rather, it is a condition of being involved, of being-in-the-world, of being together with one's fellow human beings, of active and rewarding engagement in one's everyday tasks" (113, my emphasis).

I am and what matters to me only in relation to my involvement with others. This relational ontology suggests my identity or self-interpretation is indelibly shaped by how others understand and perceive me. Psychopathology, in this regard, often creates a "stigmatized identity" (Goffman 1963) as agitation, awkward behavior, and inhibited motility and comportment disrupts the social order and the taken-for-granted flow of daily life. And this disruption is invariably mirrored or reflected back on the suffering individual. The gaze of the other leaves a stigma or mark that not only exacerbates already diminished sensory motor capacities and competencies in handling ordinary social situations; it also shapes and constitutes the sufferer's self-interpretation. This is what Heidegger means when he refers to "the real dictatorship of [*the They*]" (1927/1962: 126). The fact that existential feelings disclose how we find ourselves in a public world illuminates the ways in which others exercise a silent power over us to such an extent that they "supply the answer to the question of *who* [we are]" (128) [My emphasis].

Understanding the self in terms of being-with-others captures the way in which psychopathology should not be viewed in terms of private mental states located "inside" the head of the individual. It is, rather, a public *expression* of meaning and significance that disturbs the pre-given web of social expectations characteristic of health and normalcy. And this disturbance is often complicated by the fact that the source of psychopathology is not physically visible to others as it is with most somatic conditions. Without a wheelchair, physical lesion, or cane to point to, for example, the individual suffering from psychopathology can be further stigmatized and discredited for acting on the basis of something that is "unreal," "in your head," or worse, a "moral failing" (Aho and Aho 2008). This can result in feelings of reflexive shame and guilt, social phobia, and isolating behavior, which in turn creates a downward spiral that further undermines health (Fuchs 2003).

TEMPORALITY

Psychopathology can also distort the experience of time. On a physiological level, it can create the experience of, what Thomas Fuchs (2005) calls, "desynchronization" that disrupts the natural rhythmic equilibrium of the body as it pertains to processes such as sleep and menstrual cycles, digestion, temperature regulation, appetite, and sexual desire, and this can be extended to mood disturbances arising from bodily disunity with seasonal and atmospheric rhythms such as Seasonal Affective Disorder (SAD). On a social level, desynchronization can result in a sense of disconnection from public time as the busy demands of work and interactions with family and friends clash with lethargic motility and dulled cognitive functioning. References to feeling "overwhelmed," "unable to keep up," and "stressed" by the accelerated pace and harried obligations of modern life are common (Levine 1997, 2005). This can result in the erosion of stabilizing relationships and emotional support systems that can exacerbate the experience of isolation and loneliness, leading to feelings of "emptiness," "indifference," and "spiritual barrenness" (Aho 2007; Ulmer and Schwartzburd 1996).

In addition to the physiological and social aspects of desynchronization, there is also an existential dimension that involves the contraction or closing up of lived time, where this is understood as the horizon of sociohistorical possibilities that are open to the individual in creating his or her own identity or self-interpretation. Against the conventional view of time as a linear sequence of "now-points" that is external to us (e.g. clock-time), the phenomenological tradition introduces the idea that human existence is structured by time as a unified manifold that simultaneously stretches backward into the "past" and forward into the "future." Heidegger will refer to this manifold structure in terms of "thrown projection" in the sense that, out of the present, we are *thrown* into a specific situation (the past), and it is against the background of this situation that we press forward or *project* into future possibilities. Our temporal constitution is "ex-static" in the sense that we already "stand" (*stasis*) "outside" (*ex*) of ourselves by "running forward" (*vorlaufen*) into the future, into historically situated projects, identities, vocations, and relationships. Psychopathology disrupts this temporal unity and closes down the future as a horizon of possibilities. The result is a feeling of being trapped in "the present" (Fuchs 2005). This experience of temporal collapse is often described in terms of the "slowing-down," "dragging," or even "stopping" of time, and this makes it difficult to envision a meaningful identity or interpretation of who I might be in the future (Levine 2005; Ratcliffe 2015).

When the future contracts or closes down in this way, it can strip away the capacity for self-determination, that is, to interpret and give meaning to one's own situation. One of the distinctive features of the existential–phenomenological tradition, in this regard, is a configuration of the self as a relational tension between "facticity" ("being-in-itself") on the one hand and "transcendence" ("being-for-itself") on the other. This means humans do not act simply out of necessity arising out of the factical limitations of our physiological, sexual, or sociohistorical givenness. We are, rather, self-conscious beings that have the capacity to transcend or surpass these limitations by choosing to take a stand on them and giving them meaning. On this view, we understand who we are only in terms of the possibilities that we *project* for ourselves in the future by interpreting and taking a stand on the past that we have been *thrown* into. Psychopathology can erode away the meaning and significance of both the future and the past and, consequently, dim one's ability make or create oneself through meaning-giving choices. The future opens up not as an expansive horizon rich with affective meaning and significance but as a narrow and constricted "black hole" with possibilities that are affectively "meaningless" and "negative" (Karp 1996; Ratcliffe 2015). This means, in severe cases of temporal collapse, the very possibility of selfhood can be called into question (Aho 2014).

BIBLIOGRAPHY

Aho J. and Aho K. (2008). *Body Matters: A Phenomenology of Sickness, Illness, and Disease.* Lanham: Lexington Books.

Aho K. (2007). "Acceleration and Time Pathologies: The Critique of Psychology in Heidegger's *Beiträge.*" *Time and Society* 16(1): 25–42.

Aho K. (2014). "Depression and Embodiment: Phenomenological Reflections on Motility, Affectivity, and Transcendence." *Medicine, Healthcare, and Philosophy* 16(4): 751–759.

Dreyfus H. (1991). *Being-in-the-World: A Commentary on Heidegger's* Being and Time, *Division I.* Cambridge, MA: MIT Press.

Elpidorou A. and Freeman L. (2015). "Affectivity in Heidegger I: Moods and Emotions in Being and Time." *Philosophy Compass* 10(10): 661–671.

Fuchs T. (2003). "The Phenomenology of Shame, Guilt, and the Body in Body Dysmorphic Disorder and Depression." *Journal of Phenomenological Psychology* 33(2): 223–243.

Fuchs T. (2005). "The Phenomenology of the Body, Space and Time in Depression." *Comprendre* 15: 108–121.

Fuchs T. (2013). "The Phenomenology of Affectivity." In K. W. M. Fulford, M. Davies, R. Gipps, G. Graham, J. Sadler, G. Stanghellini, and T. Thornton (eds.), *Oxford Handbooks Online.* doi: 10.1093/oxfordhb/9780199579563.013.0038

Gadamer H. G. (1996). *The Enigma of Health.* Stanford: Stanford University Press.

Goffman E. (1963). *Stigma: Notes on the Management of Spoiled Identity.* New York: Touchstone Books.

Guignon C. (1984). "Moods in Heidegger's Being and Time." In R. Solomon and C. Calhoun (eds.), *What is an Emotion? Classic and Contemporary Readings* Oxford: Oxford University Press.

Haugeland J. (2013). *Dasein Disclosed.* Cambridge, MA: Harvard University Press.

Heidegger M. (1927/1962). *Being and Time,* trans. E. Robinson and J. Macquarrie. New York: Harper and Row.

Heidegger M. (1995). *Fundamental Concepts of Metaphysics: World, Finitude, Solitude,* trans. W. McNeill and N. Walker. Bloomington: Indiana University Press.

Karp D. (1996). *Speaking of Sadness: Depression, Disconnection, and the Meaning of Illness.* Oxford, UK: Oxford University Press.

Leder D. (1990). *The Absent Body.* Chicago: University of Chicago Press.

Levine R. (1997). *A Geography of Time.* New York: Basic Books.

Levine R. (2005). "A Geography of Busyness." *Social Research* 72: 355–370.

Ratcliffe M. (2008). *Feelings of Being: Phenomenology, Psychiatry and the Sense of Reality.* Oxford, UK: Oxford University Press.

Ratcliffe M. (2015). *Experiences of Depression: A Study in Phenomenology.* Oxford, UK: Oxford University Press.

Stanghellini G. and Rosfort R. (2013). *Emotions and Personhood: Exploring Fragility—Making Sense of Vulnerability.* Oxford, UK: Oxford University Press.

Sveneaus F. (2000). *The Hermeneutic of Medicine and the Phenomenology of Health: Steps Towards a Philosophy of Medical Practice.* Dordrecht: Kluwer.

Ulmer D. K. and Schwartzburd L. (1996). "Treatment of Time Pathologies." In *Heart and Mind: The Practice of Cardiac Psychology.* Washington: American Psychological Association.

Wrathall M. (2001). "Background Practices, Capacities, and Heideggerian Disclosure." In *Heidegger, Coping, and Cognitive Science: A Festschrift for Hubert Dreyfus. Vol. 2,* pp. 93–114. Cambridge: MIT Press.

CHAPTER 52

SELFHOOD AND ITS DISORDERS

JOSEF PARNAS AND MADS GRAM HENRIKSEN

INTRODUCTION

IF the concept of self is equated with that of the "psyche" in its common sense meaning or with that of "personality," then, trivially, all mental disorders are in some way disorders of selfhood. Therefore, a conceptual framework that defines and marks out the boundaries of these concepts is needed. The concept of the self is perhaps one of the most debated and fascinating philosophical concepts, with a remarkable recent renaissance in philosophy and psychopathology (Gallagher 2011). The literature is full of different and proliferating concepts of the self—for example, Strawson once summarized the contemporary discussions on the self within a single, academic journal, finding no less than twenty-one different concepts of the self (1999: 484).

In this essay, we first present a simplified classification of some major views on the self that can be found in modern philosophical and psychopathological literature. Subsequently, we explore how different levels or aspects of selfhood can be unstable or disturbed in different mental disorders.

CONCEPTS OF SELF

The "No Self" Doctrines

These theories comprise a vast range of claims. Some of the early, critical approaches to the self can be found in Hume, who, in his famous search for the "self," was unable to find it[1] or, in

---

[1] "For my part, when I enter most intimately into what I call *myself*, I always stumble on some particular perception or other, of heat or cold, light or shade, love or hatred, pain or pleasure. I never can catch *myself* at any time without a perception, and never can observe anything but the perception" (Hume 1888: 252; author's italics).

Nietzsche, who claimed that "The 'subject' is only a fiction: the ego of which one speaks when one censures egoism does not exist at all" (1967: 199). In twentieth-century philosophy, we find the structuralist and postmodernist proclamation of the "death" or "disappearing" of the subject (e.g. Foucault 2005). The subject or the self is here a "de-centered," passive locus of intersection of multiple historical, ideological, and socio-economical powers and discourses. Another view, predominantly originating in analytic philosophy, is to consider the self (or the "I") as a purely linguistic indexical device, bereft of any ontological thickness or of phenomenological significance. On yet another view, the Buddhist-oriented "no self" claims are, in fact, not denying individual self-experience but rather arguing that the experience of self is illusory (in a very specific sense [e.g. Albahari 2006]). From the position of phenomenological psychiatry, a common feature of the "no self" doctrines is their limited utility or even inapplicability to clinical work—are we, for example, supposed to calm a patient, expressing a terrifying lack of the sense of self, that such a sense under all circumstances is an illusory construction?

The "Experiential Self" Doctrines

The most prominent "experiential self" doctrines of our time are arguably found within phenomenology (e.g. Zahavi 2005, 2014). Notably, these doctrines have important predecessors, for example, within German idealism.[2] From a phenomenological perspective, all experience manifests in the first-person perspective as "my" experience—that is, the first-person givenness of experience implies a sense of "mine-ness," "for-me-ness," or "ipseity" that transpires through the flux of time and changing modalities of consciousness (Parnas and Sass 2011; Henriksen and Parnas 2014: 543f.). Crucially, the self, in the phenomenological sense, is not given as some kind of "object" that may show up in our experience; it is also not construed as some hypothetical substrate beneath the-stream of consciousness, somehow linking or unifying its different modalities; and, finally, the self is also not considered fully absent, unconscious, or otherwise experientially inaccessible. Rather, the phenomenological view is that the self manifests itself *pre-reflectively* as a specific mode or configuration of experience. I am always *pre-reflectively* aware of being myself and I have no need for self-reflection to assure myself of being myself (e.g. I do not need to reflect upon *who* these feelings or thoughts might belong to in order to know that it is *me*). Differently put, pre-reflective self-awareness makes self-reflection possible (Sartre 2003: 9). The reflecting (noetic) self recognizes itself in the reflected-upon (noematic) self without any need of criteria-based self-identification. Most importantly, this pre-reflective, experiential self is an intrinsic feature of experience that is operative in all forms of experience, imbuing all

---

[2] e.g. Kant writes, "I am therefore conscious of the identical self in regard to the manifold of the representations that are given to me in an intuition because I call them all together *my* representations, which constitute *one*. But that is as much as to say that I am conscious a priori of their necessary synthesis, which is called the original synthetic unity of apperception, under which all representations given to me stand, but under which they must also be brought by means of a synthesis" (1998: 248; author's emphasis). By contrast, phenomenology does not consider the self as a non-experiential, transcendental condition of possibility for experience but as a fundamental, pre-reflective feature of experience (see Zahavi's chapter on "Self" in this volume).

my experiences with an elusive, yet absolutely vital feeling of "I-me-myself" (e.g. Sass and Parnas 2003: 428f.; Hart 2009: 310; Henriksen and Nordgaard 2014: 436). This persistent, propertyless feeling of "I-me-myself" or "for-me-ness" constitutes the very "foundation" upon which richer, more complex forms of selfhood such as personhood or narrativity are constructed throughout our lives (Henriksen and Parnas 2014: 543f.). The "pre-reflective," "minimal," or "experiential" self, as the ubiquitous first-person feature of experience (Zahavi 2014), can be descriptively expanded to entail a sense of singularity, synchronic and dia-chronic self-identity, embodiment, and self–other demarcation.

THE SELF AS A PERSON OR NARRATIVE STRUCTURE

An appropriate answer to the question "Who am I?" would be something like "I am XY, with this particular age and body, these particular preferences, values, inclinations, and dispositions (including cognitive abilities, knowledge, temperamental features), and char-acter." This personal or narrative self is a product of countless interactions with other people (especially caregivers in childhood) and objects throughout life. They are partly retained in my explicit and implicit memory and partly sedimented in my dispositional reper-toire, my "habitus," as it were. My personal narrative forms what has been called an "innere Lebensgeschichte," that is, a story that I tell myself and others and that maximizes the co-herence of my personal life vicissitudes. Obviously, the personal or narrative self is heavily dependent on language and culture, and we may consider it the most complex and sophisti-cated form of selfhood.

The minimal or experiential self enters into this personal-narrative structure as a pre-condition, configuring the modes of experiential life. In other words, there is no contradic-tion or tension between the minimal-experiential self and the personal-narrative self. The narrative self has a highly complex identity-structure, which has been well captured by, among others, Ricoeur (1992), who operates with a dialectics of "ipse"-identity ("self") and of "idem"-identity ("same" [même]). Sameness ("idem-identity") can be illustrated, in ex-tremis, by the permanence or unchanging persistence of a stone; whereas selfhood ("ipse-identity" or "ipseity") implies no "unchanging core of the personality" (1992: 2). In brief, an individual remains in some sense the *same* person throughout life with a form of same-ness, whose components nonetheless change (e.g. the aging body), and where its *identity* is achieved by the interaction between the "self," the "same," and others. The self ("ipse"), in this triangle, is the unchanging first-person perspective—for example, if I keep a promise that I made twenty years ago, we can say that despite the fact that all my psychophysical charac-teristics have changed, the identity of the one "who" made the promise, that is, "me," remains intact.

DISORDERS OF SELF

Talking about "disorders" of "something" derives from a discourse in somatic medicine, where we, for example, can talk about "diseases" of the "liver." When we say "disorders" of

"X," then the "X" is envisaged as a well-demarcated "object," which is then "disturbed" in the sense of not functioning properly. However, it is difficult to replace the object "X" with the concept of "self," because the self, in the phenomenological or experiential sense, is precisely not an object, thing, or organ. As initially noted, all mental disorders may have some consequences or connotations that are reflected in some aspects or levels of selfhood. A complementary problem is linked to nosological issues. In brief, many of the contemporary diagnoses that display an epidemic-like rise in incidence (e.g. autism spectrum disorders, borderline personality disorder, and dissociative conditions) have very poor validity (Parnas 2017). Many of these issues are associated with an increasing tendency of basing a diagnosis on symptom checklists, either self-rated by the patient or ascertained through a structured, psychiatric interview (Parnas 2012; Nordgaard et al. 2012, 2013; Parnas and Bovet 2015). For the purpose of this article, we explore only the schizophrenia spectrum disorders, melancholia, other psychiatric syndromes, and personality disorders (most of which admittedly also have questionable validity). In our view, it is only in the case of schizophrenia spectrum disorders that we may truly talk about disorders of the self as a fundamental and generative feature of the illness. In the case of melancholia, we may identify certain pathologies of self-experience and certain personality characteristics (viz. *typus melancholicus* (Tellenbach 1980; Ambrosini et al. 2011)), but these manifestations seem to be mainly secondary to the underlying disorder of melancholia, which is most likely of temporality or, as Fuchs puts it, results from a desynchronization of the temporal relation of organism and environment (Fuchs 2001).

The Schizophrenia Spectrum Disorders

Systematic, phenomenologically informed empirical studies (Parnas et al. 2003, 2005; Raballo and Parnas 2012; Raballo et al. 2011; Haug et al. 2012; Nordgaard and Parnas 2014) demonstrate an altered subjective life in patients with schizophrenia spectrum disorders, reflected in the presence of certain trait-like (i.e. enduring rather than episodic), non-psychotic, anomalous self-experiences (viz. "self-disorders")—for a review of the empirical studies, see Parnas and Henriksen (2014).

In the following, we illuminate some of the central features of the altered subjective life in the schizophrenia spectrum. Typically, patients complain of feeling ephemeral, of lacking an inner "core" or "nucleus," and not knowing who they truly are. These experiences are often intermingled with a feeling of being radically different from others ("Anderssein"); a feeling that often has persisted since early childhood and which frequently is verbalized as being "wrong" (Parnas and Henriksen 2015: 237–238). It is a feeling of a difference so fundamental that it may resist further predication; it revolves around a feeling of being *ontologically or categorically different* from others and it is often a source of a profound solitude—as one patient puts it, "I looked just like every other child, but inside I was different. It is as if I am another creature that somehow ended up inside a human body" (Henriksen and Nordgaard 2014: 436). Childhood fantasies of being, say, a secrete adoptee, time-traveler, or extra-terrestrial are regular attempts to grasp this enduring, unsettling feeling.

Furthermore, patients often suffer from a failing sense of self-presence or being one with oneself (i.e. automatic, criteria-less, non-mediated, self-coincidence or "radical self-recognition" [Parnas 2007]), which often invokes more reflective forms of self-identification to reassure oneself of being oneself, for example, persistent self-monitoring in which the patients excessively takes herself as an object of reflection (a form of hyperreflexivity [Sass and Parnas 2003]). The failing saturation of self-presence (or "ipseity") allows the experiential field of immanence to become increasingly alienated and spatialized, for example, thoughts may appear as if not generated by the patient or they may be transformed into object-like entities, almost physically locatable to specific brain regions. There is a correlative, diminished sense of embodiment (e.g. the body or parts of it may feel strange, the body may feel as if it does not really fit or it may feel somehow disconnected from the mind) and of embodied presence in the shared-social world, which frequently involve a decreased ability to be affected, drawn, or stimulated by others, objects, or situations. This diminished sense of immersion may also be linked to problems with "common sense" (Blankenburg 1971), indicative of disruptions at the level of immediate preconceptual resonance or attunement with the world (Henriksen et al. 2010). Typically, such problems manifest as difficulties in grasping what is contextually relevant and appropriate and as a failing sense of what others consider self-evident (e.g. the natural evidences or the tacit axioms of social interaction). Finally, it merits attention that many patients report a variety of transitivistic experiences of permeability or blurring of self–other or self–world boundaries as well as a range of quasi-solipsistic experiences (e.g. fleeting feelings of centrality, magical thinking, and insights into layers of reality that normally are hidden from others).[3]

Generally, self-disorders appear to have been present since childhood or early adolescence and they are typically experienced in an ego-syntonic way as *modes* rather than *objects* of experience—that is, though some self-disorders, but certainly not all, may be very distressing (e.g. "Anderssein" and transitivistic experiences), self-disorders are not experienced as "foreign elements" in the patients' mental life but rather as intrinsic and habitual aspects of their existence and identity, for example, reflected in statements such as "this is just who I am" (Henriksen and Parnas 2014).[4] Self-disorders form a crucial schizophrenia spectrum vulnerability phenotype. They seem to precede, prefigure, and constrain the range of symptoms that may emerge.

The phenomenal nature of self-disorders in schizophrenia suggests that we are confronted with a disorder of the "minimal" or "experiential" self. The self-disorder here is far more fundamental than any "self-related" complaints and behaviors or characterological traits encountered in the disorders outside the schizophrenia spectrum—for example, psychological self-image or self-esteem, that is, thematized self-representational problems related at to "personal" or "narrative" selfhood.[5] At this level, the "minimal" or "experiential" self, that is, the ubiquitous first-person feature of experience, is never at stake. We have elsewhere proposed that a generative trait feature of schizophrenia is a disorder of "ipseity" or

---

[3] For rich clinical descriptions of self-disorders in schizophrenia, see Parnas and Handest (2003), Henriksen and Parnas (2012, 2017), and Henriksen and Nordgaard (2016).

[4] We have elsewhere reconceived the notion of "poor insight" in schizophrenia, suggesting that poor insight into illness is rooted in the nature of the patients' self-disorders and the related articulation of psychotic symptoms (Henriksen and Parnas 2014).

[5] Patients with schizophrenia may also exhibit self-representational problems. These are, however, largely consequential to the basic ipseity disorder. By contrast, self-representational problems alone, as encountered in, say, personality disorders, do not seem to imply any disorders of ipseity.

"minimal" self, viz. the *Ipseity-Disturbance Model* (Sass and Parnas 2003; Cermolacce et al. 2007; Nelson et al. 2014; see also Sass's chapter on "Schizophrenia as a self-disorder" in this volume). Finally, it merits attention that the notion of "ipseity disorder" does not imply something like a lack or dissolution of the "minimal" self or the first-person perspective. Rather, it indicates an instability in the normally tacit, taken-for-granted, pre-reflective sense of being a subject of awareness and action, which no longer saturates the experiential life in the usual, unproblematic way (Parnas and Henriksen 2014: 254–255).

Melancholia

Melancholia is another disorder with pronounced changes in the subjective life. However, it is important to realize from the very outset that a differential diagnosis between affective illness and schizophrenia cannot be based on the phenomenological exploration of the qualities of depersonalization that are characteristic of these conditions. Rather, it is important to consider the overall synchronic and diachronic gestalts of the disorders. Typically, melancholia is an episodic disorder in which alterations of subjectivity are state-phenomena. The most important of these changes, apart from mood, are "desynchronization" (associated with global slowing or "inhibition" of cognitive and psychomotor processes) and "corporealization" of the lived body (Fuchs 2001, 2005). There is a lag between subjective-lived time and the intersubjective-objective time, with an ensuing feeling of "not being able to . . .," that is, a kind of global insufficiency that is often associated with self-alienation. The patient may feel a sort of inner burden or obstacle, yet the "ipseity" or "for-me-ness" of experience remains intact in her self-relation—as Tatossian (2007) puts it, it is a relation of "moi à moi." In melancholia, the mental processes are slowed down with diminished and/or delayed reactivity, activity, and cognition (pseudo-dementia).

Moreover, existential time is also changed, that is, access to the future is blocked and the past relentlessly haunts the patient. The lived body loses its transparency and turns into a solid, material object, inhibiting access to the world in the sense of no longer opening it up as a realm of possibilities for action and intention (Fuchs 2005). Increasingly unable to transcend the body, the patient gradually finds herself confined within a heavy, rigid, decaying body (ibid.; Stanghellini et al. 2014). Consequently, patients typically report at variety of somatic complaints. In extremis, the profound sense of devitalization in melancholia results in the Cotard syndrome, where the patient feels dead inside (this syndrome may also be seen in schizophrenia).

In sum, we may encounter some disorders of the "experiential self" in melancholia but here they appear to be *state-phenomena, with largely intact ipseity.* These disorders are probably secondary to the disorders of mood, temporality, and embodiment.

OTHER PSYCHIATRIC SYNDROMES

Recent years have witnessed an increase in certain diagnostic categories (and a corresponding decrease in schizophrenia spectrum disorders), which, at least potentially, may involve disorders of the experiential self, for example, autistic spectrum disorders and dissociative disorders. We consider those increases to be, to a large extent, a reflection of differential-diagnostic disarray of operational psychiatric diagnosis. Thus, in many cases, what clinicians call "dissociative disorders," fulfil the diagnostic criteria for schizophrenia; similarly, those diagnosed with depersonalization typically suffer from schizotypal disorder (Parnas 2012, 2015, 2017). Moreover, the concept of "dissociation" seems to have been trivialized to any kind of mental disintegration. If "dissociation" means disintegration between mental contents and modalities, then all severe mental disorders contain an element of dissociation (e.g. a recurrent and disturbing obsession, a tendency to ruminate, or hearing a voice). In this case, the term does not contribute to psychopathological knowledge and seems vacuous. However, if "dissociation" is meant to indicate the existence of two parallel or alternating subjective streams of consciousness that are mutually unaware of each other, then dissociation is not a condition seen in psychiatric practice (Hacking 1998).

Personality Disorders

Insofar as it makes sense to use a phenomenological concept of self in the context of personality disorders, it is crucial to realize that it is the concept of "personal-narrative" self that is at stake here, not that of the "minimal" or "experiential" self. With a few exceptions, there is no phenomenological tradition of studying personality. Jung's influential "Psychological Types" (1971), written from his particular analytic point of view, contains, nonetheless, phenomenologically oriented explorations of the interplay of cognition, feelings, and general orientation such as extra- and introversion. Another, highly original approach to personality types, considering the latter as being reflective of more fundamental cognitive styles, can be found in the works of Shapiro (1965).

In the clinical context, personality disorders are the matter of clinical psychology and psychodynamic or cognitive behavior therapy. However, the very concept of "personality disorders" is unclear and it seems that psychiatry is here entangled in its own insufficiently clarified terminological history. In brief, the concept of "personality" stems from moral philosophy. In the nineteenth century, the concept of "personality" was equated with that of the "psyche." Thus, Ribot's famous textbook of psychiatry carried the title "*Les Maladies de la Personnalite*" (1884). In the twentieth century, Jaspers (1997) claims that primary delusion involves a transformation of the "whole personality," by which he means the very structures of subjectivity. The classification of Kurt Schneider (1923), which forms the root of the current DSM-5 (APA 2013) and ICD-10 (WHO 1992) classifications of personality disorders, contains categories that are in fact subsyndromic rather than reflecting pure personality types. Psychometric personality research emphasizes the following five dimensions or factors: openness, conscientiousness, extroversion, agreeableness, and neuroticism—these dimensions will be incorporated in the forthcoming ICD-11. These descriptive notions may be considered as features of the "personal-narrative" self.

Conclusion

The concept of selfhood is not derived from psychopathology and even in philosophy there is little agreement upon its significations. Thus, from a global perspective, the concept of selfhood is of little value to clinicians and researchers. This situation could be perhaps ameliorated if the concept of self underwent more rigorous conceptualization and strati-fication. However, there is one important exception to this general statement, namely the case of schizophrenia spectrum disorders. Here, it seems that the disorders of self-presence and basic self–world relation are at the very core of the illness. Already now, this knowledge is applicable in a therapeutic context and useful for diagnostic and differential-diagnostic purposes. With respect to etiological research, we see a potential for a more integrative con-ceptualization of the neurodevelopmental hypothesis of schizophrenia (Innocenti et al. 2003). Such integration needs to involve the existing insights from developmental psy-chology, psychoanalysis, phenomenology, basic neuroscience, and molecular genetics. This kind of integrative conceptualization might allow a formation of derivative, more specific hypotheses, that are testable in empirical contexts. In the current neurobiological research of symptom-substrate correlations, it is, in our view, crucial to consider the phenotypic level of schizophrenia, not as aggregation of different symptoms but rather as a trait-like alteration of the basic structures of experience.

BIBLIOGRAPHY

Albahari M. (2006). *Analytical Buddhism. The Two-Tiered Illusion of the Self.* Basingstoke: Palgrave Macmillan.
Ambrosini A., Stanghellini G., and Langer Á. I. (2011). "Typus Melancholicus from Tellenbach up to the Present Day: A Review about the Premorbid Personality Vulnerable to Melancholia." *Actas Españolas de Psiquiatría* 39: 302–311.
American Psychiatric Association (APA) (2013). *Diagnostic and Statistical Manual of Mental Disorders: DSM-5.* Arlington: APA.
Blankenburg W. (1971). *Der Verlust der natürlichen Selbstverständlichkeit. Ein Beitrag zur Psychopathologie symptomarmer Schizophrenien.* Stuttgart: Enke.
Cermolacce M., Naudin J., and Parnas J. (2007). "The 'Minimal Self" in Psychopathology: Re-examining the Self-disorders in the Schizophrenia Spectrum." *Consciousness and Cognition* 16: 703–714.
Foucault M. (2005). *The Order of Things. An Archaeology of the Human Sciences.* London, New York: Routledge.
Fuchs T. (2001). "Melancholia as a Desynchronization: Towards a Psychopathology of Interpersonal Time." *Psychopathology* 34: 179–186.
Fuchs T. (2005). "Corporealized and Disembodied Minds. A Phenomenological View of the Body in Melancholia and Schizophrenia." *Philosophy, Psychiatry, & Psychology* 12(2): 95–107.
Gallagher S. (2011). *The Oxford Handbook of the Self.* Oxford: Oxford University Press.
Hacking I. (1998). *Mad Travelers, Reflections on the Reality of Transient Mental Illnesses.* Charlottesville, London: University Press of Virginia.
Hart J. G. (2009). *Who One Is. Book 1. Meontology of the 'I': A Transcendental Phenomenology.* Berlin: Springer.
Haug E., Lien L., Raballo A., et al. (2012). "Selective Aggregation of Selfdisorders in First-treatment DSM-IV Schizophrenia Spectrum Disorders." *Journal of Nervous and Mental Disease* 200: 632–636.

Henriksen M. G., Škodlar B., Sass L. A., and Parnas J. (2010). "Autism and Perplexity: A Qualitative and Theoretical Study of Basic Subjective Experiences in Schizophrenia." *Psychopathology* 43: 357–368.

Henriksen M. G. and Parnas J. (2012). "Clinical Manifestations of Self-disorders and the Gestalt of Schizophrenia." *Schizophrenia Bulletin* 38: 657–660.

Henriksen M. G. and Nordgaard J. (2014). "Schizophrenia as a Disorder of the Self." *Journal of Psychopathology* 20: 435–441.

Henriksen M. G. and Parnas J. (2014). "Self-disorders and Schizophrenia: A Phenomenological Reappraisal of Poor Insight and Noncompliance." *Schizophrenia Bulletin* 40: 542–547.

Henriksen M. G. and Nordgaard J. (2016). "Self-disorders in Schizophrenia." In G. Stanghellini and M. Aragona (eds.), *An Experiential Approach to Psychopathology. What is it like to Suffer from Mental Disorders*, pp. 265–280. Springer.

Henriksen M. G. and Parnas J. (2017). "Clinical Manifestations of Self-disorders in Schizophrenia Spectrum Conditions." *Current Problems of Psychiatry* 18: 177–183.

Hume D. (1888). *A Treatise on Human Nature*, ed. L. A. Selby-Bigge. Oxford: Oxford University Press.

Innocenti G. M., Ansermet F., and Parnas J. (2003). "Schizophrenia, Neurodevelopment and Corpus Callosum." *Molecular Psychiatry* 8: 261–274.

Jaspers K. (1997). *General Psychopathology*, trans. J. Hoenig and M. W. Hamilton. London: Johns Hopkins University Press.

Jung C. G. (1971). *Collected Works, Vol. 6: Psychological Types*, trans. R. F. C. Hull. New Jersey: Princeton University Press.

Kant I. (1998). *Critique of Pure Reason*, trans. P. Guyer and A. W. Wood. New York: Cambridge University Press.

Nelson B., Parnas J., and Sass L. A. (2014). "Disturbance of Minimal Self (Ipseity) in Schizophrenia: Clarification and Current Status." *Schizophrenia Bulletin* 40: 479–482.

Nietzsche F. (1967). *The Will to Power*, trans. W. Kaufmann and R. J. Hollingdale. New York: Random House.

Nordgaard J., Revsbech R., Sæbye D., and Parnas J. (2012). "Assessing the Diagnostic Validity of a Structured Psychiatric Interview in a First-admission Hospital Sample." *World Psychiatry* 11: 181–185.

Nordgaard J., Sass L. A., and Parnas J. (2013). "The Psychiatric Interview: Validity, Structure, and Subjectivity." *European Archives of Psychiatry and Clinical Neuroscience* 263: 353–364.

Nordgaard J. and Parnas J. (2014). "Self-disorders and Schizophreniaspectrum: A Study of 100 First Hospital Admissions." *Schizophrenia Bulletin* 40: 1300–1307.

Parnas J. (2007). "Subjectivity in Schizophrenia: The Minimal Self is Too Small." In A. Grøn, I. Damgaard, and S. Overgaard (eds.), *Subjectivity and Transcendence*, pp. 55–70. Tübingen: Mohr Siebeck.

Parnas J. (2012). "DSM-IV and the Founding Prototype of Schizophrenia: Are We Regressing to a Pre-Kraepelinian Nosology?" In K. S. Kendler and J. Parnas (eds.), *Philosophical Issues in Psychiatry II: Nosology*, pp. 237–259. Oxford: Oxford University Press.

Parnas J. (2015). "Differential Diagnosis and Current Polythetic Classification." *World Psychiatry* 14: 284–287.

Parnas J. (2017). "Diagnostic Epidemics and Diagnostic Disarray: The Issue of Differential Diagnosis." In K. S. Kendler and J. Parnas (eds.), *Philosophical Issues in Psychiatry IV: Classification of Psychiatric Illness*, pp. 143–145. Oxford: Oxford University Press.

Parnas J. and Handest P. (2003). "Phenomenology of Anomalous Experiences in Early Schizophrenia." *Comprehensive Psychiatry* 44: 121–134.

Parnas J., Handest P., Saebye D., and Jansson L. (2003). "Anomalies of Subjective Experience in Schizophrenia and Psychotic Bipolar Illness." *Acta Psychiatrica Scandinavica* 108: 126–133.

Parnas J., Handest P., Jansson L., and Saebye D. (2005). "Anomalous Subjective Experience among First-admitted Schizophrenia Spectrum Patients: Empirical Investigation." *Psychopathology* 38: 259–267.

Parnas J. and Sass L. A. (2011). "The Structure of Self-consciousness in Schizophrenia." In S. Gallagher (ed.), *The Oxford Handbook of the Self*, pp. 521–546. Oxford: Oxford University Press.

Parnas J. and Henriksen M. G. (2014). "Disordered Self in the Schizophrenia Spectrum: A Clinical and Research Perspective." *Harvard Review of Psychiatry* 22(5): 251–265.

Parnas J. and Bovet P. (2015). "Psychiatry Made Easy: Operation(al)ism and Some of Its Consequences." In K. Kendler and J. Parnas (eds.), *Philosophical Issues in Psychiatry III: The Nature and Sources of Historical Science*, pp. 190–212. Oxford: Oxford University Press.

Parnas J. and Henriksen M. G. (2015). "Disturbance of the Experience of Self—A Phenomenologically Based Approach." In F. Waters and M. Stephane (eds.), *The Assessment of Psychosis: A Reference Book and Rating Scales for Research and Practice*, pp. 235–244. New York: Routledge.

Raballo A., Sæbye D., and Parnas J. (2011). "Looking at the Schizophrenia Spectrum through the Prism of Self-disorders: An Empirical Study." *Schizophrenia Bulletin* 37: 344–351.

Raballo A. and Parnas J. (2012). "Examination of Anomalous Self-experience: Initial Study of the Structure of Self-disorders in Schizophrenia Spectrum." *Journal of Nervous and Mental Disease* 200: 577–583.

Ribot T. (1884). *Les Maladies de la Personnalite*. Paris: Alcan.

Ricoeur P. (1992). *Oneself as Another*, trans. K. Blamey. Chicago: University of Chicago Press.

Sartre J.-P. (2003). *Being and Nothingness: An Essay in Phenomenological Ontology*, trans. H. E. Barnes. London, New York: Routledge.

Sass L. A. and Parnas J. (2003). "Schizophrenia, Consciousness, and the Self." *Schizophrenia Bulletin* 29: 427–444.

Schneider K. (1923). *Die psychopathischen Persönlichkeiten*. Leipzig/Wien: Deuticke.

Shapiro D. (1965). *Neurotic Styles*. New York: Basic Books.

Stanghellini G., Ballerini M., Blasi S., Mancini M., Presenza S., Raballo A., and Cutting J. (2014). "The Bodily Self: A Qualitative Study of Abnormal Bodily Phenomena in Persons with Schizophrenia." *Comprehensive Psychiatry* 55: 1703–1711.

Strawson G. (1999). "The Self and the SESMET." In S. Gallagher and J. Shear (eds.), *Models of the Self*, pp. 483–518. Thorverton: Imprint Academic.

Tatossian A. (2007). *La phénoménologie des psychoses*. Le Cercle Herméneutique, Collection Phéno. Paris: Vrin.

Tellenbach H. (1980). *Melancholy*, trans. E. Eng. Pittsburgh: Duquesne University Press.

World Health Organization (WHO) (1992). *The ICD-10. Classification of Mental and Behavioural Disorders*. Geneva: WHO.

Zahavi D. (2005). *Subjectivity and Selfhood. Investigating the First-Person Perspective*. Cambridge, MA: MIT Press.

Zahavi D. (2014). *Self and Other: Exploring Subjectivity, Empathy, and Shame*. Oxford: Oxford University Press.

CHAPTER 53

....

VITAL ANXIETY

....

MARÍA INÉS LÓPEZ-IBOR AND
JULIA PICAZO ZAPPINO

INTRODUCTION

....

> The great problem of present human beings is to have turned the meaning of life into problematic. That's why it is not strange that obstacles and setbacks of daily living appear wrapped in an atmosphere of anxiety. Juan José López-Ibor (1966).

ANXIETY is an ambiguous word, it is used to describe a feeling, a clinical symptom, and it is also a disorder by itself or a group of disorders (Barcia 1980; Lewis 1970).

It is a normal feeling that arises when a person believes themself to be endangered by an as yet unidentified threat or danger and, as a result of it, an increased state of alertness and exploratory attention is triggered. An emotional reaction also appears in order to protect ourselves from the danger (López-Ibor 1999).

Anxiety is a feeling and, as such, it is not just a pure psychological phenomenon. It consists also in bodily manifestations, in physiological correlates of emotions (tachycardia, blood pressure modifications, sweating, and so on). These emotions are linked to a choking sensation, oppression in the chest, and shortness of breath. Anxiety can be differentiated from anguish by feelings of inhibition (as in anguish) or on the contrary, feelings of uneasiness or nervousness (as in anxiety) (López-Ibor 1966).

It is a clinical symptom that appears in many diseases, not only in mental disorders (e.g. metabolic or cardiological conditions, cancer, and others). In medicine, symptoms are signs of an illness but in psychiatry this concept applies only partially—sometimes symptoms are the extremes of a trait conceived as dimensions, as for instance in the case of anxiety or in personality disorders. A patient suffers from an anxiety disorder when "anxiety and excessive worry (apprehensive anticipation) are present, preventing the patient from controlling the situation and when it is also accompanied by somatic symptoms such as restlessness, feeling trapped, fatigue, irritability and also persist for a while (DSM-5 2013; ICD-10 1992).

During the first half of the twentieth century the hypothesis of the origin of the meaning of anxiety was very much influenced by psychoanalytic theories (Breuer and Freud 1885-1893).

Freud changed his perspective of the concept of anxiety. Before 1926 he considered that there were two different types of anxiety: a real anxiety and a neurotic one. A real anxiety exists, it is produced by the perception of a real danger, whereas a neurotic anxiety is the consequence of the repression of the libido or the libidinous energies. After 1929 he considered that anxiety did not come from the repression of the libidinous instincts but that it was the very cause or reason of repression. Anxiety was at the very origin of psychic conflict. That is to say, he interpreted anguish almost as an adaptive reaction to a concrete situation, putting the individual in a state of alert and thus allowing them to avoid danger (López-Ibor 1966).

Neurosis was considered from a psychoanalytic point of view as an equivalent of anxiety and its symptoms secondary to it.

Freud (1967) highlighted this relationship between sadness (*traurig*), mourning (*Trauer*), and being sad (*Traurigkeit*), and the differentiation of anxiety when confronted to a danger.

Sadness is not a threat (as in anxiety) but a loss (psychic trauma, in psychoanalytic terminology) or currently stress (in the context of other research studies, defined by the feeling that one does not have control). In depression a new element is added, which is the sensation of having no escape, the feeling of not having a solution, the resignation to a *fait accompli*. If losses are changes it is because a loss has to be replaced, in a process able to maintain the psychic balance. Freud considered that anguish was the base of all neuroses, something endogenous and not reactive to any situation.

However, and at the same time, there were other theories coming from phenomenology and from existentialism that tried to explain the meaning of anxiety.

As substantiated by phenomenological and existentialist schools of thought (Kierkegaard (1957), Heidegger (1968/2002), and other philosophers, considered anxiety (*Angst* in German) as the basic radical of human condition.

For Heidegger *Angst* is the expression of the authentic existence, of *Dasein* confronting the fact of being-thrown-into-the-world.

For Kurt Schneider (1959) delusions in depressed patients are the manifestation of essential anxieties (*Ur-ängste*) of humankind: 1) the loss of health as a threat to physical integrity and survival (hypochondriac delusions); 2) economic losses as the threat of subsistence (delusions of poverty); and 3) losing the opportunity to access paradise due to a sinful existence (delusions of guilt).

ANXIETY AND ANGUISH

Anxiety and anguish share the same etymology, the Latin word *angŭstĭa*, "narrowness," "critical situation," derived from *angŭstŭs* "narrow," "strangle," "choke." Anxiety derives from the Latin *anxĭetas*, "craving," "aspiration," "worry," "embarrassment," and was introduced in modern languages through the French *anxiété*. Both *angŭstĭa* and *anxĭetas* derive from the Ancient Greek ἄγχω (*ángo*), "to strangle," "to press tight." In the course of time *angŭstĭa* and *anxĭetas* have been differentiated based on course, evolution, the presence or nature of somatic manifestations, the depth of the feeling, and other characteristics (Barcia 1980; Bomhard and Kerns 1994; Dalby 1993; *Diccionario de la lengua Española* 1970; López-Ibor 2010).

In most Roman languages *anguish* is a more profound feeling than *anxiety* and is experienced as a constriction of the throat or the chest that inhibits and hinders the activity. The expression of anxiety is related to the respiratory system, to the act of breathing, and not so much to the heart, as is the case with anguish. Anxiety conveys the impulse to liberate oneself from the threat. For that reason, the feeling of relief when anxiety has ended is a sigh (Lewis 1970–71; Dalby 1993; Eisler 1930). The philosopher Zubiri (1991), much on the same line of thought, has put the emphasis on the concept of *expectancy*.

López-Ibor (1966, 1999) has associated the words *sobrecogimiento* and *sobresalto* to two primitive defense reflexes to face a danger: the *Totstellung reflex* (death feigning reflex, death feint) present in the mimetic behavior of the animal which tries to disappear from the eyes of the predator and the *Bewegungssturm* (movement storm or tempest, instinct flurry) of poultry in the henhouse when they fly frightened by some danger. Both were described by Kretschmer (1958/1960) as reflexes underlying hysterical symptoms and López-Ibor (1966, 1965) extended the metaphor to all neurotic manifestations.

Nowadays anxiety and anguish are used to describe analogue and often interchangeable mood states. In French *anxieté* and *angoisse* were, until 150 years ago, synonymous. They share the feeling of fear being threatened by a non-identified cause (Lewis 1970–71; APA 2013; WHO 1992).

A patient described it as follows:

> I felt very bad for months, very sad and wanting to die. I'm also very nervous. I can't explain it very well . . . I would say that I have an awe, a feeling of internal restlessness that paralyzes and blocks me, doesn`t allow me to think clearly . . . It is as if I have a lump in my throat or in my stomach. Sometimes I also have palpitations and I get dizzy. And I cry a lot, but it doesn`t comfort me. I feel like this during the whole day, the only time I'm okay is when I sleep.

VITAL ANXIETY

Feelings are difficult to describe. Descartes (1637) considered them as confused thoughts, and other philosophers as rudiments of the reflective conscience before becoming conscious. Pascal (1954) started a tradition in which Schopenhauer, Nietzsche, and Freud stand out, that recovers the importance of the feelings, and of the non-rational aspects of human nature.

The concept of vital anxiety as a disturbance of vital feelings was introduced by Kurt Schneider (1959) following Max Scheler's description of four types of feelings (1972):

1. Sensory feelings (*Sinnliche Gefühle*), or feeling-sensations (*Empfindungsgefühle*) concerning specific parts of the body, such as pain, a knot in the stomach due to hunger or cold on the back from fear.
2. Vital feelings (*Lebensgefühle*), or body feelings (*Leibgefühle*) concerning body experience as a whole such as distress or wellbeing.
3. Psychic feelings (*seelische Gefühle*) or pure feelings of the Ego (*reine Ich Gefühle*), corresponding to the environment and external world. They are reactive to external circumstances such a joyfulness, enjoyment, sadness or despair.

4. Spiritual feelings (*geistige Gefühle*) or feelings of the personality (*Persönlichkeitsgefühle*),
   which are spontaneous, absolute beyond specific values, such as ecstasy or agony.

Vital feelings are those that allow us to feel our own life, in health and in illness, and
the values of the world that surrounds us. The first to use the term "vital feeling" was
Scheller—"a characteristic of cenesthesia, a vital feeling," that is to say, it is not located
nor captured with precision, nor has it a quality as marked as other sensations (quoted by
López-Ibor 1952).

López-Ibor Sr. (1950) came to the conclusion that anxiety which characterizes neurotic
disorders was a vital and not a psychic or reactive feeling, thus introducing the concept
of "vital anxiety." Vital anxiety is a vital feeling with the same characteristics as other vital
feelings such as those of well-being, discomfort, or vertigo. That is, global feelings that express our way of "being-in-the-world."

He considered that there was no disease able to reveal more of the mystery of life than
melancholy itself, claiming that "those who have been free of it, have never experienced real
suffering" (1952).

The transition between a vital or a mood feeling is important and is of great psychopathological interest. In the case of anxiety there is a *getting anxious*, an emotional reactive feeling (something has happened to me that has caused anxiety) and an anxious,
vital, non-reactive feeling (perhaps nothing has happened or nothing has happened that
we can attribute it to), and an *anxious being*, which denotes a temperamental tinge more
closely tied to personality.

Phenomenology of Vital Anxiety

Anxiety is related to our intimate relationship with ceasing to exist, with nothingness, with
the clear limits that derive from the very nature of human beings.

The purest forms of anxiety are fear of death and fear of madness (of losing control), which
are the manifestations of experiencing the threat of vanishing either physically or psychologically (Sarbin 1968).

Anxiety differs from fear in that anxiety is always felt before the unknown and fear appears
before the known, and that is why in the latter the emotional impact is less. On the contrary,
fear (*Phobos* in Greek) arises when threatened by something concrete and identified, anything can produce fear and therefore the catalog of phobias is an endless list. For Jaspers
(1958), there are a lot of people who seem to live fearlessly, because they lack imagination.

On the contrary, anxiety arises in the midst of the inexplicable, where the danger that
threatens is vague and indeterminate.

Anxiety does not appear in front of a specific object, essentially it appears in front of everything and in front of nothing, which is why we should not speak of an anxiety reaction but
rather of a situation of anxiety—one feels fear but also anxiety, every form of anxiety can be
reduced to two radicals: death or insanity.

Other authors go a step further and consider that human beings cannot live without anxiety. Gebssatel (1966) wrote: "We are as doubtful whether we really want a life without anxiety as we are certain that we want a life without fear."

The first thing we do is to seek an explanation to relieve ourselves from that anxiety, that is, to know why the illness, pain, and suffering caused by any disease is related to the threat of being ill and the possibility of death (López-Ibor 2010).

The problem of anxiety is intimately related to hope, because there is no human or psychological situation worse than despair (López-Ibor 1966).

We ask ourselves about the meaning of our illnesses, sometimes we try to link them to traumatic childhood events or previous painful experiences. The need to find a meaning for disease often comes from the need to deny transcendence. If we attribute disease to genes or to traumatic experiences or to any previous fact of life, we will not need to resort to the sense of transcendence to explain the meaning of disease.

Disease exists, and it exists because human beings are fragile, because they are "being for death" as defined by existentialists. Precisely for this reason, when human beings become sick and start asking questions, anxiety appears: "every sick person is deep down an anxious person" (Schneider 1959; Zubiri 1991; López-Ibor 2015).

What has to be done to maintain the hope of an ill person is to transform the meaning of their life, to let them go back to considering themselves belonging to the world. The world exists as long as we exist and we are in contact with it.

Normal and Pathological Anxiety

The concept of mental disorders, like many others concept in medicine, philosophy, and science, lacks a consistent definition capable of covering all situations. No definition is able to establish a precise boundary between normality and psychopathology. Psychiatric nosology has been turning around different categorical or dimensional models for the last two hundred years, and the problem is that symptoms cannot be confounded with diagnostic criteria.

The two main problems for the clinician and the researcher are the limits between normal and morbid psychological experiences; and the differences between anxiety and depression, even if these boundaries may sometimes be blurred (Yonkers et al. 1996; Angst et al. 1991).

In psychoanalysis the difference between normal and pathological anxiety was not taken into account, perhaps because Freud (1975) always wanted to make a psychopathology of daily life. Psychic anxiety cannot be equated to normal anxiety, nor can vital anxiety be equated to neurotic anxiety because vital feelings (including anxiety and sadness) are part of daily life, in which the four strata of sentimental life are or may be present, as described by Scheler (1972). Feelings are states of the self-incarnated in a corporeality (living body, incarnated soul, in our own world).

Humans, described by Heidegger (1968), live inauthentically, forgetting or ignoring what human life is, which means, we live our lives as far as possible ignoring the idea of death. But life cannot be imagined without the inexorable presence of death, disease is the image of that limit of our existence.

Normal anxiety differs from pathological anxiety in intensity, being experienced more at the psychic level, and the pathological one is somatized (with headaches, palpitations, tremors, and dizziness). It is also differentiated by its phasic evolution and by its relative independence from the environment and biographical factors (Yonkers 1996)

For López-Ibor (1965) the difference between vital and normal anxiety relied on another dimension; on the defense mechanisms they set in motion (phobias, obsessions, and conversational symptoms among others) that are not so striking in normal distress.

As Maj (2011) recently pointed out it is not always easy to establish when a depression becomes a mental disorder. He proposed three approaches: the first one is the need to take into account the context in which depression occurs; the second is that there is a qualitative difference between sadness and depression—in depression anhedonia is one of the main diagnostic criteria but it does not appear in sadness; and the third one is a pragmatic approach that considers a continuum for sadness in clinical depression.

VITAL ANXIETY AS A FORM OF NEUROSIS

The harmony of sentimental life in people suffering from a neurosis or those who are melancholic is lost, becoming dominated by vital feelings, which drown the rest (López-Ibor 1965).

The core of melancholic experience is the inability to experience or to feel sadness or what is the same: vital sadness, not reactive to daily life events. In the same way, a neurotic person is incapable of feeling anxiety, because everything is anxiety, and symptoms appear that are nothing other than the expression of the failure of their corporeality, which ceases to be silent and produces a heart that beats so hard it seems it is going to burst, lungs that prevent us from breathing, or complaints about the impossibility of doing or undoing (López-Ibor 1965, 1952).

At the beginning, patients do not articulate their distress but instead complain about headaches, trembling, or palpitations. They experience pathological anxiety not only as an uneasiness, and as a diffuse pain linked to the experience of corporality but as something tied to different parts of their own bodies. It is located in specific places (e.g. epigastrium, throat, etc.) or in more psychological aspects such as phobias. From this point of view, vital anxiety may be seen as a mixture of sensorial feeling and vital feeling.

The experience of anxiety is an experience of (sometimes unbearable) limits and when it ceases it can focus on something concrete that the subject identifies as "the cause" of anxiety. This way the appearance and creation of phobias can be understood, as phobias are a tendency to the chronification of anxiety and this anxiety itself will generate more anxiety, and the fear of anxiety is already anxiety (Angst et al. 1991).

For persons suffering from a neurotic disorder, the experience of death is lived as an "encounter with nothingness," with something that is outside, an emptiness into which the person falls. Anxiety, related to death and particularly, anxiety related to madness, or anxiety related to nothing in general, are experienced by each person in a typical and particular way. In pathological anxiety all this acquires a different nuance and is related to fear of situations, closer to everyday life events and gives rise to anxiety attacks (López-Ibor 1965).

At present, the terms anguish and anxiety are used as if they had similar meanings. In DSM-5 (2013) both would be encompassed in the concept of Generalized Anxiety Disorder (300.02), characterized by an excessive and disproportionate preoccupation, lasting for some time, with individuals feeling loss of control. Also present were daily aspects such as personal or family health, personal finances, work situation, household tasks, etc., which in principle should only trigger a consequent concern or worries. However, this way of experiencing reality generates in the person such psychic and even physical discomfort (in the form of somatizations), that it may even determine the performance of their daily activities, leading to their being unable to function with immediacy and efficiency (as their unmeasured concern demands practically all their attention), and being unable to put those thoughts aside to deal with other situations of higher priority. They also suffer from somatizaciones like tremors, cramps or muscular pains, nausea, profuse sweating, diarrhea, and other symptoms also related to stress, such as irritable bowel syndrome or cephaleas.

CONCLUSION

The term vital anxiety has passed into colloquial language as the anxiety that arises in the face of everyday events (Lewis 1970-1971). Existential philosophy speaks of "being-in-the-world," in Spanish this relationship is well understood because we have two different verbs for being (*ser* and *estar*), which make those variations of the way of being-in-the-world well understandable. Being-in-the-world, being well or being unhappy, being happy or sad or being distressed (López-Ibor 1966; Kierkegaard 1957).

In the end, anxiety and anguish are nuances of the same experience. In principle anguish is deeper, more visceral and constrictive, whilst anxiety is more related to breathing discomfort. In both cases there is fear about the dissolution of the unit and continuity of the self (anguish) and when what exists is not a fear but only a threat, anxiety appears. Anguish offers a more agonizing background, where that agony may be understood as a struggle against life itself, against disease, and against death (López-Ibor 1965).

During an anxiety attack everything is possible when control over the self is lost, and therefore anything can happen when the relationship of trust between the self and the world is lost, with patients sometimes describing sometimes that what they feel as "fear of the fear" or feeling that they are going to die.

A feeling like vital anxiety becomes pathological when mechanisms that cause a restriction of freedom and a loss of self-realization possibilities appear (López-Ibor 2015; López-Ibor 2016).

To know the meaning of anguish and anxiety helps us to know mankind. Consciousness and thought are the most specific of human functions, in which all other functions converge and are framed into. They allow us to understand what happens in the world and with oneself (consciousness) and to give it a meaning. First comes the emotional conscience and after, the reflective one, the specific human capacity to raise oneself above a situation and to consider it, taking at the same time consideration over oneself, from a distance, as Guardini said, and it is this taking distance that allows us to value our relation with the world, with ourselves, and with our history (López-Ibor 2015).

BIBLIOGRAPHY

American Psychiatric Association. (2013). Diagnostic and Statistical Manual of Mental Disorders. Fifth Edition (DSM-5).

Angst J. and Vollrath M. (1991). "The Natural History of Anxiety Disorders." *Acta Psychiatrica Scandinavica* 84: 446–452.

Baeyer W. Von. (1984). "Angst als erlebtes Bedrohtsein. Hinweis auf die Angst-Lehre des Jakob Boehme." *Nervenarzt* 55: 349–357.

Barcia R. (1980). *Primer diccionario general etimológico de la lengua española.* Madrid: Establecimiento Tipográfico de Alvarez Hermanos.

Bomhard A. R. and Kerns J. C. (1994) *The Nostratic Macrofamily: A Study in Distant Linguistic Relationship.* Berlin, New York, Amsterdam: Mouton de Gruyter.

Breuer J. and Freud S. (1893). *Studies on Hysteria. On the Psychical Mechanism of Hysterical Phenomena: Preliminary Communication.* The Standard Edition of the Complete Psychological Works of Sigmund Freud (Vol. 2). London: Hogarth Press.

Dalby J. T. (1993) "Terms of Madness: Historical Linguistics." *Comprehensive Psychiatry* 34: 392–395.

Descartes R. (1911). "The Passions of the Soul." In Haldane Rios (ed.), *The Philosophical Works of Descartes* Vol 2. London: Cambridge University Press.

Diccionario de la Lengua Española, 19th edn. (1970). Madrid: Real Academia Española.

Eisler R. (1930, reprinted 1971). *Kant Lexicon.* Anthr. 1. T. 76 (IV 188). Berlin: Mittler.

Freud S. (1976). *Letter to Richard Flatter. Psychoanalysis and Shakespeare.* New York. Octagon Books.

Gebsatell, E. von (1966) *Antropología Médica.* Madrid: Rialp.

Heidegger M. (1968/2002). "Was heisst Denken?" Gesamtausgabe, Bd. 8. Vittorio Klostermann, Frankfurt a. M. "What Is Called Thinking?" trans. J. Glenn Gray. New York: Harper & Row.

Jaspers K. (1958). *Filosofía de la Existencia.* Barcelona: Aguilar.

Kierkegaard S. (1957). *Concept of Dread,* trans. Walter Lowrie. Princeton: Princeton University Press.

Kretschmer E. (1958/1960). *Hysterie, Reflex und Instinkt [Hysteria, Reflex, and Instinkt].* New York: Philosophical Library.

Lewis A. (1970–71). "The Ambiguous Word 'Anxiety." *International Journal of Psychiatry* 9: 62–79.

López-Ibor J. J. (1952). *La Angustia Vital.* Madrid: Paz Montalvo.

López-Ibor J. J. (1965). "Basic Anxiety as the Core of Neurosis." *Acta Psychiatrica Scandinava* 41(3): 329–332.

López-Ibor J. J. (1966). *Las neurosis como enfermedades del ánimo.* Madrid: Gredos.

López-Ibor J. J. (2015). *El lenguaje de la medicina y su mutua integración con otros lenguajes. Un paradigma para la ciencia de consecuencias sociopolíticas.* Madrid: Real Academia de Doctores de España.

López-Ibor J. J., Ortiz Alonso T., and López-Ibor M. I. (1999). *Lecciones de Psicologia Médica.* Barcelona: Masson.

López-Ibor J. J. and López-Ibor M. I. (2010). "Anxiety and Logos: Toward a Linguistic Analysis of the Origins of Human Thinking." *Journal of Affective Disorders* 120(1) January:1–11.

López-Ibor J. J and López-Ibor M. I. (2013). "Paving the Way for New Research Strategies in Mental Disorders. Second Part: The Light at the End of the Tunnel." 41(2): 67–75.

López-Ibor M. I. (2016). *Depresión o tristeza; ¿Dónde está el límite?* Junio: Real Academia de Doctores de España.

Maj M. (2011). "When does a Depression become a Mental Disorder?" *British Journal Psychiatry* 199: 85–86.

Pascal L. (1954). *Obras completes.* Paris: Editions Gallimard.

Sarbin T. R. (1968). "Ontology Recapitulates Philology. The Mythic Nature of Anxiety." *American Psychology* 23: 411–418.

Scheler M. (1972). *El resentimiento en la moral. Caparros.* Barcelona: Colección Spirit.

Schneider K. (1959). *Clinical Psychopathology.* New York: Grune and Stratton.

World Health Organization (1992). *The ICD-10 Classification of Mental and Behavioral Disorders: Clinical Descriptions and Diagnostic Guidelines.* Geneva: World Health Organization.

Yonkers K. A, Warshaw M. G, Massion A. O., and Keller M. B. (1996). "Phenomenology and Course of Generalized Anxiety Disorder." *British Journal of Psychiatry* 168: 308–313.

Zubiri X. (1991). "Las fuentes espirituales de la angustia y la esperanza." *Revista Latinoamericana de Teología* 8/22: 91–97.

CHAPTER 54

HALLUCINATIONS AND PHENOMENAL CONSCIOUSNESS

AARON MISHARA AND YULIYA ZAYTSEVA

THE EARLY HEIDELBERG SCHOOL AND THE PHENOMENOLOGY OF HALLUCINATIONS

IN this chapter, we examine the problem of phenomenal consciousness and how historical contributions to the phenomenology of hallucinations, especially the early Heidelberg School (1909–1932), have relevance for our current understanding of hallucinations in schizophrenia. We will focus on the work of Mayer-Gross but will also have occasion to refer to other Early Heidelberg School members, Beringer, Gruhle, and Jaspers.

In his phenomenological analysis, Mayer-Gross examines the claim of his contemporaries that the problem of consciousness is at the heart of the enigma of hallucinations. Following Jaspers (1913a), Mayer-Gross is particularly critical of theories which do not base themselves on phenomenological data (Mishara and Schwartz 2013). That is, he contests the theories of his contemporaries, who theorize about consciousness but do not assign a proper role to the perceptual changes underlying hallucinations in schizophrenia (an argument we briefly summarize here).

Mayer-Gross may be regarded as herald of the "perceptual anomalies" approach to schizophrenia, the view that low-level perceptual anomalies play a critical role in the positive symptoms of schizophrenia, including verbal and non-verbal hallucinations, the various thought disturbances, and self-disturbances/disorders (*Ichstörungen*). The phenomenologically-oriented psychiatrists Matussek, Conrad, and Binswanger later developed this view (for reviews see Uhlhaas and Mishara 2007; Mishara 2010a; Mishara 2011; Mishara and Fusar-Poli 2013; Sterzer et al. 2016).

THE CONTESTED PSEUDOHALLUCINATION
(KANDINKSY, JASPERS, BERRIOS, AND DENING)

Following the German psychiatrist Hagen and the Russian psychiatrist Kandinsky, who himself experienced hallucinations, Jaspers (1913a) distinguishes hallucinations proper or genuine hallucinations from pseudohallucinations. While Hagen (1868) was the first to use the term "pseudohallucination" (to refer to illusory experiences falsely labeled "hallucinations"), previous variations of the concept had been circulating in nineteenth-century French psychiatry. For example, Baillarger's (1846) "psychic hallucinations" pre-date, but conceptually resemble Hagen's pseudohallucinations. They are based on involuntary images and memories and are opposed to "psychosensorial hallucinations" in which the sensory component prevails (see Berrios and Dening 1996).

The Russian psychiatrist Kandinsky[1] (Kandinsky 1880; 1890) described his own hallucinatory experiences in detail. He diagnosed himself as having *primäre Verrücktheit* (German for primary insanity), which Berrios and Dening (1996) comment, "could be translated anachronistically as 'schizophrenia-like state'").

Kandinsky (1881) defined pseudohallucinations (PHs) as "subjective perceptions similar to hallucinations, with respect to their character and vividness, but they differ because they are not experienced as having objective reality" (145).[2] PHs may accompany normal perceptions of objects, in a similar way to how memories or fantasies coexist in our consciousness with real perceptions. PHs are vivid images which are experienced as subjective, anomalous, or novel. They arise involuntarily, cannot be controlled, and change rapidly. The individual, however, may not always be able to disentangle the pseudohallucinatory image from the perceptual experience. Kandinsky writes: "In visual PHs, the image arises effortlessly in front of the person's gaze without participation of will" (133). They may be projected outside and for this reason appear to stand in front of the eyes. In auditory PHs, Kandinsky writes, "the patients sometimes state that they hear voices not with their ears but with an inner ear and call these experiences 'hearing with the soul', 'an inner voice', 'speaking the language of the soul'" (83, 84).

---

[1] Viktor Ch. Kandinsky (1849–1889) was a Russian psychiatrist and psychopathologist, who became famous for his descriptions of psychotic conditions (including his own), which were characterized by an alienation from one's perceptive, motor, and cognitive processes. He relied on a large sample of patients' clinical experiences. Kandinsky (1890) describes his own experiences with pseudohallucinations: "My pseudohallucinations are not simple, but extremely vivid images of memories and fantasies. Leaving aside their incomparably greater intensity, I find them to be different from ordinary reproduced affective ideas or other features such as their receptive feature in relation to consciousness. They are independent of the will, quite obsessive; highly sensuous and complete; they are continuous and represent a subjective experience" (311). In 1889, fearing that his psychotic symptoms were returning, Kandinsky tragically committed suicide (Lerner and Witztum 2006).

[2] Dr. Zaytseva translated the passages in Russian, and Dr. Mishara translated the German passages.

According to Kandinsky, consciousness is preserved in cases of PHs except during hypno-gogic and oneroid states. An interesting example of PHs are transparent hallucinatory images that have contours *which do not block the real objects but remain connected with them* (for in-stance, "the transparent man enters the door or gets inside through the window" (228–230).[3]

Kandinsky suggests that visual hypnagogic states in healthy people qualify as PHs. "Actually, the lively fantastic pictures experienced by healthy people before going to sleep, or in a state between sleep and wakefulness, may be characterized as PHs. These are not separate figures in the objective field of view, but complex pictures, occupying the whole visual field" (221). In contrast, panoramic hallucinations of the mentally ill during wake-fulness, or persons under hypnosis, where one feels transported into another place, are not PHs. In these cases, fantastic pictures completely replace the real environment in which the hallucinating subject dwells.

Some authors identify PHs as dominating the clinical presentation (Rybalsky 1983). The state of hallucinosis, for instance, encompasses disturbances in perception and has inner projection but is provoked by the environment. Such PHs are projected inside the head (e.g. an inner voice) or seen in the external space, sometimes referred to by the individual as being seen by the brain, not with the eyes.

Occurring against the will, PHs are experienced as independent from the conscious mind. As Kandinsky reports on his own experiences of pseudohallucination: "Appearing sponta-neously, the images can neither be changed nor expelled from consciousness" (210).

In his approach to hallucinations, Jaspers (1911, 1912, 1913a) proposed a strict distinc-tion between perception, in which the phenomenal givenness of the object is experienced as objectively present (*leibhaftig*) from representations based on imaginary constructions (what Jaspers calls imaginary, *bildhaftig*).[4] He proposed that this distinction rests on the broader opposition between perception (*Wahrnehmung*) and idea or image (*Vorstellung*). That is, perceptions generally have the character of being objectively present (*Leibhaftigkeit*), whereas the idea or representation of objects is imaginary (*Bildhaftigkeit*). Genuine or true hallucinations (*Trug-wahrnehmungen*, i.e. deceptive perceptions) are experienced as "objec-tively" present (*leibhaftig*), and may be experienced alongside real perceptions. In contrast, pseudohallucinations (deceptive images or ideas, *Trug-vorstellungen*) are experienced as im-aginary, or subjective (i.e. not real). While the former occurs in "external objective space," the pseudohallucinations occur in "inner subjective space."[5] Pseudohallucinations are not concretely real, have the character of subjectivity, and appear in inner subjective space. The

---

[3] The French author Guy de Maupassant presents a striking case of what might roughly be labeled an autoscopic "pseudohallucination" (providing we find some consensus on its definition): Suffering from terminal syphilis, he asks his friend, Bourget: "How would you feel if you had to go through what I experience? Every other time when I return home I see my double. I open the door and see myself sitting in the armchair. I know it is a hallucination the moment I see it. But isn't it remarkable? If you hadn't a cool head wouldn't you be afraid?" (Todd and Dewhurst 1955, cited by Mishara 2010b).

[4] Notably, Jaspers (1911) equates *Leibhaftigkeit* with Kadinsky's "character of objectivity" as given to phenomenal consciousness.

[5] The distinction between inner-subjective and outer-objective hallucinations is problematic for many reasons, not the least of which is the empirical data. e.g. "right-hemispheric epilepsy patients (Kamiya and Okamoto 1982) sometimes report "mental dipoplia" (i.e. the feeling of mental duality, Hughlings-Jackson 1932), which resembles the Feeling of a Presence (FOP). The invisible double may be experienced outside or inside the body and may speak with the subject from this vantage point. e.g. one

pseudohallucination has been criticized for both conceptual confusion and lack of clinical utility (Berrios and Dening 1996; Spitzer 1987).

MAYER-GROSS AND THE EARLY HEIDELBERG SCHOOL: DISRUPTION OF THE EMBODIED SELF IN ITS RELATIONSHIP TO THE HALLUCINATORY OBJECT

While Mayer-Gross acknowledges indebtedness to Jaspers in his own phenomenological approach, he opposes Jaspers's strict distinction between "genuine" versus "pseudo" hallucinations (Mayer-Gross and Stein 1928; Mayer-Gross 1932). By proposing a dialectical relationship between these terms, Mayer-Gross deconstructs Jaspers's strict opposition. Anticipating the later criticisms by Berrios and Dening (1996) Mayer-Gross observes that no matter how attractive or fashionable the term "*Leibhaftigkeit*" might have become in German psychiatry at the time, it remains ambiguous. The mere absence of Leibhaftigkeit does not properly distinguish PHs from "true" hallucinations.

Mayer-Gross cites his contemporary A. A. Grünbaum (1917), an Amsterdam psychiatrist, who describes an experience that challenges Jaspers's sharp opposition between "objective" perception (i.e. genuine hallucination) and subjective image (pseudohallucination):

Following a taxing day, Grünbaum (1917) attends a not particularly stimulating concert. He finds the conductor "boring" and experiences himself falling into a half-sleep. "I am still hearing the musical tones but now as if behind a thick wall. After shutting my eyes for a while, I see the orchestra in a most remarkable manner. The orchestra was suddenly *without distance* to my body-self (*Leib-Ich*). The sizes of the different instruments and objects were especially odd. Their dimensions appeared differently than usual. Still, their unusual sizes, being smaller or larger, did not surprise me nor put me on guard" (101).

Then, through a sudden jerk, Grünbaum is thrown back into wakefulness. He observes that "the transition back to the complete, conscious perception brought about a spatial reorganization of the entire scene ... I experienced how quickly the actual distance to the orchestra returned and how the various figures resumed their correct sizes. ... At the same time I knew that just a moment before, everything had been different" (102).

Grünbaum (1917) comments that, unlike Jaspers's definition, the "pseudohallucination" here does not occur in an "inner subjective space" which is opposed to the "external objective space" of the "perceptual (or genuine) hallucination" as Jaspers (1911, 1913a) suggests. Rather, in the pseudohallucination (in this case, hypnagogic image), there is a loss of distance between the visual image or hallucination and the body-self (*Leib-Ich*). The hallucination

---

patient heard the voice of his other self from his abdomen (Kamiya and Okamoto 1982: Case 6). The patient may also report a "double thinking" the sensation that two selves are thinking within the same subject (Mishara 2010c). There is unpublished data (from the study by Hoffman et al. 2007) that patients with schizophrenia characterize the "voices" as originating from "inside" particular parts of the body including one's own larynx, or other inner parts of the body. The reader is advised to consider the case of "reflex hallucination" described by Mayer-Gross in this contribution which suggests that the origins of hallucinations may be within one's own body, but are nevertheless no less real.

does not occur in inner subjective space, but appears, no matter how disordered, in the sur-rounding space. Grünbaum (1917) comments: "I nevertheless knew that I had the orchestra in front of me and not merely a vision" (104). That is, contra Jaspers, the experience was pervaded with its own "objective" character, its own *Leibhaftigkeit*.

Moreover, the experience "cannot be placed in specific spatial relationship to other per-ceptual objects" (Grünbaum 1917: 108). In the loss of distance, the relation between fore-ground and background is disturbed. The loss of distance between the visual image or hallucination and body-self (*Leib-Ich*) resembles – as indicated below – other anomalous relationships to the hallucinatory object including temporal, sensorimotor, and embodied processes of self.

The Loss of the Ability to Explore/Transcend the Hallucination: Spatial, Temporal, and Sensorimotor Relationships to the Hallucinatory Object

The phenomenological psychiatrist, Erwin Straus (1978; Mishara 1995) observes that we experience distance not in terms of objective space but in terms of our own momentary ability for movement. The loss of the embodied, sensorimotor relationship to the hallucina-tory object in space, time, and background (including other objects in the field) may not be specific to the pseudohallucination. Grünbaum (1917) experienced what he calls a pseudo-image (*Pseudovorstellung*) as directly related to his world (thus perceiving a world with "eyes behind the eyes").[6] By deconstructing the oppositions that characterize Jaspers's psychopa-thology, we come across a feature shared by different modalities of hallucinations in psy-chosis, that is, the loss of embodied relationship to the hallucinatory object. This disrupts the "object's" relationship to other objects in the background, as in the "fragmented" space of Grünbaum's hallucination (for more recent discussions concerning the importance of the *relationship* between hallucinator and hallucination, see Coda section, below).

---

[6] We are indebted to the very resourceful Gina Applebee, who has kindly shared the following personal communication (to Aaron Mishara, August 2017), which she has agreed to publish here. It is about how she uses a synesthesia-like process to create a stable, non-optical visual world around her: "I was totally blind by age 23, following progression of a degenerative retinal condition called S-cone syndrome. Having exercised my non-visual perception for many years prior to that final loss of retinal vision, I spent the next 5 years fully embracing and integrating those non-visual capacities without the taxing limitation of failing retinal vision. I also happened to be hallucinating blue, flickering light at that time. I spontaneously developed and subsequently refined what was initially best described as a type of synesthesia, through which I was able to see myself, objects and surfaces around me in what I experienced as a visual space. This non-optic sight is informed by my other senses (touch, hearing, etc.) in addition to my memory, knowledge and imagination. Using this non-optic sight, I am able to accurately perceive myself, others and affordances in a way that is consistent with experiences of people who have more typical visual perception." That is, Gina is able to accurately experience objects' and persons' stable locations, and related information in the environment, by what she "sees" with non-optical vision.

As suggested by Grünbaum's abrupt return to wakefulness from half-sleep, there are transitions in a self-organizing embodied, experiential field which emerge with shifting levels of consciousness (von Weizsäcker 1950a). These are efforts to maintain gestalt coherence in ongoing perception action cycle. As von Weizsäcker (director of the Heidelberg neurology clinic at the time) indicates in his sense-physiological and phenomenological experiments—well known to Mayer-Gross and the Early Heidelberg School—these transitions are rapid and ballistic in that each abrupt new organization of the surrounding field appears to emerge on its own without precedent in the prior organization. For example, Grünbaum wakens from his hypnagogic experience with a sudden jerk accompanied by a rapid recovery of spatial distance to the orchestra. Weizsäcker (1950a) calls each embodied subjective act, "improvisation." The spontaneous emergence of a new embodied field-organization sets the conditions for the total field to maintain inner coherence as a system. The strategies to maintain coherence are not consciously generated but appear to emerge effortlessly and automatically in the service of preserving the self–world relationship as coherently meaningful (see Uhlhaas and Mishara 2007; Giersch and Mishara 2017a, 2017b; Mishara 2011).[7]

As suggested, the hallucinatory object not only takes an independence from self in its spontaneous emergence, but also from the background: *there appears to be little or no relationship between the subject's body movements and how the hallucinatory object reveals itself* (see Kaminsky et al. in review). That is, the hallucination may involve a disruption of the tight coupling of perception and action. It has been hypothesized that this may be due to a discrepancy in the timing of this coupling, and/or the anomalous timing of low-level perceptual processing in very brief, millisecond durations (Giersch and Mishara 2017a, 2017b; see also Pienkos et al., 2019).

For Mayer-Gross, the hallucinations that occur in fragmentary space are highly *salient* compared to other perceptual objects (cf. Sterzer et al. 2016). That is, the features of Grünbaum's half-sleep experience are not specific to PHs (or the problem of subjective vs. actual space), but rather resemble at least some visual and multimodal hallucinations during psychosis in that they exhibit the fragmented space which Grünbaum observed in his hypnagogic hallucination. *Such fragmentation prohibits sensorimotor exploration of the hallucinatory object and, as a result, separates the hallucination from its perceptual background.* That is, to the extent that movement is unable to explore the object by viewing or experiencing it from different sides, the result is a detachment between the hallucinatory object and background. Anomalies in the timing between perception and movement may produce the fragmentation.

Mayer-Gross reports that one of his patients, early in the course of schizophrenia, not only sees (hallucinates) houses that are not there during his usual walk; he also does not see other houses, which really are there (hallucination by omission). We return to this idea when we describe the "loss of perspective" of the hallucinatory experience in our conclusions.

In his phenomenological analyses of psychosis, Mayer-Gross pays particular attention to visual and multimodal hallucinations in schizophrenia (which, he argues, share structural features with the auditory verbal/non-verbal hallucinations). In support of this approach, recent studies (e.g. Delespaul and van Os 2002; Lim et al. 2016), have indicated that when compared with unimodal auditory verbal hallucinations (AVHs), the prevalence of visual

---

[7] Interestingly, the phenomenological psychologist, D. von Uslar (1964) describes two mutually "excluding realities of the waking and dream worlds." These two worlds mutually presuppose but exclude one another in the dialectical relationship of a gestalt-circle (what von Weizsäcker (1950a) calls the "revolving door" principle, where each term presupposes but also excludes its alternative).

and multimodal hallucinations has been vastly underestimated in schizophrenia and schizo-phrenia spectrum patients.[8] On a related topic, Upthegrove et al. (2016) found that AVHs can be "experienced with additional multisensory factors, including pain, pressure and itching."

MAYER-GROSS CHALLENGES CONTEMPORARY THEORIES OF A CORE DISTURBANCE (*GRUNDSTÖRUNG*) OF SCHIZOPHRENIA

For Mayer-Gross, one cannot overestimate the role of the perceptual anomalies during the prodrome and subsequent conversion to full blown psychosis in schizophrenia. He lamented that the importance of these anomalies was being ignored by the contemporaneous trends. The prevailing view at the time assumed that it was the disruption of higher-level thought processes that was ultimately responsible for many of the symptoms of schizophrenia. Mayer-Gross countered that his contemporaries neglected the phenomenological data which indicated that there can be sensory anomalies without disturbance to thought (e.g. thought insertion, thought withdrawal, thoughts becoming loud (*Gedankenlautwerden*), which Mayer-Gross and other members of the Early Heidelberg School counted among the *Ichstörungen*). However, this same data did not support the converse view that there can be self-disturbances (as defined by the Early Heidelberg School) in higher-level cognition (as, for example, in thought insertion, thought withdrawal, somatic passivity and other "made" feelings, actions, and volitions) without some degree of anomalous perceptual experiences underlying these phenomena (a strong claim, further elaborated by Sterzer et al. 2016).

Quite the contrary, the abundance of theories at the time suggested that higher-level cognition was central and low-level perceptual processing played little or no role in schizo-phrenia. This was especially problematic when such accounts also claimed to access a theo-retical core disturbance (*Grundstörung*), from which "everything else could be derived."

Both J. Berze and C. Schneider proposed that a reduction in mental activity or conscious-ness was critical in creating the thought disturbances (as described above). Berze (1914, 1932) describes the fundamental, core disturbance (*Grundstörung*) in schizophrenia to be a "hy-potonia of consciousness," a "primary insufficiency of mental activity." The psychological *Grundstörung* is primary because the symptoms of psychosis can be derived from it. With the "hypotonia of consciousness," there is a "deficiency of the waking state," in which the usual sensations of tension (*Spannungsempfindungen*, i.e. mental tonicity) are absent. That is, reduced tone (*hypotonia*) of consciousness is the core disturbance of schizophrenia.

In a somewhat similar vein, C. Schneider (1930)[9] proposed that "thinking while falling asleep" (*Einschlafdenken*) models the mechanisms responsible for the higher cognitive

---

[8] In an experience sampling study, Delespaul and van Os (2002) found that patients with schizophrenia surprisingly experienced more visual hallucinations (62.5%) than auditory hallucinations (49.1%). Another study (Lim et al. 2016) found that lifetime prevalence of multimodal hallucinations in schizophrenia spectrum patients (53%) was nearly two times greater than all unimodal hallucinations (27%), including auditory (verbal) hallucinations (AVHs).

[9] An outspoken Nazi sympathizer, Carl Schneider, was Chair of Heidelberg Psychiatry from 1933-1946, and supplied the "scientific" rationale for the Action T4 Euthanasia program. He committed suicide while awaiting trial in prison. He is not to be confused with Kurt Schneider, who quietly opposed

disturbances in schizophrenia. However, these claims of finding a theoretical *Grundstörung* were challenged by the early Heidelberg school. Mayer-Gross, Gruhle, and Jaspers were emphatically opposed to claims of a theoretical *Grundstörung* of consciousness in schizophrenia, which could not be derived from the phenomenological data (Mishara and Schwartz 2013). In fact, Berze (1914, 1932) is himself clear that his view of the *Grundstörung* as the psychological essence of schizophrenia is theoretical: "The core disturbance (*Grundstörung*) is not available to phenomenology; it can only be inferred from the totality of the primary symptoms" (see Mishara and Schwartz 2013). Berze had observed that with a lowering of the threshold of consciousness (hypotonia), there is a lowering of individual mental acts. However, as Mayer-Gross and Gruhle indicate, Berze had not distinguished mental activity from activity generally, and thus had difficulty accounting for both the excesses of activity (often at the beginning of illness), and its reduction. Berze's activity insufficiency may well be a characteristic symptom, but by no means "the cardinal symptom" of schizophrenia. Mayer-Gross cautions that Berze's concept "loses itself completely in the theoretical."

To counter the theoretical claims of a *Grundstörung* in schizophrenia, Mayer-Gross and colleagues collected their own phenomenological data on these topics. They implemented a hypnagogic imagery study (where both a *becoming sensory* of thinking, and increased difficulty thinking (*Denkerschwerung*) were present), the mescaline model-psychosis (Beringer 1927; Mayer-Gross and Stein 1926, 1928), as well as their phenomenological analyses of symptoms from clinical cases (for discussion of hypnagogic studies and self, see Mishara 2010c; Mishara 2011).

As indicated elsewhere (Mishara, Bonoldi et al. 2015; Sterzer et al. 2016), the Early Heidelberg School (starting with Gruhle 1915) originated and developed the concept of the self-disturbances in schizophrenia (*Ichstörungen*, also called self-disorders), which eventually contributed to K. Schneider's formulation of the first-rank symptoms. In the 1920s, Beringer and Mayer-Gross used mescaline as a psychotomimetic agent to study the self-disturbances (Beringer 1927; Mayer-Gross and Stein 1926; Mayer-Gross and Stein 1928). They proposed that the self-disturbances include hallucinations, as hallucinations involve both an alienation from the perceptual world and an inability to detach (gain distance) from the hallucination. These experiences occur independently from the self's volition, and are often imposed process by foreign, omnipotent agents.

In the self-disturbances of schizophrenia and the model-psychosis (mescaline), Mayer-Gross finds the same fundamental transformations (*grundsätzlichen Abwandlungen*) of sense perception in its various modalities (visual, auditory, olfactory, gustatory, tactile, coenesthetic) and an uncoupling of perception and action:

1. Lability of threshold (*Schwellenlabilität*) (von Weizsäcker 1950a, b; Mayer-Gross and Stein 1926; Stein and von Weizsäcker 1927): There is an oversensity to stimuli in any or all of the sensory domains, that is, fine-detailed, impinging sensory experiences, a magnification of saliency often until one aspect (or view) completely occupies consciousness. This may alternate with its opposite, a "reduced ability to detect nuance, as well as dullness, emptiness, coldness, and monotonous environment, which could also indicate a change in threshold" (Mayer-Gross and Stein 1926: 370). Here there may be transitions from seeing everything as *new* and *equally important, and brightly*

the Eugenics program and was appointed Heidelberg Chair of Psychiatry (1945–1955) in an effort to rebuild Germany's medical institutions.

colored to a "pallid grey and the apocalyptic mood that the world is coming to an end" (*Weltuntergangsstimmung*) (Mayer-Gross and Stein 1926: 361). The world may be covered by a visible green "film" (reported to Aaron Mishara by a person with schizophrenia who was experiencing the early course of schizophrenia) or the *artificiality* of a stage set (Conrad 1958; Mishara and Fusar-Poli 2013), which is experienced as an alienation of the perceptual world (*Entfremdung der Wahrnehmungswelt*).

2. Patients experience fusion with their experience (difficulty to distance or distract from it) and at the same time the experience is found to be completely independent of the self's own activity or volition (passivity experiences). (Recently, this has been proposed to result from an uncoupling of automatic and controlled processing, possibly due to very early timing discrepancies (Sterzer et al. 2016; Giersch and Mishara 2017).) The changes of sensory experience are "incomparable," unlike anything experienced before. Patients and the mescaline experimental subjects have difficulty finding the descriptive vocabulary for these experiences during psychosis or psychotomimetic challenge. Gruhle and Mayer-Gross note that patients invent their own vocabulary to describe their experiences.

3. The gestalt-structure of experience may vary from minimal or absent structure to detailed, complexly elaborated experiences in any modality.[10]

4. Uncoupling of perception and action: Movements in self and others may be perceived as abnormally fast or slow. Resting objects may be seen as moving, or movements may be seen where there are none or conversely, moving objects may appear as still.

5. Hallucinating may occur in more than one modality at once, what Mayer-Gross calls a "hallucinating together of the senses" (*Zusammenhalluzinieren der Sinne*); synesthesias may be present (see Kaminsky et al. in review).

THE DEBATE WITH SCHRÖDER AND WERNICKE: ARE AUDITORY HALLUCINATIONS, THOUGHT INSERTION, AND THOUGHTS BECOMING LOUD (*GEDANKENLAUTWERDEN*) RELATED?

As indicated above, Heidelberg psychiatrists Beringer (1927) and Mayer-Gross (Mayer-Gross and Stein 1926; Mayer-Gross and Stein 1928) conducted a series of mescaline experiments to examine the phenomenology of psychotic experiences, especially the self-disturbances (*Ichstörungen*), in healthy participants. The participants included medical students and psychiatrists with the goal of becoming more able to empathize with or understand those experiences of psychotic patients that Jaspers (1913a) had labeled as non-understandable. As Jaspers emphasizes, these experiences are due to an underlying as yet unknown

---

[10] The structured verbal phrases in AVHs can lose their meaning and become more like the non-verbal akoasms. Ralph Hoffman (personal communication to Aaron Mishara, August 31, 2015), reported that when r-TMS treatment is effective, the patients sometimes experience a mitigating of the AVHs, reducing them to a kind of "mumble," or senseless gibberish. Interestingly, as Mayer-Gross observes, such akoasms may also occur before or when the AVHs begin.

neurobiological disease process, which interrupts any "understandable" development of personality (Mishara and Fusar-Poli 2013). For Mayer-Gross, the mescaline experiments were critical in that they "opened the way to explaining these non-empathizable forms of subjective experience, which, up till now, have occasioned very unsatisfactory efforts to interpret or *theoretically* understand these experiences" (Mayer-Gross and Stein 1926: 386).

Mayer-Gross's participation and observation of colleagues in the mescaline studies appear to have profoundly affected him. He repeatedly emphasizes that when we are talking about the perceptual anomalies implicated in hallucinations and the various self-disturbances, *we are talking about experiences that are difficult to articulate because they are so unlike our usual, everyday sensory experiences. The experimental mescaline participants in the mescaline model psychosis study, as also described by individuals in early psychosis, fall into a foreign, never previously experienced state.*

On the basis of his and others' experiences as participants in the mescaline studies, Mayer-Gross noted that thoughts in thought insertion (TI) are not *ascribed* to alien agency, but are rather *perceived* as alien.[11] He described a "becoming sensory" (*Versinnlichung*) in the sensory representation of thoughts (Mayer-Gross and Stein 1928; Mayer-Gross 1932). He states further that we obtain "insight into the progressive invasiveness of the thought-disturbances from the earliest sign of difficulties in concentrating . . . . These prodromal manifestations lead to a scattered emptiness of thinking, quite similar to thought withdrawal." In his careful phenomenological analysis of subtle self-perceived cognitive and other disturbances in prodromal schizophrenia and mescaline intoxication, Mayer-Gross anticipated Huber's basic-symptom concept (Mayer-Gross 1995; Mishara, Bonoldi, et al. 2015; Sterzer et al. 2016).

On the basis of his insights, Mayer-Gross finds an opponent in the Leipzig-based psychiatrist, Paul Schröder, and the latter's reliance on the celebrated neuropsychiatrist Wernicke (1906) for his theory of hallucinations. Both Schröder and Wernicke claim that thought insertion (TI) is often a precursor in the course of illness to thoughts becoming loud (GLW, *Gedankenlautwerden*) and the AVHs. Schröder concludes that TI, GLW, and AVHs are related symptoms and groups them under the unitary concept "verbal hallucinosis." Schröder (1915, 1921a,b, 1926, 1928) argues that GLW, AVHs, TI, and "the made thoughts and experiences" (Wernicke's autochthonous ideas), are *not* based on a perceptual disturbance but strictly on a verbal-linguistic one (i.e. "phonemes").

Despite the emphasis on phonemes, Schröder proposes that the critical element in this symptom-complex is a "feeling of foreignness" (*Fremdheitsgefühl*). He regards the "feeling of foreignness" as a primary, not further analyzable and not explainable original phenomenon. Its imposition on the phonemes gives these symptoms their foreign character, an "externalizing" of thoughts. Progressing in sequence from thought insertion to thoughts becoming loud and auditory verbal hallucinations, they involve "a co-speaking, a speaking before, a speaking after, a repeating, or an answering back" (Schröder 1928).

Mayer-Gross (Mayer-Gross and Stein 1928; Mayer-Gross 1932) counters that Schröder's "feeling of foreignness" as the not further analyzable original phenomenon of verbal hallucinosis is theoretical and thus, arbitrary, that is, not based on data secured by

---

[11] This point resonates with Humpston and Broome's (2015) observation: "TI is not a delusion or simply a belief: it is an experience of someone or something else's thoughts penetrating into one's head from the external, frequently accompanied by a delusional elaboration regarding the source of those thoughts and the mechanism by which they entered into the sufferer's life."

phenomenological method. He comments: "To this day we know nothing of the inner interconnectedness of these symptoms and claims *about their essence* are presumptuous. Rather, by sticking faithfully to patients' reports of subjective experience, we consistently find descriptions which clearly go back to the sensory sources . . . the perceptual anomalies in beginning schizophrenia" (323). According to Mayer-Gross, what makes the inserted thought stand out from the patient's other thoughts is not a "feeling of foreignness," but rather *the experience of individual thoughts becoming sensory* (Sterzer et al. 2016). This involves a transformed sense of what is experienced as perceptual according to a "functional transformation" (Stein and von Weizsäcker 1927; Mayer-Gross and Stein 1928; Beringer and Ruffin 1932; Weizsäcker 1950a,b). *That is, the way that the perception is given is radically altered (the "how" of the experience, which, is "incomparable" to previous perceptual experiences, i.e. a foreign, never previously experienced state).*[12]

Mayer-Gross (Mayer-Gross and Stein 1928) presents the following case as a counter-example to Schröder's theory:

> A 19 year old man (father has schizophrenia) arrived to our clinic in a highly agitated and scattered state with pronounced pressure of speech. For the past two months, he no longer goes to work. He reported the following beginning of his psychosis. During the previous night, he slept poorly. There was something uncanny in the air. Feeling restless, he whistles through the window and receives an "answer", someone whistles back. Going to the window he clearly hears children's voices, which blare out uninterruptedly in a maddening, racing manner: "Bronchitis, bronchitis, we all have bronchitis..." (the patient had been suffering from a lung infection). It seemed that someone was running down the stairs on stilts, in a manner that was so loud and threatening. From these phenomena he sharply separated the infusion (insertion) of thoughts, whereby certain names as Ford and Hindenberg came in between his own thoughts. The children's voices were by no means in his head and they had quite *surprised* him putting him in a state of intense anxiety. (454)

Contrary to Schroeder's proposed sequence of symptoms, Mayer-Gross observes the nearly simultaneous experience of akoasm (non-verbal auditory hallucinations, e.g. the "stilts" on the stairs, the whistling), verbal hallucinations (the children's voices), and thought insertion (i.e. self-disturbance). Importantly, they are not interpreted as belonging to one symptom complex (as Schröder's verbal hallucinosis), but orthogonal occurrences which, nevertheless, may involve similar neural mechanisms. The voices and akoasms "surprise," the thought insertion "interrupts," (in this case, the names Ford and Hindenburg) which involve the *disruption of context.* (We have interpreted this disruption of context as bottom-up *prediction error* in low-level sensory processing (Sterzer et al. 2016) according to what von Weizsäcker (1950 a, b; Stein and von Weizsäcker 1927) called a "functional change" in the gestalt organization of the experience. This process cannot be surmised as a generalized "feeling of foreignness" (as suggested by Schröder). The different symptoms of the self-disturbances

[12] The Early Heidelberg School's phenomenological approach described in this contribution may help shed light on some current topics in hallucinations research. e.g. there is currently great interest in individuals who experience auditory verbal hallucinations but are not distressed by these experiences, and are not in need of clinical care. It would be interesting to know (using the phenomenological method) to what extent the phenomenology of these experiences is similar, forming or not forming a continuum between groups. (See "Coda: How Does the Early Heidelberg School Contribute to Today's Phenomenology of Hallucinations?")

indicate *different levels of disruption* (lability of threshold) of the gestalt organization of the experience, a point later developed by Matussek (1952, 1953); Conrad (1958); and Binswanger (1965).

Rather than a "feeling of foreignness" which is imposed on the non-sensory linguistic phonemes in TI, GLW, and AVHs (as in Schröder's view), the experience of thinking itself is fundamentally changed. *It is not enough to say that the thinking has been made sensory, but rather the perceptual basis has itself changed, making the experience incomparable with previous sensory experience.* Mayer-Gross (Mayer-Gross and Stein 1928) gives the example of a schizophrenia patient who experiences difficulty understanding what is said around him. The words seem to be spoken backwards. Mayer-Gross interprets this to mean that *the temporal gestalt of the actual sensations of hearing has been altered.*

DEBATE WITH SPECHT ON THE NATURE OF REFLEX HALLUCINATIONS

Mayer-Gross's debate with the act theories of consciousness (e.g. Berze, C. Schneider), taken to be the core issue responsible for hallucinations, continues in more extreme form with Wilhelm Specht. A Munich psychiatrist and former assistant to Kraepelin, Specht had founded the journal *Zeitschrift für Pathopsychologie* (1912–1919) with a long list of eminent contributors at the time. Claiming to base his theory of hallucinations on Husserl, Bergson, Scheler, Lipps, and von Helmholtz, Specht (1914) locates the source of hallucinations in the mental acts and not in the intact sensory experience, which is merely misinterpreted in the act of hallucination.

Mayer-Gross acknowledges that Specht begins with the same insight that many phenomenologists have asserted: we do not perceive sensations but rather perceptual experiences, in which objects, things, persons, etc. are phenomenally given.

However this commonality ceases when Specht states that the essential matter for both perceptions and hallucination is solely the interpretive grasping act and not its perceptual content. The perceptual object remains the same whether I vary the contents by taking this or that perspective. Specht (1914) writes that in "hallucinations, it is the interpretive contents which, just as in natural perceptions, the anomaly remains entirely in the sphere of judgment, interpreting, believing, maintaining, positing, whereby the contents become falsely interpreted." Specht develops a theory which claims that hallucinations are due to misinterpretive *acts* imposed on the otherwise unchanged sensory experience. Despite changes in its modality of givenness, the sensory experience remains the same.

Here there are no qualitative nuances or variations in the sensory material. We have only a strict opposition between data being given directly in perception without interpretation and then higher judgmental acts, which arrange and misinterpret the data.

By treating the sensory component as inconsequential, Specht ignores precisely the low-level qualitative transformations of sensory givens in the perceptual processing of hallucinations, which Mayer-Gross describes in his "perceptual anomalies" approach., The Heidelberg phenomenological studies in the 1920s of hypnagogic images, the mescaline model-psychoses, and psychosis found that a loss of perspective takes place in each of these three conditions. This occurs through a disruption of the embodied relationship to the hallucinatory object(s). In A. A. Grünbaum's (1917) account of his vivid hypnagogic hallucination, we find such a loss of perspective (e.g. loss of distance). That is, the disruption of embodiment during hallucination not only includes loss of distance (spatiality), but also disturbances in temporality, and the relationship of self and others. In psychosis and the self-disturbances, "other(s)" are often asymmetrically powerful, where one's experience of pereption, action, feelings, cognition and volition are experienced as "made" and take place independently of the self's volition, etc.).

As indicated elsewhere (Uhlhaas and Mishara 2007; Kaminsky et al. in review), *the hallucinating subject is unable to vary her/his own perspective of the hallucination which, unlike usual objects, resists attempts to view the hallucinatory object from different sides, or in terms of different aspects).* Kaminsky et al. (in review) report a patient who "sees rain," a wobbling, "transparent veil," a "wall," which separates him from his surroundings. He is unable to step out into the rain and it does not change when he moves. *The fact that the rain moves with him, also indicates that he is unable to take distance from it or explore it from any other vantage point than the current one* (Kaminsky et al. in review). This case demonstrates particularly clearly how the person with schizophrenia has particular difficulty in examining the hallucinatory object through one's own exploratory movements or from different points of view. Continued phenomenological research may indicate that the inability to explore the hallucinatory object beyond one's own current perspective may be a common feature in the phenomenology of hallucinations in psychosis.

We see something similar in autoscopic echopraxia (where the double copies what the subject does). This occurs in those autoscopic hallucinations, which take over the motor system (for different subtypes of autoscopy, see Mishara 2010b). Whenever the subject turns her/his head to see the faces of the doubles (as in polyscopic heutoscopy where there are several doubles), the doubles turn their faces in the same direction, thus obstructing the patient's view. Each time the subject attempts to look at them, she/he only sees the backs of their heads as they turn in the same direction as the subject, who is unable to examine his doubles through exploratory movements.

To demonstrate how perspective is lost in psychotic hallucinations, Mayer-Gross first provides the counterexample of a delirious patient who sees gold coins on his bed. Once he reaches for the coins and finds that he cannot touch them, he corrects (transcends) his initial perspective, and no longer sees the gold pieces. But this is precisely what does not occur in the hallucinations of schizophrenia. The patient is unable to vary her/his own perspective by exploring the hallucination from other sides or aspects. Rather than making use of the additional information that becomes available by comparing information between different sense-modalities—as the delirious patient who correcting the visual hallucination by means of tactile exploration—the patient with schizophrenia fuses the information between modalities in a loss of perspective (see Wyss on loss of perspective, below). That is, the person with schizophrenia is unable to benefit by integrating the multimodal information effectively.

Here Mayer-Gross challenges Specht's account of the so-called "reflex hallucination" (first described by Kahlbaum, 1866). Akin to synesthesia, the stimulus or perceptual object in the "reflex hallucination" is correctly perceived in one sensory modality but nevertheless provokes hallucination in a second modality. Finding the term reflex hallucination based on outmoded theories, Mayer-Gross takes issue with Specht's view that the grasping of a thing in one modality triggers the hallucination in a second modality in terms of the mental act that does the transfer.

For this purpose, Mayer-Gross reports the case of an older schizophrenia patient whom he repeatedly examined on visits to the nearby Rheinau Hospital. The patient complained regularly about the inflicted tortures on her body by the hospital personnel: the cleaning of the floors in the floor above her room, the moving of furniture, the cleaning of the silver ware in the kitchen, the stirring of the soup, etc. She experienced all these noises in her body as deliberate efforts to torture her. That is, *the very real sounds of the staff's cleaning activities were experienced by her in a second sensory modality as occurring in her body*. This directly challenges Specht's view that the reflex hallucination is merely the grasping of the thing now transferred to a less familiar sensory modality through an overarching act, which occurs independently of the original perceptual material.

As a further example, Mayer-Gross cites one of the participants in the Heidelberg Mescaline study (reported by Beringer 1927):

> One believes one hears sounds and sees faces and yet, I cannot tell whether I am hearing or seeing . . . I hear scratching, harsh trumpet blasts, which are all a painful gnashing. I *am* the music, I *am* the lattice-work, whatever I see, hear, smell . . . everything which I attempt to grasp in thinking I see . . . *I saw one of my thoughts catapult out of me and merge into the lattice-work*. This is not a simile but *the sensation that something has left my body*, which at the same time is optical . . . The strange sounds are at the same time visual perceptions, jagged and angular, jagged lightning, oriental ornaments, all turning into this horrid yellow. *My body is ransacked and is, at the same time, itself.* All these things I did not think but experienced, felt, smelled, saw, and my movements were also like this. I felt, tasted, smelled the tone . . . The same occurred when I merely thought about my hands. I saw, felt, tasted my hands. Everything was so clear and certain. All critical thinking is complete nonsense in the face of the direct experiencing of the impossible.
>
> (Beringer 1927: 65; emphasis added)

Here, the "body is ransacked" in which sensory modalities and thinking collapse into one another: "The same occurred when I merely thought about my hands. I saw, felt, tasted my hands." Contra Specht, one can no longer argue that the sensory material remains the same, and it is merely the act which transfers the idea from one sensory realm to another. *The objects do not remain the same as soon as they are co-perceived in another mode of sensory processing.* Rather, in the so-called "reflex hallucinaton," each sensory domain which processes the object reciprocally shapes the object with the other participating domain, such the originally perceived object changes with the further processing in the new domain. The initially neutral kitchen or clearning utensils now take on a physiognomic quality of torture (a point later emphasized by Conrad, Matussek and Binswanger, and sometimes begins with the delusional mood in prodromal and early schizophrenia, Mishara, 2010c, 2011). As indicated above, Mayer-Gross employed a dialectical approach to psychiatric and neurologic disorders. This was in part was shaped by von Weizsäcker's presence in Heidelberg (as Director of the Heidelberg Neurology Clinic) during the time of the Early Heidelberg School of Psychiatry. In his dialectical theory of the perception action cycle, von Weizsäcker (1933, 1950a, 1950b) influenced a whole generation of phenomenological psychiatrists and phenomenologically-oriented clinicians and thinkers, including Binswanger, Blankenburg, Bujtendijk, Conrad, Ey, Gadamer, Kraus, Lang, Merleau-Ponty, Mundt, Plessner, Plügge, Straus, Tellenbach, von Bayer, T. von Uxkühl, Wyss, and countless others (see Mishara 2010c, 2011, for reviews). As von Weizsäcker, Husserl (the founder of philosophical phenomenology) examines the interrelationship between perception and action, which he finds to be critical already at the earliest stages of processing, based on "unconscious inference" (cf. von Helmholtz 1867). Husserl proposes that the passive synthesis (see Steinbock, this volume) of these very early levels of perceptual meaning occurs according to hierarchy of processing stages (see Mishara 2011; Sterzer et al. 2016). Both von Weizsäcker and Husserl observed that it is only through a tight coupling between perception and action that we are able to explore and make use of objects in our environment (see Kaminsky et al. in review).

The phenomenological psychiatrist, Wyss (Wyss 1973), who was von Weizsäcker's assistant in the Heidelberg psychosomatic clinic after the Second World War, describes a loss of perspective (what he calls "*Aperspektivität*") during dreaming and other altered states of consciousness. We think this concept is relevant to hallucinations in psychosis. In *Aperspektivität*, there is an attendant confusion between experiential modalities (perceiving (the different sensory modalities), remembering, imagining, thinking, etc.). What is meant here is not a fundamental *Grundstörung* of mental acts or consciousness but rather a failure in the ability to vary one's current perspective. With loss of perspective there is a loss of distinguishing modalities of experience (as described by the participants in the Heidelberg studies and the patients in early schizophrenia).

The ability to vary own perspective resembles Husserl's method of free-fantasy variation in which the invariant meaning remains constant across variations, or different 'aspects or "views" of the object' (for description of Husserl's phenomenological method, see Mishara 2010b, and below).

In Grünbaum's description of his hypnagogic experience, there is a loss of distance to the objects, a kind of loss of perspective in the hallucinations of half-sleep. However, as we suggest, this loss of perspective may more generally characterize hallucinations in schizophrenia. Under von Weizsäcker's influence, numerous phenomenological psychiatrists described psychosis as a failure to transcend one's current perspective. Binswanger (1957) metaphorically describes the inability to transcend one's current momentary perspective in acute psychosis as a failure to "climb" or "step" over oneself (in German *sich übersteigen*), that is, the self is an ongoing transcending of its own perspective in subjective time. Contra Specht, Mayer-Gross suggests that in the "reflex hallucination" it is not that an actual stimulation in one sensory domain triggers a stimulation in another less familiar domain for that object. It is rather that the world of objects has itself dramatically changed. As stated above, *the objects do not remain the same as soon as they are co-perceived in \another mode of sensory processing*. Thus, Mayer-Gross describes hallucination in both the mescaline psychomimetic model and in psychosis as multimodal, "a hallucinating together of the senses," in which a leakage between sensory modalities occurs in a synesthesia-like process.

In conclusion, we present a plea to scientists and clinicians, to consider methods (e.g. phenomenological psychopathology and related approaches), which take the patient's subjective experience seriously. For a long time, it was considered impossible to systematically study the patient's subjective experience, which could only be approached indirectly through scales, symptom checklists, or other measures. This does not mean that phenomenology does not contribute to such scales but it also contributes its own sort of data. In our contribution, we described a brief period in the history of phenomenological psychiatry, which has been neglected, but which provides very rich data for further phenomenological study. However as many phenomenological studies of psychopathology, the Heidelberg School approach provides novel hypotheses, which can also inform hypotheses for testing about neurocognitive mechanisms in more experimental approaches (Mishara and Sterzer 2015).

One approach is finding ways that phenomenology and neurocomputational modeling work together. For example, Sterzer et al. (2016) argue that "the phenomenon of thought insertion entails a failure of hierarchical Bayesian inference to contextualize or predict the narrative interconnectedness of thoughts. In other words, there is an imprecise representation of context and a subsequent failure to provide top-down predictions about the neural representations of thoughts. These representations are therefore experienced as being caused by external forces, much in the same way that percepts are experienced as being caused by sensory input. It is this experience of thoughts as sensations that characterizes thought insertion as a self-disturbance, in line with the phenomenological accounts of the early Heidelberg School" (2) Sterzer et al. (2016) propose that the neurocomputational mechanism underlying this "form of false inference is a reduction in the precision of prior beliefs relative to the precision in the encoding of thoughts, thus leading to increased prediction error and thus aberrant salience of thoughts. This account of thought insertion fits comfortably with explanations for delusions that are seen as a consequence of the aberrant salience of external stimuli" (2), or as we suggest here, hallucinations. Sterzer et al. (2018) write: "Predictive coding and Bayesian inference may provide a framework, linking the neurobiology of psychosis with its clinical phenomenology ... Anticipating the focus of predictive coding accounts on perceptual inference, and in line with phenomenological observations, early theories of psychosis emphasized altered perception" (e.g. Mayer-Gross) (3, 4).

Doctors Zaytseva and Mishara developed a self-disturbances questionnaire, the *Ichstörungen* Scale (IS). It is based on Mayer-Gross's phenomenological descriptions of the self-disturbances, which is arranged into categories: loss of context, experience is new/compelling (aberrant salience), reduced access/importance of autobiographical past, cognitions/emotions occur independently from self's volition, foreign agents have asymmetrical power over self, sensorimotor or perception action disturbances, thoughts becoming sensory, and anomalous body experiences. Currently the questionnaire has been piloted and applied to two ongoing studies involving patients with schizophrenia and individuals exposed to psilocybin, in both intoxicated and non-intoxicated states. The study is conducted at the National Institute of Mental Health, Klecany, Czech Republic.

Coda: How Does the Early Heidelberg School Contribute to Today's Phenomenology of Hallucinations?

As indicated above, the Early Heidelberg School's granular phenomenological approach suggests consilience with recent neurocomputational modeling. Nevertheless, the historical focus of the above contribution raises questions: How is the Heidelberg approach related to the current phenomenology of hallucinations? Does the above historical analysis contribute to, or find resonance with the newer phenomenological ways of studying the topic? Could an integrated, interdisciplinary approach which included both the older and more recent ways to phenomenologically study hallucinations pave the way to novel hypotheses for further study?

Here, we address these topics in a cursory manner. Nevertheless, it is hoped that our contribution will stimulate discussion concerning the Early Heidelberg Phenomenological School and current research:

1. What is the *relationship* between the person experiencing the voices and the "voices" themselves? Other sensory modalities or non-verbal auditory hallucinations (akoasms)?
2. *Cognitive approaches* to these topics *overlook the transformation of existence* in which the hallucinations occur.
3. The *complexity and diversity of hallucinations* across dia-gnosis, requires the phenomenological study of both clinical (need for care) and nonclinical hallucinations.
4. The last question (# 3) goes hand in hand with the need for *interdisciplinary research* and treatment, which would support different approaches listening to one another and an awareness of the diversity of individuals experiencing the hallucinations.

What is the Relationship between the Voice Hearer and AVHs and Other Modality Hallucinations?

Recent research indicates that voices have "character" (Woods et al. 2015), or are "personified" (Larøi et al. 2012). Chadwick and Birchwood (1994) describe the patient's "omnipotence appraisals" as a one-sided relationship of power attributed to the voices. They propose that the discrepancies in power that patients with schizophrenia experience with regard to their voices reflect the discrepancies they experience in actual social relationships. Individuals report their voices as omnipotent but experience these voices as benevolent or malevolent in terms of the attributions they make. That is, they employ the same attributions to their hallucinations and their experience of powerful others in their everyday social experiences. These voice hearers' appraisals reflect their experience of "subordination and low status" in their social relationships generally. Birchwood et al. (2000) write: "Our recent work has suggested that the distress arising from the activity of voices can be understood by reference to the individual's relationship with the voice, rather than voice content, topography or illness characteristics alone" (338). (See Hofmann et al. 2007 for how control/absence of control is central to the experience of the voice hearer, discussed below.) Meta-cognitive capacity can serve as a protective factor against the malevolent attributions (Connor and Birchwood 2013).

Interestingly, the Early Heidelberg School also examined the relationship between voice hearer and voices, and other types of hallucinations. They often described hallucination (AVHs, akoasms, other modalities, and multimodal) as self-disturbances involving a relationship of one-sided power, the so-called power-sphere of the self (*Machtsphäre*). Thus, they anticipated the later observations concerning the voices' omnipotent character.

Cognitive Approaches to These Topics Overlook the Transformation of Existence in which the Hallucinations Occur

In a thoughtful contribution, Raballo (2016) states that the voices involve a global transformation of self and world, where the "felt-naturalness of the psychic field seems changed" (137). This "hallucinatory transformation of the medium of consciousness" resonates with the earlier Heidelberg exploration of transformations of consciousness and self, which prepare the pathway for the phenomenal givenness of hallucinations.

Along similar lines, Larøi et al. (2010) point out that cognitive science fractionates cognitive processes rather than considering the entire subjective experience in context which undergoes transformation in psychosis. They indicate that phenomenological and cognitive approaches to hallucinations significantly differ. In the elegance and conceptual precision of cognitive studies of AVHs, there is nevertheless the danger that the "phenomenological complexity" is lost. They provide examples of how the phenomenological and cognitive approaches can be integrated in a way that mutually strengthens both. In the phenomenological approach, "the immediate experience" is not just a matter of the patient's current beliefs or attributions, but rather holistically "experienced." For the psychotic patient this involves a "changed being-in-the-world." Therefore, AVHs involve "profound transformations of self-awareness and experience." Indirectly affirming Chadwick and Birchwood's claim that AVHs involve a "relationship" of power, Larøi et al. (2010) state that hallucinations represent an intersubjective process.

Nevertheless, Stanghellini and Cutting (2003) point out that we must suspend our "common sense" views to study hallucinations phenomenologically: "Auditory verbal hallucinations (AVHs) are usually defined as perceptions of speech that occur in the absence of any appropriate external stimulus. This definition, we argue, is false. We maintain that AVHs are disorders of self-consciousness that are best understood as the becoming conscious of inner dialogue" (120). This again situates hallucinations in the phenomenological context of intersubjectivity. In contrast, however, cognitive approaches involve a "common sense" approach as its foundation and therefore, depart from phenomenological method.

For example, Birchwood and colleagues' (2000) cognitive model assumes that the same cognitive mechanisms in everyday social cognition (e.g. evolutionary rank theory, social comparison, etc.) remain intact in psychosis. However, a thorough study of the detailed phenomenology of the experience of the hallucination's omnipotence may indicate that the experience of power in psychosis may be different than the experience of disparity of power in everyday social cognition.

In an initial step, phenomenological method suspends or "brackets" everyday common sense assumptions in what is called "phenomenological re-duction." This is a "leading back" (from the Latin re-ducere) from one's current engagement with the world (naïve realism) to examine (reflectively) the "streaming-consciousness" in the here and now. This requires withholding judgment (a bracketing) concerning the researcher's beliefs or biases about current experiencing to examine how one's own subjectivity contributes to the experience (reflexivity). It attempts to overcome the naïve realism inherent in our everyday experience, the uncritical belief that what we directly see and experience is real, a world given to us naïvely and effortlessly. We remain blind to the interpretive lens through which we experience this "immediate" world, the product of implicit functioning, unnoticed biases (see Mishara 2010b; Mishara and Fusar-Poli 2013 for fuller description of phenomenological method).

Phenomenological method indicates that the "otherness" (omnipotence) in hallucinations may be completely different from our everyday experiences of others in everyday social cognition. Omnipotence may express itself as anonymous (or unseen) agents who may take over the entire perceptual field, where patients feel themselves to be "completely at the disposal" of these agents (Binswanger 1957; Straus 1958;) and/or feel their perceptions, actions, thoughts, feelings, volitions to be "made" by these agents (Kendler and Mishara in press). In such cases, *the entire field may take on a foreign, unfamiliar quality* (Conrad 1958; Mishara 2010a). The Early Heidelberg School called this an "alienation from the surrounding experiential world" (*Entfremdung der Erfahrungswelt*). Using genetic phenomenology (see entry on Genetic Phenomenology, this volume) Binswanger and others described a loosening of perceptual schemas from their perceptual-temporal background in psychosis. This impairs the ability to explore the hallucinations from different sides or aspects by means of one's own movements (as indicated above) (see Kaminsky et al. in review).

Need of care individuals are often distressed by their hallucinatory experiences but this does not mean that same schemas of relationship (intersubjectivity) apply in the naïve realism of our common sense world and the world of psychosis, suggesting two different types of relationship—namely, worldly and psychotic. Notably, this relationship goes "beyond voices" to involve akoasms (non-verbal auditory hallucinations), hallucinations in other sensory modalities (including multimodal, cross-modal, and other unimodal hallucinations). Such power relationships may be experienced through different hallucinatory modalities at once. For example, one schizophrenia patient reported (to ALM, November 2002) that martians are hurling spheres aimed at his testicles throughout the day.

The Complexity and Diversity of Hallucinations across Diagnosis Requires the Phenomenological Study of Both Clinical (Need for Care) and Non-Clinical Hallucinations

Phenomenological research examines the complexity and diversity of hallucinations (see reviews by Larøi (2006); Johns et al. (2014). The phenomenological study of such experiences also involves the comparison of those those whose voices require clinical need for care and those who experience a non-clinical hearing of voices. In a comprehensive review of AVHs across clinical and non-clinical groups, Larøi et al. (2012) comment: "One of the main characteristic features of AVHs in SZ is that individuals have little control over the onset and offset to the experience. The lack of perceived control may be crucial ... in the development of distress and in the transition between nonclinical to clinical hallucinations" (725; see also Upthegrove et al. 2016). Notably, in their phenomenological survey, Hoffman et al. (2007) also found that patients with schizophrenia reported that the most frequent characteristic that allowed them to distinguish AVHs from their own thoughts was "control." This also resonates with Chadwick and Birchwood's (1994) findings of omnipotence attribution. However, the Early Heidelberg School also resonates with Raballo (2016) that voices involve a global transformation of self and world, where the "felt-naturalness of the psychic field seems changed," which is not addressed in the cognitive studies.

Complexity/Diversity of Hallucinations Calls for Interdisciplinary Research

In a strong programmatic statement, Woods et al. (2014) indicate that phenomenology of hallucinations can be applied in an interdisciplinary context:

> One of the greatest contributions that might be made by the humanities and social sciences to the study of AVHs is in offering methods through which to conceptualize, delimit, identify, elicit, and analyze the so-called 'subjective' data that form such a central component of this research. (S247)

Jaspers's own approach to psychopathology (1913a, b) also recognized the urgency of applying both humanistic and scientific approaches to subjective data. In doing so Jaspers responds to the nineteenth-century debate between the human-historical sciences (*Geisteswissenschaften*) and the natural sciences (*Naturwissenschaften*). The former are based on the understanding of meaningful connections of mind and cultural texts; whereas the natural sciences find causal explanations between postulated natural entities. In his interactive approach to diagnosis, Jaspers used the tension between the human-historical "understanding" and natural sciences "explanation" to distinguish delusion-like ideas from primary delusions. "The new or primary in the delusion cannot be derived from some prior experience, motivation, or inner psychological connectedness in the patient. Failing to find any context that makes the patient's behavior or statements understandable, the clinician's empathic understanding falters and she/he experiences the limits of this understanding. This can only be determined interactively" (Mishara and Fusar-Poli 20: 282).

Jaspers (1913b) laments that even in his day "there is a decrease in the general level of education of psychiatrists in the human historical sciences or humanities (*Geisteswissenschaften*), and thus, failure to employ a psychology of understanding in clinical practice. As a result, the clinic has become crude and oversimplified, whereby the general desire is to do away with the humanities altogether" (336; our translation).

Phenomenology and phenomenological psychiatry have a long history of utilizing fictional literature, and other arts, as a data source in researching the conscious and unconscious structures of subjective experience: The study of literature "documents and records cognitive and neural processes of self with an intimacy that may be otherwise unavailable to neuroscience" (Mishara 2010c: 3).

For an excellent and balanced review of the diversity and richness of current approaches to phenomenology of hallucinations, see Pienkos et al. (in press).

ACKNOWLEDGMENTS

Yuliya Zaytseva is supported by the Czech Research Council (grant number AZV MH CR 17-32957A).

Bibliography

Baillarger J. (1846). "Des hallucinations." *Memories de l'Academie Royale de Medecine* 12: 273–475.

Beringer K. (1927). *Der Meskalinrausch: Seine Geschichte und Erscheinungsweise.* Berlin: Verlag Julius von Springer.

Beringer K. and Ruffin H. (1932). "Sensibilitätsstudien zur Frage des Funktionswandels bei Schizophrenen, Alkoholikern und Gesunden." *Zeitschrift für die gesamte Neurologie und Psychiatrie* 140: 604–640. doi: 10.1007/BF02864378

Berrios G. E. and Dening T. R. (1996). "The Enigma of Pseudohallucinations: Current Meanings and Usage." *Psychopathology* 29: 17–34.

Berze J. (1914). *Die primäre Insuffizienz der psychischen Aktivität.* Leipzig: Deuticke.

Berze J. (1932). "Störungen des psychischen Antriebes." *Zeitschrift für die Gesamte Neurologie und Psychiatrie* 142: 720–773.

Berze J. and Gruhle H. W. (1929). *Psychologie der Schizophrenie.* Berlin: Springer.

Binswanger L. (1957). *Schizophrenie.* Pfullingen: Günther Neske.

Binswanger L. (1965). *Wahn: Beiträge zu seiner phänomenologischen und daseinsanalytischen Erforschung.* Pfullingen: Günther Neske.

Birchwood M., Meaden A., Trower P., Gilbert P., and Plaistow J. (2000). "The Power and Omnipotence of Voices: Subordination and Entrapment of Voices and Significant Others." *Psychological Medicine* 30(2): 337–344.

Chadwick P. and Birchwood M. (1994). "The Omnipotence of Voices—A Cognitive Approach to Auditory Hallucinations." *British Journal of Psychiatry* 164(2): 190–201.

Connor C. and Birchwood M. (2013). "Through the Looking Glass: Selfreassuring Meta-Cognitive Capacity and Its Relationship with the Thematic Content of Voices. *Frontiers in Human Neuroscience* 7: 213.

Conrad K. (1958). *Die Beginnende Schizophrenie: Versuch einer Gestaltanalyse des Wahns.* Stuttgart: Thieme.

Delespaul P. and van Os J. (2002). "Determinants of Occurrence and Recovery from Hallucinations in Daily Life." *Social Psychiatry and Psychiatric Epidemiology* 37(3): 97–104.

Giersch A. and Mishara A. L. (2017a). "Disrupted Continuity of Subjective Time in the Milleseconds Range in the Self-Disturbances of Schizophrenia: Convergence of Experimental, Phenomenological and Predictive Coding Accounts." *Journal of Consciousness Studies* 24(3–4): 62–68.

Giersch A. and Mishara A. L. (2017b). "Is Schizophrenia a Disorder of Consciousness? Experimental and Phenomenological Support for Impaired Nonconscious Processing." *Frontiers of Psychology* 8: 1659. doi: 10.3389/fpsyg.2017.01659

Gruhle H. W. (1915). "Selbstschilderung und Einfühlung." *Zeitschrift Für Die Gesamte Neurologie und Psychiatrie* 28: 148–231.

Gruhle H. W. (1922). "Psychologie des Abnormen." In *Handbuch der Vergleichenden Psychologie*, pp. 3–151, ed. G. Kafka. München: Ernst Reinhardt Verlag.

Gruhle H. W. (1929). "Psychologie der Schizophrenie." In *Psychologie der Schizophrenie*, pp. 73–168 ed. J. Berze. Wien: Springer.

Gruhle H. W. (1932). "Allgemeine Symptomatologie." In *Handbuch der Geisteskrankheiten*, pp. 135–292, ed. O. Bumk. Berlin: Springer.

Grünbaum A. A. (1917). "Pseudovorstellung und Pseudohalluzination." *Zeitschrift für die gesamte Neurologie und Psychiatrie* 37: 100–109. doi:10.1007/BF02917384

Hagen F. W. (1868). "Zur Theorie der Hallucination." *Allgemeine Zeilschrift fiir Psychiatrie* 25: 1–107.

Hoffman R., Varanko M., Gilmore J., and Mishara A. L. (2007) "Experiential Features Used by Patients with Schizophrenia to Differentiate 'Voices' from Ordinary Verbal Thought." *Psychological Medicine* 38: 1167–1176.

Hughlings Jackson J. (1932). In J Taylor (ed.), *Selected Writings of John Hughlings Jackson*. London: Hodden and Stoughton.

Humpston C. and Broome M. (2015). "The Spectra of Soundless Voices and Audible Thoughts: Towards an Integrative Model of Auditory Verbal Hallucinations and Thought Insertion." *Review of Philosophy and Psychology* 1–19. doi: 10.1007/s13164-015-0232-9

Jaspers K. (1911). "Zur Analyse der Trugwahrnehmungen (Leibhaftigkeit und Realitätsurteil)." *Zeitschrift für die gesamte Neurologie und Psychiatrie* 6: 460–535.

Jaspers K. (1912). "Die Trugwahrnehmungen. Kritisches Referat." *Zeitschrift für die gesamte Neurologie und Psychiatrie* 4: 289–354.

Jaspers K. (1913a). *Allgemeine Psychopathologie*. Berlin: Springer.

Jaspers K. (1913b). "Kausale und 'verständliche' Zusammenhänge zwischen Schicksal und Psychose bei der Dementia Praecox (1913)." In *Karl Jaspers, Gesammelte Schriften zur Psychopathologie*, pp. 329–412. Berlin/Heidelberg/New York: Springer (1963).

Johns L. C., Kompus K., Connell M., Humpston C., Lincoln T. M., Longden E., . . . Larøi F. (2014). "Auditory Verbal Hallucinations in Persons With and Without a Need for Care." *Schizophrenia Bulletin* 40: S255–S264. doi: 10.1093/schbul/sbu005

Kahlbaum K. (1866). "Die Sinnesdelirien." *Allgemeine Zeitschrift für Psychiatrie und psychischgerichtliche Medizin*, 23: 56–78.

Kaminski J. A., Sterzer P., and Mishara A. L. (in revision). "Seeing Rain": Integrating Phenomenological and Bayesian Predictive Coding Approaches to Visual Hallucinations and Self-Disturbances (Ich-Störungen) in Schizophrenia. *Consciousness and Cognition*.

Kamiya S. and Okamoto S. (1982). "Double Consciousness in Epileptics: A Clinical Picture and Minor Hemisphere Specialization." In H. Akimoto, H. Kazamatsuri, M. Seino, and A. Ward (eds.), *Advances in Epileptology*, pp. 397–401. 13th Epilepsy International Symposium. New York: Raven.

Kandinsky V. K. (1880). "O gallucinaciayah. [About hallucinations]." *Meditsinskoe Obozrenie* 13: 815–824.

Kandinsky V. K. (1881). "Obsheponyatnie psihologicheskie etudi (ocherk istorii vozzreniy na dushy cheloveka i zivotnyh. [Comprehensible sketches (a sketch of the view of man and nature)]." Moskva.

Kandinsky V. K. (1890). "O Psevdohallucinatsiakh. Kritiko-klinicheskii etud. [About Pseudohallucinations, Critical-clinical Study]." St Petersburg: Isdanie EK Kandinskoi.

Kendler K. S. and Mishara A. L. (in review). The Pre-History of Schneider's First-Rank Delusions: Texts from 1810 to 1932. *Schizophrenia Bulletin*.

Lerner V. and Witztum E. (2006). "Victor Kandinsky M.D., 1849–1889." *American Journal of Psychiatry* 163: 209.

Lim H. W., Hoek M., and Deen, et al. (2016). "Prevalence and Classification of Hallucinations in Multiple Sensory Modalities in Schizophrenia Spectrum Disorders." *Schizophrenia Research* 176: 493–499.

Larøi F. (2006). "The Phenomenological Diversity of Hallucinations: Some Theoretical and Clinical Implications." *Psychologica Belgica* 46(1–2): 163–183. doi: 10.5334/pb-46-1-2-163

Larøi F., de Haan S., Jones S., and Raballo A. (2010). "Auditory Verbal Hallucinations: Dialoguing between the Cognitive Sciences and Phenomenology." *Phenomenology and the Cognitive Sciences* 9: 225–240.

Larøi F., et al. (2012). "The Characteristic Features of Auditory Verbal Hallucinations in Clinical and Nonclinical Groups: State-of-the-Art Overview and Future Directions." *Schizophrenia Bulletin* 38: 724–733.

Matussek P. (1952). "Studies on Delusional Perception. I. Changes of the Perceived External World in Incipient Primary Delusion." *Archiv für Psychiatrie und Nervenkrankheiten, vereinigt mit Zeitschrift für die gesamte Neurologie und Psychiatrie.* 189: 279–319.

Matussek P. (1953). "Studies on Delusion. II. Peculiarities of the Delusional Process Exhibited by Schizophrenic Patients in Perceiving the Essential Characteristics of Those in Contact With Them." *Schweizer Archiv für Neurologie und Psychiatrie* 71: 189–210.

Mayer-Gross W. and Stein J. (1926). "Über einige Abänderungen der Sinnestätigkeit im Meskalinrausch." *Zeitschrift für die gesamte Neurologie und Psychiatrie* 101: 354–386.

Mayer-Gross W. and Stein J. (1928). "Pathologie der Wahrnehmung. Psychopathologie und Klinik der Trugwahrnehmungen." In *Handbuch der Geisteskrankheiten*, pp. 352–507, ed. O. Bumke. Berlin: Springer.

Mayer-Gross W. (1932). *Die Klinik der Schizophrenie. Handbuch der Geisteskrankheiten*, pp. 293–578, ed. O. Bumke. Berlin: Springer.

Mishara A. L. (1995). "Narrative and Psychotherapy—The Phenomenology of Healing." *American Journal of Psychotherapy* 49(2): 180–195.

Mishara A. L. (2010a). "Klaus Conrad (1905–1961): Delusional Mood, Psychosis and Beginning Schizophrenia. Clinical Concept Translation-Feature." *Schizophrenia Bulletin* 36: 9–13.

Mishara A. L. (2010b). "Autoscopy: Disrupted Self in Neuropsychiatric Disorders and Anomalous Conscious States." In S. Gallagher and D. Schmicking (eds.), *Handbook of Phenomenology and Cognitive Science*, pp. 591–634. Berlin: Springer.

Mishara A. L. (2010c). "Kafka, Paranoic Doubles and the Brain: Hypnagogic vs. Hyper-reflexive Models of Disruption of Self in Neuropsychiatric Disorders and Anomalous Conscious States." *Philosophy, Ethics, and Humanities in Medicine (PEHM)* 5, (13): 1–37.

Mishara A. L. (2011). "The 'Unconscious' in Paranoid Delusional Psychosis? Phenomenology, Neuroscience, Psychoanalysis." In *Founding Psychoanalysis Phenomenologically*, pp. 169–197, eds D. Lohmar and J. Brudzinska. New York: Springer.

Mishara A. L. and Fusar-Poli P. (2013). "The Phenomenology and Neurobiology of Delusion Formation During Psychosis Onset: Jaspers, Truman Symptoms, and Aberrant Salience." *Schizophrenia Bulletin* 39(2): 278–286.

Mishara A. L. and Schwartz M. A. (2013). "Jaspers' Critique of Essentialist Theories of Schizophrenia and the Phenomenological Response." *Psychopathology* 46(5): 309–319. doi: 10.1159/000353355

Mishara A., Bonoldi I., Allen P., Rutigliano G., Perez J., Fusar-Poli P., et al. (2015). "Neurobiological Models of Self-disorders in Early Schizophrenia." *Schizophrenia Bulletin* 42: 874–880. doi: 10.1093/schbul/sbv123

Mishara A. L. and Sterzer P. (2015). "Phenomenology *is* Bayesian in its Application to Delusions." *World Psychiatry.* 14(2) 185–186. doi: 10.1002/wps.20213

Pienkos E., Giersch A., Hansen M., Humpston C., McCarthy-Jones S., Mishara A., Nelson B., Park S. Raballo A. Sharma J., Thomas N., Rosen C. (in press). "Hallucinations Beyond

Voices: A Conceptual Review of the Phenomenology of Altered Perception in Psychosis." Working Group Report, 4th International Consortium on Hallucination Research Meeting. *Schizophrenia Bulletin.*

Raballo A. (2016). "The Stream of Hallucinatory Consciousness: When Thoughts Become Like Voices." *Journal of Consciousness Studies* 23(7–8): 132–143.

Rybalsky M. I. (1983). *Illusii I hallucinacii. (Illusions and Hallucinations).* Maarif: Baku.

Schneider C. (1930). *Psychologie der Schizophrenen.* Leipzig: Thieme.

Schröder P. (1915). "Von den Halluzinationen." *European Journal of Neurology* 37: 1–11. doi: 10.1159/000190981

Schröder P. (1921a). "Über die Halluzinose und vom Halluzinieren (1)." *Monatsschrift für Psychiatrie und Neurologie* 49: 189–204.

Schröder P. (1921b). "Über die Halluzinose und vom Halluzinieren (2)." *Monatsschrift für Psychiatrie und Neurologie* 49: 205–220.

Schröder P. (1926). "Das Halluzinieren." *Zeitschrift für die gesamte Neurologie und Psychiatrie* 101: 599–614.

Schröder P. (1928). "Fremddenken und Fremdhandeln." *Monatsschrift für Psychiatrie und Neurologie* 68: 515–534. doi: 10.1159/000164535

Specht W. (1914). "Zur Phänomenologie und Morphologie der pathologischen Wahrnehmungstäuschungen. *Zeitschrift für Pathopsychologie, II. Bd.,* 1: 481–569.

Spitzer M. (1987). "Pseudohalluzinationen." *Forschritte Neurologie und Psychiatrie* 55: 91–97.

Stanghellini G. and Cutting J. (2003). "Auditory Verbal Hallucinations—Breaking the Silence of Inner Dialogue." *Psychopathology* 36: 120–128.

Stein H. and Weizsacker V. (1927). "Der Abbau der sensiblen Funktionen." *Deut. Zeitschr. f. Nervenheilk* 99: 1–30.

Sterzer P., Mishara A. L., Voss M., and Heinz A. (2016). "Thought Insertion as Self Disturbance (Ichstörung): A Combined Bayesian Predictive Coding, Phenomenological Approach." *Frontiers of Molecular Neuroscience.* http://journal.frontiersin.org/article/10.3389/fnhum.2016.00502/abstract

Sterzer P., Adams R. A., Fletcher P., Frith C., Lawrie S. M., Muckli L., Petrovic P., Uhlhaas P., Voss M., and Corlett P. R. (2018). "The Predictive Coding Account of Psychosis." *Biological Psychiatry* doi: 10.1016/j.biopsych.2018.05.015

Straus E. (1958). "Aesthesiology and Hallucinations." In R. May, E. Angel, and H. F. Ellenberger (eds.), *Existence,* pp. 139–169. New York: Basic Books.

Straus E. (1978). *Vom Sinn der Sinne: ein Beitrag zur Grundlegung der Psychologie,* 2nd enl. edn. Berlin: Springer Verlag.

Todd J. and Dewhurst K. (1955). "The Double: Its Psycho-Pathology and Psychophysiology." *The Journal of Nervous and Mental Disease* 122: 47–55.

Uhlhaas P. J. and Mishara A. L. (2007). "Perceptual Anomalies in Schizophrenia: Integrating Phenomenology and Cognitive Neuroscience." *Schizophrenia Bulletin* 33: 142–156.

Upthegrove R., Ives J., Broome M. R., Caldwell K., Wood S. J., and Oyebode F. (2016). "Auditory Verbal Hallucinations in First-Episode Psychosis: A Phenomenological Investigation." *British Journal of Psychiatry Open* 2(1): 88–95. doi:10.1192/bjpo.bp.115.002303

Uslar D. von. (1964) *Der Traum als Welt.* Pfullingen: Neske.

Weizsäcker V. Von. (1933). *In Der Gestaltkreis, dargestellt als physiologische Analyse des optischen Drehversuchs.* Original 1933. Edited by: Viktor von Weizsäcker. Gesammelte Schriften, Bd. 4, Frankfurt am Main: Suhrkamp; 1997: 23–61.

Weizsäcker V. Von. (1950a). *Der Gestaltkreis. Theorie der Einheit von Wahrnnehmen und Bewegen* 4. Aufl. Stuttgart: Georg Thieme Verlag.

Weizsäcker V. Von. (1950b). "Funktionswandel und Gestaltkreis." *Deutsche Zeitschrift für Nervenheilkunde* 164: 43–53.

Wernicke C. (1900). *Grundriss der Psychiatrie.* Leipzig: Verlag von Georg Thieme.

Wernicke C. (1906). *Grundriss der Psychiatrie in kliniischen Vorlestungen. Zweite revidierte Auflage.* Leipzig: Verlag von Georg Thieme.

Woods A., et al. (2014). "Interdisciplinary Approaches to the Phenomenology of Auditory Verbal Hallucinations." *Schizophrenia Bulletin* 40(4): 246–254.

Woods A., Jones N., Alderson-Day B., Callard F., and Fernyhough C. (2015). "Experiences of Hearing Voices: Analysis of a Novel Phenomenological Survey." *Lancet Psychiatry* 2(4): 323–331.

Wyss D. (1973). *Beziehung und Gestalt.* Goettingen: Vandenhoeck & Ruprecht.

CHAPTER 55

....

BODILY EXPERIENCE AND ITS DISORDERS

....

JOHN CUTTING

INTRODUCTION

ANOMALOUS experiences and beliefs concerning the body are rife in all psychiatric disorders and many neurological ones. There is a plethora of terms for them with overlapping psychiatric and neurological vocabularies.

In this chapter I aim to show the pervasiveness of bodily psychopathology and demonstrate that the profusion of terms can be whittled down to a handful of general phenomenological principles.

RANGE OF BODILY PSYCHOPATHOLOGY

The body can be anomalously experienced in respect of its shape, size, color, composition, internal spatial configuration, external location, integrity, function, belongingness, even its very existence, and in other ways. The qualities just mentioned are the commonest to emerge from a factor analysis carried out by McGilchrist and Cutting (1995) in respect of functional psychotics. Even these are a heterogeneous collection of alterations in the quality of the body as a thing among other things in the external world *and* the tacit sense of the body as a functioning organism and as a conduit between the world and ourselves.

Here are some examples:

Shape:
   'Lop-sided; right breast larger than left.'
Size:
   'My left arm feels swollen.'

Color:
  'Skin yellow.'
Composition:
  'Body a piece of canvas.'
Internal spatial configuration:
  'Arms sticking out of chest; mouth was where hair should be; two lobes of brain revolving.'
External location:
  'Face intermingled with examiner's.'
Integrity:
  'Finger went right through her and blood came out.'
Function:
  'Blood in brain polluted; stomach dead; arms gone to sleep; brain dried up.'
Belongingness:
  'Sometimes it [left arm] feels like a dead lump, like a false arm. It feels as if someone else is there with you. It feels like a dummy.'
Existence:
  'I feel as if I no longer have a right hand. I have a sense of oppression and pain.'

These extracts (Cutting 1997) give a flavor of the range involved. Table 55.1 gives a more comprehensive picture, setting out the rich vocabulary that the subject has attracted in psychiatric and neurological contexts. The plethora of such experiences in schizophrenia, for example, is barely credible. Sometimes the subject is scarcely able to delimit the boundary between his or her body and others' bodies and other things.

INCIDENCE OF BODILY PSYCHOPATHOLOGY

The incidence in schizophrenia (64%), depressive psychosis (48%), and mania (35%) is high (Cutting 1997), whereas in dementia of the Alzheimer variety it is low (1%—Burns et al. 1990), as it is in delirium (5%—Cutting 1987). No more recent comprehensive estimates of incidence are known to the author, which accords with his general view that bodily psychopathology has been under-researched in recent decades.

In non-psychotic disorders there are no reliable estimates of its magnitude. But in anorexia nervosa, for example, Bruch (1974) considered that "a disturbance of delusional proportions in the body image . . . [was] of pathognomonic significance," and Slade and Russell (1973) obtained experimental support for this. Recent studies (e.g. Nico et al. 2010) corroborate this. In hysteria anomalous awareness of the body is the essence of the condition. In anxiety, phobias, and panic disorder, the symptoms of dizziness, paraesthesia, a lump in the throat (globus hystericus), and cardiovascular and gastrointestinal experiences dominate the picture. In obsessive-compulsive disorder there is often a sense of disgust about bodily functions (von Gebsattel 1938/2012).

Neurological conditions, particularly epilepsy and brain damage, and especially if the parietal or temporal lobes are involved, are frequent causes. The incidence in subjects with an acute right-sided cerebrovascular accident is as high as 87% (Cutting 1978). In fact Gilmore et al. (1992) found it in 100% of subjects whose right hemisphere was artificially inactivated by amytal.

Table 55.1 Bodily psychopathology in psychiatric and neurological contexts

Quality affected	Psychopathological term	Meaning of term
Size	macrosomatagnosia	body part experienced as larger
	microsomatognosia	body part experienced as smaller
Shape	metamorphopsia	body part experienced as altered in shape
Spatial location	alloaesthesia	tactile experience felt elsewhere in body
	exosomesthesia	tactile experience felt outside body
Belongingness	anosognosia	denial of disability
	somatoparaphrenia	body part experienced as belonging to
	personification	someone else
	delusion of control	body part given a specific name, e.g. floppy Joe
	(passivity)	body felt as under someone else's control
Emotional attitude	anosodiaphoria	jocular minimalization of disability
	misoplegia	hatred of paralytic limb
	dysmorphophobia	sense of ugliness or inappropriate shape of
	xenomelia	body part
		hatred and wish to be rid of "normal" body part
Identifiability	finger agnosia	inability to identify fingers on request
	autotopagnosia	inability to identify any body part on request
	right–left disorientation	confusion of right and left
Existence:	phantom limb	absent limb felt as present
false positive	tactile hallucinations	non-existent tactile experiences
false negative	supernumerary phantom	multiplicity of a limb experienced
	delusional parasitosis	infestation with non-existent insects asserted
	nihilistic delusions	belief that body part no longer exists
	hemiasomatognosia	sense that half of body no longer exists
	pain asymbolia	lack of experience of pain
Function	hypochondriacal delusion	belief or sense that body part not working properly

DESCRIPTIVE BODILY PSYCHOPATHOLOGY

The convention of descriptive psychopathology requires that abnormal experience should be allocated to either hallucination, illusion, delusion, or agnosia, and any remainder lumped together as anomalous perceptual experience. This division can be found, in roughly this form, in all the main textbooks at psychopathology in the twentieth century—for example, Jaspers (1959/1963); Fish (1967); Kräupl Taylor (1979); Sims (1995); and myself (Cutting 1997). It is ripe for revision. Bodily psychopathology does not fit neatly into this five-fold division. Spitzer (1990), for example, noted that depressive bodily "delusions" did not satisfy his definition of delusion, which required that the belief was inconsistent with a consensus about some *external world* event. The definition of delusion has itself moved on from this (e.g. American Psychiatric Association 2013—DSM-5) but his comments illustrate the paradoxical situation that ensues when traditional psychopathological categories and factual psychopathological experience clash and so he had to deny statements such as "I have no bowels" any delusional status. McGilchrist and Cutting (1995) found that psychotic bodily psychopathology lay along a spectrum, with bogus sensations—"smacks," "burning feelings"—at one end, and complex, bizarre, cognitive appraisals—"Albert Rubinstein's pea in left ear"—at the other; very few were pure hallucination, illusion, agnosia, delusion, or even anomalous perceptual experience. These mismatches with the traditional categories of descriptive psychopathology indicate the need for a different approach, which is precisely what phenomenological psychopathology offers, as is discussed below.

NOSOLOGICAL SPECIFICITY OF BODILY PSYCHOPATHOLOGY

Some psychopathologists (e.g. Huber 1992; Jenkins and Röhricht 2007) have suggested that schizophrenia with prominent bodily psychopathology deserves its own nosological status, which they refer to as "cenesthetic" or "cenesthopathic" schizophrenia.

The non-belongingness of bodily experience was recognized by Kurt Schneider as characteristic of schizophrenia, and he promoted this to first-rank symptom status (Schneider 1939).

Earlier (Schneider 1920/2012), he had linked another sort of bodily experience—what he called "vital feelings," for example, knotted stomach, tension in the chest—with another psychiatric condition—endogenous depression. Although he did not use the term first-rank symptoms of endogenous depression at that time, he did consider that these vital feelings distinguished the condition from a reactive depression and normal sadness—where "psychic feelings" such as sadness predominated. Sims (1995), however, credited Schneider with having identified first-rank symptoms of an endogenous depression.

Except for hysteria and anorexia nervosa, neurotic disorders have not been accorded any specific bodily psychopathology, although some are highly suggestive of one or other condition: globus hystericus of an anxiety state in my opinion, right-sided functional complaints in depressive states (Rothwell 1994; McGilchrist and Cutting 1995), and left-sided sensory symptoms in anxiety states (O'Sullivan et al. 1992; Rothwell 1994).

PSYCHOLOGICAL ACCOUNTS OF BODILY PSYCHOPATHOLOGY

Psychological accounts of the body assume some representation in the mind of what the body is, and, further, that it is represented as a thing, like any other worldly thing. The French neurologist Bonnier (1905), the British neurologists Head and Holmes (1911), and the Austrian neuropsychiatrist Schilder (1935) all proposed a similar sort of structure for this—body image or schema, which stored what one *had* experienced and then determined what one *would* experience. The entire gamut of bodily psychopathology would thereby be deemed body image or body schema disorder.

Some bodily psychopathology does conform to this model. Phantom limb, for example, would appear to be the result of a pre-amputation body image not keeping up to date with a new situation, a scenario supported by the fact that if a subsequent cerebrovascular accident occurs in the parietal lobe, the brain region supposedly housing this body image, the phantom disappears (Head and Holmes 1911).

But some bodily psychopathology is quite counter-evidential to the notion of a single, static body image. Take anosognosia, the neurological term for a sense of non-belongingness of a body part. Fotopoulou et al. (2009) demonstrated complete and permanent recovery when their patient viewed herself in a video, and Fotopoulou et al. (2011) reported remission in two patients with somatoparaphrenia—attribution of the paralyzed limb to someone else—when they looked at themselves in a mirror. The authors attributed the improvement to the subjects' being forced to take a third-person perspective on their disability. Whatever the explanation, the experiments show that if a "body image disorder" can come and go like this there is something wrong with the notion of a single "body image," damage to which causes a set of discrete "body image disorders."

Neuropsychological Accounts of Bodily Psychopathology

In the middle decades of the twentieth century neurologists such as Brain (1941) and Hecaen and colleagues (1956) concluded that the right hemisphere was critical to the body image, as disorders such as unawareness of one side of the body (hemiasomatognosia) and dressing difficulties (dressing apraxia) were confined to those with right hemisphere damage. The situation was later revised, giving credit to the left hemisphere's provision of schematic knowledge of body parts as worldly objects. So, with left hemisphere damage this circumscribed knowledge is obliterated, leading to statements about the non-existence of body parts:

> 'It's as if I haven't any right arm and hand, but only a weight where the hand should be.'
> 'Right forearm feels different, mechanical, heavier, as if it's not there from the elbow, and in its place a feeling of uneasiness.'
>
> (Hecaen and Ajuriaguerra 1952)

The right hemisphere provides a gestalt of the entire body, stamps a sense of "myness" on experience, and is attuned to the body's spatial configuration. Subjects with right hemisphere damage:

> 'I felt as if instead of a left leg there was something that didn't belong to me, a piece of meat, as if I had no leg.'
> 'I feel as if the left leg is leaving me, and that my left eye seems to be leaving its socket.'
>
> (Hecaen and Ajuriaguerra 1952)

> 'The left half of my body has been substituted with scaffolding.'
>
> (Ehrenwald 1930)

In short, neuropsychological investigations into bodily psychopathology reveal two directions, relative to normal, in which the body is experienced: 1) shorn of its very existence as a worldly thing, replaced by sensory or vital feelings; 2) slipping away from the ambit of myness, spatially fragmenting, substituted by a worldly structure.

EXTANT PHENOMENOLOGICAL ANALYSIS OF BODILY PSYCHOPATHOLOGY

The Germans are at an advantage here, having two words for body—*Leib* and *Körper*—whereas in English and French, for example, there is only one—body, *corps*, because it turns out that only by appreciating the duality of the body, which the German terms *Leib* [living body] and *Körper* [dead, worldly, or reified body] express perfectly, can bodily psychopathology be properly understood. We shall illustrate the critical themes through the writings of three psychopathologists—Goldstein, Blankenburg, and Fuchs.

Goldstein got to the heart of the matter in his 1931 article *"Über Zeigen und Greifen"* ("On Pointing and Grasping"). The thrust of this is that the human body is both a conduit for the enactment of signs as well as an apparatus for getting—grasping—what its desires demand. This opens up a rich perspective on bodily psychopathology. Some varieties—finger agnosia (inability to point to a specified finger) and autopagnosia (inability to point to any specified body part) fall within the body's role as purveyor of signs, that is, meaning. Others—anosognosia (denial of the condition of body part), hemiasomatognosia (neglect of half body), and somatoparaphrenia (delusional elaboration of estranged limb)—are examples of body parts no longer subserving the aim of the living organism to grasp and preserve its well-being, written-off as it were.

Blankenburg's (1982) article *"Körper und Leib in der Psychiatrie"* ("Body as Thing and Body as Organism in Psychiatry") elaborates Goldstein's theme. His innovative contributions are two-fold. First he points out that the notion of body as *Körper* is relatively circumscribed: it is a thing in the world which can be externally perceived and studied scientifically. By comparison, body as *Leib* is multifaceted: he lists no fewer than seven different aspects—perspectival point in space, medium whereby sensations can be felt, agent of an "I-can" potential, locus for suffering, provider of means of self-expression, conduit between self and world, and what he calls in English "partner," by which he means a sort of honored companion of the self. Any one of these could presumably be separately dilapidated and give rise to psychopathology, but—and these are the second set of innovative remarks—he concentrates on instances of a rupture or confusion between a subject's sense of their body as *Leib* and its status as *Körper*. He sees the autistic child's preoccupation with mechanical things as an abandonment of *Leib*'s role in building up social relations and their pirouettes as treating their own body as a *Körper*-like entity which can spin round like a mechanical top. He views case reports of schizophrenics who misrecognize their face in a mirror as examples of a decoupling of their own bodily awareness through *Leib* and its *Körper* as an externally perceived thing.

In several articles, notably one in 2005, Fuchs has argued that the schizophrenic and depressive are both compromised in respect of their body's role as a catalyst for transforming the world into knowledge of this world. In schizophrenia, he maintains, there is a loss of implicit awareness of the world through the body, and, as a consequence, everything the schizophrenic does has an artificial, forced, explicit quality. By contrast, he attributes to the depressive a different kind of bodily malfunction, which results in a "reification of the lived body," that is, body becoming more thing-like, which, according to Fuchs, explains their characteristic experiences.

PHILOSOPHICAL PHENOMENOLOGY OF BODILY PSYCHOPATHOLOGY

Phenomenological psychopathology had its origins in a meeting in 1922 between Eugene Minkowski, Ludwig Binswanger, Erwin Straus, and Victor von Gebsattel. The program sketched out was anti-psychological and anti-organic (now read anti-neuropsychological) and instead embraced contemporary philosophy. In the course of their careers, Minkowski cited Bergson as his mentor, Binswanger oscillated between interpretations of Husserl and Heidegger, and Straus and von Gebsattel referred to Scheler amongst other philosophers. Jaspers (1959/1963) is not in this select group. He was a superb descriptive psychopathologist, later philosopher, but eschewed phenomenological analysis of psychopathology, whether of a Husserlian, Heidegerian, or Schelerian variety (Walker 1991).

My guide in this chapter is Max Scheler (1874–1928), whose writings on the body are concentrated in his treatise *Formalism in Ethics and Non-formal Ethics of Values* (Scheler 1913–1916/1973: 399). He too considered the body to be a dual entity—part perceiver and part perceived, partly subjective and partly objective—and recognized the philosophical implications of the German words *Leib* and *Körper* before Goldstein took this up. But there are other insights in Scheler's late philosophy (Scheler 1927–1928/1995) which have a bearing on what the body and bodily psychopathology are. Latterly he was preoccupied with a more pervasive duality of cosmic proportions, between what he called *Drang* [a surging forth of energy, including life's exuberance] and *Geist* [the facility unique to humans of, amongst other things such as objectivizing objects, knowing the essence of anything—its *Wesensein* or *Wassein*—as opposed to its coincidental properties—*zufälliges Sein*]. The body and its parts are therefore, in this respect, like any other thing in the world, known partly in the form of an essence or whatness—as a stomach, as a leg—and partly by way of a host of accidental qualities—*my* stomach in *this place now*, or *my* leg with *this* color, weight, and texture.

Much of the bodily psychopathology set out in Table 55.1 can be accommodated by assuming that the positions on the two Schelerian axes of what the body is—whose poles are 1) body as *Leib* and body as *Körper*; 2) body as *Wesensein* and body as *zufälliges Sein*—have shifted in an anomalous direction.

Let us take some examples from the Table. Somatoparaphrenia and passivity experiences, respectively the neurological and psychiatric terms for delusionally elaborated lack of myness, represent a shift toward treating a body part solely as *Körper*, a thing in the outside world, and an attenuation in its status as *Leib*, my lived body. Misoplegia and dysmorphophobia, respectively the neurological and psychiatric terms for an overly emotional attitude to a body part (deeming it inappropriately ugly or unpleasant or hating it), represent a shift in the opposite direction—accessing it as if it were some non-thing, with only its value available to knowledge and the mode of knowledge being the emotion registered. Then consider nihilistic delusions, also present in both neurological and psychiatric contexts. It was notable in Hecaen and Ajuriaguerra's cases, quoted above, that a complete disappearance of anything corresponding to a body part did not occur, but it was rather that only the essence or whatness of something was lost whereas some sort of emotion or spatial awareness remained:

> 'My right side is replaced by pain. The half corresponding to the world is abolished. Nothing exists there.'
> 'It's as if there was an emptiness vaguely on the right, that on that side everything is far away and empty.'

In our scheme, what has happened is that the essence of a body part has evaporated from the person's knowledge whereas its accidental qualities—spatiality, induced feelings—are still lively. Finally, a sizeable amount of bodily psychopathology, which are given names such as metamorphopsia, microsomatagnosia, or alloaesthesia in the neurological literature, but are lumped together as anomalous perceptual experiences in the psychiatric literature, represent an attenuation in some *zufälliges* [coincidental] quality of a correctly identified thing.

Conclusion

The range and terminology involved in bodily psychopathology is daunting. But, as promised, a phenomenological approach, following up the insights of Goldstein, Blankenburg, and Fuchs, with help from astute neuropsychologists, and critical input from one of the original trio of phenomenological philosophers, a few principles can be extracted that leave the field much clearer and more manageable. Central to my analysis is that the body is not a circumscribed entity. It is both a thing in the external world for its owner and other people and other people *and* a multifaceted agent for navigating the environment—acting on it and perceiving its richness. Bodily psychopathology reflects compromised abilities in all these areas. Some of the most bizarre and puzzling of these—nihilistic delusions (where parts of the body are deemed absent) and delusions of control (where the body loses its independence from outside influences) are plausibly, out for the first time, explained by phenomenological analysis. Max Scheler's later writing—on the nature of the essence of anything and its coincidental qualities—are the only philosophical input, known to the author, which can explain these matters. Nihilistic delusions would be, on Scheler's account, a dilapidation of essence, and delusions of control a loss of the coincidental qualities of a body—its myness and thisness.

Bibliography

Blankenburg W. (1982). "Körper und Leib in der Psychiatrie." *Schweizer Archiv für Neurologie, Neurochirurgie und Psychiatrie* 131: 13–39.
Bonnier P. (1905). "L'aschématie." *Revue Neurologique* 13: 605–609.

Brain W. R. (1941). "Visual Disorientation with Special Reference to Lesions of the Right Hemisphere." *Brain* 64: 244–272.

Bruch H. (1974). *Eating Disorders*. London: Routledge and Kegan Paul.

Burns A., Jacoby R., and Levy R. (1990). "Psychiatric Phenomena in Alzheimer's Disease." *British Journal of Psychiatry* 157: 72–94.

Cutting J. (1978). "Study of Anosognosia." *Journal of Neurology, Neurosurgery and Psychiatry* 41: 548–555.

Cutting J. (1987). "The Phenomenology of Acute Organic Psychosis: Comparison with Acute Schizophrenia." *British Journal of Psychiatry* 151: 324–332.

Cutting J. (1997). *The Principles of Psychopathology*. Oxford: Oxford University Press.

Ehrenwald H. (1930). "Verändertes Erleben des Körperbildes mit konsekutiver Wahnbildung bei linksseitiger Hemiplegie." *Monatsschrift für Psychiatrie und Neurologie* 75: 89–97.

Fish F. (1967). *Clinical Psychopathology*. Bristol: J Wright.

Fotopoulou A., Rudd A., Holmes P., and Kopelman M. (2009). "Self-observation Reinstates Motor Awareness in Anosognosia for Hemiplegia." *Neuropsychologia* 47: 1256–1260.

Fotopoulou A., Jenkinson P. M., Tsakiris M., Haggard P., Rudd A., and Kopelman M. D. (2011). "Mirror-view Reverses Somatoparaphrenia. Dissociation between First-and Third-Person Perspectives on Body Ownership." *Neuropsychologia* 49: 3946–3955.

Fuchs T. (2005). "Corporealized and Disembodied Minds. A Phenomenological View of the Body in Melancholia and Schizophrenia." *Philosophy, Psychiatry and Psychology* 12: 95–107.

Gilmore R. L, Heliman K. M., Schmidt R. P., Fennell E. M., and Quisling R. (1992). "Anosognosia During Wada Testing." *Neurology* 42: 925–927.

Goldstein K. (1931). "Über Zeigen und Greifen." *Nervenarzt* 4: 453–466.

Head H. and Holmes G. (1911). "Sensory Disturbances from Cerebral Lesions." *Brain* 34: 102–154.

Hecaen H. and Ajuriaguerra J. (1952). *Méconnaissances et Hallucinations Corporelles*. Paris: Masson.

Hecaen H., Penfield W., Bertrand C., and Malmo R. (1956). "The Syndrome of Apractognosia Due to Lesions of the Minor Cerebral Hemisphere." *Archives of Neurology and Psychiatry* 75: 400–434.

Huber G. (1992). "Cenesthetic Schizophrenia—A Subtype of Schizophrenic Disease." *Neurology and Psychiatry Brain Research* 1: 54–60.

Jaspers K. (1959/1963). *General Psychopathology*. Manchester: Manchester University Press.

Jenkins G. and Röhricht F. (2007). "From Cenesthesics to Cenesthopathic Schizophrenia: A Historical and Phenomenological Review." *Psychopathology* 40: 361–368.

Kräupl Taylor F. (1979). *Psychopathology: Its Causes and Symptoms*. London: Quartermaine House.

McGilchrist I. and Cutting J. (1995). "Somatic Delusions in Schizophrenia and the Affective Disorders." *British Journal of Psychiatry* 167: 350–361.

Nico D., Daprati E., Nighoghossian N., Carrier E., Duhumel J.-R., and Sirigu A. (2010). "The Role of the Right Parietal Lobe in Anorexia Nervosa." *Psychological Medicine* 40: 1531–1539.

O'Sullivan G., Harvey I., Bass C., Sheehy M., Toone B., and Turner S. (1992). "Psycho-physiological Investigations of Patients with Unilateral Symptoms in the Hyperventilation Syndrome." *British Journal of Psychiatry* 160: 664–674.

Rothwell P. (1994). "Investigation of Unilateral Sensory or Motor Symptoms: Frequency of Neurological Pathology Depends on Side of Symptoms." *Journal of Neurology Neurosurgery and Psychiatry* 57: 1401–1402.

Scheler M. (1913–1916/1973) *Formalism in Ethics and Non-Formal Ethics of Values.* Evanston: Northwestern University Press.

Scheler M. (1927–1928/1995). "Idealismus—Realismus." In M. Scheler, *Collected Works.* Vol. 9, pp. 183–241. Bonn: Bouvier Verlag.

Schilder P. (1935). *The Image and Appearance of the Human Body.* London: Kegan Paul, Trench & Trubner.

Schneider K. (1920/2012). "The Stratification of Emotional Life and the Structure of Depressive States." In M. R. Broome, R. Harland, G. S. Owen, and A. Stringaris (eds.), *The Maudsley Reader in Phenomenological Psychiatry*, pp. 203–207. Cambridge: Cambridge University Press.

Schneider K. (1939). *Psychischer Befund und Psychiatrische Diagnose.* Leipzig: George Thieme.

Sims A. (1995). *Symptoms in the Mind*, 2nd edn. London: W. B. Saunders.

Slade P. D. and Russell G. F. M. (1973). "Experimental Investigations of Body Perception in Anorexia Nervosa and Obesity." *Psychotherapy and Psychosomatics* 22: 359–363.

Spitzer M. (1990). "On Defining Delusions." *Comprehensive Psychiatry* 31: 377–397.

von Gebsattel V. (1938/2012). "The World of the Compulsive." In M. R. Broome, R. Harland, G. S. Owen, and A. Stringaris (eds.), *The Maudsley Reader in Phenomenological Psychiatry*, pp. 232–240. Cambridge: Cambridge University Press.

Walker C. (1991). "Delusion: What Did Jaspers Really Say?" *British Journal of Psychiatry* suppl 14: 94–103.

CHAPTER 56

THE PSYCHOPATHOLOGICAL CONCEPT OF CATATONIA

GABOR S. UNGVARI

INTRODUCTION

PECULIAR motor phenomena have been known since time immemorial (Fink and Taylor 2003). Kahlbaum (1973) is generally credited to have subsumed unusual motor behavior and related psychic symptoms under the heading of catatonia as a distinct disease entity, an attempt that was not entirely successful (Berrios 1996). Prior to Kahlbaum, a host of classical authors—Pinel, Guislain, Heinroth, Griesinger, and particularly Arndt in 1868, 1871, and 1872, to name just a few—described clinical pictures, termed as "Melancholia attonita," "Melancholie avec stupeur," or "Katalepsie und Psychose," overlapping with Kahlbaum's catatonia (Arndt 1902). Since Kahlbaum, catatonia has been an integral part of psychiatric symptomatology via magisterial descriptions by Kraepelin (1919) and Bleuler (1950), although it was thought to slowly disappear in the second part of the twentieth century. There is compelling evidence, however, that changing diagnostic practices and criteria (van der Heijden et al. 2005) and the poor recognition of catatonic symptomatology (Oulis and Lykouras 1996) were mainly responsible for the apparent "disappearance" of catatonia.

There has been an unexpected flurry of publications on catatonia over the past quarter century indicating an upsurge of interest in motor disorders in psychiatry. Disappointingly, however, the majority of the 2,983 papers appearing on Medline between 1990 and 2017 on catatonia, mostly case reports or small-scale treatment response studies, fail to address the core issues of the catatonia concept.

This is a brief, selective review of the complex problem of motor disorders in psychiatry, focusing on catatonia from a psychopathological vantage point. Details of the history, clinical presentation, neurobiology, and management of catatonia are comprehensively reviewed elsewhere (Bostroem 1928; Lohr and Wisniewski 1987; Northoff 1997; Fink and Taylor 2003; Caroff et al. 2004).

The term "motor disorders" refers to the overarching range of voluntary and involuntary movement encountered in psychiatry irrespective of their origins, ranging from drug-induced extrapyramidal symptoms to conversion symptoms such as pseudoparesis. The narrower terms "psychomotor" or "psychomotility" comprise motor symptoms likely to be related to psychic conditions: for example, psychomotor retardation associated with depressed mood. "Catatonia" represents a variety of simple motor, speech, and complex behavioral signs and symptoms that are kept together by tradition, and form loosely defined syndromes. Unless specified otherwise, "catatonia" and "catatonic syndrome" are used here interchangeably. The concept of catatonia is discussed in more detail in this article.

The following two case vignettes and the related interpretation introduce some of the issues this chapter elaborates on from a psychopathological viewpoint.

> Julius, a young man, was taken to an emergency room in a mute, motionless state. He had fled a politically troubled country, seeking asylum in the West and hoping to bring his family to live with him. Waiting for deportation after his claim for refugee status had been rejected, he was overwhelmed with mixed emotions of despair, shame, and hopelessness. Following a brief period of agitation, he suddenly became unresponsive and froze in motion. Following an organic workup in the emergency room that yielded negative results and a small dose of intravenous benzodiazepine and some comforting words, Julius fully recovered and regained his composure. The discharge diagnosis was "Catatonia."
>
> George was a sixty-four-year-old single man with a forty-year history of a psychiatric illness variously diagnosed as personality disorder, schizophrenia, and depression. Over the past forty years George had lived in social isolation, leading an itinerant lifestyle interspersed with psychiatric admissions. During his current admission, he stood in one place staring and rarely initiated conversation or answered questions. He communicated via brief handwritten notes. While standing he stroked his hair repeatedly in a uniform way for several minutes, resisting any attempts to mobilize him or change his position. There were no recent hints of him having hallucinations or delusions. George ate and slept well and maintained a low but acceptable hygienic standard. A variety of antipsychotic drugs and high dose lorazepam (12 mg/day) failed to change his overall behavior or specific motor pattern. George's latest diagnosis was also "Catatonia."

These case vignettes illustrate the deficiencies in the contemporary concept of catatonia. Apart from superficial similarities, the two presentations have nothing common, especially in terms of the time-frame, consistency, treatment response, and precipitating factors of the motor signs and symptoms. Given that both patients were diagnosed with catatonia following current diagnostic guidelines, catatonia has very broad boundaries and the term carries ambiguous clinical information.

There is another clinical issue pertinent to the psychopathology of catatonia related to George's case. Whenever his presentation was discussed in a clinical meeting, the described motor signs/symptoms were summarily dismissed as "not psychotic, only behavioral" as though his behavior and motor symptoms would not signal a fundamental change in the way he perceived and related to himself and his social environment. Although George remained consistently autistic (in Bleuler's sense) and did not allow insight into his inner world, it is safe to assume that his thinking was grossly idiosyncratic, if not profoundly delusional, and he had a distorted view of human existence in general and his own existence in particular.

THE PSYCHOPATHOLOGICAL DEFINITION
OF CATATONIA

The lack of a psychopathological definition of catatonia exemplifies the neglect of descriptive psychopathology in contemporary psychiatry. What is surprising is that modern authors do not even feel the need to find psychopathological principles to define what catatonia is. The current definitions are all non-specific, if not tautological. A few examples by authorities of the field illustrate this point: "Disturbed motor functions amid disturbances of mood and thought" (Fink 2009); "Catatonia is a syndrome of specific motor abnormalities closely associated with disorders of mood, affect, thought and cognition" (Fink-Taylor 2003); and "Catatonia is a neuropsychiatric syndrome with a unique combination of mental, motor, vegetative and behavioural signs" (Caroff et al. 2004). Only Lohr and Wisniewski (1987) have pointed out that most authors have assumed catatonia to be a "coherent, well-defined syndrome ... without ever defining exactly what it was."

None of these definitions gives guidance to the decision about what makes a neuropsychiatric sign or symptom "catatonic." As a result, the catatonic syndrome is fast being made boundless by proposals to add a range of diverse symptoms such as "prankishness" (Lohr and Wisniewski 1987), "coma" (Bender and Feutrill 2000), and "dysphagia" (Akintomide et al. 2012).[1]

Over the past hundred years, Jaspers's concept of catatonia has underpinned continental European views. Based on his broad methodological principles of understanding and explanation, Jaspers regarded catatonia as "all incomprehensible motor phenomena" (Jaspers 1963: 181) and suggested that "Somewhere between the neurological phenomena, seen as disturbances of the motor apparatus, and the psychological phenomena, seen as the sequel of psychic abnormality with the motor apparatus intact, lie the psychic motor phenomena, which we register without being able to comprehend them satisfactorily one way or the other" (Jaspers 1963: 179). "Psychic motor phenomena" were basically catatonia in Jaspers's view while "psychological phenomena" such as depressive or hysterical stupor were "not conceived to be primary motor phenomena but are actions and nodes of expressions which have to be understood" (Jaspers 1963: 179). Jaspers's psychopathological division of motor symptoms assign catatonia to the realm of schizophrenia while acknowledging that motor signs and symptoms similar to catatonia occur in a host of other psychiatric disorders.[2]

---

[1] Then, fundamental questions arise. What, other than tradition, would differentiate catatonic signs/symptoms from other motor phenomena observed in neuropsychiatry? Why is echolalia a typical catatonic symptom and palilalia not? What is the added clinical value of calling a stupor "catatonic"? Further, what is the rationale for retaining the concept of catatonia at all? If most catatonic signs and symptoms are considered to result from "either damage to the frontal lobe motor regulatory system or damage to or disruption of function in subcortical structures" (Taylor 1990), then the logical solution would be to use the diagnostic term "catatonia" only in relation to presumably specific motor disorders associated with schizophrenia as a lucid editorial suggested (Anonymous 1986).

[2] Fish's now less influential text on schizophrenia harks back to Jaspers's concept on catatonia: "Disorders of behaviour ... are often bizarre and cannot be easily understood as arising from the patient's abnormal ideas" (Hamilton 1984: 65). This is the approach followed by Kraepelin when he asserted that persistent "genuine catatonic morbid symptoms" appeared only in dementia praecox (Kraepelin 1919: 258). Kurt Schneider (1914) also came to the same conclusion following an extensive

Jaspers's definition is dynamic because it implies that, with progress in neuroscience, increasingly more signs/symptoms will move to the realm of neurology and eventually the whole concept of catatonia will be eliminated, becoming a historical footnote.[3]

The Recognition and Diagnosis
of Catatonia

The lack of its conceptual clarity is reflected in the recognition and diagnosis of catatonia that presupposes distinct and coherent descriptions of individual symptoms and syndromes for clinical practice and research. Yet, we submit that the currently available rating scales provide only crude estimations of its cross-sectional clinical picture instead of capturing the extent and depth of catatonic symptomatology. Without a firm psychopathological foundation along the lines as Jaspers suggested, the construction of rating scales remains arbitrary. While their psychometric properties, if tested, are satisfactory to excellent, their validity and clinical utility are still questionable. Thus, it is not surprising that existing rating scales differ considerably from each other in the number and definitions of symptoms and the time frame required for completing the standardized examination.

The existing seven catatonia rating scales comprise altogether fifty-four symptoms, ranging from eighteen to forty in individual scales (Sienart et al. 2011). DSM-5 (APA 2013) and ICD-10 (WHO 1992) lists twelve and nine symptoms, respectively. While the nine core symptoms (stupor, mutism, negativism, stereotypy, mannerisms, excitement, echolalia/echopraxia, posturing, and waxy flexibility) appear in all scales, in DSM-5/ICD-10 a number of additional symptoms either overlap with the core symptoms (e.g. agitation with excitement, withdrawal or refusal of oral intake with negativism or stupor) or are clearly neurological (e.g. grasp reflex or shuffling gait) or non-specific (poor compliance, affect-related behavior, or loss of initiative). Loquacity, the core symptom in at least five of the twenty-four cases described in Kahlbaum's monograph (Kahlbaum 1973: cases no. 2, 4, 7, 11, 13), appears as "increased, compulsive-like speech" in only one scale (Northoff et al. 1999). The diversity in definitions of individual symptoms for clinicians is "more than disturbing" (Sienart et al. 2011).

---

review of short-lived, catatonia-like symptoms in healthy individuals and a variety of psychiatric disorders.

[3] Jaspers's view also infers that the diagnosis of catatonia cannot be established without a neurological evaluation or the psychosocial background against which catatonia occurred. Manifestations of psychological conflicts leading to distress—still called "conversion disorder" in ICD-10 although removed from DSM-5—would not qualify as catatonia because a meaningful connection and temporal link are present between cause and consequence. (That is demonstrated in Julius's case vignette at the start of this article.) The unease with diagnosing catatonia in such clinical presentations based on superficial similarities with persistent catatonic symptoms is reflected in the creation of oxymorons such as "hysterical catatonia" (Dabholkar 1988) or "conversion catatonia" (Jensen 1984). This is not pure semantics. Enduring catatonic symptoms seen in schizophrenia differ from the fleeting psychomotor symptoms of anxiety or mood disorders not only phenomenologically (Ungvari et al. 2005; but in treatment response (Ungvari et al. 1999a) and very likely in aetiology.

The simplicity of definitions glosses over potentially important psychopathological details of individual catatonic symptoms as illustrated by the example of echolalia. The terse definitions ("mimicking another's speech" (DSM-5); "mimicking of examiner's movements/speech" (Bush et al. 1996); "reproducible (i.e. > 5 times) mimicking of other person's behaviour (echopraxia) and/or speech (echolalia)" (Northoff et al. 1999)) hide an amazingly rich symptom profile with differential diagnostic significance. In a comprehensive review, Stengel (1947) analyzed echolalia in terms of immediacy, literalness, frequency, consistency, content, propositionality, selectivity, meaningfulness, and relationship with other symptoms. "Automatic echolalia," mostly seen in catatonic schizophrenia, is immediate, literal, and non-communicatively delivered without affective changes or intellectual efforts. It may occur hours or days after the stimulus as "delayed echolalia," typically in childhood autism. "Mitigated echolalia" is a less severe variant being inconsistent in terms of literalness, immediacy, selectivity, and content, suggesting that anxiety, hostility, suggestibility, poor comprehension, and identification may play a part in its development. Mitigated echolalia is observed in aphasias, clouded consciousness, or even in fatigued healthy individuals. "Echo contamination" refers to the repeated and inappropriate intrusion of a single word just heard into the patient's speech. Loosely associated with echolalia is the "completion phenomenon" seen in transcortical aphasia and mental deficiency, when the patient automatically completes the examiner's question despite being requested not to do so. "Mental echolalia"—echolalia only in the mind—and "hallucinatory echolalia"—repeating one's own hallucinations aloud—are infrequently detected, mainly in schizophrenia. "Auto-echolalia," also called "palilalia," is a "motor disorder of speaking rather than of speech" characterized by the "involuntary repetition two or more times of a word, phrase or sentence just uttered" (Critchley 1927) with increasing speed and decreasing pitch and loudness. Palilalia appears in neurological disorders affecting the striatum and is only rarely seen in schizophrenia. The question remains whether catatonia research should continue operating with the skeleton definitions contained in the rating scales or would benefit from incorporating the observations of classical descriptive psychopathology.

Catatonic signs and symptoms wax and wane, and only longer-term, repeated observations made in different contexts allow the full clinical presentation to emerge (Kraepelin 1919). Cross-sectional examination with a rating scale cannot capture every aspect of the clinical picture; for instance, the examination schedule of the most frequently used Bush-Francis Catatonia Rating Scale (Bush et al. 1996) requires only five minutes to complete although there is a vague and controversial instruction, "Attempt to observe patient indirectly, at least for a brief period, each day" but no guidance as how to add these brief observations to the five-minute examination. In a comparison of the traditional clinical method and a rating scale-based examination of the same cohort of patients, significantly more symptoms were detected by the former method (Ungvari et al. 1999b).

Besides detection, diagnosis of catatonia is a major problem. There is no consensus on what constitutes a catatonic syndrome, or how many signs and symptoms are necessary to make this diagnosis. The presence of one to four symptoms in a variety of combinations has been proposed to diagnose catatonia (Sienart et al. 2011). The diversity of views reflects the overall uncertainty about the whole catatonia concept. There is preliminary evidence that the classical two-syndrome—retarded and excited—model of catatonia is but a rough estimate. Factor and latent analytic studies (Peralta and Cuesta 2001) have suggested four

(Kruger et al. 2003; Ungvari et al. 2009) or six (Peralta and Cuesta 2001) separate syndromes within the realm of catatonia depending on the characteristics of the patient population and the composition of the catatonic symptomatology examined.[4]

SUBJECTIVE EXPERIENCES AND THE INNER WORLD OF PATIENTS WITH CATATONIA

The stunningly bizarre motor and behavioral manifestations of catatonia demand interpretation and explanation. Kahlbaum (1973: 31–32) referred to, yet never elaborated on, the patient's "very severe physical or mental stress" and the "intense struggle that went on in his mind," as factors in the development of catatonia. Vogt (1902) made an early attempt to understand the catatonic symptomatology based on William James's psychological theory.

Psychodynamic studies of catatonia, mainly extensive case reports, provide rare insights into the workings of the catatonic individual's mind. The common thread of psychodynamic interpretations of catatonia is the assumption that it is a miscarried, but eventually successful, solution to troublesome early childhood experiences (Angyal 1950).[5]

While psychodynamic interpretations were squeezed out of mainstream psychiatry by the second part of twentieth century, the core idea of catatonia as a defence against overwhelming threat in the form of psychotic experiences and anxiety has remained. Moskowitz (2004) argued for the similarities between catatonia and animals' defensive tonic immobility from the viewpoints of cognitive neuroscience and evolutionary psychology. The treatment response of catatonia to anti-anxiety benzodiazepines provides the clinical argument in Moskowitz's hypothesis. However, only a subset of catatonic states is associated with anxiety (Northoff et al. 1996) and benzodiazepines are not a universally effective treatment (Ungvari et al. 1994), although they remain the first-line treatment option for catatonia.[6]

---

[4] The impact of ethnicity and culturally inherited patterns of expressive and reactive movements on the diagnosis of catatonia has not been extensively researched. Acute catatonic symptomatology, mainly stuporous conditions, is more frequent in developed countries or even in the offspring of patients who were born and brought up in the West (Chandrasena 1986). A recent comparative study confirmed the symptomatic difference between Indian and Welsh catatonic patients diagnosed according to the same methods (Chalasani et al. 2005). This area is a promising avenue for further research.

[5] In a brilliant case history and review of the psychoanalytic literature, Johnson (1984) listed a few partly overlapping interpretations of catatonia. Catatonia is variously conceptualized as "*a regression to an intrauterine state in which an "end of the world" fantasy is followed by an omnipotent rebirth fantasy*," as "*defiance and suppressed anger*," as an "*unresolved conflict between overly strict ego ideals and sexual and aggressive instincts*," as an attempt to "*run away from danger*" and as "*primitive attempts to avoid responsibility for willed actions, originating in early childhood experiences in which the mother is overprotective and disapproving*."

[6] In an elegant essay applying Szondi's views, Blumer (1997) asserted that the apparent disappearance of catatonia coincided with the introduction of antipsychotic drugs, which suppressed the threatening paranoia and thereby replaced the self-healing attempt of catatonia and eliminated the catatonic symptomatology related to schizophrenia. No experimental study has tried to test Blumer's hypothesis.

CONCLUSION

Catatonia remains an elusive concept. There is still no other way of approximating the defini-tion of catatonia than following Jaspers's views, which requires the clinician to delineate cat-atonic signs and symptoms from both proven neurological symptoms and psychologically determined psychomotor phenomena and behavior. Beyond these etiological assumptions, symptoms regarded catatonic must be persistent, dysfunctional, and idiosyncratic in rela-tion to the person's sociocultural environment, premorbid personality, and the current sit-uation. Simple and complex mannerisms, posturing, mundane and bizarre perseverative stereotypies, echo-phenomena, and sudden impulsive acts constitute the core elements of Jaspersian catatonia. There is little evidence that these narrowly defined signs and symptoms form sharply defined clinical syndromes or accompanied by specific affective or cognitive features (Ungvari et al. 2009).

Contemporary psychiatry pays scant attention to the subjective experiences of patients with catatonia. Traditional clinical wisdom holds that subjective experiences are not re-lated to motor symptoms (Jones 1965). Patients are sometimes amnestic to the catatonic episode while others describe the frightening delusions and/or hallucinations that made them immobile or elicited frenzied excitement. Often patients cannot give any, or only facile, explanations of the catatonic episode.[7] Studies with large samples and comprehensive meth-odology should be conducted to explore patients' experiences during a catatonic episode. Such studies would enrich our understanding of the puzzling psychomotor phenomena subsumed under catatonia.

Psychoanalysis that influenced psychiatric research and practice for decades in the twen-tieth century relied on patients' subjective experiences and their interpretations thereby contributing to the demise of descriptive psychopathology in general and the method of ob-servation in particular.

The sorry state of the catatonia concept reflects the neglect of psychopathology as a fun-damental basic science of clinical psychiatry. Mainstream psychiatry journals hardly ever publish papers on psychopathological topics; somehow it is assumed that the simplified symptom descriptions in diagnostic manuals such as in DSM-5 are the final word in psycho-pathology. Within the overall marginalization of psychopathology, motor manifestations of personality and those of the mental state have been the most overlooked in modern psy-chiatry. In clinical practice, simple movement disorders or complex behavioral patterns,

---

[7] The only systematic investigation of patients' experiences during a catatonic attack involved 24 patients (15 with psychoses, 7 with mood disorders and 2 with encephalopathy) who retrospectively completed a 14-item self-assessment scale 3 weeks after recovering from a stupor (Northoff et al. 1996). The scale covered the motor (e.g. *"I had full control over my movements"*), cognitive (e.g. *"I had many ideas in my mind"*), affective (e.g. *"I felt intense fear"*) and phenomenological (e.g. *"I felt isolated from the world"*) aspects of the catatonic episode. The items consisted of two opposing statements (e.g. *"I felt intense fear – I felt intense joy"*). The patients predominantly reported affective (overwhelming anxiety) and cognitive (ambivalence and blocked willpower) subjective experiences, although all four aspects were present in most patients. As expected, schizophrenia and mood disorder patients mainly belonged to the cognitive and affective groups, respectively. Similar studies with larger samples and more comprehensive methodology would enrich our understanding of the puzzling psychomotor phenomena subsumed under catatonia.

unless clearly drug-induced, are frequently dismissed as "it is just behavioral," as though such symptoms were not integral part of "real" psychopathology. This is a serious omission. Glossing over the behavioral/observational aspects of psychopathology deprives psychiatry of a host of phenomena that enhance our understanding of the diseased mind and refines clinical presentations for neurobiological research.

BIBLIOGRAPHY

Akintomide G. S., Porter S. W., Pierce A. (2012). "Catatonia in a Woman who is Profoundly Deaf-Mute: A Case Report." *The Psychiatrist* 36: 418–421.

Angyal A. (1950). "The Psychodynamic Process of Illness and Recovery in a Case of Catatonic Schizophrenia." *Psychiatry* 13: 149–165.

Anonymous. (1986). "Catatonia." *Lancet* ii: 954–956.

APA. (2013). *Diagnostic and Statistical Manual of Mental Disorders, Fifth Edition, DSM 5*. Washington: American Psychiatric Publishing.

Arndt E. (1902). "Uber die Gesichte der Katatonie." *Centralblatt fur Nervenheilkunde und Psychiatrie* XXV: 6–121.

Bender K. G. and Feutrill J. (2000). "Comatoid Catatonia." *Australian and New Zealand Journal of Psychiatry* 34: 169–170.

Berrios G. E. (1996). *The History of Mental Symptoms*. Cambridge: Cambridge University Press.

Bleuler E. (1950). *Dementia Praecox or the Group of Schizophrenias*, trans. J. Zinkin. New York: International University Press.

Blumer D. (1997). "Catatonia and the Neuroleptics: Psychobiologic Significance of Remote and Recent Findings." *Comprehensive Psychiatry* 38: 193–201.

Bostroem A. (1928). "Katatone Storungen. " In O. Bumke (ed.), *Handbuch der Geisteskrankheiten*. Vol. 2, pp. 134–205. Berlin: Springer.

Bush G., Fink M., Petrides G., Dowling F., and Francis A. (1996). "Catatonia. I. Rating Scale and Standardized Examination." *Acta Psychiatrica Scandinavica* 93: 129–136.

Caroff S. N., Mann S. C., Francis A., and Fricchione G. L. (2004). *Catatonia*. Washington: American Psychiatric Press.

Chalasani P., Healy D., and Morriss R. (2005). "Presentation and Frequency of Catatonia in New Admissions to Two Acute Psychiatric Admission Units in India and Wales." *Psychological Medicine* 35: 1667–1675.

Chandrasena R. "Catatonic Schizophrenia: An International Comparative Study." *Canadian Journal of Psychiatry* 31: 514–516.

Critchley M. (1927). "On Palilalia." *Journal of Neurology and Psychopathology* 18: 23–31.

Dabholkar P. O. (1988). "Use of ECT in Hysterical Catatonia." *British Journal of Psychiatry* 153: 246–247.

Fink M. (2009). "Catatonia: A Syndrome Appears, Disappears and is Rediscovered." *Canadian Journal of Psychiatry* 54: 437–445.

Fink M. and Taylor M A. (2003). *Catatonia*. Cambridge: Cambridge University Press.

Hamilton M. (1984). *Fish's Schizophrenia*, 3rd. edn Bristol: Wright.

Jaspers K. (1963). *General Psychopathology*. Manchester: Manchester University Press.

Jensen P. S. (1984). "Case Report of Conversion Catatonia: Indication for Hypnosis." *American Journal of Psychotherapy* 38: 566–570.

Johnson D. R. (1984). "Representation of the Internal World in Catatonic Schizophrenia." *Psychiatry* 47: 299–314.

Jones I. H. (1965). "Observations on Schizophrenic Stereotypes." *Comprehensive Psychiatry* 6: 323–335.

Kahlbaum K. L. (1973). *Catatonia*. Baltomore: Johns Hopkins University Press.

Kraepelin E. (1919). *Dementia Praecox and Paraphrenia*. Edinburgh: E & S Livingstone.

Kruger S., Bagby R. M., Hoffler J., and Braunig P. (2003). "Factor Analysis of the Catatonia Rating Scale and Catatonic Symptom Distribution Across Four Diagnostic Groups." *Comprehensive Psychiatry* 44: 472–482.

Lohr J. B. and Wisniewski A. A. (1987). *Movement Disorders: A Neuropsychiatric Approach*. New York: Guilford.

Moskowitz A. K. (2004). "Scared stiff: Catatonia as an Evolutionary-Based Fear Response." *Psychological Review* 111: 984–1002.

Northoff G. (1997). *Katatonie*. Stuttgart: Enke.

Northoff G., Krill W., Wenke J., Travers H., and Pflug B. (1996). "Subjectives Erleben in der Katatonie: systematische Untersuchung bei 24 katatonen Patienten." *Psychiatrische Praxis* 23: 69–73.

Northoff G., Koch A., Wenke J., et al. (1999). "Catatonia as a Psychomotor Syndrome: A Rating Scale and Extrapyramidal Motor Symptoms." *Movement Disorders* 14: 404–416.

Oulis P. and Lykouras L. (1996). "Prevalence and Diagnostic Correlates of DSM-IV Catatonic Features Among Psychiatric Inpatients." *Journal of Nervous and Mental Diseases* 184: 378–379.

Peralta V. and Cuesta M. J. (2001). "Motor Features in Psychotic Disorders. I. Factor Structure and Clinical Correlates." *Schizophrenia Research* 47: 107–116.

Schneider K. (1914). "Uber Wesen und Bedeutung katatonischer Symptome." *Zeitschrift fur diegesamte Neurologie und Psychiatrie* 22: 486–505.

Sienart P., Rooseleer J., and De Fruyt J. (2011). "Measuring catatonia: asystematic review of rating scales." *Journal of Affective Disorders* 135: 1–9.

Stengel E. (1947). "A Clinical and Psychological Study of Echo-Reactions." *Journal of Mental Science* 93: 598–612.

Taylor M. A. (1990). "Catatonia." *Neuropsychiatry Neuropsychology and Behavoral Neurology* 3: 48–72.

Ungvari G. S., Leung C. M., Wong M. K., and Lau J. (1994). "Benzodiazepines in the treatment of the catatonic syndrome." *Acta Psychiatrica Scandinavica* 89: 285–288.

Ungvari G S., Chiu H. F., Chow L. Y., Lau B. S., and Tang W. K. (1999a). "Lorazepam for chronic catatonia: a randomized, double-blind, placebo-controlled cross-over study." *Psychopharmacology* 142: 393–398.

Ungvari G. S., Chow L. Y., Leung H. C. M., and Lay B. S. T. (1999b). "Rating Chronic Catatonia: Discrepancy Between Cross-Sectional and Longitudinal Assessment." *Revista de Psiquiatria Clinica* 26: 56–61.

Ungvari G. S., Leung H. C. M., Cheung H. B. B. K., and Leung T. (2005). "Schizophrenia with Prominent Catatonic Feature ("Catatonic Schizophrenia") I. Demographic and Clinical Correlates in the Chronic Phase. *Progress in Neuropsychopharmacology and Biological Psychiatry* 29: 27–38.

Ungvari G. S., Goggins W., Leung S. K., Lee E., and Gerevich J. (2009). "Schizophrenia with Prominent Catatonic Features ("Catatonic Schizophrenia") III. Latent Class Analysis of the Catatonic Syndrome." *Progress in Neuropsychopharmacology and Biological Psychiatry* 33: 81–85.

Van der Heijden F. M. M. A., Tuinier S., Arts N. J. M., Hoogendroorn M. L. C., Kahn R. S., and Verhoeven W. M. A. (2005). "Catatonia: Disappeared or Under-diagnosed." *Psychopathology* 38: 3–8.

Vogt R. (1902). "Zur Psychologie der katatonischen Symptome." *Centralblatt fur Nervenheilkunde und Psychiatrie* XXV: 433–437.

WHO. (1992). *ICD-10. Classification of Mental and Behavioural Disorders*. Geneva: World Health Organization.

CHAPTER 57

EATING BEHAVIOR AND ITS DISORDERS

GIOVANNI CASTELLINI AND VALDO RICCA

INTRODUCTION

FEEDING and eating disorders are included into a diagnostic category, encompassing different psychopathological conditions such as Anorexia Nervosa (AN), Bulimia Nervosa (BN), Binge Eating Disorder (BED), Pica (defined as persistent craving and compulsive eating of non-food substances), Rumination Disorder, Avoidant/Restrictive food intake disorder (American Psychiatric Association 2013). All these diagnoses are defined by pathological eating behaviors combined in different patterns, and resulting in specific medical complications due to unbalanced assumption or absorption of food or purging behaviors, such as weight loss, obesity, heart or kidney failure, and haematological alterations.

When a person develops an eating disorder, nutrition is no longer anchored to its physiological meaning—which is the process to acquire food by the living organism in order to meet its dynamic needs and energy demands—and the food loses its main value of nourishment or pleasure, rather it is considered as negative and potentially dangerous. Consequently, the power supply is no longer determined by a gut feeling of hunger or satiety, but it is both quantitatively and qualitatively based on arbitrary parameters (such as rigid rules, concept of control). Therefore, patients systematically underestimate or ignore the signals of hunger and satiety to adhere strictly to their diet.

Most of the symptoms described in this chapter can be observed also in different psychopathological conditions, over the border of the category defined by the Diagnostic and Statistical Manual of Mental Disorders (DSM-5). For example, weight loss following restrictive behaviors is frequently reported in Melancholic Depression, as binge eating or *hyperphagia* are observed in several mood disorders. Body image disturbance is a transdiagnostic feature, which characterizes a plethora of different psychiatric disturbance such Body Dysmorphic Disorder, Major Depression, Social Anxiety, Gender Dysphoria,

Obsessive-Compulsive Disorder, and Schizophrenia. In order to attribute a pathological eating behavior to an eating disorder diagnosis, it is important to consider the core psychopathology related to them, and the subjective world underpinning the disorder. In other words, a phenomenological approach should take into account the reason why a young girl decides to restrict her diet, avoid specific foods, use food to manage her emotions, and begins checking compulsively her body.

In the present chapter, I will provide a schematic description of the main pathological features associated with feeding and eating disorders, with a particular attention to the psychopathological meaning of the different behaviors.

Dieting and Food Restriction

Many people begin their history of an eating disorder, by reducing or eliminating types of food from their diet, and restricting their dietary range. The way individuals decide to reduce the variability of their alimentation is quite heterogeneous and could include a real desire to lose weight by eliminating "fattening food," but can also be connected with vegetarianism, veganism, *orthorexia* (eating only "healthy food"), or specific modification of diet related to some pathologies (diabetes, food intolerance, celiac disease). An important feature of diet attempts in eating disorders is that it should be differentiated by the loss of appetite frequently observed in depression or other mood disorders. Once that dieting has started, it generally represents the core symptom of many pathological vicious cycles, also involving other pathological behaviors such as binge eating. It is also accompanied by different rituals, which sometimes characterize the whole day of the patient, such as weighing and measuring food, counting calories, eating specific food in a particular order, use a particular bowl or glass, cutting food into small pieces, disassembling foods. The so-called *forbidden foods* included junk foods and fats, carbohydrates, meat, and sweets.

Why do persons with eating disorders start dieting? Psychodynamic and cognitive perspectives highlight the relationship between body image disturbances and the restraint behaviors, as an attempt to control weight and the body (Fairburn and Harrison 2003). Adverse life events, such as sexual or emotional abuse seem to represent factors associated with the development of these behaviors (Jacobi et al. 2004; Castellini et al. 2014a, b). A phenomenological approach has recently been proposed (Stanghellini et al. 2012; 2015), individuating the core psychopathological feature of eating disorders as a disorder of lived corporeality. In this perspective, most of the symptoms arise from this core dimension. Accordingly, dieting begins as an attempt to overcome the alienation from one's own body and from one's own emotions. Indeed, many diet attempts are started to regain control of one's own emotions, for those who are not able to cope with such emotions (Ricca et al. 2012). Patients perceive dieting as the possible means to feel themselves only through objective measures and through self-starvation. Dieting is a part of the vicious cycle of maintenance of *binge eating*, as it creates a physiologic and psychological deprivation that potentiates the eventual counter-regulation of appetite, leading to this behavior.

BINGE EATING: AN OBJECTIVE OR SUBJECTIVE DEFINITION?

Binge eating is the main symptom of Bulimia Nervosa (BN) and Binge Eating Disorder (BED) and can be present also in binge/purging anorexia. In BN, it is associated with compensatory behaviors, while in BED, the compensatory behaviors are lacking or even sporadic. Frequently, the term binge eating is used to refer to a large quantity of food consumed in a short period of time, with a sense of loss of control. However, a person's definition of "large amount" is highly subjective and influenced by personal beliefs and rules, which can vary from day to day. Therefore, each attempt of finding a quantitative threshold for this behavior has been unsuccessful. Independently from the theoretical background, there is a large consensus of considering this phenomenon an inherently subjective experience and a critical underlying attribute of binge eating episodes (Castellini et al. 2012). The most accepted psychopathological and qualitative threshold for establishing a discontinuation from normalcy of the behavior is the subjective experience of lack of control, which distinguishes binge eating from *hyperphagia* (American Psychiatric Association 2013; Williamson et al. 2002). Indeed, a person can experience an *objective* episode of binge eating as well as a *subjective* one, defined as an eating episode that is not objectively large (approximately less than 500 kcalories), but that involves loss of control over eating (Cooper and Fairburn 1993; Bardone-Cone et al. 2010). The sense of lack of control over the eating behavior, can refer not just to the quantity, but also the qualitative features of food (e.g. fat, salty, forbidden), the time (eating when I'm not planning to do so), and the people involved ("I did not want to eat in front of my boyfriend"). The subjective estimation of binge eating can be determined by the personal system of values associated with food and any amount of food over a predetermined dietary rule could be perceived to be large or without control (Wolfe et al. 2009).

In a clinical setting we can assess loss of control according to questions such as: "Did you have a sense of loss of control at the time you had that meal?" "Could you have stopped eating once you started?" "Could you have prevented the episode from occurring?" Several studies have demonstrated that the experience of loss of control over eating, as opposed to the amount of food eaten, appear to be more salient for the identification of disordered eating behaviors and related distress (Tanofsky-Kraff et al. 2005; Castellini et al. 2012). This kind of observation highlights the importance of using the *subjectiveness* of the experience to understand the phenomenology of pathological eating behaviors. As well as the "large amount of food" required by the diagnostic criteria, the temporal boundary of the episode (eating in a discrete period of time, e.g. within any two-hour period) is highly subjective and can be influenced by personal beliefs and rules. The most empirically well-supported models for eating disorders propose that concerns about body image and feelings following the loss of control over eating represent maintaining factors in the vicious cycle of binge eating. The negative emotions associated with body image disturbances perpetuate the obsessive drive for thinness, which in turn leads to unrealistic dietary restraints. Binge eating occurs when dietary restraints are broken and the all-or-nothing cognitive distortions lead the individual to engage in excessive eating. Consequently, negative effects such as feelings of guilt, shame, disgust, and failure emerge and facilitate inappropriate compensatory behavior (e.g. vomiting or excessive exercise).

Accordingly, from a phenomenological perspective, the alternation of different eating behaviors can be associated with a different experience of time (Castellini et al. 2014b). For many persons with BN or BED, binge eating episode occurs in a very short period of time as a breakdown in the context of continuous control of eating habits. However, patients often report so-called *binge eating days*, during which they spend the whole time eating sweet things or *craving* or *nibbling*. The subjective perception of time during binge eating episodes is heterogeneous within patients, but generally, binge eating is experienced as a discontinuous moment in the normal time course. Sometimes, patients do not remember what they were doing, how long the episode lasted, or even what they ate. On the other hand, patients also report having planned their binge eating by buying different types of forbidden foods at the supermarket and then running to an isolated place to eat it, retreating into a mental state with an altered sense of time.

BEING IN CONTROL

Especially in anorexia and bulimia nervosa patients, the subjective perception of time appears to be interconnected with the construct of *control*. Time is perceived in different ways, on the basis of the interchange of control/loss of control phases. Indeed, the idea of lack of control over eating depends on what a person thinks is being in control of their eating. Patients always attempt to control every feature of their diet, such as the quantity and the quality of food (the so-called *orthorexia*), the timing of their meals ("never eat pasta at dinner!"), the calorie content of each item of food, but also their body, with the obsessive thoughts and repetitive behaviors included in *body checking*. This includes the frequent pinching of hands around waist, arms, or stomach, weighing themselves, and looking at themselves frequently in the mirror. The condition is not only present in eating disorder but also in body dysmorphia and obsessive-compulsive disorder.

The construct of control is mostly related to anxiety, and it has been conceptualized as anxious perception of low control over external threats and emotional reactions. Especially for anorexia nervosa patients, maintaining a sense of control by the continuous monitoring of eating and body weight and shape, and dietary restrictions can balance the subjective perception of low degree of internal control and high external control exerted by family and society (Williams et al. 1990). Therefore, for some people with eating disorders, perception of control over the body, eating habits, and physical exercise represent the way in which they can keep their emotions and relationships under control. It is noteworthy that eating disorder patients have a different perception of time, mostly depending on their limited world. Indeed, the perspective on their life is reduced to what they have eaten or the fluctuation of their body weight: the world of relationships, job opportunities, studies, and affects all fade into the background. A good example is provided by the way in which they remember periods in their life with sentences such as: "At that time I was happy, I did a lot of exercise, my nutrition was under control and I was thin . . . " or "That period was one of the worst of my life . . . I was as fat as I've ever been."

REGAIN CONTROL: THE COMPENSATORY BEHAVIORS

The compensatory behaviors occur as a way to regain control, like an attempt to restore normalcy, and clean up the sense of guilt. Patients with bulimia or anorexia nervosa generally attempt to compensate for the calories consumed by different behaviors including self-vomiting, misuse of laxatives, enemas, colonics, and the use of diuretics. Physical exercise or dieting are also used as a way to compensate the out-of-control eating behaviors. Each loss of control can be related to shame, anxiety, or depression (Wolfe et al. 2009; Castellini et al. 2012). Furthermore, compensatory behaviors are considered a way to regulate emotions in the same way as binge eating, similarly to other self-harm conducts can be associated with other psychopathological conditions such as borderline personality or mood disorders. These kinds of behaviors are particularly life-threatening as they increase the risk of heart failure, damage to the gastrointestinal system, or electrolytes alterations.

EMOTIONAL EATING: WHAT IS BEHIND BINGE EATING?

Emotional eating is defined as eating in response to a range of negative emotions such as anxiety, depression, anger, and loneliness, to cope with negative affect (Arnow et al. 1995). Different emotional states often precede the onset of binge eating as well as of purging behaviors (Dingemans et al. 2009), and frequently after these episodes there is a subsequent decrease in the negative affects (Deaver et al. 2003). According to the so-called affect-driven models, the act of eating substitutes a less aversive affective condition (e.g. guilt after binge eating) for the more aversive emotional state (e.g. depression) which preceded the binge (Stein et al. 2007). Indeed, some of the pathological eating behaviors should be considered as a consequence of a cognitive narrowing, which individuals use to escape from their awareness of negative emotional states and threats to their self-esteem.

This mechanism arises from a more general affective regulation difficulty, which is a common trait of eating disorders (Zaitsoff and Grilo 2010). However, this psychopathological feature is also associated with borderline personality disorder, mood and anxiety disorders, or different subthreshold conditions (night eating syndrome, subthreshold binge eating disorder, eating disorder not otherwise specified) (Ricca et al. 2009). Furthermore, emotion dysregulation and alexithymia are not only related with binge eating but also with restricted food consumption and compensatory behaviors, which could be interpreted as responses to regulate intense or relatively undifferentiated emotional states, to restrict the affective experience. or to take attention away from negative emotions (Castellini et al. 2012).

According to a phenomenological interpretation of emotional eating, eating disorder patients complain about being alienated from their emotions, and from the somatic responses of the body related to them (Stanghellini et al. 2012). According to this model, the cenesthetic apprehension of one's own body is the more primitive and basic form of self-awareness about one's own emotions. Indeed, patients with eating disorders often report—with different levels of insight—their difficulties in perceiving their emotions, saying they do not "feel" themselves. Feeling extraneous from one's own body may feature as a possible factor for abnormal eating patterns via emotional dysregulation and/or the dysregulation of bodily-mediated satiety responsiveness.

BODY SHAPE CONCERN AND BODY IMAGE DISTORTION: DISORDERS OF EMBODIMENT

Many academics consider the "core psychopathology" of eating disorders as basically determined by an excessive concern about body shape and weight, such that self-worth is judged largely or even exclusively in terms of satisfaction with weight and shape. Body image distortion—defined as "a disturbance in the way in which one's body weight or shape is experienced" (American Psychiatric Association 1994)—has been indicated as the psychopathological threshold between the world of eating disorders and normalcy, across a continuum of several heterogeneous features which can be found also in high-risk population or subclinical conditions. It is considered as a multidimensional pattern, including cognitive and affective components (concern and feelings about the body), perception (estimation of own body size), and behaviors related to one's own body perception (Thompson et al. 1999). Shape concerns and body image distortion severity have been associated with different long-term outcomes to treatment (Castellini et al. 2011). Body image disturbances are considered key to distinguishing between partially and fully recovered individuals and a healthier relationship with one's body may be the final hurdle in recovery (Bardone-Cone et al. 2010).

Shape concerns also have a crucial role in the vicious cycle of binge eating (Castellini et al. 2012), promoting unrealistic dietary restraint, whose violation activates an all-or-none thinking (e.g. severe restraint or complete failure). This dichotomous thinking heightens a sense of frustration, disinhibits the attempts to control food eaten, and leads to binge eating. Body uneasiness and body image disturbance are present in several psychopathological disorders such as depression and schizophrenia, as well as body dysmorphic disorder (Stanghellini 2009; Fuchs 2002). In particular, it has been observed as a core feature also in particular conditions such as gender dysphoria (Bandini et al. 2013). However, recent phenomenological approaches (Stanghellini et al. 2012) have attempted to clarify the specific significance of body image disturbance in eating disorders. According to this position, most of the pathological eating behaviors can be considered as secondary epiphenomena to a more profound pathological core, based on the relationship between lived corporeality and self-identity. In this sense, the overestimation of the importance of bodily appearance overcomes the other aspects of existence and personal identity. Persons with eating disorders are affected by a more profound disturbance consisting in disorders of the way they experience their own body (embodiment), and shape their own identity. The lived body (leib) is what allows the "belonging to the world, being in the world temporality committed" (Stanghellini et al. 2012). The primary contact with the world is the so-called field of presence, the leib with its own temporality, in which all our actions take place.

As further support to this position, it has been observed that the temporal continuity of the representation of the body is altered in patients with eating disorders. Time is no longer intentionality, and therefore it cannot be a way for being with the others in a simultaneity or in a succession temporality. Indeed, patients with eating disorders report their feeling that the body can change continuously. Time is reduced to a mere control function, in particular to be employed in control and/or loss of control of weight and eating—in other words to monitoring one's own body over time. For example, patients often make statements like: "I spend most of my time in front of the mirror to control my body," or "the perception of time depends on body control. My body is under control all the times. I fail, at times, miserably and at times I am successful, but I would like to be successful all the time," or "One morning I feel my thighs fit perfectly in my pants, another morning instead they have become huge." Clinicians should always take into consideration the situational and temporal variations of body image experiences of individuals with eating disorders. Specific situations or events activate patients' thoughts and emotions, while at other times these body image experiences are either absent or much more benign. Cash and Pruzinsky (1990) highlighted that body image must be considered as a fluid and dynamic person–situation interaction (or trans-action), and it is of note that this fluid versus static issue has long permeated much of psychology, especially the domain of personality theory. Understanding the dynamic interplay of body image and contextual events is crucial for the appreciation of body image fluidity in everyday life.

Conclusion

A phenomenological approach to eating disorders is aimed at understanding the subjective meaning of the so-called "pathological eating behaviors." In this perspective, dietary restraint or binge eating are not just symptoms challenging the lives of patients, which should be removed as soon as possible; rather they represent a "door" through which to explore the way these individuals have shaped their personal identity, around embodiment. Accordingly, a comprehensive assessment of a person with eating disorders should encompass more than the simple behavioral assessment required for a DSM diagnosis, and it should include the person's general way of perceiving their own body and their lived corporeality. Moreover, clinicians should evaluate the consequences of this core dimension on other areas of the patient's life, such as the significance of the illness and the body in intersubjective interactions as well as identity definition, space perception, and the way they experience time, associated with several features of eating disorders (such as binge eating and weight control).

An accurate psychopathological assessment in eating disorders is crucial from a clinical point of view for several reasons. First, psychopathology allows for a definition of a qualitative threshold along a continuum of severity, identifying healthy subjects from high-risk persons with abnormal eating behaviors in the general population, and non-clinical persons with abnormal eating behaviors from eating disorders in a clinical setting. Furthermore, the core features of eating disorders have been associated with different responses to psychological treatments and a different course of illness. In other words, while diagnoses do not seem to represent adequate outcome predictors, psychopathological dimensions identify subpopulations of people with eating disorders with different trajectories across time, and therefore different maintaining factors and pathogenic mechanisms.

BIBLIOGRAPHY

American Psychiatric Association. (1994). *Diagnostic and Statistical Manual for Mental Disorders.* 4th edn. Washington, DC: American Psychiatric Association.

American Psychiatric Association. (2013). *Diagnostic and Statistical Manual for Mental Disorders.* 5th edn. Washington, DC: American Psychiatric Association.

Arnow B., Kenardy J., and Agras W. S. (1995). "The Emotional Eating Scale: The Development of a Measure to Assess Coping with Negative Affect by Eating." *International Journal of Eating Disorders* 18: 79–90.

Bandini E., Fisher A. D., Castellini G., Lo Sauro C., Lelli L., Meriggiola M. C., Casale H., Benni L., Ferruccio N., Faravelli C., Dettore D., Maggi M., Ricca V. (2013). Gender identity disorder and eating disorders: similarities and differences in terms of body uneasiness. *Journal of Sexual Medicine* 10(4): 1012–1023.

Bardone-Cone A. M., Harney M. B., Maldonado C. R., et al. (2010). "Defining Recovery from an Eating Disorder: Conceptualization, Validation, and Examination of Psychosocial Functioning and Psychiatric Comorbidity." *Behaviour Research and Therapy* 48: 194–202.

Cash T. F. and Pruzinsky T. (1990). *Body Images: Development, Deviance, and Change.* New York: Guilford Press.

Castellini G., Lo Sauro C., Mannucci E., Ravaldi C., Rotella C. M., Faravelli C., and Ricca V. (2011). "Diagnostic Crossover and Outcome Predictors in Eating Disorders According to DSM-IV and DSM-V Proposed Criteria: A 6-Year Follow-Up Study." *Psychosomatic Medicine.* 73(3): 270–279.

Castellini G., Maggi M., and Ricca V. (2014a). "Childhood Sexual Abuse and Psychopathology." In G. Corona, A. E. Jannini, and M. Maggi (eds.), *Emotional, Physical and Sexual Abuse.* Heidelberg, New York, Dordrecht, London: Springer Cham.

Castellini G., Trisolini F., and Ricca V. (2014b). "Psychopathology of Eating Disorders." *Journal of Psychopathology* 20: 461–470.

Castellini G., Mannucci E., Lo Sauro C., Benni L., Lazzeretti L., Ravaldi C., Rotella C. M., Faravelli C., and Ricca V. (2012). "Different Moderators of Cognitive-Behavioral Therapy on Subjective and Objective Binge Eating in Bulimia Nervosa and Binge Eating Disorder: A Three-Year Follow-Up Study." *Psychotherapy and Psychosomatics* 81(1): 11–20.

Cooper P. J. and Fairburn C. G. (1993). "Confusion over the Core Psychopathology of Bulimia Nervosa." *International Journal of Eating Disorders* May; 13(4): 385–389.

Deaver C. M., Miltenberger R. G., Smyth J., Meidinger A., and Crosby R. (2003). "An Evaluation of Affect and Binge Eating." *Behavior Modification* 27(4): 578–599.

Dingemans A. E., Martijn C., Jansen A. T., and van Furth E. F. (2009). "The Effect of Suppressing Negative Emotions on Eating Behavior in Binge Eating Disorder." *Appetite* 52: 51–57.

Fairburn C. G. and Harrison P. J. (2003). "Eating Disorders." *The Lancet* 361(9355): 407–416.

Fuchs T. (2002). "The Phenomenology of Shame, Guilt and the Body in Body Dysmorphic Disorder and Depression." *Journal of Phenomenological Psychology* 33: 223–243.

Jacobi C., Hayward C., de Zwaan M., Kraemer H. C., and Agras W. S. (2004). "Coming to Terms with Risk Factors for Eating Disorders: Application of Risk Terminology and Suggestions for a General Taxonomy." *Psychological Bulletin* 130: 19–65.

Ricca V., Castellini G., Lo Sauro C., Ravaldi C., Lapi F., Mannucci E., Rotella C. M., and Faravelli C. (2009). "Correlations between Binge Eating and Emotional Eating in a Sample of Overweight Subjects." *Appetite* 53(3): 418–421.

Ricca V., Castellini G., Fioravanti G., Lo Sauro C., Rotella F., Ravaldi C., Lazzeretti L., and Faravelli C. (2012), "Emotional Eating in Anorexia Nervosa and Bulimia Nervosa." *Comprehensive Psychiatry*. April; 53(3): 245–251.

Stanghellini G. (2009). "Embodiment and Schizophrenia." *World Psychiatry* 8: 1–4.

Stanghellini G., Castellini G., Brogna P., et al. (2012). "Identity and Eating Disorders (IDEA): A Questionnaire Evaluating Identity and Embodiment in Eating Disorder Patients." *Psychopathology* 45: 147–158.

Stanghellini G., Trisolini F., Castellini G., et al. (2015). "Is Feeling Extraneous from One's Own Body a Core Vulnerability Feature in Eating Disorders?" *Psychopathology* 48(1): 18–24.

Stein R. I., Kenardy J., Wiseman C. V., Dounchis J. Z., Arnow B. A., and Wilfley D. E. (2007). "What's Driving the Binge in Binge Eating Disorder? A Prospective Examination of Precursors and Consequences." *International Journal of Eating Disorders* 40: 195–203.

Tanofsky-Kraff M., Faden D., Yanovski S. Z., Wilfley D. E., and Yanovski J. A. (2005). "The Perceived Onset of Dieting and Loss of Control Eating Behaviors in Overweight Children." *International Journal of Eating Disorders* 38(2): 112–122.

Thompson J. K., Heinberg L. J., Altabe M., and Tantleff-Dunn S. (1999). *Exacting Beauty*. Washington, DC: American Psychological Association.

Williams G. J., Chamove A. S., and Millar H. R. (1990). "Eating Disorders, Perceived Control, Assertiveness and Hostility." *British Journal of Clinical Psychology* 29: 327–335.

Williamson D. A., Womble L. G., Smeets M. A., Netemeyer R. G., Thaw J. M., Kutlesic V., and Gleaves D. H. (2002). "Latent Structure of Eating Disorder Symptoms: A Factor Analytic and Taxometric Investigation." *American Journal of Psychiatry* 159(3): 412–418.

Wolfe B. E., Baker C. W., Smith A. T., and Kelly-Weeder S. (2009). "Validity and Utility of the Current Definition of Binge Eating." *International Journal of Eating Disorders* 42(8): 674–686.

Zaitsoff S. L. and Grilo C. M. (2010). "Eating Disorder Psychopathology as a Marker of Psychosocial Distress and Suicide Risk in Female and Male Adolescent Psychiatric Inpatients." *Comprehensive Psychiatry* 51(2): 142–150.

CHAPTER 58

··

THE PHENOMENOLOGICAL CLARIFICATION OF GRIEF AND ITS RELEVANCE FOR PSYCHIATRY

··

MATTHEW RATCLIFFE

INTRODUCTION

PHENOMENOLOGICAL research has much to contribute to our understanding of grief. In what follows, I will illustrate this by focusing specifically on psychiatry, where there is particular need for phenomenological clarification. This need is exemplified by debates that arose in the run-up to publication of DSM-5, concerning the proposed guidelines for distinguishing grief from major depression. In DSM-IV, it is acknowledged that the symptoms of grief overlap with those of depression. However, a depression diagnosis is excluded in cases where symptoms are "better accounted for by Bereavement" (DSM-IV, TR: 356). The proposal that this clause be removed from DSM-5 proved divisive.[1] For example, Wakefield and First (2012) supported retention of a revised bereavement exclusion clause, maintaining that "bereavement-related depressions" should be distinguished from major depressive episodes in many instances where symptoms would otherwise meet the diagnostic criteria for depression. In contrast, Zisook and Shear (2009: 70–71) insisted that the vast majority of bereavement experiences do differ from experiences of major depression. Where they do not differ, their trajectories and responsiveness to treatment do not differ either. So an exclusion clause is unwarranted, given that a person can be both bereaved and depressed.[2]

---

[1] See e.g. the website of the Coalition for DSM-5 Reform: www.dsm5-reform.com (last accessed May 15, 2015). It includes details of an "Open letter to the DSM 5 Task Force." The letter addresses several concerns, including that of lowering diagnostic thresholds by removing the grief exclusion clause. An accompanying petition was signed by 15,339 people.

[2] See also Lamb, Pies, and Zisook (2010), who propose eliminating the bereavement exclusion clause but also extending DSM-IV's two-week duration requirement for major depression.

In the light of such exchanges, the need for phenomenological research is clear. If the phenomenology of "normal" or "typical" grief cannot be reliably distinguished from that of major depression, then any proposed distinction must be based on additional, non-phenomenological criteria. On the other hand, if there are significant phenomenological differences between the two, such criteria may not be required.[3] This need for phenomenological clarification is not specific to the DSM debates and applies much more widely. The questions of (a) whether and how the various forms of depression and grief are phenomenologically distinct from each other, and (b) whether any phenomenological differences are indicative of different trajectories and outcomes, are relevant to *any* attempt to classify, further understand, and respond to grief and depression, in clinical contexts and more generally.

Ultimately, DSM-5 (161) settled for something that strikes me as rather unsatisfactory. It is stated that, although a response to loss may seem "understandable or appropriate," a depression diagnosis should still be "carefully considered" where symptoms overlap. This requires "the exercise of clinical judgment," something that should take individual history and the specifics of the situation into account. In a footnote, there is also an attempt to draw some phenomenological distinctions. Grief, it is noted, tends to involve "feelings of emptiness and loss," while depression involves "depressed mood and the inability to anticipate happiness or pleasure." Positive emotions still arise during grief, while depression is more pervasive and persistent. In addition, grief usually involves retention of self-esteem, which sets it apart from the worthlessness and self-loathing more typical of depression.[4] Thoughts of dying also differ in content: the depressed person may feel that she does not deserve to live, while the bereaved person is more likely to think of joining the deceased.

Why is this unsatisfactory? The first thing to note is the frequent use of qualifiers such as "likely to," "tend to," and "generally," which appear eight times in the footnote.[5] That an instance of condition A tends to or is likely to involve symptoms *p*, *q*, and *r*, while an instance of condition B is less likely to or tends not to involve those symptoms does not facilitate a confident diagnosis of "A and not B." Furthermore, this uncertainty is unavoidable, given that the diagnostic criteria for a major depressive episode admit considerable heterogeneity. A range of different predicaments could qualify as "major depression" by meeting at least one of the two principal criteria (depressed mood and diminished interest in activity), plus at least four of seven supplementary criteria. Indeed, three of the supplementary criteria are disjunctive: weight loss or gain; insomnia or hypersomnia; psychomotor agitation or retardation (DSM-5: 160–161). By relying on permissive criteria such as these, a particular grief experience might be easy enough to distinguish from a depression experience of one or another type, but not from all the other experiences that are compatible with a major depression diagnosis.

First-person descriptions of depression and grief are often very similar to each other. In both cases, the person may report a lack of interest in activities, a sense of estrangement

---

[3] A closely related debate, which raises similar issues, concerns whether or not complicated grief should be recognized as a distinct psychiatric disorder. See e.g. Lichtenthal, Cruess, and Prigerson (2004); Zisook and Shear (2009).

[4] Loss vs. retention of self-esteem is also the principal difference emphasized by Freud in his famous essay "Mourning and Melancholia" (1917/2005).

[5] In order of appearance, they are: "likely to"; "tend to"; "may be"; "generally"; "generally"; "common"; "typically"; "generally."

from other people and social situations, feelings of meaningless and hopelessness, bodily discomfort, fatigue, and changes in the experience of time, amongst other things.[6] However, I think the apparent similarity is often symptomatic of under-description. In order to determine whether or not a grief exclusion clause is required, it is not enough to appeal to the success or failure of cursory diagnostic criteria. Where they fail, there remains the possibility that a more detailed and discriminating phenomenological analysis will succeed. I am not suggesting that we should aspire toward a neat boundary, with grief on one side and major depression on the other: boundaries will always be blurred and there will be plenty of in-between cases. Hence a degree of idealization is inevitable. However, this does not prohibit robust phenomenological distinctions. That there are cases falling in between A and B need not detract from the claim that A and B are structurally very different, any more than the existence of grey detracts from the distinction between black and white. And the ability to make clear, principled phenomenological distinctions can aid one in determining whether a given case is more like one or the other. Thus, as Pies (2012) points out, an "in depth understanding" of the phenomenology is needed, of a kind that "symptom checklists" do not facilitate. I have no doubt that many clinicians are already operating with something like this, in a way that has not yet been codified. However, this in itself is not a reason to dismiss the need for explicit phenomenological work, at least on the assumption that it is a good thing to be able to communicate the basis for one's clinical decisions and to formulate shared standards for diagnosis.

In addressing the phenomenology of grief, it is important to keep two issues distinct: (i) whether and how typical grief differs from major depression and other psychiatric conditions; (ii) where and how the line should be drawn between normality and pathology. Even if typical grief could be distinguished from all forms of psychiatric illness, it might still be regarded as pathological according to one or another criterion (e.g. Wilkinson 2000). The phenomenological question is not only distinct from but also importantly prior to the question of pathology. If we want to assess whether or not a condition is pathological, it helps to have a good grasp of what that condition is. So lack of clarity over whether and how it is distinct from something else is not a good starting point. Phenomenology therefore has an important role to play in refining our sense of what the relevant phenomena actually are, given that neither grief nor depression are currently conceived of in wholly non-phenomenological terms.

In the remainder of this article, I will take some preliminary steps toward a comparative phenomenological analysis. This will involve sketching three important differences between experiences of "typical" grief and major depression:

1 Grief involves losing systems of possibility, while depression involves losing access to kinds of possibility.
2 Grief involves dynamic perspective-shifting, whereas depression involves an inability to shift perspective.
3 Grief involves a sustained ability to relate to and feel connected with other people, the capacity for which is substantially diminished in depression.[7]

---

[6] All of these themes are present in autobiographical accounts of grief, such as those cited in this article. They also feature prominently in first-person accounts of depression (Ratcliffe 2015).

[7] These same differences, along with several others, are mentioned by Lamb, Pies, and Zisook (2010: 23). In grief, they note, a sense of connectedness to others remains, as does the sense that things

In both grief and depression, 1 to 3 should not be construed as separable components of experience that just happen to accompany each other, and neither is the relationship between them a causal one. They are inextricable aspects of a unitary structure; each implies the others. I concede that major depression is heterogeneous, a point that I have addressed at length elsewhere (Ratcliffe 2015). The same applies to grief; even "typical grief" no doubt encompasses a range of subtly different (and perhaps, in some cases, substantially different) kinds of experience. So, when describing the phenomenology of typical grief, there is inevitably a degree of abstraction and simplification. Even so, depression experiences have in common a pervasive sense of isolation, lack of dynamism, and loss of possibility.[8] This can be contrasted with the underlying structure of "normal" or "typical" grief, and—I will add—"complicated" grief. DSM-5's remarks on comparative phenomenology are admittedly suggestive of the relevant phenomenological differences and can no doubt aid differential diagnosis. But there remains the risk of superficially similar symptom descriptions obscuring profound differences in how a person relates to the world as a whole and to other people, and of different descriptions obscuring commonalities. Phenomenological analysis provides insight into underlying structural differences between grief and depression experiences, thus facilitating a more discerning interpretation of first-person reports. What I will say here is very much a starting point, and it is somewhat schematic. My aims are to illustrate the role that phenomenological research can play here, and to sketch some potentially fruitful themes to explore, rather than to finish the job.[9]

Projects and Possibilities

Profound grief involves what I will call "loss of a system of possibilities." Nearly all of one's projects and pastimes can depend for their intelligibility on a relationship with a particular person. When one is confronted by that person's irrevocable absence, they collapse. Consider the event of losing a partner. Person A's activities may implicate her partner, B, in a range of ways. In a case of goal-directed action, A might do something because B has asked her to do it, because B needs her to do it, because B cares about the outcome, so that B can accomplish something else, so that a life shared with B is sustained or enhanced, and so forth. In many cases, it is not "I" who does something alone, but "we" who do it together for reasons that are "ours." It is "we" who care about a given outcome, "we" who have made and continue

---

will or at least could get better. And what I will say about perspective-shifting can be related to their observation that grief comes in waves, while depression is ever-present. I elaborate on these themes in a way that complements their approach. But I further maintain that these three aspects of experience are to be understood in terms of a single, unified phenomenological structure, in grief and in depression.

[8] Of course, they can share various other symptoms as well, such a lethargy and bodily discomfort. However, for current purposes, I suggest that a selective emphasis on isolation, stasis, and loss of possibility is a fruitful one.

[9] A detailed comparative analysis will also need to include a more discriminating account of the kinds of experience encompassed by "major depression" (Ratcliffe 2015). In addition, grief will need to be considered in relation to various other psychiatric categories, such as post-traumatic stress disorder. Individual and cultural differences in the expression, experience, and interpretation of grief (including religious interpretation) will also need to be addressed at length.

to affirm certain commitments, "we" who depend on each other's support to get things done. This dependence is not restricted to goal-directed activities and the larger projects in which they are embedded. Take the case of going to a cinema simply to enjoy a film. Here too, B may be implicated throughout. Enjoying the film involves a sense of watching it *with* B and sharing in an experience. The two parties may interpret the film together, while they watch it and also afterwards. Even when B is not present, A may think about how B would react to the film, and A's enjoyment of it may stem, in part, from being able to tell B about it afterwards and construct an appraisal of it in conversation with B. More generally, how a situation matters to A and the kinds of action it demands from her are symptomatic of cares and concerns that only make sense given her relationship to B. The point extends to how the world *appears* to A and the degree to which she feels comfortably immersed in it. Regardless of whether or not we want to insist that specifically *sensory* perception of our surroundings incorporates a sense of how things matter to us, it is plausible to maintain that we *experience* our surroundings as significant, as mattering, in a range of ways. We do not ordinarily need to explicitly infer the significance of a situation from a prior experience of it. Given different sets of projects, cares, and concerns, an entity or situation might appear practically salient to us in any number of ways—as something that could enhance or interfere with a project, as interesting, enticing, exciting, disappointing, or threatening.

A wholesale collapse of practical meanings would therefore involve experiencing the world and one's practical relationship to it in a profoundly different manner, and this is exactly how experiences of bereavement are often described. One loses a system of significant possibilities that was previously integral to the experienced world and served to regulate one's activities, thus making it "impossible for us to actively engage in the world just as we had before the death" (Attig 2004: 350). For this reason, Carse (1981: 6) describes grief as a "cosmic crisis." Our lives, he says, can be so bound up with the lives of others that they "scarcely belong to us." In the event of a particular person's death, a system of possibilities that operated as a backdrop to meaningful activity is lost and the world is profoundly different.[10] This is a prominent theme in every autobiographical account of grief that I have come across, and is something that people express in a variety of ways (e.g. Didion 2005, 2011; Hemon 2013; Humphreys 2013; Lewis 1966; Nussbaum 2001; Riley 2012). For example, Oates (2011: 176) writes, "Without meaning, the world is *things*. And these things multiplied to infinity." Her account emphasizes how, when one grieves, entities in general appear bereft of the practical meanings they once had. Everything therefore looks strange, somehow different. Instead of being greeted by objects and situations that are relevant in the light of one's concerns, one encounters bare, indifferent "things."

All of this appears markedly similar to losses of possibility that feature in first-person accounts of depression. However, there is a distinction to be drawn between losing a "system of possibilities" and losing access to "types of possibility." For instance, no longer being able to hope for something or other differs from no longer being able to entertain an attitude of the kind "hope." The type of grief experience I have described involves the former. One no longer finds things significant in the ways one did, and one can no longer sustain a system of hopes

---

[10] This is sometimes described in terms of lost "assumptions." Something that one habitually presupposed, took for granted, and came to depend upon is lost: "When somebody dies a whole set of assumptions about the world that relied upon the other person for their validity are suddenly invalidated" (Parkes 1998: 90).

that depended upon one's relationship with the deceased. It could even be that a system of possibilities is eroded to such an extent that all hopes with a specific content, the hope for *this* and the hope for *that*, are lost. Even so, one remains capable of finding things practically significant, capable of hoping. At the very least, what endures is an inchoate sense that life could one day be better than it currently is.[11] The point applies equally to goal-directed projects, enjoyable pastimes, and so forth.

What people with diagnoses of major or severe depression often describe is superficially similar to this but importantly different: an experience of losing the capacity for hope or for certain kinds of hope, of losing the ability to find anything significant in one or another way. As with grief, this permeates how one experiences and relates to the world. But there is a sense of stasis, inescapability, irrevocability, which sets it apart from losing a system of possibilities. Hence there are two qualitatively different ways in which life might seem pointless and activities meaningless. One could lose a token *system* of possibilities, of a kind that sustains specific projects and patterns of activity, or one could lose phenomenological access to *types* of possibility, to the sense that anything ever could be relevantly different from the present in a good way, that any project ever could be sustainable. First-person accounts of clinical depression generally indicate the latter:

> When I'm depressed life never seems worth living. I can never think about how my life is different from when I'm not depressed. I think that my life will never change and that I will always be depressed. Thinking about the future makes my depression even worse because I can't bear to think of being depressed my whole life. I forget what my life is like when I'm not depressed and feel that my life and future is pointless.
> When depressed I feel I have no future and lose any hope in things improving in my life. I just feel generally hopeless.
> There seemed to be no future, no possibility that I could ever be happy again or that life was worth living.
> Life will never end, or change. Everything is negative. I lose my imagination, in particular, being able to imagine any different state other than depression. Life is a chore.[12]

Having "no future" is also a prominent theme in many accounts of grief, but there is a difference between an inchoate, uncertain future that is bereft of possibilities one previously took for granted and a future that no longer incorporates the possibility for any kind of positive change.[13] It can be added that the experience of losing a system of possibilities in grief *is* at the

---

[11] This corresponds to what Lear (2006) calls "radical hope." See Ratcliffe (2015: chapter 4) for a discussion of radical hope in grief, and its absence in depression.

[12] These testimonies were obtained via a questionnaire study, conducted as part of the 2009–12 AHRC- and DFG-funded project "Emotional Experience in Depression: A Philosophical Study." For a detailed discussion of the questionnaire, see Ratcliffe (2015: chapter 1).

[13] Hence grief and depression can also involve different alterations in the structure of temporal experience. I have argued elsewhere that temporal experience in depression, like depression itself, is highly variable. Nevertheless, there is a difference between inhabiting a world where the future offers no prospect of significant change (or no prospect of positive change, at least) and feeling "lost," insofar as the future is no longer experienced in the light of a specific system of projects. This difference, amongst others, serves to distinguish temporal experience in many (but not all) cases of grief from experiences of time that are more typical of depression (Ratcliffe 2015: chapter 7). For further discussion of temporal experience in depression, see also Fuchs (2013). For a wider-ranging discussion of the varieties of temporal experience in psychiatric illness, see e.g. Minkowski (1970).

same time the experience of a particular person's irrevocable absence. The deceased was not simply a worldly entity that one cared deeply about (and continues to care deeply about) but also a condition of intelligibility for a world that was once taken for granted, for a system of significant possibilities that were once integral to the experienced environment. The death of these possibilities is inextricable from the death of the person; a singular experience is both localized and all-enveloping. This combination of specificity and generality is, in my view, of considerable philosophical interest. It is commonplace in philosophy to distinguish between intentional states that have a specific object, such as perceiving or remembering something in particular, and diffuse states that have a much more general object, such as the world as a whole, or perhaps no object at all. For instance, we might distinguish an emotion of fearing something specific from a more enveloping feeling or mood of anxiety. Yet a *singular experience* of grief is focused upon the loss of a particular person and, at the same time, amounts to a profound change in how one experiences and relates to the world as a whole. So grief does not confirm to a distinction between specifically focused and more diffuse experiences.

Despite the all-enveloping structure of grief, it does not involve loss of access to kinds of possibility (at least not to the same kinds of possibility that are lost in depression). There is a difference between no longer finding a wide range of entities and situations significant in a particular way and experiencing the world as altogether bereft of a certain kind of significance. In the latter case, nothing appears significant in that way and it also seems that nothing ever could. The world of grief therefore has a particularity to it that the world of depression lacks. Even where an experience of depression does seem to have a specific object, the alteration in one's sense of the possible is further-reaching and not implied in the same way by that object. Of course, it might be objected that major depression is also diagnosed in certain cases where systems of possibility, rather than types, are lost. This is surely so, but one could respond that it should not be. These two broad kinds of predicament are qualitatively different in structure. If major depression does accommodate both, then the category needs to be applied in a more restrictive or discerning way, thus distinguishing depression experiences where certain types of possibility are lost from superficially similar experiences, including many of those that arise during grief.

Perspective-shifting

The contrast between losing systems and types of possibility points to a further difference between grief and depression: experiences of grief have a process structure that depression lacks. To quote C. S. Lewis (1966: 50), "I thought I could describe a *state*; make a map of sorrow. Sorrow, however, turns out to be not a state but a process." Of course, it can be added that depression has a process structure too. Even if the world is experienced as bereft of the potential for meaningful, positive change, people still become depressed, recover from depression, fall back into depression, and experience different degrees or kinds of depression in succession. But my emphasis here is on the phenomenology: grief is *experienced* in a more dynamic way. The world of severe depression is experienced as unchanging and inescapable; one cannot adopt a perspective outside of it; one cannot relive or imagine something that one could contrast with it. Grief, on the other hand, involves intensified interaction between contrasting and often conflicting perspectives. It is not the case that someone dies and a system of possibilities vanishes instantaneously. The bereaved person continues to antic-ipate things in a habitual, practical way, drifting into patterns of activity and thought that somehow implicate the deceased. These are then disrupted by the dawning recognition of loss. There is what we might call an *experience of negation*: one habitually anticipates certain things and is then confronted by the impossibility of one's expectations ever being fulfilled. Hence there is an ongoing tension between competing ways of finding oneself in the world, different perspectival structures:

> Later, at the motel, I stand in the darkened living room and stare out at the dark ocean—a stretch of beach, pale sand—vapor-clouds and a glimpse of the moon—the conviction comes over me suddenly *Ray can't see this, Ray can't breathe* . . . As I've been thinking, in restaurants, staring at menus, forced to choose something to eat. *This is wrong. This is cruel, selfish. If Ray can't eat* . . .

> (Oates 2011: 244)

Furthermore, the bereaved person continues to remember what the world was *like* before the death. She can also imagine a counterfactual world where the death has not occurred. So her current predicament is experienced as contingent; it could have been otherwise. We should not conceive of these conflicting and contrasting perspectives as fully separate from each other; it is not simply that perspective *a* follows *b*, which follows *c*. Perspectives overlap, interact, and are reshaped in the process. Peter Goldie makes an insightful comparison with free indirect style in literary narratives and elsewhere, a way of writing that combines in-ternal and external perspectives on a situation, usually those of author and character. He proposes that autobiographical memory involves a psychological analogue of this, some-thing that is especially salient in grief:

> When you grieve, you often look back on the past, on your time together with the person you loved, knowing now what you did not know then: that the person you loved is now dead, and that you now know the manner and time of the dying . . . autobiographical narra-tive thinking can reveal or express both one's internal and external perspective on one's tragic loss, so that these two perspectives are intertwined through the psychological correlate of free indirect style.

> (Goldie 2012: 65–66)

Hence the gulf and the conflict between the world at time 1 and the world at time 2 is inte-gral to the experience. When recalling time spent with the deceased, memories are infected with the present. Yet they also include a sense of one's current perspective as a contingent one, as something that differs in a profound way from how things once were and how they might have been. Goldie (2012) further proposes that the narratives one constructs and revises during grief are inextricable from the grieving process and give it a meaningful unity. Grief is partly constituted by a variably coherent, dynamic story that envelops, connects, and reshapes the various different perspectives. It is plausible, in my view, to construe this nar-ration process in terms of the negotiation and reconciliation of perspectives. In contrasting past with present and re-narrating one's memories in the light of the present, one fosters coherence, a sense of past and present as quite different and yet integrated into a unitary per-spective upon one's life.

Depression, in contrast, involves a substantially diminished ability to shift perspectives in this way. One cannot "see outside"; things could not be otherwise. One might remember *that* things were not always like this, but one cannot rekindle a sense of what it was like or imagine what it would be like for them to be different. Lack of access to types of possibility applies not only to current experiences of and thoughts about one's surroundings but also to memories, imaginings, and expectations. Hence the narratives of those who are currently depressed often lack the movement between points of view that we find in first-person accounts of grief and in autobiography more generally. Byrom Good (1994: 153–155) observes that illness narratives usually include "multiple perspectives and disparate points of view, all representing aspects of the narrator's experience and the possibility of diverse readings of what had happened and what the future might hold." The point applies equally to grief. Indeed, given the gulf between before and after, the divergent points of view are especially "disparate" in grief. But Good goes on to note that this structure, this "quality of subjunctivity and openness to change," is absent from "narratives of the tragic and hopeless cases." Grief thus involves a sense of contingency (it was otherwise; it could have been otherwise) that is lacking in depression. This is not to suggest that depression, insofar as it involves a more profound loss of possibility, must also involve greater distress. The grieving person is capable of imagining a world where the death did not happen. She might run through events in agonizing detail, wonder how they could have turned out differently, and think about what she might have—or not have—said and done. Moreover, the contrast between the world as it was and the world she now inhabits is ever-present to her, in the guise of habitual dispositions to act, ways of seeing things, and ways of thinking that she lapses into and then experiences as negated. A dining table that appears to her as it would have done were B alive, as though B were there for dinner tonight, there to talk through the day's activities over a bottle of wine and a meal, is then recognized as somehow illusory; its qualities shift. The transition between these experiences adds up to a painful feeling of absence, lack, or negation, which differs from a more pervasive and constant sense of absence that arises in depression. This is not to deny that depression also involves *feelings* of absence. For instance, one might remain able to *anticipate*—in some way—experiencing certain types of possibility, even though one is unable to experience them. Consequently, one is constantly confronted by a world that appears lacking. Even so, these two broad kinds of absence-experience are quite different in character.

INTERPERSONAL CONNECTION

Altered experiences of, and relations with, other people are implied throughout what I have so far described. In grief, projects collapse (to varying degrees) because they depend on a relationship with a particular person. And the interplay between competing perspectives involves a continuing recognition of what it is to relate to someone in that kind of way. In the case of depression, it is not so much that a specific relationship is lost; the sense of being able to enter into a *type* of interpersonal relation is eroded. There is a sense of insurmountable isolation from people in general: "when we experience everyday sorrow, we generally feel—or at least are capable of feeling—intimately connected with others. . . . In contrast, when we experience severe depression, we typically feel outcast and alone" (Pies 2008: 3). This isolation is inseparable from a sense of the world as bereft of possibilities for meaningful action. Almost all of our activities implicate other people in some way. Without any prospect of the relevant kinds of interpersonal relation, these activities become unsustainable.

I do not wish to imply that, following bereavement, a person continues to "feel connected" to people in general. She may feel profoundly isolated from everyone or almost everyone. Nevertheless, there remains an enduring sense of connection with the deceased. The "continuing bonds" literature makes a convincing case for the view that typical or normal grief does not—or at least need not—involve ultimately "letting go" of the deceased, ceasing to address her, relate to her, feel connected to her. Continuing relations with the dead are ubiquitous and healthy. Rather than "disengaging" from the relationship, it is renegotiated to varying degrees and in different ways (Klass, Silverman, and Nickman (eds.) 1996). There are several aspects to this. For instance, one might continue to communicate with the deceased, something that may or may not include an experience of reciprocity. It is also frequently observed that the bereaved engage in "searching behaviours" (e.g. Parkes 1998: chapter 4). Furthermore, when one habitually anticipates or actively seeks out the deceased, one may find him. Sensed presence experiences are not uncommon, and a range of more specific sensory perceptual experiences can also arise (Rees 1971). Indeed, it has been reported that, in some cultures, perceptual or perception-like experiences of the deceased follow spousal bereavement in up to 90% of cases (Keen, Murray, and Payne 2013). It is debatable whether, when, and why such reactions should be regarded as pathological.

On the other hand, grief also involves repeated confrontations with the absence of the deceased. There is thus a complicated, dynamic interplay of presence and absence, involving habitual anticipation and its negation, perceptual and quasi-perceptual experiences of presence and absence, and a sense that the world as a whole is somehow lacking (Ratcliffe 2016). But, throughout all of these experiences, one retains the capacity to enter into a *type* of second-person relation with others, of a kind that involves feelings of connection, mutual recognition, and sharing. What is lacking and recognized as lacking is the ability to relate to a particular individual, at least in the way one once did. Depression experiences, in contrast, involve an experienced inability to enter into that *kind* of relation with other people, to "feel connected" to anyone:

> They seem far away, hard to relate to them.
> Nobody understand or loves me.
> There is the realisation you have never connected with anybody, truly, in your life. Family are self centred and shaming, either ignore comments which don't fit with their picture of how things should be going or they decide that shaming you into "pulling yourself together" will sort it out.
> I feel detached from them.
> People change from being people who I love and am connected with to being hosts of a parasite—me. I can't see why anyone would like me want me love me.[14]

Of course, a depression narrative may emphasize a relationship—or lack thereof—with one or more specific individuals. But there is also a wider-ranging change in the structure of interpersonal experience, an inability to enter into kinds of second-person relation that more usually sustain one's projects and imbue one's world with meaningful possibilities.

However, it should be added that some grief experiences similarly lack the dynamism described earlier; the predicament can seem static, permanent. There is a global sense of disconnection from other people and even from activities that did not depend upon the

---

[14] These testimonies were obtained via a questionnaire study. See n. 7 for details.

deceased in any obvious way. But although such experiences—sometimes labeled as "complicated grief"—seem to involve a loss of possibility akin to that of depression, they are importantly different in structure. The stasis of depression involves feeling unable to relate to others, whereas the stasis of grief can be symptomatic of a resolute and unwavering second-person relationship with a specific individual, the deceased. There is an enduring interpersonal connection, of a kind that detaches the grieving person from the world of the living, from any sense of significant temporal change, from shared temporality. As Riley (2012: 60, 21) writes, "in essence you *have* stopped. You're held in a crystalline suspension. . . . I tried always to be there for him, solidly. And I shall continue to be."[15] Nussbaum (2001: 82–83) offers this insightful remark:

> We might add that what distinguishes normal from pathological mourning is, above all, this change of tense: the pathological mourner continues to put the dead person at the very center of her own structure of goals and expectations, and this paralyzes life.

So, while the world of depression is static and bereft of meaningful pastimes partly because one experiences oneself as incapable of certain kinds of second-person relation, the world of so-called "complicated" grief (one kind of complicated grief, at least) is similarly static but has a very different underlying structure: stasis is attributable to one's continuing to relate to a specific individual in a certain way, rather than failing to relate to anyone in that way.[16]

That said, there are other grief experiences that *do* involve a pervasive sense of being unable to relate to other people in general, of a kind that is close to or indistinguishable from interpersonal experience in depression. I am thinking, in particular, of "traumatic grief" (e.g. Neria and Litz 2004). This is sometimes identified with "complicated grief," but differs from what I have just described. A central theme is the pervasive loss of what we might call "affective trust" in things and, more specifically, in other people.[17] A sense of security that was once presupposed as a backdrop to meaningful activities and to one's relations with other people is disturbed. Nothing and nobody is encountered in quite the same way as before.

---

15 See also Ratcliffe (2016) for a more detailed discussion of Riley's account.

16 One might wonder whether and to what extent the kinds of experience I have described are specific to personal grief. Perhaps the break-up of a relationship, the loss of a job, one's children growing up and leaving home, or moving to an unfamiliar country can all similarly involve losing systems of possibility, oscillating between conflicting perspectives and yearning for interpersonal relationships that are no longer available. Although there are considerable similarities between bereavement experiences and experiences associated with other kinds of loss, I think there is something distinctive about grieving over the death of another person. One is confronted with the prospect of *irrevocable* loss and absence. The experienced interplay between presence and absence, and the way in which one continues to relate to someone who has died, thus have a distinctive character (Ratcliffe 2016). However, I am willing to concede that there are at least some cases where a person grieves in this way over the death of a non-human animal.

17 More generally, I want to maintain that the kinds of phenomenological change I have described in both grief and depression are essentially, although not exclusively, "affective" in character. Feelings, I argue, are not generally experiences of the body in isolation from the environment; they also shape how we experience and relate to our surroundings and to other people. At least some instances of grief involve alterations in what I have elsewhere called "existential feeling," a felt sense of reality and belonging that is presupposed by all intentional states with specific or even very general contents. I construe shifts in existential feeling in terms of changes in the *kinds* of possibility that one is open to (Ratcliffe 2008, 2015). Hence it might seem that typical grief does not involve a change in existential feeling, while depression and some forms of complicated or traumatic grief do. However, I would not

One is vulnerable before people in general, in a way that interferes with the abilities to enter into second-person relations that involve a sense of connectedness, to embark upon projects that depend on others for their sustenance, and to contemplate the possibility of a future that departs in positive ways from the present. With this basic sense of confidence, trust, or safety gone from the world, *types* of possibility are lost (including that of experiencing and relating to other people in certain ways), rather than just systems of possibility (Ratcliffe, Ruddell, and Smith 2014).

So experiences of grief can differ markedly, depending on how one relates to others, to the living and the dead. And, in some cases, the difference between grief and depression is greater than in others. Nevertheless, an informative phenomenological distinction (admittedly one that involves substantial idealization and allows for borderline cases) can be made between losing specific individuals, along with associated systems of possibility, and losing types of possibility. This distinction may not track current diagnostic practice but, if that is the case, phenomenological research can contribute to a case for revision.

INTERPERSONAL RELATIONS AND SELF-REGULATION

I have focused principally on experiential differences between grief and depression. However, I also think there are lessons to be learned from studying the phenomenology of grief that apply equally to depression and various other psychiatric illness categories. Reflecting upon the structure of grief serves to make salient the extent to which the regulation of our experiences, thoughts, and activities depends upon specific individuals and other people in general. Profound grief inevitably involves some degree of detachment from mundane, everyday, norm-governed interactions with other people. But projects and pastimes prove resilient to the extent that continuing relations with others hold them in place and assist one in negotiating changes. In addition, the narratives that we construct around our experiences are influenced by interactions with others, and often co-constructed. It follows that the course of a grieving process depends, to a significant extent, on how the bereaved person relates to others and on how they relate to her.[18] Studying the phenomenology of grief thus serves to illustrate the—often insufficiently acknowledged—extent to which the experienced world, our sense of rootedness within it, and our ability to act in meaningful ways all depend upon other people. A fully developed account of the various ways

---

want to insist that typical grief is bereft of "existential changes." In fact, I think that certain aspects of the experience, such as a pervasive loss of confidence or sense of helplessness are plausibly interpreted in that way. Rather, my claim here is that typical grief does not involve an existential change *of the same kind* as that found in depression. If it is accepted that grief sometimes or always involves changes in existential feeling, the dual nature of grief—its specificity and generality—complicates my account of these feelings by problematizing my contrast between specifically directed intentional states and non-specific, pre-intentional existential feelings; it might turn out that a singular experience can be both. An interesting question to address is whether this duality is specific to the interpersonal realm, whether only a person can be both an entity in one's world and a condition for one's world.

[18] See Sbarra and Hazan (2015) for a recent discussion of how emotional experience is interpersonally regulated in grief.

in which experience, thought, and activity are interpersonally regulated may prove equally illuminating when seeking to better understand all those cases of psychiatric illness where social isolation and estrangement from others are prominent themes. I am increasingly of the view that J. H. van den Berg (1972: 105) was right in remarking that "loneliness is the nucleus of psychiatry."

ACKNOWLEDGMENTS

Thanks to Matthew Broome, Andrea Raballo, and Giovanni Stanghellini for helpful comments on an earlier version.

BIBLIOGRAPHY

American Psychiatric Association. (2000). *Diagnostic and Statistical Manual of Mental Disorders* (4th edn, text revision). Washington: American Psychiatric Association.

American Psychiatric Association. (2013). *Diagnostic and Statistical Manual of Mental Disorders* (Fifth Edition). Washington: American Psychiatric Association.

Attig T. (2004). "Meanings of Death Seen Through the Lens of Grieving." *Death Studies* 28: 341–360.

Berg J. H. van den. (1972). *A Different Existence: Principles of Phenomenological Psychopathology*. Pittsburgh: Duquesne University Press.

Carse J. P. (1981). "Grief as a Cosmic Crisis." In O. S. Margolis, H. C. Raether, A. H. Kutscher, J. B. Powers, I. B. Seeland, R. DeBillis, and D. J. Cherico (eds.), *Acute Grief: Counseling the Bereaved*, pp. 3–8. New York: Columbia University Press.

Didion J. (2005). *The Year of Magical Thinking*. London: Harper Perennial.

Didion J. (2011). *Blue Nights*. London: Fourth Estate.

Freud S. (1917/2005). "Mourning and Melancholia." In *On Murder, Mourning and Melancholia*, trans. S. Whiteside, pp. 201–218. London: Penguin.

Fuchs T. (2013). "Temporality and Psychopathology." *Phenomenology and the Cognitive Sciences* 12: 75–104.

Goldie P. (2012). *The Mess Inside: Narrative, Emotion, & the Mind*. Oxford: Oxford University Press.

Good B. (1994). *Medicine, Rationality and Experience: An Anthropological Perspective*. Cambridge: Cambridge University Press.

Hemon A. (2013). *The Book of my Lives*. London: Picador.

Humphreys H. (2013). *True Story: The Life and Death of My Brother*. London: Serpent's Tail.

Keen C., Murray C., and Payne S. (2013). "Sensing the Presence of the Deceased: A Narrative Review." *Mental Health, Religion & Culture* 16: 384–402.

Klass D., Silverman P. R., and Nickman S. L. (eds.) (1996). *Continuing Bonds: New Understandings of Grief*. London: Routledge.

Lamb K., Pies R., and Zisook S. (2010). "The Bereavement Exclusion for the Diagnosis of Major Depression: To Be, Or Not to Be." *Psychiatry* 7(7): 19–25.

Lear J. (2006). *Radical Hope: Ethics in the Face of Cultural Devastation*. Cambridge MA: Harvard University Press.

Lewis C. S. (1966). *A Grief Observed*. London: Faber & Faber.

Lichtenthal W. G., Cruess D. G., and Prigerson, H. G. (2004). "A Case for Establishing Complicated Grief as a Distinct Mental Disorder in DSM-V." *Clinical Psychology Review* 24: 637–662.

Minkowski E. (1970). *Lived Time: Phenomenological and Psychopathological Studies*, trans. N. Metzel. Evanston: Northwestern University Press.

Neria Y. and Litz B. T. (2004). "Bereavement by Traumatic Means: The Complex Synergy of Trauma and Grief." *Journal of Loss and Trauma* 9: 73–87.

Nussbaum M. C. (2001). *Upheavals of Thought: The Intelligence of Emotions*. Cambridge: Cambridge University Press.

Oates, J. C. 2011. *A Widow's Story*. London: Fourth Estate.

Parkes C. M. (1998). *Bereavement: Studies of Grief in Adult Life*, 3rd edn. London: Penguin Books.

Pies R. (2008). "The Anatomy of Sorrow: A Spiritual, Phenomenological, and Neurological Perspective." *Philosophy, Ethics, and Humanities in Medicine* 3(17): 1–8.

Pies R. (2012). "After Bereavement, Is it Normal Grief or Major Depression? The PBPI: A Potential Assessment Tool." *Psychiatric Times* February 21.

Ratcliffe M. (2008). *Feelings of Being: Phenomenology, Psychiatry and the Sense of Reality*. Oxford: Oxford University Press.

Ratcliffe M. (2015). *Experiences of Depression: A Study in Phenomenology*. Oxford: Oxford University Press.

Ratcliffe M. (2016). "Relating to the Dead: Social Cognition and the Phenomenology of Grief." In D. Moran and T. Szanto (eds.), *The Phenomenology of Sociality: Discovering the 'We'*, pp. 202–215. London: Routledge.

Ratcliffe M., Ruddell M., and Smith B. (2014). "What is a Sense of Foreshortened Future? A Phenomenological Study of Trauma, Trust and Time." *Frontiers in Psychology* 5 (Article 1026): 1–11.

Rees W. D. (1971). "The Hallucinations of Widowhood." *British Medical Journal* 4: 37–41.

Riley D. (2012). *Time Lived, Without Its Flow*. London: Capsule Editions.

Sbarra D. and Hazan C. (2015). "Coregulation, Dysregulation, Self-Regulation: An Integrative Analysis and Empirical Agenda for understanding Adult Attachment, Separation, Loss, and Recovery." *Personality and Social Psychology Review* 12: 141–167.

Wakefield J. C. and First M. B. (2012). "Validity of the Bereavement Exclusion to Major Depression: Does the Empirical Evidence Support the Proposal to Eliminate the Exclusion in DSM-5?" *World Psychiatry* 11: 3–10.

Wilkinson S. (2000). "Is 'Normal Grief' a Mental Disorder?" *Philosophical Quarterly* 50: 289–304.

Zisook S. and Shear K. (2009). "Grief and Bereavement: What Psychiatrists Need to Know." *World Psychiatry* 8: 67–74.

CHAPTER 59

....

GENDER DYSPHORIA

....

GIOVANNI CASTELLINI AND MILENA MANCINI

AROUND the question of gender dysphoria, there are still many unclear aspects, and limited information. For example, for many people, the terms "gender" and "sex" are used interchangeably, and thus incorrectly. In recent years, there has been a great deal of attention on the gender question, and from a psychopathological and nosographic point of view, many steps forward have been taken, but there is still much to do.

Gender is a social combination of identity, expression, and social elements related to masculinity and femininity. It includes gender identity (self-identification), gender expression (self-expression), social gender (social expectations), gender roles (socialized actions), and gender attribution (social perception). This concept is strictly related to the term of gender identity. It is an individual's internal sense of being male, female, both, neither, or something else. In other words, gender identity is the subjective experience of membership to a gender. This subjective sense of belonging to a given gender is generally taken for granted by most of the persons.

Gender identity is part of our general identity, and provides a sense of continuity of the self. Interrogatives on this aspect of our life are barely present in our consciousness—at least in ordinary circumstances. Exceptions are represented by stages of development such as adolescence, or by some categories of persons who do not identify themselves with the dichotomous categories male/female. The debate on gender identity has recently broken into the consciousness for psychopathology, increasing interrogation from different perspectives, including medicine, psychology, anthropology, and ethics. In very general terms, is the philosophical issue of gender identity is: 1) the existence of only two diametrically opposed genders or either–or categories—male and female merely defined in terms of anatomical characteristics; 2) if the differences between men and women follow these binary, dichotomous and stable categories.

In the present chapter, we will resume the historical trajectory of gender definition, emphasizing the importance for psychopathology of a different perspective on gender than the common definition provided by Western culture. We will first offer a brief description of the concepts of gender identity, sexual orientation, gender role, and gender dysphoria. Our approach is coherent with the dimensional view proposed by the DSM board (American Psychiatric Association, 2013), as well as by LGBT (lesbian, gay, bisexual, transgender, queer, and/or questioning individuals) movements. This position considers gender dysphoria and transsexualism as positions on a gender variants continuum. We assume gender heterogeneity and aim to understand how persons who are dysphoric about their gender experience themselves (their body) and the way they are looked at by other persons, and finally how these affect their own sense of identity. Every psychological, medical, or surgical treatment should come as consequences of this understanding of "what is it like" to suffer from gender dysphoria. This is an opposite view with regard to the rigid anatomical perspective, which reduces transgender to individuals who are in the wrong body and must "rectify" this error with hormonal treatment or surgical intervention.

GENDER DYSPHORIA VERSUS DISORDER OF GENDER

Since 2013, the board for DSM-5 (American Psychiatric Association 2013) decided that gender identity disorder no longer exists. The dichotomous perspective that identified a stigmatizing threshold between normalcy and pathology was replaced by a dimensional characterization of the distress that may accompany the incongruence between one's experienced or expressed gender and one's assigned gender. Indeed, there are individuals who have an uncertain or confused gender identity, or are transitioning from one gender to the other, who do not fit into this dichotomous scheme. The extreme of this continuum is represented by gender dysphoria, defined as the distress that may accompany the incongruence between one's experienced or expressed gender and one's assigned gender (American Psychiatric Association 2013). For gender dysphoric persons, the primary source of suffering is the sense of dissonance with the gender assigned to one's anatomical sexual characteristics.

Conversely, gender dysphoric persons are characterized by a strong and persistent identification with the opposite sex, discomfort with their own sex, and a sense of inappropriateness in the gender role of that sex (American Psychiatric Association 2013). GD subjects experience a cognitive state in which their physical body contrasts with their self-perceived identity (Gooren 2006), and which can be a source of deep and chronic suffering (Gooren 2011). Transgender persons perceive their gender identity as incongruous with their body, and therefore experience the desire to develop a gender role consistent with their gender identity.

The gender dysphoria condition highlights the dichotomy and the contradictions of the postmodern society between a physical reality (anatomical body) and the mental reality (gender identity) (Winter 2003). Therefore, a main issue in this area is what makes us male or female. For those persons who are not clearly classified as he or she, the Western world has coined the word "transgender." Indeed, the natal anatomic view of gender has been the mainstream view in most developed countries. According to this perspective the determinant of our sex identity is based on our external anatomy, and persons should grow up with a gender role that matches their anatomy, and those who deviate from these "rules" are seen as mentally disordered.

Clinicians should be aware that gender-atypical does not always underly a pathological condition, rather it refers to somatic features or behaviors that are not typical (in a statistical sense) of individuals with the same assigned gender in a given society and historical era.

For behavior, gender-nonconforming is an alternative descriptive term. As for all the other clinical conditions included in the DSM, mental health professionals should consider taking care of persons with gender atypical features only when they identify an individual's affective/cognitive discontent with the assigned gender, the so-called dysphoria.

The identification with a pole of the gender dimension or alternatively the hetorogeneity of self-gender perception vary according with different cultures and countries. For example, gender fluidity was reported by 4.6% of males and 3.2% of females in Netherlands (Kuyper and Wijsen 2014) and by 35% of persons in Israel (Joel et al. 2013). Within transgender persons, 25% defined themselves as non-binary gender (Harrison et al. 2012).

The Descriptive Level: Definition of Gender Identity, Gender Role, and Sexual Orientation

In light of the above considerations, it is necessary to provide a definition of a) gender identity, b) gender role, and c) sexual orientation.

Gender Identity: How Do We Develop the Sense of Gender Membership?

Gender membership is a fundamental component of our general identity. It is part of the so-called "sexual identity," which is a mosaic concept, including not just gender identity, but also biologic gender, sexual orientation, as well as gender role. The term "gender" originally related to one's belonging to a specific category of persons. The Latin word *gens* referred to Roman families, which were large groups of persons related to each other sharing the same name (e.g. gens Iulia to which Julius Caesar belonged). Now "gender" refers to the subjective belonging to the categories of male, female, or an alternative gender. This concept was first introduced in the psychosexual development model proposed by Masica et al. (1971), who first described persons with discrepancies between biological sex and gender identity.

Biological or chromosomal sex is actually binary (i.e. the presence of a Y or X chromosome). However, what is between this first step of psychosexual development and the adult sexual identity is much more complex than a binary divide. The chromosomal sex influences the determination of the gonadal sex, in differentiating the bipotential gonadal ridge into either testes or an ovary (Jost et al. 1973). Across the gestational period, under the effect of different hormones, external genitalia become defined and visible. Masculinization induced by testosterone determines closure of the urethral folds and development of the prostate and scrotum (Migeon and Wisniewski 2003), while in women the "road" of feminization is toward development of the uterus, fallopian tubes, and the distal portion of the vagina. Then the feminine genital tubercle develops as a clitoris, the urethral folds form the labia minora and the labioscrotal swellings give rise to the labia majora (Achermann and Hughes 2008). From this time the morphology of external genitalia allow our family to establish our masculine/feminine name and the so-called "assigned gender." It is clear how this anatomic idea of gender has been conceptualized in a binary, dichotomous manner with a male gender identity at one pole and a female gender identity at the other pole.

For most people the sense of being male or female is congruent with anatomical/morphological sex. Also, it is commonly assumed that gender is univocally and linearly dependent on chromosomes X or Y. However, there are several conditions, such as disorders of sex development (DSD), which challenge the relationship between chromosomal gender and gender identity. For example, persons reporting 5alpha-reductase-2 deficiency spend their life until late adolescence trusting in their feminine identity, while they have masculine (XY) chromosome (Cohen-Kettenis 2005). Modern medicine attempted to find valid ways of managing gender identity and further intervention on DSD, without a common consensus.

This kind of observation demonstrates the lack of a univocal correspondence between biological gender and gender identity. Moreover, according to Money and his colleagues (1955, 1968) and the first postulation of his psychosexual model, gender identity is not innate, rather it is dynamic process which results from the continuous integration between biological changes, cultural influences, and experiential steps through life. Indeed, there are individuals who have an uncertain or confused gender identity or who are transitioning from one gender to the other, without fitting into a dichotomous scheme.

The age for gender identity (i.e. an individual's personal sense of self as male or female) development is still matter of debate. Freud assumed that gender identity becomes stable with the resolution of the Oedipus complex, and a child acquires a stable gender identity when he identifies himself with the same sex parent. However, nowadays scientists tend to put the onset of gender identity at a more precocious age. Gender identity usually develops by age three, remaining stable over a person's lifetime (Giordano 2012).

How We Act Our Gender: The Gender Role

The term "gender role" describes the behaviors, attitudes, and personality traits that a society, in a given culture and historical period, designates as masculine or feminine, that is, more "appropriate" for, or typical of, the male or female social role (Lawrence and Zucker 2012). Gender role represents the public manifestation of our gender identity, and the way our gender identity is defined through the gaze of the others.

The concept of gender role can be interpreted in the light of the construct of social identity or more exactly "social role," which includes participant roles, positions, relationships, reputations, and other dimensions of social personae, which are conventionally linked to epistemic and affective stances (Ochs 1993). Social role related to identity is multiple and varied, describing individual representations that embody particular social histories built up through, and continually recreated in, one's everyday experiences (Bucholtz and Hall 2005). Moreover, it is acknowledged that individuals belong to varied groups and so take on a variety of identities as defined by their membership of these groups. In our use of language, we represent a particular identity at the same time that we construct it. One of the more prominent positions on social identity is Anthony Giddens's theory of structuration (1991). According to Giddens, individual agency is a semiotic activity, a social construction, "something that has to be routinely created and sustained in the reflexive activities of the individual." In our locally occasioned social actions, we, as individual agents, shape and at the same time are given shape by what Giddens refers to as social structures. In our actions, we draw on these structures and in so doing recreate them and ourselves as social actors. The repeated use of social structures in recurring social practices in turn leads to the development of larger social systems, "patterns of relations in groupings of all kinds, from small, intimate groups, to social networks, to large organizations" (Giddens 1991).

Indeed, gender role is a social construct which depends on the historical period and cultural influences, which define what is commonly accepted as being appropriate for masculine or feminine identity (Zucker 2000). Across history, the heterogeneity of gender role expressions showed the need for self-definition of gender variant persons who attempted to present themselves as non-dichotomically defined. Transgender people are finding creative and constructive ways out of their situation, expanding the possibilities for language and identities, and overcoming the limitation of sociocultural traditional models (Kulick 1999). Transgender persons attempted to reconstruct the world around them by the power of a new language; a language relating to bodies, ways of dressing, and also words. For example, different terms have been adopted for the necessity of non-gender definition such as androgynous, mixed gender, pangender. Gender fluidity has been expressed as bi-gender, gender fluid, pangender, while absence of gender has been defined as A-gender, gender neutral, non-gendered (Bockting 2008) (see Table 59.1). The transgender world is characterized by continuous linguistic innovation (Castellini 2016), as an act to challenge a world that has not provided membership categories for them. Many words have been invented and adopted by transgender persons to define themselves, including *gendertrash, spokensherm,* and *genderqueer* (Kulick 1999). Words such as *femisexuals, mascusexuals, transhomosexuals* have also been coined, demonstrating great creativity in the language of transgender persons (Kulick 1999). These examples suggest an attempt among transgender people to transcend grammatical gender and reconfigure language to express their subjectivities and desires.

One of the contributions that work on transgenderism can offer to sociolinguistics and anthropology is a focus on the relationship between language and the lived body. Transgenderism contributes to an affirmation of the permeability of gender boundaries. Several studies have been undertaken regarding the language of transgender persons and the adoption of stereotypical speech, that is, a way of speaking that helps to promote the appearance of appropriately sexed corporeality. For example, it has been noted that transgender females generally use more tag questions (i.e. questions appended at the end of statements, like "this is silly, isn't it?") and the so-called "empty adjectives" like lovely and precious (Kulick 1999). On the other hand, transgender males are told to use a certain aggressive style and to tell people what they want instead of asking it, to help them pass as men. Sociolinguistic theories (Bourdieu et al. 1970; Bourdieu 1980; Giddens 1991) focused on the relationship between the process of identity construction and language. Their research is concerned with the ways in which individuals use language to co-construct their everyday worlds and, in particular, their own social roles and identities and those of others.

Table 59.1 Glossary of terms relating to gender

REDEFINING GENDER*

Agender (also non-gender)	Person not identifying with any gender and they can be categorized as man or woman or neither. Characterized by the feeling of having no specific gender.
Androgynous	A person who may appear with masculine and feminine traits or as neither male nor female, or as in between male and female. It is a non-traditional gender expression.
Bigender	A person who identifies with both genders and/or who has a tendency to move between masculine and feminine gender-typed behavior depending on context.
Bisexual	A person attracted to males/men and females/women. This attraction may be on an emotional, physical, or sexual level, and it may be not equally split between genders, and there may be a preference for one gender over others.
Cisgender	A person whose gender identity matches the biological sex they were assigned at birth. It is based on the physical sex.
FTM or F2M (Female-to-Male)	Term used to identify a person who was designated a female sex at birth and currently identifies as male, or identifies predominantly as masculine. They often live as a man. This includes a heterogeneous range of experiences, such as: (1) self-identification as men or male, (2) self-identification as transsexual, transgender men, transmen, female men, new men, or FTM. In many cases, these persons reject all definition and some people prefer the term MTM (male-to-male) to underscore the fact that although they were assigned female at birth, they never had a female gender identity.
Gender binary	The idea that there are only two diametrically opposed genders or either-or categories—male and female, based on sex assigned at birth. It is a cultural belief that does not consider the membership of a gender as a continuum or spectrum of gender identities and expressions. This idea is limiting for those who do not fit neatly into the either-or categories.
Gender conforming	Gender expression is consistent with cultural norms. Therefore, man is masculine and woman is feminine.
Genderfluid	A gender identity where a person shifts between man/masculine and woman/feminine, or falls somewhere along this spectrum. A person may identify with 1) neither or both female and male; 2) experiences a range of femaleness and maleness, with a flow between genders; 3) consistently experiences his/her gender identity outside of the gender binary.
Gender nonconforming	Gender expression is inconsistent with cultural norms expected for that gender. Specifically, boys or men are not "masculine enough" or are feminine, while girls or women are not "feminine enough" or are masculine. Gender nonconforming is often inaccurately confused with sexual orientation. For example, not all transgender people are gender nonconforming, and cisgender people may also be gender nonconforming. This term may be used in tandem with other identity.

(continued)

Table 59.1 Continued

Genderqueer	An umbrella term for people whose gender identity is not included within the binary of female and male, is between or beyond genders, or is some combination of genders.
Intersex	Term to describe someone with a disorder of sexual development, one who is born with sex chromosomes, external genitalia, and/or an internal reproductive system that is not considered "standard" or normative for either the male or female sex. This term is frequently confused with transgender, but the two are completely distinct.
Intergender	A person whose gender identity is between genders or a combination of genders.
LGBTQ	Acronym used to refer lesbian, gay, bisexual, transgender, queer, or/and questioning individuals. Often seen as LGBT or LGBTQ.
MTF or M2F (Male-to-Female)	Term used to identify a person who was designated a male sex at birth and currently identifies as female, lives as a woman, or identifies as feminine. This includes a broad range of experiences: (1) men who identify as women or female; (2) as transsexual, transgender women, transwomen, male women, new women, or as MTF. In many cases, these persons prefer the term FTF (female-to-female) to underscore the fact that though they were assigned male at birth, they never had a masculine gender identity.
Non-binary (gender)	Describes a spectrum of gender identities and expression that is outside of or beyond two traditional concepts of male or female. Term include "agender," "bigender," "gender-queer," "gender fluid," and "pangender."
Pangender	This term concerns a non-binary gender defined as including all genders and not being exclusively man or woman. It refers to a person whose gender identity is comprised of many gender identities and/or expressions.
Transgender (TG)	An umbrella term describing a person whose gender identity does not match the biological sex assigned to birth. It refers to anyone who transcends the conventional definitions of man and woman and whose self-identification or expression challenges traditional notions of male and female. This term includes two categories: (1) transgender man (or Transman)—a woman who identifies as a man (see also FTM); (2) transgender woman (or Transwoman)—a man who identifies as a woman (see also MTF).
Transsexual	A person whose gender identity is different from their designated sex at birth and who has had hormonal or surgical interventions to change their body to be more aligned with their gender identity.

*Sources:
– JAC Stringer of The Trans and Queer Wellness Initiative (2013) JAC (at): http://www. TransQueerWellness.org
– *Teaching Transgender Toolkit*, by Eli R. Green and Luca Maurer: http://www.teachingtransgender.org/

What I Like: The Sexual Orientation

In clinical practice with gender dysphoria, we often have to deal with the general public's ignorance regarding gender identity/dysphoria. It is quite common, for example, for people to confuse gender dysphoria with homosexuality. Even though these two concepts are mutually correlated, gender identity and sexual orientation do not represent the same construct. Sexual orientation refers to the sex of the person to whom an individual is erotically attracted. It comprises several components, including sexual fantasy, patterns of physiological arousal, sexual behavior, sexual identity, and social role. Scientific studies demonstrating the healthy, adaptive functioning of the great majority of gay and lesbian adults paved the way toward removal of homosexuality as an illness from the DSM in 1973 (Bayer 1981). Therefore, homosexuality is now recognized as a non-pathological variant of human sexuality.

A relevant issue is represented by the so-called cross-gender behaviors among children and young adolescents. The diagnosis of gender dysphoria in children is controversial (Meyer-Bahlburg 2010). Several different categories of gender discordance, each characterized by a unique developmental trajectory, have been described (Steensma and Cohen-Kettenis 2011). They differ in regard to whether gender discordance emerges in childhood, adolescence, or adulthood; whether the gender discordance is persistent or transient; and whether there is a post-transition homosexual or heterosexual orientation. In follow-up studies of pre-pubertal boys with gender discordance—including many who are not being treated for mental health issues—the cross-gender tendencies usually fade over time and do not persist into adulthood, with only 2.2% (Green 1987) to 11.9% (Zucker and Bradley 1995) continuing to experience gender discordance. Rather, 75% become homosexual or bisexual in fantasy and 80% in behavior by age nineteen; some gender-variant behavior may persist (Zucker and Bradley 1995; Zucher et al. 1993). The desistance of gender discordance may reflect the resolution of a "cognitive confusion factor," (Zucker and Bradley 1995; Zucher et al. 1993) with increasing flexibility as children mature in thinking about gender identity and realize that one can be a boy or girl despite variation from conventional gender roles and norms.

While sexual orientation is no longer considered a matter for medical or psychological interventions, it is true that non-heterosexual persons or other sexual minorities often report psychopathological disturbances related to their condition. One of the possible explations for this could be the relationship with stigma and discrimination. Homophobia was originally defined by Weinberg (1973) as "the dread of being in close quarters with homosexuals," and many theorists (Herek 1984; Weinberg 1973) have emphasized that homophobia has to do with the personal discomfort and fear that heterosexuals may experience when associating with gay men and lesbians.

DIFFERENT PERSPECTIVES ON GENDER VARIANTS

Gender variants are not a novelty of modern society. In the art of the Renaissance there would be a sort of hesitation before the difference between the categories of male and female. In Renaissance painting, there was an indeterminacy of sexual identity, for example, Leonardo's effeminate men and Michelangelo's virile women (Ferrari 2003). The history of art reports a plethora of gender fluidness or uncertainty, such as the hermaphrodite statues in the Hellenistic period, Ribera paintings of the seventeenth century, or the Sultane Reine of the painter Vien. In contemporary art this hesitation, the ability to swing your identity, seem to reappear with force reaching the extreme limit of the iconography transgender. The photographer Nan Goldin shows in his photos the impossibility of precise identification of the nude in sexuality. From the naked to the represented object there is always the start of sexual identity movement, an endless shift of identity. In the phase of the passage from the naked to the represented object, the nude is shaped like the endless transit of sexual identity.

Contrary to the anatomical position, the psychosocial perspective maintains that the sex category into which we are placed at birth is simply a first guess as to what identity we will later assume, and that it is possible to grow up with a gender that does not match that original sex category (Winter 2003). Therefore, "transgender" should be considered as an aspect of human diversity rather being considered a disorder, deviance, or at worst depravity. The conflict between these two perspectives is a serious matter of concern for transgender persons, involving the discrepancy between identity and the name written in a passport, social welfare rights, marrying and parenting rights, even the search for a job.

The anthropological perspective allows us to consider the ways in which culture shapes and is itself shaped by the activities and understandings of people, from the most intimate of bodily concerns to the most global of economic systems. Indeed, there are different ways in which sexuality and gender are understood in other cultures and, in so doing, can underscore the importance of disengaging concepts of sex from those of gender (James 1998). This area highlights the importance of the social context in shaping our understanding of gender as something that is not given, but rather learned. In many parts of the world male and female are not seen as the only possible gender identities, and they need not to be regarded as mutually exclusive. Indeed, some peoples recognize the possibility of a third gender, and in Western societies, until the late eighteenth century, popular and medical science assumed that there was only one gender. This interpretation suggests that gender identity may be a more important marker of personhood and self-identity than anatomical sexual identity. However, when it comes to how to respond to individuals whose gender role and identity is manifestly at odds with their physical body and appearance, most groups or societies are at a loss. So fundamental is the need for clarity about who is male and who is female that those who demonstrate apparent uncertainty (or indeed express a perplexing certainty) are viewed with alarm (Wilson 1998).

There is no universal patterning of tasks or behaviors according to sex. For example, in some societies men may adopt more nurturing kinds of behavior than women, while women adopt more aggressive roles (Mead 1935). An interesting example is represented by *Hijras* in India, a religious community of men who dress and act like women and for whom commitment to the role of *hijra* is signified through their impotence as men, an impotence usually achieved through the act of castration. As children they often have interest in playing with girls, with wearing female rather than male clothing and using eye make-up. Gilbert Herdt notes that central to *hijra* identity is their in-betweenness, their being neither man or woman is what being *hijra* is (Herdt 1996). The idea that a person's identity arises out of his/her sense of who he/she is and how he/she presents to the world is more widespread in those countries that are least influenced by Judeo-Christian or Western psychiatry. Among them is Thailand, which is overwhelmingly Buddhist (Rompjampa 1973).

Languages reflect how the issue of gender identity is differently managed across cultures. For example, the Thai language fails to distinguish between sex and gender. One word, *phet*, says it at all. The word is so versatile it can even be used for "sexuality." Moreover, Thai culture allows for the possibility that there may be more than two sexes and genders; thus, for example, the common term for transgender is *phet tee sam*, the third gender (Winter 2003). On the contrary, the linguistic consequences of the anatomic view are evident in the English-speaking world. For example, male-to-female persons are generally called transsexual males or male transgenders, regardless of their perceived female identity. Indeed, many male-to-female persons refer to themselves as transgender females not males. A first consequence of this linguistic discrepancy is marriage: even though male-to-female persons are often attracted to males they may not be able to marry them, since in a number of Western countries this qualifies as a same-sex marriage and is illegal. Moreover, transgender persons may find it difficult to get a job simply because their gender identity and appearance fail to match their official documents. In Italy, the anatomic perspective is so strong that to get a new "legal" gender identity, persons must undergo a genital reassignment surgery intervention. In other words, they must sterilize themselves to adopt an (official) gender identity that resembles their perceived identity. Also, transgender persons can be victims of the anatomical perspective, as many of them say that they were "born transgender" but now they are male or female.

The conflict between the two views (natal anatomical versus psychosocial) is nowhere more evident than it is in the names given to the surgical operations in which a person's genital are removed (Winter 2003). In English, the mainstream name is "sex reassignment surgery." The connotation is one of moving away from the sex to which one properly belongs. In contrast, many transgenders talk about "sex confirmation surgery," the connotation being moving toward the sex they always should have been.

The anatomic view is so represented in Western culture that the less-informed public finds it difficult to distinguish between gay and transgender persons. Considering sexual orientation, the anatomic view allows the statement that male-to-female persons should be considered as homosexuals. However a male-to-female person who is attracted to men generally feels female, and may have felt like this as long as she can remember, often pre-dating any feelings of sexual attraction. Conscious that her attraction toward men is consistent with her feelings of identity, she sees herself as heterosexual. She probably sees her partner's attraction to her in the same light, as indeed he might.

CLINICAL EXAMPLES

Two Different Life Trajectories: From Francesco to Luisa and from Marco to Camilla

Luisa, born Francesco, perceives her objective body as an impediment for her life realization. This was true the day she asks for help at the Gender Clinic but also continued after medical and surgical treatments. Our impression was that these difficulties were due to her long experience of discrimination and perceived extraneousness to the world. The first day of acceptance to the clinic she stated:

> I cannot stand my body anymore, it is between me and my life . . . I spent 23 years waiting for this moment. Now I want hormones and surgery as soon as possible. My dream is to wake up one day, and to be a woman.

Luisa gave up her job, because she believed that a person can only exist in the eyes of others, as totally a man or a woman. She did not want to appear a clown; she desired to erase all traces of masculinity from her body. Luisa experienced her first cross-gender behaviors when she was five years old. She sometimes wore feminine clothes, and reported marked cross-gender identification in role-playing, as she always acted as a mother or a bride. Her father was clearly against her "abnormal" feminine behaviors, and often stigmatized them. Luisa told the clinicians:

> Luckily my puberty started late. Because this period was a living hell. I had my first relationship with a gay person. I could not bear him to look at or touch my genitals. At age 12, my body began to change . . . first hairs, the testicles became enlarged and I had my first erection.

During adolescence, Luisa realized for the first time that she had been born in the wrong body. Luisa hated her body in such a way that she reported several dysfunctional diet attempts, throughout her life:

> Women have a lean and slim body and mine is always so cumbersome. I do not go looking for a job because they do not want to look me like a freak. I do not want to be seen as a tranny. I want to be Luisa. You always have to justify your existence, how do you put in a CV a name that has nothing to do with your appearance. I waited 20 years without a boyfriend, I lost many years which are important to study or to build a profession. Hormone therapy has led to the reduction of body hair, loss of spontaneous erections, breast growth. I'm not happy, you can still see the signs of my male body . . . broad shoulders, a beard that despite the laser treatment does not go away. I cannot go around like that. I must continue to bandage the penis and cover it. While in elementary school I was in a secure environment, in junior high and high school, things change. Teachers always invited me to wear "more appropriate attire." I started to avoid the male companions . . . Violent games, the jokes, and stuff like that. Spending time alone with some companions. The rest of the guys called me "faggot", or a drag queen and consider me strange. During this time my father began to verbally attack me . . . I got to the stage where I felt it was better if I'd never been born. At the same time I suffered the worst humiliation of my life. A group of classmates gathered around me after school and began to laugh at me, the way I walked, dressed . . . someone even kicked me. Friends and classmates did nothing. And since then I stopped going to school.

Camilla, born Marco, spent her adolescence living either as a man either as a woman. She accepted her life trajectory and she referred to a family environment of tolerance and protection against stigma. At the end of hormonal treatment she was completely satisfied. Sometimes she goes out dressed as a woman, especially at night. She works as a physiotherapist in a neutral appearance. When she asked for help at the clinic in Florence she wished to change her documents, but not to undergo a genital reassignment. Camilla started dressing in women's clothes. She usually played with her mother, who had fun with her and encouraged her to try and play cross-gender roles. Since early adolescence she always imagined herself as a girl or as a neutral individual, adopting either male or female names.

> The first hair, the first erections did not cause me hardship but a feeling that something foreign to me was happening to my body. I do not consider myself gay. Gays are those that go

with people of their own sex. I do not consider myself belonging to the male gender, but perhaps not entirely to the female. My mother always told me I do not care if you like men or women, if you want to be a man or woman. I would like to change some things in my body, make it less masculine . . . I do not know, however, if I want to go ahead. I'm so happy . . . I finally feel that something is changing inside of me. Even just the idea of not having more male hormones in the body makes me feel good. I removed his beard. The penis does not particularly bother me since I no longer have erections. I got a job as a hairdresser. I want to make an identity change without surgery. When I walk around I feel that people do not look at me anymore like a man.

Conclusion: Gender Dysphoria as a Subjective Condition of Non-Belonging

These two life trajectories of gender variant persons may demonstrate that different environmental factors may influence the sense of non-belonging of gender dysphoric individuals. A Western anatomic perspective that hardly accepts heterogeneity, fluidity, and uncertainty may increase the sense of non-membership of transgender persons.

Western psychiatry considers gender dysphoria to be a psychiatric disorder by pointing out that it is rare, and it represents abnormality (Winter 2003). The only treatments that are typically considered in Western countries are hormone therapy or surgery. However, a large proportion of transgender persons want to live in their actual condition without undergoing any medical or surgical intervention (Conway 2011). While the recognition of gender dysphoria as a disorder may allow access to state insurance and medical services, as well as legal protection against discrimination, most transgender persons see themselves not as disordered but rather as part of human diversity. Gender dysphoric individuals often state that their minds are fine but that they were born in the wrong body, and their mental problems are the consequences of reactions from family, friends, and society.

Contrary to the anatomical position, the psychosocial perspective maintains that the sex category into which we are placed at birth is simply a first guess as to what identity we will later assume, and that it is possible to grow up with a gender that does not match that original sex category (Winter 2003). Therefore, "transgender" should be considered as an aspect of human diversity rather being considered a disorder, deviance, or at worst depravity. The conflict between these two perspectives is a serious matter of concern for transgender persons, involving the discrepancy between identity and the name written in a passport, their social welfare rights, their rights to marry and become parents, even the search for a job.

Bibliography

Achermann J. C. and Hughes I. A. (2008). "Disorders of Sex Development." In H. M. Kronenberg, S. Melmed, K. S. Polonsky, and P. R. Larsen (eds.), *Williams Textbook of Endocrinology*, 11th edn. pp. 783–848. Philadelphia: Elsevier Saunders.
American Psychiatric Association. (2013). *DSM-5: Diagnostic and Statistical Manual for Mental Disorders*, 5th edn. American Psychiatric Press, Washington, DC.
Bayer R. (1981). *Homosexuality and American psychiatry: The Politics of Diagnosis*. New York: Basic Books.

Bockting W. O. (2008). "Psychotherapy and the Real-Life Experience: From Gender Dichotomy to Gender Diversity." *Sexologies* 17(4): 211–224.

Bourdieu P. (1980). *Questions de sociologie*. Paris: Minuit.

Bourdieu P., Passeron J. C., and Chamboredon J. C. (1970). *Le Métier de sociologue, Mouton-Bordas, Paris, 1968; Zur Soziologie der symbolischen Forme*. Frankfurt: Suhrkamp.

Bucholtz M. and Hall K. (2005). *Identity and Interaction: A Sociocultural Linguistic Approach. Discourse Studies*. London-Thousand Oaks, CA-New Delhi: SAGE Publications.

Castellini G. (2016). "Language of Self-Definition in the Disorders of Identity." *Journal of Psychopathology* 22: 39–47.

Cohen-Kettenis P. T. (2005). "Gender Change in 46, XY Persons with 58-reductase-2 Deficiency and 179-hydroxysteroid dehydrogenase-3 Deficiency." *Archives of Sexual Behavior* 34: 399–410.

Conway L. (2011). "How Frequently Does Transsexualism Occur?" Article posted on June 4, 2011. http://ai.eecs.umich.edu/people/conway/TS/TSprevalence.html

Ferrari F. (2003). *La pelle delle immagini, Jean-Luc Nancy*. Torino: Bollati Boringhieri editore.

Giddens A. (1991). *Modernity and Self-Identity. Self and Society in the Late Modern Age*. Cambridge: Polity Press.

Giordano S. (2012). *Children with Gender Identity Disorder, a Clinical, Ethical and Legal Analysis*. London and New York: Routledge.

Gooren L. (2006). "The Biology of Human Psychosexual Differentiation." *Hormones and Behavior* 50: 589–601.

Gooren L. (2011) Clinical practice. Care of transsexual persons. *New England Journal of Medicine* 364: 1251–1257.

Green R. (1987). *The "Sissy-Boy Syndrome" and the Development of Homosexuality*. New Haven: Yale University Press.

Harrison J., Grant J., and Herman J. L. (2012). *A Gender Not Listed Here: Genderqueers, Gender Rebels, and Otherwise in the National Transgender Discrimination Survey*. Los Angeles, CA: eScholarship, University of California.

Herdt G. (1996). "Introduction. Third Sexes and Third Genders." In G. Herdt (ed.), *Third Sex, Third Gender: Beyond Sexual Dimorphism in Culture and History*, pp. 1–24. New York: Zone Books.

Herek G. M. (1984). "Attitudes Toward Lesbians and Gay Men: A Factor Analytic Study." *Journal of Homosexuality* 10: 1–21.

James A. (1998). "The Contribution of Social Anthropology to the Understanding of the Atypical Gender Identity in Childhood." In D. Di Ceglie (ed.), *A Stranger in My Body. Atypical Gender Identity Development and Mental Health*, pp. 81–83. London: H. Karnak Books Ltd.

Joel D., Tarrasch R., Berman Z., Mukamel M., and Ziv E. (2013). "Queering Gender: Studying Gender Identity in "Normative" Individuals." *Psychology & Sexuality* 5: 291–321.

Jost A., Vigier B., Prepin J., and Perchellet J. P. (1973). "Studies on Sex Differentiation in Mammals." *Recent Progress in Hormone Research* 29: 1–41.

Kulick D. (1999). "Transgender and Language. A Review of the Literature and Suggestions for the Future." *A Journal of Lesbian and Gay Studies* 5: 605–622.

Kuyper L. and Wijsen C. (2014). "Gender identities and Gender Dysphoria in the Netherlands." *Archives of Sexual Behavior* 43: 377–385.

Lawrence A. A. and Zucker K. J. (2012). "Gender Identity Disorders." In M. Hersen and D. C. Beidel (eds.), *Adult Psychopathology and Diagnosis*, 6th edn, pp. 601–635. Hoboken, NJ: Wiley.

Masica D. N., Money J., and Ehrhardt A. A. (1971). "Fetal Feminization and Female Gender Identity in the Testicular Feminizing Syndrome of Androgen Insensitivity." *Archives of Sexual Behavior* 1: 131–142.

Mead M. (1935). *Sex and Temperament: I: Three Primitive Societies*. New York: Norton.

Meyer-Bahlburg H. F. L. (2010). "From Mental Disorder to Iatrogenic Hypogonadism: Dilemmas in Conceptualizing Gender Identity Variants as Psychiatric Conditions." *Archives of Sexual Behavior* 39: 461–476.

Migeon C. J. and Wisniewski A. B. (2003). "Human Sex Differentiation and Its Abnormalities." *Best Practice & Research Clinical Obstetrics & Gynaecology* 17: 1–18.

Money J., Hampson J. G., and Hampson J. L. (1955). "Hermaphroditism: Recommendations Concerning Assignment of Sex, Change of Sex and Psychologic Management." *Bulletin of the Johns Hopkins Hospital* 97: 284–300.

Money J., Ehrhardt A. A., and Masica D. N. (1968). "Fetal Feminization Induced By Androgen Insensitivity in the Testicular Feminizing Syndrome: Effect on Marriage and Maternalism." *Best Practice & Research. Clinical Obstetrics & Gynaecology* 123: 105–114.

Ochs E. (1993). "Constructing Social Identity: A Language Socialization Perspective." *Research on Language and Social Interaction* 26: 287–306.

Romjampa T. (1973). "The Construction of Male Homosexuality in the Journal of the Psychiatric Association in Thailand." Paper presented in the Third International Conference of Asia Scholars, Singapore.

Steensma T. D. and Cohen-Kettenis P. T. (2011). "Gender Transitioning Before Puberty?" *Archives of Sexual Behavior* 40(4): 649–650. doi:10.1007/s10508-011-9752-2

Weinberg G. (1973). *Society and the Healthy Homosexual*. New York: St. Martin's Press.

Wilson P. (1998). "Development and Mental Health: The Issue of Difference in Atypical Gender Identity Development." In D. Di Ceglie (ed.), *A Stranger in My Body. Atypical Gender Identity Development and Mental Health*, pp. 1–9. London: H. Karnak Books Ltd.

Winter S. J. (2003). "Language and Identity in Transgender: Gender Wars and the Case of the Thai Kathoey." Conference paper presented at the Hawaii Conference on Social Sciences, Waikiki.

Zucker K. J. (2000). Book Review: A Guide to America's Sex Laws. *Archives of Sexual Behavior* 29(3): 300–301.

Zucker K. J., Bradley S. J., Sullivan C. B., Kuksis M., Birkenfeld-Adams A., and Mitchell J. N. (1993). "A Gender Identity Interview for Children." *Journal of Personality Assessment* 61: 443–456.

Zucker K. J. and Bradley S. J. (1995). *Gender Identity Disorder and Psychosexual Problems in Children and Adolescents*. New York: Guilford Press.

CHAPTER 60

....

HYSTERIA, DISSOCIATION, CONVERSION, AND SOMATIZATION

....

MARIA LUÍSA FIGUEIRA AND LUÍS MADEIRA

INTRODUCTION
....

DISSOCIATION, conversion, somatization, and hysteria are symbols deployed to describe an assorted range of phenomena and mechanisms that are conceptually and historically intertwined and which can be organized together. The puzzling situation of how little is still known about them is witnessed in their Anglo-Saxon depiction as "medically unexplained symptoms." Their prognosis and treatment strategies (Brand, Lanius, Vermetten, Loewenstein, and Spiegel 2012) also suggest they are two-edged diagnoses, at first delineated by the absence of other, organic, disorders causing the symptoms (e.g. limb paralysis despite no evident acute vascular brain disorder or depersonalization without features of a major depressive disorder). The second edge is the fact that they reflect anxiety as a foundation feature leading to most pharmacotherapies being ineffective (Brand, Classen, McNary, and Zaveri 2009) and that the patient might suffer from an underlying personality disorder which only responds to long-term psychotherapy. Indeed, these diagnoses involve stigma and discrimination on the part of mental health providers who find such patients annoying and frustrating (or, at least, dissatisfying) (Freidl, Spitzl, Prause, Zimprich, Lehner-Baumgartner, Baumgartner et al. 2009).

It would be an arduous (or perhaps impossible) task to compile and depict in a short chapter all the phenomena entailed in hysteria (including the features of a "hysterical" personality), the assorted manifestations linked with conversion and dissociation, and the neurological and physical symptoms (and signs) which have not yet been medically explained. The reader will therefore find herein, an up-to-date discussion on the range of symptoms and their organization in these fields, concepts, and current disagreements, including descriptions of experiences given as examples. For the purpose of understanding the matter more clearly, the chapter is divided in three sections: (1) hysteria, (2) dissociation, and (3) conversion and somatization.

HYSTERIA

Hysteria (and its uses in psychiatry, including *hysterical* personality) is a "term that is best abandoned"; the term was relevant in psychiatric nosology and psychopathology until the 1980s, when it was dropped in favor of the concepts of conversion (e.g. Steinberg, Rounsaville, and Cicchetti 1990), dissociation (e.g. World Health Organization 1992), and the rise of the somatoform and somatization phenomena and categories. Reasons for doing away with the term include the psychoanalytical influences from which psychiatry has attempted to distance itself and, as pointed out above, the profoundly entangled prejudice surrounding this uncomfortable (peer-to-peer) diagnosis, one that is incommunicable (to patients). Hysteria includes a great array of symptoms (in extremis, all symptoms not otherwise explained) from screaming, seizures, limb paralysis, stupor, mutism to skin lesions. They are often thought by the interviewer to be exaggerated or theatrical and therefore collide with the nature of symptoms in psychiatry and medicine (interpersonally experienced as real). First coined in 1795, by Ferriar (cited by Mace 1992), the expression "hysterical conversion" responds to the baffling situation where biochemistry, structural neuroimaging, and electrophysiology (and all state of the art complementary exams) fail to explain the present physical (mostly neurological) symptoms (despite the definition, we have now several studies attempting to shed light into the neurobiology and neuroscience of conversion and somatization—Broome 2004; Vuilleumier 2014; Perez, Dworetzky, Dickerson, Leung, Cohn, Baslet et al. 2015). Yet of all literature on hysteria, that of the psychoanalytical school it is particularly vast (headed by Freud's contribution whose input and critical appraisal can be found in Mace 1992a, 1992b) and in neurology (where a distinction of functional from the neurological symptoms is necessary (Lynn and Rhue 1994)). These authors have put forward the following theories to explain such symptoms (which are also speculative): (1) that hysteria is "psychological," sustaining a (certainly outdated) dualist account of the mind–brain and that "hysteria behaves as though anatomy did not exist" (Freud and Breuer 1985/1966: 169) or that (2) hysterical symptoms are inchoate symptoms of a neurological disorder whose manifestation only occurs later in its natural history, again a theory based on little empirical evidence. The first account is grounded in Freud's "revolutionary" considerations (and method) that a *reason* (and not a cause) could account for the symptoms which would be located in the psychological realm. Although the specifics changed throughout his work, he accredited the importance of trauma which would also constitute a major line of research (see also the seminal contribution by Charcot 2013), the relevance of sexuality, libido, and erotogenesis (see Benedikt 1868: 48–54) and secondary gain (the possibility of unconscious and seemingly unrelated gain after the situation). The latter is connected with the extent to which research has been carried out on conversive symptoms in neurology (which share a different background knowledge), thus showing the limited impact on prognosis and scenario. Moreover, today, no explanation has yet been given for the full range of symptoms presented; the fact remains that subjects with these symptoms differ markedly from those with factual physical/neurological (and psychiatric) symptoms as well as those which simulate diseases. The next section introduces dissociation which is a discrete field of research with its own history and conceptual input.

UNDERSTANDING DISSOCIATION

The counterparts of dissociative phenomena can be traced back through time, far before those belonging to *hysteria*; they may be found in the depictions of pre-historical ecstatic experiences and of demonic possessions and exorcisms during the Inquisition. Yet the use of the words "association" and "dissociation" emerged only in the nineteenth century in medicine, having had two meanings. The first meant the possibility of "unconscious" occurrences where "the patients' memory, imagination and perception is changed or sometimes lost as if dissociated from their personal consciousness" (Abercrombie 1832). This consideration was seized upon by psychoanalysts and localizationists and was key to "the possibility of double consciousness" (Wigan 1985)—further considered grounds for "multiple personalities." The second term, dissociation, means the "separation of mental functions usually integrated and consciously accessible—a disintegration that involve either/both memory, identity, perception, emotions and will" (Spiegel and Cardeña 1991). This perspective refers to a disruption of mental functions—in trauma studies, this latter idea would become the main meaning—a patient not knowing who he is or losing parts of his memory despite the remaining elements of consciousness working correctly.

Yet, several conceptual ambiguities undermine these definitions including the discussion about what dissociation stands for, whether dissociation should only be considered in subjects with mental disorder, and what dissociative phenomena could be unpacked further. The first question refers to dissociation being considered both a *mechanism* (*epistemology*) and a *symptom* (*phenomenology*) or a *category* (*nosology*) in itself. Examples of dissociation as a mechanism include all the functional neurological symptoms (similes of neurological symptoms without any organic basis) taken as "dissociative symptoms" whereby "dissociative mechanisms" are involved—for example, a burning sensation in the foot with no evidence of skin and neuronal damage, would suggest to the neurologist that the explanation lies in *dissociation/conversion*.

Dissociation also represents phenomena with an anxious or depressive explanation/mechanism—for example, a patient who complains of being "depersonalized," "void," and "numb, as if he can't feel" when he becomes anxious or depressed. Depersonalization would be aptly considered in such depressive and anxious states and would be an example of a dissociative phenomenon. An important distinction would be to consider them as a state or a trait—dissociation relevant to state occurs over a limited period of time while if it occurs as a trait, it would have been present ever since childhood or adolescence. The relevance of this feature includes further implications as to its meaning as a symptom (see Parnas, Moller, Kircher, Thalbitzer, Jansson, Handest et al. 2005).

Yet, dissociation also refers to nosological categories (including three categories) as is the case of the depersonalization category in the DSM-5 (American Psychiatric Association 2013). This category constitutes a cluster of symptoms with an individualized clinical construct, prognosis, and treatment strategies. The possibility that the label attributed to depersonalization may be used to signal both a symptom and a category, provides the key to explaining several misconceptions in clinical practice and research.

The second challenge considered above, concerns the disagreement about whether these phenomena are psychopathological (occurring only in patients with mental disorders) and if the counterparts occurring in the population are qualitatively different (and therefore do not receive the same label), or whether there are counterparts in the general population where dissociative phenomena are widespread and are only different in quantity/relevance in mental disorders. The latter position leads to several considerations, such as whether dissociation could even be adaptive—for example, depersonalization occurring during stressful events or sadness reducing the magnitude of the experienced emotion—or a voluntary experience—for example, a person attempting to escape from the boredom or tedium of a moment allows the mind to drift into other contents and later realizes that s/he was not really "there" for a while. Yet, the extent of distress that depersonalization may represent in depressive episodes or the nature of the derealization that occurs in psychosis and schizophrenia are also suggestive of a qualitative difference which needs further exploration (see further detail in Dell and O'Neil 2010). Irrespective of former considerations, these phenomena have been studied in (1) burn-out-like periods (Mayer-Gross 1935), (2) after prolonged sleep (Bliss 1959), (3) hallucinogenic toxicosis (Fleming 1936), (4) severe melancholic episodes (Kraus 2002; Fuchs 2005), and (5) schizophrenic passivity experiences (Langfeldt 1960). The discussion of a quantitative or a qualitative difference between "pathological" and "non-pathological" dissociation is linked with the latter of the above considerations—of a possible phenomenological complexity where a detailed enquiry could shed light on the differentiation of individual sorts of dissociative phenomena. If we take derealization, a good example of how a subjective symptom may be phenomenologically complex, we come to the conclusion that it is a subjective, self-conscious experience and refers to different depictions—for example, forms of derealization could include being "lost to understanding the meaning of other persons' behaviours" or "feeling that reality has new meanings which are mysterious." Consequently, a detailed examination might unpack these phenomena into a larger range of experiences and give rise to discussing whether some dissociative phenomena are trans-nosological or if this phenomenological detail could help identify the particulars of each situation. Another example is the comprehensively detailed forms of depersonalization (see the EASE interview in Parnas, Møller, Kircher, Thalbitzer, Jansson, Handest et al. 2005) that allows for a special set of phenomena to be identified which pinpoint the particularity of schizophrenic subjectivity. Recently, with regard to anxiety disorders, a clinical study has taken this into consideration and has attempted to obtain further knowledge about the different sorts of dissociative maladies in anxious subjects (Madeira, Carmenates, Costa, Linhares, Stanghellini, Figueira et al. 2017).

A brief incursion into the history of dissociation shows segregated waves of research (according to changes in the interest shown in the field), for example, a decline in the early twentieth century and a resurgence in the 1970s. Dissociative symptoms are considered in various psychiatric categories (anxiety disorders are a clear example of where several categories may show symptoms); moreover, there are major categories in dissociation, particularly in the DSM-5: depersonalization/derealization disorder, dissociative amnesia (with or without fugue), and dissociative identity disorder (American Psychiatric Association 2013). Depersonalization and derealization have been discussed by Griesinger and Dugas, whose seminal accounts point to a core disturbance in the way that experiences and thoughts are undertaken by the Self. See an extensive discussion in Dell and O'Neil (2010) and their original depictions "as if each of my senses, each and every part of myself was separated from me and couldn't offer me any feeling, my eyes see and my spirit has perception but the sensation of what I see is absent" (Griesinger as cited by Sierra 2009: 8) and the "alienation of personality, a state where thoughts and acts become strange to the self" (adapted from Dugas and Moutier 1911). Yet today, gathered under the general scope of the whole umbrella, it is possible to identify particular experiences constituting the depersonalization umbrella.

First, changes in the accessibility of feelings ranging from a loss of expressing emotions owing to boredom: "I just cannot feel when I'm bored, every experience becomes grey and bleak and I long to recover that sense of feeling," to severe disturbances in self-esteem happening in major depression: "the worst is not the suffering but the lack of all feelings; I cannot even cry; there was a time where I could but now I feel as if I have lost all feelings and this is the most miserable I ever felt."

Secondly, where experiencing reality is concerned, it includes an awareness of foreignness or unreality in the person's setting and means changes when calling upon perception and tuning into the world. A clear depiction of these changes is the feeling of perplexity in psychosis "everything is strangely new. I have never experienced this, new senses and intense meanings. I cannot cope with all that is new and mysterious; my thoughts rush along in the attempt to feel and make sense of all this" (seminally operationalized in Conrad 2013). A recent depiction of a particularly meaningful derealization experience is contained in the Truman Symptoms (Fusar-Poli, Howes, Valmaggia, and McGuire 2008) which appear relevant in the ultra-high risk for psychosis (see clinical research in Madeira, Bonoldi, Rocchetti, Brandizzi, Samson, Azis et al. 2016), when experiencing others as if they were actors in a show.

Furthermore, changes in the somatic bodily experience which might include changes in immediate bodily control such as in being ashamed "I cannot move myself despite my longing to disappear, my body becomes heavy and open to everyone to see and even penetrate my existence," or a sense of disembodiment or loss of feeling about implicitly having a bodily presence (see this topic in Fuchs and Schlimme 2009; Stanghellini 2009). There also changes in experiences involving thought (and its processes) that can range from difficulty in concentrating "my head feels as if it's filled with cotton wool," to feeling the pressure of thoughts rushing beyond understanding, as if "my head was constantly being overwhelmed" (the Examination of Anomalous Self-Experience checklist provides a large range of disturbed thought process; Parnas, Moller, Kircher, Thalbitzer, Jansson, Handest et al. 2005).

Lastly, there are also assorted forms of detachment from oneself and the world, ranging from the subject feeling that s/he is constantly under self-observation (and actual out-of-the-body experiences where the subject feels as if s/he is on the outside), to forms of detachment from the world as if a barrier prevents actual contact with reality or a feeling of changed bodily control as if the body has become a robot. A relevant contribution (cited earlier) comes in the recent accounts on depersonalization/derealization that indicate their role as core schizophrenic experiences including "a disturbance of first person perspective, the loss of natural evidence, an increased introspection, forms of hyper-reflexivity" (Parnas, Moller, Kircher, Thalbitzer, Jansson, Handest et al. 2005).

Dissociative amnesia and fugue comprise several phenomena including moments of absorptive-imaginative stance with partial or complete objective and subjective amnesia. Yet these gaps in the awareness or the memory of one's behavior or experiences might trouble the subject because there is no controlling his behavior or there is interference with his general functioning and activities by his having no memory of performing some tasks—for example, worrying and returning home because he thought he had forgotten to take his children to the nursery and then realizing that he had performed this task without being aware of having done so. Some studies suggest that these symptoms are concurrent with stress or traumatic events including PTSD (Serra, Fadda, Buccione, Caltagirone, and Carlesimo 2007) while others suggest they happen according to particular personality traits (Leong, Waits, and Diebold 2006), out of the blue or even partially in voluntary moments (e.g. in absorbed skilful coping or multitasking). Many of these subjects are unaware of their memory loss until someone tells or asks them about it. After this, the experience becomes a subjective awareness of memory loss which can be localized, selective, or generalized. In the first case, the memory about the events is lost only momentarily and the absence of these data can be unconscious until later on (not immediately following the event). Usually this or these moments are clearly demarcated in his biography. Selective amnesia involves segregated memory loss of particular features (e.g. the knowledge of autopsychic time and space orientation) and yet memory is preserved for other elements during that period. Lastly, in generalized amnesia, there is (usually) a sudden onset of the loss of personal information, skills, or knowledge about the world which constitutes the incapacity to retrieve one's identity in biographical details. In the DSM-5, dissociative amnesia can coincide with fugue—a situation where the subject acts in an unexpected and yet purposeful and personally coherent way. These periods might be short and he may miss work, or they can include longer periods where he travels to another city gets himself a new name and identity and is unaware of the changes in his life. When the fugue period comes to an end, these subjects may find themselves anxious, perplexed, ashamed, and even frightened about not remembering what happened during such a period. The end can happen suddenly with no interference of external family, friends, or colleagues although it may also come about through their confrontation.

The category of dissociative identity disorder is the modern account of the old "multiple personality disorder" and refers to the emergence of behaviors (and personality traits) distinct from the person's usual bearing—as if some (or all) subjects' actions, speech and demeanors were involuntarily made anew (beyond their control) (Maiese 2015). These features are followed by different grades of amnesia—subjects may be completely unaware of the large range of symptoms while others partially recall these states and characterize them as intrusions, influences, and interactions by behaviors, thoughts, illusions, and hallucinations as well as the disorganization of lived in space and time. Phenomenologically, it is a heterogeneous category including several states whose overall significance for psychiatry is problematic (for diagnostic and treatment reasons) (see another all-encompassing discussion in Dell and O'Neil 2010).

It is also possible to consider dissociative symptoms such as those observed and diagnosed by neurologists, which occur in isolated form and have neither a neurological diagnosis nor an organic account, such as migraine and epilepsy (clinical samples in Baker, Hunter, Lawrence, Medford, Patel, Senior et al. 2003; Serra, Fadda, Buccione, Caltagirone, and Carlesimo 2007). For the first type, the concept of dissociation finds its own meaning as the "absence of structural neurological disease" and sustains the designation of "functional neurological symptoms." It implies that there are no changes in neuroimaging and biochemical exams which can be accredited to the described experience and observed behavior. The diagnosis of a dissociative reason in neurology relieves the neurologist about the possibility of a "true neurological cause" and patients are often discharged from ambulatory treatment and allocated psychiatric resources. Yet, ominous disorders may reveal dissociative experiences including ones such as derealization, depersonalization, amnesia, and fugue as well as show all the likely signs and symptoms of migraine, epilepsy, and stroke. The prevalence of disso-ciative disorders and/or symptoms in patients with a diagnosis of stroke, is still unknown. Yet its study could help us to find important aspects of dissociation in neurology, for in-stance, in transient ischemic attacks (TIA), dissociative symptoms could lie in either origin, and a symptom could follow localized vascular damage, thus further clarifying the neuro-psychiatric organization of dissociative symptoms. Also, and in the case of migranous and epileptic origins, several mechanisms have been proposed—for instance, depersonalization and derealization are particularly common in temporal epilepsy (together with dissociative amnesia which can also ensue). The neurological explanation for these symptoms should be excluded (by psychiatrists and neurologists) before considering a dissociative cause. Moreover, researchers should bear in mind that the localization or representation in the brain of a neuropsychiatric symptom does not imply the same for a psychiatric practitioner.

The idea of a "dissociative mechanism" server as the link between dissociation and con-version/somatization could mean that psychological symptoms can be transformed into physical symptoms due to *lack of* mentalization.

SOMATIZATION AND CONVERSION

As mentioned above, somatization and conversion are linked to the idea of transforming a "psychological" element or issue into a "physical" phenomenon (symptom). Conversion symptoms are sometimes placed under the umbrella of dissociation so as to include other sorts of neurological symptoms (motor and deficit, sensorial, convulsive, and an assorted mixture) that have no justifiable organic cause. Yet, somatization is usually segregated from dissociation and constitutes a broader field of research which, despite being akin to disso-ciation, has been historically concurrent with it. The term was proposed by Wilhelm Stekl and Pierre Janet to consider mental and emotional suffering expressed as bodily symptoms (see Janet 1977). Today, the category differs and it is accepted that it may be accompanied by anxiety or disordered mood diagnosed according to standard criteria. Furthermore, it is also believed that they (i.e. somatization and dissociation) do not share an inverse rela-tion to feelings—the more someone somatizes something, the less he experiences it emo-tionally. Not only is somatization broader, but it also establishes particular intersections with other research fields in psychiatry such as psychosomatic medicine and liaison psychi-atry. Conversion and somatization symptoms should be considered separately from their categories: as mentioned earlier, these symptoms can occur in isolated form in several mental disorders (e.g. depression or personality disorders). Yet there are categories with a particular clinical history and treatment. These diagnoses should be considered only after excluding all other disorders (including neurological or psychiatric disorders) if the presentation includes somatization (plus pain) and neurological symptoms (mostly referring to con-version symptoms). The clinician should bear in mind some suggestive features including prior conversions, preceding emotional stress, anxiety, or dysphoria or symptoms that are presented indifferently (*belle indifference*) if the subject has particular personality traits, if there is apparent secondary gain or if there is improvement upon suggestion or sedation (Purtell, Robins, and Cohen 1951; Gatfield and Guze 1962; Perley and Guze 1962; Slater 1965; Raskin, Talbott, and Meyerson 1966; Bishop and Torch 1979; Watson and Buranen 1979).

Yet the same sources suggest that when taking into account the prior history of conversion, any of these elements might be unreliable in a differential diagnosis. Moving toward modern psychiatric nosology we have observed a simplification of Guze's original fifty-nine criteria for Briquet's Syndrome to the thirty-seven DSM-III symptoms and later, into the four sorts of items of DSM-IV (four bodily, two gastrointestinal, one pseudoneurological, and one sexual). ICD criteria for somatization disorder show little agreement with these DSM criteria which, together with the fact that many of these experiences and behaviors are culture-specific, make diagnosis treacherous outside the Western world. Due to the uniformity of culturally influenced personality traits, it seems that analyzing temperament and character might help diagnosis (see TCI in Cloninger 1987, 1993). While multidimensional personality traits appear to be involved in somatization and conversion disorder there is no specific personality associated with them. Somatization seems to be related to high harm avoidance and low self-directedness—cluster C personality features (see TCI, Cloninger 1993) while conversion and dissociation are related to high novelty-seeking—cluster B personality features. Low self-directedness and cooperativeness seem to run the risk of dissociation particularly if they express high novelty-seeking while somatization occurs in subjects showing high harm avoidance (see Mulder and Joyce 1997). Robbins and Kirmayer (2009) attempt three operational definitions of somatization (1) high levels of functional somatic distress, (2) hypochondriasis, and (3) patients showing current major depression or anxiety.

Together the diagnostic criteria for hysteria, conversion, and dissociation appear to be discrepant (suggesting historical uncertainties and quandaries), insufficient (unreliable and lacking validity and prognostic significance), and of little practical use (e.g. the psychiatric concept as used by neurologists, and the impossibility of using it to explain to patients what they are experiencing). A part of the problem lies in the assortment of concepts used in these fields (clinical and research) which include (among others) "somatization," "conversion," "hysterical," "functional symptoms," "psychogenic," "somatoform," and "dissociative." To some extent, they represent overlapping clinical features and at other times, they are used outside their conceptual field. Additionally, the use of these terms is dubious as (1) for hysteria psychiatry has made a determined effort to remove this label, most of these patients are referred to neurologists who use a different terminology and the diagnosis cannot be used in practice (with the patient) as it is pejorative and (2) the same is the case with somatization where the practical distinction as regards conversion is not all that simple (as physical versus neurological does not stand and perhaps the meaningful clinical distinction is merely between the acute symptoms (needing referral to emergency wards) and the gradual onset of symptoms (seen by general physicians)).

Extensive research effort has allowed several breakthroughs and "there is a growing body of evidence linking the dissociative disorders to a trauma history, and to specific neural mechanisms" (Spiegel, Loewenstein, Lewis-Fernández, Şar, Simeon, Vermetten et al. 2011) and led to (an evidence-based) reorganization of the dissociative category in the DSM-5 (Spiegel, Lewis-Fernández, Lanius, Vermetten, Simeon, and Friedman 2013). Despite the developments of recent interest and reaching a new definition in our diagnostic manuals, research in the area continues to be lost in the operationalization of subjectivity (essential) and is still unable to make full sense of what are considered "unexplained symptoms." Perhaps a necessary first step is researching the phenomenology of these symptoms (phenomenological psychopathology) to further our knowledge on their specificities and differences, possibly richer detail could allow unpacking into new, assorted, or enhanced symbols—the latter being essential for translational (and clinical) studies.

BIBLIOGRAPHY

Abercrombie J. (1832). *Inquiries Concerning the Intellectual Powers and the Investigation of Truth*. New York: J. and J. Harper.

American Psychiatric Association. (2013). *Diagnostic and Statistical Manual of Mental Disorders (DSM-5®)*. Arlington American Psychiatric Publishing.

Baker D., Hunter E., Lawrence E., Medford N., Patel M., Senior C., et al. (2003). "Depersonalisation Disorder: Clinical Features of 204 Cases." *The British Journal of Psychiatry* 182: 428–433.

Benedikt M. (1868). *Elektrotherapie*. Vienna: Tendler.

Bishop E. R. and Torch E. M. (1979). "Dividing 'Hysteria': A Preliminary Investigation of Conversion Disorder and Psychalgia." *The Journal of Nervous and Mental Disease* 167: 348–356.

Bliss E. L. (1959). "Studies of Sleep Deprivation—Relationship to Schizophrenia." *Archives of Neurology & Psychiatry* 81: 348–359.

Brand B. L., Classen C. C., McNary S. W., and Zaveri P. (2009). "A Review of Dissociative Disorders Treatment Studies." *The Journal of Nervous and Mental Disease* 197: 646–654.

Brand B. L., Lanius R., Vermetten E., Loewenstein R. J., and Spiegel D. (2012). "Where Are We Going? An Update on Assessment, Treatment, and Neurobiological Research in Dissociative Disorders as We Move Toward the DSM-5." *Journal of Trauma & Dissociation* 13: 9–31.

Broome M. R. (2004). "A Neuroscience of Hysteria?" *Current Opinion in Psychiatry* 17: 465–469.

Charcot J.-M. (2013). *Clinical Lectures on Diseases of the Nervous System* (Psychology Revivals). Routledge.

Cloninger C. R. (1987). "A Systematic Method for Clinical Description and Classification of Personality Variants." *Arch Gen Psychiatry* 44: 573–588.

Cloninger C. R. (1993). "A Psychobiological Model of Temperament and Character." *Arch Gen Psychiatry* 50: 975.

Conrad K. (2013). *Beginning Schizophrenia: Attempt for a Gestalt-analysis of Delusion*. Cambridge: Cambridge University Press.

Dell P. F. and O'Neil J. A. (2010). *Dissociation and the Dissociative Disorders*. New York: Routledge.

Dugas L. and Moutier F. (1911). *La Dépersonnalisation*. Paris, Felix Alean.

Fleming G. W. T. H. (1936). "Mescaline and Depersonalization." (Journal of Neurology and Psychopathy xvi: 193).

Freidl M., Spitzl S. P., Prause W., Zimprich F., Lehner-Baumgartner E., Baumgartner C., et al. (2009). "The Stigma of Mental Illness: Anticipation and Attitudes Among Patients with Epileptic, Dissociative or Somatoform Pain Disorder." *International Review of Psychiatry* 19: 123–129.

Freud S. and Breuer J. (1895/1966). *Studies On Hysteria*. New York: Avon Books.

Fuchs T. (2005). "Corporealized and Disembodied Minds: A Phenomenological View of the Body in Melancholia and Schizophrenia." *Philosophy, Psychiatry, & Psychology* 12: 95–107.

Fuchs T. and Schlimme J. E. (2009). "Embodiment and Psychopathology: A Phenomenological Perspective." *Current Opinion in Psychiatry* 22: 570–575.

Fusar-Poli P., Howes O., Valmaggia L., and McGuire P. (2008). "'Truman' Signs and Vulnerability to Psychosis." *The British Journal of Psychiatry* 193: 168 (Just one page)

Gatfield P. D. and Guze S. B. (1962). "Prognosis and Differential Diagnosis of Conversion Reactions." *Disease of the Nervous System* 23: 623–631.

Janet P. F. (1977). *The Mental State of Hystericals*. Washington DC: University Publications of America.

Kraus A. (2002). "Melancholie: Eine art von depersonalisation. Affekt und affektive Stoerungen." In T. Fuchs and C. Mundt (eds.) *Affekt und affektive Storungen*, pp. 169–186. Paderborn: Schoningh.

Langfeldt G. (1960). "Diagnosis and Prognosis of Schizophrenia." *Proceedings of the Royal Society of Medicine* 53: 1047–1052.

Leong S., Waits W., and Diebold C. (2006). "Dissociative Amnesia and DSM-IV-TR Cluster C Personality Traits." *Psychiatry (Edgmont)* 3: 51–55.

Lynn S. J. and Rhue J. W. (eds.) (1994). *Dissociation: Clinical and Theoretical Perspectives*. New York, NY, USA: Guilford Press.

Mace C. J. (1992a). "Hysterical Conversion. I: A History." *The British Journal of Psychiatry* 161: 369–377.

Mace C. J. (1992b). "Hysterical Conversion. II: A Critique." *The British Journal of Psychiatry* 161: 378–389.

Madeira L., Bonoldi I., Rocchetti M., Brandizzi M., Samson C., Azis M., et al. (2016). "Prevalence and Implications of Truman Symptoms in Subjects at Ultra High Risk for Psychosis." *Psychiatry Research* 238: 270–276.

Madeira L., Carmenates S., Costa C., Linhares L., Stanghellini G., Figueira M. L., et al. (2017). "Basic Self-Disturbances beyond Schizophrenia: Discrepancies and Affinities in Panic Disorder—An Empirical Clinical Study." *Psychopathology* Mayer-Gross W. (1935). "On Depersonalization." *British Journal of Medical Psychology* 15: 103–126.

Maiese M. (2015). "Dissociative Identity Disorder and the Fragmentation of the Self." In *Embodied Selves and Divided Minds*, pp. 183–226. New York: Oxford University Press.

Mulder R. T. and Joyce P. R. (1997). "Temperament and the Structure of Personality Disorder Symptoms." *Psychological Medicine* 27: 99–106.

Parnas J., Moller P., Kircher T., Thalbitzer J., Jansson L., Handest P., et al. (2005). "EASE: Examination of Anomalous Self-Experience." *Psychopathology* 38: 236–258.

Perez D. L., Dworetzky B. A., Dickerson B. C., Leung L., Cohn R., Baslet G., et al. (2015). "An Integrative Neurocircuit Perspective on Psychogenic Nonepileptic Seizures and Functional Movement Disorders." *Clinical EEG and Neuroscience* 46: 4–15.

Perley M. J. and Guze S. B. (1962). "Hysteria—The Stability and Usefulness of Clinical Criteria: A Quantitative Study Based on a Follow-up Period of Six to Eight Years in 39 Patients." *New England Journal of Medicine* 266: 421–6

Purtell J. J., Robins E., and Cohen M. E. (1951). "Observations on Clinical Aspects of Hysteria; A Quantitative Study of 50 Hysteria Patients and 156 Control Subjects." *Journal of the American Medical Association* 146: 902–909.

Raskin M., Talbott J. A., and Meyerson A. T. (1966). "Diagnosis of Conversion Reactions. Predictive Value of Psychiatric Criteria." *Journal of the American Medicine Association* 197: 530–534.

Robbins J. M. and Kirmayer L. J. (2009). "Attributions of Common Somatic Symptoms." *Psychological Medicine* 21: 1029–1045.

Serra L., Fadda L., Buccione I., Caltagirone C., and Carlesimo G. A. (2007). "Psychogenic and Organic Amnesia. A Multidimensional Assessment of Clinical, Neuroradiological, Neuropsychological and Psychopathological Features." *Behavioural Neurology* 18: 53–64.

Sierra M. (2009). *Depersonalization*. New York: Cambridge University Press.

Slater E. (1965). "Diagnosis of 'Hysteria'." *British Medical Journal* 1: 1395–1399.

Spiegel D. and Cardeña E. (1991). "Disintegrated Experience: The Dissociative Disorders Revisited." *Journal of Abnormal Psychology* 100: 366–378.

Spiegel D., Loewenstein R. J., Lewis-Fernández R., Şar V., Simeon D., Vermetten E., et al. (2011). "Dissociative Disorders in DSM-5." *Depression and Anxiety* 28: 824–852.

Spiegel D., Lewis-Fernández R., Lanius R., Vermetten E., Simeon D., and Friedman M. (2013). "Dissociative Disorders in DSM-5." *Annual Review of Clinical Psychology* 9: 299–326.

Stanghellini G. (2009). "Embodiment and Schizophrenia." *World Psychiatry* 8: 56–59.

Steinberg M., Rounsaville B., and Cicchetti D. V. (1990). "The Structured Clinical Interview for DSM-III-R Dissociative Disorders: Preliminary Report on a New Diagnostic Instrument." *American Journal of Psychiatry* 147: 76–82.

Vuilleumier P. (2014). "Brain Circuits Implicated in Psychogenic Paralysis in Conversion Disorders and Hypnosis." *Neurophysiologie Clinique/Clinical Neurophysiology* 44: 323–337.

Watson C. G. and Buranen C. (1979). "The Frequencies of Conversion Reaction Symptoms." *Journal of Abnormal Psychology* 88: 209–211.

Wigan A. L. (1985). *A New View of Insanity: The Duality of Mind*. Reprint. Malibu: Joseph Simon.

World Health Organization. (1992). *The ICD-10 Classification of Mental and Behavioural Disorders*. Geneva: Diamond Pocket Books (P) Ltd.

CHAPTER 61

OBSESSIONS AND PHOBIAS

CLAIRE AHERN, DANIEL B. FASSNACHT,
AND MICHAEL KYRIOS

INTRODUCTION

THIS article examines the phenomenology of two particular unwanted intrusive experiences—phobias and obsessions. Both are repetitive, uncontrollable, and are recognized to originate from within the person. The concept of phobias and obsession can be both a distinct emotional state, a central symptom of a disorder, or part of an entire range of psychiatric disorders. Both phobias and obsessions can involve almost any situation, and may occur to a minor degree in almost anybody. The chapter begins by characterizing phobias as an experience associated with fear; an intense concentration of anxiety to specific situations or stimuli. Two common and disabling phobic conditions, social phobia and agoraphobia, are then presented. The chapter then describes the varied phenomenology and emotions associated with obsessions. While anxiety is often an emotional state in obsessions, pathological doubt, particularly about moral self-worth, is also argued to be a central feature in the experience of obsessions.

PHOBIA

The experience of fear is a typical, evolutionary important sensation, which helps individuals learn to avoid or manage dangerous situations and objects (Marks and Nesse 1994). However, in extreme cases, individuals experience "a fear of an imaginary evil or an undue fear of a real one" (Rush 1798). Phobic fear is an intense and persistent anxiety, disproportionate to the actual threat. Individuals describe this fear to be beyond voluntary control—even in the face of reason—and often go great lengths avoiding feared situation (Marks 1969). Phobias are largely categorized according to the source of the anxiety-provoking stimuli as either external (e.g. agoraphobia, social or animal phobias, phobias related to stimuli in the environment) or internal (e.g. illness, obsessions, worries) (Marks 1969).

Social phobia, for instance, can be considered an excessive variant of shyness. The individual fears behaving unacceptably in a social situation, and that such "misbehavior" will lead to disastrous consequences (e.g. losing face or ridicule from others) (Clark and Wells 1995). A strong desire to convey a favorable impression of oneself in social situations, paired with excessive self-consciousness, leads the social phobic to experience themselves negatively "as a social object" (Clark 2001: 407). The overestimated likelihood and/or severity of embarrassment or humiliation makes socially anxious individuals avoid social situations. They may also avoid associated cues during such social interactions (e.g. avoiding eye contact), followed by extensive rumination after social encounters (Hofmann 2007). While some individuals experience a physiologically intense fear reaction in specific performance-orientated situations (e.g. public speaking, signing documents), others feel embarrassment and shame in social situations (Hofmann, Alpers, and Pauli 2009). Together, these factors create an overwhelming feeling of separateness and strangeness in one's social environment.

> Lidia, thirty-six years, recalled that she was "always shy" as a child, preferring to play alone and draw. Her last significant relationship ended six years ago. Lidia and her ex-partner had slowly developed their relationship over many years, but ultimately Lidia felt that her social anxiety "put a burden" on the relationship. Lidia felt "too awkward" to try face-to-face dating, but was active in an online group chat and had developed a close connection with one of the other members who lived in another country.
>
> Lidia created a successful online business, which enabled her to work independently, however the business increasingly required her to make telephone calls. Lidia dreaded these calls; she felt she "knew" that others could sense her anxiety through her trembling voice. Lidia feared that she was misrepresenting her product, and so she would procrastinate from making phone calls, or avoid them altogether.

Derived from Greek origins and meaning "fear of the market place," agoraphobia often includes a fear of social ridicule from others. However, it is not a distinct single fear of social interactions but rather a collection of avoidance responses to multiple feared stimuli related to the need to escape or feel safe. The term describes a varying combination of anxiety including fear of being in an exposed place, or being unable to receive help (e.g. in an enclosed space, or crowded, remote areas), with individuals commonly fearing that they are noticeable and socially unacceptable to others. Agoraphobic fears occur in many combinations and usually are associated with other symptoms such as panic attacks, feelings of depersonalization, depression, and also obsessions (Marks 1987), as the individual vigilantly monitors their bodily sensations as the principal means to assess how safe they feel in their world (Trigg 2013). The agoraphobic individual tends to have a "fixed safety base" (e.g. home) often marked by its familiarity rather than actual safety from being alone and helpless; moving away from this base is associated with increasing anxiety and avoidance behavior.

> Noel, fifty-four years, lives with his wife and adult daughter. Eighteen months previously he had a fall at home, surgery on his hip, and a lengthy recovery. Despite his doctor's insistence that he could return to work, and that work would improve his physical rehabilitation, Noel felt unsteady and "weak." On his first attempt to drive after surgery, Noel recalled quickly feeling tense and light headed, and he returned home almost immediately.
>
> Even though Noel was often alone, for days at a time, he felt comfortable in his home. Noel's doctor noted that he would see him in the waiting room, hours before his appointment was scheduled. Noel had recently been driving more frequently but did not drive to "new places" on his own, asking his daughter to chaperone him to his first session.

OBSESSIONS

Obsessions involve the experience of unwanted, intrusive, and uncontrollable thoughts, images, or urges (Jaspers 1997). Obsessional intrusions are invasive to the flow of consciousness, occurring against one's will as unpleasant and unwanted disturbances. Both the content and process of the obsession is experienced as unacceptable and distressing. This leads to a secondary defensive component in attempting to control and avoid the fears associated with the obsession (von Gebsattel 1954). Although obsessions can take a variety of forms, most commonly they are experienced as unwanted and intrusive thoughts (Rachman 2003). For example, an individual may have the obsessive thought that "I could kill everyone in the car if I just swerved into oncoming traffic" or "Am I catching germs from this?" Other less frequent forms of obsessions, images, and urges are just as repugnant and objectionable (e.g. unwanted images of incestuous acts, the urge to push someone in front of an oncoming train).

Intrusive thoughts in the general population and in obsessional patients do not differ in their occurrence or content, but in the appraisal of the intrusions. Most people are able to generally ignore or dismiss unwanted intrusions that enter into our consciousness as irrelevant, unhelpful, and superfluous to requirements. For the obsessive individual, however, the intrusion is taken as evidence that these thoughts reveal some personal meaning about the person's true self as "mad, bad, dangerous—or all three" (Rachman 2003: 6). Obsessions are therefore distressing to the individual for stressing and contradicting one's sense of self. Clark (2004) argues that one of the key features of obsessions is that they are experienced to be inconsistent with the core values of the self. Yet, given that the majority of the population experience intrusive phenomena, how is it that only certain people will make misappraisals of the meaning of their intrusions?

Aardema and O'Connor (2007) propose that obsessions are distressing for representing a feared possibility for who a person is, or might become. In particular, fears of moral self-standing are often central to deriving threat from one's own thoughts, albeit experienced as unwanted and intrusive, and provoking unease in one's self–world interactions. Obsessions can be experienced as significant markers of moral standing (Rachman 1997), or even as morally equivalent to unacceptable actions (Shafran, Thordarson, and Rachman 1996). This leads the individual to inflate the significance of their thoughts and try to suppress such thoughts as a way of disproving one's moral unacceptability (Bhar and Kyrios 2007; Guidano and Liotti 1983) and resolve "contradictory aspects of a single self" (Kempke and Luyten 2007: 293).

Moreover, negative moral interpretations can be made even when the content of obsessions does not involve moral themes such as sex, religion, or ethics. For instance, one individual judged her obsessions regarding symmetry to be morally unacceptable because they were "crazy" (O'Neill 1999). Another who had thoughts of harming his two-year-old son found his obsessions distressing because of the implications that he was an inherently evil person (O'Neil, Cather, Fishel, and Kafka 2005). This individual was driven to hold his son after an intrusion, not to ensure that his son was safe but to reassure himself that he was not evil and was able to resist "temptation."

> Nate is a twenty-six-year-old married engineer living with his wife and newborn son. Four months prior to presenting for treatment, Nate observed a humorous discussion led by

colleagues at work about unusual fetishes. While he found the conversation uncomfortable, he rationalized "it didn't mean anything, so I thought that was it." However, later that evening while bathing his son, Nate reported a horrifying image of performing a sexual act on his son. As well as being highly distressed by the content of these repugnant images, Nate experienced shame and disgust at himself for having such thoughts, and feared that he may be a latent pedophile; "What father does this? . . . what sort of person does this?!"

Empirical research also supports that obsessional individuals are more likely to make negative moral inferences about themselves based on their intrusions, that their "feared self" is significantly more likely to consist of bad and immoral traits (Ferrier and Brewin 2005), and that obsessions reflect a fear as to who the person might be or might become (Aardema et al. 2013). Similarly, Doron, Moulding, Kyrios, and Nedeljkovic (2008) demonstrated that "sensitivity" in the self-referent domain of morality (i.e. perceiving morality as important to self-worth, but concurrently feeling inadequate in this domain) is linked to obsessive-compulsive disorder (OCD), but not to other anxiety disorders.

Sensitivity in moral self-worth has also been associated with overestimating threat, and an inflated sense of being pivotally responsibility for preventing harm, or trying to prevent harm (Doron et al. 2008). For the individual experiencing obsessions, the world is generally experienced as unsafe. The individual experiences a constant state of unease as the potential for threat seems to lurk everywhere, even in those places generally deemed innocuous (Straus 1938). The associated moral imperative to respond is therefore strong as the obsessive individual fears the guilt from not behaving responsibly (Mancini and Gangemi 2004), attributing greater importance to errors of omission than errors of commission (Salkovskis 1985). However, the overestimation of personal responsibility intensifies the potential severity of any harmful consequence. Thus, the obsessive individual assesses the severity of detrimental consequence as high, being unable to ignore intrusions, which compel the obsessive individual to devote immediate attention to reducing the threat thereby promoting a spur to action (Wroe and Salkovskis 2000).

Nate did not share the experiences with his wife for fear that she would take his son away from him, and he avoided being left alone with his son, or helping with bathing and changing. Instead, Nate became hyper-responsible in caring for his son by compulsively cleaning his bottles and checking the locks on his son's window, which over time, generalized to cleaning and checking the whole house. Upon his wife's requests that Nate spend more time with their son, he disclosed his unacceptable fears and with her unwavering support and reassurance, Nate was able to help with their son. However, the thoughts remained and although he doubted their validity, he could not completely dismiss them, as he could "never be sure" that he would not act on them. The insatiable doubt tormented him, prompting excessive vague reassurance-seeking from his wife. Although his obsessions were highly distressing and his compulsions disabling, the shame associated with his experiences meant that Nate did not initially disclose his obsessional symptoms, instead presenting for a fear of flying.

The obsessive individual desires certainty that their actions have had the necessary ability to absolve responsibility and threat. The desire for absolute certainty leaves the obsessive individual suspicious, because when there is room for error, there is room for doubt. The overarching uncertainty stems from a pathological doubt about the order of the world and basic assumptions that we normally take for granted (von Gebsattel 1954). For instance, normally we trust that our house will not be crushed by a random meteor and feel assured in the small numbers that suggest that it is a minute possibility. In contrast, the obsessive individual focuses on the marginal possibility of such an event making it real and threatening. O'Connor and Robillard (1995) further suggest that individuals experiencing obsessions doubt their own sensory information. Instead of examining the available evidence in what they can see, they fear what they cannot see. Indeed, OCD has been associated with deficits in non-verbal information (see Muller and Roberts 2005 for a review), and low confidence in their memory and related processes (e.g. decision-making, concentration, and attention; Nedeljkovic and Kyrios 2007). The distrust in available sensory information leads one to favor the subjective and emotional narrative that arises from the content of their obsessions.

Where we can normally trust in those things that we cannot be absolutely certain, the obsessive individual maintains an intense quest for certainty, leading to meticulousness and a pursuit of perfection. Objective evidence that one would normally deem sufficient is considered as not good enough. Thus, obsessional individuals continue to attune to the minutiae and at the expense of the bigger picture, spending excessive time to finish the task at hand. As it is impossible to complete tasks perfectly within the confines of an objective clock-time, the individual frequently feels overwhelmed and suffocated. Alternatively, they may experience a rush as they perceive themselves able to successfully, albeit temporarily, ward off their threats. However, the pursuit of perfection further propels the individual into deeper obsession.

Any temporary sense of omnipotence is however wiped out by an inability to control (or appraise) intrusive thoughts. Widely recognized as one of the distinguishing features of obsessions is that the individual has insight; they are aware that their intrusive thoughts come from within, that they are unreasonable, and that they have voluntary control over their actions (Clark 2004; Jaspers 1997). Nevertheless, they feel compelled, unable to resist, and that a response is inevitable (Straus 1938). Moreover, the individual recognizes the arbitrary and nonsensical nature for their obsession; one individual compulsively washed his hands to resolve contamination from outside his house, and yet he comfortably shared his bed with his pet dog who is housed outside during the day. This incongruence between the individual's rational thought and emotive experience is not only frustrating, confusing, and anxiety-provoking, but also associated with a deep sense of shame (de Haan, Rietveld, and Denys 2013; von Gebsattel 1954). In an effort to control approval from others, the individuals tend to conceal their obsessions, and present for treatment after suffering for a prolonged period.

Although insight is widely considered important for distinguishing obsessions from an overvalued idea or delusion (de Haan et al. 2013), some scholars suggest that OCD may be better characterized as a belief disorder. Obsessive individuals are prone to inferential confusion, a faulty reasoning process whereby the individual mistakes a small hypothetical possibility for a real probability (Aardema, Emmelkamp, and O'Connor 2005). As lamented by Dalle Luche and Iazzetta (2008), "the compulsive adherence to an incoercible doubt represents an equivalent to the delusional absolute certainty: the doubt is the psychotic feature of the phobic-obsessives" (148).

CONCLUSION

Both fear and intrusions can be considered typical human experiences. It is the intrapersonal management of these experiences however, that leads to persistence and magnification of subjective distress, intrusiveness of symptoms, and hence, dysfunction. The anxiety in phobia creates an intense feeling of vulnerability in one's environment, and overwhelming urges to avoid the particular stressful situation. Obsessions also may incorporate intense anxiety and avoidance. This chapter suggests that obsessions incorporate uncertainty in moral self-worth, pathological doubt, an inflated sense of responsibility, shame, and guilt. This experience provokes unease in one's self–world interactions, leading the obsessive individual to an intense quest for certainty and perfection, ultimately propelling the individual into deeper obsession.

BIBLIOGRAPHY

Aardema F., Emmelkamp P., and O'Connor K. (2005). "Inferential Confusion, Cognitive Change and Treatment Outcome in Obsessive–Compulsive Disorder." *Clinical Psychology & Psychotherapy* 12(5): 337–345.

Aardema F., and O'Connor K. (2007). "The Menace Within: Obsessions and the Self." *Journal of Cognitive Psychotherapy* 21: 182–197.

Aardema F., Moulding R., Radomsky A. S., Doron G., Allamby J., and Souki E. (2013). "Fear of Self and Obsessionality: Development and Validation of the Fear of Self Questionnaire." *Journal of Obsessive-Compulsive and Related Disorders* 2(3): 306–315.

Bhar S. and Kyrios M. (2007). "An Investigation of Self-ambivalence in Obsessive-Compulsive Disorder." *Behaviour Research and Therapy* 45(8): 1845–1857.

Clark D. A. (2004). *Intrusive Thoughts in Clinical Disorders: Theory, Research, and Treatment.* New York: Guilford Press.

Clark D. M. (2001). "A Cognitive Perspective on Social Phobia." In W. R. Crozier and L. E. Alden (eds.), *International Handbook of Social Anxiety: Concepts, Research and Interventions Relating to the Self and Shyness*, pp. 405–430. New York: John Wiley.

Clark D. M. and Wells A. (1995). "A Cognitive Model of Social Phobia." In R. Heimberg, M. Liebowitz, D. A. Hope, and F. R. Schneier (eds.), *Social Phobia: Diagnosis, Assessment and Treatment*, pp. 69–93. New York: Guilford Press.

Dalle Luche R. and Iazzetta P. (2008). "When Obsessions are Not Beliefs: Some Psychopathological-grounded Observations about Psychotherapy with Severe Phobic-obsessive Patients." *Comprendre* 16-17-18: 141–157.

de Haan S., Rietveld E., and Denys D. (2013). "On the Nature of Obsessions and Compulsions." *Modern Trends in Pharmacopsychiatry* 29: 1–15.

Doron G., Moulding R., Kyrios M., and Nedeljkovic M. (2008). "Sensitivity of Self-beliefs in Obsessive Compulsive Disorder." *Depression and Anxiety* 25(10): 874–884.

Ferrier S. and Brewin C. R. (2005). "Feared Identity and Obsessive-compulsive Disorder." *Behaviour Research and Therapy* 43(10): 1363–1374.

Guidano V. and Liotti G. (1983). *Cognitive Processes and Emotional Disorders.* New York: Guilford Press.

Hofmann S. G. (2007). "Cognitive Factors that Maintain Social Anxiety Disorder: a Comprehensive Model and its Treatment Implications." *Cognitive Behaviour Therapy* 36(4): 193–209.

Hofmann S. G., Alpers G. W., and Pauli P. (2009). "Phenomenology of Panic and Phobic Disorders." In M. M. Antony and M. B. Stein (eds.), *Oxford Handbook of Anxiety and Related Disorders*, pp. 34–46. New York: Oxford University Press.

Jaspers K. (1997). *General Psychopathology*. Baltimore: The John Hopkins University Press.

Kempke S. and Luyten P. (2007). "Psychodynamic and Cognitive-behavioral Approaches of Obsessive-compulsive Disorder: Is it Time to Work through Our Ambivalence? *Bulletin of the Menninger Clinic* 71(4): 291–311.

Lipton M. G., Brewin C. R., Linke S., and Halperin J. (2010). "Distinguishing Features of Intrusive Images in Obsessive-compulsive Disorder." *Journal of Anxiety Disorders* 24(8): 816–822.

Mancini F. and Gangemi A. (2004). "Fear of Guilt from Behaving Irresponsibly in Obsessive-compulsive Disorder." *Journal of Behavior Therapy and Experimental Psychiatry* 35(2): 109–120.

Marks I. (1969). *Fears and Phobias*. New York: Academic Press.

Marks I. (1987). *Fears, Phobias and Rituals: Panic, Anxiety, and Their Disorders*. New York: Oxford University Press.

Marks I. and Nesse R. (1994). "Fear and Fitness: An Evolutionary Analysis of Anxiety Disorders." *Ethology and Sociobiology* 15: 247–261.

Muller J. and Roberts J. E. (2005). "Memory and Attention in Obsessive–compulsive Disorder: A Review." *Journal of Anxiety Disorders* 19(1): 1–28.

Nedeljkovic M. and Kyrios M. (2007). "Confidence in Memory and Other Cognitive Processes in Obsessive-compulsive Disorder." *Behaviour Research and Therapy* 45(12): 2899–2914.

O'Connor K. and Robillard S. (1995). "Inference Processes in Obsessive-compulsive Disorder: Some Clinical Observations." *Behaviour Research and Therapy* 33(8): 887–896.

O'Neill S. A. (1999). "Living with Obsessive-compulsive Disorder: A Case Study of a Woman's Construction of Self." *Counselling Psychology Quarterly* 12(1): 73–86.

O'Neil S. E., Cather C., Fishel A. K., and Kafka M. (2005). "'Not Knowing if I was a Pedophile . . .'—Diagnostic Questions and Treatment Strategies in a Case of OCD." *Harvard Review of Psychiatry* 13(3): 186–196.

Rachman S. (1997). "A Cognitive Theory of Obsessions." *Behaviour Research and Therapy* 35(9): 793–802.

Rachman S. (2003). *The Treatment of Obsessions*. Oxford: Oxford University Press.

Rush B. (1798). "On the Different Species of Phobia." *The Weekly Magazine of Original Essays, Fugitive Pieces, and Interesting Intelligence*, 1: 177–180.

Salkovskis P. M. (1985). "Obsessional-compulsive Problems: A Cognitive-behavioural Analysis." *Behaviour Research and Therapy* 23(5): 571–583.

Shafran R., Thordarson D. S., and Rachman S. (1996). "Thought-action Fusion in Obsessive Compulsive Disorder." *Journal of Anxiety Disorders* 10(5): 379–391.

Straus E. (1938). "Ein Beitrag zur Pathologie der Zwangserscheinungen." *Monatsschrift für Psychiatrie und Neurologie* 98: 61–101.

Trigg D. (2013). "The Body of the Other: Intercorporeality and the Phenomenology of Agoraphobia." *Continental Philosophy Review* 46(3): 413–429.

von Gebsattel V. E. (1954). *Die Welt des Zwangskranken; Prolegomena einer medizinischen Anthropologie*. Berlin: Springer.

Wroe A. L. and Salkovskis P. M. (2000). "Causing Harm and Allowing Harm: A Study of Beliefs in Obsessional Problems." *Behaviour Research and Therapy* 38(12): 1141–1162.

CHAPTER 62

THOUGHTS WITHOUT THINKERS

Agency, Ownership, and the Paradox of Thought Insertion

CLARA S. HUMPSTON

INTRODUCTION

WHEN we think, how do we know the thoughts are ours? Furthermore, how do we know we are the thinkers of such thoughts? The vast majority of us would never even consider asking these questions because nothing is more taken for granted, nothing defines our autonomy as an individual more than the feeling that we are in charge of our thinking processes, our emotions, and actions. As a result, questions like these are almost "reserved" to the realm of philosophical investigation which the layperson would likely view as far-fetched and esoteric. However, extraordinary as it may sound, this feeling of being able to think freely and being "in charge" is actually a luxury to some.

I am speaking of individuals who have experienced thought insertion and other forms of thought interference (e.g. thought withdrawal, broadcast), which are classed as "first-rank" symptoms of schizophrenia spectrum psychoses and hence have special diagnostic significance (see the article on first-rank symptoms in the current volume). These symptoms quite physically rob the individual of their ability to think their own thoughts and also the feeling of being the thinker. As such, questions about thinking are no longer limited to the world of philosophical enquiry and have indeed become a constant theme, or even a "reality" for the individual afflicted with psychosis. The implications of losing one's ability to generate and control thoughts are also immense, often causing great pain and suffering to the individual and sometimes (albeit far less commonly) even leading to forensic consequences (Mullins and Spence 2003). But how could thought interference possibly happen in the first place, other than when explained as disorders of the brain and nothing else? Surely any "rational person" would never endorse such absurd experiences as a part of "external reality"?! Assertions of this kind are made far too readily by clinicians and researchers alike, often without pausing for a moment to ponder the meaning and significance beyond the symptoms as treatment targets.

The main focus of the current essay is thought insertion from a phenomenological perspective. I aim to discuss some of the current theories of thought insertion and address it not only as a psychotic symptom but also as a fundamental disturbance of one's self, which both challenges and forms one's reality; further, perhaps in contrary to the current medical definition of thought insertion, I will put forward the argument that the experience of thought insertion alone does not always constitute a delusional belief. I will then consider the relationships between thought insertion and other psychotic phenomena (in particular auditory–verbal hallucinations) and finally, theoretical implications of viewing thought insertion on a spectrum of self-disturbances.

The Subjective Experience of Thought Insertion

Of all the available first-person accounts of schizophrenia and related psychoses (such as those published in *Schizophrenia Bulletin* as a regular feature of the journal, e.g. Payne 2012; Timlett 2012), there are actually very few direct descriptions about what it is like to experience inserted thoughts; examples of thought insertion are more frequently found in older clinical reports, such as this often-used quote from Mellor (1970):

> I look out of the window and I think the garden looks nice and the grass looks cool, but the thoughts of Eamonn Andrews come into my mind. There are no other thoughts there, only his . . . He treats my mind like a screen and flashes his thoughts on to it like you flash a picture.

The reason for the lack of first-person narratives (i.e. written by sufferers themselves) could be that thought insertion often occurs in florid psychotic states which, when recalled during phases of remission, may no longer possess the salience and immediacy of the original experience; however, this example from Payne (2012) offers an insightful and poignant summary:

> Here is a related conundrum: are you in control of your own thoughts? It sounds like a very odd question, but it's at the core of the experience of schizophrenia.
> A dying person who is normal, even a person in front of a firing squad, has choices.
> A psychotic person is less, even minimally, in control of his thoughts.

It is interesting how she formulated thought (dis)ownership as a question rather than a statement ("are you in control?") and viewed it as "the core of schizophrenia"—if Mellor's vignette is a textbook case of thought insertion as a delusion, Payne's account to a certain extent challenges the notion of delusional conviction and perhaps whether thought insertion is a delusion at all (I will later argue that the answer is not clear-cut). If one is able to question the delusional nature of a thought or belief, by default that thought will no longer qualify as a delusion at least in an orthodox psychiatric sense, which defines thought insertion as "the delusion that certain thoughts are not the patient's own but implanted by an outside agency" (Gelder, Harrison, and Cowen 2006: 12). Does this imply that once someone starts to question the veracity of the experience, the experience will automatically "disqualify" as a delusion or even disappear altogether? However, as Payne points out in the next two sentences, a psychotic person is still "minimally in control of his thoughts." This creates a paradox: if one cannot lose control over one's thoughts unless they are delusional, then the mere realization that these lost thoughts are in fact one's own would disqualify them from being delusional. Labeling thought insertion as a delusion thus becomes the consensus as it is seemingly the most convenient method to solving the paradox but such an explanation by no means captures the entirety of the experience. Indeed, thought insertion is perhaps more of an *experience* than just a belief, delusional or not. More recently, evidence from both quantitative and qualitative research has emerged to support the notion that the boundaries between sensory experience and belief (at least in psychosis) are much more blurred than previously speculated (Jones and Luhrmann 2015; Rosen et al. 2016). Thought insertion is of no exception—maybe its paradoxical nature is best considered as a complex combination of both perception and belief formation which has lost the senses of agency and ownership of thought.

AGENCY AND OWNERSHIP OF THOUGHT

In order to fully appreciate the complexity of thought insertion, I will first discuss some of the current philosophical theories (and limited empirical evidence from neuropsychological studies) of the phenomenon in question. It is widely acknowledged that "normal" or one's own thoughts are immune to error through misidentification relative to the first-person pronoun (the immunity principle): that is, "when a speaker uses the first-person pronoun ('I') to refer to him or herself, she cannot make a mistake about the person to whom he or she is referring" (Gallagher 2000; Shoemaker 1968). This means that when one uses "I" as in "*I* think *my* thoughts"; they cannot possibly be referring to anyone else by saying "I." It may seem obvious or even pedantic to stress the importance of the first-person pronoun but the distinction of "I" is essential to thought insertion. For the person experiencing thought insertion, it is not just "*I* don't think *my* thoughts" but also "these thoughts that occur in *my* mind are not *mine*." Many theorists agree that these two statements differentiate two important concepts, namely the senses of agency and ownership: agency refers to the sense that I am the one who is causing or generating an action, whereas ownership is defined by the sense that I am the one who is undergoing an experience (i.e. the experience belongs to me, voluntary or not; Gallagher 2000).

Thought insertion is considered to violate the immunity principle (and also the "Cartesian principle," see Billon 2013) because in thought insertion the decision of when to use "I" does not come naturally: in fact, some argue that the patient's sense of agency has diminished but the sense of ownership is left intact. In other words, the individual misattributes the agency to someone else while recognizing the thoughts are in their own mind and they are the "owner" or even "container" of the inserted, external thoughts. But the very act of misattributing agency implies volition and deliberation which borders on the realm of the "judgment" or agency (Synofzik, Vosgerau, and Newen 2008) and not just a "sense" which is often far more minimal and basic, sometimes even possessing sensory qualities: some patients report knowing the exact location and feeling the associated tactile sensation of external thoughts entering their head (Mullins and Spence 2003). The same explanation may be applied to ownership: I argue that only because inserted thoughts occurs within a mind (sense of ownership), they do not always have to belong to the mind (judgment of ownership) in which they are found (Bortolotti and Broome 2009; Humpston and Broome 2016).

One may regard this as yet another paradox because the externality of inserted thoughts is only accessible through the first-person perspective. Given that when thoughts are obtained through introspection ("privileged access") they will automatically integrate into one's direct and taken-for-granted self-knowledge and hence are inseparable from the rest of one's subjectivity, something like thought insertion becomes naturally implausible and such implausibility adds to the falsehood that is central to the current definition of a delusion. However, if one separates the process of thinking from the thoughts that are produced, the paradox of thought insertion may become a little less daunting. It is true that the "I" from the immunity principle acts as a prerequisite of thinking, but it can also act as a mere metaphor. The individual experiencing thought insertion adopts the position of "I" without endorsing the first-person nature of "I" due to the constraints of language and not personal choice. The personal choice is that it is *not* "I" who thinks these thoughts; because of the loss of "I," it cannot possibly act as the causal agent of any thought in the first place. Therefore, I posit that in thought insertion, the only process left intact is the judgment of ownership and not the sense of ownership whereas both the sense and judgment of agency are severely damaged.

Neuropsychological theories and empirical studies have also offered support for the differentiation between agency and ownership; the most influential theory about the feeling of agency in intentional motor acts is perhaps the comparator model (e.g. Frith 2012; Blakemore, Wolpert, and Frith 2002) which, as some may argue, focuses on the minimization of prediction error when comparing expected and outcome states of an action. If the error signal is large, the sense of agency is attributed externally as in self-initiated actions there is no or only minimal "mismatch" between what is the desired motor consequence and what is the actual sensory feedback (however, this process might not be applicable to the sense of ownership: see Sato and Yasuda 2005). This model nicely explains phenomena such as passivity experiences or made actions (also a first-rank symptom of schizophrenia), but is the process of thinking also a motor act? Some theorists have indeed argued in favor of this notion, suggesting a "feeling of thinking" (Campbell 1999; Gerrans 2015) in terms of imagined action and inner (imagined) speech. However, even if the act of thinking does follow the same pattern as initiating (inner) actions, the act of ascribing thinking to another agent cannot be fully accounted for by large error signals. For example, why would one attribute the agency of thought to that particular agent and not simply anything "non-self"? I suggest that this lack of explanation actually provides support for a duplex or two-factor account of thought insertion.

THOUGHT INSERTION AS A DUPLEX PROCESS

The two-factor account of delusion formation (Davies, Breen, Coltheart, and Langdon 2001) is not a new concept, in particular its application to monothematic delusions such as the Capgras delusion (where the affected individual holds the belief that someone close to them has been replaced by an imposter). However, for complex delusional systems often found in schizophrenia, it is extremely difficult to formulate a single unifying theory to capture the heterogeneity of delusions. The kind of two-factor account I am proposing here is in fact not about delusion formation—indeed, I do not consider thought insertion as *entirely* a delusion—but for thought insertion as a duplex process involving both sensory experiences and alterations in reasoning.

Phenomenological investigations have established striking similarities between what is sensory and what is a thought or belief in the subjectivity of psychotic experiences. The Husserlian phenomenological tradition, for example, requires the formal suspension (epoché) of prior taken-for-granted assumptions about the nature of a given experience under investigation (see Broome et al. 2012: 14) which is inevitably at odds with the definitions, formulations, and diagnostic judgments adopted by many psychiatrists even before speaking with the patient. Instead, by adopting an ontological neutrality, the patient's first-person experience will come to the forefront and becomes the only centrality without the constraints of any predefined explanatory theory.

Orthodox psychiatric accounts about the seemingly clear-cut distinctions between a hallucination and a delusion, for example, are "not what the textbooks describe" (Jones and Shattell 2016: 769). Patients with psychosis feel their experiences are beyond that which language and words can adequately express and as a result use many metaphors to try and convey what is in essence indescribable (but not incomprehensible). What the patient senses and what they think are almost one and the same, with patients reporting localized thoughts in a particular part of their brain and also "soundless voices" or "a sense of being spoken to" rather than literally hearing a voice with acoustic qualities through their ears. With these theoretical and practical challenges to our "ordinary" understanding of psychopathology in mind, I posit that we should avoid the terminology "delusion of thought insertion" but instead simply call it "thought insertion" and when there is an associated delusional elaboration about the source of the inserted thoughts, "delusions *in* thought insertion."

Of course, many may argue a change of one proposition (what does it matter whether it is delusion "of" thought insertion or delusion "in" thought insertion?) is merely a game of lexicon; furthermore, surely no one can *actually* receive external thoughts from without, it is physically and scientifically impossible so it *must* be a delusion no matter how much analysis we do! Still, how can anyone tell if an experience is an *actual* experience without being the experiencer? Just like no one can "literally" have thoughts that are not theirs, it is also a fact that no one can entirely take over another person's perspective—to the experiencing individual, however, the feeling of having external thoughts (and indeed, any other aspect of unusual phenomena) is extremely real and salient, perhaps even more real than consensual reality due to the saliency. Psychotic symptoms are not "real" by nature of external observation, yet they can be more literal and concrete than anything else to the person with psychosis, often with their whole experiential field dominated by a single absorbing mental event whilst feeling detached from external reality (Perona-Garcelán et al. 2008, 2012). Therefore, the first stage of thought insertion (and related aspects of psychosis) is likely a basic and generative sensory experience of "finding" or "feeling" thoughts entering one's mind from external space.

This very sensation of "receiving" thoughts being forced into one's mind is undoubtedly a highly salient and sometimes disturbing event, and any delusions that ensue are almost one's natural need to explain the experience, one's instinctive search for meaning. Yet such meaning cannot possibly be found by ordinary logic, given how extremely unusual the original experience is—hence "calling for" an equally extraordinary explanation as the second stage of thought insertion, often by delusional means. Even the essential indexical "I" of thinking only acts as a mere prerequisite of an *assigned* thinker, in order for the individual to formulate the sentence by which they try and describe the feeling to another. Using the first-person pronoun serves the purpose of communication by, rather than representation of, the agent possessing the inserted thoughts.

Let us consider the following three sentences:

    i) "This thought is not mine."
   ii) "This thought is given to me/thought by person X."
  iii) "This thought has been transmitted to me by X via a device in my brain."

The first sentence, however bizarre it may sound, is a statement based on an observation that a foreign thought has entered one's subjective space because the thought is somehow different from the background of the subject's own thoughts (against personal values, interests and history, for example). This is to assume that one can readily differentiate which thoughts belong to the self and which do not by the process of introspection, thus an ability to either self-ascribe them as one's own or discard them as alien, which is again not usually a conscious effort as most would take their thinking processes with a certain "mineness" and givenness. Hence I argue that it is the lack of "mineness" and not always a delusional elaboration that "completes" the phenomenon of thought insertion (Humpston and Broome 2016).

The second sentence has a clear target and focuses on an external agent: person X. Now the subject has begun to try and explain where the thought comes from and after some logical or illogical inferential deliberation, has decided on person X. One could say the "level" of a delusion is more applicable to this second sentence. On the other hand, the third sentence may be considered "the most delusional" due to its sheer bizarreness and implausibility yet the experience behind this conclusion may not be any less real only because there is a stronger, more detailed elaboration.

THE ROLE OF DELUSIONAL ELABORATION

As detailed in the previous section, there are levels of how "delusional" a given explanation may be, regardless of the original generative experience. However, there is no way of telling whether the original experience is the same across individuals because the individual has to verbalize the experience in question first. If the only expression of such a bizarre and unsettling mental event is a delusional elaboration, no matter how remote from what realistically could happen, surely the elaboration itself carries meaning and significance for the individual. Assuming the experience of sensing or receiving external thoughts is indeed universal, the heterogeneity of the explanation that ensues serves as a reminder of how a delusion arises not only from alternations in brain function, but is also shaped if not defined by factors both unique to the individual and common to their social and cultural environment (Larøi et al. 2014; Luhrmann, Padmavati, Tharoor, and Osei 2015). For example, individuals in Western industrialized countries may be more likely to attribute thought insertion and related thought interference/alien control phenomena to "influencing machines" (Hirjak and

Fuchs 2010) whereas individuals in less industrially developed countries may attribute the same phenomena to witchcraft or demonic possession.

Nevertheless, all types of delusional elaboration for thought insertion have one common feature: they reflect the intrinsic need to search for meaning, as a human being, after an un-explainable yet highly perplexing and salient event. This search for meaning is separate from one's rich imagination since psychosis, I argue, is not simply "imagined" because even the act of imagining is no longer a willed action, but an automatic process that has gained autonomy and spontaneity whilst losing privacy and first-person authority. The perceptualization of imagination (Rasmussen and Parnas 2014) significantly accentuates the reality of internally generated events and the contrast between the "realness" of this externalization and the orig-inal perplexity caused by thought insertion is not something anyone could easily ignore. As a consequence, a (delusional) meaning is attached to the external nature of the experience and this meaning is reinforced as long as the experience itself maintains externality. On the other hand, once a delusional elaboration has fully formed, it may become incorrigible and the individual may defend the delusional meaning with anything they view as supporting evidence, hence reinforcing the explanation through processes such memory consolidation.

Could it be that although the individual did not actively "choose" or even endorse the delu-sional ideation at first, the meaning it offers causes the individual to "latch onto" the same ex-planation because no matter how frightening the delusion is, at least it reconciles the even more frightening experience of thought insertion and provides some kind of "comfort" and sense of purpose at the same time? I think this is very much a probable reason for delusional conviction and maintenance—being able to identify the person or "the organization" sending the external thoughts could be much more preferable to living in constant uncertainty and perplexity, even if one may never be able to resolve the paradoxical nature of thought insertion. The fear of losing one's control over, and integrity of, one's innermost thoughts is unspeakable, but once there is a target, an "enemy," one could at least in theory redirect the fear to something more "real" than oneself at the cost of being unreal to everyone else in the external world.

RELATIONSHIP WITH
AUDITORY–VERBAL HALLUCINATIONS

I will now discuss how thought insertion is intertwined with another important aspect of psychosis, namely auditory–verbal hallucinations. As argued previously, I strongly believe that any experience—let it be a "normal" experience or a psychotic "symptom"—should not, and cannot be viewed in isolation from other experiences. This is not simply because experiences often tend to occur simultaneously, but also because, in order to achieve a "complete" phenomenology, we rely on the integration of all inputs from our current ex-periential status. Even something very basic, such as a faint smell, can trigger a stream of memories or influence behavior, which in turn creates more experiences for the individual. Schizophrenia and its key positive symptoms discussed here are of no exception: although they constitute a syndrome which is by no means independent from other syndromes in psychiatric nosology, each symptom is interrelated with another and together they weave the picture of the patient's subjective experience. As Fletcher and Frith (2009) posit in their review, "how one experiences something at a basic sensory level is dependent on one's know-ledge of it (expressed in terms of its predictability) . . . each experience is affected by what one believes" (52). On this basis they continue to propose a Bayesian approach to explaining pos-itive symptoms: "the extent to which one updates what one believes is affected by how that experience adds to it. This is, of course, the insight captured by Bayes' theorem."

The Bayesian framework posits that the processing of information depends on both prior or top-down knowledge, expectation, and experience in the face of current or bottom-up (often sensory) inputs which acts as an iterative process to minimize the discrepancy (i.e. prediction error) between them (Corlett et al. 2009). Whilst the current essay will not discuss in detail this approach, it sheds some light on how belief and experience are interdependent, rather than independent entities. For example, inserted thoughts could be traced back to one's own thoughts but also linked with "soundless voices" (see below) and "true" auditory–verbal hallucinations. With thought insertion being the result of the loss of agency and own-ership by one's own thinking processes, these externalized thoughts subsequently re-enter the subject's inner psychological space as alien without regaining the senses of agency and ownership. This re-entering process could be immediate, because thoughts cannot exist—at least not for very long—without a "container" or a thinker. An analogy of thought insertion would be that it is almost like an autoimmune disease of thought: produced from the mind, but because of a loss of vital properties (senses of agency and ownership) they are targeted (and attacked) as foreign invaders by the mind itself. This account is compatible with the theory that self-disturbances in schizophrenia act as a "generative disorder" (Cermolacce, Naudin, and Parnas 2007) or Minkowski's "trouble générateur."

Furthermore, "soundless voices" could be the in-between step or mediator between thought insertion and "true" auditory–verbal hallucinations; once the subject *assigns* a voice-like quality (whether it is actually audible or not) to their external thoughts, it pushes the equilibrium equation toward a "hallucination" because if the subject already perceives thought insertion as "soundless voices," it is only natural that other qualities (e.g. sound) nor-mally associated with voices ensue conceptually and perhaps also perceptually. Therefore, I think that thought insertion and auditory–verbal hallucinations share an interdependent relationship and the property of which is largely reliant on second-order judgments and attributions.

The notion of "soundless voices," albeit (again) paradoxical, is in fact nothing new; as summarized by Jones (2010), Bleuler described "vivid thoughts" which were called voices by his patients. However, there has been no investigation as to whether these very vivid thoughts are inserted or external thoughts. Auditory–verbal imagery can appear extremely real even in non-clinical populations (McGuire et al. 1996), yet in these groups the agency and ownership of their verbal imagery remain intact and very few fail to distinguish verbal imagery from actual sensory perceptions. Nevertheless, in patients with schizophrenia the majority can also distinguish their voices from "real" auditory perceptions (Miller 1996) whilst believing in the "reality" of their voices. It may be that the patients are sentient to the *realities* of both their voices and external speech, but what is the key feature which sets apart the two equally prominent realities? Once again, I think the answer lies in the sense of "mineness" which demarcates "my reality" from "external reality." It is ironic how the actual loss of "mineness" (i.e. thought insertion and auditory–verbal hallucinations) can create the patient's reality ("my reality") while all at the same time being experienced as if they come from without ("external reality").

I stress again that these phenomena cannot be interpreted in isolation; it may seem confusing or paradoxical at first glance but in order to capture the complexity of their phenomenology, it is inevitable in my opinion that the components of the totality of experience relate to one another. I argue that "soundless voices" are not synonymous with, or equivalent to, thought insertion even though they share similarities in phenomenology; instead, thought insertion can act as a precursor to "soundless voices" via the process of secondary appraisal and elaboration. Assuming the definition of "true" auditory–verbal hallucinations is theoretically and empirically valid (i.e. the subject really hears sound in auditory–verbal hallucinations), soundless voices, by definition, can become "true" auditory–verbal hallucinations if and when they gain acoustic qualities or audibility. By this definition (albeit problematic perhaps) soundless voices are primordial hallucinations (I have decided to avoid the term "pseudohallucinations" as I think it undermines the subjective reality of the experience) without sensory features and are not identical to thought insertion. They can be viewed as the intermediate state between thought insertion and "true" auditory–verbal hallucinations (Humpston and Broome 2016).

CONCLUSION

In this article I have discussed the nature of thought insertion as a result of a loss of ownership and agency over thought, which often acts as a generative phenomenon to delusion formation but which does not always qualify as a delusional belief by itself. I understand it may be somewhat controversial to argue for a non-delusional account for extraordinary mental events such as thought insertion, and I am aware some may argue that by "validating" the reality of thought insertion one might inadvertently intensify the delusional conviction of an individual with psychosis and therefore impede recovery. However, I also believe that in order to fully comprehend thought insertion it is essential to view it from the perspective of the experiencer. If and when a delusion forms as a result of thought insertion, the delusion in question needs to be considered in conjunction with, but not instead of, the original generative experience of what is subjectively an event of finding external thoughts in one's mental space (actual or metaphorical) and objectively an event of losing the senses of agency and ownership of these thoughts. I have also argued that thought insertion needs to be considered in continuity with other symptoms of disrupted self-awareness on the schizophrenia spectrum, in particular auditory–verbal hallucinations with and without sound ("soundless voices"), which are in fact be transdiagnostic and reach beyond psychotic symptoms alone (although this calls for further analysis).

Taken together, however, my intention has never been to necessarily disentangle the paradoxes of thought insertion altogether but to offer a new angle to understanding them; one may have to admit that the very nature of thought insertion precludes a unifying account and come to the conclusion that some paradoxes are fascinating simply because they remain paradoxical no matter how deeply one attempts to analyze and solve their mystery. Thought insertion perhaps is one such mystery—but one must not be discouraged from continuing the endeavor, for it is these unsolvable questions that power one to further the enquiry into the bizarre, intriguing, and surprisingly understandable human experience that we call psychosis. Although the aim of the phenomenological approach is never to completely explain the mechanisms underpinning unusual experiences like thought insertion, and a complete epoché may not always be possible, it can nevertheless assist with, and significantly contribute to, one's efforts in constructing a more accurate and complete descriptive "picture" of psychopathological experiences (McCarthy-Jones et al. 2013). Perhaps the key implication for practice is that by shedding one's own judgments and assumptions about reality or "normality," the clinician would be able to listen more carefully to the expressions of the experiencing individual whose reality is no less real than one's own, which is of course the foundation of any strong therapeutic alliance.

BIBLIOGRAPHY

Billon A. (2013). "Does Consciousness Entail Subjectivity? The Puzzle of Thought Insertion." *Philosophical Psychology* 26(2): 291–314.

Blakemore S. J., Wolpert D. M., and Frith, C. D. (2002). "Abnormalities in the Awareness of Action." *Trends in Cognitive Sciences* 6(6): 237–242.

Bortolotti L. and Broome M. (2009). "A Role for Ownership and Authorship in the Analysis of Thought Insertion." *Phenomenology and the Cognitive Sciences* 8(2): 205–224.

Broome M. R., Harland R., Owen G. S., and Stringaris A. (eds.) (2012). *The Maudsley Reader in Phenomenological Psychiatry*. Cambridge, UK: Cambridge University Press.

Campbell J. (1999). "Schizophrenia, the Space of Reasons, and Thinking as a Motor Process." *The Monist* 82(4): 609–625.

Cermolacce M., Naudin J., and Parnas J. (2007). "The 'Minimal Self' in Psychopathology: Re-examining the Self-disorders in the Schizophrenia Spectrum." *Consciousness and Cognition* 16(3): 703–714.

Corlett P. R., Frith C. D., and Fletcher P. C. (2009). "From Drugs to Deprivation: A Bayesian Framework for Understanding Models of Psychosis." *Psychopharmacology* 206(4): 515–530.

Davies M., Breen N., Coltheart M., and Langdon R. (2001). "Monothematic Delusions: Towards a Two-factor Account." *Philosophy, Psychiatry, & Psychology* 8(2): 133–158.

Fletcher P. C. and Frith C. D. (2009). "Perceiving is Believing: A Bayesian Approach to Explaining the Positive Symptoms of Schizophrenia." *Nature Reviews Neuroscience* 10(1): 48–58.

Frith C. (2012). "Explaining Delusions of Control: The Comparator Model 20 Years On." *Consciousness and Cognition* 21(1): 52–54.

Gallagher S. (2000). "Philosophical Conceptions of the Self: Implications for Cognitive Science." *Trends in Cognitive Sciences* 4(1): 14–21.

Gelder M., Harrison P., and Cowen P. (2006). *Shorter Oxford Textbook of Psychiatry*. Oxford: Oxford University Press.

Gerrans P. (2015). "The Feeling of Thinking: Sense of Agency in Delusions of Thought Insertion." *Psychology of Consciousness: Theory, Research, and Practice* 2(3): 291.

Hirjak D. and Fuchs T. (2010). "Delusions of Technical Alien Control: A Phenomenological Description of Three Cases." *Psychopathology* 43(2): 96–103.

Humpston C. S. and Broome M. R. (2016). "The Spectra of Soundless Voices and Audible Thoughts: Towards an Integrative Model of Auditory Verbal Hallucinations and Thought Insertion." *Review of Philosophy and Psychology* 7(3): 611–629.

Jones N. and Luhrmann T. M. (2015). "Beyond the Sensory: Findings from an In-depth Analysis of the Phenomenology of 'Auditory Hallucinations' in Schizophrenia." *Psychosis* 8(3): 191–202.

Jones N. and Shattell M. (2016). "Not What the Textbooks Describe: Challenging Clinical Conventions About Psychosis." *Issues in Mental Health Nursing* 37(10): 769–772.

Jones S. R. (2010). "Do We Need Multiple Models of Auditory Verbal Hallucinations? Examining the Phenomenological Fit of Cognitive and Neurological Models." *Schizophrenia Bulletin* 36(3): 566–575.

Larøi F., Luhrmann T. M., Bell V., Christian W. A., Deshpande S., Fernyhough C., et al. (2014). "Culture and Hallucinations: Overview and Future Directions." *Schizophrenia Bulletin* 40(Suppl 4): S213–S220.

Luhrmann T. M., Padmavati R., Tharoor H., and Osei A. (2015). "Differences in Voice-hearing Experiences of People with Psychosis in the USA, India and Ghana: Interview-based Study." *The British Journal of Psychiatry* 206(1): 41–44.

McCarthy-Jones S., Krueger J., Larøi F., Broome M., and Fernyhough C. (2013). "Stop, Look, Listen: The Need for Philosophical Phenomenological Perspectives on Auditory Verbal Hallucinations." *Frontiers in Human Neuroscience* 7: 127.

McGuire P. K., Silbersweig D. A., Wright I., Murray R. M., Frackowiak R. S., and Frith, C. D. (1996). "The Neural Correlates of Inner Speech and Auditory Verbal Imagery in Schizophrenia: Relationship to Auditory Verbal Hallucinations." *The British Journal of Psychiatry* 169(2): 148–159.

Mellor C. S. (1970). "First Rank Symptoms of Schizophrenia. I. The Frequency in Schizophrenics on Admission to Hospital. II. Differences between Individual First Rank Symptoms." *British Journal of Psychiatry* 117: 15–23.

Miller L. J. (1996). "Qualitative Changes in Hallucinations." *The American Journal of Psychiatry* 153(2): 265–267.

Mullins S. and Spence S. A. (2003). "Re-examining Thought Insertion." *British Journal of Psychiatry* 182(4): 293–298.

Payne R. (2012). "Night's End." *Schizophrenia Bulletin* 38(5): 899–901.

Perona-Garcelán S., Cuevas-Yust C., García-Montes J. M., Pérez-Álvarez M., Ductor-Recuerda M. J., Salas-Azcona R., et al. (2008). "Relationship between Self-focused Attention and Dissociation in Patients with and without Auditory Hallucinations." *The Journal of Nervous and Mental Disease* 196(3): 190–197.

Perona-Garcelán S., García-Montes J. M., Ductor-Recuerda M. J., Vallina-Fernández O., Cuevas-Yust C., Pérez-Álvarez M., et al. (2012). "Relationship of Metacognition, Absorption, and Depersonalization in Patients with Auditory Hallucinations." *British Journal of Clinical Psychology* 51(1): 100–118.

Rasmussen A. R. and Parnas J. (2014). "Pathologies of Imagination in Schizophrenia Spectrum Disorders." *Acta Psychiatrica Scandinavica* 131(3): 157–161.

Rosen C., Jones N., Chase K. A., Gin H., Grossman L. S., and Sharma R. P. (2016). "The Intrasubjectivity of Self, Voices and Delusions: A Phenomenological Analysis." *Psychosis* 8(4): 357–368.

Sato A. and Yasuda A. (2005). "Illusion of Sense of Self-agency: Discrepancy between the Predicted and Actual Sensory Consequences of Actions Modulates the Sense of Self-agency, But Not the Sense of Self-ownership." *Cognition* 94(3): 241–255.

Shoemaker S. S. (1968). "Self-reference and Self-awareness." *The Journal of Philosophy* 65(19): 555–567.

Synofzik M., Vosgerau G., and Newen A. (2008). "Beyond the Comparator Model: A Multifactorial Two-step Account of Agency. *Consciousness and Cognition* 17(1): 219–239.

Timlett A. (2012). "Controlling Bizarre Delusions." *Schizophrenia Bulletin* 39(2): 244–246.

SECTION FIVE

LIFE-WORLDS

SECTION EDITORS: ANTHONY VINCENT
FERNANDEZ AND GIOVANNI STANGHELLINI

CHAPTER 63

THE LIFE-WORLD
OF PERSONS WITH
SCHIZOPHRENIA
Considered as a Disorder of Basic Self

LOUIS SASS

INTRODUCTION

THE idea that a disorder of self might be at the core of schizophrenia or schizophrenia-spectrum disorders is not a new hypothesis. In his classic *General Psychopathology*, first published in 1913, Karl Jaspers (1963: 121f.) presents loss of the *Cogito* (of the "mineness" or "I-quality" of experience) as the most prominent source of that essential strangeness that, in his view, actually *defines* the schizophrenic condition. Emil Kraepelin (1971: xvi), the father of modern psychiatric nosology, had already pointed to this feature of what he termed *dementia praecox*: "There is simply no ego there" (*Da ist ein Ich einfach nicht mehr da*). In recent decades this notion has come once again to the fore, in the hypothesis of an ipseity-disturbance or disorder of basic, core, or minimal self—of the very experience of existing as a subject of experience or agent of one's own actions.

Sass and Parnas (2003) formulated this foundational disorder of core self or ipseity (derived from *ipse*, Latin for "self" or "itself") as having three interrelated aspects, and argued that, taken together, these can account for all the major symptoms of schizophrenia (Sass 2014a): 1) hyperreflexivity and 2) diminished self-presence—together with a correlated 3) disturbance of "grip," "hold," or "grasp" on the cognitive/perceptual world. This ipseity-disturbance hypothesis is currently the most influential formulation in phenomenological psychopathology of schizophrenia—which, in turn, is the disorder that has received the most attention by phenomenologically oriented specialists.[1]

The ipseity-disturbance hypothesis has generated much scholarship and research. Of crucial importance are attempts to operationalize the concept and determine that it is, indeed, distinctive of persons in the schizophrenia spectrum. Below I will review this important

[1] This chapter incorporates some passages from several previous publications, including Sass (2014a; 2017: appendix), Sass and Borda (2015). I thank Mads Henriksen and Greg Byrom for helpful comments.

research, which mainly relies on a qualitatively rich, semi-structured interview called the EASE: Examination of Anomalous Self-Experience (Parnas et al. 2005), and has been described in detail elsewhere. The focus of this chapter will, however, be on theoretical work, together with some quasi-empirical research, that attempts to investigate the underlying nature of "self-disorder" in more depth through 1) offering theoretical clarification by considering its different, interlocking aspects as well as what may be its distinctive pathogenetic forms or stages (primary versus secondary); 2) investigating it in a comparative context; and 3) discussing its possible correlates on the neurobiological or neurocognitive plane.

Self-disorder is a crucial but difficult concept, easily misunderstood or oversimplified. It requires not only empirical validation but also conceptual analysis and comparative investigation in light of various analogies.

THE IPSEITY-DISTURBANCE MODEL

Three Aspects

As noted, the ipseity-disturbance model of schizophrenia postulates that the fundamental disturbance or *"trouble générateur"* of this illness or set of illnesses is a disturbance of "core" or "minimal" self—also known as "ipseity" (Nelson, Parnas, and Sass 2014a; Sass 2014a; Sass and Parnas 2003; Sass et al. 2011). The term ipseity (synonymous with "core self," "basic self," or "minimal self") refers to the crucial sense of self-sameness, of existing as a subject of experience *or subject pole* that is alive and at one with itself at any given moment, *serving as a vital center point of subjective life*. One person who suffered from schizophrenia, the writer Antonin Artaud, spoke of what he called "the essential illumination" and this "phosphorescent point"—thereby referring to a vital and illuminating center-point that he equated with the "very substance of what is called the soul," and described as a prerequisite for avoiding "constant leakage of the normal level of reality" (Artaud 1976: 169, 82; Artaud 1965: 20). The so-called *autobiographical* self or *narrative* continuity concerns a less foundational level (Gallagher 2011; Parnas and Henriksen, this volume); and although disturbances at this level certainly occur in schizophrenia, they are less *distinctive* of schizophrenia (also found in dissociative identity disorder and borderline personality) and not likely to be strongly pathogenetic (Parnas and Sass 2011).

As noted, ipseity disturbance can be described in terms of three essential and interlocking aspects.

1) Hyperreflexivity refers to an exaggerated self-consciousness, a coming-to-focal-or-explicit-awareness of processes and phenomena that would normally remain in the implicit background of experience, where they would normally be "inhabited" or experienced (tacitly) as part of oneself, but that now come to be experienced as having an alien quality (e.g. kinesthetic and proprioceptive bodily sensations; the verbalizations inherent in our inner speech or thought) (Sass 1992; Sass et al. 2011; Henriksen et al 2015).[2]

---

[2] The awareness we normally have of our bodies (the normal "lived body") is, writes Gurwitsch (1964: 302, describing Merleau-Ponty's views), "not . . . knowledge in thematized form. [Rather] an inarticulate and indistinct familiarity completely devoid of positional and disclosing consciousness."

2) Diminished self-presence (a.k.a. diminished self-affection) refers to a decline in the experienced sense of being a subject of awareness or agent of action—of existing, we might say, in the first-person perspective. This experience of one's *own* presence as a conscious, embodied subject is so fundamental that any description risks sounding empty or tautological; yet its absence can be acutely felt: "I was simply there, only in that place, but without being present," said one patient (Blankenburg 1971); another felt overwhelmed by "total emptiness . . . as if I ceased to exist" (Parnas et al. 2005).

3) Disturbed grip or hold on the cognitive-perceptual world refers to disturbances of spatio–temporal structuring of the experiential field, and of the clarity of such crucial experiential distinctions as perceived versus remembered versus imagined. It is assumed that such disturbances of grip or hold are grounded in abnormalities of the embodied, vital, experiencing self, which normally serves as a constituting and orienting background for experience of the world (Merleau-Ponty 2012 re "hold" or "prise"; Sass 2004, 2014a).

Disorders of ipseity help to account for the "bizarre" and characteristically schizophrenic quality of various symptoms. An example would be the kinds of delusions that are typical of schizophrenia patients. These involve, in addition to altered *cogito* (an obvious self-related feature), also certain alterations in the general look and feel of the perceptual field that constitute the delusional mood (a manifestation of disturbed grip), and a characteristic combination of certitude with inconsequentiality—of certitude re the delusion together with its irrelevance for real-world action (a manifestation of a certain quasi-solipsism associated with altered ipseity) (Sass and Byrom 2015a).

Interdependence of the Three Aspects

The three aspects are intimately interlinked, and should perhaps be understood more as aspects of a single whole than as separate but interacting processes. (It should be noted, however, that this aspects versus processes distinction may itself be exaggerated and somewhat misleading—subject as it is to the deficiencies of all attempts to capture subjectivity in definite concepts largely deriving from other domains (see Fink 1995: 97f.; Sass 2014b.)[3]

Consider hyperreflexivity and diminished self-presence. On superficial consideration, these two phenomena might seem mutually contradictory, perhaps even psychologically incompatible—since one involves *heightened* self-consciousness, the other a form of *diminished* self-awareness. But phenomenological consideration suggests that they are better understood as not only compatible but even mutually complementary. Whereas hyperreflexivity emphasizes how something normally tacit becomes focal and explicit, diminished self-affection emphasizes a complementary or equiprimordial aspect of the *very*

---

[3] The difficulty of talking of such issues is well recognized by Eugen Fink, Husserl's closest associate, who warned against "seduction by mundane meanings" (1995: 97f.). In Fink's view, every attempt to speak of "the transcendental" necessarily encounters conflict and contradiction. This is due to the gap between the intended, transcendental sense of words as used in phenomenology (which aims at subjectivity itself) and the mundane or natural sense, grounded in the "natural attitude," whence they derive their original sense.

same process: the fact that what once was tacitly lived (e.g. kinesthetic sensations of lived body, inner speech as basis of thinking) is no longer being inhabited as a medium of taken-for-granted ipseity or basic selfhood.

A second form of interdependence is exemplified by the relationship between hyperreflexivity-together-with-diminished-self-presence, on one hand, and, on the other, the concomitant mutations in experience of the world termed disturbed grip. One might refer here to a "world-shaping relation" (Taylor 1993) between a certain kind of lived body or corporeally grounded subjectivity, and the experiential world that it constitutes.

Forms of ipseity characterized by hyperreflexivity and diminished self-presence would imply, and in a sense *constitute*, a certain fragmentation, disorganization, and fading in the field of awareness. This is because distracting and normally irrelevant forms of self-experience (think of emerging kinesthetic sensations and inner speech), together with a diminished sense of being a vital witnessing presence, would undermine the coherence, equilibrium, or sheer presence of one's experience of the world—thereby accounting for the "constant leakage of the normal level of reality" to which Artaud referred in the quotation above.

Normal self-presence, with its balance of tacit and explicit, is, in fact, a necessary condition for the experience of appetite, vital energy, and point of orientation—all crucial for allocating significance and associated salience. It is, after all, vital self-presence that normally grounds human motivation and organizes our experiential world in accord with needs and wishes, thereby giving objects their "affordances" (Gibson 2014)—their decisive importance as obstacles, tools, objects of desire, and the like. It is, one might say, a matter of "mattering"—of constituting a lived point of orientation and the correlated pattern of meanings and hierarchies of significance that make for a coherent and significant world. Absent this vital self-presence, with the orientation and sense of reality it anchors, the entire framework for assigning salience is likely to be disrupted—for then there can be no clear sense of goal-directedness, or associated differentiation of means from goal, no strong reason for certain objects to occupy the focus of awareness while others recede, no reason for attention to wend outward toward the world rather than inward toward hyperreflexive awareness of one's own body or processes of thinking (Sass and Parnas 2003: 436).

The intimate relationship between these three aspects of ipseity disturbance illustrates the "intentional intertwining" or "mutual implication by meanings" that Husserl identified as the "essence of conscious life" (1977: 26). The three manifestations of ipseity disturbance likewise illustrate what Merleau-Ponty (2012: 195) described as "internally linked" aspects of experience and behavior that "manifest a single typical structure" and stand in a relationship of "reciprocal expression."

Primary and Secondary Forms of Anomalous Self-Experience

I have pointed out the *interdependence* or even *complementarity* of the three aspects of ipseity disturbance. It is also important to consider a certain heterogeneity *within* each one of these aspects—in particular the distinction between *primary* and *secondary* factors. (This is a largely *diachronic* issue, having to do mainly with developments over time—as opposed to the *synchronic* complementarity just discussed.)[4] Some forms of ipseity disturbance may be more fundamental in a pathogenetic sense (and more neurobiologically determined) in the sense of occurring in a largely passive, automatic, and non-volitional fashion. Others may be more consequential or compensatory, sometimes having a quasi-intentional flavor (albeit with neurobiological correlates). Later I shall describe how an understanding of this primary versus secondary distinction is relevant for a neurobiological account of schizophrenia.

Hyperreflexivity, for example, cannot be reduced to an exaggeration of "introspective" or "top-down" awareness of an essentially intellectual or volitional nature (Sass et al. 2011). The more general phenomenon of hyperreflexivity does *include* such processes, which are more active and might be termed "*reflective*" in nature, but more central to this concept (and likely to be more pathogenetically primary) is "*operative* hyperreflexivity," which involves processes that are generated automatically and passively experienced (re "operative intentionality" versus "act intentionality," see Merleau-Ponty 2012: 18). This more primary, spontaneous "popping-out" of phenomena (e.g. kinesthetic sensations, fragments of inner speech) would engage attention, thereby motivating further, more intense, but pathogenetically secondary forms of attentive scrutiny, including reflective and defensive forms. These latter, secondary forms may well become quasi-automatized. They are likely to be counterproductive, exacerbating abnormal salience and associated fragmentation. Indeed they—like the primary factors—may well be *necessary* (but not sufficient) features for the development of a true schizophrenic syndrome (Sass 2003; 2014a).

Diminished self-presence—decline in the experienced sense of existing as a living and unified subject of awareness or agent of action (Sass and Borda 2015; Sass et al. 2011)—can also occur in both *primary* and *secondary* fashion, the latter involving defensive or even intentional or quasi-intentional processes. For an analogy from outside the schizophrenia spectrum, consider the depersonalization characteristic of depersonalization disorder or PTSD (post-traumatic stress disorder), which is almost universally understood as involving a *defensive*, and in this sense secondary, dissociative reaction to traumatic situations (Noyes and Kletti 1977; Simeon and Abugel 2006).

Depersonalization disorder patients complain of loss of emotions and of feelings of estrangement or detachment from their own mind and body as well as from the external world (Sierra and David 2011). This clinical picture—involving forms of diminished self-presence generally assumed to be defensive in nature—resembles many of the self-anomalies experienced in schizophrenia (Sass et al. 2013b), and may, in fact, offer a close parallel to the secondary dimension of many cases of schizophrenia. This is particularly relevant given recent recognition of the contributory etiological role, in schizophrenia, of external stressors and sources of anxiety, including sexual or physical abuse, cultural dislocation, and social defeat, but also given the unsettling or traumatic experience of psychosis itself, or of derived factors resulting from treatment settings (e.g. physical or pharmacological restraint, coercive inpatient treatments) (Myin-Germeys and van Os 2007; Matheson et al. 2014)—all of which could elicit dissociative reactions as one major form of defense.

---

[4] The synchronic/diachronic distinction largely corresponds with Husserl's distinction between static and genetic phenomenology (the latter including what he termed "motivational" issues) (Husserl 1999).

Volitional (or largely volitional) instances of ipseity disturbance are afforded by the processes of intense introspectionist psychology—which is clearly a secondary form involving *reflective* hyperreflexivity (Sass et al. 2013a) (and which might also be termed hyperreflectivity)—and of Eastern meditation techniques expressly dedicated to appreciating the illusory nature of the self (clearly a secondary form of diminished self-presence). Both processes are accompanied by alteration of one's experience of external reality, including derealization with dimming of the emotional valence of the world. It is clear, then, that *secondary* forms of both hyperreflexivity and diminished self-presence and hyperreflexivity (i.e. "hyperre*flection*"—in these cases *outside* schizophrenia) will cause or be accompanied by mutations not only in self-experience but also in a person's grip on the world. (It is relevant here to consider the potential dangers of meditative practices, which can apparently be stressful and perhaps pathogenic for some vulnerable individuals (see Rocha 2014.)

Research on Anomalous Self-Experience

Empirical Studies

Most empirical investigation of the ipseity-disturbance model in recent years has employed the Examination of Anomalous Self-Experience (EASE) (Parnas et al. 2005), a semi-structured interview format now translated into nine languages. The EASE is a qualitatively rich, fifty-seven-item interview that operationalizes and quantifies the ipseity-disturbance model and is designed to detect sub-psychotic experiences. Many EASE items largely target one or another aspect of the (highly interdependent) ipseity disturbance. Thus Items 2.1 and 2.16 (referring to: Diminished sense of basic self, Diminished initiative) imply diminished self-affection. Items 1.7 and 2.6 (Perceptualization of inner speech or thought, Hyperreflectivity) suggest hyperreflexivity of some kind. Items 1.10 and 2.12 (Inability to discriminate whether an experience is perception/fantasy/memory, Loss of common sense/perplexity) indicate disturbed "hold" or "grip" on the world. Still other EASE items (e.g. 4.1: Confusion with the other) more clearly imply two or more aspects.

There have been numerous studies using the EASE (or EASE-proxies). They are broadly supportive of the ipseity-disturbance hypothesis, showing that disturbance of ipseity or minimal self:

- is far more prominent in schizophrenia than in psychotic disorders outside the schizophrenia spectrum, such as bipolar disorder with psychosis, or than in heterogeneous clinical samples;
- aggregate selectively in those at risk for schizophrenia, either in genetic relatives or in prodromal individuals;
- strongly predicts future onset of schizophrenia spectrum disorders in non-psychotic clinical populations and in those at high risk for psychosis;
- characterizes schizophrenia spectrum disorders independently of the intensity or presence of frank psychotic symptoms, given that it occurs in both psychotic schizophrenia spectrum disorders and schizotypal disorder;

- increases in relation to symptomatic expression along the schizophrenia spectrum in a large genetic linkage sample; and
- correlates with social dysfunction; and also with suicidality (more strongly than do positive symptoms)—thereby suggesting that concern about distorted and diminished forms of basic self-experience may contribute crucially to the particular kind of despair to which such patients are prone. (For supporting references re all the above, see Nelson et al. 2014a; Parnas and Henriksen 2014; Parnas, Raballo, Handest et al. 2011.)

Anecdotal/Theoretical and Quasi-Empirical Studies

I turn now to more theoretically oriented, exploratory studies that use the EASE by relying on quasi-empirical and sometimes anecdotal evidence. These have compared schizophrenic self-alterations with subjective changes in psychotic depression and mania, but also in depersonalization disorder and heightened forms of introspection. Unlike the above-mentioned empirical work, the purpose here is less to establish the specificity of self-disturbance to schizophrenia, or its overall degree, than to clarify the internal structure and pathogenetic role of the ipseity disturbance in the schizophrenia spectrum and elsewhere.

Schizophrenia and Affective Psychoses

As already noted, the classic psychopathological distinction between schizophrenia and affective psychosis is largely supported by EASE results—which show dramatically lower EASE scores in bipolar disorder and in non-schizophrenic psychotic syndromes than in schizophrenia (Parnas and Henriksen 2014). Still, it is well known that affective psychosis *can* sometimes be difficult to distinguish from schizophrenia, and that affect-disorder patients do sometimes manifest anomalies that are at least *reminiscent* of disturbances of ipseity or basic self—including (some would claim) apparent "first-rank symptoms" and other "mood-incongruent" features (Peralta and Cuesta 1999). It seems worthwhile, therefore, to look beyond the quantitative EASE findings cited above in order to consider whether certain kinds of self-disturbance might nevertheless be found in affective disorders.

In an exploratory study, accounts from the literature on phenomenological psychopathology, together with published reports from patients with schizophrenia, mania, and psychotic depression, were examined with respect to the five EASE dimensions: A) cognition and stream of consciousness, B) self-awareness and presence, C) bodily experiences, D) demarcation/transitivism, and E) existential reorientation (Sass and Pienkos 2013a). The methodology had a tripartite/dialectical structure: After considering more obvious *differences* between schizophrenia and affective disorders, some striking *similarities* or *affinities* between the two conditions, including self anomalies, were noted. Finally, more subtle but fundamental *differences* between schizophrenia and mood disorders were explored.

There are in fact some important, self-related anomalies, described in the EASE, that do seem to be reasonably common in mania or psychotic depression and appear in the published accounts. Thus the "feeling of having no feeling," which is common in melancholia (Jaspers 1963; Stanghellini 2004), may resemble EASE 2.4: Diminished presence. Manic feelings of mystic union may resemble EASE 4.5: Other transitivistic phenomena (e.g. "a pervasive feeling of being too open or transparent"). However, what were *not* observed were what seem to be certain more *severe and disruptive* dislocations of self or self/world boundaries: for example, 4.1: Confusion with the other, or solipsistic experiences like 5.3: Feeling as if the subject's experiential field is only extant reality (e.g. "as if only objects in his visual field existed"). Clear instances of EASE 1.2: Loss of thought ipseity—in which the patient feels that "certain thoughts [are] deprived of the tag of mineness"—appeared to be very rare if not absent in mania and psychotic depression. These findings support some little-known but interesting, earlier attempts to refine the "first-rank symptoms of schizophrenia" in more precise, even perhaps pathognomonic terms (Koehler 1979).

Schizophrenia, Depersonalization, and Introspectionism

One may also wonder about affinities and differences between schizophrenia and certain specific conditions, psychopathological or otherwise, that, though *outside the schizophrenia spectrum*, might nevertheless demonstrate, in especially clear form, some key features of altered ipseity—namely, hyperreflexivity or diminished self-presence. Such studies are potentially relevant for the modeling of possible pathogenetic processes.

One study focused on what is perhaps the purest instance of diminished self-affection in psychopathology: depersonalization disorder (Sass et al. 2013b). A sister study focused on what would seem to be a pure instance of hyperreflexivity (or, at least, of hyper*reflectivity*): the method and orientation of self-observation adopted by "introspectionist" psychologists of the early twentieth century such as E. B. Titchener (1912; Sass et al. 2013a). It should be noted that both these conditions would seem to involve largely *secondary* forms of ipseity anomaly. Whereas the self-reflection of introspectionism is volitionally initiated and intentionally driven (a clear example of *reflective* hyperreflexivity or hyper*reflectivity*), the loss-of-self in depersonalization is generally assumed to involve, not *operative* (primary) diminished self-presence, but a goal-directed (albeit not consciously initiated) process of psychological defense.

These exploratory, quasi-empirical studies applied EASE categories either to published descriptions of depersonalization experiences (case reports, autobiographical accounts) or else to published introspectionist reports (experiments recorded by trained introspective observers in psychological experiments). Although the presence of EASE-type experiences in these conditions indicates that ipseity disturbance is not entirely *unique* to schizophrenia, it also suggests that such disturbance might well constitute an important *trouble générateur* in schizophrenia—given that these pure (albeit secondary) forms of hyperreflexivity or diminished self-presence do indeed generate experiences that mimic many of the characteristic experiences of schizophrenia.

Since these comparative studies do not allow for *quantitative* ratings of *average* levels of self-disturbance in these populations, they do not permit us to say whether self-disturbance is *equally prominent* as in schizophrenia. Results do show, however, that the majority of EASE items were in fact easily found in both depersonalization disorder (72% of the items) and the introspection accounts (77%), thereby indicating considerable experiential overlap with the schizophrenia spectrum.

Some of the EASE items found in these two studies were not surprising: diminished self-presence (e.g. EASE 2.1: Diminished sense of basic self) is, after all, an obvious aspect of depersonalization, while alienating self-reflection (e.g. EASE 1.7: Perceptualization of inner speech or thought) might well be expected in the introspectionist stance. There was, however, also considerable crossover: thus, items indicating hyperreflexivity were common in depersonalization patients; items indicating diminished self-affection were common in introspectionist subjects. This crossover is consistent with the interdependence of hyperreflexivity and diminished self-affection postulated by the ipseity-disturbance model.

Also noteworthy was the presence, in both groups, of disturbed cognitive or perceptual "hold" or "grip" on the world, as indicated by, for example, loss of common sense/perplexity (EASE 2.12), disturbed time-experience (EASE 1.14), and attentional disturbances (EASE 1.12). All these findings are consistent, incidentally, with Sass's (1992; 2017) earlier work on "madness and modernism": namely, his demonstration that what he termed the "*hyperreflexivity*" and "*alienation*" of literary and artistic "modernism" (mainly in works of the twentieth-century artistic and intellectual avant-garde) parallel, in important respects, most of the key symptoms of schizophrenia. ("Alienation," in his usage, is closely akin to the depersonalization/derealization of diminished self-affection: Sass 2017: preface.)

It is important, however, to consider not just *affinities* but also *discrepancies*: viz. EASE items that were *not* endorsed in depersonalization or introspection. It is reasonable, after all, to expect significant *differences* between persons whose self-anomalies derive largely from such defensive or quasi-intentional factors (secondary factors), versus those whose abnormalities are likely to be more grounded in involuntary or *operative* ones (primary factors).

Some of the EASE items are quite subtle or may sometimes seem to overlap, rendering interpretation somewhat difficult. Nevertheless, some patterns are suggested. It is noteworthy that EASE items indicating feelings of passivity and alienation (e.g. 1.7: Perceptualization of inner speech or thought, 2.2.2: Distorted first-person perspective involving "constant self-monitoring") and alienation or fading of self and world (2.4: Diminished presence) generally seemed prominent in depersonalization and introspection as well as in schizophrenia (affinities). However, items more suggestive of severe *dislocation, erosion*, or *dissolution* of first-person perspective (such that self and other can seem fused or confused) tended to be absent from either depersonalization or introspection (discrepancies). These latter (the discrepancies) included, for example, EASE 2.9: Identity confusion, 3.9: Mimetic experience, 4.2: Confusion with one's specular image, also 1.16: Discordance between intended expression and the expressed.

The affinities—experiences found in depersonalization and introspection *as well as* schizophrenia—might be considered to be consistent with heightening or recognizing aspects or features of the *normal* self or subject—which does, after all, have its paradoxical aspects. (The philosopher Sartre, e.g. describes normal subjectivity as a "nothingness" that nevertheless experiences itself as distinct from its objects.) By contrast, the latter, discrepancy experiences (found *only* in schizophrenia) may suggest collapse of more "transcendental" or constituting structures of experience: for example, of the very polarity of subject versus object/other, or of the most foundational sense of one's distinctness as a *subject* of experience.

Two Additional Empirical Studies

A Panic Disorder Study

The findings from a recent empirical study of panic disorder patients largely corroborate those from the studies of introspection and depersonalization just discussed—and in this case based on actual EASE interviewing. In the panic disorder study, trained interviewers carried out

EASE interviews with forty-seven hospitalized panic disorder patients and forty-seven healthy controls (Madeira, Carmenates, Costa et al. 2017a, 2017b). A key purpose was to clarify what might—or might not—be specific to the schizophrenia spectrum domain. The study showed that anomalous self-experiences (as defined in the EASE) can indeed be prevalent in panic disorder, including disturbances of self-awareness, body experience, and thought. The distribution of EASE items and sub-items in the panic disorder sample was heterogeneous, however.

The panic disorder sample was found to have a much higher EASE scores than those found in previous EASE studies of bipolar psychosis or of groupings of miscellaneous non-schizophrenia spectrum mental disorders, but lower than scores found in previous EASE studies of schizophrenia spectrum patients. Panic disorder patients showed many common forms of derealization and depersonalization—perhaps involving more "secondary" and defensive psychological processes. They tended however to lack indicators suggesting truly profound distortion of the normal "transcendental" conditions of consciousness (i.e. as concerning the very constitution of subjective life or "basic self") that might constitute a more "primary" factor in schizophrenia. In this sense these subjects appear similar to those with depersonalization disorder or engaged in introspection. Overall, the findings support the ipseity-disturbance or basic self-disturbance model of schizophrenia, while also indicating the need for careful phenomenological exploration of self-anomalies in order to distinguish certain "psychotic-like phenomena" found in a variety of diagnoses (typically involving various forms of depersonalization and derealization) from those that seem characteristic of true psychotic or schizophrenic conditions.

An Empirical Study of the Effects of Introspection

The potential effects of secondary forms of alienating self-consciousness (*reflective hyperreflexivity*) were directly demonstrated in a ground-breaking experimental study from the 1970s. Hunt and Chefurka (1976) subjected healthy people to a state of isolation and inactivity and, using methods modeled on classical introspectionism (e.g. Titchener 1912), directed them to attend to their "immediate subjective state," thereby inducing a reflective form of hyperreflexivity. Resulting experiences closely resembled psychedelic phenomena as well as schizophrenic symptoms: subjects reported sensory hypersensitivity, depersonalization and derealization, perceptual anomalies with "felt portentousness," feeling watched by a room that seemed somehow alive, aloneness and detachment, and ideas of reference, together with "mental daze" involving "cognitive disorganization" or "blank empty awareness." More recently, Petitmengin et al (2009) showed that a reflective focus on normally pre-reflective levels of awareness is associated with diminished agency and body ownership, permeable ego boundaries, and ineffability.

Such findings have implications for the conceptualization of psychological forms of treatment, implications consistent with the self-disorder model of schizophrenia (Škodlar et al. 2013): it suggests, in particular, 1) the possible *danger* of encouraging forms of alienating self-reflection that might have the iatrogenic effect of *exacerbating* hyperreflexivity and alienation (some variants of Cognitive Behavior Therapy (CBT) or Acceptance and Commitment Therapy (ACT) treatment may run this risk), and also 2) the potentially reintegrative and *curative* effects of encouraging engagement with practical action and in non-threatening forms of social interaction.

Summary

We see, then, that schizophrenic self-disorder is a complex phenomenon that requires careful theoretical analysis as well as empirical investigation and comparative study. Overall, the essential disturbances of normal ipseity captured by EASE items seem to be more characteristic of schizophrenia than of most other abnormal conditions. They are not, however, *unique* to schizophrenia, given that some aspects can occur in severe affective disorder and can even be quite prominent also in depersonalization disorder and the introspectionist stance—as well as in an anxiety disorder sample of panic disorder patients; also there are striking analogues from modernist and postmodernist literary and artistic production—cultural domains in which acute self-consciousness and alienation play a central role. We have also seen, however, that the most severe disruptions of self may be more rare or even absent outside schizophrenia.

Neither the concept of ipseity nor that of ipseity disturbance seems, then, to be a purely unitary concept. Ipseity disturbance is neither a simple quantifiable dimension nor some mysterious x-factor that cannot be further analyzed. Ipseity disturbance does have a holistic, gestalt-like quality; also, it may come in degrees. Yet it is also possible, indeed necessary, to consider its structure or component aspects, especially if one seeks to explore its variability and pathogenesis, and also its neural correlates—which is the topic to which we now turn.

NEUROCOGNITIVE DIMENSIONS

Historical Background and Theoretical Concerns

It is important to recognize that the ipseity-disturbance model, and perhaps especially the notion of hyperreflexivity, seems to conflict with the most dominant, *traditional*, overall ways of conceptualizing neurobiological factors in severe psychopathology.

Madness has, since ancient times, largely been conceived as a decline of higher or more rational faculties of mind, including abstraction and self-consciousness, often with concomitant emergence of more primitive, concretistic, or Dionysian/passionate (instinct-dominated) forms of subjective life. This is true of the biological accounts that came into prominence in the nineteenth and early twentieth centuries and have remained highly influential ever since—for example, in the work of Emil Kraepelin on *dementia praecox*, of Kurt Goldstein on concreteness or loss of the "abstract attitude," of Freud on regression to "primary process" thinking, and also in the somewhat earlier writings of Hughlings Jackson and Maudsley (Sass 1992: appendix).

Hughlings Jackson, who was inspired by the evolutionism of his time, saw mental illnesses, both neurologic and psychiatric, as consequences of a disintegration of the higher mental processes involving volition, control, self-consciousness, and reasoning, together with an associated release of impulsive and instinct-driven behavior patterns or automatisms emerging from "lower" or more primitive and emotion-dominated levels of the nervous system. Maudsley, perhaps the most important British psychiatrist of his time, wrote in 1874 of the surprising "mindlessness" that, he believed, exists even "at the back of what looks like very partial mental disorder" (Berrios 1985; Clark 1981: 284–286; Sass 1992: appendix). Such visions—emphasizing deficit and/or primitivity—hardly seem consistent with the forms of hyperconsciousness, derealization, devitalization, or self-alienation emphasized in the ipseity-disturbance model.

A second feature of the traditional reductionistic version of the neurobiological model is the assumption of unidirectional causality and an associated denial or neglect of the pathogenetic relevance of psychological factors. By the end of the nineteenth century this had become practically an official dogma: "It is not our business, it is not in our power," wrote Maudsley, "to explain *psychologically* the origin and nature of any of [the] depraved instincts" manifested in typical cases of insanity. The alienist's purpose was only to observe and classify, since the "explanation, when it comes, will come not from the mental, but from the physical side" (Clark 1981: 271). Such a view tends to deny the importance of secondary factors involving defensive processes motivated by particular subjective experiences, especially those that might sometimes involve volitional or semi-volitional reactions on the patient's part.

The neurobiological abnormalities found in schizophrenia in recent decades have frequently been interpreted in accord with these traditional reductionistic models—that is, as constituting the underlying neural substrate or source of the lowered mental level or diminished higher-level control (suggestive of dementia and sometimes regression) that is ascribed to these conditions. However, careful consideration of the basic self-disturbances described above might inspire one to doubt such views, and to search for a theoretical account more congruent with the clinical realities recognized in phenomenological psychopathology. Interestingly, the most recent neurocognitive models of schizophrenia are, in fact, quite consistent with the ipseity-disorder view—and with the neurocognitive accounts endorsed or suggested in Sass's phenomenological account (1992: appendix; 2017: appendix).

Recent Neurocognitive Models

Consider, for example, "salience dysregulation," the notion that key schizophrenic symptoms involve abnormalities, both neural and psychological, in how particular stimuli emerge into focal awareness. The limbic-system overactivity this involves (which largely implicates hippocampal abnormalities) was associated, not long ago, with a supposed dominance of "primitive" mental tendencies and memories (Andreasen 1986: 39, 43; 1988: 1382), or with "overwhelming instinctual forces" and a loss (reminiscent of Kurt Goldstein's views) of the capacities for abstraction, logical reasoning, and independent judgment (Weinberger 1987: 661–666; Goldberg et al. 1987: 1013). Now, however, it tends to be related—far more plausibly—to forms of hyperconsciousness that can result in a fragmented (and I would say, quasi-surrealist) vision of external reality and a focal awareness of kinesthetic and proprioceptive sensations that implies an alienated experience of the one's own lived body (Nelson et al. 2014c; Sass 1990; Sass 2017: appendix; Sass and Borda 2015).

Another neurocognitive trend found in schizophrenia—the absence of normal prefrontal dominance previously termed "hypofrontality"—was previously associated with a general loss of higher cognitive capacities: with a "dementia of the prefrontal type" akin to Goldstein's concept of "concreteness" or loss of the abstract attitude (Goldberg et al. 1987: 1013). More recent models speak, however, of failure to suppress activation of the Default-Mode Network

(DMN). This suggests that such absence of prefrontal, executive dominance actually subserves forms of consciousness that are free-floating and abstract, hypothetical rather than literal, and introspective rather than practical in nature—all quite consistent with the ipseity-disturbance model and the notion of hyperreflexivity in particular (Sass and Borda 2015; Sass and Byrom 2015b).

Similar points could be made about the "source-monitoring" abnormalities that seem to underlie first-rank symptoms in schizophrenia: rather than conceiving these abnormalities as indicating decline of the capacity for "metarepresentation," as has been suggested (Frith 1992), one may view them as involving hyperreflexive tendencies to take one's own lived body as an object of awareness, and thus to fail to inhabit the body in the tacit and automatic manner that is required for normal forms of real-world oriented activity (Nelson et al. 2014b).

Still another approach to schizophrenia focuses on abnormalities of brain laterality. Here too, much of the evidence does not, in fact, favor the traditional irrationalist or reductionistic models previously proffered, but points rather to the diminished capacity for spontaneous and context-bound forms of cognition (often accompanied by a compensatory reliance on inappropriately deliberate or rational faculties) that occurs with a relative decline of right-hemisphere activation or dominance (McGilchrist 2009).

We see, then, that recent neurobiological research on schizophrenia and current models does not implicate the decline of intelligence, rationality, or self-conscious awareness—or the regression or instinct-domination—assumed by many traditional theories. The evidence is actually more compatible with theoretical models postulating dysfunctional hyper-awareness, a loss of normal spontaneity or embeddedness, or even, at times, a kind of hypertrophied rationality divorced from lived body and practical context.

The key to explaining schizophrenia does not, however, seem likely to be contained in any single neurocognitive theory. Indeed it is probable that schizophrenia is a heterogeneous illness: not a disease entity in which all cases have the same etiology, but more of a final common pathway (itself somewhat heterogeneous) to which a variety of different causal factors—or combinations of factors—may lead.

Primary and Secondary Factors

Of particular importance for neurocognitive modeling of schizophrenic pathogenesis is the distinction between "primary" versus "secondary" factors. One needs to ask, for example, whether certain forms of hyperreflexivity or diminished self-presence or disturbed "grip," for instance, might have a more primary, basic, perhaps affliction-like quality, and be prominent from early in life, whereas other forms—more reactive, reflective, or even quasi-volitional in nature—might develop later as *sequelae* or defensive reactions to these more foundational problems (Sass 2017: appendix).

It is noteworthy that most research on the above-mentioned neuro-level correlates has concerned patients whose disorder is well established, and shows mainly that the neural correlates *accompany* the psychological trends or symptoms in question. This leaves open the possibility that the psychological trends just discussed—such as hyper-scrutiny (associated with salience dysregulation) or withdrawal from an action-orientation (associated with abnormal default-mode or DMN activation)—could be occurring in a largely "secondary" way, perhaps as a consequence of, or defensive reaction to, some more basic disruption of experiential life.[5] There is, in any case, a related but alternative hypothesis that can perhaps claim stronger evidence in support of its potentially "primary" pathogenetic status. This is the notion of disturbed "perceptual integration," which has been found in schizophrenia patients and also (to a milder degree) in children, still relatively normal, who are at high risk for, or will later develop, schizophrenia spectrum disorders (Borda and Sass 2015; Gamma et al. 2014; Parnas et al. 1996; Postmes et al. 2014; Silverstein and Keane 2011).

Perceptual integration refers to the synthesizing of information from different sense modalities, such as visual and auditory, and perhaps especially between interoceptive and exteroceptive processes, such as kinesthesia/proprioception and visual perception. Disturbance of perceptual integration (perceptual *dys-integration*, we might call it) would be consistent with the presence of "basic symptoms"—the subtle but persistent disruptions of perceptual, motoric, affective, and cognitive life found in people prone to schizophrenia, and which can be interpreted as involving subtle disturbances of self-experience (Klosterkötter et al. 2001; Schultze-Lutter 2009). Disruption of this integration may be related to the disturbed "connectivity" of various brain networks, which is certainly characteristic of schizophrenia (Brent et al. 2014; Manoliu et al. 2013).[6]

It is not difficult to conceptualize why successful perceptual integration would be crucial in the development of normal minimal or basic self-experience (*ipseity*): such integration contributes not only to the unity of object perception but also to the (closely related) sense of being grounded as a living corporeal presence or organizing viewpoint on the world. Indeed, the neural circuitry of perceptual integration might well constitute, in large measure, the neural foundation of basic self-experience and the capacity to differentiate self from other (Brent et al. 2014).[7]

It seems plausible, then, that perceptual dys-integration might underlie foundational, primary, or "operative" forms of disruptive hyperreflexivity, diminished self-presence, and disturbed cognitive/perceptual "grip" on the world, together with associated "basic symptoms" (Borda and Sass 2015). Other forms, more reactive or defensive in nature, might come into prominence somewhat later in the causal sequence (Sass and Borda 2015). The forms of hyperreflexivity or diminished self-presence associated, for instance, with withdrawal from practical activity, hypervigilance, or diminished spontaneity might be largely reactive or defensive, more associated with shifting attitudes or orientations to experience, and perhaps more variable in nature (albeit also grounded in more intrinsic neurocognitive abnormalities mentioned above). It seems obvious, after all, that each of the psychological orientations

---

[5] We should not, however, *rule out* a more causally fundamental status, which is entirely possible. Some of these psychological tendencies and neural correlates discussed above sometimes do occur independently of, and prior to, psychotic episodes (e.g. Winton-Brown et al. 2014); each could involve some inborn or other basic propensity. On the close intertwining of defenses with temperamental or cognitive dispositions, see Shapiro, *Neurotic Styles* (1965).

[6] This dysconnectivity may involve abnormalities in medial/lateral prefrontal cortex, or perhaps insular cortex—which plays an important role in integrating interoceptive and exteroceptive perceptual processes as well as in vital emotions and desires that affect the lived body and sense of core self.

[7] In one study (Lenggenhager, Tadi, Metzinger et al. 2007), participants subjected to "multisensory conflict" (conflicting visual and somatosensory input) had a schizophrenialike experience, feeling "as if a virtual body seen in front of them was their own body and mislocaliz[ing] themselves toward the virtual body, to a position outside their bodily borders."

associated with the above-mentioned specific hypotheses (withdrawal, hypervigilance, diminished spontaneity) could at least be exacerbated or diminished in accord with willful, quasi-intentional, or defensive actions or attitudinal orientations on the part of the subject; in this sense they are best conceived not as pure defect states but as existing in a gray zone between act and affliction.

One or more of these latter, perhaps secondary factors (which could themselves be potentially overlapping) might be *necessary* for the development of schizophrenia, but perhaps not *sufficient* in the absence of a more fundamental disturbance of basic integration and selfhood. It should be noted, however, that although perceptual dys-integration may well be a necessary factor, it alone *also* seems unlikely to provide a *sufficient* condition—given that it can be found in other conditions and does not always lead to schizophrenia. Some combination of factors—but perhaps not always the same *balance* of factors—is probably required for that (admittedly) rather heterogeneous "final common pathway" that we term "schizophrenia."

Primary factors relevant to self-disturbance might well be more decisive in so-called "poor premorbid" patients or cases with early or "insidious" onset, who are often dominated by negative symptoms and "nonparanoid" features. Secondary factors might be more crucial for cases with more acute onset and better premorbid functioning, and with more prominent positive and perhaps especially dissociation-like symptoms, as well as for acute exacerbations later in the course of illness. (For discussion of two pathways to psychosis, one more endogenous, the other trauma-driven, see Kilcommons and Morrison 2005.)

It is well known that symptoms of schizophrenia can fluctuate dramatically, sometimes in association with the patient's personal attitude or orientation (Bleuler 1982) but at other times having a more random quality (see Matthysse et al. 1999 re *dialipsis*). It is difficult to square such variability with many current cognitive models of schizophrenia, whether modular or molar.

One advantage of the ipseity-disturbance hypothesis is that it is more compatible with this fluctuating nature of schizophrenia symptoms, across time and situation. "Self-affection" is akin to an affect-state in which the sense of vital existence may wax or wane in conjunction with one's prevailing perspective, orientation, or attitude toward the world. The diverse forms of self-consciousness captured by "hyperreflexivity" would be similarly variable, given they involve forms of attention, which obviously shift and transform. The self is not, after all, something one just *happens* to be aware of: its existence is inextricable from processes of self-awareness (implicit and otherwise) *by which* it is constituted. It is understandable, then, that ipseity might be unstable in schizophrenia, at times relatively stable but at other times turning "wobbly" in the words of one patient, whose "vantage point," what she called the "solid center from which one experiences reality," would become "fuzzy" at times, "break[ing] up like a bad radio signal" or eroding "like a sand castle . . . sliding away in the receding surf" (Saks 2007). A fundamental or operative vulnerability would exist in tight interaction with more secondary processes that are more variable over time.

There is need for research that explores the variable nature of various neurocognitive and neurobiological trends. Such research would manipulate and investigate the effects of changing mental orientation or stance (e.g. of adopting a withdrawn/introspective versus practical focus, of scrutiny versus a spontaneous orientation) in both schizophrenic and normal subjects. The purpose would be to determine the extent to which various phenomena—including the anomalous experiences described in the EASE, as well as such cognitive abnormalities as salience dysregulation, perceptual fragmentation, mind-wandering, and disturbed sense of agency (or their milder equivalents), *together, in some studies, with their neural correlates*—might alter in accord with such changes. Here it would be useful to supplement the EASE, which focuses on *self*-experience, with semi-structured interview studies that concern alterations of *world*-experience—including mutations of time, space, other persons, and general atmosphere. These latter alterations are targeted in the recently published, sister interview format called the EAWE: Examination of Anomalous World Experience (Sass, Pienkos, Škodlar et al. 2017; Sass, Pienkos, and Fuchs 2017; see also Sass and Pienkos 2013b; Sass 2014a).

It is entirely plausible that such alterations would occur. As noted above, past studies already show that mere adoption of an intensely introspective/detached orientation toward experience, on the part of normal subjects, can bring about certain "psychedelic" or psychotic-like forms of perceptual experience akin to what occurs in schizophrenia (see Research on Anomalous Self-Experience section re Hunt and Chefurka 1976). It would be surprising if neuro-level abnormalities were not also produced, at least to some degree, by shifting attitudes or orientations on the subject's part. In this respect such abnormalities may be subject to (though not entirely the product of) varying, defensive, or even intentional or quasi-intentional factors—of the kind that are inherent in depersonalization defenses, introspectionism, and perhaps forms of meditative practice.

The research I am recommending should not, of course, *dichotomize* act versus affliction, but rather recognize the ambiguous, interwoven nature of actual psychological life in both pathological and normal contexts. Such research could help to clarify the complex syntheses of primary and secondary factors in the pathogenesis of schizophrenia. Its potential relevance for devising treatments to alleviate abnormal tendencies could be considerable.

Concluding Remark

This proliferation of theoretical possibilities may seem excessive to some *devotés* of the scientific principle of Occam's razor. But Occam's razor favors the simplest formulation *that is adequate to the phenomena to be explained.* An adequate model of schizophrenia may need to postulate shared disturbances of core-self experience that nevertheless follow a variety of distinct pathways, and occur in various forms. Such a model is preferable to unidimensional alternatives, given its ability to account for the distinctive yet highly diverse and varying types of experiential and neurocognitive abnormalities that have been documented in research on schizophrenia. It may be that just this sort of theoretical labor is what is required if we hope to emerge from the relative stagnation—now widely recognized (e.g. Hyman 2012)—into which research on schizophrenia has fallen.

Bibliography

Andreasen N. (1986). "Is Schizophrenia a Temperolimbic Disease?" In N. Andreasen (ed.), *Can Schizophrenia be Localized in the Brain?* pp. 37–52. Washington D.C.: American Psychiatric Press.

Andreasen N. (1988). "Brain Imaging: Applications in Psychiatry." *Science* 239: 1381–1388.

Artaud A. (1965). *Artaud Anthology*. San Francisco: City Lights Books.

Artaud A. (1976). *Antonin Artaud: Selected Writings*, ed. S. Sontag. Berkeley: University of California Press.

Berrios G. E. (1985). "Positive and Negative Symptoms and Jackson." *Archives of General Psychiatry* 42: 95–97.

Blankenburg W. (1971). *Der Verlust der Naturlichen Selbstverstandlichkeit: Ein Beitrag zur Psychopathologie Symptomarmer Schizophrenien*. Stuttgart: Ferdinand Enke Verlag.

Bleuler M. (1982). "Inconstancy of Schizophrenic Language and Symptoms." *Behavioral and Brain Sciences* 5: 591.

Borda J.-P. and Sass L. (2015). "Phenomenology and Neurobiology of Self Disorder in Schizophrenia: Primary Factors." *Schizophrenia Research* 169: 464–473.

Brent B. K., Seidman L. J., Thermenos H. W., Holt D. J., and Keshavan M. S. (2014). "Self-Disturbances as a Possible Premorbid Indicator of Schizophrenia Risk: A Neurodevelopmental Perspective." *Schizophrenia Research* 152: 73–80.

Clark M. J. (1981). "The Rejection of Psychological Approaches to Mental Disorder in Late Nineteenth-Century British Psychiatry." In A. Scull (ed.), *Madhouses, Mad-Doctors, and Madmen: The Social History of Psychiatry in the Victorian Era*, pp. 271–312. Philadelphia: University of Pennsylvania Press.

Fink E. (1995). *The Sixth Cartesian Meditation: The Idea of a Transcendental Theory of Method*. Bloomington: Indiana University Press.

Frith C. D. (1992). *The Cognitive Neuropsychology of Schizophrenia*. East Sussex: Psychology Press.

Gallagher S. (2011). "Introduction: A Diversity of Selves." In S. Gallagher (ed.), *The Oxford Handbook of the Self*, pp. 1–30. Oxford: Oxford University Press.

Gamma F., Goldstein J., Seidman L., Fitzmaurice G., Tsuang M., and Buka S. (2014). "Early Intermodal Integration in Offspring of Parents with Psychosis." *Schizophrenia Bulletin* 40: 992–1000.

Gibson J. J. (2014). *The Ecological Approach to Visual Perception: Classic Edition*. New York: Psychology Press.

Goldberg T. E., Weinberger D. R., Berman K. F., Pliskin N. H., and Podd M. H. (1987). "Further Evidence for Dementia of the Prefrontal Type in Schizophrenia." *Archives of General Psychiatry* 44: 1008–1014.

Gurwitsch A. (1964). *The Field of Consciousness*. Pittsburgh: Duquesne University Press.

Henriksen M. G., Raballo A., and Parnas J. (2015). "The Pathogenesis of Auditory Verbal Hallucinations in Schizophrenia." *Philosophy, Psychiatry, and Psychology* 22(3): 165–181.

Hunt H. T. and Chefurka C. M. (1976). "A Test of the Psychedelic Model of Altered States of Consciousness." *Archives of General Psychiatry* 33: 867–876.

Husserl E. (1977). *Phenomenological Psychology: Lectures, Summer Semester, 1925*, trans. J. Scanlon. The Hague: Martinus Nijhoff.

Husserl E. (1999). "Static and Genetic Phenomenological Method." In E. Husserl, *The Essential Husserl: Basic Writings in Transcendental Phenomenology*, ed. D. Welton, pp. 316–321. Bloomington: Indiana University Press (an excerpt from Husserl's *Analyses Concerning Passive and Active Synthesis*).

Hyman S. E. (2012). "Psychiatric Drug Discovery: Revolution Stalled." *Science Translational Medicine*. 4(155): 155cm11.

Jaspers K. (1963). *General Psychopathology*. Chicago: University of Chicago Press.

Kilcommons A. M. and Morrison A. P. (2005). "Relationships Between Trauma and Psychosis: An Exploration of Cognitive and Dissociative Factors." *Acta Psychiatrica Scandinavica* 112: 351–359.

Klosterkötter J., Hellmich M., Steinmyer E. M., and Schultze-Lutter F. (2001). "Diagnosing Schizophrenia in the Initial Prodromal Phase." *Archives of General Psychiatry* 58: 158–164.

Koehler K. (1979). "First Rank Symptoms of Schizophrenia: Questions Concerning Clinical Boundaries." *British Journal of Psychiatry* 134: 236–248.

Kraepelin E. (1971). *Dementia Praecox and Paraphrenia*, trans. R. M. Barclay. Huntington: Robert E. Krieger.

Lenggenhager B., Tadi T. Metzinger T., et al. (2007). "*Video ergo sum*: Manipulating Bodily Self-Consciousness." *Science* 317: 1096–1099.

Madeira L., Carmenates S., Costa C., Linhares L., Stanghellini G., Figueira M. L., and Sass L. (2017a). "Basic-Self Disturbances Beyond Schizophrenia: Discrepancies and Affinities in Panic Disorder. An Empirical Clinical Study." *Psychopathology* 50(2): 157–168. doi: 10.1159/000457803

Madeira L., Carmenates S., Costa C., Linhares L., Stanghellini G., Figueira M. L., and Sass L. (2017b). "Rejoinder to Commentary: 'Panic, Self-Disorder, and EASE Research: Methodological Considerations." *Psychopathology* 50(3): 228–230. doi:10.1159/000477371

Manoliu A., Riedl V., Doll A., Bauml J. G., Muhlau M., Schwerthoffer D., Scherr M., Zimmer C., Forstl H., Bauml J., Wohlschlager A., Koch K., and Sorg C. (2013). "Insular Dysfunction Reflects Altered Between-Network Connectivity and Severity of Negative Symptoms in Schizophrenia During Psychotic Remission." *Frontiers in Human Neuroscience* 7: 216.

Matheson S. L., Shepherd A. M., Pinchbeck R. M., et al. (2014). "Childhood Adversity in Schizophrenia: A Systematic Meta-Analysis." *Psychological Medicine* 43: 225–238.

Matthysse S., Levy D. L., Wu Y., Rubin D. B., and Holman P. (1999). "Intermittent Degradation in Performance in Schizophrenia." *Schizophrenia Research* 40: 131–146.

McGilchrist I. (2009). *The Master and his Emissary: The Divided Brain and the Making of the Modern World*. New Haven: Yale University Press.

Merleau-Ponty M. (2012). *The Phenomenology of Perception*. trans. D. A. Landes, 1945. London: Routledge (French pagination, in margins, cited above).

Myin-Germeys I. and van Os, J. (2007). "Stress-Reactivity in Psychosis: Evidence for an Affective Pathway to Psychosis." *Clinical Psychology Review* 27: 409–424.

Nelson B., Parnas J., and Sass L. (2014a). "Disturbance of Minimal Self (Ipseity) in Schizophrenia: Clarification and Current Status." *Schizophrenia Bulletin* 40: 479–482.

Nelson B., Whitford T. J., Lavoie S., and Sass L. (2014b). "What are the Neurocognitive Correlates of Basic Self-Disturbance in Schizophrenia?: Integrating Phenomenology and Neurocognition. Part 1 (Source Monitoring Deficits)." *Schizophrenia Research* 152: 12–19.

Nelson B., Whitford T. J., Lavoie S., and Sass L. (2014c). "What are the Neurocognitive Correlates of Basic Self-Disturbance in Schizophrenia?: Integrating Phenomenology and Neurocognition. Part 2 (Aberrant Salience)." *Schizophrenia Research* 152: 20–27.

Noyes R. and Kletti R. (1977). "Depersonalization in Response to Life-Threatening Danger." *Comprehensive Psychiatry* 18: 375–384.

Parnas J., Bovet P., and Innocenti G. M. (1996). "Schizophrenic Trait Features, Binding, and Cortico-Cortical Connectivity: A Neurodevelopmental Pathogenetic Hypothesis." *Neurology Psychiatry and Brain Research* 4: 185–196.

Parnas J., Moller P., Kircher T., Thalbitzer J., Jansson L., Handest P., and Zahavi D. (2005). "Ease: Examination of Anomalous Self-Experience." *Psychopathology* 38: 236–258.

Parnas J., Raballo A., Handest P., Jansson L., Vollmer-Larsen A., and Saebye D. (2011). "Self-experience in the Early Phases of Schizophrenia: 5-Year Follow-Up of the Copenhagen Prodromal Study." *World Psychiatry* 10: 200–204.

Parnas J. and Sass L. (2011). "The Structure of Self-Consciousness in Schizophrenia." In S. Gallagher (ed.), *The Oxford Handbook of the Self*, pp. 521–546. Oxford: Oxford University Press.

Parnas J. and Henriksen M. G. (2014). "Disordered Self in the Schizophrenia Spectrum: A Clinical and Research Perspective." *Harvard Review of Psychiatry* 22: 251–265.

Peralta V. and Cuesta M. J. (1999). "Diagnostic Significance of Schneider's First-Rank Symptoms in Schizophrenia: Comparative Study Between Schizophrenic and Non-Schizophrenic Psychotic Disorders." *British Journal of Psychiatry* 174: 243–248.

Petitmengin C., Bitbol M., and Nissou J. M. (2009). "Listening from Within." *Journal of Consciousness Studies* 16: 252–284.

Postmes L., Sno H. N., Goedhart S., van der Stel J., Heering H. D, and de Haan L. (2014). "Schizophrenia as a Self-Disorder Due to Perceptual Incoherence." *Schizophrenia Research* 152: 41–50.

Rocha T. (2014). "The Dark Night of the Soul." *The Atlantic*, June 25.

Saks E. (2007). *The Center Cannot Hold*. New York: Hyperion.

Sass L. (1990). "Surrealism and Schizophrenia: Reflections on Modernism, Regression, and the Schizophrenic Break." *New Ideas in Psychology* 8: 275–298.

Sass L. (1992). *Madness and Modernism: Insanity in the Light of Modern Art, Literature, and Thought*. New York: Basic Books.

Sass L. (2003). "'Negative Symptoms', Schizophrenia, and the Self." *International Journal of Psychology and Psychological Therapy* 3: 153–180.

Sass L. (2004). "Schizophrenia: A Disturbance of the Thematic Field." In L. Embree (ed.), *Gurwitsch's Relevancy for Cognitive Science*, pp. 59–78. New York: Springer.

Sass L. (2014a). "Self-Disturbance and Schizophrenia: Structure, Specificity, Pathogenesis (Current Issues, New Directions)." *Schizophrenia Research* 152: 5–11.

Sass L. (2014b). "Explanation and Description in Phenomenological Psychopathology." *Journal of Psychopathology* 20: 366–376.

Sass L. (2017). *Madness and Modernism: Insanity in the Light of Modern Art, Literature, and Thought—Revised Edition*. Oxford: Oxford University Press.

Sass L. and Parnas J. (2003). "Schizophrenia, Consciousness, and the Self." *Schizophrenia Bulletin* 29: 427–444.

Sass L., Parnas J., and Zahavi D. (2011). "Phenomenological Psychopathology and Schizophrenia: Contemporary Approaches and Misunderstandings." *Philosophy, Psychiatry, and Psychology* 18: 1–23.

Sass L. and Pienkos E. (2013a). "Varieties of Self Experience: A Comparative Phenomenology of Melancholia, Mania, and Schizophrenia, Part I." *Journal of Consciousness Studies* 20: 103–130.

Sass L. and Pienkos E. (2013b). "Space, Time, and Atmosphere: A Comparative Phenomenology of Melancholia, Mania, and Schizophrenia, Part II." *Journal of Consciousness Studies* 20: 131–152.

Sass L., Pienkos E., and Nelson B. (2013a). "Introspection and Schizophrenia: A Comparative Investigation of Anomalous Self Experiences." *Consciousness and Cognition* 22: 853–867.

Sass L., Pienkos E., Nelson B., and Medford N. (2013b). "Anomalous Self-Experience in Depersonalization and Schizophrenia: A Comparative Investigation." *Consciousness and Cognition* 22: 430–441.

Sass L. and Borda J.-P. (2015). "Phenomenology and Neurobiology of Self Disorder in Schizophrenia: Secondary Factors." *Schizophrenia Research* 169: 474–482.

Sass L. and Byrom G. (2015a). "Phenomenological and Neurocognitive Perspectives on Delusion. *World Psychiatry* 14: 164–173.

Sass L. and Byrom G. (2015b). "Self-Disturbance and the Bizarre: On Incomprehensibility in Schizophrenic Delusions." *Psychopathology* 48: 293–300.

Sass L., Pienkos E., and Fuchs T. (eds.). (2017). "Special Topic Issue: Other Worlds: The Examination of Anomalous World Experience (EAWE)." *Psychopathology* 50(1): 3–104.

Sass L., Pienkos E., Škodlar B., Stanghellini G., Fuchs T., Parnas J., and Jones N. (2017). "EAWE: Examination of Anomalous World Experience." *Psychopathology* 50(1): 10–54.

Schultze-Lutter F. (2009). "Subjective Symptoms of Schizophrenia in Research and the Clinic: The Basic Symptoms Concept." *Schizophrenia Bulletin* 35: 5–8.

Shapiro D. (1965). *Neurotic Styles*. New York: Basic Books.

Sierra M. and David A. S. (2011). "Depersonalization: A Selective Impairment of Self-Awareness." *Consciousness and Cognition* 20: 99–108.

Silverstein S. M. and Keane B. P. (2011). "Perceptual Organization Impairment in Schizophrenia and Associated Brain Mechanisms; Review of Research from 2005–2010." *Schizophrenia Bulletin* 37: 690–699.

Simeon D. and Abugel J. (2006). *Feeling Unreal: Depersonalization Disorder and the Loss of Self.* New York: Oxford University Press.

Škodlar B., Henriksen M. G., Sass L., Nelson B., and Parnas J. (2013). "Cognitive-Behavioral Therapy for Schizophrenia: A Critical Evaluation of its Theoretical Framework from a Clinical-Phenomenological Perspective." *Psychopathology* 46(4): 249–265.

Stanghellini G. (2004). *Disembodied Spirits and Deanimated Bodies*. Oxford: Oxford University Press.

Taylor C. (1993). "Engaged Agency and Background in Heidegger." In C. Guignon (ed.), *The Cambridge Companion to Heidegger*. pp. 317–336. Cambridge: Cambridge University Press.

Titchener E. B. (1912). "Description vs Statement of Meaning." *American Journal of Psychology* 23: 165–182.

Weinberger D. R. (1987). "Implications of Normal Brain Development for the Pathogenesis of Schizophrenia." *Archives of General Psychiatry* 44: 660–669.

Winton-Brown T., Howes O., Stone J., et al. (2014). "Dissecting Dopamine, Salience, and the Risk of Psychosis." *Early Intervention in Psychiatry* 8: 37.

CHAPTER 64

THE LIFE-WORLD OF PERSONS WITH MOOD DISORDERS

THOMAS FUCHS

INTRODUCTION

PHENOMENOLOGICAL psychopathology has a long tradition of describing and analyzing the subjective experience of affective disorders, in particular, melancholic depression. These analyses have mostly focused on dimensions such temporality, spatiality, embodiment, personality, or identity (Straus 1928; Gebsattel 1928; Tellenbach 1980; Kraus 1987; Stanghellini 2004; Fuchs 2000, 2005). However, the dimension of time has always played a particular role, pointing to the close connection of mood disorders with the temporality of existence. This chapter is based on the assumption that disturbances of temporal experience may indeed be considered the foundational disturbances of affective disorders, even if they equally manifest themselves in the patient's bodily, spatial, and intersubjective experience.

The connection between affectivity and temporality has already been discussed in 'The Experience of Time and its Disorders' (Fuchs, this volume, chapter 49). The major results may be summarized as follows:

- On the most basic level, the temporal continuity of conscious experience is established by the linking of retention, presentation, and protention (cf. Husserl's analysis of internal time-consciousness, Husserl 1969). However, lived time is also constituted by the dynamics of *conation*—that means drive, striving, urge, or impulse—which are generally directed toward the future (e.g. toward the fulfillment of thirst, hunger, sexual desire, or other goals of drives). Conation is also influenced by feelings of *bodily vitality* such as freshness, vigor, or agitation on the one hand, and tiredness, exhaustion, or apathy on the other hand. These basic bodily states are equally connected to variations of lived time (as visible, e.g. in agitation versus lethargy).
- *Mood states and existential feelings* (Ratcliffe 2008) do not only permeate and color the experiential field, but always have a temporal dimension as well. Thus, boredom results from

a mismatch between drive and interest on the one hand, and lacking possibilities for attention and action on the other. As is well known, boredom makes time-conscious or explicit as a sluggish flow. Furthermore, melancholy or nostalgia are moods related to a painfully missed past, whereas longing is related to a desired future. On the contrary, in diffuse anxiety the future is felt as an impending danger or doom. Finally, elation and euphoria are accompanied by an acceleration, dysphoria, and depression by a retardation of lived time.

- *Emotions* are linked to temporality as well. Thus, desire, hope, or fear are directed toward an anticipated future; in surprise, fright, or shame the present is experienced in an intrusive way, whereas sadness, grief, or guilt feelings are bound to the past. Since emotions are always related to the self and its maintenance (Depraz 1998; Slaby and Stephan 2008), they manifest the general structure of "concern" (*Sorge*), to use Heidegger's term, as the fundamental condition of human existence in time. Moreover, from an embodied point of view, emotions (from the Latin *e-movere*, "to move outward") are kinetic, dynamic forces, that means motivations for movement and action that project the person toward the world and the future (Sheets-Johnstone 1999; Slaby et al. 2013; Fuchs 2013b; Fuchs and Koch 2014).

- Finally, the intersubjective dimension of affectivity may also be conceived in terms of temporality, namely as attunement or *synchronization* and "detuning" or *desynchronization*. On the one hand, emotions and mood states may be shared with others in intersubjective presence or *contemporality* (Minkowski 1933/1970; Fuchs 2013a). This is the case in pre-reflective intercorporeality, bodily resonance, empathy, or in the flow of joint action, usually accompanied by a basic feeling of being attuned and connected with others. On the other hand, *acceleration* of one's own time as in hypo-manic or manic agitation leads to a desynchronization from others, expressed in feelings of impatience, irritation, or aggression. On the contrary, grief or unresolved guilt feelings are equivalent to a partial desynchroniziation in the sense of *retardation* or remanence. This culminates in depression as a loss of basic contemporality, experienced as a feeling of disconnectedness, exclusion, and isolation from others.

As can be seen, a phenomenological approach to affectivity regards conation, mood, existential feelings, and emotions as a fundamental dimension of existence, which crucially influences the experience of a person's present, past, and future as well as intersubjective temporality. This becomes particularly obvious in mood disorders such as depression and mania.

THE PHENOMENOLOGY OF DEPRESSION

Focusing on severe or melancholic depression, I will give a two-level account which describes it on the one hand as the result of an intersubjective desynchronization, and on a deeper level as a disturbance of conation or "vital inhibition."

Vulnerability and Premorbid Situation

Phenomenological psychopathology has not only conceptualized depression itself as a disturbance of lived time—I only mention the most significant contributions by von Gebsattel

1928; Minkowski 1933/1970; Straus 1947; Binswanger 1960; Tellenbach 1980; Tatossian 1983; Fuchs 2001, 2013a; Gallagher 2012; Stanghellini 2004; and Stanghellini et al. 2017. Phenomenology has also elaborated the peculiar personality structure and form of existence which creates a disposition to the illness. The most important contribution consists without doubt in Tellenbach's concept of the "Melancholic Type" (*Typus Melancholicus*) which is marked by traits such as conscientiousness, orderliness, rigidity, overadaptation to social norms, and by dependent and symbiotic tendencies in interpersonal relationships (Tellenbach 1980; Kraus 1987). This type has been found in numerous studies to be the most frequent variant of premorbid personalities in patients with major depression (v. Zerrsen and Pössl 1990; Mundt et al. 1997; Kronmüller et al. 2002; Stanghellini et al. 2006). Its structure may also be interpreted in terms of an *existential vulnerability* (Fuchs 2013c): The Melancholic Type is particularly sensitive with regard to situations consisting in inevitable transitions, role changes, and losses—for example, divorce, bereavement, loss of employment, but also becoming a parent, a demanding promotion in one's job, children moving out of the home, retirement, etc. In addition, the patients try to avoid by all means any situation where guilt or falling short of one's duties become inescapable. Overall, they shrink back from confrontation with the basic conditions of existence like decision, guilt, separation, isolation, and finiteness.

Thus, it is ultimately the unavoidable progress and transience of life itself which for the Melancholic Type becomes an existential threat. Being implicitly aware of this vulnerability, the patients seek to protect themselves by what may be called *existential defence mechanisms* (Fuchs 2013c). Trying to avoid fundamental changes, holding oneself within the boundaries of the established order, clinging to close relationships, and avoiding any guilt—all this has the deeper sense of a protection against the transitoriness, but also the inevitable "mineness" and loneliness of an autonomous existence. This is why the Melancholic Type strives for continuous harmony, social concord, and punctual delivery of duties. He must owe nothing to anyone since his identity essentially depends on the role which society has assigned to him, not on self-determination and autonomy (Kraus 1987). However, sooner or later this rigid defence structure proves precarious. If individuals with such a personality structure once fall short of their duties, if they experience unjustified rejections or the loss of significant others, then their world literally collapses. They find themselves in what Karl Jaspers (1925) called a *limit situation*, that means, a situation where one's fundamental expectations and assumptions about oneself and the world prove illusory.

Importantly, Tellenbach already characterized the premorbid or triggering situation of depression typical for the Melancholic Type in temporal terms, namely by the notions of "remanence" (lagging behind one's duties or demands) and "inclusion" (rigid fixation on established orders or relationships, unability to transcend one's narrow role identity). Such situations may also be conceived as a *desynchronization* (Fuchs 2001): Unable to hold pace with the course of events and the demands of the situation, the patient falls back in relation to the shared or intersubjective time. An inability to grieve plays an important role for this desynchronization: giving up familiar role patterns and attachments seems too threatening or too painful so that the patient remains stuck in the past. The depressive illness may thus be regarded as resulting from a limit situation which overburdens the patient's capacities of coping, adaptation, and change.

However, it should also be noted that the proportion of Melancholic Types in depressed patients seems to have been decreasing over the last three decades, whereas other, in particular narcissistic personalities, now play a far greater role (Ronningstam 1996; Schröder 2005; Twenge and Campbell 2008; Twenge and Foster 2010). Their depression, in contrast, is mainly caused by a failure of achievement, on the background of too high aspirations regarding individual performance and success. Feelings of guilt are increasingly replaced by feelings of insufficiency and also by hypochondriac fears regarding one's own bodily performance. With these patients, depression results not from an experience of loss or a sense of guilt, but from the perceived discrepancy between a culturally inflated self-image, social demands on achievement, and the individual's actual self-realization or performance. Thus, a desynchronization or lagging behind is found here as well, but the major existential threat is no longer guilt or separation as in the Melancholic Type, but the narcissistic *shame* that arises from missing one's goals (Ehrenberg 2010: 128ff.).

Regardless which personality type with its specific vulnerability is taken into account, the notion of desynchronization also points to the social conditions of an ever accelerated society which favors a "remanence" of individuals and, with its demands on continous increase in performance and self-optimization, may lead to a "weariness of the self" (Ehrenberg 2010). Here lies one of the major origins of disorders which were formerly called "exhaustion depression," but now have received the less stigmatizing designation of "burn-out syndrome." They are marked by a spiral of excessive demands on oneself and growing psychophysical exhaustion. At the beginning we usually find an extension of working time, with the goal to keep pace with external demands. This results in a loss of the daily structure and the natural rhythms of exertion and regeneration. Despite ever more straining their will, the patients experience increasing inefficiency, followed by frustration, inner emptiness, and fatigue to the point of a psychophysical breakdown and finally of full-blown depression. A case example may illustrate this:

> A 34-year-old patient fell ill with a severe depression. Having completed his business studies and an MBA with top degrees, he had signed up with a prestigious international management consultancy and worked 60 to 80 hours a week, thus more and more losing his friends except his girlfriend whom he only met on weekends. For a project in the USA he commuted between the continents, allowing himself no more than 5 hours sleep per night. When he nevertheless received a "non-sufficient" performance assessment by his superior, this came as a shock. From that day on, the job became a torment for him, causing increasing doubts in its meaning, severe sleeping disorders and growing exhaustion. He had the feeling of only functioning like a machine and looking at himself from the outside. At the culmination of his social withdrawal, his girlfriend separated from him, which he did not even experience as painful. Two weeks later he collapsed at a business meeting and was subsequently admitted to a psychiatric ward. His depression was characterized by predominant feelings of failure and shame, constant self-accusation and an experience of bodily decay. (Own clinic, T. F.)

The patient's life plan was characterized by a rigid orientation toward professional achievement at the cost of interpersonal relationships. His efforts of continuous self-acceleration converged with the demands of an accelerated society, but overburdened the ressources of the body, which may only be cyclically regenerated (Fuchs 2018). The illusion of a continuous narcissistic assent collapsed with the offending assessment, which thus functioned as a limit situation. From now on, an increasing desynchronization developed, connected with a sense of depersonalization, and finally led to the depression.

Psychopathology of Depression

Desynchronization of the Body

As we have seen, desynchronization may be regarded as a major triggering situation of depression. The illness itself now corresponds to a switch from a social and existential to a *biological* desynchronization on a vital level, that means to a partial decoupling between organism and environment. The perceived limit situation may thus be regarded as a "switching point" which induces a reaction of the entire organism, namely a psycho-physiological slow-down or *stasis*.[1] At the physiological level, we find a disturbance of biorhythms such as the neuro-endocrine cycles, the menstrual cycle, circadian temperature rhythms, and the sleep/wake cycle (Wehr and Goodwin 1983). Moreover, the loss of drive, appetite, libido, interest, and attention manifest a general reduction of the *conative-affective dynamics* of the body that is normally directed to the environment and toward the future.

This manifests itself, on the one hand, in psychomotor inhibition, a slowing-down of action as well as thought, and in an overall deceleration of lived time (see next section). On the other hand, it is also expressed in an increasing rigidity and retardation of the lived body, which loses its fluid functioning and makes itself felt in heaviness, exhaustion, oppression, and general constriction (Fuchs 2005; Ratcliffe 2013; Stanghellini et al. 2017). The stagnation of bodily functions thus results in what may be called a *reification* or *corporealization* of the lived body (Fuchs 2005), which occurs in connection to the temporal deceleration. The body is no longer a transparent medium of one's relation to the world but rather appears as a burden or an obstacle. Patients experience their bodily functions as slowed down or blocked; in extreme cases, this culminates in depressive stupor, in which a loss of conation, a petrification of the body, and a standstill of experienced time are combined. The basis for this is the convergence of lived body and lived time in the primary conative dynamics of life.[2]

The psychomotor inhibition and loss of drive also affects the patient's lived space: external goals withdraw in the distance; they lose both their attraction and attainability. The objects are no longer at the disposal of the patient's body as a matter of course. Thus, lived space as a space of possibilities or affordances shrinks (Fuchs 2007; Ratcliffe 2015: 103). The patient can no longer easily transcend the body's boundaries—which is what we implicitly do when desiring things, reaching for them, walking toward our goals, thus anticipating the immediate future. Time and space, as we can see, are interconnected: Anticipation of what is possible or what is to come, and the extension of space around us are one and the same thing. For the depressed person, however, the peripersonal space is no longer embodied; there is a

---

[1] From a sociobiological point of view, depression may also be regarded as an evolutionary protective mechanism in situations of social stress or defeat which consists in a psycho-physiological block or paralysis, in passive-submissive behavior toward other members of the tribe, and which dispenses the individual temporarily from social demands and competitive situations (see Bjorkqvist 2001; Gilbert 2006, 2016).

[2] It should be remarked that there are also mixed states with felt constriction despite still remaining drive and conation, usually called "anxious" or "agitated depression." In these, patients experience a feeling of drivenness or urgency without any escape (Ratcliffe 2012).

gap between the body and its surroundings. This in turn reinforces the bodily constriction and enclosure which was mentioned before.

Intersubjective Desynchroniziation

Thus, an inhibition of lived time and conation is the hallmark of severe depression, as phenomenological psychopathology has pointed out; we will look at this in more detail now. Following Straus (1928), in melancholic or endogenous depression the "ego-time" of the movement of life gets stuck, whereas the "world time" goes on and passes by. This can be expressed as a retardation of inner time, depending on the reduced conation, and a resulting desynchronization from the outer or world time.

Accordingly, in a number of experimental studies depressive persons have been shown to experience a time dilation, that is, they estimated given time intervals to be longer than the objectively measured time (Bech 1975; Kitamura and Kumar 1982; Münzel et al. 1988; Mundt et al. 1998; Bschor et al. 2004; Mahlberg et al. 2008). On the other hand, Thönes and Oberfeld (2015), in a more recent meta-analysis, reported no significant differences in time perception tasks between depressed patients and normal controls, while confirming the significance of subjective time retardation. Here, it might be necessary to distinguish severe from mild and moderate depression, as confirmed by the study of Münzel et al. (1988), who found a measurable time dilation in endogenous depressives, but not in neurotic and reactive depressives.[3]

In any case, it should be emphasized that the inhibition of inner time is not only an individual experience, but connected to the *social desynchronization*, as expressed by the following patient:

> My inner clock seems to stand still, while the clocks of the others run on. In everything I do I am unable to move forward, as if I am paralyzed. I lag behind my duties. I am stealing time. (Own clinic, T. F.)

All the patients' attempts to keep up with events and obligations fail and reinforce their feeling of remanence, resulting in an increasing decoupling from intersubjective contemporality. To this is added a loss of *intercorporeal resonance* and affective attunement (Fuchs 2013b): Whereas conversations are normally accompanied by an exchange of expressions and by a tacit synchronization of gestures and gazes, the patients' countenance remains frozen, and their attunement with others fails. They are no longer capable of being moved and affected by things, situations, or other persons, even their relatives. Painfully they experience their lifelessness and rigidity in contrast to the dynamics of life going on around them. In his autobiographical account, Solomon describes his depression as "a loss of feeling, a numbness, [which] had infected all my human relations. I didn't care about love; about my work; about family; about friends . . ." (Solomon 2001: 45).

Based on an embodied account of emotions (Niedenthal 2007; Fuchs and Koch 2014), the lack of emotional life may be derived from the rigidity and corporealization of the lived body: Without bodily resonance, emotions may no longer be expressed or felt. Moreover, since emotions are also *motivating* forces, their lack contributes to the disturbance of

---

[3] For a neurophenomenological account of desynchronization of inner and world time, investigating its possible neurophysiological correlates in somatomotor and sensory brain networks, see Northoff et al. 2017.

conation and the overall retardation of temporality. The resulting state, often described by the patients as a "feeling of not-feeling," can also be regarded as an *affective depersonalization* (Fuchs 2000; Kraus 2002; Stanghellini 2004): As the basic sense of self is bound to bodily self-affection, the failure of conative-affective dynamics is accompanied not only by a loss of contemporality with others but also by a profound self-alienation.

Alteration of Future and Past

While the alterations described so far mainly affect the intersubjective present, we now look at the dimensions of future and past.

Since conation provides the propulsive energy that directs us toward the future, its lack results in a retraction of the future as a space of anticipated possibilities. This concerns the immediate bodily capacity of action as well as the pursuit of longer-term projects:

> It became impossible to reach anything. Like, how do I get up and walk to that chair . . . To get out of bed at midday was an ordeal. I felt that I had nothing to look forward to, no interest in anything—in short I felt totally apathetic.
>
> (Lott 1996: 246–247)

What remains is an empty volition that is unable to set the body in motion and to engage in longer-term plans. Moreover, without the recurrent cycles of need and satisfaction, or anticipation and fulfillment, the cyclical structure of lived time is increasingly replaced by a linear, homogeneous time that the patient cannot engage in and shape (Fuchs 2018). Thus, on the one hand, the future is blocked, on the other hand it turns into an empty "flight of time" irreversibly running toward death. This uninhibited rule of linear time is illustrated by two further quotations:

> I am only waiting for the day to come to an end—another meaningless day, merely a further step towards death.
>
> (Own clinic, T. F.)

> The fact that symphonies come to an end frightened me. The way a piece of music moves towards its end in accordance with an inner logic and even hurries towards it in an irreversible sequence—that was the course of my life, and what happened in the past is unalterable, irrevocable.
>
> (Kuiper 1991: 168; own translation)

Future thus loses its character of openness, possible novelty or surprise. Instead, it becomes as a mechanical process leading to an inevitable end, which is known from the past, or to some inescapable calamity. It adopts itself the perfect tense and thus becomes *the future perfect*, especially in the form frequently used by patients in their complaints: the feared event (ruin, punishment, death) *will then have certainly taken place.* As Minkowski already observed, without one's own impetus toward the future, "the whole of becoming seems to rush toward us, a hostile force which must bring suffering" (1970: 188). The future is thus obstructed, occupied by an already impending and determined doom.

A complementary change is found in the experience of the *past.* Since progress toward the future is blocked, the patients are also unable to close up and leave behind their past experiences. "The more the inhibition increases and the speed of inner time slows down, the more the determining power of the past is experienced" (Straus 1928). As Kuiper writes in his self-report of a psychotic depression:

> What has happened can never be undone again. Not only the things go by, but also possibilities pass by unused. If one does not accomplish something in time, it is never done any more ... The real essence of time is indelible guilt.
>
> (Kuiper 1991: 155, 162; own translation)

Frequently, mistakes made long ago are then experienced as if they had just been committed—a paradox, which Kimura has expressed as a continuing perfect tense instead of the preterite.[4] In the perfect, the past is not actually over, it can no longer be forgotten and becomes a facticity accumulated in the present. "I understand that the time may be past, but the past is still present as an accusation," is Kuiper's description (1991: 156). Guilt is thus reified and cannot be obliterated in the future through the development of relationships to others: "One has said things which cannot be made unsaid; one can no longer escape from what one has done" (own clinic, T. F.). Since reparation or change are deemed impossible, the future subjunctive, as Binswanger remarked (1960: 26f.), withdraws into the past and becomes past subjunctive, an empty possibility of lamenting: "*if only I had done (not done) this.*" Such typical phrases manifest the vain attempt to retrieve the lost scope of possibilities in the past, yet with the obvious result of merely increasing the burden of regret and guilt.

Transition to Delusion

With increasing inhibition, the basic movement of life comes to a standstill. The depressive has fallen out from contemporality and literally lives in another, sluggish time—usually expressed in the complaint that time stretches in a tormenting way. This reified, spatialized time can be subdivided in the way that, normally, only physically measurable time can be. This becomes manifest in the not infrequent appearance of iterative or compulsive symptoms:

> I sit at home noticing that time moves forward agonizingly slowly. Another moment, still another moment ... At times, I actually have to count the seconds, from one to five, one to five, again and again—completely meaningless. (Own clinic, T. F.)

As Minkowski remarked, counting moments of objective time may create a mechanical forward movement. "This progression, or rather this illusion of progression, comes to fill in for the weakening dynamism" (Minkowski 1970: 299). If life no longer unfolds and grows in the temporal stream of self-realization or "becoming" (Gebsattel 1928), it remains an empty sequence of moments: "Time degenerates into mere succession when our ability to fulfil time falters," writes Theunissen (1991: 304). No longer able to live and shape time actively, the depressive patient succumbs, powerless, to its mechanical dominance.

Complete desynchronization from intersubjective time is marked by the transition into *melancholic delusion*. It can be understood as the explicit manifestation of the disturbed conative temporalization at the implicit level: Past and future have now been finally fixated, frozen into the perfect tense of irreversible guilt, and in the future perfect of certain ruin, decay, or death.

---

[4] Bin Kimura, *Time and Self*, Tokyo 1982; quoted after Kobayashi 1998: 168.

At the same time, a return to the shared contemporality with others has become unimaginable. They are separated from the patient by an abyss and can no longer be reached. With the loss of contemporality the flexibility of perspective-taking is lost as well, since this is essentially based on an open future allowing for alternatives to one's convictions. The patient, however, is forced *to equate his self with his current experience* (Kraus 1991): "It has always been and will always be like this"—to be told anything different must be an illusion. Even the explicit memory of a recovery from an earlier depression remains abstract for the patient and does nothing to change the hopelessness of the present situation. The same is true of his past integrity which was nothing but a sham in view of his actual depravity—it was only a pretense, a fraud.

Depressive delusions may thus be described as "frozen realities"—beliefs and convictions which result from the freezing of self-temporalization and which resist any change or intersubjective allignment of perspectives. In this sense, hypochondriac delusions can be understood as being rooted in abnormal bodily experiences that manifest the stagnation of bodily functions and are considered irreversible. Delusions of guilt express the experience of irrevocably falling behind one's duties, of not being able to forget, of being constantly forced to remember one's past mistakes. Finally, in Cotard's syndrome or nihilistic delusion the patient feels as if he were already dead and had to exist in this state forever (Enoch and Trethowan 1991). The standstill of lived time has become absolute, resulting in an eternity of the present. However, this is obviously the opposite of the mystical "nunc stans" in which the fleeting course of time is suspended by a fulfilled present:

> I do not exist any more. When someone speaks to me, I feel as if he were speaking to a dead person.... I have the feeling of being an absent person. In sum, I am a walking shadow. (Quote of a patient by Minkowski 1970: 328)

The sense of reality that goes missing in Cotard's syndrome may be considered as being ultimately based on the synchronization of self and world, brought about, above all, through intercorporeality and contemporality: reality is at its basis always a *shared* reality (Varga 2012; Fuchs 2013b). Nihilistic delusions thus manifest the extreme of a derealization that results from the loss of affective attunement to a shared world.

Finally, depressive suicides may also be regarded as the consequent realization of the overall standstill of time and loss of intersubjective contemporality. Although this is only rarely experienced in the extreme form of Cotard's syndrome, it nevertheless already comes near to an experience of death. On the one hand, suicide then realizes or literally "executes" this experience; on the other hand, it also means the last perceived possibility to escape the tormenting state of frozenness by an act of will—paradoxically speaking, to restore the future for one last time with the intention to anihilate it once and for all.

Before looking at possible therapeutic strategies that may be derived from this account of depression, we will first look at the temporality of chronic depression and mania.

Chronic Depression

Chronic depression is a frequent phenomenon: about 30% of depressions are classified as chronic, or as Persistent Depressive Disorder according to DSM-5, that is, lasting for at least two years (Rush et al. 1995; Blanco et al. 2010; APA 2013). Chronic depression may occur either as primary dysthymia or result from a major depression that does not completely remit (Chronic Major Depressive Disorder, CMDD). It is usually characterized by a milder degree of somatic symptoms such as inhibition, weight loss, and vital disturbances; in other words, conation is less affected than mood and emotions.

Nevertheless, the subjective suffering may even be more pronounced than in acute and severe depression. In CMDD, this is mainly due to a secondary neurotic development: On the one hand, the repeated experience of failure and disappointment regarding a hoped-for remission leads to increasing resignation and despair. A diminished and miserable life seems to be the inevitable prospect for all further future. In this way, depressive mood, so to speak, maintains and reinforces itself with increasing duration. On the other hand, secondary consequences of depression may contribute to the chronification, such as loss of one's job, attrition and disruption of relationships, stigmatization and social exclusion, but also a secondary gain derived from the patient role and a fixation on one's illness. In all these respects, the patients' relation to themselves, their stance-taking toward their own condition becomes a major component of the illness itself, even more pronounced than in acute depression.

Although the experience of implicit or inner time in chronic depression is not necessarily slowed down as it is in severe depression, patients usually experience a uniformity and sameness of past, present, and future—as it were, a monotonous landscape of dejection and failure: "This is how my life has always been, and how it will remain in the future." In this landscape of futility, ultimately nothing has significance—everything just passes. As Minkowski explains, "it is in the orientation of our life toward the future which gives it a meaning, a direction: when this orientation is missing, everything seems to amount to the same thing, seems stupid, without rhyme or reason . . ." (Minkowski 1970: 303), and this is what chronically depressed patients describe.

Moreover, low self-esteem, self-fulfilling prophecies of failure, and increasing feelings of hopelessness constitute vicious circles that maintain the illness. Patients withdraw from social contacts in resignation or mute accusation, and they often discourage their relatives, friends, and caregivers by their lamenting behavior. Not infrequently, rejective, devaluating, or even hostile attitudes may emerge. This secondary development is obviously different from the Melancholic Type personality which is mainly oriented toward social attunement, harmony, and compliance with the demands of others. In the background, there is often a developmental history of early trauma and psychological insults (emotional or sexual abuse, neglect, or other kinds of maltreatment) that has lead to a lifetime pattern of interpersonal avoidance and distrust. This pattern now significantly impedes the remission of the depression and has to be addressed by specific psychotherapeutic approaches (see e.g. McCullough 2010; McCullough et al. 2011).

THE PHENOMENOLOGY OF MANIA

Mania is obviously the antithesis of depression. The depressive heaviness, inhibition, and retardation is replaced by lightness, disinhibition, and acceleration. The lived body, instead of its constriction in depression, is characterized by a *centrifugal expansion*, which is due to an increase of vital drive and connation, and accompanied by a general sense of power and appropriation. The body seems to have lost all resistance that normally impedes acting out every impulse immediately. Accordingly, the patient's lived space is extended, abounding with possibilities and affordances that all seem attractive and promising. However, mania is not so much a state of happiness and cheerfulness, but rather a state of superficial elation, often experienced with feelings of flying or floating. One may speak of a "vital euphoria," since the manic mood is not due to a primary narcissistic grandiosity, but mainly to the excess of drive, energy, and conation. On the other hand, mania may also display the well-known "mixed states," characterized by emotional lability and rapid shifts between euphoria, dysphoria, and irritability (Swann et al. 1993; Henry et al. 2007; Fernandez 2014). This points out that the crucial alteration in mania consists in the excess of conation, while the resulting mood states may vary to a certain extent, depending not least on the resistance which the patients meet in their environment, but also on an imminent shift to a depressive phase.

Regarding temporality, we find the opposite type of desynchronization as compared to depression, namely an *acceleration* and thus, a partial decoupling of the inner time from the world time.[5] Accordingly, manic action is characterized by restless hustle and agitation; the patients only fleetingly enter into contact with the world and others (Binswanger 1960, 1964; Alonso-Fernandez 1982). The present is never enough, but virtually marked by what is still missing or what would be possible; the interest is always distracted in favor of the next-to-come. Whereas depressive patients keep lamenting over missed opportunities of the past, manic persons are constantly ahead of themselves, addicted to the seemingly unlimited scope of possibilities. The future cannot be awaited and expected, but must be assailed and seized immediately. Impatience leaves no ease for pursuing long-term goals. The past, on the other hand, is forgotten as soon as new alluring options and possibilities emerge; commitments are betrayed in favor of a more enticing future.

All this leads to a momentary life, consisting of isolated "nows," not allowing for a sustained development and conclusion of projects. The manic mode of existence is volatile, playful, and provisional; both the past and the long-term future lose their influence on the present (Figueira and Madeira 2011). If one project fails, half a dozen other plans take its place at once, resulting in a spinning round on the spot without actual efficacy. In so doing, manic persons neglect the natural rhythms which oppose their acceleration: They repress the cyclic time of the body in favor of a homogeneous, linearly accelerated time (Fuchs 2018). They disregard the needs of their body, deny it the necessary sleep, and ignore the signs of beginning exhaustion. The body is thus exploited mercilessly and turned into a mere vehicle of the inflated drive. The rhythmic, and as such also retarding, moment of existence is no longer perceived, but rather repressed or overrun.

If we turn to *intersubjectivity*, we find the patients bustling around in dispersed attention, without being able to take a specific interest in others. Though the manic person constantly approaches and seizes them, he soon loses his interest once they do not participate, and no deeper affective connection results. The patient's euphoria feigns affection, but actually remains a fixed state of empty cheerfulness. Since the component of *receptivity* in contact with others is lacking, all encounters cannot establish satisfaction and fulfillment. Lack of distance and disinhibition, often a sexualized behavior to the point of promiscuity, may have a

---

[5] This acceleration of lived temporality may be experimentally verified: In studies on time estimation, hypo-manic and manic patients ususally experience a shortening of time periods (Bschor et al. 2004; Mahlberg et al. 2008).

destructive effect on personal relationships. Frequently, the manic episode leaves behind a mess of job loss, debts, or divorce.

In sum, in mania the movement of life is accelerated and overtakes the external, social, or world time. Manic patients thus live over their means and exhaust their biological and social resources to the point of depletion and breakdown. Even though they may not realize this immediately for lack of self-criticism, the disillusionment after the manic episode is all the more profound and may often contribute to a sudden fall from mania into depression. In the long term, the upheavals of bipolar disorder cause a recurrent disruption of the steady course of one's life (Jamison 1996) and may even lead to a fragmentation of narrative identity:

> If you are manic-depressive, your life has no continuity any longer. What could be narrated as a more or less consistent story before, disintegrates in retrospect into unconnected areas and fragments. The illness has blown up your past, and to an even greater extent it threatens your future. With every manic episode, your life as you knew it becomes more impossible. The person who you thought to be and to know does not possess a firm foundation any more. You can no longer be sure of yourself.
>
> (Melle 2016: 113)

The repeated experience of becoming "a completely different person" may thus severely undermine one's sense of authenticity and diachronic identity. It certainly calls not only for long-term medication, but also for a continuous and trusting therapeutic relationship that is able to help patients distinguish between different states of self, to bridge periods of self-loss, and to compensate for the recurrent social desynchronization caused by the illness.

Conclusion: A Resynchronizing Therapy

In this chapter, I have described depression as a desynchronization of the individual from the shared contemporality, which turns into a physiological desynchronization of organism and environment. As an inhibition of vitality, it proceeds to impair the conative basis of experience. The loss of goal-oriented capacities of the body, of drive, appetite, and desire are equivalent to a slowing-down of lived time to the point of its standstill.[6] As a result, time emerges explicitly and in reified form, in particular as a reification of the past and the future. Thus the guilt, the losses, and failures gain dominance over the future and its possibilities. No longer able to live time actively, the depressive person succumbs to its dominance. Melancholic delusion is the utter manifestation of the decoupling from common time. The various affective, cognitive, sensorimotor, and social symptoms of depression, despite not always having time as their manifest theme, are thus traced back to an underlying disturbance of lived time. In mania, on the other hand, we find largely opposite, but equally detrimental connections between conation, temporality, and intersubjectivity.

---

[6] It may be of interest to note that in a comparative study of major depressive and schizophrenia patients, Stanghellini et al. (2017) found that in MDD, unlike in schizophrenia, there is no disarticulation or fragmentation of time-experience (i.e. no disorder of the temporal synthesis of protention, presentation, and retention) but a disorder of conation or "inhibition of becoming." On this important difference, see also Fuchs 2013a.

From this point of view, the treatment of affective disorders should have the aim to restore and support the failing processes of synchronization. Apart from biological approaches, a psychosocial "*resynchronizing therapy*," which I shortly outline for depression, should take into account the following guidelines (Fuchs 2014):

(1) The first requirement would be a spatial and temporal frame creating a legitimate re-covery period for the patient, a "time-out" so to speak, during which he or she can gradually readapt to the common social course of time with as little pressure as pos-sible. This will often require hospitalization. In this phase of treatment the aim is to loosen the rigidity of bodily restriction and anxiety, which is achieved by psychotropic medication, relaxation techniques, and moderate bodily exercise, but also by the relief of everyday tasks that overburden the patient's capacities.

(2) Secondly, it is important to give rhythm to everyday life, that is, to emphasize repe-tition and regularity in the structure of the day and week. This cyclical temporality helps the patient to gain a stand against the fleeting, linear time and to support the resynchronization of internal and external rhythms (Fuchs 2018).

(3) A careful activation therapy may support the patient's orientation toward future goals, however modest. This may be stressful at first, since the patient's own, appetitive mo-tivation is still missing and each action is in immediate danger of not satisfying his or her high demands on achievement. It is therefore important to explain to the patient that the intentional arc alone, which he draws in planning and execution, is enough to extend his sensorimotor space again und to re-establish his directedness toward the future.

(4) From this follows the principle of "optimal resynchronization": The patient should experience a degree of activation and stimulation appropriate to his present state, so that the empty time is filled again without, however, causing a relapse into uncoupled time by forced rehabilitation. The image of a gear-change suggests itself here, where different levels of synchronization are chosen according to the present capacity.

(5) After the remission of acute depression, it becomes important to further the psycho-logical and social processes of resynchronization whose failure have contributed to the onset of illness, above all, processes of grief and role change. This will usually be con-tinued in outpatient psychotherapy.

These guidelines may be combined with different psychotherapeutic approaches, which are certainly among the most important means of ultimately re-establishing intersubjective contemporality.

BIBLIOGRAPHY

American Psychiatric Association. (2013). *Diagnostic and Statistical Manual of Mental Disorders (DSM-5)*. Arlington: American Psychiatric Publishing.

Alonso-Fernandez F. (1982). "Space and Time for the Manic Person." In A. J. J. de Koning and F. A. Jenner (eds.), *Phenomenology and Psychiatry*. New York: Grune & Stratton.

Bech P. (1975). "Depression: Influence on Time Estimation and Time Experience." *Acta Psychiatrica Scandinavia* 51: 42–50.

Binswanger L. (1960). *Melancholie und Manie*. Pfullingen: Neske.

Binswanger L. (1964). "On the Manic Mode of Being-in-the-world." In E. Straus (ed.), *Phenomenology, Pure and Applied*, pp. 131–132. Pittsburgh: Duquesne University Press.

Bjorkqvist K. (2001). "Social Defeat as a Stressor in Humans." *Physiology & Behavior* 73: 435–442.

Blanco C., Okuda M., Markowitz J. C., Liu S. M., Grant B. F., and Hasin D. S. (2010). "The Epidemiology of Chronic Major Depressive Disorder and Dysthymic Disorder: Results from the National Epidemiologic Survey on Alcohol and Related Conditions." *Journal of Clinical Psychiatry* 71: 1645–1656.

Bschor T., Ising M., Bauer M., et al. (2004). "Time Experience and Time Judgment in Major Depression, Mania and Healthy Subjects. A Controlled Study of 93 Subjects." *Acta Psychiatrica Scandinavica* 109: 222–229.

Depraz N. (1998). "Can I Anticipate Myself? Self-affection and Temporality." In D. Zahavi (Ed.) *Self-awareness, Temporality, and Alterity*, pp 83–97. Dordrecht: Kluwer.

Ehrenberg A. (2010). *The Weariness of the Self. Diagnosing the History of Depression in the Present Age*. Montreal: McGill University Press.

Enoch M. D. and Trethowan, W. H. (1991). *Uncommon Psychiatric Syndromes*, 3rd edn. Bristol: John Wright.

Fernandez A. (2014). "Reconsidering the Affective Dimension of Depression and Mania: Towards a Phenomenological Dissolution of the Paradox of Mixed States." *Journal of Psychopathology* 20: 414–422.

Figueira M. L. and Madeira L. (2011). "Time and Space in Manic Episodes." *Dialogues in Philosophy, Mental and Neuro Sciences* 4: 22–26.

Fuchs, T. (2000) *Psychopathologie von Leib und Raum*. Darmstadt: Steinkopff.

Fuchs T. (2001). "Melancholia as a Desynchronization. Towards a Psychopathology of Interpersonal Time." *Psychopathology* 34: 179–186.

Fuchs T. (2005). "Corporealized and Disembodied Minds. A Phenomenological View of the Body in Melancholia and Schizophrenia." *Philosophy, Psychiatry & Psychology* 12: 95–107.

Fuchs T. (2007). "Psychotherapy of the Lived Space. A Phenomenological and Ecological Concept." *American Journal of Psychotherapy* 61: 432–439.

Fuchs T. (2013a). "Temporality and Psychopathology." *Phenomenology and the Cognitive Sciences* 12: 75–104.

Fuchs T. (2013b). "Depression, Intercorporeality and Interaffectivity." *Journal of Consciousness Studies* 20: 219–238.

Fuchs T. (2013c). "Existential Vulnerability. Toward a Psychopathology of Limit Situations." *Psychopathology* 46: 301–308.

Fuchs T. (2014). "Psychopathology of Depression and Mania: Symptoms, Phenomena and Syndromes." *Journal of Psychopathology* 20: 404–413.

Fuchs T. (2018). "The Cyclical Time of the Body and its Relation to Linear Time." *Journal of Consciousness Studies* 25: 47–65.

Fuchs T. and Koch S. (2014). "Embodied Affectivity: On Moving and Being Moved." *Frontiers in Psychology. Psychology for Clinical Settings* 5: Article 508, 1–12.

Gallagher S. (2012). "Time, Emotion, and Depression." *Emotion Revue* 4: 127–132.

Gebsattel E. von. (1928). "Zeitbezogenes Zwangsdenken in der Melancholie." *Nervenarzt* 1: 275–287.

Gilbert P. (2006). "Evolution and Depression: Issues and Implications." *Psychological Medicine* 36: 287–297.

Gilbert P. (2016). *Depression: The Evolution of Powerlessness*. London/ New York: Routledge.

Henry C., M'Bailara K., Desage A., et al. (2007). "Towards a Reconceptualization of Mixed States, Based on an Emotional-reactivity Dimensional Model." *Journal of Affective Disorders* 101: 35–41.

Husserl E. (1969). *Zur Phänomenologie des inneren Zeitbewusstseins*. Husserliana X, Nijhoff, Den Haag, trans. J. Brough ("On the Phenomenology of the Consciousness of Internal Time"). Dordrecht: Kluwer Academic Publishers (1991).

Jamison K. R. (1996). *An Unquiet Mind. A Memoir of Moods and Madness*. London: Picador.

Jaspers, K. (1925). *Psychologie der Weltanschauungen*. 3rd edn. Berlin: Springer.

Kitamura T. and Kumar R. (1982). "Time Passes Slowly for Patients with Depressive State." *Acta Psychiatrica Scandinavia* 65: 415–420.

Kobayashi T. (1998). *Melancholie und Zeit*. Basel/Frankfurt: Stroemfeld.

Kraus A. (1987). "Rollendynamische Aspekte bei Manisch-Depressiven." In K. Kisker, et al. (eds.), *Psychiatrie der Gegenwart*, Vol. 5, pp. 403–423. Berlin/ Heidelberg/ New York: Springer.

Kraus A. (1991). "Der melancholische Wahn in identitätstheoretischer Sicht." In W. Blankenburg (Ed.) *Wahn und Perspektivität*, pp. 68–80. Stuttgart: Enke.

Kraus A. (2002). "Melancholie: eine Art von Depersonalisation?" In T. Fuchs and C. Mundt (eds.), *Affekt und affektive Stoerungen*, pp. 169–186. Paderborn: Schoeningh.

Kronmüller K.-T., Backenstrass M., Kocherscheidt K., Hunt A., Unger J., Fiedler P., and Mundt Ch. (2002). "Typus Melancholicus Personality Type and the Five-factor Model of Personality." *Psychopathology* 35: 327–334.

Kuiper P. C. (1991). *Seelenfinsternis. Die Depression eines Psychiaters*. Frankfurt/M: Fischer.

Lott T. (1996). *The Scent of Dried Roses*. London: Viking.

Mahlberg R., Kienast T., Bschor T., and Adli M. (2008). "Evaluation of Time Memory in Acutely Depressed Patients, Manic Patients, and Healthy Controls Using a Time Reproduction Task." *European Psychiatry* 23: 430–433.

McCullough J. P. (2010). "CBASP, the Third Wave and the Treatment of Chronic Depression." *Journal of European Psychotherapy* 9: 169–190.

McCullough J. P., Lord B. D., Martin A. M., Conley K. A., Schramm E., and Klein, D. N. (2011). "The Significant Other History: An Interpersonal-Emotional History Procedure Used with the Early-onset Chronically Depressed Patient." *American Journal of Psychotherapy* 65: 225–248.

Melle T. (2016). *Die Welt im Rücken*. Berlin: Rowohlt.

Minkowski E. (1933). *Le temps vécu*. Paris: d'Arey. Engl. trans. (1970) *Lived Time: Phenomenological and Psychopathological Studies*. Evanston: Northwestern University Press.

Mundt C., Backenstrass M., Kronmüller K. T., Fiedler P., Kraus A., and Stanghellini G. (1997). "Personality and Endogenous/Major Depression: An Empirical Approach to Typus Melancholicus." *Psychopathology* 30: 130–139.

Mundt C., Richter P., van Hees H., and Stumpf T. (1998). "Zeiterleben und Zeitschaetzung depressiver Patienten." *Nervenarzt* 69: 38–45.

Münzel K., Gendner G., Steinberg R., and Raith L. (1988). "Time Estimation of Depressive Patients: The Influence of the Interval Content." *European Archives of Psychiatric and Neurological Sciences* 237: 171–178.

Niedenthal P. M. (2007). "Embodying Emotion." *Science* 316: 1002–1005.

Northoff G., Magioncalda P., Martino M., Lee H. C., Tseng Y. C., and Lane T. (2017). "Too Fast or Too Slow? Time and Neuronal Variability in Bipolar Disorder—A Combined Theoretical and Empirical Investigation. *Schizophrenia Bulletin* 44: 54–64.

Ratcliffe M. (2008). *Feelings of Being. Phenomenology, Psychiatry and the Sense of Reality.* Oxford: Oxford University Press.

Ratcliffe M. (2012). "Varieties of Temporal Experience in Depression." *Journal of Medicine and Philosophy* 37: 114–138.

Ratcliffe M. (2013). "A Bad Case of the Flu? The Comparative Phenomenology of Depression and Somatic Illness." *Journal of Consciousness Studies* 20: 198–218.

Ratcliffe M. (2015). *"Experiences of Depression. A Study in Phenomenology."* Oxford: Oxford University Press.

Ronningstam, E. (1996). Pathological narcissism and narcissistic personality disorder in Axis I disorders. *Harvard Review of Psychiatry* 3: 326-340.

Rush A. J., Laux G., Giles D. E., et al. (1995). "Clinical Characteristics of Outpatients with Chronic Major Depression." *Journal of Affective Disorders* 34: 25–32.

Schröder, A. (2005). Der Narzisstische Typus als pathoplastische Variante der Primär-persönlichkeit unipolar Depressiver. Eine empirische Studie über die Zunahme narzisstischer Persönlichkeitszüge in der zweiten Hälfte des 20. Jahrhunderts. Heidelberg: Med. Dissertation Universität.

Sheets-Johnstone M. (1999). "Emotion and Movement. A Beginning Empirical-Phenomenological Analysis of Their Relationship." *Journal of Consciousness Studies* 6: 259–277.

Slaby, J. and Stephan, A. (2008). "Affective intentionality and self-consciousness." *Consciousness and Cognition* 17: 506-513.

Slaby J., Paskaleva A., and Stephan A. (2013). "Enactive Emotion and Impaired Agency in Depression." *Journal of Consciousness Studies* 20: 33–55.

Solomon A. (2001). *The Noonday Demon: An Atlas of Depression.* London: Vintage Books.

Stanghellini G. (2004). *Disembodied Spirits and Deanimatied Bodies: The Psychopathology of Common Sense.* Oxford: Oxford University Press.

Stanghellini G., Bertelli M., and Raballo A. (2006). "Typus Melancholicus: Personality Structure and the Characteristics of Major Unipolar Depressive Episode." *Journal of Affective Disorders* 93: 159–167.

Stanghellini G., Ballerini M., Pesenza S., Mancini M., Northoff G., and Cutting J. (2017). "Abnormal Time Experiences in Major Depression: An Empirical Qualitative Study." *Psychopathology* 50: 125–140.

Straus E. (1928). "Das Zeiterlebnis in der endogenen Depression und in der psychopathischen Verstimmung." *Monatsschrift für Psychiatrie und Neurologie* 68: 640–656.

Straus E. (1947). "Disorders of Personal Time in Depressive State." *Southern Medical Journal* 40: 254–259.

Swann A. C., Secunda S. K., Katz M. M., et al. (1993). "Specificity of Mixed Affective States: Clinical Comparison of Dysphoric Mania and Agitated Depression." *Journal of Affective Disorders* 28: 81–89.

Tatossian A. (1983). "Dépression, vécu dépressif et orientation thérapeutique." In Collectif (ed.), *La maladie depressive*, pp. 277–293. Paris: Ciba.

Tellenbach H. (1980). *Melancholy. History of the Problem, Endogeneity, Typology, Pathogenesis, Clinical Considerations.* Pittsburgh: Duquesne University Press.

Theunissen M. (1991). *Negative Theologie der Zeit*. Frankfurt: Suhrkamp.

Thönes S. and Oberfeld D. (2015). "Time Perception in Depression: A Meta-Analysis." *Journal of Affective Disorders* 175: 359–372.

Twenge, J. M. and Campbell, S. M. (2008). Generational differences in psychological traits and their impact on the workplace. *Journal of Managerial Psychology* 23: 862-877.

Twenge, J. M. and Foster, J. D. (2010). Birth cohort increases in narcissistic personality traits among American college students, 1982–2009. *Social Psychological and Personality Science* 1: 99-106.

Varga S. (2012). "Depersonalization and the Sense of Realness." *Philosophy, Psychiatry, & Psychology* 19: 103–113.

Wehr T. A. and Goodwin F. K. (1983). "Biological Rhythms in Manic-depressive Illness." In T. A. Wehr and F. K. Goodwin (eds.), *Circadian Rhythms in Psychiatry*, pp.129–184. Pacific Grove, California: Boxwood.

Zerssen, D. von and Pössl, J. (1990). The premorbid personality of patients with different subtypes of an affective illness: Statistical analysis of blind assignment of case history data to clinical diagnoses. *Journal of Affective Disorders* 18: 39-50.

CHAPTER 65

THE LIFE-WORLD OF THE OBSESSIVE-COMPULSIVE PERSON

MARTIN BÜRGY

INTRODUCTION

THE development of international classification systems has ended the "Babylonian confusion" in the language used in psychiatry and has led to reliable diagnoses (Müller 1986). Yet, the descriptive classifications lack any real connection to the aetiology of the conditions, which reduces their therapeutic relevance. According to Andreasen, there are increasing problems with the validity of psychiatric diagnoses caused by the lack of competence in phenomenology. This is due, in particular, to the reduction of psychiatric diagnosis to the use of checklists of symptoms (Andreasen 2007). These problems are also reflected in the current diagnostic classification of obsessive-compulsive disorder.

The phenomenological method, however, remains a necessary precondition for being able to approach the patient's experience in as objective a manner as possible, and for being able to record this precisely, and to differentiate and describe it. Together with its importance for the validity of psychiatric diagnoses, it is at the same time important for psychotherapy and pharmacotherapy and the further development of biological approaches (Akiskal 2006; Fuchs 2002; Nelson et al. 2009). Phenomenology fundamentally means, however, placing the focus of attention on the human subject, which is more than its biological and psychological functions. Compared with the analytical methods of the natural sciences, and because this method is rooted in philosophy and anthropology, attention is always directed to the entirety of the person and to the synthesis of the individual findings (Mezzich 2007; Schmidt-Degenhard 2011).

The present chapter is a phenomenological investigation of obsessive-compulsive conditions. It is structured on three levels: from the static understanding, via the genetic understanding, to the hermeneutic understanding as initially described by Jaspers. It starts with a succinct account of these three levels of understanding. Against this background, the chapter explores the relationships between the description, genesis, and meaning of symptoms and investigates the life-world of people with obsessive-compulsive disorder. These findings are illustrated on the basis of a case study.

THREE LEVELS OF "UNDERSTANDING"

In *General Psychopathology*, we encounter three different ways of understanding, which Jaspers continued to modify from the first edition of 1913 up to his final revision of the last edition of 1959 (Jaspers 1913, 1959). Here, understanding always means "the conception of the psychological which is gained from within" (1959), which has an impressive immediacy, and which is developed in a methodical sequence of levels. The first level is that of "static understanding," which focuses the direct experience of the patient in the here and now and which is classed as being descriptive phenomenology. The second level is that of "genetic understanding," in which an attempt is made to put oneself in the patient's shoes in order to investigate how psychological phenomena arise from one another. The "empathetic understanding" was initially presented by Jaspers as a stand-alone method, but it was later logically subsumed under the genetic understanding. Jaspers initially still called his third stage "understanding and interpreting," but he later renamed this as "seizing the totality." By this he meant that research, which has as its subject the individual and the specific, cannot succeed without an orientation to the whole, and thus to a certain extent also without an orientation to meaning and sense. The movement from the individual to the whole, for example, from individual phenomenon to the total experience of the person or from the individual symptom to the ideal-typical unity of the mental disorder, is completed in the hermeneutic circle (Spitzer 1985). I will refer to this third level of understanding as "hermeneutic understanding." These three ways of understanding described here are built on one another and are intertwined. The further understanding is removed from the direct object of experience and the more it brings into focus the genesis or the entirety of the person and the illness, or the general points underlying it, the more interpretive and speculative, but also the more complete, the findings will be. This methodological procedure has not yet been fully realized in relation to mental illnesses. Even the two major case studies by Tellenbach on melancholy (Tellenbach 1971) and by Blankenburg on schizophrenia (Blankenburg 1971) lack this methodological order. In his later work on "*Phenomenology as the Foundational Discipline of Psychiatry*" (*Phänomenologie als Grundlagendisziplin der Psychiatrie*) in 1991 Blankenburg wrote: "For the future, it's an important task to bring descriptive, genetic and hermeneutical phenomenology into a close connection with one another (Blankenburg 1991: 99). (Compare: Stanghellini, chapter on Phenomenological psychotherapy, in this Handbook.)

THE STATIC UNDERSTANDING

The static understanding focuses on direct experience in the investigative situation and therefore represents the highest level of evidence. A review of the phenomena, which is as unbiased as possible, as required by Husserl, is complemented by the targeted checking of diagnostic assumptions that have developed historically and which lead the investigation.

The first description of a patient with an obsessive compulsion—in this case, a fear of touching—is provided by Esquirol in 1839. He emphasizes the two characteristics of the constant fight against the obsessive thoughts whilst at the same time maintaining the insight into their ridiculousness (Esquirol 1839). In the German-speaking countries it was v. Krafft-Ebing who introduced the concept of obsession in 1867. However, he used this term to describe a compulsion which the melancholy state of mind exercises on perceptions (v. Krafft-Ebing 1867). In an 1868 lecture to the Berlin Medical-Psychological Society, Griesinger described three patients who had obsessive ideas which were not supported by affect (Griesinger 1868). Westphal was, in 1877, the first person to provide a definition of compulsion, to cover the phenomena described by Griesinger, and this definition, though it has since been modified, remains valid to this day:

> By obsessive ideas, I mean those ideas which, with otherwise normal intelligence and without being determined by an emotional or affect-like state, appear in the mind of the person affected by them, against and contrary to their will and which they cannot remove, such that these ideas prevent and intersect with the person's normal course of ideas. These ideas are always experienced by the person as being abnormal and alien to him and as being ones which he would oppose, were he in full control of his consciousness.
>
> (Westphal 1877: 669)

In his work, "*Conceptual Investigation into Compulsion*" (*Begriffliche Untersuchung über den Zwang*) in 1939, Schneider explicitly disputes the work of Westphal and arrives at a "core definition" which is linguistically simpler and extremely sharp, and which later found its way into his *Clinical Psychopathology*: "We speak of compulsion when a person is unable to displace contents of his consciousness even though he finds these to be nonsensical or experiences them to be dominating his thoughts without good reason to do so" (Schneider 1939: 23–24). With this formulation, Schneider created not only the preconditions for making a differential diagnostic delimitation between delusional and affective disorders, but also an orientation for the diagnostic exploration of obsessive-compulsive disorders which has remained valid until the present day. His definition was accepted into the psychiatric classification systems even though it has since undergone further modifications.

The tenth edition of the *International Classification of Diseases* (ICD-10) (Dilling et al. 1991) places obsessions (intrusive or obsessive thoughts) and compulsions (compulsive actions) in a relationship of equal value. The fourth edition of the *Diagnostic and Statistical Manual of Mental Disorders* (DSM-IV) (APA 1994), by contrast, allocates obsessive-compulsive disorders to the category of anxiety disorders, which implies a dynamic relationship between primary obsessions (usually obsessive thoughts), which create anxiety, and secondary compulsions (usually compulsive actions), which serve to control the anxiety (Kapfhammer 2008). DSM-5 (APA 2013) does indeed set aside the subordination of the obsessive-compulsive disorders to the category of anxiety disorders and it introduces degrees of insight into the foolishness of the compulsions, but it retains the structure of conditions in relation to obsessions and compulsions (Ehret and Berking 2013). Schneider (1939) had already formulated this relationship between primary and secondary compulsions: an item of the contents of consciousness intrudes to which the "I" then adopts a position. Schneider maintained his descriptive position, and this is presumably why he never made any reference to the works of Binder, which were heavily influenced by psychoanalysis, and who, a few years previously, had characterized the primary compulsion as being the actual "disturbing psychism" which is followed by the "defence psychism" (Binder 1936). In a phenomenological approach to obsessive-compulsive disorder, I have above all pointed to the differential diagnostic significance of the distinction between primary and secondary compulsions. While, on the behavioral level, it is usually only non-specific symptoms (especially washing and checking compulsions) that stand out, an investigation of the primary phenomena can allow the distinction between delusional thoughts and obsessions to be made (Ballerini and Stanghellini 1989; Bürgy 2007).

The organization of the obsessive-compulsive phenomena described found its way into the further differentiation of obsessive-compulsive symptoms. Despite their great formal similarity, obsessive-compulsive symptoms can vary widely in their phenomenology. One advance in this field is provided especially by the factor-analytical differentiation of subtypes (Bloch et al. 2008; Leckman et al. 2010). Working on the basis of the four main subtypes, Hoffmann and Hofmann have produced some exemplary phenomenological work on the threat and defense sides of obsessive-compulsive conditions (Hoffmann and Hofmann 2004). This not only further limits the importance of anxiety in obsessive-compulsive disorder, but it also allows a deeper insight to be gained into the primary and maintaining phenomena.

1. Compulsive checking: The perceived threat to the individual, which is at the root of compulsive checking, is that *feeling of incompleteness* which Janet was the first to describe in relation to obsessive-compulsive disorder in 1903 (Ecker and Gönner 2006). In an act of defense, this primary feeling is externalized and symbolically fought against. There is therefore, for example, no end to the checking of electrical appliances and plug sockets because neither the person's affect nor his insight arrives at the conclusion that the action has been completed. The patient suffers from the conviction that there is a permanent threat emanating from him, which always seeks and finds new contents.

2. Compulsive repetition, compulsive orderliness, and obsessive thoughts: These are all related to the threat posed to a person by his thoughts about blasphemy, his own serious misdeeds, illness, dirtiness, contamination, and shame in relation to his own person or body. Compulsive repetition and compulsive orderliness are attempts to neutralize this threat. The disturbance phenomenon at the root of this behavior is not, for example, the fear that a fire could break out or that a close relative could be harmed in an accident, but rather the fear that one could have *caused* the fire or the accident oneself and without noticing this. This kind of thinking is magical thinking and indicates the person has deficiencies in his self-perception. His consciousness and his attentiveness are not reliable.

3. Washing, polishing, and cleaning compulsions: A thorough examination of the roots of these phenomena shows that they are not based on a fear of the threat of contamination but rather on *disgust* at the thought of potentially touching or having touched the objects in question. A closer examination of the fear of contamination and illness shows that this is merely a secondary rationalization of a primary, overpowering sensitivity to disgust. As a representative of the German phenomenological-anthropological school, v. Gebsattel had already described the "disgust-phobia of the obsessive-compulsive person" in 1954 and he stated that this was the original cause of compulsive washing (v. Gebsattel 1954).

4. Collecting and hoarding: Compulsive collecting and hoarding relates to objects of relatively low value, which over the course of time fill living spaces, making them unusable
for the purposes of actually living. Secondary rationalizations for this type of behavior
are thriftiness or providing for times of emergency. The patient feels an intimate connection with the objects for which he is responsible and to which he in part ascribes
mental sensations. The defensive aspect of these behaviors is to create a sense of security against the threat posed by *dissolution* and *emptiness* by indulging in this "hoarding
behavior." Different authors have therefore attributed the origins of this phenomenon
to a "disorder of the self" or to a "weakness in the integration of the I" (Lang 1986;
Quint 1988; Bürgy 2001).

The common feature in all these experiences remains the *sense of incompleteness* in relation to one's own person, feelings of not being present in a legitimate or complete way,
that actions cannot be completed and of running the risk of harming others. Hoarding and
collecting can be seen as attempts to deal with a person's own incompleteness and emptiness, in the same way as washing, polishing, and cleaning are attempts to fend off feelings of
disgust, and fear of confusion and disintegration. The depersonalization experience plays a
special role in actions which cannot be completed, in the phobic avoidance of a "disgusting
substance," in the magical thinking surrounding ideas of harming other people and in the
ever-more intrusive and pressing obsessive thoughts. The following description of acute clinical decomposition of obsessive-compulsive disorder includes factors of all four subtypes.

CASE STUDY ON STATIC UNDERSTANDING

A twenty-four-year-old student, Ms A., had a diagnosis of obsessive-compulsive disorder
for at least four years. She was admitted as an inpatient at a psychiatric unit for the first time
because her fears had become uncontrollable. Ms A. reported that in the run-up to her admission to the clinic, she visited her grandmother, her father's mother, in the nursing home,
who suffered terrible pains in her hip. She went on to say that the nursing staff initially gave
her grandmother Paracetamol and later on "strong Pregabalin." She reported that while her
grandmother was taking the medication she said to her, "I am taking this for you." This led Ms
A. to develop a sense of deep responsibility and guilt. Because of this she felt unable to go into
the nursing home to see her grandmother again because she was afraid that she had injured or
even killed her grandmother. She felt embarrassed to say this but she could not get rid of the
feelings of anxiety and guilt, even though she knew that this was nonsense. The compulsions
got the upper hand over her. She said that when she went to the nursing home she ought to
have been thinking the right way about it and that she should not have had any frightening
images in her mind, for example, that there was a knife sticking into her grandmother and
that everything was covered in blood. The more she felt herself to be under pressure, the more
urgent these intrusive images and thoughts became, the more she had to keep checking and
the more insecure she became. She wasn't able to speak to her parents because she feared that
this would lead to her receiving the news of her grandmother's death. She said that she no
longer felt safe and that she had a strange feeling that she was going mad. She took refuge in
the clinic, because she was afraid her grandmother would die. She reported that she feared

becoming contaminated with the "sticky and disgusting nature of her grandmother" when she was with her parents or her boyfriend. She was overwhelmed with washing, disinfecting, and checking things and had felt "as though she was detached" from herself.

Because of her pronounced depersonalization and desultory thinking, it took a few days before proper evidence for Ms A.'s accounts of her experience could be found. Her presentation of her current life-world made it easier to discern the extent of her compulsions. She portrayed two life-worlds which were strictly separated from one another: "A normal world and a world of compulsions." When she was at home with her parents she avoided everything. She had her own little room there which her parents were not allowed to enter, which she constantly washed. She entered it after completing a particular ritual, as though entering a canal lock, and did not want to leave it again. She also reported that she had a perfectly planned cleaning ritual for whenever she returned to her own room at the college where she was studying. This involved her own litter bin, bags, and clean bathing shoes so that she would not bring any part of her boyfriend or parents into her flat with her. She felt that her hand washing, showering, and cleaning her room helped her to create distance and to calm her feelings down. When her feelings became too strong and confused, she no longer felt "herself," she felt that she became detached from her body and became a real robot. She always met her boyfriend outside of her flat or at her parents' home and only had sex with him in a hotel where everything was hygienic and sterile. Her female friends were allowed to visit her in her flat because they weren't contaminated. She led a very normal student life with them, which was not affected by her compulsions.

THE GENETIC UNDERSTANDING

Genetic understanding follows as the second level of understanding and investigates the question as to how obsessive symptoms develop or how these emerge from the patient's personality and their life-story. It is usually recorded retrospectively and is therefore of lesser evidential value than the static understanding. The triggering situation is given prominent importance in this interface.

Up until the 1980s, the view had stubbornly persisted that a compulsive character was the personality basis for the development of obsessive-compulsive disorder (Bürgy 2005a). Kretschmer, Jaspers, and Schneider had, however, already pointed out that sensitive personality traits were a prerequisite of obsessive-compulsive disorder. Kretschmer writes in his book on "*Physique and Character*" in 1921: "The sensitive person is thin-skinned, impressionable but restrained and processes experiences sustainably. He has a long-lasting hidden affective tension, is ethically sensitive and ambitious, feeling unsure of himself, he tends to feelings of guilt and hides behind an asthenic façade a pronounced, if also inhibited wish to assert his own will" (Kretschmer 1977: 183). In 1986 Lang extended the psychoanalytic concept of compulsive neurotic symptoms as representing an unconscious form of conflict resolution by the addition, on a social level, of the concept of a compulsively neurotic person as an "inhibited rebel," (Lang 1986). These hypotheses are supported by the results of comorbidity studies which show that in 51–75% of cases of obsessive-compulsive disorders there is also a personality disorder from Cluster C of the DSM-IV classification. Cluster C can be described as follows: A tendency to be easily offended by criticism and rejection, the exaggeration of potential problems, continuous tension and anxiety, a feeling of helplessness and dependency, enormous separation anxieties, excessive conscientiousness, a lack of flexibility, and passive aggression (Csef 2001; Zaudig 2011).

The question remains, however, as to how symptoms of obsessive-compulsive disorder develop on the basis of this personality typology. In the classical psychiatric literature there are two basic approaches to the genesis of compulsion. On the one hand, for authors like Kraepelin, Aschaffenburg, Störing, and v. Gebsattel, the focus is on the genesis of affect. In the other approach compulsion is seen as being a disorder of thought content and is therefore moved closer to delusion. This approach is found in the works of authors like Westphal, Binder, and Schneider (Bürgy 2005b). Freud was one of the first researchers who attempted to combine these two positions. In his 1909 work, *"Notes on a Case of Obsessional Neurosis"* (*Bemerkungen über einen Fall von Zwangsneurose*), he described the primary battle between two strongly contradictory feelings, especially between love and hate, which leads to strong feelings of insecurity, ambivalence, weakness of will, and to the creation of neurotic symptoms in the form of symbolic compulsive actions. As a secondary effect, the obsession becomes isolated from the affect so that in the case of obsessive-compulsive disorder virtually no affect is present (Freud 1909). Binder felt that the cause of the start of compulsion resulted from a failure of integration and v. Gebsattel traced it back to the disintegration of affects (Binder 1936; v. Gebsattel 1968). v. Gebsattel describes in subtle casuistry the case of a man with a washing obsession who fails "to integrate the feeling of disgust into the structure of the person." Affect and cognition are always closely associated with one another. Hoffmann and Hofmann also stress the importance of the intensity of feelings and the confusion between them at the start of the illness. The person will, above all, experience affects such as pain, grief, loneliness, anxiety, disgust, and rage (Hoffmann and Hofmann 2004). In some of my works I have described the situation which triggers the obsessive-compulsive condition as follows: At the root of obsessive-compulsion the person feels a deeply anchored sense of insecurity and anxiety and the associated inner tension, and also has inadequately differentiated affects. By this I mean that the person has a poorly developed ability to identify, express, and communicate affects. In a situation in which a person feels emotionally overwhelmed, there is a confusion of conflicting affects, which encloses the person within a vicious circle of feelings of powerlessness, helplessness, and isolation. These strong affects are attached to a biographically charged, external object in order to subdue the inner chaos, while compulsive actions, in addition, represent attempts to re-establish the control which has been lost. The strengthening of defenses against these, however, does not bring calm to the person but instead serves to further build up the obsessive-compulsive symptoms so that these do not stop (Bürgy 2005b).

This original confusion is countered by behavioral therapy, producing a therapeutic differentiation of emotions, the establishment of a sense of reality, and the activation of the self-system which includes all the person's previous experiences, feelings, convictions, and values, as well as the constitution of an active I-subject (Hoffmann and Hofmann 2010).

CASE STUDY ON GENETIC UNDERSTANDING

Ms A. reported that her father himself also suffered from compulsions, for example, he filed everything "in a million different folders" and that he too did not let anyone else touch his washing. She said that when she was younger, if people did not behave the way he wanted them to he would react angrily and torment the person concerned. He had been jealous and controlling toward her mother and her mother had felt lonely and had cried a lot. Ms A. had therefore become her mother's confidante very early on. She used to comfort her mother and had developed a keen sense for when there was about to be an argument between her mother and her father. She had always been oversensitive and able to tell when one of her brothers or sisters had a problem and even if something bad happened to someone. That was why she had the feeling that she was responsible for stressful situations and why she felt that she was at the mercy of these situations. When she was asked if she had had any early symptoms of obsessive-compulsive disorder, she said that even as a child she had filled up her pockets with cash till receipts as these were important to her. She had also hoarded her clothes and could not bear to be parted from them. She could not bear the feelings that these objects were irretrievable, of being separated from them, nor the feelings of emptiness. Her brothers, aged twenty-three and thirty-one, were healthy but her sister, who was thirty-six, suffered from touch phobia.

Ms A. described the triggering situation for her current symptoms as follows: It had all begun with the death of the first of her grandmothers to die, her mother's mother. She said that she had been very close to her grandmother and been with her at her death and had felt very guilty about her death. Her grandmother had had a stroke and after that Ms A. had visited her every day for months. She had tried to keep her grandmother alive by sending her thoughts and strength. She had felt that she was only allowed to think good thoughts and that she must not let her go. She said that she became increasingly afraid that she would lose her grandmother. She also had ever worsening mental images of her grandmother's death in her head. She said that she noticeably lost the ability to control these thoughts. She said this had been Hell for her and represented an enormous responsibility and increasing fear and guilt. Ms A. said that when her grandmother finally died, she still felt very close to her. This feeling comforted her. In the farewell room, however, she had once again experienced feelings of anxiety and guilt, that she had failed, and that she had killed her grandmother by her own thoughts. When she was pressed toward the coffin by the large numbers of people at her grandmother's funeral, she felt a strong feeling of disgust welling up in her. Her aunt had then also touched her hands which served to further increase her feeling of disgust. She reported that her feelings became completely confused and had increased to a "massive fear of being annihilated," as though death could be passed on to her. This is why she had begun to wash everything. This had helped her to keep these feelings at a distance. She said the washing made the feelings subside until she no longer experienced herself, and she finally also became dissociated from her own body and then felt like a robot. She was embarrassed to talk about it and was afraid that people might laugh at her. She knew that her fears were much too far-fetched.

Ms A. went on to report that it was also after this event that she had begun to clean and disinfect everything. She had tried to dispose of the material which was contaminated with disgust and to keep it away from her. This had developed into a situation in which she "lived in two worlds," which she constantly had to keep apart from one another. She really could not stop all her cleaning tasks. She reported that she found it particularly difficult to separate herself emotionally from her parents and from her boyfriend. She felt that her compulsions would therefore also help to create this distance from them. She said that she was simply not able to carry so much ballast around with her. She also said that although she naturally wanted to lead a normal life, she did not know whether she would ever be able to give up this need to be separate from them.

THE HERMENEUTIC UNDERSTANDING

The third level of understanding, the hermeneutic understanding, aims at highlighting the *philosophical and anthropological dimension of meaning and sense* of the symptoms of compulsion. This approach has the least amount of evidence in sensual experience. It is more interpretive and speculative, but it is able to combine symptoms described descriptively and genetically as if in a common bond with one another in regard to their meaning.

The primary threatening aspect in compulsion is characterized by an inner state, which can be described as a confusion of affect including the fear of dissolution, a sense of incompleteness, a threatening experience of disgust and depersonalization. v. Gebsattel attempted to summarize all the different ways of experiencing threat and specified them, above all, as immobility, a tendency to remain in the same state, relative lack of emotion, severe isolation and a directionless, free-floating character (v. Gebsattel 1954). As a consequence of the defensive aspects of this condition, the person develops an inability to complete actions. v. Gebsattel therefore describes the anthropological dimension of obsessive-compulsive disorder as a *discontinuation of a person's personal development in time*. Time and life come to a standstill and the future is switched off. v. Gebsattel describes the consequences of this disruption to personal development as follows: "For the obsessive-compulsive person, what has happened in the past does not take the form of a completed action, it assails him as something uncompleted and overwhelms him with symbols of impurity, dirtiness and death" (1954: 144). The standing still of time, with the associated loss of the future, leads to the theme of death in obsessive-compulsive disorder.

In 1938, Straus published the autobiographical account of a female patient whose compulsive washing developed from an original fear of death, which was only secondarily displaced, and always in external respects, into the experience of disgust (Straus 1938). In 1965, Skoog found unsettling death motifs in more than 70% of obsessive-compulsive patients who were specifically asked about this (Skoog 1965). And, in 1972, Schwidder found that the fear of a death which could occur at any time was the central fear of people with obsessive-compulsive disorder (Schwidder 1972). The topic of death is still important in current publications for people with obsessive-compulsive disorder. Conventional symbols of death, such as crosses, people in mourning clothes, hearses and cemeteries, etc. create a strong feeling of unease in people with obsessive-compulsive disorder as well as the magical expectation that a disaster will happen. The fear of decay, illness, and death, mixed with disgust is regularly hidden behind compulsive washing (Hoffmann and Hofmann 2017).

Probably the most intensive and most differentiated treatment of the death motif is that of the Göttingen psychiatrist Meyer. In Meyer's opinion, the phobic element which already manifests itself in the initial phase of compulsive neurosis points to the avoidance of death, which is always immanent in life, and thus to what v. Weizsäcker called a "life which is unlived" (Meyer 1973, 1975). Meyer classified obsessive-compulsive disorder as being a *thanatophobic* neurosis (Meyer 1982) and thus provided an interpretation which is also found in the structural-anthropological approach of Lang. Lang takes up Freud's idea of the special importance of the death-wish in obsessive-compulsive disorder. Using the example of Shakespeare's dramatic character Lady Macbeth, he develops the significance of compulsive washing in obsessive-compulsive disorder as a defense against guilt and death (Lang 1998).

The fear of dying and death is to be found in many of the fears of an obsessive-compulsive: the fear of dead creatures, of corruptible matter, of dirt and dust, and the fear of anything which is definitive, unrepeatable, or unpredictable in life. And this fear of death is also hidden behind hopeless and exhausting battles, extreme caution, care, and vigilance. These security systems are used to fend off a more primal experience, which cannot be fully relinquished in the present moment with all its dangers and possibilities.

Lived Time

It is initially possible to detect the person's change in their experience of time from their symptoms. Control actions, repetitive actions, ordering, washing, and cleaning, as well as collecting and hoarding, all represent the struggle of sensitive people against the disintegration of their affects or emotions, against feelings of disgust, and against their experience of incompleteness and emptiness. The compulsive symptoms slow down lived time. In the most extreme cases, this leads to patients coming to a complete standstill and to attempts to return to the past. The obsessive-compulsive person's own experience of life cannot be freed from feelings of guilt, sin, and failure. His ability to develop his own opportunities in life, to be dynamic and creative, and to develop bold plans or utopian ideals for the future is inhibited. He is less active in taking up and shaping the possibilities for growth and development which are present in his own life. His fear of death is overwhelming. Faced with the fact of his own death one day, he experiences a fear of dying without really ever having properly lived. This explains why symbols of death come to have such a magical significance for him. He feels that the possibilities in his own life are being controlled by an unpredictable fate, rather than by his own life and his life is constantly under threat of being choked off by a plethora of precautionary and security measures, which he takes to protect himself.

Lived Space

The obsessive-compulsive person lives in a confined space and between two worlds, between contamination and normality, control and behaving in a natural way, egocentrism and responsibility/guilt. He is highly sensitive and irritable, and loses the feeling for himself quickly because of other people. He also needs protection and space for retreating from other people in order to be able to control the demands placed on him by the outside world. His inner and outer worlds are inadequately separated from each other. He quickly begins to experience the outside world as being threatening and he soon becomes convinced that he has damaged someone in the outside world without anyone having noticed it. He experiences his own incompleteness as well as feelings of emptiness, guilt, and disgust. His feelings of incompleteness and emptiness show that his sense of self is overwhelmed in his contact with the environment. Here the feelings of guilt are linked to his relationship to the needs of others and feelings of disgust describe fears that he may be penetrated by an alien and disgusting substance, that the obsessive-compulsive person will lose themselves, become totally disintegrated, and die off. Ms. A lives in her own private and smallest possible space, surrounded by contaminated materials. From time to time she seeks to break out, to go on holiday, and to seek out places other than that in which she experiences compulsions and outside of her bland normality. It is then that she feels really free and alive. She then has no more thoughts of death and her fear of death.

Lived Body

The obsessive-compulsive person's sensitivity and irritability in their own experience of themselves also leads to a fear of close physical contact or contamination. This represents a fear of being penetrated by a foreign substance, that one's self will be lost, dissolved, and drained away. The obsessive-compulsive person will generally maintain physical distance from others and fears contamination and defilement. He needs time to build up trust and a sense of security. He finds it easier to establish feelings of closeness and wanting to make contact with others from within himself, than to let himself be moved by something which is external to him. His weak sense of self makes him maintain a physical distance from others in order to keep the forces of death and disintegration under control. Ms A. rarely tried to break out and escape from her state of torpidity. She did sometimes, however, seek to do this by dancing but she preferred to dance alone and, in doing so, she maintained her distance from others.

Lived Otherness

The obsessive-compulsive person normally likes to bury himself in his everyday routine, in normality and inconspicuousness. He does not, however, initially experience the new, the unknown, and the unusual as being contaminated. It is only when he gets closer to others and, in particular, in his relationships that his "otherness" can be fully seen. It is only when he gets close to people and things that the fears of contamination, depersonalization, and disintegration, and of facing a deadly threat develop. He always keeps his distance, remains hidden and aloof in order to remain alive and to maintain a barrier between himself and death. He seeks to bring all those close to him under his control and thus, in effect, to neutralize them. This means that the obsessive-compulsive person's own individuality as expressed, in particular, in spontaneous gestures, is at risk of being hidden or completely lost.

CASE STUDY ON HERMENEUTIC UNDERSTANDING

In much of Ms A.'s experience there is the fear of finitude and death. In reply to the question about what the death meant for her, Ms A. said for her, death was more important in relation to other people; she thought about their deaths and her own responsibility and guilt for them. She felt that she should not be allowed to harm anyone through her bad thoughts. This was why the idea of "the last thought" was so important to her, particularly on New Year's

Eve, because it was something which could not be corrected, and that time is passing, year after year. She said that for her there was something like a battle to make sure she had "the right last thought," and this was associated with guilt about failure if it was not "the correct thought." She felt that with each passing year she was getting further away from the paradise where everything had once been good. Her mother had told her that at the time of her birth she had not wanted to come out of the womb. She often felt as if she would rather be in a "Wonderland" where everything is good and where, in her opinion, there would be no more pain or guilt.

She said that she hated cemeteries and undertakers' businesses and that she always got sick if she had to drive past them. Crucifixes and crosses always made her feel guilty about the things which she did wrong and about her bad thoughts. Crosses reminded her of her blasphemous thoughts, such as, for example, about peeing in the church, and of how imperfect she is and that there had been one person living on the earth who had managed to live his life without being guilty of anything.

Ms A. had originally also sought to prevent the death of her grandmother, magically by energy transfer, as well as by controlling her destructive thoughts. When her grandmother died, she began to experience feelings of a loss of control, guilt, and despair. Her fear of the death of her grandmother, and the initial feelings of closeness to her grandmother after her death, became transformed into a threat that her grandmother's death could be transposed onto her. She suddenly began to experience fear of the "disgusting penetrating substance," of disintegration and oblivion. She tried to control death and keep it at a distance by her never-ending washing and checking compulsions and by separating off her compulsive worlds from the real world. It is clear that the trigger situation, the fear of her own death, was hiding behind the concern and anxiety about her grandmother. This thantophobia accordingly underlies the disturbance side and the compulsive actions represent a projective defense mechanism against this.

Conclusion

We first undertook to describe the structure of compulsion, using the static understanding. The disturbance or threat side was reviewed, together with the underlying feelings of guilt, incompleteness, emptiness, and disgust, which follow the never-ending attempts to neutralize it on the defending and coping side, including the experience of depersonalization. The case study relating to Ms A. shows, in particular, the interpersonal dimension of feelings of responsibility and guilt, the fear that the boundaries between the inside and the outside are lost and that the idea of killing someone becomes real. The defense against frightening perceptions is performed by completing checking actions, which minimize fear and lead to depersonalization. The separating off of compulsive worlds creates further interpersonal distance.

The genetic understanding highlights the lack of differentiation of the affects, as well as the inner tension, which are both rooted in a personality which is deeply prone to being unsettled and is at the same time inhibited, and its biographical development. The person's sense of being overwhelmed in the trigger situation leads to confusion of conflicting affects, which build up in a vicious circle of powerlessness, helplessness, and isolation, and become attached to a biographically charged external object. The defending against the object does not lead to any feeling of calm but instead reinforces the symptoms of compulsion. In Ms A. we find a highly irritable personality who, because of her biographical development, is oriented toward the perception of other people and one which is also characterized by her particular feelings of responsibility and guilt. In the trigger situation, her sense of responsibility for the life of a particularly close person reaches such a pitch that the actual death of that person leads to confusion of affect and fear of dissolution. Her own fear of death is triggered and projected onto the "disgusting substance" and onto the washing and checking compulsions, and, together with the separation of these worlds of compulsion from the real world, represent defenses against this fear.

The hermeneutical understanding therefore portrays the fear of death and defense against it, thus highlighting the basic anthropological dimension of obsessive-compulsive disorder and its significance and meaning. The thanatophobic obsessive-compulsive person attempts to stop time and impermanence and thus rapidly falls victim to the pressure of his passing and unlived life. Ms A. experiences her fear of death above all in the trigger situation in which her compulsive coping strategies are combined to form a meaningful unity. She is confronted everywhere with impermanence, her hopeless struggle, and her insurmountable feelings of guilt. For her, time is running out, paradise was lost through her birth and it becomes ever more distant with each passing year of her life.

The disturbance of the threatening side of the compulsion therefore permeates all levels of her understanding up to her fear of death, which becomes ever more apparent, and which is not significantly ameliorated by living a meaningful life. Static, genetic, and hermeneutic dimensions of understanding can be associated with, and related to one another in the hermeneutic circle. It is clear from the case of Ms A. that she is really trying to complete her task of personal development, which is bound up in compulsion: To differentiate herself from others, to delegate responsibility where appropriate, to live her own life, to accept what is irreplaceable in the course of time, as well as the threat of death, and to reintegrate the separated worlds of her normal everyday life. This creates both an analytical ordering of the obsessive-compulsive symptoms as well as their synthetic combination in the totality and purposefulness of the person, which, according to Jaspers, always remains open and incommensurable (Jaspers 1959).

BIBLIOGRAPHY

Akiskal H. S. (2006). "The Necessity of Integrating Phenomenology and Neurobiology in Bipolar Disorder." *Journal of Affective Disorders* 94: 1.

American Psychiatric Association. (1994). *Diagnostic and Statistical Manual of Mental Disorders: DSM-IV*. Washington DC: American Psychiatric Association.

American Psychiatric Association. (2013). *Diagnostic and Statistical Manual of Mental Disorders: DSM-V*. Washington DC: American Psychiatric Association.

Andreasen N. C. (2007). "DSM and the Death of Phenomenology in America: An Example of Unintended Consequences." *Schizophrenia Bulletin* 33: 108–112.

Ballerini A. and Stanghellini G. (1989). "Phenomenological Questions about Obsession and Delusion." *Psychopathology* 22: 315–319.

Binder H. (1936). "Zur Psychologie der Zwangsvorgänge." In H. Binder, *Ausgewählte Arbeiten (Selected Works) (1971)*, S. 221–317. Band 1. Bern: Huber.

Blankenburg W. (1971). *Der Verlust der natürlichen Selbstverständlichkeit. Ein Beitrag zur Psychopathologie symptomarmer Schizophrenien.* Stuttgart: Enke.

Blankenburg W. (1991). "Phänomenologie als Grundlagendisziplin der Psychiatrie." *Fundamenta Psychiatrica* 5: 92–101.

Bloch M. H., Landeros-Weisenberger A., Rosario M. C., Pittenger C., and Leckman J. F. (2008). "Meta-analysis of the Symptom Structure of Obsessive-Compulsive Disorder." *American Journal of Psychiatry* 165: 1532–1542.

Bürgy M. (2001). "The Narcissistic Function in Obsessive-Compulsive Neurosis." *American Journal of Psychotherapy* 55: 65–73.

Bürgy M. (2005a). "Psychopathology of Obsessive-Compulsive Disorder. A Phenomenological Approach." *Psychopathology* 38: 291–300.

Bürgy M. (2005b). "Zur Psychopathologie des Zwangs. *Zeitschrift für klinische Psychologie.*" *Psychiatrie und Psychotherapie* 53: 213–229.

Bürgy M. (2007). "Obsession in the Strict Sense. A Helpful Psychopathological Phenomenon in Differential Diagnosis between Obsessive-Compulsive Disorder and Schizophrenia." *Psychopathology* 40: 102–110.

Csef H. (2001). "Zwang und Persönlichkeit." *Persönlichkeitsstörungen* 5: 81–90.

Dilling H., Mombour W., and Schmidt M. H. (eds) (1991). *Internationale Klassifikation psychischer Störungen: ICD-10.* Bern: Huber.

Ecker W. and Gönner S. (2006). "Das Unvollständigkeitsgefühl. Neuentdeckung eines alten psychopathologischen Symptoms bei Zwangserkrankungen." *Nervenarzt* 77: 1115–1122.

Ehret A. M. and Berking M. (2013). "DSM-IV und DSM-V: Was hat sich tatsächlich verändert?" *Verhaltenstherapie* 23: 258–266.

Esquirol E. (1839). *Des maladies mentales considérées sous les rapports medical, hygiénique et médico-legal.* Paris: Bailliére.

Freud S. (1909). "Bemerkungen über einen Fall von Zwangsneurose." In *Gesammelte Werke*, Band 14, S. 379–463. Frankfurt: Fischer (1941).

Fuchs T. (2002). "The Challenge of Neuroscience: Psychiatry and Phenomenology Today." *Psychopathology* 35: 319–326.

Griesinger W. (1868). "Über einen wenig bekannten psychopathischen Zustand." *Archiv für Psychiatrie und Nervenkrankheiten* 1: 626–635.

Hoffmann N. and Hofmann B. (2004). *Expositionen bei Ängsten und Zwängen.* Beltz: Weinheim Basel Berln.

Hoffmann N. and Hofmann B. (2010). *Zwanghafte Persönlichkeitsstörung und Zwangserkrankungen.* Berlin, Heidelberg: Springer.

Hoffmann N. and Hofmann B. (2017). *Wenn Zwänge das Leben einengen.* 15. Auflage. Berlin, Heidelberg: Springer.

Jaspers K. (1913). *Allgemeine Psychopathologie.* Berlin: Springer.

Jaspers K. (1959). *Allgemeine Psychopathologie.* 7. Auflage. Berlin: Springer.

Kapfhammer H.-P. (2008). "Zwangsstörung. In: Möller H.-J., Laux G., and Kapfhammer H.-P. (eds), *Psychiatrie und Psychotherapie.* Band 2. 3. Auflage, S. 633–658. Heidelberg: Springer.

Kretschmer E. (1977). *Körperbau und Charakter.* 26. Auflage. Berlin: Springer.

Lang H. (1986). "Zur Struktur und Therapie der Zwangsneurose." *Psyche* 11: 953–970.

Lang H. (1998). "Ätiologie und Aufrechterhaltung der Zwangsstörungen aus psychodynamischer Sicht." In Ambühl H. (ed.), *Psychotherapie der Zwangsstörungen*, S. 23–30. Stuttgart, New York: Thieme.

Leckman J. F., Denys D., Simpson H. B., Mataix-Cols D., Hollander E., Saxena S., Miguel E. C., Rauch S. L., Goodman W. K., Philips K. A., and Stein D. J. (2010). "Obsessive-Compulsive Disorder: A Review of the Diagnostical Criteria and Possible Subtypes in Dimensional Specifiers for DSM-V." *Depression and Anxiety* 27: 507–527.

Meyer J. E. (1973). *Tod und Neurose*. Göttingen: Vandenhoeck & Ruprecht.

Meyer J. E. (1975). "Die Todesthematik in der Entstehung und im Verlauf von Zwangsneurosen." *Zeitschrift für Psychotherapie und medizinische Psychologie* 25: 124–128.

Meyer J. E. (1982). *Todesangst und das Todesbewußtsein der Gegenwart*. 2. Auflage. Berlin, Heidelberg, New York: Springer.

Mezzich J. E. (2007). "Psychiatry for the Person: Articulating Medicine's Science and Humanism." *World Psychiatry* 6: 1–3.

Müller C. (ed.) (1986). *Lexikon der Psychiatrie*. 2. Auflage. Berlin, Heidelberg, New York, London, Paris, Tokyo: Springer.

Nelson B., Fornito A., Harrison B. J., Yücel M., Sass L. A., Young A. R., Thompson A., Wood S. J., Pantelis C., and McGorry P. D. (2009). "A Disturbed Sense of Self in the Psychosis Prodrom: Linking Phenomenology and Neurobiology." *Neuroscience and Biobehavioural Reviews* 33: 807–817.

Quint H. (1988). *Die Zwangsneurose aus psychoanalytischer Sicht*. Berlin, Heidelberg: Springer.

Schmidt-Degenhard M. (2011). "Anthropologische Aspekte psychischer Erkrankungen." In Möller H.-J., Laux G., and Kapfhammer H.-P. (eds), *Psychiatrie, Psychosomatik, Psychotherapie*, Band 1, 4. Auflage, S. 383–396. Berlin, Heidelberg: Springer.

Schneider K. (1939). "Begriffliche Untersuchung über den Zwang." *Allgemeine Zeitschrift für Psychiatrie und ihre Grenzgebiete* 112: 17–24.

Schwidder W. (1972). "Klinik der Neurosen." In Kisker K. P., Mayer J. E., Müller C., and Strömgren E. (eds), *Psychiatrie der Gegenwart*, Band II/1. 2. Auflage, S. 351–415. Berlin, Heidelberg, New York: Springer.

Skoog G. (1965). "Onset of Anacastic Conditions. A Clinical Study." *Acta Psychiatrica Scandinavica Supplement* 184: 1–82.

Spitzer M. (1985). *Allgemeine Subjektivität und Psychopathologie*. Frankfurt: Haag & Herchen.

Straus E. (1938). "Ein Beitrag zur Pathologie der Zwangserscheinungen." *Monatsschrift für Psychiatrie und Neurologie* 98: 61–81.

Tellenbach H. (1971). *Melancholie: Problemgeschichte, Endogenität, Typologie, Pathogenese, Klinik*. Berlin: Springer.

v. Gebsattel V. E. (1954). "Die Welt des Zwangskranken." In *Prolegomena einer medizinischen Anthropologie*, S. 74–128. Berlin: Springer.

v. Gebsattel V. E. (1968). "Die anakastische Fehlhaltung." In *Imago Hominis*, S. 173–199. Salzburg: Müller.

v. Krafft-Ebing R. (1867). *Beiträge zur Erkennung und richtigen forensischen Beurteilung krankhafter Gemütszustände für Ärzte, Richter und Verteidiger*. Erlangen: Enke.

Westphal C. (1877). "Über Zwangsvorstellungen." *Berliner Klinische Wochenschrift* 46: 669–672.

Zaudig M. (2011). "Heterogenität und Komorbidität der Zwangsstörung." *Nervenarzt* 82: 290–298.

CHAPTER 66

THE LIFE-WORLD OF PERSONS WITH HYSTERIA

GUILHERME MESSAS, RAFAELA ZORZANELLI,
AND MELISSA TAMELINI

"The passion of hysteria is only a name, yet diverse and uncountable are the ways it encompasses."

Galen (*De locis affectibus* (8.413.15–414.16))

INTRODUCTION

HYSTERIA has a unique position within psychopathology, as it seems to harbor imprecisions and conceptual indecisions of this discipline. Its definition was never consensual, and the flaws in its understanding reveal much of the epistemological avatars that have guided psychopathology, and consequently psychology and psychiatry, throughout this century and the previous one.

Throughout history, the concept of hysteria has been connected to a range of behaviors and psychological states marked by drama, mystery, or falsity (Kraus 2007). Hysteria was understood as a plurality of somatic manifestations that were difficult to decipher, ranging from exaggerations in emotional expression, gestures, and mimicry, to paresthesia, involuntary movements, or even the complete loss of consciousness associated with convulsive seizures. This rich symptomatic expression of suffering and physical symptoms, combined with the absence of anatomical and pathophysiological markers, has established lasting controversies around its conception. In nineteenth-century France, where its modern roots are found, the concept of hysteria already evoked disputes over its legitimacy. While Charcot and the Salpêtrière school were striving to demonstrate the relevance of the construct, the Nancy school, represented by Bernheim, argued that the state of the Salpêtrière hysterics was due to suggestion and did not exist outside of that circumstance (Trillat 1986; Bogousslavsky 2011).

Such discussions of the nature of hysteria have never been closed in psychiatry. However, after the development of psychoanalytic theory, they seem to have given way to a consensus.

Hysteria was central to the development of Freud's theory, and his understanding of the phenomenon, supported by the postulate of the unconscious, eventually prevailed in culture.

The psychoanalytic orientation also guided the official classifications of psychiatry until the 1980s. At that time, the desire to build a definitive and absolutely reliable classification system within the field of psychiatry emerged with vigor. In this context, the errant construct of hysteria seemed problematic. Its troubled course in the field of psychiatry, on one hand, denounced the fragility of the scientific ambitions mentioned above and, on the other, gave way to an understanding too closely connected to psychodynamic theories. Thus, with the stroke of a pen, hysteria was banned from official psychiatric classifications after 1980 with the publication of the *Diagnostic and Statistical Manual of Mental Disorders*—DSM-III (APA 1980).

If we briefly revisit the changes throughout the various editions of the manual, we will observe that in DSM-I (APA 1952) the category closest to the hysterical phenomena appeared with the denomination of conversion reaction. In DSM-II (APA 1968), it was grouped under the new diagnosis of hysterical neurosis, echoing the concept of hysteria of the psychodynamic theories. In DSM-III (APA 1980), the new category becomes Somatoform disorders, divided into several sub-categories (somatization disorder, undifferentiated somatoform disorder, pain disorder, and somatoform disorder not otherwise specified). In DSM-IV (APA 1994), the modifications focused on changes in the list of criteria for inclusion in the category of somatoform disorders. In its most recent edition, DSM-5 (APA 2013), several changes were made: the category of conversion disorder was delimited with more detailed criteria; the category of somatic symptoms disorder (SSD) is created, combining those of somatization disorder and somatization disorder not otherwise specified; the pain disorder and body dysmorphic disorder sub-categories were removed and hypochondriasis was renamed as illness anxiety disorder and redefined (Moldovan et al. 2015). This DSM-5 proposal, in line with the principles of DSM-III, specifying subtypes of a larger category— whose gestalt could be compared with hysteria—was not immune to controversies either, especially regarding the coherence of these divisions as parts of a whole (Mayou et al. 2005; Starcevic 2006; Regier 2007).

This historical "decline" of hysteria in the field of psychiatry has diverse interpretations. Micale (1993) notes that the diagnosis of hysteria and its various formulations underwent a radical process of nosological remodeling in the twentieth century, and would be disappearing if not entirely gone. Neither historians nor clinicians, however, agree on the disappearance of hysteria (Stone et al. 2008). Lewis considers hysteria one of those diseases "which has had a sentence of death passed upon them more than once, yet they obstinately survive" (1975: 9). There is evidence that it is the medical interest in this entity—inhabiting "the no-man's land between these two specialties [neurology and psychiatry]" (Stone et al. 2008: 12)—that has disappeared, not the phenomenon itself. Thus, assuming the clinician's insistence on recognizing the existence of hysteria in diverse contexts and in a manner impervious to the current epistemological dispositions, it is necessary to seek a methodological framework that will give it anthropological support. Although the developments of the classical notion of hysteria are marked by a persistent conceptual indefinition, an essential core of the lived hysterical world can be identified in a consistent manner in the clinical experience.

The understanding of hysteria as an anthropological unit can only come about through the investigation of the essential structures of human existence. Thus, it is within the framework of phenomenological psychopathology, the most advanced modality of psychopathological science (Stanghellini 2009), that are found the methodological tools for a deep psychopathological dissection of the hysterical person.

Throughout the chapter, we will trace a course demonstrating the essential unity of the fundamental structures of the hysterical human existence, unfolded in its main anthropological conditions of possibility: temporality, spatiality, embodiment, and identity. The adjective "anthropological" indicates that the level at which this phenomenon occurs is not that of the integration of the self, that is, the ontological level, which is necessary for the personality to be constituted as an ontological unity in time and space and for it to have a competent body to express life as meaning (Merleau-Ponty 1945/2012). The ontological level "determines existence in general" (Binswanger 1958: 191) and precedes and functions as a condition of possibility of the anthropological level. Characteristics of hysteria do not take place in the constitution of the self (Charbonneau 2010), but in the loss of a healthy balance of its transcendental anthropological proportions. To better elucidate hysteria, we will compare the hysterical condition with other conditions that may be confused with it, or that, by being opposite, may aid in its elucidation. Finally, we will briefly present a dialectical perspective of the phenomenology of hysteria, which takes into account the fundamental ambiguity of human existence.

THE PHENOMENOLOGICAL UNDERSTANDING OF THE ESSENTIAL CORE OF HYSTERIA

The act of phenomenological understanding seeks to reveal fundamental elements of the existential reality that are stable enough to be identified in other similar cases in pathological or non-pathological situations. This essential core must necessarily be found in every phenomenological manifestation studied.[1] In the case of hysteria, from what we have seen previously, this identification gains even greater relevance, since the multiplicity of symptoms of the condition casts doubt even on its anthropological and psychopathological validity. The following reflections on the hysterical essence observe a criterion of descending importance for its understanding.

Interpersonality: Relational Hypo-Sufficiency

The best-known essential definition of hysteria goes back to Jaspers, formulated in his famous sentence: ". . . crave to appear, both to themselves and others, as more than they are and to experience more than they are ever capable of" (1997: 443). This definition, never entirely rejected by other phenomenological psychopathologists, contains much of what is meant

[1] The phenomenological strategy of searching for the essence of psychological experiences is not undebatable, since other researchers consider ideal types or prototypes as the main object of phenomenology (Fernandez 2016). Moreover, the search for a fixed object as the aim of the phenomenological procedure is also disputable (Messas et al. 2017).

by hysteria, although the Jaspersian conception of phenomenology has been limited to the descriptive layer of experience, leaving out the investigation of the structuring pre-reflexive layer (Messas 2014). The importance given by the author of *General Psychopathology* to "appear before the other" is fundamental to the understanding of hysterical experiences.[2] It is by means of a more detailed analysis of this definition that we will arrive at the central function of otherness in the constitution of hysteria.

Hysteria is based on an experience of imbalance between the poles of interpersonality. There is an anthropological disproportion (Blankenburg 1982) between the importance of the pole of the I and that of the pole of the other, with priority given to otherness.[3] Hysterical experiences have as their fundamental presupposition the existence of an extremely powerful, we may even say, omnipotent other. The exaggerated expressiveness of the hysterics or their typical dramaticity (Charbonneau 2007) is based, in contrast with what Jaspers thought, on this fragility of the I, exposed in an excessive way to the existential supremacy of the other. As the other manifests herself, in the eyes of the hysteric, in a totipotent way, and shows herself unshakeable in her self-sufficiency, a mobilization is required from the hysterical person to remove the other from indifference and draw her to herself. With this, the hysterical person seeks to achieve some balance for his insufficient I. The central relevance of this interpersonal characteristic led Schneider, in his classic work *Clinical Psychopathology*, to reject the use of the term hysteria for one of his psychopaths, giving preference to the more explicit and descriptive notion of "Psychopaths in need of esteem" (Schneider 2007).

Hysterical relational hypo-sufficiency also supports the fact that the hysterical existence can take many forms, following the general lines of culture and the behavioral possibilities in the social and historical moment, being sometimes an expression of existential protest (Jonckheere 2009: 71). As a result, when hysteria enters the field of interest in psychopathology, it was a mainly female clinical manifestation, provoked by a supposedly repressed sexual urge. However, phenomenologically, one should not understand a mechanism of repression of female sexual desire—or even of any other desire—as the basis for the anthropological understanding of hysteria because hysteria is also a masculine anthropological condition (Charbonneau et al. 2015). The logic is the reverse: hysteria seeks to pre-reflexively identify themes, identities, and behaviors that are capable of producing movement and attention in the other. If, in a particular relationship, in a specific cultural period, such as the end of the nineteenth century, the sexual theme is the most powerful in the mobilization of the other, that will be the theme to gain hysterical existence. If, in another relation, the trigger of possible mobilization is different, hysteria takes on another of its thousand forms.

In the life-world of hysteria, the existential movement is the mobilization of everything that can remove the hysterical I from its position of inferiority and hypo-sufficiency, granting it, even if falsely, a position of centrality. Thus, hysterical consciousness is a consciousness of exaggeration, theatricality, and staging (Charbonneau 2007). It is precisely in

---

[2] The Jaspersian definition extends the "appear before" to the I of the hysterical person itself. Later, in this text, we will defend how this modality of appearance may be reduced to "appear before the other."

[3] We consider, throughout this chapter, that the style of the anthropological disproportion in hysteria determines strong interpersonal polarities. Consequently, hysteria may be better understood in terms of the polarity I–Other (however, with a view to reading flow, we will only use the notions of "I" and "other") than in terms of self-modifications. In hysteria, the role of the self is limited to enhancing the above mentioned polarity.

the theater that the human dramas are emphasized through a caricatural expressiveness. In order for the central themes of human life to be detached from the monotony of everyday life, they must be clothed with a pretense that is paradoxically the affirmation of truth.

The relational hypo-sufficiency of the I determines that the insertion of the hysterical person in the world depends too much on the meanings and values that the other imprints on the world, or that the hysteric believes the other imprints on the world. From this derives the seduction typically associated with hysteria, since to seduce means to seize and to offer, immediately and expressively, that which, for the other, has value. Another proof of this anthropological subjugation of the hysterical I to the meaning imposed by the other is hysterical suggestibility (Charcot 1888). The hyper-valuation of the other also underlies the cases of fantastic pseudology. In these, a representative fantasy, originally aimed at capturing the attention of the other, is taken to ultimate consequences, dominating the weakened I of the hysteric, who comes to believe in his own mental constructions. This belief in the unreality of facts is radically different from a schizophrenic delusion, because of the existential dimension in which they occur (Charbonneau 2010). If schizophrenic pathologies occur at the ontological level of the constitution of the self (Fuchs 2007), the experiences of the hysterical world are limited to the anthropological level, in which the primary constitution of the self is not compromised. Likewise, hysterical alterations, even when assuming supposedly psychotic characteristics, continue to have the other as a tacit end to which their clinical manifestations turn (Sigmund 1997). Hysteria is subjugated to the sense emanating externally from the values and desires of the other, and as such is capable of capturing an integral sense, unlike what occurs in schizophrenia. To return to the classic example of nineteenth-century female hysteria, from the perspective of incipient psychoanalysis: hysteria resulted from the impossibility of conscious emergence of a morally intolerable psychic content. Now, for a content to be—even if unconsciously, within the psychodynamic model—intolerable, it must already be fully meaningful in advance. It is, therefore, legitimate to say that meaning floods the hysteric. Hysteria is the flooding of a meaning which has as primary source the meaning of the world given by the other. Consequently, from the anthropo-phenomenological point of view, it is illegitimate to speak of hysterical psychosis (Sigmund 1997). More precisely, as the author points out, the severe alterations of hysteria must be considered as pseudopsychoses.

We have seen how hysteria is based on the domination of the I by the excess of meaning coming from the other. This existential condition can also be understood as the expression of a singular heteronomy. Kraus coined the term heteronomy to define the domination of melancholic existence by the rules of the collectivity; for him, melancholia would be in opposition to hysteria (2007), although this clear anthropological distinction can be lost in a purely semiological analysis (Kraus 1985). The melancholic would be heteronomous because she would allow herself to be entirely determined by the rules of the collectivity, incorporating the totality of her I into the collectively determined role. There is nothing to contradict in this deep perception of melancholy in its relations with the other and the collectivity. However, it is worth noting what Kraus means by heteronomy. For the author, the meaning determining the melancholic experience is the meaning of the norms and social roles established by culture. In this sense, for the melancholic, both her own I and the I of others are pre-reflexively perceived as heteronomous, since both must be governed by a norm that, established by the collective, transcends both. Perhaps it would be more accurate, in this case, to speak in terms of collective heteronomy, since the notion of heteronomy in itself can be more comprehensive. Hysteria also appears to be characterized by a different modality of heteronomy. In it, heteronomy seems to be singular, that is, the other that is considered pre-reflexively is an exclusive, personalized, private, and heroic individual, representing a power that goes beyond conventional social norms. This excellence by which the other is experienced by the hysteric makes her primarily the object of passion, the typical feeling of sublime and irreproducible relationships. The uniqueness of the heteronomy of the hysteric other makes the hysterical person normally interested in persons holding or presumed to hold positions of power. The other is intended by the hysterical person as unique in its meaning-giving power. This characteristic also makes the hysterical person different from the maniac, with which he could be confused, in his contempt for social conventions. The manic person, however, has a strong, egocentric ego (Sass and Pienkos 2015) that addresses the world, whereas in hysteria, as we have seen, the I is frail and hypo-sufficient.

Rovaletti examines in depth this singularity of the other as experienced in hysteria, of which a heroic and therefore painful role is required. She affirms that "pure and simple desire would humiliate [the hysteric] and cause her horror, but on the other hand she would find no charm in respect that was only respect" (1999a: 6). The other, endowed of excessive importance by the hysterical person must, at the same time, be restricted in her role (Sutter 1983). On one hand, if she allows herself to freely express her desire over the hysterical person, she is repelled by having acted unilaterally, transforming the hysterical person into an object. On the other hand, an integral respect, by which the hysterical person is treated as a single being and endowed with her own desire, disqualifies the relation. Respect, in a way, mitigates the intensity and especially the effectiveness of the other's power. The hysterical I needs to identify its totipotent other as a continuous power, as a Nietzschean superman beyond morality. The hysterical person needs the other in a way that is perfectly pictured in the famous phrase quoted by Simone de Beauvoir, echoing a familiar one: "I would like giants and all I find is men" (2011: 417). Thus, an insoluble paradox marks the relations of the hysterical I with its other. The Nietzschean hero demanded by the hysterical person—and in which she is transformed as a reflection—is regulated by a mixture of strength and candor, practically impossible to achieve. It is as if hysterical seduction needed to invoke the heroism of the other to be protected by it. However, to do so and attain its full protection, it needs to know the other in her extreme limits. The typical case of this situation is the hysterical erotic seduction in which the hysterical person does not have an effective sexual purpose. Seduction serves as certification for the other to be able to desire deeply, reducing the hysterical person to the condition of an object, but at the same time maintaining a position of respect in which the hysterical I is embraced in its frailties. This paradox of hysterical relationships, as you can imagine, is at the root of many relational difficulties.

Another factor hindering the establishment of in-depth interpersonal relationships is hysterical immaturity, given by the continued state of hypo-sufficiency and interpersonal disproportion. The maturity of the personality is based on a presupposed possibility of attributing to any person the same existential potentials and limitations that the own subject has, in which the relational poles are able to alternate their value according to the context. In the case of hysteria, as the I fixates itself on a less-value condition if compared to others of which it depends to exist (or from which it cannot free itself), it is not competent to carry out the alternation leading to maturity, preventing its consciousness from living the experiences that arise from this alternation.

Thus, affectively, the hysteric is dominated by immature feelings, often taken as "childish," and which determine, as a reflection on the other, attitudes of discontent and even irritation. Usually idealized by the hysterical person, the excessive value of the other leaves the impression of being based on false and even invasive feelings. The impression of sentimental falseness that the hysterical person promotes originates in the exaggeration that each affection or feeling contains, precisely because they are oriented to the mobilization of the other. A state of subjugation can result from this interpersonal hypo-sufficiency, causing hysterical relations to sometimes assume a perverse face. Perversity as such, however, in which subjugation is rooted in the desire to nullify the other, lies at the opposite pole of hysteria. The hysterical person just seeks to keep the other powerful in a state of attention and availability.

For this reason, the positional exaggeration conferred by the hysteric on the other must also merit investigation from the experiences lived by this other by means of affective resonance (Messas 2010). Affective resonance is an indispensable tool for a diagnosis, as advocated by Minkowski and his notion of "diagnostic par pénétration" (1995). To the experiential exaggeration of the hysteric corresponds a discomfort in the other, experienced, more often than not, as an invasion of her privacy or an outrage to her authentic availability. Often within a relationship, the hysterical person seeks to go beyond the limits determined by social conventions and attract the other into a zone of intimacy, many times with the proposal of relational themes of embarrassing content or performing acts of evident seduction. The embarrassment—or irritation and disbelief—occasionally experienced by the partners in their relations with hysterical people is the corresponding affective face of the interpersonal pressure that the hysterical person places upon them. Hysteria is a dramatic scene requiring the active participation of the observer, usually invading his personal availability. A hysterical interpersonality is a unilateral decree, dictating a full and intense form of relationship— often without the assumption of the intimacy that is essential to a relationship. Occasional intense feelings, produced in the interpersonal relationship involving the hysterical person can have a flavor of inauthenticity, as already pointed out by Jaspers (1997) and Kraus (2007). This inauthenticity presupposes the inability of the hysterical feeling to actually touch the other. The hysterical person always falls short of herself, exalting her states and themes of consciousness to imitate a relational equality that cannot be attained. This hysterical sentimentality may occasionally seem to the inattentive observer or an observer who is only concerned with the descriptive layer of behavior as an inflation of the I—they "appear, ... to themselves more than they are ..." (Jaspers 1997: 443). However, a more comprehensive analysis accurately identifies the opposite state: the apparently narcissistic experiences of hysterical vanity lie in phenomenological compensation (Minkowski 1995), a mechanism aimed at rebalancing the inequality in which it exists, and that drives its impotent I to live near fragmentation as we shall see below. Strictly speaking, the hysterical person does not believe or disbelieve in herself, but is dominated by a set of feelings or behaviors that end up oppressing her to such a degree that it no longer makes sense to measure the situation in terms of belief or disbelief, truth or lie, authenticity or inauthenticity.

Temporality

Given that relational hypo-sufficiency is the essential anthropological core of hysteria, temporality is characterized by the presence of the other as the attracting and conducting pole of experience. Thus, temporality in hysterical existences is usually marked by the preponderance of elements connected to the present. Since what matters is the other, temporality is determined by a constant updating of the life-world, dependent on the presence or absence of the other. Every time there is a change of the other with whom the hysterical person relates, there is a re-updating of parts of her personality, making her unstable. This instability is born of an excessive valence of the present, since the hysterical person lives "unhindered" from the elements of retention of the past and the indeterminacies of the future. This is the aspect of temporality that can best meet the impositions of hysterical interpersonality. It is important to notice that, although there is a preponderance of the present, we are not faced with a constitutive change of temporality, or a disintegration of lived time, that is typical of schizophrenia (Fuchs 2013). The exaggerated relevance of the present can justify possible substance abuses and other behaviors marked by a fleeting and volatile instant (Kimura 2005).

Spatiality

Spatiality is the transcendental framework fundamental to the existential movement and the understanding of the hysterical essence. The hysterical movement in the world is based on situations that, from the spatial point of view, are marked by

a) Centrality-peripherality. The hysterical person divides the lived space in terms of the dialectic centrality-peripherality. Hysterical relations always occur as a movement in which the center must necessarily be occupied by someone who determines a peripheral position to the other. As we have seen above, in a deeper level of analysis, the other will always be the center of experience, situated on a stage of maximum visibility and value. However, the above-mentioned anthropological mechanism of phenomenological compensation makes the hysterical person deceptively appear to occupy the relational center. This vicarious occupation occurs through the production of intense emotions, the elevation of the colors of the emotions contained in an interrelational act, and is based, according to Blankenburg, on the need to overcome failures in the constitution of the I (1974).

b) Anthropological distance. Hysteria is an experience of primordial distance, of incapacity for a true approach. Distance is the matrix that allows the scenic visibility of the hysterical person. The hysterical person does not base her relationships on an approach by which a fertile relationship is consolidated into a dual unity. On the contrary, the heroic other of the hysteric must be kept at a distance, just so that her heroism is not reduced to human banality. The strength with which the hysterical person depends anthropologically on her heroic other is sustained by the distance maintained from the other. The visuality of hysterical behavior, its mannerisms, sentimental affectations, and extroversion, eventually depend on a distance for their effectiveness. For this reason, the romantic and idealized passion is the most characteristic feeling of the hysterical person. Romantic passion occurs in the absence of the beloved object, in its distance in time (the idealization of lost and impossible loves, for example) and in space (the romanticization of other cultures or societies, in which one could find a heroic person to love). The occasional excessive approximation of the hysteric with the other, leading to intimacy, could remove the brightness of the relationship.

Embodiment

Embodiment will also serve the anthropological core of hysteria. Thus, corporeality tends to serve as a tool for expression and compensation of this fundamental core. Hysterical intensity, understood as compensation for the fundamental hypo-sufficiency of the I, can be well expressed in the domains of the body. The exaggeration of the hysteric can be marked, for example, by subordination to the dictates of fashion and by the excessive use of corporal expression, reaching, in more intense cases, a condition of mannerism. It is an instrumentalized body (Blankenburg 1974) and excessively placed as a function of the eyes of the other. For this reason, the bodily complaints of the hysterical person tend to be indeterminate and changeable (Kraus 1996), varying according to desires perceived in the other. The embodiment of the hysterical person is traversed more by passive suffering than by active elaboration. Physical suffering appears in chronic pain, fibromyalgia, chronic fatigue, etc., or in excessive care for the body (e.g. rigorous diets, or an intense routine of exhausting physical exercise, aiming at becoming a perfect object of desire). Both the painful embodiment and that which seeks perfection can remove the existence of its own authenticity.

Social Identity

In hysteria, the way the I relates to its partial identities is marked by detachment. Kraus (2007) examined the hysterical mode of existence from the point of view of the dialectic between the I and its identity. Following a Sartrean perspective, he argues that the defining factor of the hysterical person is her low adherence to social identities. As opposed to the melancholic, who clings exaggeratedly to her partial identities, becoming hypernomic, the hysterical person adheres only superficially and tangentially to the partial identities, becoming hyponomic. The hysterical person is able to understand the social roles at her disposal, but she cannot keep up with them. The hysteric easily takes two paths, that of transience and that of deformity.

i. Hysterical hyponomy makes each identity role dominant in consciousness for a short time, soon being replaced by another. This is why the hysterical person seems to cry convulsively in one moment to, immediately after, faced with another relational situation, laugh comfortably, leaving the observer with the impression of deceit. This is not a question of the falsification of feelings, but of their transience. The excessive rapidity of their succession causes each of them to be experienced superficially. This superficiality may reach such a point that the hysterical person itself is no longer able to control the role it plays; in these situations, the hyponomic heteronomy makes the role itself dominate the hysterical person, configuring the dissociative states in which there seems to be another I controlling her actions. Here again we find a paradox in the hysterical form of being: dissociative semiology is the clinical form of an autonomous heteronomy, a control of the I by another hidden I, which acts according to its own laws, as a character.

ii. This other I can, therefore, become a character that dominates the author herself, in a parody of Pirandello's play (1921). The hysterical person, being dominated by a partial identity that does not linearly follow the demands of social roles, deforms it, transforming her existence into social caricatures, as postulated by Charbonneau et al. (2015). Thus, hysterical behavior is established like that of a buffoon, a Don Juan, etc., types that were previously literary and idealized rather than actually existing in social everyday life. The hysterical person, also from the point of view of identities, lives in a world of imagination and distortion. ·

Hysterical Anthropological Fragmentation

The notes made so far are capable of guiding the psychopathological understanding of the continuous manifestations of the personality of the hysterical person, such as exaggeration in expressions, seduction, and drama. However, for the understanding of semiologic dissociative elements (i.e. acute or sub-acute traits marked by the disappearence of psychic elements such as memory and identity), or somatic elements such as paresis, anesthesia, or sensory loss (as in hysterical blindness or deafness), it becomes necessary to elucidate the second transcendental existential foundation of hysteria: fragmentation.

The "negative" clinical findings are also based on the excessive presence of the other as the source of a dictatorial meaning to which the I feels imprisoned and on which it depends. The inability to exit the situation of relational hypo-sufficiency, in certain critical situations in which there is an increase in relational tensions, rises to the point of triggering another phenomena of hysteria: anthropological fragmentation. Hysteria, in its dissociative and conversive patterns, is characterized by the anthropological modifications in dimensions that are vital for the existence as follows.

Temporality

When hysterical fragmentation is in place, temporality is marked by the partial discontinuity of the present in its relations with the past. This fragmentation of the present assumes two forms that are usually connected. The first has as a characteristic the suppression of the experiential continuity of some recent fact, of great significance, coming directly from the interpersonal relations. The most typical case of this form of hysterical fragmentation is post-traumatic dissociation, in which, although existence continues to move in the world, in general, according to its previous pattern, the exact mnemonic segment connected to the other disappears from the hysterical consciousness. This temporal gap, however, paradoxically represents the excessive presence of an aggressive punctual action of the other in the hysterical consciousness, which is not capable of integrating it into the total flow of its existence, producing a discontinuity that affects only a portion of the anthropological integrity of the hysterical person. The same existential foundation explains the classic hysterical *belle indiférence*. In hysterical temporality, the other is preserved as absence; in schizophrenia, on the other hand, the other submerges in the figure of an anonymous world—the Dreadful (Binswanger 1957)—or of a threat that does not come from the conversations between the I and the other.

This partiality, which depletes relevant segments of the present (Chammond 1992), can lead to the second form of the temporal fragmentation of hysterical existence, the exaltation of manneristic behaviors (Charbonneau et al. 2015). Hysterical mannerism is the manifestation on the surface of consciousness of the replacement of the genuine temporality of biography by a behavioral atypicality, created only to fill the gap left by fragmentation. Mannerist types created by hysteria are not anchored in an integral temporality, in which the future is the consequence of the present. Thus, the types of hysterical mannerism do not favor the construction of a web of relationships: they do not go beyond the exaltation of a colorful and temporally inconsequential present. This fragmented present, because it is not based on the roots of the biography itself, also has volatility as a consequence. In certain cases, some of these mannerist hysterical experiences may take on the appearance of absolute dyscontrol, which at first makes them almost indistinguishable from a psychotic picture, although, as we have seen, they occur in different existential dimensions. The temporality of hysteria, therefore, even in its fragmentation, continues to be driven by the other.

Mercurial Spatiality

The fragmentary spatiality of hysteria turns the experiential field into a mercurial soil, ready to dissolve at any moment. The fragmentation of lived spatiality assists in the differential recognition of hysteria in relation to mania and melancholia. The state of maniacal exaltation fully and coherently compromises all the partial functions of consciousness; in relation to mania, hysterical excitation tends to be more discontinuous, with abrupt and sometimes contradictory emotional variations among them, showing dependence on the relation with the observer (Sigmund 1997). Melancholy, although semiologically opposed to mania, from the point of view of the unity of its spatiality, seems to be similar. The melancholic experiences reach the whole of existence, whereas in hysteria any depressive findings are not total (Kraus 1985), they shake only part of the functions of consciousness, as in the aforementioned *belle indiférence*.

Puzzle Corporeity

The fragmentation of the hysterical world acts directly in corporeity, that is, in the experience of the lived body (Zutt 1963). The inability to maintain biographical temporality causes the body to lose its characteristics as an instrument for the realization of a life-project, becoming the passive stage of failure in the anthropological integrity of the experiences. Hysterical conversion presents to the other an I dethroned of its own body and eager for reintegration of possession. This reintegration can only occur by the direct action of the other, observed classically in the influence of hypnosis on the hysterical cases. The difference in being a body and having a soma (Fuchs & Schlimme, 2009) is clear in hysterical experiences. The soma, physical body (*Körper*) that silently supports existence, is ordered by the rules of physiology. The lived body (*Leib*) is ordered by the idiosyncratic representations of each person: it is an instrument of its field of signification in the world (Merleau-Ponty 2012). In the hysterical person, there is a fragmentation of the lived body, a situation in which it becomes the repository of the impossibilities of signification of the hysterical consciousness. The meaning of a situation of which the I participates and to which it must react, if intolerable for the hysterical person, is drained into the lived body. However, as seen in conversions, it cannot be found in the lived body either. There it arises only as a denial of the power of the I, as motor fragility or sensory anesthesia. This meaning dissolved in the fragmentation of the unity of the lived body calls for a reunification. This reunification is given by the language of the totipotent and heroic other. There is, as a central characteristic of hysteria, the possibility of the behavior of the hysterical person being interpreted by the observer. The other is the giver of language, the agent capable of translating the disembodied expressiveness of the hysterical person into a reunified meaning. The hermeneutic function of the observer of the hysteria is equivalent to that of someone who assembles a puzzle. In this puzzle, each piece, isolated, does not seem to have an autonomy of meaning. Once connected, as if by magic, the pieces gain integral meaning. In the same way, the hysterical person experiences in himself/herself a meaning that cannot be expressed as a result of an existential weakness that needs the other to find its narrative (Rovaletti 1999b).

An Anthropology of Hysteria: Dialectic and Existence

The maintenance of the concept of hysteria is, in a sense, a symbol of the preservation of interpersonality as a primordial instrument for the construction of phenomenological diagnoses. Hysteria can only be defined from an interpersonal perspective, in which the observer tries to connect the patient's scattered experiences into a unity of meaning (Giorgi 2009). This general unity, regardless of its diversity of presentation, may be termed hysteria, if by that concept we mean a mode of being-in-the-world that can be experienced by all people at some point in their lives. Moments in which the foundations of adulthood depend heavily on the giving of meaning provided by a meaningful other. Therefore, hysteria is a general anthropological essence, participant, more actively or passively, of any and all human experience, and should not be understood as a pathology in the strict sense of the word. Hysteria, as a tyranny of the heteronomous meaning, can only be identified by an act of knowledge founded on an epistemology of interpersonality that allows it to be understood as an anthropological direction of meaning (Binswanger 1956), susceptible to a high degree of conceptual indetermination (Depraz et al. 2011). This indeterminacy does not mean that hysteria cannot be differentiated from conditions that are also expressed in the interpersonal world, and especially from borderline existence. We believe that despite possible similarities in the emotional presentation, drama and relevance of the pole of the other, in the life-world of borderline persons we have a distinct anthropological essence, characterized by meaninglessness of life and "and empty intentionality" (Stanghellini and Rosfort 2013: 173), whereas in hysteria the intentionality has the other as its main goal. Can we, departing from this, postulate a constructive existential value for hysteria? Could one suppose that an involuntary and radical subordination to the other might lead to some existential advantage? The possible positive value of hysterical experiences seems to lie in the stabilization of the existence of the hysterical person in the power of the other, in the construction of a hierarchical relationship that can, at certain moments in life, or even definitively, make viable a life that, without such support, would not find paths for its own authenticity. Hysterical experience— notably in the personalities marked by the anthropological essence of hysteria—shows that existential authenticity should not be understood exclusively as a position of autonomy of the I in relation to the other. The examination of hysteria shows that to exist in an authentic manner is also possible through a hierarchical existence in which the other is irreplaceable and anthropologically necessary. As we shall see below, this statement is not an apology for tyranny or subordination. It is the opposite.

The anthropological value of hysteria can also be understood from another perspective. Hysteria, by establishing a special dual relationship, in which the other primarily, and the I secondarily, break the norms of conduct consolidated in the social roles of culture, may possess a value of creative insubordination. Hysteria would be the battering ram of a possible renewal of society's patterns of experience and behavior (Blankenburg 1974; Dorr-Zegers 2008). Hysteria is, from this perspective, anti-melancholia, with its behaviors of adherence to tradition. The hysterical person, with his supposed sentimentality and inauthenticity, not only leads to breaking the boundaries of the habitual, but somehow induces the other to do so, seducing him to undertake experiences on the limit of herself. Jointly, the hysterical relational duality may be a form of Dionysian refusal of the tradition enshrined in laziness and in the indulgence of habits naturalized by unreflective repetition. Hysteria is an unexamined uprising that, at a second stage, claims for a reflection on the very ordering of life and social relations. Here again, hysteria diverges anthropologically from mania: mania has the appearance of rupture, with its jocular irreverence; however, it is no more than a conservative exaltation of the I, by means of inflation of the self. Hysteria is, in a sense, a creative distortion of the anthropological proportions of the interpersonality, which makes and invites the other to make life a constant paroxysm, hoping that the repetition of an existential fiction can lead life to the experience of brilliance and passion, regardless of risking annulment in the abysses of the vital falsification. Hysteria makes us face, like no other anthropological condition, the dilemmas of human renewal.

Hysteria, anthropologically, reveals the Sartrean bad faith (1943) of which human identity is composed and which it needs to transcend its own facticity, but in which it risks becoming incarcerated. The capacity for transcendence and renewal belongs to the human being, but in hysteria it is revealed more clearly by the force of mobilization of the other. This mobilization of the other and the I, although partially inauthentic, detaches the individuals from the community background in which they are rooted. From this detachment, two trajectories can be established: one of them passes through the rejection of the collective against the excessively singular individual; in the other, the novelty it contains can offer the collective new forms of existence. Forms that, initially inauthentic, by the use and repetition, gradually become authentic for all. It is this anthropologically hysterical function that inspires the artists who, breaking the conventions of their time, launch the history of society to new paths. In short, we could say that the anthropological essence of hysteria is the human dialogue between voluntary servitude (Boétie 2002) and Nietzsche's superman. A radical and profoundly human dialogue, which resists time and changes in classificatory framings.

BIBLIOGRAPHY

APA. (1952). *Diagnostic and Statistical Manual of Mental Disorders*, 1st edn. Washington, DC: American Psychiatric Association.

APA. (1968). *Diagnostic and Statistical Manual of Mental Disorders*, 2nd edn. Washington, DC: American Psychiatric Association.

APA. (1980). *Diagnostic and Statistical Manual of Mental Disorders*, 3rd edn. Washington, DC: American Psychiatric Association.

APA. (1994). *Diagnostic and Statistical Manual of Mental Disorders*, 4th edn. Washington, DC: American Psychiatric Association.

APA. (2013). *Diagnostic and Statistical Manual of Mental Disorders*, 5th edn. Arlington, VA: American Psychiatric Publishing.

Beauvoir S. (2011). *The Second Sex*, trans. C. Borde and S. Malovany-Chevallier. New York: Vintage Books.

Binswanger L. (1956). *Drei Formen missglückten Daseins: Verstiegenheit, Verschrobenheit, Manieriertheit*. Tübingen: Max Niemayer Verlag.

Binswanger L. (1957). *Schizophrenie*. Pfüllingen: Neske.

Binswanger L. (1958). "The Existential Analysis School of Thought." In R. May, E. Angel, and H. F. Ellenberger (eds.), *Existence: A New Dimension in Psychiatry and Psychology*, pp. 191–213. New York: Basic Books.

Blankenburg W. (1974). "Hysterie in anthropologischer Sicht." *Praxis der Psychotherapie* 19: 262–273.

Blankenburg W. (1982). "A Dialectical Conception of Anthropological Proportions." In A. De Koonig and F. Jenner (eds.), *Phenomenology and Psychiatry*, pp. 35–50. London: Academic Press.

Boétie E. (2002). *Le Discours de la Servitude Volontaire*. Paris: Petite Bibliothèque Payot.

Bogousslavsky J. (2011). "Hysteria After Charcot: Back to the Future." In J. Bogousslavsky, *Following Charcot: A Forgotten History of Neurology and Psychiatry*, pp. 137–161. Basel: Karger.

Chammond J. (1992). "Pénibles devenirs dans les névroses. Hystérie, la temporalité close." *Cliniques méditeranéennes* 35/36: 75–90.

Charbonneau G. (2007). *La situation existentielle des personnes hystériques: intensité, centralité et figuralité*. Société d'anthropologie phénoménologique et d'Hermeneutique Générale. Paris: Vrin.

Charbonneau G. (2010). *Introduction à la Psychopathologie phénoménologique*. Paris: MJM Fédition.

Charbonneau G., Schmit P.-E., and Ordono R. (2015). "L'homme et son hystérie: Anthropologie et psychologie de l'hystérie masculine." In G. Charbonneau, P.-E. Schmitt, and R. Ordono (eds.), *Le Cercle Herméneutique*, pp. 24–25. Paris: Vrin.

Charcot J. M. (1888). *Leçons du mardi à la Salpêtriére*. Progrès medicale, Paris: Tomo I. Lecrosniew & Babe.

Depraz N., Varela F., and Vermersch P. (2011). *À l'épreuve de l'expérience. Pour une pratique phénoménologique*. Bucarest: Zeta Books.

Dörr-Zegers O. (2008). "Personality Disorders from a Phenomenological Perspective." *Actas Esp Psiquiatr* 36(1): 10–19.

Fernandez A. V. (2016). "Phenomenology, Typification, and Ideal Types in Psychiatric Diagnosis and Classification." In R. Bluhm (ed.), *Knowing and Acting in Medicine*, pp. 39–58. Lanham, MD: Rowman & Littlefield International.

Fuchs T. (2007). "The Temporal Structure of Intentionality and Its Disturbance in Schizophrenia." *Psychopathology* 40: 229–235. doi: 10.1159/000101365

Fuchs T. (2013). "Temporality and Psychopathology." *Phenomenology and The Cognitive Sciences* 12(1): 75–104. doi: 10.1007/s11097-010-9189-4

Fuchs T. and Schlimme J. E. (2009). "Embodiment and Psychopathology: A Phenomenological Perspective." *Current Opinion in Psychiatry* 22(6): 570–575. doi:10.1097/YCO.0b013e3283318e5c

Giorgi A. (2009). *The Descriptive Phenomenological Method in Psychology. A Modified Husserlian Approach*. Pittsburgh: Duquesne University Press.

Jaspers K. (1997). *General Psychopathology*. (M. W. Hamilton & J. Hoenig) Baltimore: Johns Hopkins University Press.

Jonckheere P. (2009). *Psychiatrie Phénoménologique: Tome 2*. Argenteuil: Le Cercle Herméneutique.

Kimura B. (2005). *Scritti di psicopatologia fenomenologica*. Roma: Giovanni Fioriti Editore.

Kraus A. (1985). "Phänomenologie pseudohysterischer Verhaltens-und Erlebnisweisen Melancholischer." *Fortschritte der Neurologie-Psychatrie*. 53: 469–475.

Kraus A. (1996). "Pseudohysterie Melancholischer." In G. Seidler (ed.), *Hysterie heute. Metamorphosen eines Paradiesvogels*, pp. 131–143. Stutgart: Ferdinand Enke Verlag.

Kraus A. (2007). "Modes d´existence des hystériques et des mélancoliques." In P. Fédida and J. Schotte (eds.), *Psychiatrie et existence*, pp. 231–246. Grenoble: Éditions Jérôme Millon.

Lewis A. (1975). "The Survival of Hysteria." *Psychological Medicine* 5: 9–12. doi: 10.1017/S0033291700007169

Mayou R., Kirmayer L. J., Simon G., Kroenke K., and Sharpe M. (2005). "Somatoform Disorders: Time for a New Approach in DSM-V." *American Journal of Psychiatry* 162(5): 847–855.

Merleau-Ponty M. (2012). *Phenomenology of Perception*, trans. D. Landes. London, New York: Routledge.

Messas G. (2010). "A Phenomenological Contribution to the Approach of Biological Psychiatry." *Journal of Phenomenological Psychology* 41: 180–200. doi: 10.1163/156916210X532117

Messas G. (2014). "O sentido da fenomenologia na Psicopatologia Geral de Karl Jaspers." *Psicopatologia Fenomenológica Contemporânea* 3(1): 23–47.

Messas G., Tamelini M., and Cutting J. (2017). "A Meta-analysis of the Core Essence of Psychopathological Entities: An Historical Exercise in Phenomenological Psychiatry." *History of Psychiatry*, doi: 10.1177/0957154X17715414

Micale, M. S. (1993) "On the 'Disappearance' of Hysteria: A Study in the Clinical Deconstruction of a Diagnosis." *Journal of the History of Science Society* 84: 496–526.

Minkowski, E. (1995). *Le temps vécu*. Paris: Presses Universitaires de France.

Moldovan R., Radu M., Băban A., and Dumitraşcu D. L. (2015). "Evolution of Psychosomatic Diagnosis in DSM. Historical Perspectives and New Development for Internists." *Romanian Journal of internal Medicine* 53(1): 25–30.

Pirandello L. (1921). *Sei personaggi in cerca d´autore*. Firenze: R. Bemproda & Figlio—Editori.

Regier D. A. (2007). "Somatic Presentations of Mental Disorders: Refining the Research Agenda for DSM-V. Editorial." *Psychosomatic Medicine* 69: 827–828.

Rovaletti M.-L. (1999a). "La histeria o la tentativa extrema del ser como exhibición." *Revista Chilena de Neuropsiquiatría* 37: 83–90.

Rovaletti M.-L. (1999b). "La histeria; una condición humana hecha de pura ceremonia." *Revista Chilena de Neuropsiquiatría* 37: 91–99.

Sartre J.-P. (1943). *L´être et le néant*. Paris: Gallimard.

Sass L. and Pienkos E. (2015). "Faces of Intersubjectivity: A Phenomenological Study of Interpersonal Experience in Melancholia, Mania, and Schizophrenia." *Journal of Phenomenological Psychology* 46(1): 1–32.

Schneider K. (2007). *Klinische Psychopathologie. 15 Auflage*. Stuttgart, New York: Georg Thieme Verlag.

Sigmund D. (1997). "Phänomenologie der hysterischen Pseudopsychosen. *Fortschritte der Neurologie-Psychatrie* 65: 387–395.

Stanghellini G. (2009). "The Meanings of Psychopathology." *Current Opinion in Psychiatry* 22(6): 559–564. doi: 10.1097/YCO.0b013e3283318e36

Stanghellini G. and Rosfort R. (2013). "Borderline Depression. A Desperate Vitality." *Journal of Consciousness Studies* 20(7–8): 153–177.

Starcevic V. (2006). "Somatoform Disorders and DSM-V: Conceptual and Political Issues in the Debate." *Psychosomatics* 47(4): 277–281.

Stone J., Hewett R., Carson A., Warlow C., and Sharpe M. (2008). "The 'Disappearance' of Hysteria: Historical Mystery or Illusion?" *Journal of the Royal Society of Medicine* 101(1): 12–18. doi: 10.1258/jrsm.2007.070129

Sutter J. (1983). *L'anticipation*. Paris: Presses Universitaires de France.

Trillat É. (1986). *Histoire de l'hysterie*. Paris: Seghers.

Zutt J. (1963). "Über den tragenden Leib." In J. Zutt (ed.), *Auf dem Wege zu einer antropologischen Psychiatrie. Gesammelte Aufsätze*, pp. 416–426. Berlin, Göttingen, Heidelberg: Springer Verlag.

CHAPTER 67

THE LIFE-WORLD OF PERSONS WITH BORDERLINE PERSONALITY DISORDER

GIOVANNI STANGHELLINI AND MILENA MANCINI

INTRODUCTION

BORDERLINE personality disorder (BPD) is a highly variegated clinical constellation of abnormal phenomena characterized by unstable mood, behavior, and relationships. Despite different approaches emphasizing different aspects of BPD, there is general agreement about the fact that its principal features are the following: 1) emotions tend to be intense and rapidly shifting; 2) relationships tend to be conflicted and stormy; 3) there may be impulsive, self-destructive, or self-defeating behaviors; 4) there is a lack of a clear and coherent sense of identity.

In this chapter, we describe BPD from the angle of the emotions displayed by these persons. We assume that their existence oscillates between dysphoria and anger: dysphoric mood is a permanent trait, and angry affect is an intermittent state. Since dysphoria and anger generate two different life-worlds to borderline persons, our descriptions will include two distinct configurations: the dysphoric life-world and the life-world of anger. The world of dysphoria is characterized by a painful experience of incoherence and inner emptiness, a feeling of uncertainty and inauthenticity in interpersonal relationships, and an excruciating sense of futility and inanity of life. But it also entails a sense of vitality, although a disorganized, aimless, and explosive one. In the world of anger the vague and confused sense of self and others is suddenly replaced by a clear, although elementary normative, universe in which it is painfully obvious to the borderline person who is "good" and who is "bad." This sudden feeling of infallible righteousness helps the borderline person find his lost identity in a world that momentarily regains its structure and meaning.

In the following section we provide a comprehensive analysis of the value-structure of persons with BPD. They live under the spell of a *frustrated normativity* (Stanghellini and Rosfort 2013a), driven by the value of authenticity thus entering into collision with the ethical norms or social conventions that structure and organize our interpersonal world and the hypocrisy and inauthenticity of the pallid emotions by which other persons live.

EMOTIONS IN BORDERLINE PERSONS

There are two basic emotions characterizing the life-world of borderline persons: *anger* and *dysphoria*. Before we proceed with the description of these, it is appropriate to briefly introduce a distinction between *affects* and *moods* (Stanghellini and Rosfort 2013a; see also Rosfort's chapter on *Emotions,* this volume). *Affects* are focused and possess a specific directedness. They are felt as motivated, more determinate and articulated than moods. Affects normally do not open up a horizontal awareness, but occupy all my attentional space. This is the case with anger. *Moods,* on the contrary, are unfocused. They do not possess a specific directedness and aboutness. They are felt as unmotivated. Moods do not direct us to anything specific in our relation to the environment, and we are not able to put our finger on what exactly causes our particular mood.

Anger is an *affect* triggered by a personal offense and as such it often motivates a desire for retaliation. Anger may entail assaultive behavior which summons these affects as a sinister shadow. Despite its complex cognitive, personal, and social aspects (Solomon 2007), anger is, in most cases, a readily identified emotion because of its rather clear behavioral manifestations such as increase of muscle tension, scowling, grinding of teeth, glaring, clenching of fists, changes of arm position and body posture (Tavris 1989).

The characterization of *dysphoric mood* requires more attention because of its more subdued manifestation and less direct connection to behavioral patterns. Dysphoria manifests itself as a prolonged, unmotivated, indistinct, and quasi-ineffable constellation of feelings that convey a nebula of vague impulses, sensations, and perceptions that permeate a person's whole field of awareness. The psychological and psychopathological characterization of dysphoria is quite difficult because of its subdued manifestation and loose connection to definite behavioral patterns. It is an oppressive, and sometimes unbearable, mood. In its etymological roots the word "dysphoria" (*dysphoros* = hard to bear) is quite polysemous, nearly overlapping "bad mood" in very general terms, vaguely defining an emotional condition in which a person is heavily oppressed, and in which that person may either react and show his feelings, or passively suffer and submit to them (Stanghellini 2000; Stanghellini and Rosfort 2013a). Phenomenal characterizations of dysphoria mainly focus on its being felt as a burden one cannot get rid of because it is not external to one's own self. It is an obstacle to movement and, at the same time, it may generate impatience, restlessness, and an incoercible impulse to move away without a definite goal. It is also experienced as an uncomfortable feeling characterized by being painful and sorrowful, as well as discontented and indignant (see Rossi Monti and D'Agostino's chapter *Dysphoria in Borderline Person*, this volume). This complexity elicits opposite kinds of movement such as inaction/action, resignation/resistance, suffering/retaliation (Stanghellini and Rosfort 2013a, 2013b). Also, in dysphoria, the normal distinction between self and other is blurred. No particular action is dictated by dysphoric mood. On the contrary, it complicates the relation between feeling and action because it introduces doubts and questions. Dysphoria is a mood that consists of a purely noetic act without a noematic target. In BPD existence, noematic representations do not function as a dispositive "to control the noetic act so that it does not deviate from its relationship with life" (Kimura 2000: 88; our translation). This characterization tallies perfectly with the experience that borderline persons have of their own dysphoric mood: an untamed source of vitality, a disturbing and an exuberant force, creative and destructive at the same time, a vigor that brings life as well as annihilation.

In the borderline person's existence there is a dialectic between dysphoria and anger:

- Dysphoria is the *background mood trait* characterizing persons with borderline personality disorder (Stanghellini and Rosfort 2013b). It is the long-lasting and profound emotional tonality or basic temperament in which the borderline person is enmeshed, and as such it influences both the voluntary and involuntary aspect of her perceptions and actions. This emotional state is saturated with a brimming constellation of feelings without any explicit object or target.
- Anger is an *acute intermittent state*. Angry outbursts, emanating from the dysphoric background, are typically accompanied by feelings of shame and humiliation and may generate acute micro-psychotic episodes during which the borderline person may develop paranoid symptoms, including transitory persecutory delusions in which the persecutor is typically a significant other (the patient's partner, relative, or therapist, for example).
- Dysphoria can also be an *acute intermittent state* during which their dysphoric mood intensifies, culminating in a painful paralysis of action characterized by feelings of spleen, boredom, despair, emptiness. This may entail tormenting ideas of meaninglessness, persecutory guilt, and, in the most severe cases, suicidal ideation.

There are other emotions that may have a special importance in the experience of borderline persons, namely, *boredom* and *shame*.

Boredom

Boredom is a mood characterized by a pervasive lack of interest in everything. The entire world is monotonous, and this monotonousness cannot be analyzed by the person into further elements, but encloses the surroundings, things as well as persons, in a vague and unarticulated way: the world as a whole "seeps towards me from the globe like a cosmic fog, deadening my mind, slackening my will, and depleting me of energy" (Smith 1986: 191). While bored, the world-whole is just happening and is a blankness that endures. Lived space is an indifferent extension, devoid of salience, offering no directions, moribund. It conveys a feeling of meaninglessness and *finis vitae*. Lived time is an oppressing stillness. One's movements remain stuck in indecisiveness. The other is distant, meaningless, annoying.

Heidegger (1995) recognizes three forms of boredom: (1) being bored *with* something (or to be sick of something) (*Gelangweiltwerden von etwas*), (2) being bored *by* something (*Sichlangweilen bei etwas*), and (3) profound boredom (*tiefe Langweile*). Each form of boredom is distinguished from the others in terms of its relation to how time passes (see also Freeman and Elpidorou 2015).

The first form of boredom is our pre-theoretical understanding of boredom. It occurs when we are bored with some person, object, or state of affairs that causes annoyance. It arises, quoting Heidegger's example, while waiting at the station for our train which is already delayed, and communications are not encouraging because we don't know when the train is going to arrive. The second form of boredom is both more profound and slightly more complicated. In it, *there is no determinate person or object that is boring*. Rather, we are bored by something indeterminate and unfamiliar: something that has the character of "I know not what" (Heidegger 1995: 114), and that Heidegger ultimately identifies with the passing of time itself—not in the form of time dragging, as in the first form of boredom, but rather in the sense of *time standing still*. Heidegger's example of this form of boredom is attending a dinner party, on our own volition, in an attempt to kill time. At the party, the food, company, and music are all pleasant. And yet, when we reflect upon the evening and situate it in terms of what was interrupted in order to attend the party and of what is coming in the next days, it dawns on us that we were bored all this time after all. Our own decision to partake in such a predictable, and *in retrospect* dull, event results in an emptiness: the party does not fulfil us.

Profound boredom is the third and deepest form of boredom. It is an extreme and over-whelming experience in which everything bores us and, unlike the first form of boredom, there is no point in fighting it. In profound boredom we stand without any concerns and interests. Profound boredom strips away all identifying characteristics, history, or projects; beings as a whole withdraw, they lose all significance. In profound boredom, absolute indifference overtakes us and we become insignificant, as does our surrounding environment. This form of boredom thus renders us "an undifferentiated no one" by disclosing to us a world with no meaning or significance (Heidegger 1995: 135).

In the borderline existence, the boredom implicated is of the third kind. Here, boredom shares with dysphoria the same temporal structure (monotonousness) and an analogous feeling of bluntness. Indeed, in boredom as well as in dysphoria the world, other people, and oneself just happen and are void of significance. The disappearance of meaning and significance that people with borderline personality disorder experience in boredom is correlated with temporality. Total indifference means that nothing carries future prospects for us and that nothing relates and gives meaning to our past. Indeed, in borderline boredom, all three temporal dimensions of *Dasein* (past, present, and future) blend together and it is this "unarticulated unity" that entrances *Dasein* (Heidegger 1995: 148). What bores us is not any specific entity or state of affairs; rather, it is time (as originary temporality) itself. Time bores us by entrancing and binding us. So, in this way, the mind goes blank. Nothing has a sense. The borderline person goes around in circles, and in a purposeless way.

Shame

Whereas boredom is a mood that stymies my mind and dulls my attention, *shame* is an affect that awakens and focuses my attention. When I feel ashamed, I am aware of being seen by another person whose gaze uncovers a part of who I am, usually a part that makes me feel embarrassed, dishonored, and humiliated (Stanghellini and Rosfort 2013a, 2013b). Lived space in shame has a centripetal character as one experiences a feeling of centrality. I feel my body naked, deprived of any protection, soiled. The other is in a dominant position, a watcher or a witness. Lived time comes to a fixation in an instant that grows to infinity. My identity is constantly threatened by the instability brought about by humiliation.

The effect of shame is that it reduces the complexity of the person that I am to one single aspect of it: when I feel ashamed, I think that for the other I am *nothing but* that specific feature of the complexities of who I am. In shame, I feel that my whole self disappears, while that detail—the *stain*—of my self that made me feel ashamed becomes over-conspicuous and takes center-stage. Shame reveals to me my selfhood as an object for another; or shame is, as Sartre writes, "shame of *self*; it is the *recognition* of the fact that I *am* indeed that object which the Other is looking at and judging" (Sartre 1956: 261). The others are piercing gazes that nail me to what awakened my feeling of shame: an act or an omission, or some failing or defect, which elicited contempt, derision or avoidance from other people. Shame means to be utterly exposed to the present, to the painful presence of devaluating gazes, to annihilating disdain and contempt (Fuchs 2003).

The feeling of shame—Scheler argues (2012; see also Cutting 2009a, 2009b)—belongs to the *clair-obscure* of human nature. For our unique place within the structure of the world and its entities is between spirituality and animality. Shame is the revelation of the nature of the human being: the basic condition for the feeling of shame to occur is only given when the light of consciousness is existentially bound up with the living organism and shines down on the inner life. To the origin of the feeling of shame there belongs something like an imbalance and disharmony between the sense and the claim of spiritual personhood and embodied animal needs. It is only because the human essence is tied up with a "lived body" that we can get in the position where we can feel shame.

THE LIFE-WORLD OF DYSPHORIA

Dysphoria and anger engender very different kinds of existential orientation, thereby enacting very different configurations of the life-world that borderline persons live in.

Time

There are two main time features in the life-world of dysphoria. The first is *monotony*. Time can be experienced as a tedious, wearing, dull cloud in which past, present, and future are not clearly separable. The second is *instantaneity*. Time is experienced as an absolute "now" into which the person, her identity, and history collapse.

We have seen this first feature of borderline temporality while describing profound boredom. In profound boredom one feels stripped away from all identifying characteristics, history, or projects. It renders one "an undifferentiated no one" and discloses a world with no meaning or significance. In boredom, nothing matters to us, nothing attracts us, there is nothing to which we can relate. The world, other people, and oneself just happen and are void of significance.

To the dysphoric person, the "now" is a *pure present*, lacking extension into the future (*protention*) and into the past (*retention*). Presenting themselves independently from past and future, they cannot feel the "length" of these nows, as it is possible with a present that develops out of the past and is directed toward the future. Each now moment thus becomes an infinity. This kind of absolute "now" has no temporal delimitation, no historical determination, and no linguistic-symbolic articulation. This isolated "now" is not able to carry any kind of relation to, or become an integrated part of, the narrative identity of the dysphoric person. In these moments, an acute feeling of despair, that is, discordant directions of intentionality leading to a paralysis of thinking and action, accompanies dysphoria. This "transitory present" has no depth. "It lacks the fulfilment which only originates from the integration of past experience and anticipated future" (Fuchs 2007: 381).

Yet in the life-world of dysphoria the absorption in the present moment quite paradoxically does not just convey feelings of void and monotony, but also thrilling experiences of instantaneity. Time in the life-world of dysphoria is punctuated by "islands of feast" in a stagnant "ocean of spleen" (Kane 2001: 214). It is being "dead for a long time" interrupted by transient, vanishing, volatile moments of intensity. Dysphoria is punctuated with moments of excitement during which one's blind vitality finds its fulfillment. This side of time-experience is called by Bin Kimura (1992) *intra festum*. As in the atmosphere of a feast, here we find the irruption of spontaneity and ecstasy, oblivious of the past and the future. Blind spontaneity is the opposite of voluntary autonomy as the rapture of ecstasy is the opposite of engaged care. Moreover, dysphoric persons are unable to cope with the flux of immediateness; this flux becomes paroxysmal, immediateness chaotic. The borderline person is immersed in the *intra festum* and experiences a short circuit of selfhood in front of the paroxysm of chaotic immediateness. The absolute "now" is the night of the self and the disintegration of personhood. In dysphoric temporality there is no separation, no space in between the "now" and the person: the person collapses into her "now" (Stanghellini and Rosfort 2013a).

Thus, the present moment is *momentary* in the sense that it is lived as evanescent and fleeting. But next to this volatile and empty character of temporality, sometimes the events are not just momentary, but also *momentous*, that is, overwhelmingly significant. The present moment can be spasmodic, urgent, clamant. Events—including the appearing of a person in the room, someone's way of moving, the tone of his voice—may acquire an offensive, thing-like physiognomy, and become intruding. Borderline persons can be overly sensitive to minimal social stimuli, like the other's facial expressions that pass unobserved by the majority of people. Typically, the patient is not capable of integrating these "spasms" of hyper-awareness in a fluent and attuned relationship with the other person. Instead of contributing to the development of an exchange of feelings and views between oneself and the other, they stand out as islands of immediateness, leaving no space between oneself and the other, and between oneself and one's own overwhelming insights.

Dysphoric persons, therefore, live in a restricted temporal horizon and are scarcely aware of a future or a past. They appear inconstant, voluble, "moody," often prey to emotional crises. They also appear to be trapped in present stimuli, so that, for instance, their therapeutic conversation is often a mere catalogue of recent events. Their awareness is captivated by the present moment, as if they were unable to switch off the stimuli that are coming from the environment or from their own body. These sensations may appear irrelevant or meaningless to an external observer, but for borderline patients themselves they are abnormally important and amplified. This phenomenon cannot be explained as abnormal arousal, as it is the case with anxious patients. A further feature of temporal discontinuity is the so-called "traumatic system" (Meares 2000) that will be analyzed in the section on narrative and limit-situation section.

Space

Dysphoria has a horizontal absorption in the sense that it attends to the world as a whole, not focusing on any particular object or situation. No particular action is dictated by dysphoric mood. On the contrary, it complicates the relation between feeling and action because it introduces doubt, hesitation, and questions. It entails a kind of paralysis of action and thinking, but not a static one, rather a frenzied, disconcerting paralysis.

Dysphoric space is usually experienced as indifferent extension, a space devoid of salience that offers no directions and no way out. We find an apparently similar phenomenon describing lived space in persons with schizophrenia. The basic difference between these two is that whereas in the schizophrenic mood lived space conveys a feeling of unreality, in borderline persons it conveys a feeling of meaninglessness. Furthermore, when dysphoria turns into boredom, the surrounding world is "moribund" (Stanghellini and Rosfort 2013a).

Body

The emotional fragility or stable instability experienced by borderline persons while inhabiting the dysphoric life-world is caused by a raw, unmediated bodily vitality that does not accommodate to pre-reflective intentional structures or cognitive efforts. Their dysphoric mood is characterized by extreme presence of a primary, bodily force that fragments the intentional structure of the lived body, exposing a brutal vitality, a mere body entirely at the mercy of the basic biological values that nourish and to some extent orient human emotional life. There is little possibility for action in this kaleidoscopic universe of raw feelings. Objects become unfocused and intentional structures crumple under the intensity of this emotional pressure. The intimate sense of being an embodied self is eclipsed by the sense of having an intimidating body. This chaotic vitality, being devoid of intentional structure and content, desperately seeks an object, mostly a person, at which to direct its surplus of energy. This means that the dysphoric person feels the presence of a spontaneous energy without any clear direction or target. It is emotional energy that throws itself at the other with an overwhelming intensity. Often, this impulse takes on a sexual form. This power is a violent spasm that takes control of the body and takes the representation of oneself to pieces, reducing it to an assemblage of disordered emotions and drives. However, it is also a power that expresses an encouraging vitality seducingly in touch with invigorating sensations.

The sense of void is very common in borderline depression or in the micro-depressive episodes which may punctuate the borderline person's daily existence. These are the episodes during which deep feelings of depersonalization add up to the permanent lack of a stable, integral identity. Sensations of emptiness, numbness, fragmentation, vanishing of one's own self are typically accompanied by feelings of abandonment and aloneness. Precisely because dysphoria as a mood cannot be easily modulated, the only possible control is sought outside of the mind. This relief can be achieved by acting on the environment and transforming it with violence. Yet, self-harm is the most typical way to find relief from the torment of the inner tension of dysphoria (Rossi Monti and D'Agostino 2014). Self-mutilations might represent a means of reducing the tension. Cutting represents another attempt to modulate or staunch a negative and oppressive mood condition, precipitating it in a place that has a name and is objectifiable, delimited, and so also "curable" (Rossi Monti and D'Agostino 2014). It is as if the body could be a concrete and visible sort of drain for overwhelming emotions.

Self

Dysphoric mood brings about a formless sense of one's own self. The development of a co-hesive and continuous sense of self depends upon a special form of dialogue (Stanghellini 2016) that is lacking in the borderline person's life-history. A non-linear, associative, and ap-parently purposeless form of dialogue, whose topic may at first glance seem banal. It is like a game, since it is apparently aimless. Or like an atmosphere, because it can be extremely dif-ficult to answer questions about what is actually going on here or what we are really talking about. Intimacy is the basic emotion involved in this kind of conversation. Intimacy, Meares (2000) explains, is not to be equated with confession or unrestrained revelation. Rather, it is a feeling of "aloneness-togetherness" in which this special kind of conversation is embedded, such as having a peculiar warmth or a form associated with a sense of well-being. Intimacy fundamentally depends upon the sharing of one's own inner experience with another.

Moreover, the integrity of the self can be damaged by traumatic experience. The kind of trauma at issue here is not only sexual abuse or some form of violent behavior, but rather takes the form of an invalidating environment. An invalidating environment is one in which communication of private experiences is not met by appropriate responses. Instead of being validated, private experiences are trivialized, their expression is discouraged, and emotions (especially painful emotions) are disregarded. The kind of trauma that may jeopardize the development of a warm and intimate sense of self is the absence of recognition (Stanghellini and Rosfort 2013a).

Other Persons

At the heart of borderline persons' drama resides the excruciating experience of the other. The main concern of the borderline person is to achieve a sense of recognition. The other is indispensable for living and its absence makes the presence of the self impossible. The other is experienced as absent when she is not totally present. Her absence, or incomplete pres-ence, is often the reason for feelings of non-recognition and desperate loss of selfhood. The other who does not donate her entire self is an inauthentic other. The other is also the source of aching shame, since her gaze is permanently experienced on the razor's edge between rec-ognition and humiliation.

In synchrony with the drastic fluctuation of feelings, there is an instability in the appear-ance of other persons. In the life-world of dysphoria, others may appear as mere shadows. The other is experienced as indefinite, indeterminate, indistinct, ill-defined. All these qual-ities that the dysphoric person perceives in other persons express in semi-sensorial terms the unintelligibility of the other. The indefiniteness of the other worsens in acute dysphoric-depressive episodes during which the other may become opaque: fuzzy, blurred, caliginous, cloudy, foggy, grey, hazy. When the dysphoric mood turns into anger, the other changes from being opaque to being tenebrous: he is ambivalent, evasive, obscure, puzzling, un-explicit, and suspect (Stanghellini and Rosfort 2013a).

Something of the desperate and frustrated energy of the dysphoric mood is transferred to the intentional structures of the interpersonal relation. The borderline person longs for intense, passionate relationships. It is all-or-nothing. This immensely intense character of the interpersonal relationships makes them highly vulnerable. The slightest change in the emotional atmosphere, a wrong word, a delay, and the borderline person feels attacked or humiliated, and reacts with anger.

THE LIFE-WORLD OF ANGER

Time

As we have seen in describing the life-world of dysphoria, borderline persons live unhistorically, bound to a transitory present without depth (Stanghellini and Rosfort 2013a). The dysphoric person is absorbed in an unmediated instantaneity (Kimura 1992): a pure or absolute now devoid of past and future. This is also the case with anger, although with some relevant differences.

Anger makes a person identify completely with her momentary state of mind, unable to gain a distance from the present situation, torn by emerging impulses. In anger, borderline persons are completely absorbed by the phenomenon that agitates them. When a person is angry, a relevant feature of the world (usually threatening her personal existence and the value she attaches to it) captivates her, irrupts into her field of awareness without her having decided to turn her attention to it. She becomes fixated on the object of her anger, and all her attention is captured by it.

Space

Significant transformations in the experience of space may occur in relation to the complexity of emotions that characterize the borderline existence. In the life-world of anger, events are described as "wounding," "biting," "stinging." Someone's remark may be felt as "caustic," "corrosive"; her behavior "raw," "sharp." Changes in lived space make it possible to experience someone's comportment as piercing; the piercing metaphors arise from alterations of lived space (Stanghellini and Rosfort 2013a).

In general, the physiognomy of things in the life-world of borderline persons reflects the fluctuation in lived time between evanescence and urgency: things show themselves on the edge between melting and blasting. Whereas in dysphoria space is an indifferent extension devoid of salience and offers no directions and movement remain stuck in the indecisiveness of juxtaposition, in the life-world of anger space offers no protection. Space is a bee-line between the angry person and the person who offended her. The offending one gains an absolute centrality around which everything else dissolves.

Body

In the grip of the anger the body is impregnated by it. A numb and empty body becomes a body filled with anger, that is, a bodily self that can finally feel itself, a strong and hard embodied self that repays the suffered insults—but at the cost of losing its humanity, and thus wrecking the fragile dialectic of selfhood and otherness constitutive of personhood. It is a bodily self that is insensitive to the voice and the face of the other person, a self without innocence. The body merely becomes a "state" of wild emotional tension bringing the person to destruction.

Self

Anger tends to preserve and maintain a precarious cohesion of the self (Pazzagli and Rossi Monti 2000: 223). In this perspective, anger is to a certain extent a self-defining emotion. This is the case for the borderline person's anger, which seems to be situated at the point where an intention swings into its opposite: fragile doubts about oneself and the other into incorrigible convictions, moral indignation into the dishonor of aggression, the fire of love into the stake of intolerance (Stanghellini 2000). This is indeed the place of emotions like shame and humiliation that pave the way to the outburst of anger. The life-world of shame to a certain extent parallels that of anger. The experience of humiliation precedes the experience of anger. I feel seen by another person whose piercing gaze nails me to a part of myself that makes me feel humiliated. I feel my body deprived of any protection and at the same time dirtied. Yet shame, as compared to dysphoria, is a feeling that restores a sense of self-identity and self-recognition, although confined to a negative part of one's self. The effect of shame is that it reduces the nebula of feelings conveyed by dysphoria to one single feature: *my stain*. Reducing my identity to my defect, it restores a primitive sense of selfhood.

Anger may come as a reaction to shame, and in this case, the person may lose her opportunity to contact and recognize that part of herself that the other's gaze has revealed. When shame turns into anger we forget that we must feel shame because of our being a continuous movement and a transition in which the gaze of the other serves to acknowledge our limitations and to come to terms with our *guiltless guilt* (Scheler 2012).

Anger tends to preserve and maintain a precarious cohesion of the self, in the sense that venting one's anger is a way of feeling alive and of affirming one's right to exist as the unique person that one is. In anger episodes, the vague and confused sense of values and norms that characterizes dysphoric existence is suddenly replaced by a crystal clear, although elementary normative, universe in which it is painfully obvious to the borderline person who is "good" (oneself) and who is "bad" (the other). This sudden feeling of infallible rightfulness helps the borderline person to find his or her lost identity in a world that momentarily regains its structure and meaning.

Other Persons

First of all, anger is the means through which the borderline person reacts to every minimal break in empathy: anger emerges when the person feels that the other will not fulfill her basic need for recognition. Anger makes the other clearly visible, strongly characterized, and standing out very distinctively. It allows a switch from the state of vagueness where the other is blurred and ambiguous to a condition in which the other is crisp and clear. In this sense, anger has a "centripetal" role, coagulating the emotional dispersion that characterizes dysphoria. Furthermore, anger defends from the pain of separation and loss: a mind kept busy by angry fantasies is still clinging to what it has lost (Rossi Monti and D'Agostino 2014). In the light of anger, which dissipates the hazy atmosphere of dysphoria, the other suddenly comes into focus as a persecutor. The gaze of the other mercilessly lays bare the patient's inner insufficiency and thus makes her feel humiliated. So, the sense of identity established by anger is highly unstable due to the fact that the cohesion brought about by anger is constantly threatened by the instability brought about by humiliation. Moreover, feelings of abandonment, or lack of attention, acceptance, help, protection, reciprocity, support—or in short, lack of *recognition*—are typical in the borderline traumatic existence. The dysphoric person looks primarily in the direction of the other. It is the other who is guilty, since he or she acted out of voluntary intention. These feelings may kindle acute emotional states characterized by, resentment and indignation. The self-other relationship may take the form of a transitory persecutory delusion (Stanghellini and Rosfort 2013a, 2013b).

NARRATIVE SELF AND LIMIT SITUATION

As we saw above, borderline persons lack "object constancy" in the sense of being able to retain a positive image of significant others in spite of temporary separation or rejection. The result is what Fuchs (2007) has called a fragmentation of the narrative self: a shifting view of oneself, with sharp discontinuities, rapidly changing representations of oneself and the others and an underlying feeling of inner emptiness. There is no sense of continuity over time and across situations, no concept of self-development that could be projected into the future, but only an endless repetition of the same emotional states, creating a peculiar a-temporal mode of existing. The patients often rapidly change their goals, jobs, and friends as well as their convictions; they are unable to commit themselves to a set of self-defining volitions, enduring relationships, and long-term aspirations (Westen and Cohen 1993).

Temporal integration and narrative identity are closely intertwined. Narrative identity implies a meaningful coherence of the personal past, present, and future. This meaningful coherence is the product of an enduring labor striving to make one's life coherent and to fill it with meaningful behavior. Narrative identity is different from mere constancy or sameness, since it is a temporal relation to oneself by remaining faithful to one's commitments, promises, and responsibilities in front of other people (Ricoeur 1992: 118). It also requires the capacity of self-determination by forming durable second-order volitions, at the price, if necessary, of repression or conflicts. Borderline persons lack the capacity to form enduring second-order volitions, in the light of which present impulses could be evaluated and selected.

An essential feature of the borderline persons' life-world is that typically these persons are not able to distance themselves from present events. The present moment irrupts without mediation into the existence of borderline persons. Borderline persons are not able to liberate themselves from what they are suffering right now: there is no separation between the now experience and the borderline person. The incapacity to distance oneself from an event, to take a stance in front of it, to integrate it into a narrative sequence and by doing so to give a personal meaning to it, are defining characteristics of trauma. A trauma is an event that the person is not able to appropriate, that is, to integrate in her narrative identity. Our existence is moved forward by what happens in our life. Events happen to us as a part of involuntary otherness involved in a human life, and we appropriate these events, or we define ourselves in opposition to these events; but no matter how we relate ourselves to these events, our sheer relation, our position-taking, instills personal meaning in them, and by this activity we affirm our selfhood. The event becomes a traumatic event, it becomes pathogenic, when it does not kindle the dialectic of narrative identity—rather, it arrests the historicity of existence (Stanghellini and Rossi Monti 2009a, 2009b).

The typical trauma in the existence of borderline persons involves a special of relational trauma or "limit situation." Limit situation (German: *Grenzsituation*) is a concept developed by Jaspers (1919) to conceptualize situations with specific toxicity for a given kind of vulnerable individual. Fuchs (2013) has used this concept to elaborate "existential vulnerability." Jaspers defined limit situations as antinomies inevitably given in human existence: fight, guilt, finality, suffering. Limit situations are characterized by "inevitable antinomies which prevent a person from going on as usual. A personal solution is necessary to accustom which implies change or development." A limit situation is any of certain situations in which a human being is said to have "differing experiences from those arising from ordinary situations" (Mundt 2014).

Borderline persons live out a traumatic existence because their now moments are pure presentification, lacking protention and retention. Also, they are incapable of distancing themselves from the present experience and by doing so to take a different stance toward it, that is, to view their present from a different angle (Stanghellini and Rosfort 2013a). This is the nature of the existential vulnerability of borderline persons that finds its counterpart in specific limit situations characterized relational trauma.

The frequency of traumatic experiences is significantly higher than in other personality disorders or in depression. However, clinicians should not automatically assume that present traumatic experiences are re-enactments of early traumatic experiences. Correale (2007) advises clinicians to transfer the focus of attention during therapy sessions from the search of early psychological adversities to the *daily traumas* suffered by these patients. This is not to deny the importance of child abuse or neglect in the pathogenesis of this condition. Rather, it is a way to meet the patients' need to recount their traumatic existence, and to enhance the patients' capacity to describe their experiences and reflect upon them by placing them in time and history. This, of course, will also improve the clinician's understanding of what is actually going on in the patient's life-world. We suggests focusing on what we call "traumatic sequence," performing with the patient a kind of slow-motion recollection of the daily traumatic events that constellate her existence. Typically, the traumatic sequence includes four steps:

1. The traumatic experience usually originates in the context of a traumatic relationship. The borderline person conceives of partnerships as the encounter between two spontaneities, not regulated by any sort of internal or external *nomos* (Stanghellini and Rosfort 2013a). Furthermore, she requires the other to be present and loyal, and capable of recognition, that is, a source of validation. In addition, presence, loyalty, and recognition must be accompanied by the other's spontaneity, being free from social conventions and acting according to the vital impulses of the present moment.
2. The traumatic sequence typically starts with an unexpected event of disappointment and disillusion. The other does something (or fails to do something) and thereby hurts the borderline person's sensibility. The borderline patient may notice, for example, that

while waiting for her boyfriend she was overwhelmed by a quasi-ineffable variety of bad moods, characterized on the cognitive level by a state of dissonance and indecision. She could not construct any consistent and stable explanation of her boyfriend's behaviour: "What's going on?", "Is he stuck in traffic?", "Did he have a car accident?", "Did he forget about our appointment?", "Was he distracted by something or someone else?", "Another woman?", "Is that an ambiguous way of letting me down?", and so on. This is an initial to *situate* her emotions, that is, to recognize and relate them to the present situation, to understand them as one's own personal way of being attuned to that given situation. Borderline persons fail to see in their emotional reactions the involuntary *manifestation of otherness*, that is, the re-enactment of one's past and the manifestation of one's character. Thus, they fail to engage in a proper "hermeneutics of the *I am*" (Stanghellini and Rosfort 2013a).

3. Emotional dissonance is prodromal to a phase of despair. While she was waiting for her boyfriend, her thinking completely collapsed. She could make no decision at all. She was in a kind of psychic paralysis. She felt that events are random, reality uncontrollable, the behavior of other persons unintelligible, and the whole world nonsensical. The outside world, as well as her own actions and reactions, were lived as though they were entirely out of control and unpredictable. Despair may be the ingress into dissociation, which is often considered a desperate defense or adaptation to traumatic experiences. In the state of dissociation there is a collapse of the capacity of mentalization. Dissociation may imply amnesia, and therefore this phase may be absent in the patient's spontaneous recollection of the traumatic sequence.

4. The last step of the traumatic sequence is a mechanical, routine interpretation of the traumatic event. The borderline person typically assumes one of the following stereotyped roles: victim, perpetrator, bystander.

Victim. She may identify with the role of the *victim*, and in this case feel passively involved and totally without responsibility for what happens. 'I am the victim, the other is the perpetrator'. It is the other who is guilty, since he or she acted out of voluntary intention. From this self-other relationship can emerge emotional states characterized by anger, resentment, and indignation until they could take the form of a transitory persecutory delusion. Usually, the persecutor is a significant other. This makes the persecutory delusions of borderline persons radically different from paranoid delusions in persons with schizophrenia, which typically involve anonymous others. Furthermore, borderline persons are more vulnerable to developing feelings of shame. A mixture of anger plus shame may trigger transitory persecutory delusions in borderline persons, and especially delusions of reference, which typically arise in the type of borderline persons who are particularly vulnerable to narcissistic rage associated with feelings of humiliation.

Perpetrator. She may admit she misbehaved. Nonetheless, she thinks she cannot be held entirely responsible. It was for her a sort of reflex, an automatic response she simply could not control: 'I am bad, but I am not guilty because it's not my fault'. Indeed, borderline persons seldom develop feelings of guilt or guilt delusions as melancholic persons do. When she takes up the role of perpetrator, she may feel prey of a kind of "guiltless guilt." In this case, guilt is neither placed on a flesh-and-blood other (e.g., one's partner) nor on an anonymous other (as is the case with schizophrenic delusions of alien control). Guiltless guilt is the experience of the influx in one's life of an uncontrollable destructive force that comes from within. Borderline persons are the witnesses of an ultimate truth: they feel the alienating power of the involuntary, that is, of the otherness that is constitutive of our personhood.

Bystander. Here, the borderline person is a merely passive spectator of the ineluctable and unpredictable events. She feels she cannot decide, control, or change the course of her life: 'It always goes like this. This happened again. I can do nothing to avoid it'. She feels prone to develop feelings of impotence and helplessness, and to conceive of life as nonsensical. Oppressed with tedium, her mind becomes a mirror that reflects the ineluctability of the world and her own powerlessness, that is, the futility of existence. The world and life itself simply is, it just happens. Tedium may be interrupted by cynical, sarcastic, or auto-sarcastic remarks. In this case, neither is the other construed as a perpetrator nor is the self felt as dominated by otherness. The responsibility is on sheer life itself, on its inescapable as well as unpredictable nature. Borderline persons construe themselves as the bystanders of their tragic destiny.

The relationships of borderline persons are often traumatic. Limit situations always originate in the context of traumatic self–other relationships. The main reason for this is that an essential feature of the fabric of the human self that is missing in the life-story of borderline persons. This is the issue of the other's recognition and of intimacy. Both are missing in the circumstances that Meares (2000) calls the "invalidating trauma." The main reason for this is that the two main sources of recognition are missing in the life-world of borderline persons: the other as a partner in their intimate relationships, and the other a companion in their inner conversation. The others are means to satisfy our own need for recognition. This is not the case for borderline persons who feel victimised by their partners. Yet this need for other-recognition can be mitigated by self-recognition. The borderline persons' acute need for the other's recognition is a consequence of their lack of self-recognition. The latter is essentially based on the presence, in one's "intimate conversations," of an implicit other who would understand our actions and projects, to whom we could tell our life story. This implicit presence of the other presupposes early experiences of secure relationships to relevant others. In the case of borderline persons, an implicit other with whom one can share an intimate conversation, as well as a secure relational pattern, is radically lacking.

VALUES IN BORDERLINE PERSONS

The desperate vitality inherent in dysphoria engenders an intense need to satisfy the affective, biological values brought about by vigorous feelings of being alive. These values run counter to and often clash with the ethical norms and social rules that structure the world in which we all live, provoking a frustrated sense of worthlessness and inanity. The emotional intensity does not allow bordeline persons to distance themselves from what they feel here and now, and therefore they are not able to understand their feelings in the light of the values that constitute their own life-world. They live under the spell of what we may call a *frustrated normativity* (Stanghellini and Rosfort 2013a). The norms by which the borderline person is driven are not the ethical norms or social conventions that structure and organize our interpersonal world. Rather, borderline persons refuse such conditions, thus entering into collision with what they consider the hypocrisy and the inauthenticity of the pallid emotions by which other persons live. The borderline person cannot—or will not—let his bouts of energy be restricted by or conformed to the needs of other people, ethical norms, or social conventions, all of which he considers inauthentic and therefore as an unwarranted challenge to his truly natural being, his spontaneity.

This kind of emotionally frustrated normativity can be the initial cause of borderline depression. It is the presence of a vitality that merely strives to affirm its own emotional intensity, to satisfy its own rudimentary feelings of being alive and the anonymous values revealed and engendered by these feelings, without any regard for the ethical or social norms that govern the world in which the borderline person desperately tries to live. Feelings are the most important values in the borderline person's life-world. Social norms are deemed inauthentic values because they disregard the intimate feelings of the person whose behavior they are meant to inform and orient. The incapacity to distance oneself from one's own feelings means that the borderline person is not capable of appropriating those very feelings in the light of the norms that are part of being a person in a world shared with other persons. She is condemned simply to live the intense but disrupted life of her feelings. The norms, ethical as well as social, that allow us to distance ourselves from our feelings and needs in the light of our care for living "a good life" with other people are merely viewed as annoying attempts to drain the vitality that sustains the borderline world. The normative frustration experienced by borderline persons continuously generates desperate attempts to maintain their vitality in the face of what they consider to be the encumbering strictures and platitudes of everyday life.

The values that are at play in the interpersonal world of borderline persons are directed to achieve goals like "to belong/to be accepted/to draw close and enjoyably reciprocate with another/to converse in a friendly manner, to tell stories, exchange sentiments, ideas, secrets/to communicate, to converse/to laugh and make jokes" (Kane 2001: 234–235). These goals are felt by borderline persons as standard, basic aspirations of what, with Meares (2000), we may call intimacy, but these aspirations are often unrealistic and almost unattainable.

The borderline person's values not only clash with the norms and conventions that rule our interpersonal world; they are also in conflict with one another. The borderline person requires the other to be present and loyal, and capable of recognition, that is, a source of validation. In addition, presence, loyalty, and recognition must be accompanied by the other's spontaneity, being free from social conventions and acting according to the vital impulses of the present moment. Furthermore, the borderline person is not capable of autonomy in the sense of establishing a coherent enough representation of herself and remaining faithful to it, and thus takes to an extreme the value of spontaneity. They conceive of partnerships as the encounter between two spontaneities, not regulated by any sort of internal or external *nomos*: "to be free from social restrictions/to resist coercion and constriction/to be independent and act according to desire/to defy convention" (Kane 2001: 234).

The borderline person postulates as essential to life what is unstable and fleeting par excellence: the immediate encounter with the other, the encounter between two desires. The imperatives shouted at the other are the following: "Spontaneously fulfil my desire with your own desire!" and "Stay here! Do not abandon me! Keep on burning with an inexhaustible desire!" Need for recognition and fear of abandonment force the borderline person to insatiably aspire to a sort of emotional osmosis with the other. The other is needed as a source of recognition. The absence of the other makes the presence of the self impossible. The other's absence, or incomplete presence, is often the reason for feelings of un-recognition and desperate loss of selfhood. The absent other, or the other who does not donate his entire self, is an abandoning other and an inauthentic other.

We know how an encounter based on these needs (immediacy and authenticity) can be unrealistic and almost unattainable. Furthermore, the borderline's desire conceals the difference between oneself and the other, and between one's desire for love and love in its actuality. In short: between an idealized form of love and the actual relationship with the other person. What the borderline person idealizes is not the other, but Love itself. What the borderline person considers to be her most non-renounceable value is indeed her innermost symptom. The borderline existence is a dangerous shelter that meets its defeat because it postulates as non-renounceable in life what is more alien and inaccessible to it, what in life itself is unstable and fleeting par excellence: the immediate encounter with the other, the encounter between two desires.

BIBLIOGRAPHY

Correale A. (2007). *Area traumatica e campo istituzionale*, 2nd edn. Rome: Borla Edizioni.

Cutting J. (2009a). "Scheler, Phenomenology, and Psychopathology." *Philosophy, Psychiatry & Psychology* 16(2): 143–159.

Cutting J. (2009b). "Psychopathologists and Philosophers." *Philosophy, Psychiatry & Psychology* 16(2): 175–178.

Freeman L. and Elpidorou A. (2015). "Affectivity in Heidegger II: Temporality, Boredom, and Beyond." *Philosophy Compass* 10(10): 672–684.

Fuchs T. (2003). "The Phenomenology of Shame, Guilt and the Body in Body Dysmorphic Disorder and Depression." *Journal of Phenomenological Psychology* 33(2): 223–243.

Fuchs T. (2007). "Fragmented Selves: Temporality and Identity in Borderline Personality." *Psychopathology* 40(6): 379–387.

Fuchs T. (2013). "Existential Vulnerability: Toward a Psychopathology of Limit Situations Psychopathology" 46(5): 301–308.

Heidegger M. (1995). *The fundamental Concepts of Metaphysics: World, Finitude, Solitude*. Bloomington and Indianapolis: Indiana University Press.

Jaspers K. (1919). *Psychologie der Weltanschauungen*. Berlin: Springer.

Kane S. (2001). "4.48 Psychosis." In S. Kane (ed.), *Complete Plays*, pp. 203–246. London: Methuen.

Kimura B. (1992). *Écrits de psychopathologie phénoménologique*, trans. J. Bouderlique. Paris: Presses Universitaires France.

Kimura B. (2000). *L'Entre. Une approche phénoménologique de la schizophrénie*, trans. C. Vincent. Grenoble: Éditions Jérôme Millon.

Meares R. (2000). *Intimacy and Alienation: Memory, Trauma and Personal Being*. London: Routledge.

Mundt C. (2014). "Jaspers' Concept of 'Limit Situation': Extension and Therapeutic Applications." In T. Fuchs, T. Breyer, and C. Mundt (eds.), *Karl Jaspers' Philosophy and Psychopathology*, pp. 169–178. Heidelberg: Springer.

Pazzagli A. and Rossi Monti M. (2000). "Dysphoria and Aloneness in Borderline Personality Disorder." *Psychopathology* 33(4): 220–226.

Ricoeur P. (1992/1990). *Oneself as Another*, trans. K. Blamey. Chicago: University of Chicago Press; *Soi-même comme un autre*. Paris: Éditions du Seuil.

Rossi Monti M. and D'Agostino A. (2014). "Borderline Personality Disorder from a Psychopathological-dynamic Perspective." *Journal of Psychopathology* 20: 451–460.

Sartre J.-P. (1956/1943). *Being and Nothingness: A Phenomenological Essay on Ontology*, trans. H. E. Barnes. New York: Philosophical Library.

Scheler M. (2012). *Person and Self-value: Three Essays*. Berlin: Springer Science & Business Media.

Smith Q. (1986). *The Felt Meanings of the World: A Metaphysics of Feeling*. West Lafayette: Purdue University Press.

Solomon R. C. (2007). *True To Our Feelings: What Our Emotions Are Really Telling Us*. Oxford: Oxford University Press.

Stanghellini G. (2000). "The Doublets of Anger." *Psychopathology* 33(4): 155–158.

Stanghellini G. (2016). *Lost in Dialogue*. Oxford: Oxford University Press.

Stanghellini G. and Rossi Monti M. (2009a). *Psicologia del patologico: Una prospettiva fenomenologica-dinamica*. Milano: Raffaello Cortina Editore.

Stanghellini G. and Rossi Monti M. (2009b). "Explication or Explanation?" *Philosophy, Psychiatry & Psychology* 16(3): 237–239.

Stanghellini G. and Rosfort R. (2013a). *Emotions and Personhood: Exploring Fragility—Making Sense of Vulnerability*. Oxford: Oxford University Press.

Stanghellini G. and Rosfort R. (2013b). "Borderline Depression: A Desperate Vitality." *Journal of Consciousness Studies* 20(7–8): 153–177.

Tavris C. (1989). *Anger: The Misunderstood Emotion*. Revised Edition. New York: Simon and Schuster.

Westen D. and Cohen R. P. (1993). "The Self in Borderline Personality Disorder: A Psychodynamic Perspective." In Z. V. Segal and S. J. Blatt (eds.), *The Self in Emotional Distress: Cognitive and Psychodynamic Perspectives*, pp. 334–368. New York: Guilford Press.

CHAPTER 68

....

THE LIFE-WORLD OF PERSONS WITH DRUG ADDICTIONS

....

GILBERTO DI PETTA

THE PHENOMENOLOGICAL APPROACH
....

WHAT sense is there at this moment in time in proposing a phenomenological approach to addiction, which is such a varied psychopathological and human condition, when empirical research is centered entirely on the collection, analysis, and elaboration of measurable and verifiable models? The psychosocial hypotheses of the last century, which supplied different interpretations of the social context and the addictive personality, seem to have lost their bite. No psychosocial model is able to help explain the tremendous diffusion of various forms of drug abuse among the general population. Both the models of family and of society have undergone a great change in the last fifty years. However, there is no psycho-social parameter that is closely linked in any way to the explosion and multiplication of drug abuse. Furthermore, the psychosocial models have been lacking in any attempt to set up therapeutic protocols that aim at recovering the individual and helping him to overcome drug abuse. It has not been possible to repeat the success achieved by the neurobiological approach, which substitutes one drug with another (e.g. heroin–methadone) in the treatment of drug abuse. The study of receptors and ligands has not kept up with the incredible proliferation of synthetic drugs, for which, at this time, no substitute exists. The spread in the abuse of non-pharmacological additives has made the use of drugs that can contrast the effect of each substance virtually impossible. The typical present-day drug addict is a polyabuser, in whose brain it is practically impossible to pinpoint where the behavioral and neuropsychic effects of any single drug take place. Nowadays the world of addiction is highly differentiated with synthetic and recreational substances being used alongside the more traditional drugs. And other addictions have come to exist besides drug addiction—gambling, shopping, sex, the Internet, etc. Some eating disorders can also be considered a form of addiction. It is obvious that in the field of neuropsychiatry the effects of chemical agents like drugs are completely different from behavioral disorders caused by gambling or the Internet. The psychiatric effect of drugs has been compared to synthetic psychoses, which are considered to be esogenic psychosis, having a very different psychopathological structure from the schizophrenic and affective psychosis of more standard psychoses.

The question of the phenomenological approach should be explained. The phenomenological-existential approach is first and foremost philosophical, and is based on philosophical thinkers such as Buber, Dostoevsky, Frankl, Heidegger, Husserl, Jaspers, Kierkergaard, Nietzsche, Sartre, Tillich, and others. It is concerned with the understanding of people in relationship to the world in which they live and with the individual's search for what it means to be alive. It is committed to exploring questions about living and dying. The phenomenological approach, due to its inclination to grasp the intrinsic nature of phenomena, tends to form a common denominator which is in opposition to the proliferation of normal addictive behavior and is a sort of typical style of life of the addicted person, independently of a whole series of differential factors (personality, chemical or behavioral addiction, psychiatric complications). Phenomenology attempts to understand the "how" of each phenomenon, that is, the way in which it happens independently of its causes. For the doctor, a profound understanding of the way in which the phenomenon of addiction is formed represents a step into the patient's world. It allows the doctor to work together with his patient toward a better understanding of the patient's problems and thus clears the way for successful treatment. This may seem rather simplistic when compared to the approach of empirical research which is very careful to analyze and elaborate all the possible variables. However, having the chance to view a unitary perspective is a great help since it allows the doctor to have an immediate overall picture, and this is especially useful when meeting the patients since the characteristic of these patients, which is based entirely on "all and now," certainly does not provide much time for the working out of a therapeutic relationship. If the doctor manages to break through the patient's "addictive bubble" in the first meeting, he will then be able in some measure to appreciate the patient's intentionality. In turn this will allow the doctor to help steer his patient away from the polarization of his intentionality toward the object of his addiction, thus setting up the premise for a therapeutic relationship. When the doctor first meets the patient the most important thing for him is to achieve something on which to build up a contact with his patient from the very beginning rather than focus on the neurobiological determiners and the personological configurations of the patient. Because the addict's world is a purely sensorial world based primarily on perception, any attempt at a more rational approach is not likely to prove successful. Any dropping out from the treatment at this stage would have dramatically negative consequences for the patient, both physically and psychosocially. The more an addict becomes socially integrated, the less apparent are those elements that derive from social degradation and the consideration of being a social outcast. Thus the catastrophic downward curve of their existence is reflected and dangerously amplified in their position in society.

Toward the end of their existential journey and of their drug addiction the lives of people, who were apparently quite different beforehand, flow together into a common dimension of loss. This is a sort of common destiny. Any initial difference disappears and what emerges is the phenomenon in its common denominator. The collapse of existence, cleared of its a priori formal structures of space and time, becomes evident. The knowledge of the constitution of "the life-world" of the addict is fundamental not only for any transformative approach that attempts to tackle the problem, but also for any attempt to reinstate the treatment, the world-project, the constitution of the other. In 1927 Heidegger, in *Being and Time*, defined "care" (*Sorge*) as a fundamental existential dimension. According to Heidegger we are human insofar as we take care of something, or someone, including oneself. The "world-project" is built around the concept of taking care, or the reaction to the "being-thrown-into-the-world" by being born, with the differing future prospect which allows the individual to express his own individuality. The anthropological-phenomenological definition of the addict can begin from a context which is the exact opposite of this: negligence, the *loss of care*, and as a result the loss of a world-project built around the treatment. The phenomenological approach is particularly successful when it has something on which to build upon. Giving positive results when it can begin from a relationship with those patients who are particularly unwilling to enter into any kind of relationship whatsoever, having been continuously rejected and having become accustomed to a nomadic existence, which has profoundly undermined their own personality.

THE ADDICTIVE WORLD

It would be wrong to consider the complexity of the addictive experience exclusively in psychological terms (intrapsychic and interpersonal conflict) or, as is becoming more common, exclusively in neurobiological terms (circuits of pleasure). The phenomenological approach extends above all to a horizon of an anthropological nature (Weizsaecker 1967; 1968), interpreting the addictive phenomenon as a result of the deep crisis of the own being-there (*Dasein*) that has unhinged the *being-in-the-world* of the postmodern subject. Drugs and other narcotic substances have in fact been used since human life began on the planet, accompanying us in our rituals for sacred occurrences, when we went to war, in love, and during Dionysian frenzies. The fact that these substances, which have been present for thousands of years, have represented a medical epidemiological problem only since the last decades of the last century implies that the cultural ritualization of their use is no longer applicable. This change has occurred at the same time as the development of techniques of synthesis of those drugs and of the explosion in mass communication. For the doctor who has been trained to think phenomenologically, faced with the world of drug addicts he is dealing with *tracing* all that remains of those beings he encounters: human beings who have lost their defining personalities, beings that are simply either *integrated* or *disintegrated*, beings who are either "in" or "out," inhabiting vagabond worlds, living clandestine lives, wherever they are and whatever they do remaining forever transitory, temporary fragments of lived life and consciousness: when the doctor comes face to face with them, he too is forced to become a wanderer, without any roots, almost obliged to be as much an interpreter of postmodern restlessness as his patients.

There is an invisible thread that, on the edge of nothingness, ties together the passion for drugs/drug addiction and lived experiences like boredom (*Noia, Langweiligkeit, Spleen*), emptiness, angst, and pervasive and intense anger (*Verstimmung, Hubris*): these features constitute both the psychopathology of the addict as a man living on the edge and unmistakable features found in contemporary philosophy (Heidegger, Sartre, Camus) and modern literature (Baudelaire, Musil, Joyce, Kafka). Mythical heroes of the generations belonging to the second half of the twentieth century—short-lived bright stars like James Dean, Jim Morrison, Kurt Cobain, all of whom embodied the impossibility/incapacity/inability of living their own not-to-be-found dimension, losing their lives at the very moment of their maximum, yet still immature, splendor. This balancing on the edge of the abyss connects, albeit from a distance and through the deformed effect of the reproducibility of the masses, the existence of drug addicts to the tragic destinies of figures like Keats, Shelley, Byron, or Werther and Ortis, or Michaelstaedter, the bohemians and the *scapigliati* who experienced the *fin de siècle* weariness of over one hundred years ago, like Corazzini, Campana, Gozzano. All figures who have left us, both in their works and in the example of their short lives and their untimely deaths on the threshold of adulthood, the tragic sense of their inability to adapt to the modern world.

With the final sunset over both the rural and industrial world, the traditional cities which had been the historical framework of modern industrial and bourgeois civilization, gave way to the infinite series of no man's land that characterizes modern cities and their outskirts. The current metropolitan *topos* is by its own definition a "nowhere"—a discontinuous and confused untidy succession of abandoned post-industrial wasteland, shopping centers, areas which are out of bounds and delimited, without history or sense. These places have no sense of meeting or of relationships between people, no cafés or places to walk and talk, no love or death. This is the background where the drug addict unequivocally realizes the figure of *being-in-the-crisis* as *being-in-the-wreck* or *being-in-nothingness*. In the heart of darkness of one of the deepest holes of contemporary nihilism the addict's existence might represent the place where the last battle is being fought to save all that makes man what he is, without all the historical encrustations on which the traditional idea of being-man were founded, and which have gradually been abandoned.

The first generation that embraced the consumption style of the heroin addict emerged in the West in the 1960s and 1970s. The failure of the youth movement's demonstrations, the subversive terrorist acts committed by extremists together with the return to a quiet bourgeois existence of many of the instigators of the revolutionary movement provided the ex-hippies with an alibi to completely destroy themselves. In this way opiates/narcotics met the need to alleviate the pain and anger of all those who had experienced the "season of illusions" and witnessed the failure of social reform and the consequent return to selfish interests and conformity. The world that had restored bourgeois ideals and forced them on the survivors of a counter-culture could not be accepted. Thus, needles, spoons, distilled water, and lemon became the instruments of a rite of passage. The first time it was normal for someone else to administer the drugs, thereafter you would do it on your own. Pulling your belt tightly round your arm with your teeth, passing the needle or "sword" from one to another for a shot, you found yourself on the threshold of a new and fantastic discovery. The whole world became indifferent and you became indifferent to the progressive and unstoppable deconstruction and degradation of your own life. Today almost no one from this first generation is still alive. Nearly all have succumbed to overdoses or AIDS.

What else remains for adolescents today apart from the noisy silence that fills up the boring everyday routine of adults? The night. How is night time experienced? How are its spaces organized? How are those empty intervening metropolitan spaces filled? Or rather, how do all those needs/requests that are suppressed by everyday culture express themselves? Who are the figures, the characters, and what processes do they set off, for example, in the world of nightclubs some of which are referred to in slang as being *borderline*, because they are the home of extreme *on-the-edge* effects? What then are the behavioral combinations or the experiential, symptomatological, and psychopathological clusters that emerge from the miscellany of these chronically a-structured personalities, trapped in a sort of continuous present? All of this is associated with a vision of one's own life as being ensnared in the instant of an atemporal present, where nothing has any meaning other than the emergent moment that is, compared to what is continually being taken away from the senses because it is disappearing; where one's own life is seen as being separated from any working objective or pretext for responsibility; and where the only sense/sensation/feeling that remains, after all the needs for survival have crumbled, is either of panic or undirected ludic; where everything that you do is either an action or is not carried out because any idea of planning for the future is impossible.

The turning-point for this second generation of new addicts who do not consider themselves real drug addicts at all, is to be found in their search for the experience of a high (or a buzz) which leads them to use a mixture of drugs. The tragic outcome of the lifestyle of these polyabusers seems to confirm that human beings are not mature enough to live in complete freedom, where freedom also means being free from the symbolic forms that ritualize and ceremonialize all the ups and downs of life. At this point the drug addict, surpassing the narrow medical world, sets out the *ontological* problem of the freedom of man in the world.

The analysis that phenomenology carries out at the base of consciousness and of experience and of the addict's world, in this playing by ear, beyond the disintegration of categories, captures the eternal instant, the disappearance of the past as a memory and of the future as a project, the transformation of cyclical time into linear time. The drug addict's craving after a meaning among the ruins left behind by his addiction, almost caused by the emptiness of non-sense, is met. The doctor and the patient, both wayfarers among the ruins of the world, become traveling companions in the difficult search for a meaning which at this point has become a common objective

From the phenomenological point of view, the addict appears as a tragic figure devoured by his own boundless appetite, dominated by a grandiose and unlimited picture of himself, condemned forever to follow his erratic consciousness. He will continuously and without success keep searching in the crepuscular *nirvana* of the high for his lost presence, profoundly and irredeemably damaged in its emphatic relation with the world, exposed to the misery of its continuous failure and faced with the insignificance of everyday reality compared to his artificial paradise.

Today, while the more accredited approaches appear to be experiencing increasing difficulty, the phenomenological approach permits the doctor to work in conditions that allow him to have satisfactory visibility of both the patient and his path to recovery, as well as allowing him to apply himself successfully to the continuing relationship while at the same time maintaining contact with the patient despite the inconstancy and the chronicity of the various problematic situations. Once again "treatment," "the world," "the project," "lived space," "lived time," "the situation," "the lived body," "conscience," "destiny," and "freedom" are all essential in order to enable any kind of favorable encounter with anyone who, like all addicts, has either lost himself completely or is in the process of doing so. Borgna, in 1978, published a seminal paper entitled "La tossicomania come esperienza psicoterapeutica" ("Drug Addiction as a Psychotherapeutic Experience"), which is of extraordinary relevance. Indeed, it can be considered the groundwork for all subsequent research on the subject. The essential aspects of this paper can be summarized as follows:

1) Drug addiction is an experience that is deeply inherent to the human experience. Or rather, drug addiction is a possibility inscribed in the destiny of every one of us.
2) The feeling of "emptiness" is the core of the drug addict's experience.

3) Being able to relate to the drug addict is only possible outside the professional role and after having abandoned every certainty.
4) The discovery in the drug addict's world of a distinctive feature of our time: the loss of the sense of the world.

An article entitled "L'esperienza del *Leib* sessuale nei tossicodipendenti" ("The Experience of the Sexual *Leib* in Drug Addicts) was published by Callieri in 1993. "It seems to be the case that the heroin-addicts are lacking in any ability to effectively plan their lives because they consider their bodies simply as being an obstacle, or rather, as an inexhaustible source of urgent needs. They can remain a presence, while rarely taking part" (Callieri 1993: 75). Thus, the physical body (*Körper*) takes the place of the lived body (*Leib*) in drug addicts, and all meaningful communication with others breaks down, leaving room only for the barest of superficial exchanges. The addict's sexuality tends to remain within the closed circle of *being-high* and functions in the present living exclusively for the next fix. The encounter for the *body-I-have* is reduced to a mere risk. The body is at the disposal of another body, occasional epiphenomenon of life/existence. What is missing entirely is "that which is beyond," the *encounter* with another body seen as one's own opening up toward the other body. The osmosis between sexuality and existence is completely absent here due to the coagulation or even cicatrizing effect of *craving* (the compulsive desire for drugs). It is almost as if a single longing has summed up and absorbed all the others resulting in the loss of *We-ness*.

ADDICTIVE BEING-IN-THE-WORLD: GENERAL FEATURES

The life-world of drug addicts is conditioned by the presence or absence of narcotic substances. These substances, or the behavior resulting from drug abuse while they are being used, totally absorb the patient's intentional consciousness and modify its spatial-temporal structure. Since the patients during their lives are not always under the influence of drugs, or totally involved with their addiction, it follows that their state of intentional consciousness varies according to how much the object of their addiction has influenced their lived experience/life. Therefore we can summarize the way in which the patients experience addiction fundamentally in the following three dimensions:

1) When the patient is directly under the effect of drugs or when his resulting behavior is caused by the addiction. This is a passive dimension. Whereas in normal conditions we have a natural relationship with the surrounding world, and our common sense is the obviously pre-reflexive result of this situation, under the influence of a drug intoxication we lose this stable contact with reality (*Selbstverstaendlich*) and, as a result, suffer from an intense *in*stability, which we can identify with the term *floating* world.
2) When the object of addiction is not present. This is the phase of abstinence or craving, and is characterized by the lack of the substance and the resulting irrepressible longing to have it. In this phase the patient undergoes an intentional polarization, which is both absolute and specific, on how to get his hands on the drugs again. The addict's purpose

is polarized by his desired objective. Everything else is excluded or considered only as tools which can help achieve the final goal.

3) When the patient is desensitized to the substance or the addictive behavior. This is the phase when the problem becomes chronic, in which the effects of the addictive behavior have faded, though the patient is not yet able to live a normal life. He is apathetic, indifferent, abulic, lacking in will-power and the world seems grey to him. This is the dimension of the frozen world-of-life.

THE FLOATING LIFE-WORLD:
EYELIDS LIKE A SETTING SUN

What precisely do addicts mean when they say: "I am high"? What is the psychopathological meaning of this state of consciousness which for them represents a sort of steady-state? (Cargnello, Callieri, & Morselli, 1962) described a condition of "twilight calm" in subjects who experienced LSD, after the hallucinatory state. On this base, we can consider the experience of a *high* as an equivalent of the *twilight state* of consciousness. In the classic description by Jaspers (1913) and Schneider (1959), the *twilight state* of consciousness is a restriction of the field of consciousness. In the *twilight state* of consciousness there is no dramatic alteration of arousal. The field of consciousness, furthermore, can still spread itself. The *twilight state* of consciousness is a sort of threshold between the light of reality and the shadow of dream and psychosis. The *twilight state* of consciousness promotes illusions, delusions, hallucinations. Depersonalization and derealization are normal experiences in the *twilight state* of consciousness, in which it is more likely that transitional phenomena occur, from basic symptoms to final full-blown psychotic phenomena (Kolsterkoetter, 1988; Gross, Huber, Kolsterkoetter, & Linz, 1987). Addicts experience this vulnerable condition every day, every month, every year. The perception of reality in addicts is discontinuous and incomplete and this *twilight state* becomes a sort of normal way of life. This state of consciousness is like a display that is continuously turned on and off, short flashes appear and disappear. Because of instability the *twilight state* becomes a transitional state.

Making eye contact with a drug addict who has taken drugs inevitably reveals his eyes to be "*les yeux en coucher de soleil*" (eyelids like a sunset). In that instant, while his experience has been swallowed up by the nirvana of the flash or the kaleidoscopic dizziness of a high, we who are standing in front of him, no longer exist for him. The world tends to disappear. His intentionality is completely "floating," the world around is only perceived weakly and intermittently. There is no longer any *noema* present in the patient's awareness, only a *noesis* which melts into the hazy line on the horizon. On the other hand the fantastic interior experience is sharply in focus and, if sedatives are involved, there is a kind of fusion with the ocean, while if stimulants are used there is a kaleidoscope of shining photons and hypercolors. The floating world is characterized by splitting, vibration, and a multiplication of images which can be both sequential or overlapping. There exists a violent twilight state of consciousness in patients who are suffering from the effects of drugs and are, consequently, in the situation of a *floating* world. Their lived body has become disjointed. Their senses have started to become something like a wild kaleidoscope. The lived space is haemorrhagic and the perception is of a loss of space, of being nowhere. Lived time is liquid and indefinite. "Life appears as if it were only a moment, freed and released from the present and the future" (Beringer 1927).

There is no present, no past, no future. Having lost the connection of interior time all the drug addict has left is the transient moment of satisfaction. However, no sooner has the drug addict achieved a moment of pleasure than it suddenly vanishes and he is condemned to impulsive and compulsive repetition. When the patient experiences a high, he feels so absorbed in the present that he is no longer able to see the future. No longer being able to experience the past and having lost touch with the future, the patient ends up being unable to grasp the present. "The addict is trapped in this repetition with no chance of moving forward" (Gebsattel 1954: 35). The instantaneity, the pure instant, is the gap between the last dose and the next one: the liquid instant of "the high" rules. The moment of altered consciousness and the time of the depthless instant dominate everything else. Thus, the patient is trapped in a sort of circular liquidity of lived time, and suffers the pure illusion of linear movement. This state of consciousness or this way of being can overlap with a manic state, although they are in fact very different conditions. The manic appears hyperactive, while the addict is passive during this moment of bliss. The instant that the drug addict experiences is dilated and swallows both past and future, while that of the manic is an instant that is being continually projected into the future freed from the past. The manic feels himself as being omnipotent, while the drug addict wallows in a feeling of blissful impotence.

THE WORLD OF CRAVING: A CIRCULAR CHAIN

What exactly happens in the state of acute drug deprivation? The acute withdrawal (the "cold turkey" syndrome) is a state of real discomfort. The patient's existence is centered around where the pusher is—the exact square, the road, the underpass. An acute and intolerable sense of emptiness continues to get ever more urgent. Anger, irritability, and loneliness are the dominant emotions that inundate the addict's state of mind. There is a contrast between the cold space of substance craving which can be defined with the word "absence," and the hot space of substance enjoying which can be defined with the word "presence." When the patient experiences craving both past and future have been lost. The past is reduced exclusively to "the last time in which I have taken drugs." Everything is manipulated and everyone is reduced to being an obstacle in the way of the addict's only remaining relationship—with the drugs he takes. The relapse and the nostalgia are strictly related to the experience of craving. The memory of the pleasure deriving from the drug is unforgettable. Intentionality, in this experience of craving, is totally directed to the search for substances. All the behavior is drug-oriented. Generally the patient is very active in order to find the drug as soon as possible. They always need more and more substances in order to feel themselves still alive. Often only a relapse can represent the way out from this terrible condition. Circular time is the temporal structure of craving: a chain which links the past and the future, continually displacing the past into the future, the future into the past.

THE FROZEN WORLD-OF-LIFE: LIKE SNOWMEN

On the other hand, following chronic drug tolerance, which results in the desensitization of substances, we have a sort of intentional dramatic seizure of the world, which we can call the *frozen* world. In the encounter with a chronic addict, an examiner will encounter the following: an empathy failure; boredom; emptiness; lack of meaning; loneliness; isolation. The lived time, space, body, and other existential parameters differ enormously in comparison with the same parameters of the floating world. Following chronic intoxication, the patient's consciousness becomes viscous, and the lived body is blocked—now he finds himself in the state we call the *frozen* world. The body is modified at a neurobiological level by a chemical graft which inserts a relevant new artificial element into the lived body. The object body (*Körper*) is the vehicle of powerful substances which can successfully alter all sensations and perceptions, and the whole world-experience, reducing the addict's self into nothing more than a denatured, mineralized body (*Körper-ding*). His intentionality is coagulated, time is insular and has been reduced to a pure frozen present without past and without future until the complete loss of the passing of time is experienced. Others have become unattainable objects which are lifeless, like unattainable distant snowmen. Tragically these patients become mere bystanders to their own existence. In order to feel themselves still alive they need more and more substances. But after years and years of addicted life, the effect of those substances has started to wear off. There is tolerance, habit, ineffectiveness, along with a progressive destruction of both the existential background and the existential network, as well as a development in progressive psychopathology and brain injury. *Being-in-nothingness* can became the typical state of addicts in the frozen condition. In this case, the frozen condition has become a sort of terminal point in the existence of addicts.

THE PARADISE LOST: THE DEATH OF THE FEELING

It is necessary to differentiate this state from other ordinary states of depression. In fact, if we examine "depressive states" in addicted people a paradox emerges: does something like "depression" in addictive persons actually exist? We find several depressive-like conditions: the end of the "honeymoon," the chronic state of abstention, the chronic abuse as the drug becomes increasingly ineffective. In these conditions the addict's life is meaningless, without colors, without taste, without smell, without emotions. The chronic pain of the addict is not the same thing as depression. In addition, the end dose of methadone or buprenorphine puts the patient in an uncomfortable situation. During psychotherapeutic treatment, the patient can encounter a lack of motivation. On the other hand, during community treatment or in prison, these patients, deprived of drugs, appear similar to patients suffering from depression. When the patient manages to resist a relapse he lives a sort of depressed lucidity: this is the sign of detoxification. The structure of a lived time experience in these addiction-related situations is completely different from the structure of lived time in normal life and in a depressive experience. In depression the lived time is trapped in an irremovable past, which blocks the flow of time toward the present and the future. In these addicted-related conditions the essential characteristic is the reduction of the present into an island without past and without future. The final collapse of the addictive "Dasein" is a sort of being-in-nothingness. The crisis of the temporal-spatial vortex eventually and inevitably leads to the "blow of the vacuum" (*le coup de vide*): the experience of unreality or no self-experience. The total collapse of the world is the final result of the breaking down of the temporal and spatial structure of "being-there" ("Dasein") (Binswanger 1958). All addictions lead to the final collapse of the *Being-in-the-world-with-others* structure, and many addicts remain without the spatial-temporal dimension, thus making it virtually impossible for them *to stay in a space-with-others* and *to project themselves in time.*

THE THERAPEUTIC ENCOUNTER WITH THE DRUG

A doctor who meets an addict has to be without any prejudices and has to do his best to make contact both with the emotional nucleus of the person he has in front of him and with the "drug experience." This has to be done at the same time, though separately. The person who is talking in front of him is not merely a person who is a patient. He is also in a certain sense the drug itself. The doctor, therefore, makes contact both with the person and with the drug. The first thing he has to do is to make the drug into something akin to an experience endowed with a sense. The relationship that exists between the patient and the drug to which he is addicted is not a relationship between a free mind and a free object. The *bond* that ties the drug addict to the drug represents a distortion both of time and space, which is able to deform his whole world. Whatever idea the doctor has as regards the drug, it cannot in any way coincide with the drug the patient describes. If the doctor does acquire an adequate understanding of the substance in question and manages to look at it, at least in part, with the eyes of his patient, and in part with his own ability, he cannot avoid sharing a respect for the drug in a similar way to the psychiatrist who respects the delusion when his patient finally makes it clear to him. This explication or *revelation* of the delusion is always a gift that the patient makes to the doctor, it is the revealing of a hidden secret. The doctor must not forget that the patient has dedicated a great part of his life to the drug in question, ending up with having emptied himself out completely because of it. The drug is an overwhelming passion, a total and exclusive love, to which the patient has given everything. He has nothing else and he is nothing else. Having completely identified himself with the drug he has inevitably canceled himself out. He has thrown himself headlong into it just as a man can throw himself into the void. The drug is the precipitate of the last identity that the patient has left. If the drug has become a mask, then the patient has in turn become the drug. This means that if we want to talk about the drug then we have to talk about the patient's self. Nothing at all can come between the patient and the drug. They coincide with each other. Only the meeting with the doctor can demarcate the boundary between the subject and the drug. The doctor's first task is to create an *epoché* (a bracketing or suspension) once he has stopped considering the drug merely as a chemical agent and has started to consider it as a vital element: the element that characterizes the addict's life-world. The drug, therefore, represents the meeting place. It follows then that the objective is that of creating this together with the patient, or rather, to recreate this together in order that a part of the subjectivity of the doctor contaminates the remaining subjectivity of the patient.

The patient should stand up at the end of the meeting feeling that he has been speaking *to* someone who has finally understood the drug, and has therefore stopped underestimating it. The idea the patient has of the drug, and which remains with him after he has left the doctor, is no longer the same idea he had before meeting the doctor. It is an idea of the drug that remains powerful, but also necessarily includes fragments of the other person's idea. If the doctor has been able to create in his own consciousness the idea of the drug through the eyes of the patient, then, in a collateral way, the patient cannot avoid finding himself having a new idea of the drug as seen through the doctor's eyes. This is something that never occurred during the pseudo-sharing experience with other drug addicts. As a result of this the first crack will appear in the dyadic-symbiotic drug-patient crystal, with the introduction of the doctor's subjectivity. At this point the patient starts to feel confused, while at the same time a newly kindled desire to meet the doctor again will start to appear. A wish to see that person again who has made the addict feel something new. That presence (*Dasein*) which has caused this new sensation. Deep down the addict still remains on the hunt for feelings. Meanwhile the doctor will have managed to wrongfoot his patient's prejudice with regard to all those people who don't take drugs and are therefore not able to understand him. In this way, the doctor has succeeded in initiating a process that is the opposite of the action of the drug over the patient: drugs petrify a patient's consciousness, making it inorganic/lacking in coherence/disorganized while the doctor subjectifies the drug, makes it coherent/organized—he responsibilizes it, he humanizes it, thus successfully reclaiming a part of the patient for humanity (Zutt 1963). This resurfacing of the "you," purposefully triggered in the patient's "ego" by the doctor, troubles/agitates/upsets the patient so much so that it almost achieves an effect comparable/similar to that of the drug itself.

Most importantly of all the doctor should be ready to hem in the void, to reach the core of the patient's life, because that is where anything that is left of the patient (even if it is nothing more than an inner strength) can still be found. This phenomenology of the first contact is experienced with great intensity, and that which continues after the encounter, also out of the setting, has been called "point blank phenomenology" (Di Petta 2004). Basically, it is about entering into the inclination of the other person, in other words being able to make a direct contact. This is made possible above all through the use of one's own personal resources rather than professional ones, and yet runs the risk of *losing* the patient through having revealed yourself rather than losing him anyway though remaining within the norms. For this to be successful it is necessary to have already achieved great freedom of movement, which in turn derives from an extremely disciplined training.

A Lived Time Psychotherapy: The Dasein-group Analysis

Dasein-group analysis (Di Petta 2006) represents a further development in the theoretical phenomenological and existential frame applied to addicted patients who are also mentally ill. Dasein-group analysis is a powerful form of therapy that focuses on concerns rooted in human existence (Binswanger, 1957), giving movement to the blocked time the addicts suffer. *Pathicity* (Straus 1930; 1978) allows an access into the patient's time-experience (Minkowski 1971). This phenomenological approach to the psychotherapy of addicts has been applied[1] in those addiction centers with everyday contact with patients, and has always given rise to an intense emotional atmosphere. In many of these patients the human sense of identity is lost even where there is no psychotic symptomatology. In these cases, the only way to survive is to achieve vital contact with another person, feeling empathy for the emotional, affective dimension of another person. The "epoché" (Husserl 1965) is the preliminary condition of this setting. Especially when this requires the doctor to abandon his own role. The lived experiences mix freely in a totally emotional context. Subsequently within the group the shared emotions reveal a truly meaningful lived dimension, made up of pain and pleasure, helplessness and happiness, loneliness and nearness, anger and friendship: a sort of "fundamental affective position" (Heidegger's *Befindlichkeit*, 1927). This group approach is centered on the search for an authentic intersubjective encounter, as the crucial embodied event (Binswanger, 1963) This condition, which happens *face-to-face* between two human beings in the middle of the group, is the necessary step for any subsequent cure. The phenomenological background has been extremely useful especially in the close encounter (*face-to-face*) with the patient, who is respected more as a real person than as just another clinical case. These experiences in the emotional context of the phenomenological group freely mix with each other, producing change and transformation in all participants. The passage from initial negative emotions to final positive emotions in each group session is crucial. It is like a journey from helplessness to hope, from pain to light, from loneliness to intimate nearness. The doctor here is not outside the group, but completely inside it. Both the doctor and the patient abandon their roles and are in the phenomenological group as human beings *body-to-body, existence-to-existence*, as persons who love, cry, feel, without the barrier that exists between *therapists* and their *patients* (Binswanger, 1942) From being *one-next-to-another* (*Nebeneinandersein*) and from being *one-in-front-of-another* (*Voreinandersein*) to *being-one-with-another* (*Miteinandersein*). This gives them the chance to live in a space and time in which it is not important to answer the question, "who am I?" but the questions "what do I feel?" and "how do I feel?" Starting from a common emotional hinterland, in which we can find our lost parts, in which we can give to others the parts they have lost, in which we can find our own internal experience, and in which there is the chance to look for and discover these parts which are still alive.[2] The group participation is open to everybody, no matter what his condition. Anyone from anywhere is admitted to this new kind of group. At the end of the group session it is evident that not even heroin is able to calm anyone more than a warm hug between two human beings; and that life itself is a greater excitement than cocaine.

---

[1] One of the most important ideas of phenomenology, in fact, is the deep union between the subject, other people and the world-of-life. This idea offers an enormous transforming potentiality, which is very useful in a modified setting of group psychotherapy.

[2] Beyond the language of medicine and psychology the essence of psychotic experience, e.g. remains something that cannot be explained, even if it is possible to perceive it. Phenomenological language in this case must adapt itself to the heart of the lived experience.

Bibliography

Beringer K. (1927). *Der Mescalinrausch*. Berlin: Springer.

Binswanger L. (1942). *Grundformen und Erkenntnis Menschlichen Daseins*. Zurich: Niehans.

Binswanger L. (1957). *Daseinsanalyse und Psychotherapie*. Zurich: Speer.

Binswanger L. (1958). "Daseinsanalyse, Psychiatrie, Schizophrenie." *Schweizer Archive Neurologie Psychiatrie* 81: 1–8.

Binswanger L. (1963). *Essere nel mondo*. Roma: Astrolabio.

Borgna E. (1978). "La tossicomania come esperienza psicoterapeutica." *Psichiatria Generale e dell'età evolutiva* 3: 127–137.

Callieri B. (1993). "L'esperienza del Leib sessuale nei tossicodipendenti." *Attualità in Psicologia* 8: 5–9.

Cargnello D., Callieri B., and Morselli G. E. (1962). *Le psicosi sperimentali*. Milano: Feltrinelli.

Di Petta G. (2004). *Il mondo tossicomane, fenomenologia e psicopatologia*. Milano: Franco Angeli.

Di Petta G. (2006). *Gruppoanalisi dell'esserci: tossicomania e terapia delle emozioni condivise*. Milano: Franco Angeli.

Gebsattel E. von. (1954). "Zur Psychopathologie der Sucht." In *Prolegomena einer medizinschen Anthropologie*, pp. 220–227. Berlin: Springer.

Gross G., Huber G., Klosterkoetter J., and Linz M. (1987). *BSABS. Bonner Skala für die Beurteilung von Basissymptomen*. Berlin-Heidelberg-New York: Springer.

Heidegger M. (1927). *Sein und Zeit*. Tubingen: Niemeyer.

Husserl E., (1965/2004). *Idee per una fenomenologia pura e per una filosofia fenomenologica*, trans. E. Filippini. Torino: Einaudi.

Jaspers K. (1913). *Allgemeine Psychopathologie*. Berlin: Springer

Klosterkoetter J. (1988). *Basissymptome und Endphänomene del Schizophrenie*. Berlin: Springer.

Minkowski E. (1971). *Il tempo vissuto. Fenomenologia e psicopatologia*. Torino: Einaudi.

Schneider K. (1959/1983). *Psicopatologia clinica*, trans. B. Callieri. Roma: Città Nuova.

Straus E. (1930). *Vom Sinne der Sinne*. Berlin: Springer.

Straus E. (1978). *Geschehenis und Erlebnis*. Berlin: Springer.

Weizsaecker V. von. (1967). *Pathosophie*. Goettingen: Vandenhoeck & Ruprecht.

Weizsaecker V. von. (1968). *Der Gestaltkreis. Theorie der Einheit von Warnhemen und Bewegen*. Stuttgart: Georg Thieme.

Zutt J. (1963). "Zur Anthropologie der Sucht." In *Auf dem Wege zu einer Anthropologischen Psychiatrie*, pp. 423–430. Berlin: Springer.

CHAPTER 69

THE LIFE-WORLD OF PERSONS WITH AUTISM

FRANCESCO BARALE, DAVIDE BROGLIA,
GIULIA ZELDA DE VIDOVICH, AND
STEFANIA UCELLI DI NEMI
Translated by Martino Rossi Monti

INTRODUCTION

AUTISM is a generalized developmental disorder that occurs early in life due to an alteration in the neurobiological foundations of intercorporeality and intersubjectivity. In autism, the role of biological factors is already evident in early stages of development and has a direct impact on clinical conditions. As a result, interpersonal relationships and basic social learning are dramatically impaired. Nonetheless, autistic people often develop—at a very early stage—a peculiar way of experiencing the world sensorially and perceptually (Lai 2014; Barale and Ucelli 2006a). In general, autism can be defined as an atypical form of existence in which the biological prerequisites allowing a "normal developing" child to harmonize with its caregivers through an "embodied" mimetic attunement and to implicitly and spontaneously absorb meanings, codes, and rules, are gravely compromised. In other words, autism can be seen as a form of existence that develops from a fragile or absent "natural self-evidence" with respect to human interactions. Despite these difficulties, however, sensory-perceptual worlds of some kind do emerge in autistic people, albeit each with its own particular features: autism, therefore, is not the "empty fortress" described by Bruno Bettelheim (1967), but rather a "full weakness," so to speak. These existential worlds involve an original difficulty in harmonizing with others, and are often difficult to grasp or imagine for those who live outside of them (Barale and Ucelli 2006b).

Autistic conditions are extremely heterogeneous in many respects. As a rule, they are not confined to childhood, but last a lifetime, while their existential developments can take many forms. In fact, adult clinical cases provide ample evidence of the variability of the syndromic construct at the etio-pathogenetic level, as well as the plurality of hypothetical nuclear aspects and phenomenal expressions of the disorder (Barale et al. 2009). Autism can be associated with mental retardation, while language, if present, is often compromised or atypical. When cognitive skills are intact (but they are often irregular and peculiar) and language is not impaired (at least at the morphostructural level), it is usual to speak of high-functioning autism.

KANNER AND ASPERGER

Working contemporaneously but independently of each other, Leo Kanner (1943) and Hans Asperger (1944) described an infantile syndrome that they labeled "autistic"—a Bleulerian term until then employed only in the context of schizophrenic disorders. Kanner identified some key features that reappeared, in different ways, in the subsequent categorial definitions of autism: isolation, need for repetition, and the so-called "islets of ability."

Autistic isolation is the direct expression of an original social weakness, a difficulty in engaging in spontaneous interaction. As such, it cannot be classified as a secondary phenomenon, a defensive withdrawal. It is certainly true that, in the course of its development, autism also leads to a condition of withdrawal and to a "secondary" isolation. From the very start, the difficulty in grasping the meaning of other people's actions and deciphering them (which, depending on the cases, can be more or less severe), in sustaining mutual relationships and developing spontaneous social skills, are a source of enormous frustration and dismay. Hence there arise feelings of humiliation, powerlessness, social fear, and an increasing defensive withdrawal—in other words, everything that constitutes the secondary dimension of autism. However, those who have extensive familiarity with people suffering from more or less severe forms of autism can often appreciate the level and persistence of their need for communication, their atypical and unhappy sociability, and the amount of joy usually accompanying episodes of successful interaction and emotional exchange (Barale and Ucelli 2006a).

An entire empirical literature shows that there is no such thing as a biologically grounded lack of social needs in autistic people. In fact, such needs, which are an essential ingredient of humanity, can be clearly identified, even though they are hindered by impairments in "primary intersubjectivity" (Trevarthen 1998, 2003, 2005) and manifest themselves in atypical, dysfunctional, and often paradoxical ways. A fundamental concept must be introduced here: autism cannot be conceived purely in terms of "deficit" nor can it be captured by simple definitions or reduced to all-or-nothing formulas based on the presence or absence of this or that function, be it cognitive, linguistic, or affective.

Sameness was described by Kanner as an intolerance to change and as a particular need to cultivate repetitive interests, sometimes bizarre ones, or to persevere in repetitive motor actions. The problem of repetitive behaviors is as complex in autism as in psychic life in general, and intersects in complex ways with the problem of isolation and obsessive compulsiveness. Autistic repetitive behaviors are heterogeneous and manifest themselves at different levels of complexity, stretching from simple stereotyped actions and increasingly elaborate routines to forms of withdrawal into often sophisticated areas of interest. Depending on the degree of complexity, such behaviors can serve different functions. In many cases, however, repetition fulfils basic needs of organization, which are particularly pressing in the context of existential worlds deprived of "natural self-evidence" and characterized, as we shall see, by a fragile predictability. Those who inhabit such worlds describe them as "a confusing interacting mass of events, people, places, sounds and sights. . . . Set routines, times, particular routes and rituals all help to get order into an un-bearably chaotic life" (Joliffe 1992).

Islets of ability are areas of competence of various kinds (visual-spatial, mathematical, musical, etc.): they can be either ordinary skills simply preserved in the context of a ge-neral disability and "central coherence" weakness, or they can be peculiar (in some cases extraordinary) ones. This particular feature of autism has played an important role in re-search both because areas of discontinuous competence express aspects of subjectivity that are important to understand and appreciate, and because its study (especially in the context of a "central coherence" deficit model) has increased our knowledge of the functioning of the autistic mind.

Drawing from the Bleulerian tradition as well as the German temperament psycho-pathology, Asperger isolated and described in detail four cases of infantile "autistic psy-chopathy" out of a much larger series of cases. Asperger's descriptions emphasized the sociopathic side of the disorder and focused on the children's difficulty in empathizing and grasping the emotional world of the other. The descriptions included a sharp differentiation between preserved aspects of language (phonology, syntax, semantics) and compromised areas (subtle interpersonal communicative skills, prosody, tone, pragmatics, and so on). To be sure, Kanner's and Asperger's optimistic prognostic pictures were proven wrong by late twentieth-century scientific advancements. However, their groundbreaking observations continued to play a foundational role in understanding autism. The stress they put—through an objectifying, but also participatory and open, observation—on the existence of preserved and crucial worlds of experience in autistic people can still be a source of inspiration for researchers.

Interlude. Autism and Schizophrenia: The Changing Fortunes of a Controversial Relationship

When confronted with such a unique condition of self-isolation, both Kanner and Asperger resorted to the Bleulerian term "autistic" in order to describe it. Considering the options available at the time, this was probably the most reasonable scientific term to adopt. This choice, however, came with some powerful implications. We will mention just two of them: 1) the link between autism and schizophrenia (which is in line with a tradition that goes back to the early twentieth century and Sante De Sanctis's notion of dementia praecocissima); 2) the implicit inclusion of autism within the general paradigm of Freudian Sexualtheorie. This paradigm, which dominated psychoanalytic psychopathology for the first half of the twentieth century, viewed psychopathological conditions as forms of fixation/regression to different stages of psychosexual development (the more severe the condition, the more primitive the stage). "Autism is nothing but Freud's autoeroticism without Eros": Eugen Bleuler's explicit definition of autism shows how indebted he was to the idea of explaining psychopathological organizations as fixations/regressions to increasingly archaic stages of development (in this case, to the so-called "autoerotic" stage) (Bleuler 1911). This approach was in line with what Karl Abraham, a pupil of Freud's, was theorizing in those years (Barale and Ucelli 2001).

The fact that modern theories of autism emerged in the context of a radical crisis of the foundational assumptions behind the very term "autism" may seem paradoxical. The term did survive, but both its main implications were abandoned in the last decades of the twentieth century. The "divorce" between autism and schizophrenia will be discussed later. The crisis of the paradigm of Sexualtheorie in psychopathology cannot be addressed here.

However, there is another paradox in the history of the relationship between autism and schizophrenia: the last decades of the twentieth century—when research on the foundations of autistic disorder flourished—witnessed a parallel decline of the notion of "autism" in the understanding of schizophrenia. In fact, in the past thirty years, autism has been the most notable absentee in definitions of schizophrenia. The reasons behind this decline, which was somewhat inevitable given the all-encompassing project that dominated psychiatry over the past decades, cannot be discussed here. This project was guided by the neo-Kraepelian idea of focusing on the objective evidence of symptoms in order to purify the operational criteria from any subjectivity and preliminary psychopathological hypothesis. As a result, in the DSM, autism has come to play a marginal role in the categorization of schizophrenia: it is hesitantly admitted to describe only schizophrenic conditions characterized by a dramatic "social withdrawal." This way, one of the glorious notions of the psychiatry of yesteryear was emptied of most of its epistemic force.

History, however, can be cunning, and often paradoxically so. In subsequent developments, both conditions (schizophrenia and autism) came to be seen as heterogeneous and rooted in neurodevelopmental impairments. Gradually, research has highlighted significant areas of overlap, with respect to genetic contribution to basic vulnerability as well as some developmental aspects. It is likely that research on the workings of the autistic mind and on its correlation with an impairment in primary intersubjectivity (Zahavi 2005) will lead to a resumption and improvement of research on schizophrenia and its essentially "autistic" dimension. This time, however, the terms are reversed: as a construct, autism is no longer an offshoot of theories of schizophrenia nor is it confined to the old conceptual framework; rather, it is now capable of generating knowledge useful to illuminate certain aspects of schizophrenic experience.

SOME RECENT MODELS FOR AUTISM

What happened to the Kannerian notion of autism once detached from its psychopathological matrix? However flawed, this matrix still provided this theoretical construct with some coherence. Deprived of its roots, in the late '70s "autism" was redefined in behavioral terms as a condition of objective alteration in three operationally definable symptomatic domains: impairment in social interaction, linguistic and non-linguistic abnormalities in communication, and restricted and stereotyped patterns of behavior and interest. Devoid as it is of psychopathological organizers, this definition immediately appears too inclusive and generic. Epidemiological evidence, however, validate the syndromic coherence: there is a statistically significant co-presence of alterations in the three domains (Wing 1979). All the later nosographic descriptions, which we cannot discuss here, followed the same pattern of "de-psychopathologization."

The consequence of this trend was that the construct increasingly lost its specificity, especially when compared to the original descriptions of the disorder. A diagnostic hyper-inclusivity predictably followed, due to the many variations in expression and severity of abnormalities detectable in the three too-generically-defined symptomatic domains. Finally, in recent times, we have witnessed the emergence of the idea of an autistic "spectrum" in which countless combinations find their proper place: the spectrum comprises the classic Kannerian traits (isolation, obsessive repetition, etc.), but also different conditions, including the most nuanced ones. It is clear that there is a growing and increasing recognition of the heterogeneity of the disorder.

We cannot, however, follow this story or explore its numerous implications, as it is still largely unfolding. What should be stressed, however, is that this change in perspective had the merit of removing historical prejudices and misunderstandings, thereby fostering the growth of scientific knowledge, in particular as regards the neurobiological underpinnings of autistic developments. At the same time, however, the definition of autism (or, better, of "autisms") purely in terms of behavioral dysfunctions, the absence of psychopathological organizers, and the resulting diagnostic hyper-inclusivity, generated at least two main problems: 1) on the side of research, a difficulty in defining more precise correlations with biological bases; 2) more generally, an increasing neglect of the autistic "worlds" and autistic subjective experience, as if autism was simply a set of maladaptive behaviors waiting to be treated and modified, irrespective of the understanding of such worlds.

Let us now go back to the attempts to understand autistic experience or to identify what is common to the many different forms of autism included in the "spectrum." This shared element would mean that the term "autism" could still indicate something "typical" and could not be reduced to a sort of "administrative category" (Gillberg 1995) within which to group very heterogeneous conditions that only share a generic impairment (with very different degrees of gravity) at some behavioral level. As such, this category would no doubt be destined to dissolve with the growth of knowledge capable of identifying, within it, more specific correlations. During the last two decades of the twentieth century, however, some new explanatory models emerged from the ruins of the psychogenic model. From different perspectives, these models have tried to organize and integrate the clinical and neurobiological evidence in pursuit of a consistent definition of the multiform functioning of the autistic mind. Among these, it is worth mentioning the Theory of Mind Mechanism (TOMM Baron-Cohen 1985, 1995, 2006; Leslie 1987); the Affective Contact Deficit Hypothesis (Hobson 1989, 1993); the Weak Central Coherence Theory (Frith 1989; Happè 1994, 1997); the Executive Dysfunction Hypothesis (Damasio 1978; Russell 1997); the Defective Cognitive and Affective Integration Theories (Brothers 1989, 1995; Sigman 1995); the Imitative Models (Gopnik 2000) and the Enactive Mind from Actions to Cognition model (Klin 2003 Gallagher 2015a).

None of these models, however, has been able to provide a complete picture of autism. On the other hand, all have produced important empirical evidence and have contributed to a better understanding of autistic worlds, which is essential if we want to provide the right treatment in the appropriate context. The sources of inspiration behind these lines of research were different, as were the notions of "social cognition" they promoted. Their respective difficulties led to the hybridization of models and fields of research. Somehow, however, a common ground was eventually reached. Each from its own perspective, these models have shown that what is at stake in autism—in different ways and degrees—are the species' innate and pre-programmed preconditions allowing a spontaneous inclusion within the context of primary intersubjectivity (Zahavi and Parnas 2003). All these lines of research share this view, whatever their model for the development of "social cognition" might be ("simulationist," "interactive," or "theory-of-mind"—Gallagher 2015). Indeed, findings coming from such different studies, if observed from a complexity perspective, clearly show that the problem of autism concerns precisely the integration of attentional, cognitive, and affective factors and the neurofunctional networks underlying such integration.

In what follows, however, we will not discuss these models and their different pathogenic hypotheses about neurodevelopment, but rather, we will explore the experiential world of autistic people by trying to adopt their peculiar "point of view."

TEMPORALITY AND SAMENESS

In Kanner's observations, obsessive need for repetition and immutability was listed among the key traits: the particular relationship that autism entertains with temporality did not escape his attention. Autistic persons feel the constant need to keep internal and external events in check. Indeed, the obsessive dimension of autism is one of the unsolved problems of current research (in contrast with non-autistic obsessive disorders, medications very rarely provide relief). Obsessive behaviors, which from the outside appear irrational or bizarre, should be understood as attempts to reorganize a space–time continuum that otherwise would seem to slide into chaos. In this sense, bringing things to a halt might limit entropy or loss.

In some cases, routine and restriction of psychomotor intentionality (up to and including stereotypy) seem to be conditions for the existence of any experience at all, because they provide it with limits and meaning. The inflexibility of both rituals and areas of interest does represent a diagnostic criterion, but remains one of the least understood aspects of autism even in recent models, despite its importance at the subjective level and as regards the patterns of communication and relationship regulated by it. In the context of a fragile balance, crises are often triggered by disruptions of sameness or frustration resulting from the disappointed expectation that things should follow a precise temporal order. Often, anything that bursts suddenly and unexpectedly into the autistic existence cannot be integrated and generates intense anxiety, which usually manifests itself, especially in non-verbal individuals, through so-called "problem behaviors" (which are equally expressive of many other kinds of distress).

The few descriptions "from within" that we possess show that the anancastic dimension of autism cannot be equated with the egodystonic experience typical of obsessive individuals. On the contrary, in the absence of alternative strategies of orientation and organization, and in an interpersonal world deprived of "natural self-evidence" and predictability, anancastic behaviors represent a grid/cage/container perceived as absolutely necessary in the face of a potential experience of chaos, confusion, and fragmentation. In its most dramatic manifestations, such experience is felt as a catastrophic threat to the stability of the borders between the self and the world. In this sense, Temple Grandin's famous "squeeze machine" can be reinterpreted precisely as a remedy to such feeling (Grandin 1995).

In autism, this crucial aspect of temporality is connected to the difficulty in developing fluid "forward models" of experience. In normotypical developments, every intentional and motor sequence, whether in the "incoming" or "outgoing" mode, implies a "programming-representation" of the sequence, which is a sort of anticipation of its consequences. In a way, this "pre-vision" is nothing but a particular instance of the general and mutual co-implication of the three dimensions of temporality: the future, the present, and the past. As such, it also has specific neurophysiological correlates: the anticipatory representations of goal-directed actions and of the embodied self in action (both one's and the interlocutor's self actually) are continuously processed in the prefrontal cortex and, as the sequence unfolds, processed and re-elaborated in the frontal-limbic-cerebellar circuits. These representations not only precede and regulate the execution and/or understanding of goal-directed sequences, but are also reshaped in the course of the sequences, which in turn they contribute to reshaping. "Anticipatory models" of experience are therefore indispensable for a fluid, dynamic, and open interaction between the self and the world.

Long before these aspects had received neurophysiological confirmation (Jeannerod 1994) and had been studied primarily in the context of the executive functions deficit model, the great clinician Margaret Mahler (1968), who had no scientific knowledge of the matter, brilliantly grasped this particular aspect of autism: "these children seem to have no intuition of the future," she wrote; their experience does not seem to be "future-oriented," as if the consequences of their and other people's actions could not be predicted. Therefore, in autism, exchanges between the self and the world follow rigid and unmodifiable patterns: immediate responses cannot be inhibited or adjusted according to the circumstances. Self- and context-oriented reflection—namely, the immediate and pre-reflective apperception of the embodied self in its interaction with the world—cannot maintain their fluidity and openness, and this affects the feeling of agency too.

In autism, the difficulty in integrating large neurological circuits (the "central coherence deficit," if you will) is reflected in a particular impairment in the experience of time. In fact, the disruption of the flow of intentional movement is connected to what has long been called, without further specification, the deep "dyspraxic core" of autism (Mahler 1968). This autistic feature is particularly evident and relevant in the world of interpersonal interactions because of the mentioned difficulty in automatically recognizing, "attuning" with, and spontaneously adjusting to the feelings of others. In reality, however, this issue concerns the dimension of intentionality as such. On the whole, we are faced here with a crucial question. Any encounter with autistic worlds, but also any attempt to engage in a habilitation program or build "autism friendly" settings, will inevitably collide with a number of obstacles: a restricted form of experience, a low predictability of the world, and a strong need for sameness. All these aspects must be understood and taken into account: obviously, the idea is not to take them as immutable factors, but to open the way to new forms of meaningful, lived experience and communal activities without triggering dramatic disruptions of psychological homeostasis.

THE PERCEPTUAL ARTICULATION OF EXPERIENCE

The study of autistic perceptual experience has a long and controversial history. Converging empirical findings point to a deficit in the integrated functioning comprising attention, perception, apperception, and integration of internal and external sensory stimuli. Attention, eye fixation, and object preference patterns have been thoroughly investigated in populations at risk and in prospective studies, in an attempt to identify early and reliable pre-dictive markers of autism. For example, research has been conducted on the peculiarities of eye fixation patterns (Merin 2007), on the lack of preferential eye contact (Jones 2008), and on the preference for geometric rather than human shapes (Pierce 2011).

Instances of both over- and under-arousal in autism have been carefully described: in over-arousal, disproportionate responses are triggered by seemingly insignificant stimuli and details (one example is hypersensitivity to sounds, noises, and minimal environmental changes); in under-arousal, by contrast, individuals show a certain disinterest for interac-tive and relational stimuli. An unclear distinction between the animate and the inanimate had already emerged in Kanner's seminal descriptions, where patients displayed a tendency to prefer interaction with inanimate rather than animate objects. Hyper-selective attention, difficulties in the shifting of attentional focus, and sensory modulation dysfunctions often stand out very clearly and have given rise to interpretative disputes. Are these features "pri-mary" atypias correlated to a nuclear aspect of the disorder, or are they consequences of sec-ondary adaptations? Can they be defined as a global deficit or are they limited to certain types of stimuli and specific forms of attention?

Clinical and neurophysiological findings are in this sense contradictory (O'Riordan and Plaisted 2001; (Williams 2005), but seem to point to a transmodal problem as regards sen-sory domains, a problem correlated to atypical patterns of neocortical connectivity and af-ferent processing—a "central coherence" deficit, if you will—often characterized by local hyperactivity and long distance hypoconnectivity. In any case, the peculiarity of perceptual experience has a strong impact on the organization of autistic existential worlds. Here as well it seems that a dynamic element is missing, namely a form of attention that, in the in-teraction with the animate and inanimate world, is capable both of focusing on irrelevant aspects of experience and effortlessly ignoring them, in a constant process of reorganiza-tion. Autistic experience seems almost immune to distraction and hardly sensitive to other people's views. As a result, one can sometimes encounter a startling observational and dis-criminating capacity, to the point where even minor details and differences are registered. Absolute pitch and the ability to piece together picture-less, white jigsaw puzzles are among the peculiarities of autistic perceptual organization.

In the context of such an idiosyncratic experience of the world, stress has been put on the impairment in social perception and especially on joint attention deficits (Sigman 1986). "Proto-declarative" gestures generally develop in the first half of the second year of life: through them, the child controls and directs the attention of the interlocutor to an ob-ject of joint attention. These gestures are therefore essential for the construction of a shared framework of meaning. Their absence is one of the best-known indicators of potential risk of developing autism. Equally idiosyncratic, in autism, is the so-called lived distance: "Beyond the physical and geometrical distance existing between me and all things"—Merleau-Ponty has written—"a lived distance links me to things that count and exist for me, and links them to each other. At each moment, this distance measures the 'scope' of my life. Sometimes between me and events there is a certain leeway (Spielraum) that preserves my freedom without the events ceasing to touch me. Sometimes, however, the lived distance is at once too short and too wide: the majority of events cease to count for me, whereas the nearest ones consume me. They envelop me like the night, and they rob me of individuality and freedom" (Merleau-Ponty 1945/2013: 299).

AFFECTIVITY AND RECIPROCITY

Affectivity is historically one of the most misunderstood aspects of autism: at first, it was confined to psychogenic theories of cold parenting and, later on, to variations on the theme of autism as "lack of emotions." In fact, autistic subjects do establish emotional ties with the external world and sometimes express extreme feelings in response to emotional and relational atmospheres. Autistic affectivity appears to oscillate constantly between the poles of the excessive and the defective, the "too much" and the "too little." Impaired functionality of natural mechanisms of regulation, modulation, communication, and mimic recognition exposes autistic people to often chaotic and extreme emotional experiences, which are dealt with by relying on private strategies of organization.

Clara C. Park (2001), writing about her daughter, has left us an eloquent description of these enigmatic extremes of ecstasy and despair, which have forced her and her husband to continually put things in doubt and question both the events and the network of affective meanings in which they were immersed. Some things catch the attention of autistic people because of their novelty, others because they are a confirmation of a previous expectation or state of anguish. To a certain extent, this is the case for everyone, but in autistic people this dynamic unfolds through associations and private emotional codes that cannot be grasped from the outside. In the words of Clara Park: "But what good did it do to know that a lighted window had disrupted the darkness of the building across the street?" (Park 2001). Affections and emotions are there, but the idiom is private. To approach an autistic world requires a patient deciphering and communal creation of alternative styles of expression.

The apparent refusal to communicate (through echolalia, prolonged silence, or problem behaviors) has its own semantics and points to emotional worlds difficult to penetrate but nonetheless present. In her books, essays, and conversations with Oliver Sacks, Temple Grandin has stressed that exchanges of affection appear to her as incomprehensible and regulated by mysterious subtleties (Grandin 1995): for her, to explore interpersonal worlds is equivalent to deciphering structures, codes, and mysterious life forms, as "an anthropologist on Mars" would do (Sacks 1995). However, there are also forms of life and experience that cannot be grasped and learned from the outside, as it happens with a foreign language. They are embedded in us from birth and stem from an original experiential core and "intercorporeal" sharing. It is precisely within this core that something, in autistic developments, seems to have gone wrong. Affectivity, language, and inter-human communication somehow form a shadowy area where different concepts overlap and get mixed up and where our understanding of autism "from the outside" is faced with its aporias and challenges.

The "affective contact" deficit could be reconsidered in terms of "original reciprocity": from the start, communication exchanges are characterized, on the one side, by reciprocity and, on the other, by some tension and a resulting pleasure in mutual recognition. Since the '70s, studies have shown impaired recognition of facial expressions of emotional states in autistic individuals: it was on the basis of such evidence that the original affective deficit model of autism was elaborated. Indeed, something seems not to be working at the level of primary intersubjectivity. There appears to be no given background for the emergence of an interpersonal self within a world of shared meanings. What is lacking is an "initially quite atheoretical, implicit, and prereflexive self-evidence, an automatically-given background of meaning which works as an intersubjective matrix providing meaning and a sense of reciprocity. In non-autistic individuals, this self-evidence gradually expands and allows them to navigate their way almost automatically in the inter-human world as in their natural environment, an environment which they have somehow pre-comprehended from the beginning" (Barale and Ucelli 2006b: 108–109).

Imitation plays a key role in these processes: primary imitation gradually gives way to increasingly complex and less "echo-like" imitative skills. It is no coincidence that imitation is a traditional topic of research in autism. A few years after Kanner's studies, Edward Ritvo was the first to give a clinical description of imitation deficits in autistic children (Ritvo 1953). Later on, Rogers and Pennington systematically studied these deficits and, drawing from Daniel Stern's conceptualizations (Stern 1985), speculated that an original imitative deficit could be hampering self–other mapping processes. Early imitative processes, which are spontaneous and pre-representational, are also fundamental for development of affective attunement as described by Stern and for "intercorporeal dialogue" with the caregivers. Peter Hobson (1989) has done extensive research in this area. A Canadian prospective study of a population of children at genetic risk has shown that deficits in imitation precede the emergence of clear autistic symptoms (Zwaigenbaum 2005. These findings (confirmed by neuroimaging studies) have fostered methods of intervention focused on supporting embryonic capacities for imitative interaction, which is considered the true driving force behind the development of social skills (Meltzoff 2000).

In reality, this issue is both complex and controversial. However, it is reasonable to suppose that some kind of imitative deficit might deprive autistic children of basic information about other people's worlds and possible connections between internal states and behaviors. Imitation implies feeling what the other feels. This, in turn, is the prerequisite for the development of a capacity to form an internal representation of that feeling, namely of a meta-representational capacity. The plurality of mimetic desires typical of human beings is in turn closely associated with the problem of identification and social recognition. The complexity of simulation and imitation processes is reflected on bonding functions and affective relationships between the self and the other. Alexandre Kojève (1947) reminded us that mimesis—namely a desire for the other's desire—is the form of reciprocity on which social recognition is grounded. In the last two decades, neuroscience of mirror systems has provided empirical confirmation of these insights, opening the way for research on alterations in embodied simulation across the autistic spectrum (Gallese 2006; Oberman 2007).

INTENTIONALITY AND INTERCORPOREALITY

"I cannot reach my baby": these were the words of the mother of one of the autistic children observed by Kanner. "He walks as if he is in a shadow," Kanner suggestively remarked, somehow echoing the mother's dismay at the emotional detachment of her enigmatic son (Kanner 1943). Seemingly self-evident aspects of experience can appear, in fact, as mute and enshrouded in mystery. It is interesting to note that the difficulty in perceiving and representing the other's intentionality is bidirectional: it affects both those who try to approach the world of an autistic person and the autistic person herself.

From whatever scientific perspective we decide to address the problem—be it through the lenses of the affective contact deficit hypothesis, the empathy deficit, the executive functions deficit, or the central coherence deficit—it is clear that this problem concerns the core foundations of human intentionality: here lie the processes allowing one to perceive (or, better, "to feel," thanks to the body as a "tacit cogito," as Merleau-Ponty put it) both one's and other people's actions as "goal-oriented" and as rooted in a common ground, and to modulate them accordingly. This leads to the development of a sense of self as an "intentional agent" actively immersed in a set of goal-oriented and identifiable exchanges. The sense of "mineness" of experience, objects, and desires becomes altered in a universe where the boundaries between the self and the other, the accidental and the intentional, the physical and the mental, tend to blur. In this sense, even the frequent misuse of pronouns (the lack of "I" and the use of the third person to refer to oneself) discloses the complex constellations of meaning typical of autistic subjectivity and agency.

Intercorporeality comes well before mind reading and the attribution of mental states (Gallese 2007): it is a direct, pre-representational form of understanding of the other, rooted in the body and in the activation of specific neural systems through "intentional attunement." Deficits in psychomotor coordination and fluency (and therefore, to varying degrees, in intercorporeality) had already been described in the first observations of autistic children, especially by Asperger. Often, the body appears as if hindered by an obstacle and trapped in a postural clumsiness or afflicted by an almost imperceptible dissonance. These peculiar body-states correlate in a complex way with difficulties in intercorporeal attunement, which is the pre-verbal foundation of communication between people. These aspects contributed to the development of the idea of the "dyspraxic core" of autism.

Recent findings have confirmed such difficulties in intercorporeal organization in individuals with autism, highlighting important aspects and neurophysiological mechanisms. In typical developments, intentional sequences "incarnate" from the very start in their own psychomotor organization and kinematics both their "what" (i.e. the action itself) and their "why" (i.e. the intention underlying the action). This applies both to "incoming" processes (i.e. understanding the meaning of other people's sequences), and "outgoing" ones (i.e. sequence execution). In other words, the same motor sequence—for example, reaching out to grasp a glass of water—can have quite different "whys": drinking, moving the glass, throwing water on the interlocutor, and so on. In normotypical developments, the "what" and the "why" are inherently inscribed from the beginning in the kinematic organization of the intentional sequence, which is different in the three cases mentioned above. Specific mirror systems apparently ensure the gestalt, immediate, and pre-reflective recognition of the "embodied meaning" of intentional sequences. From the very beginning, conversely, in autistic developments there is a difficulty in inscribing both the "what" and the "why" in the understanding and execution of intentional sequences. In the case of high-functioning autism, the "what" and "why" of intentional sequences are rather "superimposed" from the outside: they do not intrinsically belong to the psychomotor and immediate organization of sequences, which, however, lack such intrinsic coherence anyway. These recent findings are extremely relevant from a practical point of view, especially when integrated in the modalities with which autistic patients are approached and interventions and habilitation programs are initiated. However, as it happens with other features of autism, even this one is not entirely "static" or "global." The ability to incarnate and recognize the "why" in intentional sequences is not always absent, nor is it immutable: in fact, contexts of intense and shared practical activity may allow its emergence (Boria et al. 2009).

CONCLUSION

We have described some characteristics of the world of autistic people, which suggest, despite the extraordinary diversity of conditions covered by this term, some essential common traits. These common elements concern fundamental aspects of human intentionality, such as the preconditions of social relatedness. The different "autisms" are forms of existence that, for various biological reasons, develop from a fragile natural self-evidence of the inter-human world, from an original intercorporeal and interpersonal weakness. However, worlds of some kind do emerge from such conditions, with peculiarities that we must try to understand, if we want to relate to them and arrange appropriate contexts and interventions.

In conclusion, it is worth emphasizing a point once again: autism is not conceivable purely in terms of "deficit." None of its aspects can be explained away through clear-cut definitions or "all-or-nothing" formulas on the basis of the presence or absence of this or that function, be it cognitive, linguistic, or affective (Lord and McGee 2001). As we have seen, for example, the development of imitative capacities is not entirely absent, but, rather, atypical. A similar consideration applies to the recognition and communication of emotions. There are indeed numerous signs of atypical sociability and "need for sociability" (Knobloch and Pasamanick 1975;); the recognition of the "why" of intentional sequences is not statically absent, but can be stimulated by intense and shared practical activity (Boria et al. 2009).

To think of autistic worlds as instantiations of simple "deficits" is no less serious a mistake than to embrace the old psychogenic theory, according to which autism was simply a "consequence" of cold parenting. The various models we have described were developed in the psychological laboratory. However, it has long been noted that there is a discrepancy between what is seen in the laboratory and what is observable in ecological contexts. Therefore, some have emphasized the necessity to expand both observations and "naturalistic" interventions beyond the confines of the laboratory. Artificial strategies adopted by high-functioning subjects in the laboratory, for example, do not match "spontaneous" capacities. Even more interestingly, in "natural" and "autism friendly" contexts—where the peculiar needs of autistic people are accommodated—one can often observe not only "islets" of ability, but also surprising oscillations in the same abilities and disabilities, so that unsuspected capacities sometimes emerge. As Uta Frith remarked, in autism a deficit is never either static or global (Frith 1989). Therefore, we must get used to the idea that "autisms" are not pure deficits, but atypical developments or "full weaknesses" where all the ingredients of humanity are somehow present, although in atypical and dysfunctional combinations. In these unique existential worlds, where nothing is purely defective, the incapacity to perceive and experience the other is never total or irrevocable.

Translated from the Italian by Martino Rossi Monti.

Bibliography

Asperger H. (1944). "Die 'Autistischen Psycopathen' im Kindesalter." *Archiv fur Psychiatrie und Nervenkrankheiten* 117: 76–136.

Barale F. and Ucelli di Nemi S. (2006a). "Voce Autismo cosiddetto 'infantile' (disturbo autistico)." In F. Barale, et al. (eds.), *Psiche. Dizionario storico di psicologia, psichiatria, psicoanalisi e neuroscienze*, vol. 1, pp. 117–124. Torino: Einaudi.

Barale F. and Ucelli di Nemi S. (2006b). "La debolezza piena. Il disturbo autistico dall'infanzia all'età adulta." In S. Mistura (ed.), *Autismo. L'umanità nascosta*, pp. 51–206. Torino: Einaudi.

Barale F., et al. (2009). "L'autismo a partire dalla sua evoluzione nell'età adulta: nuove conoscenze, criticità, implicazioni riabilitative." *Noos* 15(3): 257–291.

Barale F. and Ucelli di Nemi S. (2001). "Alle fonti delle concezioni psicodinamiche delle psicosi. Karl Abraham e la psichiatria del suo tempo." *Rivista di Psicoanalisi* 4: 693–709.

Baron-Cohen S. (1995). *Mindblindness. An Essay on Autism and Theory of Mind*. Cambridge, MA: MIT Press.

Baron-Cohen S. (2006). "The Hyper-systemizing, Assortative Mating Theory of Autism Progress." *Neuro-Psychopharmacology & Biological Psychiatry* 30: 865–872.

Baron-Cohen S., Leslie A. M., and Frith U. (1985). "Does the Autistic Child Have a 'Theory of Mind'?" *Cognition* 21: 37–46.

Bettelheim B. (1967). *The Empty Fortress: Infantile Autism and the Birth of the Self*. New York: Free Press.

Bleuler E. (1911). *Dementia praecox oder Gruppe der Schizophrenien*. Leipzig-Wien: Deuticke. (New edition with an introduction by B. Küchenhoff). Psychosozialverlag, Gießen, 2014.

Boria S., et al. (2009). "Intention Understanding in Autism." *PloS One* 4(5): e5596.

Brothers L. (1989). "A Biological Perspective on Empathy." *American Journal of Psychiatry* 146: 10–19.

Brothers L. (1995). "Neurophysiology of the Perception of Intentions by Primates." In M. S. Gazzaniga (ed.), *The Cognitive Neurosciences*, pp. 1107–1115. Cambridge, MA: MIT Press.

Damasio A. R. and Maurer R. G. (1978). "A Neurological Model for Childhood Autism." *Archives of Neurology* 35: 777–786.

Frith U. (1989). *Autism: Explaining the Enigma*. Oxford: Blackwell.

Gallagher S. and Varga S. (2015a). "Social Cognition and Psychopathology: A Critical Overview." *World Psychiatry* 14(1): 5–14.

Gallagher S. and Varga S. (2015b). "Conceptual Issues in Autism Spectrum Disorders." *Current Opinion in Psychiatry* 28(2): 127–132.

Gallese V. (2006). "La molteplicità condivisa. Dai neuroni mirror all'intersoggettività." In S. Mistura (ed.), *Autismo. L'umanità nascosta*, pp. 207–270. Torino: Einaudi.

Gallese V. (2007). "Before and Below "Theory of Mind": Embodied Simulation and the Neural Correlates of Social Cognition." *Philosophical Transactions of the Royal Society B-Biological Sciences* 362(1480): 659–669.

Gillberg C. (1995). *Clinical Child Neuropsychiatry*. Cambridge: Cambridge University Press.

Gopnik A., Capps L., and Meltzoff A. N. (2000). "Early Theories of Mind: What the Theory Can Tell Us about Autism." In S. Baron-Cohen, et al. (eds.), *Understanding Other Minds: Perspectives from Autism and Cognitive Neuroscience*, pp. 50–72, 2nd edn. Oxford: Oxford University Press.

Grandin T. (1995). *Thinking in Pictures*. New York: Doubleday.

Happè F. (1994). *Autism: an Introduction to Psychological Theory*. London: UCL Press.

Happè F. (1997). "Central Coherence and Theory of Mind in Autism: Reading Homographs in Context." *British Journal of Developmental Psychology* 15: 1–12.

Hobson R. P. (1989). "Beyond Cognition: A Theory of Autism." In G. Dawson (ed.), *Autism: Nature, Diagnosis and Treatment*, pp. 22–48. New York: Guilford.

Hobson R. P. (1993). "The Emotional Origins of Social Understanding." *Philosophical Psychology* 6: 227–249.

Jeannerod M. (1994). "The Representing Brain: Neural Correlates of Motor Intention and Imagery." *Behavioural Brain Sciences* 17(2): 187–245.

Joliffe T., Lakesdown R., and Robinson C. (1992). " Autism, a Personal Account." *Communication* 26(3): 12–19.

Jones W., Carr K., and Klin A. (2008). "Absence of Preferential Looking to the Eyes of Approaching Adults Predicts Level of Social Disability in 2-Year-Old Toddlers with Autism Spectrum Disorder." *Archives of General Psychiatry* 65(8): 946–954.

Kanner L. (1943). "Autistic Disturbance of Affective Contact." *Nervous Child* 2: 217–250.

Klin A., Jones W., Schultz R., and Volkmar F. (2003). "The Enactive Mind, or from Actions to Cognition: Lessons from Autism." *Philosophical Transactions of the Royal Society B-Biological Sciences* 358(1430): 345–360.

Knobloch H. and Pasamanick B. (1975). "Some Etiologic and Prognostic Factors in Early Infantile Autism and Psychosis." *Pediatrics* 55(2): 182–191.

Kojève A. (1947). *Introduction à la lecture de Hegel. Leçons sur la "Phénoménologie de l'esprit" professées de 1933 à 1939, à l'Ecole des hautes études, rèunies et publiées par Raymand Queneau.* Paris: Gallimard.

Lai M. C., Lombardo M. V., and Baron-Cohen S. (2014). "Autism." *Lancet* 383(9920): 896–910.

Leslie A. M. (1987). "Pretense and Representation: The Origins of a Theory of Mind." *Psychological Review* 94: 412–426.

Lord C. and McGee J. (eds.). (2001). *Educating Children with Autism Spectrum Disorders: Report of the Committee on Early Intervention in Autism.* Washington, DC: National Academy of Sciences.

Mahler M. (1968). *Infantile Psychosis.* New York: International Universities Press.

Meltzoff A. N. and Prinz W. (eds.) (2000). *The Imitative Mind: Development, Evolution, and Brain Bases.* Cambridge: Cambridge University Press.

Merin N., Young G. S., Ozonoff S., and Rogers S. J. (2007). "Visual Fixation Patterns during Reciprocal Social Interaction Distinguish a Subgroup of 6-Month-Old Infants At-Risk for Autism from Comparison Infants." *Journal of Autism and Developmental Disorders* 37(1): 108–121.

Merleau-Ponty M. (2013). *Phenomenology of Perception*, trans. D. A. Landes. London: Routledge. (*Phénoménologie de la Perception*. Paris: Gallimard, 1945).

Plaisted, K. C. (2001). Reduced generalization in Autism. An alternative to Weak Central Coherence. In J.A. Burack T. Charman (Eds), The Development of Autism: Perspective from Theory and Research (pp 139–169). Mahwah, NJ: Laurence Erlbaum Associates.

Oberman L. M., Pineda J. A., and Ramachandran V. S. (2007). "The Human Mirror Neuron System: A Link between Action Observation and Social Skills." *Social Cognitive & Affective Neuroscience* 2(1): 62–66.

Park C. (2001). *Exiting Nirvana: A Daughter's Life with Autism.* Boston, New York, London: Little, Brown and Company.

Pierce K., Conant D., Hazin R., Stoner R., and Desmond J. (2011). "Preference for Geometric Patterns Early in Life as a Risk Factor for Autism." *Archives of General Psychiatry* 68(1): 101–109.

Ritvo E. R. and Provence S. (1953). "Form Perception and Imitation in Some Autistic Children: Diagnostic Findings and their Contextual Interpretation." *Psychoanalytic Study of the Child* 8: 155–161.

Russell J. (1997). *Autism as an Executive Disorder.* Oxford: Oxford University Press.

Sacks O. (1995). *An Anthropologist On Mars: Seven Paradoxical Tales.* New York: Knopf.

Sigman M., Mundy P., Sherman T., and Ungerer J. (1986). "Social Interactions of Autistic, Mentally Retarded and Normal Children and their Caregivers." *Journal of Child Psychology and Psychiatry* 27(5): 647–655.

Sigman M., Yirminya N., and Capps L. (1995). "Social and Cognitive Understanding in High-Functioning Children with Autism." In E. Schopler and G. B. Mesibov (eds.), *Learning and Cognition in Autism,* pp. 159–176. New York: Plenum Press.

Stern D. N. (1985). *The Interpersonal World of the Infant.* London: Karnac Brooks.

Trevarthen C. (1998). "The Concept and Foundations of Infant Intersubjectivity." In S. Bråten (ed.), *Intersubjective Communication and Emotion in Early Ontogeny,* pp. 15–46. Cambridge: Cambridge University Press.

Trevarthen C. (2003). "Infant Psychology is an Evolving Culture." *Human Development* 46: 233–246.

Trevarthen C. (2005). "Action and Emotion in Development of the Human Self, Its Sociability and Cultural Intelligence: Why Infants Have Feelings Like Ours." In J. Nadel and D. Muir (eds.), *Emotional Development,* pp. 61–91. Oxford: Oxford University Press.

Williams D. L., Goldstein G., Carpenter P. A., and Minshew N. J. (2005). "Verbal and Spatial Working Memory in Autism." *Journal of Autism and Developmental Disorders* 35(6): 747–756.

Wing L. and Gould J. (1979). "Severe Impairments of Social Interaction and Associated Abnormalities in Children: Epidemiology and Classification." *Journal of Autism and Childhood Schizophrenia* 9: 11–29.

Zahavi D. (2005) *Subjectivity and Selfhood: Investigating the First-Person Perspective.* Cambridge, MA: MIT Press.

Zahavi D. and Parnas J. (2003). "Conceptual Problems in Infantile Autism Research: Why Cognitive Science Needs Phenomenology." *Journal of Consciousness Studies* 10(9–10): 53–71.

Zwaigenbaum L., Bryson S., Rogers T., Roberts W., Brian J., and Szatmari P. (2005). "Behavioral Manifestations of Autism in the First Year of Life." *International Journal of Developmental Neuroscience* 23(2–3): 143–152.

CHAPTER 70

EATING DISORDERS AS DISORDERS OF EMBODIMENT AND IDENTITY

GIOVANNI CASTELLINI AND VALDO RICCA

EATING DISORDERS: WHAT IS BEHIND PATHOLOGICAL BEHAVIORS?

EATING disorders (EDs) are defined as psychiatric syndromes, characterized by a persistent disturbance of eating or eating-related behaviors, that result in the altered consumption or absorption of food and that significantly impair physical health or psychosocial functioning. According to a behavioral level of assessment, the fifth edition of the Diagnostic and Statistical Manual of Mental Disorders (DSM-5) divides the category of Feeding and Eating Disorders into pica, rumination disorder, avoidant/restrictive food intake disorder, anorexia nervosa, bulimia nervosa, and binge-eating disorder (American Psychiatric Association 2013). However, overcoming this position, the phenomenological perspective takes into account the subjective perception of one's own body and behaviors, and the system of significance and values related to them. Furthermore, several authors support a dimensional rather than categorical approach, which appears to be more coherent to this perspective, and allows for the description of a more complex pattern of eating disorder symptomatology, which is shared by all the main diagnoses. Finally, the temporal instability of the DSM diagnoses, and the substantial crossover between them, support adopting dimensional models (Castellini et al. 2011; Milos et al. 2013).

Indeed, diagnostic categories seem to differ between them, only in terms of state-dependent symptoms, such as weight loss (anorexia nervosa vs bulimia nervosa), purging behaviors (bulimia nervosa vs binge eating disorders) binge eating (differentiating subtypes of anorexia nervosa). However, from a phenomenological perspective it is important to understand why patients with EDs decided to change their eating habits, why their weight became the core of their entire life, and why available psychological treatments often reduce the pathological behaviors but scarcely challenge the core psychopathology.

According to these observations, there is general agreement in considering behavioral anomalies—which are required for DSM diagnosis—as secondary epiphenomena to a more profound psychopathological core, defined by excessive concerns about body shape and weight (Fairburn and Harrison 2003). In particular, patients with EDs overvalue their body shape and weight. Furthermore, the body image disturbance has been associated with a more profound disturbance consisting in disorders of the way persons experience their own body and shape their personal identity (Stanghellini et al. 2012). In other words, whereas most people evaluate and define themselves on the basis of the way they perceive their performance in various domains, patients with EDs judge their self-worth largely, or even exclusively, in terms of their shape and weight and their ability to control these aspects of their body.

The psychopathological core, rather than behavioral abnormalities, plays a crucial role in the onset and persistence of these disorders. Indeed, it has been associated with different responses to psychological treatment in several reports, and some authors have pointed out that the threshold to define the full recovery process might be body shame, appearance schemas, and thin-ideal internalization. Therefore, these may be fruitful targets of intervention among those on a recovery trajectory.

Moreover, the lived world of people with EDs can include a distorted perception of space and time. Several behaviors and cognitive distortions can be derived from a basic sense of spatial metamorphosis that is deeply associated with the disorder of corporeality. In the same way, the perception of time in ED patients appears to be connected with the temporal discontinuity of the representation of one's own body, and the need for predictability of one's own life, which is achieved/failed according to control of eating and weight.

In line with this perspective, a comprehensive assessment of persons with EDs should include: the way of perceiving one's own body and lived corporeality, the significance of the illness and the body in inter-subjective interactions, as well as the personal identity definition, spatial perception, and the way of experiencing time associated with several ED features (such as binge eating or weight control).

Eating Disorders as Disturbance of Self-identity

According to several psychological theories, persons with EDs are characterized by a dysfunctional system for evaluating self-worth. Whereas most people evaluate and define themselves on the basis of a variety of domains of life (e.g. the quality of their relationships, work, parenting, sporting ability, etc.), people with EDs judge themselves largely, or even exclusively, in terms of their body shape as well as their eating habits, and their ability to control weight (Fairburn 2010).

From a psychodynamic perspective, Hilde Bruch (1982) suggested that the dissatisfaction with the body image that characterizes persons with EDs reflects a maladaptive "search for selfhood and a self-respecting identity." Stern (1985) emphasizes that feeding is a vital activity for the construction of the self, as it serves as a framing environment and allows face-to-face contact with the caregiver via the phenomenon of "affective attunement," an essential step toward the development of a narrative self and a sense of identity. Also, within the cognitive model, self-concept is defined as a set of knowledge structures about the self that originate from the cognitive products of the person's interaction with the social world. These aspects are important for the development of self-schemas that shape the individual's social interactions (Markus et al. 1985).

From a cognitive point of view, the self-concept is defined as a set of knowledge structures about the self that originates from the cognitive products of the person's interaction with the social world. These aspects are important for development of self-schemas that shape the individual's social interactions (Markus 1977). The literature in this field has provided two main constructs to pertaining one's own identity, which have been proposed as maintaining factors of EDs: severe clinical perfectionism and core low self-esteem (Fairburn 2010). Clinical perfectionism is a system for self-evaluation in which self-worth is judged largely on the basis of striving to achieve demanding goals and success at meeting them (Shafran et al. 2002). Perfectionism is well-known to be frequently observed in patients with ED (Sassaroli et al. 2011). In this case, "perfectionism" is not the same as "obsessionality," at least in phenomenological terms. The former is a personality trait, that is present in obsessive-compulsive personality as well in other mental disorders (e.g. eating disorders), whereas the world of the obsessive largely differs from the one of persons affected by eating disorders. There is often an interaction between the two forms of psychopathology with the patient's perfectionist standards being applied to the attempts to control eating, shape, and weight, as well as other aspects of life (e.g. performance at work or sport). Regarding the core of low self-esteem, most patients with EDs have an unconditional and pervasive negative view of themselves that is seen as part of their permanent identity. These patients show particularly pronounced negative cognitive processing biases, coupled with over-generalization, with the result that any perceived "failure" is interpreted as confirmation that they are failures as people thereby reaffirming their overall negative view of themselves (Fairburn et al. 1993). Moreover, in a psychodynamic perspective, impairments in overall identity development and the failure to establish multiple and diverse domains of self-definition have been considered the core pathoplastic mechanism of EDs (Stern 1985; Sands 1991; Goodsitt 1997; Malson 1999; Piran 2001).

Stanghellini et al. (2012) provided a phenomenological interpretation of the core psychopathology of EDs based on a disturbance of self-identity. According to this hypothesis, in persons with EDs the disturbance of the experience of one's own body is interconnected with the process of shaping their personal identity. The cenesthetic apprehension of one's own body is the more primitive and basic form of self-awareness, and patients with EDs often report—with different extents of insight—difficulties in perceiving their emotions and that they do not "feel" themselves (Piran 2001). Indeed, feeling oneself is a basic requirement to achieve an identity and a stable sense of one's self (Stanghellini et al. 2014). Therefore, for persons prone to symptomatology of EDs, the identity is no longer a real psychic structure that persists beyond the flow of time and circumstances. The experience of not feeling one's own body and emotions involves the whole sense of identity. This causes us to deprive ourselves of our existence as a being-for-itself and instead learn to falsely self-identify as a being-in-itself (Sartre 1992). Therefore, there is the need to resort to one's own body weight as a viable source of definition of the self, as patients often report: "Sometimes, the emotions I feel are extraneous to me and scare me"; "I see myself out of focus, I don't feel myself." From an empirical point of view, the relationships between abnormal eating behavior and self-construct or identity in EDs has already been investigated (Norbø et al. 2006). For example, Nordbø documented that anorexic persons may explain their behavior as a tool for achieving a new identity Skarderud (2007 showed that for some persons with ED, changing one's body is a means of changing one's identity. They want to change, and changing one's body serves as both a concrete and a symbolic tool for such ambitions. Thus, shaping oneself is a "concretised metaphor" (Stanghellini et al. 2012), establishing equivalence between a psychic reality (identity) and a physical one (one's body shape). As suggested by Surgenor et al. (2003), looking into the different ways persons with ED construe their own self, especially in relation to their disorder and therapy, has strategic implications for the therapeutic endeavor.

The Questionnaire IDEA (IDentity and EAting Disorders): an Instrument to Measure Disorders of Self-identity

Recently, based on a phenomenological perspective, a questionnaire named IDEA (IDentity and EAting disorders) has been used to assess and validate abnormalities in lived corporeality and personal identity (Stanghellini et al. 2012). The questionnaire was developed based on the following conceptual areas: feeling oneself through the gaze of the other, defining oneself through the evaluation of the other, feeling oneself through objective measures, feeling extraneous from one's own body, feeling oneself through starvation, defining one's identity through one's own body, feeling oneself through physical activity and fatigue. Theoretically, the questionnaire assumed that most pathological eating behaviors and features are a consequence of the severity of abnormal bodily experiences and an identity disorder. The authors demonstrated that the questionnaire was able to identify relevant psychopathological phenomena that are closely related to the specific anomalies of ED patients measured with commonly-adopted psychometric instruments. In particular, the subscales showed a different pattern of association with the features of EDs. Feeling oneself through the gaze of the other and defining oneself through the evaluation of the other was associated with overvalued thoughts regarding body shape. A measure of alienation from one's own body and emotions, and feeling extraneous from one's own body, significantly correlated with concerns about weight and body shape. Finally, feeling oneself through objective measures and feeling oneself through starvation were associated with overvalued thoughts regarding weight and eating concerns and with dietary restriction, respectively. In line with these results, some characteristic ED behaviors, such as starvation and the fixated checking of objective measures, might be interpreted as an alternative coping strategy aimed at feeling oneself for those patients who are unable to feel themselves cenesthetically. These results were confirmed for patients reporting anorexia nervosa, bulimia nervosa, and binge eating disorder (Stanghellini et al. 2012). Moreover, it was also applied beyond the boundaries of the DSM diagnostic categories, and abnormal bodily experiences were observed not just for "over-threshold" ED patients. First of all, it was tested in a large population of university students who did not suffer from EDs (Stanghellini et al. 2014). IDEA appeared to be able to identify vulnerability in subjects without full-blown EDs but with abnormal eating patterns. Moreover, the questionnaire provides a numerical threshold to discriminate clinical vs non-clinical populations. Indeed, in people who develop clinically relevant EDs, extraneousness from one's own body is a phenomenon that is significantly more manifest and penetrant than in people who display over-threshold, but non full-blown abnormal eating patterns. This could represent the first step to demonstrate that IDEA is able to identify candidate experiential intermediate phenotypes that express a gradient of vulnerability from healthy to clinical persons with EDs. Finally, the questionnaire was applied to morbidly obese patients, which is a population at high risk of developing ED behaviors (Castellini et al. 2014). The vulnerability to ED behaviors such as binge eating appeared to be associated with abnormal bodily experiences in a dimensional pattern. In this study, authors also found that abnormal bodily experiences measured by IDEA represented the psychological underpinning of the relationship between binge eating behaviors and impulsivity. A mediation model clarified that not impulsivity in itself, but the presence of impulsivity in persons affected by abnormal bodily experiences, may lead to ED psychopathology and abnormal eating behaviors. Authors concluded that the disturbance in the lived corporeality may represent the core vulnerability trait underlying the association between personality traits such as impulsivity and the development of eating disorders features.

The Lived Body in Persons with Eating Disorders

The process of personal identity development has been considered as deeply interconnected with lived corporeality, and with representation of one's own body. Indeed, according to a neurobiological perspective, the experience of the body is the original anchor of our developing sense of the self (Kinsbourne 2002). The mind continues to mature until it can represent and reflect upon its own contents. The self becomes abstracted from the body and it is intellectualized as the self-conscious mind. However, the felt self and its body background continue to frame whatever is the current focus of attention. During the developmental period, every person structures his or her own primitive form of self-identity around the progressive building and discovering of the body image. Although there is no definite consensus on the concept of body image (Gallagher 2006), it has become clear that the body image is neither completely innate nor completely constructed out of experience and learning. Body image is considered as a multidimensional pattern, which includes cognitive and affective components (concerns and feelings about the body), perception (estimation of body size), and behaviors related to the perception of one's own body (Thompson et al. 1999). It has been defined as the picture of the body that is formed in the mind (Schilder 1950) or "a system of perceptions, attitudes and beliefs pertaining to one's body" (Gallagher 2006). For a more accurate psychopathological definition, it is important to distinguish between different dimensions of embodiment, such as body schema, body image and lived body, although no consensus concerning terminology has yet emerged (Gallagher 2006). The concept of body image should be clearly differentiated from body schema, which is "a system of sensory-motor capacities that function without awareness or the necessity of perceptual monitoring" (Gallagher 2006). According to Head (1926), the body schema is a model/representation of one's own body that constitutes a standard along which postures and body movements are judged. This representation can be considered the result of comparisons and integration at the cortical level of past sensory experiences (postural, tactile, visual, kinesthetic, and vestibular) with current sensations. This gives rise to an almost completely unconscious "plastic" reference model that makes it possible to move easily in space and to recognize the parts of one's own body in all situations.

Several studies have demonstrated the importance of concerns related to the body (e.g. shape, weight) in determining different courses of EDs, in terms of response to treatment and long-term outcome (Fairburn et al. 2003; Castellini et al. 2011). Patients with EDs typically overvalue their body shape and weight; body image disturbances may be the key to distinguish between partially and fully recovered individuals and a healthier relationship with one's body may be the final hurdle in recovery (Bardone-Cone et al. 2010). In particular, it has been suggested that body image distortion—defined as "a disturbance in the way in which one's body weight or shape is experienced" (American Psychiatric Association 1994)—represents a specific trait of EDs, which allows distinguishing between affected ED patients and normal subjects, across a continuum of severity of several psychopathological domains.

The relationship between body image and identity has been postulated by Allamani and Allegranzi (1990) who refer to body image as "a complex psychological organization which develops through the bodily experience of an individual and affects both the schema of behaviour and a fundamental nucleus of self-image."

In recent studies, which advance the phenomenological perspective mentioned above, Stanghellini et al. (2012, 2015) demonstrate that the core psychopathology in EDs is related to a dimension of embodiment named "lived-body-for-others." According to these findings, persons with EDs experience the body first and foremost as an object being looked at by another, rather than cenesthetically or from a first-person perspective. This is also related with a feeling of extraneousness from their own body, and with a constant attempt to define themselves through pathological behaviors such as starvation or fixated checking of objective measures. Such behaviors may operate as coping strategies aimed at being able to experience the self in some way for those who are unable to feel themselves cenesthetically.

This position draws from the background of Sartre's philosophy, which defines the process of self-structuration across life by drawing on the progressive consciousness of one's own lived corporeality. From a phenomenological perspective, there is a distinction between lived body (*Leib*) and physical body (*Körper*), or body-subject and body-object. The first is the body experienced from within, my own direct experience of my body in the first-person perspective, myself as a spatiotemporal embodied agent in the world; the second is the body thematically investigated from without, from a third-person perspective, for example as viewed by natural sciences such as anatomy and physiology (Husserl 1912–1915; Merleau-Ponty 1996). The body can be apprehended in the first-person perspective as the body-I-am. This is the cenesthetic apprehension of one's own body, the primitive experience of oneself, the basic form of self-awareness, or the direct, unmediated experience of one's own "facticity," including oneself as "this" body, its form, height, weight, color, as well as one's past and what is actually happening. First and foremost, we always have an implicit acquaintance with our own body from the first-person perspective. The lived body turns into a physical, objective body whenever we become aware of it in a disturbing way. Whenever our movement is somehow impeded or disrupted, then the lived body is thrown back on itself, materialized or "corporealized." It becomes an object for me. Having been a living bodily being before, I now realize that I have a material (impeding, clumsy, vulnerable, finite, etc.) body (Fuchs 2002). In addition to these two dimensions of corporeality, Sartre emphasized that one can apprehend one's own body also from another vantage point, as the body when it is looked at by another person. When I become aware that I or, better, my body, is looked at by another person, I realize it can be an object for that person. Sartre calls this the "lived-body-for-others." "With the appearance of the Other's look," writes Sartre, "I experience the revelation of my being-as-object." The result is a feeling of "having my being outside . . . [the feeling] of being an object" (Sartre 1992). Thus, one's identity becomes reified by the gaze of the other, and reduced to the external appearance of one's own body. The phenomenological concept of lived body must also be differentiated from the body image, as the immediate experience of one's body (the layer of kinesthetic sensations), and not a representation of it (Husserl 1912–1915; Merleau-Ponty 1996; Stanghellini 2012). The lived body is my own direct experience of my body from a first-person perspective, of myself as a spatiotemporal embodied agent in the world.

Anomalies with embodiment have already been posited as central domains of several mental disorders, including schizophrenia (Stanghellini 2008) manic-depressive disorders (Fuchs 2002), and body dysmorphic disorder (Morris 2003). Abnormal attitudes toward one's own corporeality, and difficulties in the definition of one's own identity, have been proposed as the core features of these disorders. In subjects with a proneness to pathological eating behaviors, the body is no longer the essential experience of being-in-the-world, but a prison which represents the only way to define themselves.

The body becomes the means to get in touch with their own emotions. Accordingly, these are sentences often reported by ED patients: "Having my weight under control makes me feel in control of my emotional states"; "If my measurements remain the same over time I feel that I am myself, if not I feel I am getting lost."

From a neurobiological perspective, brain activation in response to the view of one's own body involves extensive circuitry including dorsolateral prefrontal, supplementary motor, insular, inferior parietal (representation of one's own body schema), fusiform (human face recognition process), occipitotemporal (the so-called "extrastriate body area") and cingulate regions. Moreover, body image distortion has been associated with a specific activation pattern that includes the inferior parietal lobule and the dorsolateral prefrontal cortex (DLPFC) (Pietrini et al. 2011). The DLPFC represents an intriguing neurobiological correlate for psychopathological domains, given the functions associated with this brain region. It is part of corticostriatal loops, which contribute not only to executive functions but also to the regulation of emotional impulses mediated by limbic and paralimbic structures (Lévesque et al. 2003) by means of enhancing the tendency of individuals to suppress aversive emotional states (Miller & Cohen 2001). Furthermore, it may represent the biological underpinning of the link between body image and identity disturbance in EDs. Indeed, the DLPFC has long been considered a key component of a network subserving awareness of self and metacognitive evaluation of the self (Johnson et al. 2002). Therefore, in EDs specific activation of DLPFC in response to body image distortion tasks could suggest that the oversized body stimuli can be considered highly relevant for self-evaluation (Castellini et al. 2013).

THE OTHER

Clinicians often report that ED patients define themselves through the gaze of other persons: "For me it's very important to see myself through the eyes of the others"; "The way I feel depends on the way I feel looked at by the others"; "Sometimes I focalize myself through the gaze of the others." As previously stated, a specific alteration of lived corporeality can be detected in patients with EDs, and represents the psychopathological dimension underpinning the commonly observed body image disturbance. More specifically, persons with proneness to the symptoms of EDs showed a predominance of one dimension of embodiment, namely the lived-body-for-others, which is a concept proposed by Sartre (1992). In addition to the body-subject and body-object dimensions of corporeality, Sartre emphasized that one can apprehend one's own body even from another point of view, as one's own body when it is looked at by another person. Thus, one's identity becomes reified by the gaze of the other, and reduced to the external appearance of one's own body. Therefore, the lived body is no longer direct, first-personal experiential evidence, but it is an entity that exists as viewed from an external perspective (Sartre, 1992). This means that the other becomes the mirror in which one can perceive oneself. The comprehension of the profound uneasiness of lived corporeality of EDs—leading to the sense of alienation from one's own body and from one's own emotions—should be integrated with an exaggerated concern to take responsibility for the way one appears to others, as well as the possibility of feeling oneself only through the gaze of the other, through objective measures and through self-starvation (Stanghellini et al. 2014). This interpretation overcomes the general position of the alloplastic personality frequently observed in subjects with EDs. According to this perspective, for persons with EDs the other is no longer an interlocutor with which to engage an intersubjective co-creativity relationship, but is the one who confirms my existence, my being-in-the-world. The gaze of the other becomes the unique way through which we are aware of our own presence. It is as the mirror in which we see ourselves and feel ourselves.

THE LANGUAGE OF BODY AND EATING

In some way, eating and feeding disorders represent an example of psychopathology of postmodernity, in which language changes and innovations mirror the fluidity of cultural transformations and their impact on the representation and significance of the body. The dimension of feeling oneself through the gaze of the other and defining oneself through the evaluation of the other can be integrated in the concept of public consciousness. Public self-consciousness, as opposed to private self-consciousness, includes all those qualities of the self that are formed in other people's eyes. In fact, persons with ED have a tendency to think of those aspects of the self that are matters of public display, rather than attending to more covert, hidden aspects of the self, for example, one's privately held beliefs and feelings (Scheier and Carver 1985).

Indeed, the language adopted by persons with EDs to define themselves is often exclusively based on terms regarding objective evaluation of their body, such as *large* or *thin, fat* or *slim*, the way dresses fit around their body, or the proportion of space their body occupies in a room. In most cases, the terms fat or slim transcend objective measures and regard the moral value of the person: fat means lacking control of one's instincts, of little worth, and weakness. The use of the word hunger is often present in the speech of persons with EDs to express their difficulty in defining their emotions (alexithymia) and sensations, which, again, they perceive as extraneous and dangerous. In the diaries of persons with EDs we can find expressions such as: "I came back home after a terrible day where it all went wrong . . . I realized I have an irresistible hunger . . . " The quality of food transcends its association with taste and can be viewed as a dysfunctional way of expressing and modulating emotions: salty and full-bodied foods seem to predominate in moments of anxiety, while the sweet, warm, soft or liquid prevail in conditions of sadness: "I want the food that I swallow to be something cuddly ... sweet after so many things to love ... " (Todisco and Vinai 2007). The term, "pleasure" reported in their diaries often does not have anything to do with what we generally consider to be pleasure, because it is often equated with the reduction of emotional distress. That is, "pleasure" often arises in these disorders from anesthetic conditions regarding emotions and visceral sensations, or, in persons with anorexia nervosa, from the perception of hunger during starvation periods.

Concepts of control, starvation, and loss-of-control binge eating have taken on different meanings according to the cultural and historical context. In fact, in ancient Greek and Roman cultures—which identified balance as the highest value for a person—the ideal for eating was that of measure, the absence of voracity (Montanari 1989). On the contrary, in Celtic and Germanic cultural traditions the big eater was considered a positive and valiant person (Montanari 1979). In the Germanic mythology and poems of chivalry, the image of the brave warrior was even that of a strong man, greedy, insatiable, and able to swallow huge quantities of food and beverages (Montanari 1993). Relevant differences also existed between the Mediterranean and Continental Europe, as demonstrated for example by opposite rules across the monastic orders. The monastic rules in North Europe were harsh and strict, marked by fasting and penance, while in the South (those developed by Benedict of Norcia, for example) were characterized by a greater sense of balance closer to the Roman culture (Montanari 1988). During the medieval era, binge eating was in fact a privilege of the nobility, in light of widespread constant fear of hunger (Montanari 1993). Regarding semantic and moral values, while nowadays the notion of fat among persons with EDs is synonymous with weak, incompetent, and inefficient, in the Middle Ages fat was something desirable: a "fat cheese offered to Charlemagne was described as something delicious" (Bianchi 1980). The term fat also had a positive connotation in aesthetics and even in politics. Being fat was a sign of wealth and nutritional well-being; so it meant not only beautiful but also rich and powerful: for example in the Florence of the Middle Ages, the upper class was called *popolo grasso* (fat people) (Montanari 1993). The value of thinness as a symbol of efficiency and productivity appeared only in the eighteenth century, especially in relation to the emergence the bourgeoisie and Puritanism, as opposed to old Europe (Barthes 1970). Gradually, industrialization allowed access to adequate food consumption for a wider population. Therefore, the notion of the "binge" lost its positive meaning, and the fear of hunger was replaced by the fear of loss of control (De Garine and Pollock 1995).

Nowadays, it is important to consider the role of language and symbols adopted by the media, and their effects on the pathogenesis of EDs. Not only do the media glorify a slender ideal, they also emphasize its importance, and the importance of appearances in general, and they glorify slenderness and weight loss and emphasize the importance of beauty and appearances (Spettigue and Henderson 2004). A number of studies have documented the trend of increasing thinness in *Playboy* centerfolds, Miss America contestants, and fashion models between the 1950s and the 1990s (Garner et al. 1980; Wiseman et al. 1992). The multi-billion dollar beauty industry depends on a strong emphasis on the value of beauty and appearances for women, because this supports a consumption-based culture in which the answer for any problem can be achieved by purchasing advertised products for improving one's appearance (Thomsen et al. 2001). In another survey, middle-aged women were asked what they would most like to change about their lives, and more than half of them said "their weight" (Kinsbourne 2002). The pervasive body dissatisfaction is so widespread in Western countries that authors coined the term "normative discontent" (Oliver-Pyatt 2003). The role of media in the development of body dissatisfaction and eating disorder symptomatology was supported by a recent naturalistic experiment conducted in Fiji (Becker et al. 2002). Until recently, Fiji was a relatively media-naïve society with little Western mass-media influence. In this unique study, the eating attitudes and behaviors of Fijian adolescent girls were measured prior to the introduction of regional television and following prolonged exposure. The results indicate that following television exposure, these adolescents exhibited a significant increase in disordered eating attitudes and behaviors.

How are these epidemic phenomena related to identity? Nordbø et al. (2006) suggest that pathological eating behavior represents a tool for achieving a new identity. Skarderud (2007) showed that for some persons with EDs, changing one's body is a tool for becoming another person. They want to change, and changing one's body serves as both a concrete and a symbolic tool for such ambitions. Thus, shaping oneself is a "concretized metaphor," establishing an equivalence between a psychic reality (identity) and a physical one (one's body shape). As suggested by Surgenor et al. (2003), looking into the different ways persons with EDs construct the self, especially in relation to their disorder and therapy, has strategic implications for the therapeutic endeavor.

According to the different perspectives presented here, language impacts the experience and definition of the body, which is related to the construction of identity. EDs are conditions in which the process of self-identity construction is interfered with by a profound uneasiness toward one's own body. EDs schematize the relationship among language, body, and identity, as they are ways in which people feel a disturbance of the implicit connection between *Leib, Körper*, and body-for-others, and this causes disturbances in identity. Societal and cultural norms and values, particularly as expressed in language and symbols, may exacerbate this identity split and the distress felt by such individuals, by limiting the opportunities for self-expression: in EDs, this is by having a limited definition of beauty and ideal body.

In EDs, the definition of the body can offer a kind of "materialized metaphor" that may be used to shape identity, and patients remain entrenched in the limitations of their corporealized language, which limits the expression of their own identity.

SUBJECTIVE PERCEPTION OF SPACE IN EATING DISORDERS

Several behaviors and cognitive distortion often taken into account by the psychiatric and cognitive literature can be derived from a basic sense of spatial metamorphosis that is deeply associated with the disorder of corporeality. Patients with EDs with a severe clinical condition often have been reported to say: "I cannot step through the door," "I take a lot of space when I'm in a room," "My body does not fit into my clothes." Indeed, individuals with EDs perform repetitive, often time-consuming, and compulsive behaviors such as long hours of lifting weights, excessive mirror checking or avoidance, comparing one's appearance with that of others, seeking reassurance about the perceived weight fluctuation, skin picking, camouflaging the perceived changes of the space they feel to occupy (e.g. with hair, makeup, body position, or clothing), frequent clothes changing and frequent body measuring. Although the goal of such behaviors is to diminish the anxiety provoked by the body image concerns, these behaviors often increase and maintain anxiety.

The cognitive literature generically ascribes these behaviors to a body image disturbance. However, the disturbance of body image in EDs cannot simply be ascertained from a somatosensorial alteration, or a failing of the integration of somatic sensations at different levels. According with the identity disturbance of EDs, we can expand the disorder of lived corporeality in terms of space occupied by the body. Therefore, persons with EDs report an extreme polarization of the continuum represented by the sentence: "I am the space that my body occupies." Bonnier (1893) proposed that the space is the unifying element to define the various somatic and visceral sensations. Therefore, the mental representation of one's body is first a spatial representation. In this model, the body schema is the mental representation of topography that allows us to first know the space we occupy and that allows us the orientation with respect to the external environment and the various parts of our body. In line with this position, Fisher and Cleveland (1969) address the issue of body image primarily in terms of bodily boundaries, and the body helps to create a sense of individuality in each of us, especially in terms of space. Generally speaking, body image boundaries coincide with those of the physical surface of the body. For persons with EDs, spatiality loses the anthropological feature with "I'm in the skin of my body." Being in this sense does not mean being "here" or "there" (the basic form of self-experience—sense of existing as a subject of awareness—rooted in one bodily experience), but just being "here" where I occupy a place, a space. Thus, the space become smaller, and becomes too tight to contain my body.

SUBJECTIVE PERCEPTION OF TIME
IN EATING DISORDERS

Time in patients with EDs is often perceived in different ways *coherently* with their subjective world related to body experiences and eating behaviors. A phenomenological assessment for EDs must include the subjective perception of time to understand the meaning of the so called "pathological eating behaviors." Every human experience is configured on experience of time. Indeed, the stream of consciousness comprises an ensemble of experiences that is unified both at any given time and over time. The temporal continuity of the representation of the body is altered in patients with EDs. Time is no longer intentionality, and therefore it cannot be a way for being with the other in a simultaneity or in a succession temporality. Merleau-Ponty (1996) dedicates one of the most important parts of his lecture about the lived body (*Leib*) to be considered as "belonging to the world, being in the world temporality committed." He focuses on the temporal dimension since the structure of the world is the temporality, following the approach of Husserl's consciousness of inner time. In this sense, the primary contact with the world is the so-called field of presence, the *Leib* with its own temporality, in which all our actions take place.

Patients with EDs always report the feeling that the body can change continuously. Time is reduced to a mere control function, and in particular to be employed in control and/or loss of control of weight and eating—in other words to monitoring one's own body over time.

Specific situations or events activate patients' thoughts and emotions, while at other times these body image experiences are either absent or much more benign. The subjective perception of time in ED patients appears to be connected with the temporal discontinuity of the representation of one's own body, and the need for predictability of one's own life, which is achieved/failed according to control of eating and weight. For example, there can be activating contexts such as a public party. Persons' beliefs entail self-evaluative social comparisons in which they look extremely fat, and they infer that others at the party notice how fat they are. Diaries often used as a self-monitoring strategy of treatment can describe activators of body image dysphoria, and capture such prototypical and troublesome body image states. For the therapist and client alike, this is clinically useful in the process of beginning to understand the essentially scripted nature of the client's experiences.

BIBLIOGRAPHY

Allamani A. and Allegranzi P. (1990). "Immagine corporea: dimensioni e misure. Una ricerca clinica." *Archivio di Psicologia Neurologia Psichiatria* 2:171–195.

American Psychiatric Association. (1994). *Diagnostic and Statistical Manual for Mental Disorders* (4th edn.) Washington, DC: American Psychiatric Press.

American Psychiatric Association. (2013). *Diagnostic and Statistical Manual of Mental Disorders* (5th edn.) Washington, DC: American Psychiatric Association.

Bardone-Cone A. M., Harney M. B., Maldonado C. R., et al. (2010). "Defining Recovery from an Eating Disorder: Conceptualization, Validation, and Examination of Psychosocial Functioning and Psychiatric Comorbidity." *Behavior Research and Therapy* 48: 194–202.

Becker A. E., Burwell R. A., Herzog D. B., Hamburg P., and Gilman S. (2002) "Eating Behaviours and Attitudes Following Prolonged Exposure to television Among Ethnic Fijian Adolescent Girls." *British Journal of Psychiatry* 180(6): 509–514.

Bonnier P. (1893). *Vertige*. Paris: Masson.

Bruch H. (1982). "Anorexia Nervosa: Therapy and Theory." *American Journal of Psychiatry* 139: 1531–1538.

Castellini G., Lo Sauro C., Mannucci E., et al. (2011). "Diagnostic Crossover and Outcome Predictors in Eating Disorders According to DSM-IV and DSM-V Proposed Criteria: A 6-year Follow-up Study." *Psychosomatic Medicine* 73: 270–279.

Castellini G., Polito C., Bolognesi E., et al. (2013). "Looking at My Body. Similarities and Differences Between Anorexia Nervosa Patients and Controls in Body Image Visual Processing." *European Psychiatry* 28: 427–435.

Castellini G., Stanghellini G., Godini L., et al. (2014). "Abnormal Bodily Experiences Mediate the Relationship between Impulsivity and Binge Eating in Overweight Subjects Seeking for Bariatric Surgery." *Psychotherapy and Psychosomatics*; 84(2):124–126.

De Garine I. and Pollock N. J. (1995). *Social Aspects of Obesity*. London: Gordon and Breach Publishers.

Fairburn C. G. (2010). "Cognitive Behavior Therapy and Eating Disorders." *Psychiatric Clinics of North America* 33: 611–627.

Fairburn C. G., Peveler R. C., Jones R., et al. (1993). "Predictors of Twelvemonth Outcome in Bulimia Nervosa and the Influence of Attitudes to Shape and Weight." *Journal of Consulting and Clinical Psychology* 61: 696–698.

Fairburn C. G., Cooper Z., and Shafran R. (2003). "Cognitive Behaviour Therapy for Eating Disorders: A 'Transdiagnostic' Theory and Treatment." *Behavior Research and Therapy* 41: 509–528.

Fairburn C. G. and Harrison P. J. (2003). "Eating Disorders." *Lancet* February 1; 361(9355): 407–416. Review.

Fisher S. and Cleveland S. E. (1969). "The Body Image Boundary Construct: A Study of the Self-steering Behavior Syndrome." *Journal of Projective Techniques and Personality Assessment Volume 34, 1970 - Issue 6* 33: 318–321.

Fuchs T. (2002). "The Phenomenology of Shame, Guilt and the Body in Body Dysmorphic Disorder and Depression." *Journal of Phenomenological Psychology* 33: 223–243.

Gallagher S. (2006). *How the Body Shapes the Mind*. Oxford: Oxford University Press.

Garner D. M., Garfinkel P., Schwartz D., and Thompson M. (1980). "Cultural Expectations of Thinness in Women." *Psychological Reports* 47: 484–491.

Goodsitt A. (1997). "Eating Disorders: A Self-psychological Perspective." In D. Garner and P. Garfinkel (eds.), *Handbook of Treatment for Eating Disorders*, pp. 205–228. New York: Guilford Press.

Head H. (1926). *Aphasia and Kindred Disorders of Speech*. London: Cambridge University Press.

Husserl E. (1912–1915). *Ideen zu einer reinen Phaenomenologie und phaenomenologische Philosophie. II. Phaenomenologische Untersuchungen zur Konstitution*. Den Haag: Nijhoff.

Johnson S., Baxter L., Wilder L., et al. (2002). "Neural Correlates of Self Reflection." *Brain* 125: 1808–1814.

Kinsbourne M. (2002). "Brain and Body Awareness." In T. F. Cash and T. Pruzinsky (eds.), Body Image: A Handbook of Theory, Research, and Clinical Practice. Guilford Press London.

Lévesque J., Eugène F., Joannette Y., et al. (2003). "Neural Circuitry Underlying Voluntary Suppression of Sadness." *Biological Psychiatry* 53: 502–510.

Malson H. (1999). "Women under Erasure: Anorexia Bodies in Postmodern Context." *Journal of Community & Applied Social Psychology* 9: 137–153. 41.

Markus H. (1977). "Self-schemata and Processing Information about the Self." *Journal of Personality and Social Psychology* 35: 63–78.

Markus H., Smith J., and Moreland R. (1985). "Role of the Self-concept in the Perception of Others." *Journal of Personality and Social Psychology* 49: 1494–1512.

Merleau-Ponty M. (1996). *Phenomenology of Perception* [1940], trans. C. Smith. New York: Humanities Press.

Miller E. K. and Cohen J. D. (2001). "An Integrative Theory of Prefrontal Cortex Function." *Annual Review of Neuroscience* 24: 167–202.

Milos G. F., Baur V., Muehlebach S., and Spindler A. (2013). "Axis-I Comorbidity Is Linked to Prospective Instability of Diagnoses Within Eating Disorders." *BMC Psychiatry* 7; 13: 295.

Montanari M. (1979). *L'alimentazione contadina nell'alto Medioevo*. Napoli: Liguori.

Montanari M. (1988). *Alimentazione e cultura nel Medioevo*. Roma-Bari: Laterza.

Montanari M. (1989). *Convivio. Storia e cultura dei piaceri della tavola dall'Antichità al Medioevo*. Roma-Bari: Laterza.

Montanari M. (1993). *La fame e l'abbondanza*. Roma-Bari: Laterza.

Morris K. J. (2003). "The Phenomenology of Body Dysmorphic Disorder: A Sartrean Analysis." In K. W. M. Fulford, K. J. Morris, J. Z. Sadler, et al. (eds.), *Nature and Narrative*.

An Introduction to the New Philosophy of Psychiatry, pp. 171–185. Oxford: Oxford University Press.

Nordbø R. H, Espeset E. M, Gulliksen K. S, et al. (2006). "The Meaning of Self-starvation: Qualitative Study of Patients' Perception of Anorexia Nervosa." *International Journal of Eating Disorders* 39: 556–564.

Oliver-Pyatt, W. (2003). *Fed Up!* New York: McGraw-Hill.

Pietrini F., Castellini G., Ricca V., et al. (2011). "Functional Neuroimaging in Anorexia Nervosa: A Clinical Approach." *European Psychiatry* 26: 176–182.

Piran N. (2001). "Reinhabiting the Body." *Feminist Psychology* 11: 172–176.

Sands S. (1991). "Bulimia, Dissociation, and Empathy: A Self-psychological View." In C. Johnson (ed.), *Psychodynamic Treatment of Anorexia Nervosa and Bulimia Nervosa*, pp. 34–50. New York: Guilford Press.

Sartre J. P. (1992). *L'être et le neant* [1943], trans. *Being and Nothingness*. New York: Washington Square Press.

Sassaroli S., Apparigliato M., Bertelli S., et al. (2011). "Perfectionism as a Mediator between Perceived Criticism and Eating Disorders." *Eating and Weight Disorder* 16: 37–44.

Scheier M. F. and Carver C. S. (1985). "The Self-Consciousness Scale: A Revised Version for Use with General Populations." *Journal of Applied Social Psychology* 15: 687–699.

Schilder P. (1950). "The Image and Appearance of the Human Body: Studies in the Constructive Energies of the Psyche." New York: International University Press.

Shafran R., Cooper Z., and Fairburn C. G. (2002). "Clinical Perfectionism: A Cognitive-Behavioural Analysis." *Behavior Research and Therapy* 40: 773–791.

Skarderud F. (2007). "Eating One's Words, Part I. 'Concretised Metaphors' and Reflective Function in Anorexia Nervosa—An Interview Study." *European Eating Disorder Review* 15: 163–174.

Spettigue W. and Henderson K. (2004). "Eating Disorders and the Role of the Media." *The Canadian Child and Adolescent Psychiatry Review* 13(1):16-9.

Stanghellini G. (2008). *Psicopatologia del senso commune*. Milano: Raffaello Cortina Editore.

Stanghellini G., Castellini G., Brogna P., Faravelli C., and Ricca V. (2012). "Identity and Eating Disorders (IDEA): A Questionnaire Evaluating Identity and Embodiment in Eating Disorder Patients." *Psychopathology* 45(3): 147–158.

Stanghellini G., Trisolini F., Castellini G., Ambrosini A., Faravelli C., and Ricca V. (2015). "Is Feeling Extraneous from One's Own Body a Core Vulnerability Feature in Eating Disorders?" *Psychopathology* 48(1): 18–24.

Stern D. (1985). *The Interpersonal World of the Infant: A View from Psychoanalysis and Developmental Psychology*. New York: Basic Books.

Surgenor L. J., Plumridge E. W., and Horn J. (2003). "'Knowing One's Self' Anorexic: Implications for Therapeutic Practice." *International Journal of Eating Disorders* 33: 22–32.

Thompson J. K., Heinberg L. J., Altabe M., et al. (1999). *Exacting Beauty*. Washington, DC: American Psychological Association.

Thomsen S. R., McCoy K., and Williams M. (2001). "Internalizing the Impossible: Anorexic Outpatients' Experiences with Women's Beauty and Fashion Magazines." *Eating Disorders* 9: 49–64.

Todisco P. and Vinai P. (2007). *Quando le emozioni diventano cibo. Psicoterapia cognitiva del binge eating disorder*. Torino: Edizioni Libreria Cortina.

Wiseman C. V., Gray J. J., Mosimann J. E., and Ahrens A. H. (1992). "Cultural Expectations of Thinness in Women: An Update." *International Journal of Eating Disorders* 11: 85–89.

SECTION SIX

CLINICAL PSYCHOPATHOLOGY

SECTION EDITORS: MATTHEW R. BROOME
AND PAOLO FUSAR-POLI

CHAPTER 71

FIRST-RANK SYMPTOMS OF SCHIZOPHRENIA

LENNART JANSSON

UNTIL recently, the Schneiderian first-rank symptoms (FRS), a group of psychotic symptoms, have held emblematic significance for making the schizophrenia diagnosis. In ICD-10 the presence of one FRS for one month suffices for establishing the diagnosis, and in DSM-IV the presence of one such symptom during a one-month active phase. Frequently, we not only hear their presence being advanced as an argument for the diagnosis, but even their absence as an argument against it. Empirical studies now seem to indicate that they are non-specific and, accordingly, they are losing importance. In this chapter we will explore the FRS, their rise and fall in clinical psychiatry, and their significance for the diagnosis of schizophrenia.

THE HISTORICAL BACKGROUND

Nineteenth-century psychiatry knew the phenomena of FRS, but failed to provide sufficiently detailed definitions and demarcation of them. This task was accomplished by Kraepelin in his textbook of psychiatry (1915), and by Jaspers in his *General Psychopathology* (1997). One example of the early descriptions is Haslam's nosography of a psychotic patient published in 1810, in which extensive experiences of influence caused by an "air loom" are the most salient features (López-Ibor and López-Ibor 2014).

Symptoms of schizophrenia later known under the name of FRS are frequently mentioned in classic psychiatric textbooks. Kraepelin (1919) describes a wide range of hallucinatory phenomena in dementia præcox (schizophrenia), and among these, voices of people speaking about the patient (9), voices making remarks about the thoughts and the doings of the patient (10), and the patient's own thoughts appearing to be spoken aloud, which Kraepelin finds "quite specially peculiar to dementia præcox" (12). Thoughts being spoken aloud become "common property." Still more characteristic of this disease he finds the feeling of one's thoughts being influenced (12), "plundered, organized and published." Experiences of the body being laid hold of, "twisted" (12), "vivisected" (27), etc., result in a conviction in the patient of becoming "the sports of all sorts of influences" (16). Indifferent remarks and chance looks appear suspicious to the patient (31) and give rise to idiosyncratic interpretations, for example, a fern in a buttonhole indicating war.

Similarly, Bleuler (1950) refers to patients with schizophrenia believing that they are influenced by hostile forces, for example, by the means of "mysterious apparatus and magic" (118); cases in which paresthesias are believed to be caused by other people are mostly schizophrenic (303). The phenomenon of thoughts being heard (Gedankenlautwerden) occurs only very rarely in other psychoses, he notes (300). These, too, are pre-Schneiderian descriptions of FRS.

Kurt Schneider published a list of FRS in his 1950 textbook, *Klinische Psychopathologie* (KP), translated into English as *Clinical Psychopathology* (CP) in 1959. The motivation for promoting certain clinical symptoms of psychosis to first-rank status was the following:

> Among the many abnormal modes of experience that occur in schizophrenics, there are some which we put in the first rank of importance, not because we think them to be "basic disturbances" but because they have this special value in helping us to determine the diagnosis of schizophrenia as distinct from nonpsychotic abnormality or from cyclothymia. (CP: 133)

Thus, he did not consider these symptoms as fundamental or generative for the symptomatology of schizophrenia the same way as Bleuler's basic symptoms. The background for his first-rank approach was the pragmatic composition of clinical guidelines for general practitioners in a booklet titled *Psychischer Befund und psychiatrische Diagnose (Beiträge zur Psychiatrie)* (PB) [*Psychic Symptoms and Psychiatric Diagnosis (Contributions to Psychiatry)*] (Schneider 1939).

His emphasis on these symptoms was not based on empirical evidence but rather on clinical experience and theoretical considerations as he considered them as expressive of underlying ego-disturbances (Bürgy 2011):

> Among the basic attributes of psychic experience, certain disturbances of the sense of identity are highly specific for schizophrenia. By these we mean disturbances of the sense of "I," "me and mine," which consist in feeling that what one is and what one does have passed under the direct influence of others. These disturbances have already been considered earlier, and have been demonstrated with reference to thinking, feeling, impulse, and will, and have been spoken of in connection with thought-withdrawal and the influencing of thought, feeling, impulse (drive), and will.
>
> (Schneider 1959: 120)

Elaborating Jaspers's model of the "consciousness of the self" he found the ego-disturbances, or self-disorder (Parnas et al. 2005), to be constitutive of these symptoms of schizophrenia. The disturbance of the sense of "I" or "me and mine," often referred to as a loss of mineness, is an aspect of Jaspers's loss of consciousness of activity according to this model.

Following a number of editions of PB until the mid-1940s, Schneider reused its content in his textbook, published after his appointment as professor of psychiatry in Heidelberg (replacing Carl Schneider, the Nazi professor who committed suicide in 1946, following his internment). And accordingly, FRS came to obtain a prominent place in German psychopathology. British psychiatry still being under strong German influence, the FRS found their way into the Present State Examination in the 1960s (PSE; Kendler 2009; Wing et al. 1974). Actually, its CATEGO-derived core schizophrenia class, S+, is defined from the presence of FRS (and of other delusions and auditory hallucinations).

The introduction of operationalism in nosology also saw a need for specific, well-defined criterial symptoms. Schneiderian first-rank symptoms, already incorporated in the PSE, seemed like perfect candidates because of their "first-rank importance." They made their first appearance in pre-DSM-III operational Research Diagnostic Criteria (RDC; Spitzer et al. 1978) as

> Thought broadcasting, insertion, or withdrawal . . . Delusions of being controlled (or influenced) . . . Auditory hallucinations in which either a voice keeps up a running commentary on the subject's behaviors or thoughts as they occur, or two or more voices converse with each other.

Not yet named FRS in RDC, these phenomena made their way into the diagnostic algorithms of DSM-III and DSM-III-R, reaching their acme of significance as FRS in DSM-IV, in which just one such symptom is needed for the diagnosis of schizophrenia.

DSM-5 (2013) became the turning point: here, FRS no longer form part of the diagnostic criteria and are just mentioned in passing in the text. Previous to the publication, the evidence against the pathognomonic status of the FRS seemed to accumulate; for example, FRS are also found in patients with affective disorders. Furthermore, the prevalence of FRS in schizophrenia differs considerably across studies, and they do not seem to affect the outcome. Thus, a critical review of thirty-five years of FRS studies by Nordgaard et al. (2008) does "not allow for either a reconfirmation or a rejection of Schneider's claims about FRS," and, therefore, the authors recommend that the FRS be de-emphasized in the next revisions of the diagnostic systems.

FRS were indeed mentioned in the text of pre-operational ICD-8, but just like in DSM they found their way into the diagnostic criteria of operational ICD-10, and like DSM-IV they achieved a pathognomonic status, one such symptom present for one month sufficing for the diagnosis of schizophrenia. The FRS are omitted as a separate criterion in ICD-11, and disturbances of self-experience in turn are highlighted.

THE DEFINITION AND DEMARCATION OF FRS

Schneider's FRS consist of *three areas of psychopathology*: delusional perception, phenomena of passivity or influence, and certain verbal-acoustic hallucinations. The basic psychopathology governing these phenomena are self-disorders like self-alienation, transitivism, and solipsism. These phenomena being well known for clinicians, Schneider contributed only sketchy descriptions in his writings, a fact allowing ample and divergent interpretation by later writers (Koehler 1979).

1. *Delusional perception (DP)*, never part of the DSM criteria, but still comprised by the ICD-10 definition of FRS, is an area of psychopathology which is largely ignored by present-day

clinicians. Schneider, referring to the works of Jaspers and Gruhle, gives the following definition (104):

> Delusional perception (DP) takes place when some abnormal significance, usually with self-reference, is attached to a genuine perception without any comprehensible rational or emotional justification.

Schneider emphasizes the two-component (*zweigliedrig*) nature of DP, the one component being the neutral perception, the other one the "groundless" (*ohne Anlaß*) delusion which apparently cannot be inferred from the otherwise unaffected perception. This simplified model, which has formed the basis for the PSE operational definition of DP, fails to convey the psychological essence of the experience. However, Schneider writes that it cannot be derived from any particular emotional state but often from a delusional atmosphere termed "delusional tension" by Gruhle and the "preparatory field" by Schneider himself. This atmosphere is often an experience of oddness which gains the essence of something significant but, according to Schneider, does not offer content to the delusion.

DP belong to the class of primary delusions examined by Jaspers (1997: 98ff.; Kraus 2014). Originating in the experiential structure of schizophrenia, they are vividly given, pathic rather than gnostic by nature, and not yet fully thematized. The elaboration of delusional content is referred to as a secondary delusion. Jaspers distinguishes between these true, primary delusions and delusion-like ideas as seen in other, for example, affective, psychoses. Parnas (2004) terms the former group *autistic-solipsistic delusions*, informed by the autistic and solipsistic aspects of schizophrenic experiencing. The convincing pathic givenness of primary delusions explains the often contradictory explanatory account given by the patients, conflicting with their level of intelligence and their life experiences.

Matussek (1987) and Conrad (1958) expound the psychology of DP. In beginning (paranoid) schizophrenia Conrad often finds a psychological tension, for example, between external obstacles and personal wishes. A delusional mood evolves as a change in the physiognomy of the surrounding world, a stage he names the *trema* (i.e. "stage fright"). In this state the patient is alarmed by the emergence of strangeness, where things no longer form reliable and familiar background for everyday experiencing but begin to vibrate from a disconcerting presence (Génnart 2011: 292). According to Matussek, there is a loosening of the natural perceptual context, for example, a railway station with all the objects belonging there, and an expanded prevalence of the "essential properties" of the perceptual objects. These properties are detached from their specific context and "encircle" the object like a cloud. By way of an accentuation of the physiognomy of the environment, single isolated aspects come to the fore and acquire intrusive experiential quality, a phenomenon called intrusive derealization (Matussek 1987; Gross et al. 2008; Parnas et al. 2005). This is the starting point of a delusional, referential interpretation, DP, the salient feature of Conrad's next stage of schizophrenia, the *apophany*.

2. *The experiences of influence* (or passivity phenomena), counted among the FRS by Schneider (CP: 133–134), are:

> the experience of influences playing on the body (somatic passivity experiences); thought-withdrawal and other interferences with thought; diffusion of thought; delusional perception and all feelings, impulses (drives), and volitional acts that are experienced by the patient as the work or influence of others.

Schneider considers the common structure for these phenomena to be transitivistic, representing "the 'lowering' of the 'barrier' between the self and the surrounding world, the loss of the very contours of the self." Thus, they represent the self-disorders included in Bleuler's fundamental symptoms in the context of disorders of the "person" or "ego" (1950: 143–147). The phenomena here are psychotic experiences, as they are accompanied by explanatory delusions as to who or how. However, pure transitivistic experiences may be non-psychotic (or at least only near-psychotic), for example, as an unpleasant experience of confusing oneself with one's interlocutor (Parnas et al. 2005), not to be counted as FRS.

In the RDC (as we saw above), and in DSM, these phenomena have been reduced to delusions. DSM-III refers to them as a "belief or experience" (182), but in the diagnostic criteria for schizophrenic disorder (188) only as a "bizarre delusion." In DSM-5 they are mentioned in the Glossary of Technical Terms under "delusions" (819–820). This implies that the demonstration of a transitivistic experience is no longer viewed as a prerequisite for rating the phenomena.

The diagnostic criteria for schizophrenia of ICD-10 comprise the presence of thought insertion, thought withdrawal, thought broadcasting, and delusions of control, influence, or passivity, clearly referred to body or limb movements or specific thoughts, actions, or sensations. Thus, there is a differentiation between the listed thought phenomena and the remaining phenomena considered delusions. PSE and SCAN manuals, acting as the glossaries of ICD-10, have sections on "experiences of thought disorder" and "replacement of will" (SCAN 1999: chapter 18) mostly defined as experiences. SCAN even differentiates between thought broadcast proper and delusions of thoughts being read, the latter including explanatory delusions to thought broadcast but also delusions related to expansive delusions, not covered by the FRS.

3. The last area of psychopathology to be included in the FRS consists of certain *verbal-acoustic hallucinations*:

> . . . hearing one's own thoughts (or thoughts being audible), voices conversing one with another, and voices that keep up a running comment on the patient's behavior.
>
> (CP: 96)

Schneider's definition of the first of these phenomena, audible thoughts, is rather hazy, and his examples are of little use, for example, "I hear my own thoughts. I can hear them when everything is quiet." Perceptualization of inner speech, usually acquiring an acoustic quality, is a frequent phenomenon in schizophrenia spectrum patients. What is usually meant by audible thoughts as an FRS is a psychotic transitivistic superstructure in which the patient has an experience of other people being able to perceive his thought, a phenomenon closely related thought broadcasting. Some psychopathological manuals like the PSE and SCAN emphasize that the thoughts should sound aloud, "almost so loud that someone standing nearby could hear them" (SCAN 1999), an unfortunate criterion as it neglects the altered spatial structure of schizophrenic experiencing (Henriksen et al. 2015), in which the distance does not always matter (also reflected in the so-called extracampine hallucinations, hallucinations beyond the sensory field). What is most important is the experience of thoughts being publicly disclosed. Near-psychotic borderline cases are frequent, in which the patient fears that others might perceive his thoughts, well aware of the impossibility.

Voices conversing one with another, and voices keeping up a running comment on the patient's behavior are covered by DSM-IV (285) and ICD-10 (Green Book: 64). Here, these voices are not restricted to third person addressing (i.e. by "he" or "she"). Of course, conversing voices are heard in the third-person, but commenting voices not necessarily so: some patients do hear a voice commenting on their behavior in the second person ("you").[1] However, some manuals such as PSE and SCAN, define commenting voices as third-person hallucinations. "Third-person voices" are often used as a synonym for FRS-hallucinations, which is incorrect as there are examples that do not belong here (e.g. voices criticizing the patient in the third person).

The running comments are continuous, neutral descriptions of the patient's acts, like "now he is reading a newspaper," but the very word, "comment," tempts to a different interpretation, namely critical remarks, for example, "she is ugly," which is not covered by Schneider's definition.

FRS constitute continua of psychopathological phenomena (Koehler 1979). Thus, passivity phenomena, originating in transitivism, can be traced from passivity mood—the mood of being somehow in a passive, dangerously exposed position, at the mercy of the world (Parnas et al. 2005)—through intermediate phenomena like combinations of depersonalization and experiences of control or influence to clear-cut FRS. Klosterkötter (1992) expounds the stepwise development of psychopathology in beginning schizophrenia from basic symptoms (step 1, non-psychotic subjective experiences) as "initial deficiencies" via intermediate phenomena (step 2, more specific basic symptoms closely related to self-disorders) to FRS, a development named "transition sequence." So, cognitive disturbance of movement leads to autopsychic depersonalization and eventually to experiences of will being influenced.

THE DIAGNOSTIC SIGNIFICANCE OF FIRST-RANK SYMPTOMS

Evidence against the pathognomonic significance of FRS for the diagnosis of schizophrenia seems to accumulate (Nordgaard et al. 2008). They are reported to be present in many other diagnostic categories than schizophrenia: affective and non-affective psychosis, and even non-psychotic states like neurosis and personality disorder. This latter claim is absurd, as FRS, psychotic symptoms by definition, do not belong in non-psychotic disorders. Their clinical significance has been questioned by the findings in genetic and prospective studies, too.

However, a number of circumstances interfere with these negative conclusions. The first of these is the definition of the FRS themselves. As demonstrated by Koehler (1979), there are many conflicting definitions due to Schneider's rather ambiguous descriptions of the phenomena. As we saw, passivity phenomena have been redefined as delusions in DSM, thereby neglecting their transitivistic nature, which Schneider regarded as their core

---

[1] We have even met a patient hearing a commenting voice in the first person ("I"), "pretending to be me."

phenomenon. Furthermore, different authors do not agree on which phenomena to include in the FRS (Koehler 1979).

Second, studies examining the affinity of FRS to schizophrenia are based on differing definitions of schizophrenia, another neglected area (Nordgaard et al. 2008). Historically, there are in the neighborhood of forty definitions of this disease (Jansson and Parnas 2007), all differing with regard to criteria of duration, psychopathological content (e.g. inclusion/ exclusion of affective symptoms), sex ratio, and other demographic features, etc. The correspondence between each of these definitions and the core gestalt of schizophrenia, made up by its autistic structure or "basic mood," is quite unknown. Thus, the claim that FRS are found outside schizophrenia, may depend on the delimitation of the schizophrenia concept in question. Some schizophrenia definitions (e.g. DSM-IV and ICD-10) include FRS in their diagnostic criteria rendering the question of the affinity of FRS to schizophrenia almost tautological.

Due to all these conceptual and methodological difficulties FRS are losing their status as pathognomonic symptoms of schizophrenia, already accomplished by DSM-5, in which they are relegated to rank-and-file hallucinations and delusions, a fate to all appearances befalling them in ICD-11, too. In a generation or so we can, therefore, expect clinicians to forget the FRS, as was earlier the case with schizophrenic autism. However, although the concept of FRS is disappearing from ICD-11 (WHO 2019), too, the passivity phenomena will still play a role in the diagnostic criteria. These phenomena are listed among the core symptoms of schizophrenia under the term, disturbances of self-experience. The examples given in brackets are: the experience that one's feelings, impulses, thoughts, or behaviour are under the control of an external force. Disturbances in self-experience, or self-disorders (Parnas et al. 2005), are indeed core phenomena of schizophrenia, and emphasizing these disorders in ICD-11 will hopefully serve to increase the interest among clinicians and researchers for the experiential structure of this disease as a counterpoise to the less specific psychotic phenomena listed in the diagnostic criteria of, for example, DSM-5. A growing body of empirical evidence is accumulating pointing to the specific quality of self-disorders for the diagnosis schizophrenia spectrum disorders (e.g. Haug et al. 2012; Raballo and Parnas 2011) and for the prediction of schizophrenia spectrum diagnoses (Parnas et al. 2011). There is already evidence of psychotic symptoms of schizophrenia, including FRS, emerging from the self-disorders (cf. Koehler's continua (1979) and Klosterkötter's transition sequences (1992), mentioned above). More qualitative research is needed to map out the development of FRS but the necessary prerequisite is the sophistication of the psychopathological concepts beyond the operational definitions of the prevailing diagnostic manuals and psychopathological instruments, and Nordgaard et al. (2008) also recommend the application of a phenomenological perspective in future studies aiming at validating FRS as diagnostic features.

BIBLIOGRAPHY

Bleuler E. (1950). *Dementia Praecox or the Group of Schizophrenias*. New York: International Universities Press.

Bürgy M. (2011). "Ego Disturbances in the Sense of Kurt Schneider: Historical and Phenomenological Aspects." *Psychopathology* 44: 320–328.

Conrad K. (1958). *Die beginnende Schizophrenie. Versuch einer Gestaltanalyse des Wahns.* Stuttgart: Thieme.

Génnart M. (2011). *Corporéité et présence. Jalons pour une approche du corps dans la psychose.* Argenteuil: Le Cercle Herméneutique Éditeur.

Gross G., Huber G., Klosterkötter J., and Linz M. (2008). *BSABS—Bonn Scale for the Assessment of Basic Symptoms.* Maastricht-Herzogenrath: Shaker Verlag.

Haug E., Lien L., Raballo A., Bratlien U., Øie M., Andreassen O. A., Melle I., and Møller P. (2012). "Selective Aggregation of Self-Disorders in First-Treatment DSM-IV Schizophrenia Spectrum Disorders." *The Journal of Nervous and Mental Disease* 200: 632–636.

Henriksen M. G., Raballo A., and Parnas J. (2015). "The pathogenesis of auditory verbal hallucinations in schizophrenia: a clinical-phenomenological account." *Philosophy, Psychiatry & Psychology* 22: 165–181.

Jansson L. and Parnas J. (2007). "Competing Definitions of Schizophrenia: What can be Learned from Polydiagnostic Studies?" *Schizophrenia Bulletin* 33: 1178–1200.

Jaspers K. (1997) *General Psychopathology.* Baltimore and London: John Hopkins University Press.

Kendler K. S. (2009). "An Historical Framework for Psychiatric Nosology." *Psychological Medicine* 39: 1935–1941.

Klosterkötter J. (1992). "The Meaning of Basic Symptoms for the Genesis of the Schizophrenic Nuclear Syndrome." *The Japanese Journal of Psychiatry and Neurology* 46: 609–630.

Koehler K. (1979). "First Rank Symptoms of Schizophrenia: Questions Concerning Clinical Boundaries." *British Journal of Psychiatry* 134: 236–248.

Kraepelin E. (1915). *Clinical Psychiatry. A Textbook for Students and Physicians.* London: The Macmillan Company.

Kraepelin E. (1919). *Dementia Præcox and Paraphrenia.* Edinburgh: Livingstone.

Kraus A. (2014). "Karl Jaspers on Primary Delusional Experiences of Schizophrenics: His Concept of Delusion Compared to That of the DSM." In T. Fuchs, et al. (eds.), *Karl Jaspers' Philosophy and Psychopathology.* New York: Springer Science+Business Media.

López-Ibor J. J. and López-Ibor M. I. (2014). "Romanticism and Schizophrenia. First Part: The Recency Hypothesis and the Core Gestalt of the Disease." *Actas Espanolas De Psiquiatria* 42: 133–158.

Matussek P. (1987). "Studies in Delusional Perception." In J. Cutting and M. Shepherd (eds.), *The Clinical Roots of the Schizophrenia Concept. Translations of Seminal European Contributions on Schizophrenia,* pp. 89–103. Cambridge: Cambridge University Press.

Mellor C. S. (1970). "First Rank Symptoms of Schizophrenia." *British Journal of Psychiatry* 117: 15–23.

Nordgaard J., Arnfred S. M., Handest P., and Parnas J. (2008). "The Diagnostic Status of First-Rank Symptoms." *Schizophrenia Bulletin* 34: 137–154.

Parnas J. (2004). "Belief and Pathology of Self-awareness. A Phenomenological Contribution to the Classification of Delusions." *Journal of Consciousness Studies* 11: 148–161.

Parnas J., Møller P., Kircher T., Thalbitzer J., Jansson L., Handest P., and Zahavi D. (2005). "EASE: Examination of Anomalous Self-Experience." *Psychopathology* 38: 236–258.

Parnas J., Raballo A., Handest P., Jansson L., Vollmer-Larsen A., and Sæbye D. (2011). "Self-experience in the Early Phases of Schizophrenia: 5-year Follow-up of the Copenhagen Prodromal Study." *World Psychiatry* 10: 200–204.

Raballo A. and Parnas J. (2011). "The Silent Side of the Spectrum: Schizotypy and the Schizotaxic Self." *Schizophrenia Bulletin* 37: 1017–1026.

SCAN. (1999). *Schedules for Clinical Assessment in Neuropsychiatry, Version 2.1, Glossary.* Geneva: World Health Organization.

Schneider K. (1939). *Psychischer Befund und psychiatrische Diagnose.* Leipzig: Thieme.

Schneider K. (1950). *Klinische Psychopathologie.* Stuttgart: Thieme.

Schneider K. (1959). *Clinical Psychopathology.* New York and London: Grune & Stratton.

Spitzer R. L., Endicott J., and Robins E. (1978). "Research Diagnostic Criteria: Rationale and Reliability." *Archives of General Psychiatry* 35: 773–782.

WHO—World Health Organization. (2019). ICD-11. Retrievable from: http://icd.who.int

Wing J. K., Cooper J. E., and Sartorius N. (1974). *The Measurement and Classification of Psychiatric Symptoms.* Cambridge: Cambridge University Press.

CHAPTER 72

....

SCHIZOPHRENIC DELUSION

....

ARNALDO BALLERINI

INTRODUCTION

RETHINKING schizophrenia seems to be a top-priority task for clinical psychopathology and psychiatric nosography today, given the doubts that many of us harbor about the definition and delineation of the concept itself as schizophrenic illness, its autonomy, and its limits. In this chapter I address the relation that may or exist not between delusion and the syndrome that we can still call schizophrenia.

Wolfgang Blankenburg (1971) writes that phenomenological and *Dasein*-analytical research has been accused of attending above all to paranoid psychoses, but very little to those syndromes that from the beginning are much more pronouncedly *deficient*. It is true that in phenomenological and *Dasein*-analytical research delusion has been largely in the forefront because of the many points of support it can offer to interpret the schizophrenic world. Yet, just as it happens for the whole complex of phenomenological research, current *Dasein*-analytical research too tends to go back from full-blown symptoms like delusions to a more subtle phenomena. As an example, Kimura Bin in his autobiography says, "My gaze rested more on autism than on delusion, more on the structure of experiencing than on the contents experienced, and more on the crisis of the selfhood of the I in *aida* with others than on the disorder of the solipsistic I" (Kimura Bin 1992). For him, human beings, and they alone, have had to take on during their development the difficult task of integrating the gap between two levels of subjectivity: being a member of human society and a unique individual self. From the phenomenological standpoint, schizophrenia represents a "pathology of being oneself in relation to others" (Kimura Bin 1992).

Certainly, the association delusion-schizophrenia is an impasse into which the concept of schizophrenia has historically dragged us. But it must be observed first of all that the concept of delusion pertains to the semantic universe of psychopathology, while the concept of schizophrenia belongs to that of nosography. There has never been, and perhaps will never be, a complete overlapping of the two spheres, the two fields of research, which utilize different "organizers" (Ballerini and Stanghellini 1991) and, all in all, operate with purposes that are not identical, despite the project which illuminates the work of Kurt Schneider (1950) to base the nosographical category "schizophrenia" on exclusive psychopathological foundations, such as first-rank symptoms, and among these delusional perception.

LOOKING FOR THE CORE OF SCHIZOPHRENIAS

The great synthesis made by Kraepelin (1889) brought together under the name of *Dementia Praecox* disparate syndromes, from hebephrenia to delusional syndromes, on the principle of similar outcomes, fatally destined to a chronic condition of disintegration similar to dementia. Kraepelin himself at a certain point distinguished these syndromes from paraphrenia, since in the latter there are conspicuous chronic delusions which nonetheless do not evolve toward a state of decline or toward a pervasive hermetic closure of the sufferer into his own idiosyncratic world.

In the century that has passed since then, a long sequence of studies have been carried out on the outcomes of the illness described by Kraepelin, and later united by E. Bleuler (1911) into the concept of "group of schizophrenias." Even if Bleuler was not much more optimistic than Kraepelin about the outcome of schizophrenias, his shift of emphasis onto the dynamic-psychological mechanisms of the disorder, and his idea that in any case it was a question of a kind of "affective dementia" and not a cognitive one, encouraged the investigation of possible prognoses entailing some sort of reversibility. One of the most accurate evaluations of the factors influencing the course and outcomes of schizophrenia is the one conducted many years ago as part of the international study these aspects of schizophrenia (WHO 1979): of the forty-seven probable predictors analyzed, the most powerful predictor of a negative course is the pre-psychosis condition of deficient integration into social and sexual life. It is not difficult to see in this empirical observation a reference to possible autistic traits in the personality before the onset of illness.

Bleuler's thesis was that the core of the group of schizophrenias was a disorder of association. The thesis affirming that the primary and essential phenomenon characterizing schizophrenic syndromes is the splitting of the mind has been shown to be quite vague in its clinical application, to the point of expanding, as has happened in the past, the boundaries of schizophrenia virtually *ad libitum*, in a sort of evaporation of the concept itself.

The next attempt, markedly coherent in terms of methodology and radical in its linearity, was certainly that of K. Schneider who asserted that a diagnosis of schizophrenia is a diagnosis of the state and not of the course, whatever it might be, and that it is to be founded on Jaspersian psychopathology, that is to say, on the study of the patient's subjective experiences. It is this study that has led to the identification of some *Erlebnisse* considered typical, and that have been translated on a semiological level as "first-rank symptoms." The impact that this way of thinking has had and continues to have in the clinical diagnosis and treatment of schizophrenias is enormous, because of the epistemic rigor that characterizes it, and the "first-rank symptoms" have become a part of every diagnostic system of schizophrenia, whether directly or "camouflaged." Schneiderian psychopathology of schizophrenia excludes from the defining features of schizophrenia the linear progress toward chronic states, abolishing in this way at least what had been "Kraepelin's principle." It also excludes the fundamental role that the associative disorder had had in Bleuler's definition of schizophrenia and its outcomes. "Lesser degrees of 'being unhinged' (*Zerfahren*) in thought and language can be found everywhere," Schneider wrote (1950). Yet first-rank Schneiderian symptoms, or symptoms that closely resemble these, are also present in the circle of manic-depressive psychoses, especially in the so-called "mixed" states or rapid swings between mania and major depression.

Autism (Not Delusions) as
the Core of Schizophrenia

After the failure of the effort of a large part of contemporary psychiatry to define the schizophrenic disorder according to operational criteria, the thesis prevailed that no symptom is in and of itself pathognomonic of schizophrenia and that "schizophrenic-ness" derives from an overall context perceived by the observer and in which the various symptoms are immersed. That is to say, that what is relevant to grasp the core of schizophrenia is the peculiar atmosphere that typically colors the various symptoms. This approach is aimed at an intuitive kind of knowledge, a sort of pre-categorial grasping or feeling. To this approach the concept "autism" is not simply a symptom in the patient, but also a subjective feeling in the observer.

This is the type of program we would truly need in order to adapt Bleuler's insight about autism to the clinical understanding of schizophrenia. But up to now it has been the case that the very essence of autism, which makes it a different and specific way of being, disappeared when the attempt was made to transcribe it into defining categories, characteristics observable within the sphere of natural experience. Parnas and Bovet (1991), for example, reveal themselves to be well aware of this methodological risk when they write that autism "disintegrates" in the descriptive-objectivist model of medicine and that it defies every operational formulation.

It seems that we are condemned to a sort of vicious circle in which the symptoms with a high degree of reliability (e.g. certain delusional or hallucinatory experiences) turn out to be not specific or reflect the construct validity of the schizophrenia concept, or at any rate secondary, and moreover do not necessarily transmit the essence of the pathology of the spectrum of the schizophrenic condition; while more global phenomena, like autism, seem more specific, and more precursory, but lose, at least in part, their validity as diagnostic tools when they are delineated in objective-behavioral symptoms. Naturally, the patient does not talk about autism per se. Yet persons with schizophrenia can make us perceive their problematic position, their lived experience of "*ontological*" (and not simply "ontic-existential") insecurity compared to the naturalness of others and their "shared sense" of the real world. This dramatic lack of the pre-cognitive and pre-verbal grip which is manifested in the lack of common sense. The disorder of attunement with the world of everyday life, the evanescence of the "vital contact with reality," finds in autism its most salient point right in the relationship with other people. It is this aspect that, all in all, permits schizophrenia to be described as a "pathology of encounter."

Minkowski's concept of "vital contact with reality" can be traced back to a famous statement by Husserl (1936): within the vital flow of intentionality of which the life of a subject-I consists, every other I is already, from the beginning, intentionally involved on the path of empathy and the empathetic horizon. Besides, it has been noted that the loss of intersubjective obviousness, which leaves the schizophrenic (or pre-schizophrenic) person so often and so dramatically at the mercy of the drift of "perplexity" and "hyperreflexivity," takes on pathological relevance because of its forced disproportion and invasive spread. Binswanger (1956) adopts the term *Verschrobenheit* (a term that can be translated as eccentricity or queerness, that according to the Oxford Concise Dictionary perhaps originates from German *quer*, meaning oblique or thwart; another option would be bizarreness) to describe a way of being which he saw as largely superimposable onto the concept of autism. A number of the most recent studies (see Parnas et al. 1982, Parnas and Jorgensen 1989; Parnas et al 1998, Parnas 2012) maintain that traces of the "complex" represented by autism and its being inextricably connected to self-disorders can be seen in the pre-schizophrenic personality and in the spectrum of schizophrenic disorders, and sometimes even in blood relatives who are not ill. If we consider autism to develop where an "empirical" Ego attempts to make up for the defeat of the foundation of the "transcendental" Ego, the course of schizophrenia can commence when psychotic states of consciousness meet with a person marked by this fragility.

The hypothesis that emerges from all this is the following: autism could be the specific factor that ultimately makes schizophrenic symptoms, like delusions, *schizophrenic*, immersing the psychopathological phenomena into that particular "atmosphere" so often evoked when discussing schizophrenia.

THE AUTISTIC "TAINT" CHARACTERIZING SCHIZOPHRENIC DELUSIONS

One thing is certain: in practice, a clinician begins to think that *that* delusion is of the schizophrenic kind when certain aspects emerge that lend a particular "atmosphere" to it. These aspects can belong to the content of delusion; for example, when in the subject of persecutory delusion, persecutors are more faceless groups, agencies, or associations than individual identifiable persons, this is a feature that makes it more likely to be of the schizophrenic kind. This sends us back to the defective constitution of the Self and of the Other as subjects, and the homogenization and relative abstraction of the persecutors reflects not only their inaccessibility and distance as individuals, but seems to favor the emergence of universal and ontological elements that prevail over worldly elements (Bovet and Parnas 1993).

It is well known that the *contents* of delusions can vary according to the patient's cultural and historical milieu (Agresti 1959). Where once reference was more often made, for example, to possession, magic, etc., now the reference is more often to electronic devices. The change is particularly evident in schizophrenic delusion, as opposed for instance to melancholic delusion, highlighting that schizophrenia concerns "the historicalness of *Dasein*" (Binswanger 1960) compared to melancholy, so that—Binswanger continues—every schizophrenic has, so to speak, his own schizophrenia in relation to his own life-history and the alternatives that derive from that, while the melancholic has the melancholy of all melancholic persons, that is to say, he suffers from a generic threat of *Dasein* (including guilt, ruin, and physical illness).

In the meantime perhaps we should distinguish between "contents" and "themes" of delusion: it is the former that change culturally, while the latter continue to send us back to the fundamental schizophrenic problem of the altered or deficient foundation of intersubjectivity and the individuation of the Self. This is what leads to delusion, which expresses and at the same time attempts to make up for this deficit, a "metaphysical quality" (Bovet and Parnas 1993). Kraus (1994) has called attention to the way delusional ideas with a "technical" *content* (a pronounced presence of electronic media in the delusion) are found above all in schizophrenia and how this points us to an abnormal "permeability" of the

I–World boundaries and thus to the experiences of outside action. This is perhaps the trans-cultural *theme* of schizophrenic delusion: the feeling of uncertain and blurred Self–World relationship—the very theme of schizophrenic autism.

Another typical theme of schizophrenic delusions is genealogy or one's origin and na-ture. Not infrequently, too, delusional ideas which seem peculiarly schizophrenic emerge in the sphere of the problem of the individual's origins (Ballerini 2005). Delusion about one's genealogy can however assume different contents (e.g. being a descendant of the Czar, or the belief that one is Napoleon) as was the case in the last centuries; although the con-tent may change through the ages, nonetheless the theme that can be found in the back-ground in many patients with schizophrenia is the concern with one's origin alluding to the schizophrenic's central problem of identity: the constitution of identity of the I based on being oneself also in relation to others. Racamier (1980) argues that the node of the schiz-ophrenic imaginary universe (the "ghost of self-generation"), would contain the possibility of telling us something about the constitutive moment of schizophrenia, so different from the paranoiac *romance*: not simply an ontic discourse about one's noble ancestors, but an on-tological one about one's very nature as a non-human being—sometimes referred to as the "bizarreness" of schizophrenic delusions. Thus the content (or the fragments of content) of a schizophrenic delusion tells us of autism, that is, of an ontological catastrophe, the crisis of "Who" which seems central in the disastrous psychotic courses which we call schizophrenia.

Another fundamental characteristic of schizophrenic delusions is their *form*, further pre-cise features which characterize them rather than delusions in general. In schizophrenic delusions a personal, relevant meaning becomes manifested; to this meaning the patient gives the value of evidence, of a penetrating sign coming from a higher reality, lived in an atmosphere which appears to the observer, but not to the subject, as one of great receptive passivity of the meanings emanating from objects. The basic problem is if a structure of being-delusional exists that is specific to being-schizophrenic. The anthropological device of "revelation," by means of which new "truths" appear to consciousness, defines perhaps the "primary" delusion (as is the case with delusional perceptions) as opposed to the delusion-like ideas, centered conversely on the device of "confirmation" of a blunted affect and an intol-erance of ambiguity, more than defining a specifically schizophrenic delusion. Nonetheless Kraus's analyses (1982, 1983), delineate a way of being in delusion, which certainly is closer than any others to a delusional world such as is most typically present in a schizophrenic. Kraus underlined how these differences in the various ways of being delusional are par-ticular evident with respect to "delusional certainty": whereas in manic-depressives this is marked by "intolerance of ambiguity" leading to the adoption of a unilateral way of thinking; in persons with schizophrenia the "delusional certainty" has precisely the traits of revelation, in that there appear "new formations which take the place of reality."

We can return to the topic of the relationship between delusion as "confirmation" or conversely as "revelation," paying special attention to the processes that lead to the actual-ization of meanings, as Stanghellini and Ballerini proposed (1992): the change in the rela-tionship between subject and object. A proportion exists in normality between the sense of being the author of the world's meanings and what the world's objects seem to reveal to us by themselves, and every excited state or rigidly fixed idea shifts this proportion. It is with the dramatic and extreme vanishing of the I's activity and I's total passivity that things are experienced as emanating meanings that impose themselves as a *Diktat*, a penetrating sign coming from a higher reality, lived in an atmosphere experienced by the patient in a state of total passive receptiveness.

Many of us have never believed that schizophrenia can be defined only by means of "objectifiable," conventional symptoms, and this is accompanied by great caution in making a diagnosis of schizophrenia, especially on the part of those who do not identify schizophrenia with primary delusion.

And yet we can perhaps find warning clues, more than in the phenomenon of delusion in general, in particular thematic-formal aspects of delusion, which mark the crisis of the obviousness of the ontological foundation of the Self and the World, that is to say, of selfness in intersubjectivity. The essential point here, for the schizophrenic, is the possibility, along the course of an ante-festum temporality, to achieve in the future the possibility of an I capable of being itself in the intersubjective dimension, warding off the risk of alienation to not-I.

BIBLIOGRAPHY

Agresti E. (1959). "Studio delle varianti cliniche dei temi e dei contenuti deliranti in epoche diverse. Confronto dei vari tipi di delirio a distanza di circa un secolo." *Rivista di patologia nervosa e mentale*. 80: 845–865.

Ballerini A. (2005). *Caduto da una stella. Figure della identità nella psicosi*. Rome: Giovanni Fioriti Editore.

Ballerini A. and Stanghellini G. (1991). Organizzatori Nosografici e Organizzatori Psicopatologici. In: *Nosografia e Transnosografia*. Atti del II Congresso Nazionale della Società Italiana di Storia della Psichiatria, Siena 21–23 March 1991.

Binswanger L. (1956). *Italian translation: Tre forme di esistenza mancata*. Milan: Il Saggiatore, 1964.

Binswanger L. (1960). *Italian translation: Melanconia e Mania*. Turin: Boringhieri, 1971.

Blankenburg W. (1971). *Italian translation: La perdita della evidenza naturale*. Milan: Cortina, 1998.

Bleuler E. (1911). *Italian translation: Dementia praecox o il gruppo delle schizofrenie*. Roma: La Nuova Italia Scientifica, 1985.

Bovet P. and Parnas J. (1993). "Schizophrenic Delusions: A Phenomenological Approach." *Schizophrenia Bulletin* 19: 579–597.

Husserl E. (1936). *Italian translation: Idee per una fenomenologia pura e per una filosofia fenomenologica*. Turin: Einaudi, 1965.

Kimura B. (1992). *Italian translation: Scritti di psicopatologia fenomenologica*. Roma: Giovanni Fioriti Editore, 2005.

Kraepelin E. (1889). *Italian translation: Trattato di psichiatria*. Milan: Vallardi, 1907.

Kraus A. (1982). "Identity and Psychosis in the Manic-Depressive." In A. J. J. De Koning and F. A. Jenner (eds.), *Phenomenology and Psychiatry*, 201–216. London, Toronto, Sydney: Academic Press.

Kraus A. (1983). "Schizoaffective Psychoses from a Phenomenological-Anthropological Point of View." *Psichiatria Clinica* 16: 265–274.

Kraus A. (1994). "Phenomenology of the Technical Delusion in Schizophrenics." *Journal of Phenomenological Psychology* 25: 51–69.

Parnas J. (2012). "The Core Gestalt of Schizophrenia" *World Psychiatry* 11(2) (June): 67–69.

Parnas J., et al. (1982) Behavioral precursors of schizophrenia spectrum. A prospective study. *Archives of general psychiatry* Jun; 39(6):658–664.

Parnas J. and Jorgensen A. (1989). "Pre-morbid Psychopathology in Schizophrenia Spectrum." *British Journal of Psychiatry* 155: 623–627.

Parnas J. and Bovet P. (1991). "Autism in Schizophrenia Revisited." *Comprehensive Psychiatry* 32(1): 7–21.

Parnas J., et al. (1998). "Self-Experience in the Prodromal Phases of Schizophrenia: A Pilot Study of First-Admissions." *Neurological Psychiatry and Brain Research* 97–106.

Racamier J. P. (1980). *Italian translation: Gli schizofrenici.* Milan: Cortina, 1983.

Schneider K. (1950). *Italian translation: Psicopatologia clinica,* 4th edn. Roma: Giovanni Fioriti Editore, 2004.

Stanghellini G. and Ballerini A. (1992). *Ossessione e Rivelazione.* Turin: Bollati Boringhieri.

Weitbrecht H. J. (1957). "Zur Frage der Spezifitaet psychopathologischer Symptome." *Fortschritte Neurologie – Psychiatrie* 25: 41–56.

World Health Organization (WHO) (1979). *Schizophrenia: An International Follow-up Study.* Chichester, UK: John Wiley & Sons.

CHAPTER 73

....

DELUSIONAL MOOD

....

MADS GRAM HENRIKSEN AND JOSEF PARNAS

INTRODUCTION

THE clinical concept of delusional mood or atmosphere (*Wahnstimmung*) denotes a psychopathological syndrome that tentatively may be defined as a global, diffuse, ominous feeling of something (not yet defined) impending. Since delusional mood often precedes delusion formation, it has also been labeled "the predelusional state." The significance of delusional mood or the predelusional state was already noted by several nineteenth-century psychiatrists.[1] However, there is no empirical-epidemiological data on its frequency; thus, we are not able to rule out that the majority of delusions in schizophrenia are preceded by elements of delusional mood, but there is no data to this effect. Although delusional mood is listed in some psychopathological assessment tools like the Present State Examination, the contemporary diagnostic manuals (ICD-10 and DSM-5)[2] make no reference to delusional mood and often it risks slipping "under the radar," that is, being unnoticed or perhaps misinterpreted, for example, as manifestations of anxiety or depression, which, as we will see, are in fact frequent manifestations of delusional mood. Delusional mood is only rarely detected in routine clinical work. Detection of delusional mood requires an in-depth psychopathological interview, focusing upon the pre-onset features of the patient's subjective experiences, which rarely happens in a standard, routine clinical setting. When detected, it is typically in patients with well-defined, abrupt onset of psychosis, who are able to give an account of their experience of incipient psychosis.

In this article, we explore how patients usually experience delusional mood, we account for its central features, and we seek to elicit certain typical phases that tend to lead to the crystallization of primary delusion. First, we examine Jaspers's description of delusional mood, which illuminates several of its key features. Jaspers, however, does not explore these features in any detail, so to provide a comprehensive account of delusional mood, we must go beyond Jaspers, seeking to unfold what is only implicitly present in his description. Second,

---

[1] For a dense, yet comprehensive description of the conceptual history of delusional mood, see Berrios (1996: 115–125).

[2] *International Classification of Diseases*, 10th revision (WHO 1992) and *Diagnostic and Statistical Manual of Mental Disorders*, 5th edn. (APA 2013).

we examine Conrad's notion of "trema," which offers important contributions to the study of delusional mood.[3] Initially, it merits attention that we are not exploring the predelusional state of *psychosis* generally but of *schizophrenia* specifically, that is, we are exploring a particular "mood" from which primary delusion may arise (Jaspers 1997: 98f.; cf. Berrios 1996: 125). Moreover, we neither suggest that delusional mood is *always* clinically detectable prior to the emergence of delusion nor that the presence of delusional mood *necessarily* leads to delusion formation. In other words, we assume that delusional mood may occur episodically and recede spontaneously without leading to the emergence of primary delusion. In some patients with schizotypal disorder, we may observe brief, psychotic-near experiences that possess the structure of delusional mood.

PHENOMENOLOGY OF DELUSIONAL MOOD

"Something is going on; do tell me what on earth is going on . . . How do I know, but I'm certain *something is going on*" (Jaspers 1997: 98; author's italics).[4] This famous quote from a patient of Sandberg's illuminates core features of the experience of delusional mood. Patients are somehow certain that "something" is going on or that "something" is about to happen. Still, the more precise nature of this "something" eludes their grasp; it has not yet taken form or materialized into something more concrete, into a proper "object" so to say. The transformation of this perplexed state of atmospheric insecurity into a definable object marks the very onset of psychosis, viz. delusion formation (e.g. "I'm under surveillance," "I'm being tested," etc.). This puts delusional mood in a central position—as Conrad puts it, "Here we refer to the most important concept of classical psychiatry, i.e. delusional mood, which signifies the peculiar borderland between normal and psychotic experience" (2002: 83).[5] In delusional mood, Jaspers argues, patients "feel uncanny ['*unheimlich*'] . . . Everything gets a *new meaning*. The environment is somehow different" (1997: 98; author's italics). He specifies that perceptual content remains unchanged in itself and yet everything appears in the light of a subtle, all penetrating, uncertain, and uncanny change, "something is in the air" (ibid.). Jaspers also argues that the "delusional atmosphere with all its vagueness of content must be unbearable. Patients obviously suffer terribly under it and to reach some definite idea at last is like being relieved from some enormous burden" (ibid.). Finally, quoting Hagen, Jaspers

[3] Conrad's book, *Die beginnende Schizophrenie* (2002), has not been translated into English. All quotations from this book are our translations. For an English translation of selected parts of Conrad's book, see Broome et al. (2012: 176–193).

[4] In the original quotation, the patient does not herself use the adverb "certain" ("*gewiß*"). Yet, her phrasing strongly suggests that although she does not know what is going on, she has do doubt that something is in fact going on ("Es ist was los, sag mir doch, was ist denn los . . . Ja ich weiß es ja nicht, aber es *ist doch etwas*" [Jaspers 1973: 82; author's italics]). Later, we explore this quality of certainty in delusional mood.

[5] Research on anomalous self-experiences (i.e. self-disorders) in schizophrenia draws the validity of the distinction between normal experience, delusional mood, and psychotic experience into question. Already in the "normal" or "premorbid" mode of experience, patients experience a variety of self-disorders, which destabilizes their experiential life and makes them vulnerable to schizophrenia spectrum disorders (for a review, see Parnas and Henriksen 2014).

notes that patients feel that "they have lost grip on things, they feel gross uncertainty which drives them instinctively to look for some fixed point to which they can cling" (ibid.). This fixed point, lending perspective, stability, certainty, and frequently also some form of ease, is the delusion.

Jaspers's description, though dense and underdeveloped, offers important clues for unraveling the complexities of the phenomenon of delusional mood. First, it is a "mood" ("*Stimmung*"), not an emotion or affect. Roughly put, emotions and affects typically have intentional objects (e.g. we are glad about *something*, happy for *someone*, etc.), whereas moods have no distinct intentional objects. Their intentional directedness, if we can speak of one, is more global and diffuse (e.g. if we are sad, everything appears to us in the light of sadness).[6] In Heideggerian terms, we could say that moods constitute "an irreducible background that determines the way the world is disclosed to us" (Henriksen et al. 2010: 361; cf. Heidegger 2007: 172–179) or, as Ratcliffe puts it, moods "constitute a kind of anchor that ties us to the world and opens it up as a meaningful realm of deliberation and action" (2002, 298). In delusional mood, the world appears strangely, yet indefinably different. Events or objects lose their natural sense of familiarity, purposefulness, and coherence, and the world itself becomes increasingly uncanny ("*unheimlich*," literally meaning "non-homely")—that is, the patient no longer feels at home or at ease in the world.

Second, the subtle, all penetrating change ("*alles durchdringende Veränderung*") imbues everything with a "new meaning." Jaspers does not explain this claim; he only states that the content of perception remains unchanged. In our view, which is inspired by Heidegger (2007), Conrad (2002), and Matussek (1987), the "new meaning" arises not from changes in perceptual experience per se but rather from a global, gestaltic change.[7] Thus, the coffee mug in front of me still appears to me as a coffee mug; its meaning is in itself unaltered. Rather what seems to be changed is the overarching meaning structure ("*Bedeutsamkeit*"), that is, the world as a practical and functional context in which objects are embedded and from which they receive their meaning (Heidegger 2007: 114–122; Gennart 2011: 292). In delusional mood, the context's mutually implicative referential functions are somehow loosened or weakened, decontextualizing singular perceptual elements from their ordinary, contextual embeddedness and enabling new, unfamiliar meanings to emerge alongside the familiar ones (cf. Matussek 1987: 90). For example, the casual look of a stranger in the street or the tone of voice of a waitress could indicate that they "know" what is going on; the manufacturer's print on the coffee mug could be a sign pointing to the nature of the impending, etc. Eventually, the patient may experience that objects, events, or others, as Fuchs puts it, no longer "present" themselves in the phenomenological sense of the term, but "only *pretend* to be just themselves" (Fuchs 2005: 136; author's italics), leaving an impression of a strange, unreal, artificial, or staged world—a typical form of derealization in schizophrenia (Jansson 2015: 64–65).

---

[6] For details on the distinction and relationship between emotions/affects and moods, see Stanghellini and Rosfort (2013: 163–166).

[7] The "basic symptom" approach has identified subtle perceptual disturbances prior to psychosis onset, e.g. sensory over alertness, micro- and macropsies, and derealization (see domain C.2; Gross et al. 1987: 68–82). In our view, these disturbances do not reflect "disorders of perception" per se but rather alterations of pathic-noetic pole of experience.

Third, "do tell me what on earth is going on," the patient said. This complaint may be taken to indicate that she suspects or begins to suspect that someone actually knows what is happening but intentionally is withholding this crucial piece of information from her. Experiences of self-reference is regularly an inherent part of the clinical picture of delusional mood, that is, the patient becomes aware that whatever is going on or is about to happen is somehow directly linked to or has special significance for her. Jansson offers the following paradigmatic example of primary self-reference in schizophrenia—"She felt that everybody was looking at her *for no reason*" (2015: 57; our italics). The emphasis is critical, that is, the patient's feeling that others are looking at her is not motivated by or carries traces of underlying or preceding mental states such as feelings of insecurity, inferiority, guilt, paranoia, etc. In other words, her experience of others looking at her is *primary* in the sense that the immediately sensed link between her and others is psychologically irreducible.[8] In delusional mood, this self-referential awareness, that is, the awareness that whatever is going on or about to happen is intimately tied to the patient, separates the patient from others and puts the patient in a unique, central position in the world; increasingly, it seems as if everything turns around the patient—a manifestation of a quasi-solipsistic, existential stance.

Eventually, suspiciousness and mistrust permeate the entire life world. In this perplexed state, the patient struggles to make sense of her experiences. Desperately, she searches for solutions or answers, seeking that "fixed point" that can explain what is going on and which she is almost destined to cling to. Notably, Ey (1973) called the cognitive efforts in this search for meaning and explanation for the "psychotic work" ("*le travail psychotique*"). Through the patient's "psychotic work," the atmospheric uncertainty of the delusional mood, combined with the revelatory (apophantic) givenness of the primary delusional experience, is eventually cognitively elaborated into specific delusional contents or "objects" (Conrad 2002).

Fourth, it is well established that primary delusions in schizophrenia (i.e. delusional perception and delusional ideas)[9] are imbued with a sense of absolute, apodictic certainty ("*Gewißheitsbewußtsein*"). However, as Müller-Suur points out, "even in the so-called delusional mood, where the situation is characterized by a consciousness of uncertainty ['*Bewußtsein der Ungewißheit*'] and anxiety, this consciousness of uncertainty ['*Ungewißheitsbewußtsein*'] in schizophrenics is *absolutely certain*" (1950: 45; our italics). Of course, the patient does not know what is going on, but she has not a shred of a doubt that something is in fact going on. Thus, delusional mood is an emblematic stage for the formation of primary delusional phenomena. According to Müller-Suur, the depth and quality of experiential certainty is a distinctive feature of schizophrenia. Where the formation of non-schizophrenic delusion begins with suspiciousness in the pre-psychotic stage ("does that perhaps mean something?"), which only gradually solidifies the delusional conviction in a progressive and inferential fashion, the formation of delusion in schizophrenia is already in the delusional mood, in the midst of all its uncertainty and vagueness, permeated by a strong sense of certainty ("that means something!") (ibid.).

---

[8] While non-primary types of self-reference can be encountered in other mental disorders as well, "the primary type is seen exclusively here" (Jansson 2015: 58), i.e. in the schizophrenia spectrum disorders.

[9] See Jaspers (1997: 98–104); Schneider (1950: 106–117); or Conrad (2002: 88–184) for a discussion of these forms of primary delusion in schizophrenia.

So far, we have sought to unfold the complexities of delusional mood implied in Jaspers's description. In the following, we explore Conrad's notion of "trema," which includes delusional mood as one of its temporally more advanced features but which also entails a more comprehensive outlook at the late prodromal experiential and existential changes in incipient psychosis.

THE "TREMA"

In his seminal book *Die beginnende Schizophrenie* (2002), Conrad combines phenomenology and gestalt psychology in an analysis of 107 patients with schizophrenia.[10] On the basis of this material, Conrad elicits a stage model of incipient schizophrenia, comprising the "trema" (the near-psychotic phase), the "apophantic" and "apocalyptic" phases (psychosis), the consolidation, and the residual state. For the purpose of this article, we discuss only the "trema" and its features.

Conrad adopts the notion of "trema" from the world of theatre, where it signifies the actor's "state of tension" ("*Spannungszustand*") before going on stage (2002: 42), to emphasize how the near-psychotic phase is experienced by patients.[11] This heightened state of tension has the effect of restraining the psychic total field ("*Gesamtfeld*") by raising mental barriers that enclose and limit the individual's mind and freedom. Unlike the actor or athlete who may decide not to perform, the patient cannot leave this changed, restrained psychic field. Unable to escape and with pressure accumulating and mental barriers continuing to rise, the patient is inevitably pushed toward the critical point. Following Conrad's conception of the dynamics of the psychic field, the pressure may only decrease and the mental barriers fall once the critical point is crossed. This crossing, however, is never neutral; it allows for only two outcomes: victory or defeat, increase or decrease of self-esteem (2002: 43). The kernel of the critical point gravitates around experiences of something decisive impeding. This particular feature of the "trema," Conrad, following Jaspers, calls "delusional mood." Delusional mood is, however, often preceded by or, more correctly, intertwined with other features of the "trema" (2002: 87), including *an increase of basic affective tone* ("*erhöhten Bodenaffektivität*"), *indications of guilt or depressive-like states*, and *mistrust*. To elicit these three features of the "trema," we bring, in the following, our translation of a selected extract of Conrad's textbook example (2002: 21–38). For this purpose, we

[10] Epidemiologically, the sample is quite selective, comprising only soldiers (men), admitted to the military hospital in 1941–42 after exposure to various stressors in the context of the Second World War. These patients tend to present with an acute onset of psychosis. By contrast, more insidious or less flamboyantly psychotic forms of schizophrenia (e.g. hebephrenia) are not discussed.

[11] "Trema" is usually translated into or equated with "stage fright" (e.g. Mishara 2010), which refers to the anxiety or fear that may arise in actors before performing in front of an audience or, more precisely, before the evaluating looks of others. However, "stage fright" is far too narrow a term to capture what is at stake in the notion of "trema." Conrad is partly to blame for this misconception, because, when introducing the concept, he makes the reference to the case of the actor. However, he also clearly states that "trema is not always identical to anxiety" and that, e.g. "the tension before a sporting match is also trema," which is typically dominated by joy or excitement (2002: 42). Thus, the core of the "trema" is the heightened state of tension.

have intentionally have left out major parts of the textbook example, concerning the fully formed psychotic experiences, etc.

> While living with his parents [at the age of 18; approximately two years earlier], Rainer reports that he had the impression that they reproached him for supporting him for so long. This "pressure" led him to drop out of high school and take a job at the tax authority, which he didn't really want and which also prevented him from pursuing the military career he desired. He later joined the RAD ("Reich Arbeits-Dienst", i.e. the national work force) and was deployed in southern France, building roads and cutting down trees. From the very moment he was deployed, he felt under pressure, as if an extraordinary work effort was expected from him. For some time, he had the impression that "something was in the air", but he couldn't tell what it was. Then "rumors" spread, sort of in the background, that he, as the only one, would be promoted to scout leader. No names were ever mentioned but it was clear to him that he would be chosen. For this reason, the others suddenly became very hostile toward him. During a break, the bags of bread were not in proper shape and his superior told him, "Bring in it order. You are responsible to me"; a hint of his upcoming promotion. Similar hints occurred constantly.
>
> He didn't talk to the others, as he feared their envy. 2–3 days passed. The others looked strangely at him and acted all but friendly toward him. From conversations, he soon realized that he would get a special "role" during the night, perhaps he would be taken into the open and burn marked with a symbol of hammer and sickle. He decided to stay awake that night and resist. From the creaking of the floorboards and the beds, he could clearly hear, how they tried to sneak up on him. He jumped out of bed to attack his opponent but there was none. As soon as he lay down, they started to sneak up on him again, and all the time he had to jump up. When the guards entered the room, he immediately sensed that they were "instructed". They found him near the stove and gave him a warning. When they later that night again found him standing by the stove instead of lying in his bed, he was locked in the guardroom. It was quite clear that they "knew". Returning to his barrack in the morning, everybody "knew" and he felt surrounded by a hostile atmosphere. Even his best friend asked him, "quite innocently", what was wrong. Everybody was dissembling. Undoubtedly, they wanted to see how he reacted.
>
> Rainer later explains his time in the RAD as a preparation period, where he was being tested for a military career as officer (2002: 22–24).

First, a slightly increased basic affective tone is already detectable in Rainer's impression that his parents "reproached" him, which caused enough pressure and mental barriers to make him change his planned career path; he quit high school and took a job at the tax authority. Conrad notes that the parents did not reproach him and they were in fact disappointed with his hasty decision to leave school (2002: 41). Later, when deployed, the already increased basic affective tone intensifies significantly—he now feels "under pressure," as if something extraordinary is expected of him, eventually culminating in the experience of something crucial impeding, something intimately related to himself.

According to Conrad, a frequent manifestation of the increased basic affective tone is the so-called "crazy actions" ("*Unsinnige Handlungen*"), which often leave us baffled. According to Conrad, "crazy actions" should be grasped within the context of the patient's altered psychic field. These seemingly incomprehensible actions can, at least partly, be understood as attempts to overcome an unbearable, inner tension or pressure by a gross violation of the given situational context and its rules (2002: 66). Conrad offers several examples of "crazy actions" (2002: 63–69). We will only mention one, namely that of a twenty-four-year-old sergeant, Hiltfried K., who, as his troops' advance stopped in the vicinity of Paris, took his service vehicle and, breaking explicit orders, drove with some privates under his command to Paris to show them the beauty of the city and to instill in them respect of the enemy's culture—an incredible transgression of the German military discipline, which made the sergeant's behavior appear completely "mad" in the eyes of his superiors (2002: 68). Prior to the incident, the sergeant's behavior had been impeccable, but for long he had felt "a terrible tension" and he was utterly disappointed in his comrades who plundered during the troops' advance.

Second, the increased basic affective tone often manifests with a tonality of guilt, anxiety, potentially fear of death or depression (2002: 69) but also occasionally of anticipatory excitement, euphoria, or manic-like loss of inhibition (2002: 73). In the case of Rainer, Conrad argues that feelings of guilt must have accompanied the impression of his parents' "reproach"; otherwise it seems unlikely that he would have changed his career plans (ibid.). In other patients, guilt feelings are far more prominent. Conrad offers another example:

> One patient (case 88), who once had a relationship and intercourse with a widow, cannot stop ruminating about whether or not she might report him for having infected her with a venereal disease. Admittedly, he had never had a venereal disease but he could not be absolutely sure. He had no idea why she should now wish to destroy him but he assumed it was a revenge for him calling off the relationship. These ruminations rendered him unable to sleep or work. A few weeks later, he developed severe psychosis with self-reference, believing that disguised policemen were monitoring him in the ward (2002: 74).

Such experiences of guilt, which, most importantly, are *not* motivated by any offense that may explain the presence and persistence of guilt, are, according to Conrad, indicative of a changed structure of experience. The patient seems to experience a kind of chasm, dividing and even isolating him from others and the shared world. As Conrad puts it, "in horror, the patient feels that he has lost the possibility of a 'we', the sense of community. In the most dreadful way, he is banished to his own world. The possibility of crossing ['*Überstieg*'] is drawn into question, almost already lost" (2002: 73). A few aspects merit explication: i) the chasm is not a mental barrier, similar to those we described above, which can be torn down or penetrated, for example, by a "crazy action"; ii) the chasm is far more absolute, unbridgeable as it were, separating the guilty from the innocent; and iii) though invisible to others, the chasm "is unforgettable to the guilty" (2002: 70–71). Conrad seems to suggest that traces of such a profound separation from the shared world can be found in nearly all forms of "trema" (2002: 73). This observation coheres with ideas found elsewhere in phenomenological psychopathology, for example, in Binswanger, who argues that the core of schizophrenia, in the case of Ellen West, consists in an irreconcilable breach between her own, private world ("*Eigenwelt*") and the shared-social world ("*Mitwelt und Umwelt*") (Binswanger 1958; cf. Stephensen and Henriksen 2017); or, in Henriksen and Parnas (2014), who argue that many patients with schizophrenia adopt "a double ontological orientation . . . which refers to the predicament (and ability) of simultaneously living in two different worlds, namely the shared-social world (i.e. the natural ontological attitude) and a private, psychotic world (i.e. a solipsistic ontological attitude)" (Henriksen and Parnas 2014: 544).

Third, mistrust is the final feature of the "trema," characterized also by the increased basic affective tone. "It is not *what* people do or say that affect us but rather what they do *not* say or what they do behind our backs; what they intend to do, what they hide, what they talk about when we are not around" (Conrad 2002: 80; author's italics). As already noted, perceptual contents remain unchanged in themselves. By contrast, the change, springing from this pervasive, all-piercing form of mistrust, consists in the *"loss of the background's neutrality"* (ibid.; author's italics). Usually, the background lurks unnoticed in the periphery of our experiential field, but in the "trema" it may take on "entirely different properties" (ibid.). In the state of mistrust, anything eluding one's grasp or thematic focus of attention becomes "a barrier," loaded with an atmospheric quality of hostility or aggression. This is aptly illustrated in the case of Rainer, who describes how others looked strangely at him, acted unfriendly toward him, were envious, dissembling, etc. Even his best friend's "innocent question" regarding Rainer's wellbeing was by no means innocent, that is, it had an ulterior motive, etc. Conrad also describes how another patient "behind his comrades harmless utterances surmised envy and a wish to supplant him from his position" (ibid.).

The final feature of the "trema," viz. the delusional mood, is of course intimately connected to the increased state of basic tension, experience of guilt and so forth, and the mistrust—"it [all] figures at once in this peculiar mood; everything which we for didactical concerns have described separately" (ibid., 87). Conrad's own description of delusional mood draws considerably on and does not substantially differ from that of Jaspers, and therefore we do not explore it further here.

Conclusion

The formation of primary delusion is often preceded by an increase of basic affective tone, followed by an atmosphere of apprehension, free-floating anxiety, guilt, or depression (occasionally of elation or ecstasy), perhaps of something impending, "something in the air." The delusional mood becomes increasingly self-referential; whatever is going on or about to happen is directly linked to the patient. Eventually, the world may come to be experienced as staged, artificial, or unreal. Dislocated from the shared-social world by an unbridgeable chasm, mistrust and suspiciousness permeate the life-world and the patient seeks actively to decipher what on earth is going on, striving to find some solution or explanation to this unbearable, tense state of ontological insecurity, exposure, and confusion. Finally reaching that "fixed point" marks the onset of psychosis. Notably, patients with psychotic symptoms are regularly mistrustful and suspicious, for example, harboring doubts about the identity of their perpetrators or the magnitude of their surveillance. These forms of atmosphere of suspiciousness may occur in all delusional conditions, that is, delusional disorder or psychotic affective disorder. Thus, a patient who feels persecuted and finds the presence of a policeman on the street corner as a part of his persecution is not experiencing delusional mood. Therefore, once delusions have crystallized, it no longer makes sense to speak of a delusional mood.

The phenomenological exploration of delusional mood and incipient psychosis in schizophrenia suggests that the psychotic "content" (primary delusion) only materializes and takes its clearly, object-like status (noematic form) on the basis of an initially global and diffuse state of atmospheric, pathic tension, which has no clear and distinctive subject-object intentional structure (Griffero 2014). Through the "psychotic work," the atmospheric uncertainty of delusional mood, with its extreme poverty of clearly demarcated noematic elements, combined with the apophantic givenness of the primary delusional experience, is eventually cognitively elaborated into specific delusional contents, now acquiring a clear form of a noematic "object" (e.g. a "theme"). In this regard, the psychotic "object" is *sensu stricto* secondary to or derived from the primary delusional experience.

BIBLIOGRAPHY

American Psychiatric Association (APA). (2013). *Diagnostic and Statistical Manual of Mental Disorders*, 5th edn. (DSM-5). Washington: APA.

Berrios G. E. (1996). *The History of Mental Symptoms. Descriptive Psychopathology Since the Nineteenth Century*. New York: Cambridge University Press.

Binswanger L. (1958). "The Case of Ellen West," trans. W. M. Mendel and J. Lyons. In R. May, E. Angel, and H. F. Ellenberger (eds.). *Existence. A New Dimension in Psychiatry and Psychology*, pp. 237–364. New York: Basic Books.

Broome M. R., Harland R., Owen G. S., Stringaris A. (2012). *The Maudsley Reader in Phenomenological Psychiatry*. New York: Cambridge University Press.

Conrad K. (2002). *Die beginnende Schizophrenie. Versuch einer Gestaltanalyse des Wahns*. Bonn: Edition Das Narrenschiff im Psychiatrie-Verlag.

Ey H. (1973). *Traite des hallucinations, Tome I et II*. Paris: Masson.

Fuchs T. (2005). "Delusional Mood and Delusional Perception—A Phenomenological Analysis." *Psychopathology* 38: 133–139.

Génnart M. (2011). *Corporéité et présence. Jalons pour une approche du corps dans la psychose*. Argenteuil: Le Cercle Hermeneutique.

Griffero T. (2014). *Atmospheres: Aesthetics of Emotional Spaces*, trans. S. Sanctis. Farmham: Ashgate.

Gross G., Huber G., Klosterkötter J., and Linz M. (1987). *Bonner Skala Für die Beurteilung von Basissymptomen*. Berlin/Heidelberg: Springer Verlag.

Heidegger M. (2007). *Being and Time*. Oxford: Blackwell.

Henriksen M. G., Škodlar B. Sass L. A., and Parnas J. (2010). "Autism and Perplexity: A Qualitative and Theoretical Study of Basic Subjective Experiences in Schizophrenia." *Psychopathology* 43: 357–368.

Henriksen M. G. and Parnas J. (2014). "Self-disorders and Schizophrenia: A Phenomenological Reappraisal of Poor Insight and Noncompliance." *Schizophrenia Bulletin* 40: 542–547.

Jansson L. (2015). "Near-psychotic Phenomena in a Clinical Context." In F. Waters and M. Stephane (eds.), *The Assessment of Psychosis. A Reference Book and Rating Scales for Research and Practice*, pp. 55–74. New York: Routledge.

Jaspers K. (1973). *Allgemeine Psychopathologie*, 9th edn. Berlin: Springer Verlag.

Jaspers K. (1997). *General Psychopathology*, trans. J. Hoenig and M. W. Hamilton. London: Johns Hopkins University Press.

Matussek P. (1987). "Studies in Delusional Perception." In J. Cutting and M. Shepherd (eds.), *The Clinical Roots of the Schizophrenia Concept*, pp. 89–104. Cambridge: Cambridge University Press.

Mishara A. L. (2010). "Klaus Conrad (1905–1961): Delusional Mood, Psychosis, and Beginning Schizophrenia." *Schizophrenia Bulletin* 36(1): 9–13.

Müller-Suur H. (1950). "Das Gewissheitsbewusstsein beim schizophrenen und beim paranoischen Wahnerleben." *Fortschritte der Neurologie, Psychiatrie, und ihrer Grenzgebiete* 18(1): 44–51.

Parnas J. and Henriksen M. G. (2014). "Disordered Self in the Schizophrenia Spectrum: A Clinical and Research Perspective." *Harvard Review of Psychiatry* 22(5): 251–265.

Ratcliffe M. (2002). "Heidegger's Attunement and the Neuropsychology of Emotion." *Phenomenology and the Cognitive Sciences* 1: 287–312.

Schneider K. (1950). *Klinische Psychopathologie*. Stuttgart: Georg Thieme Verlag.

Stanghellini G. and Rosfort R. (2013). *Emotions and Personhood. Exploring Fragility—Making Sense of Vulnerability*. Oxford: Oxford University Press.

Stephensen H. B. and Henriksen M. G. (2017). "Not Being Oneself: A Critical Perspective on 'Inauthenticity' in Schizophrenia." *Journal of Phenomenological Psychology* 48: 63–82.

World Health Organization (WHO). (1992). *The ICD-10. Classification of Mental and Behavioural Disorders: Clinical Description and Diagnostic Guidelines*. Geneva: WHO.

CHAPTER 74

···

DELUSION AND
MOOD DISORDERS

···

OTTO DOERR-ZEGERS

INTRODUCTION

THE problem of delusion in mood disorders has drawn less attention than delusion in schizophrenic patients, probably due to the lack of diversity, since they are always the same topics: guilt, poverty, and somatic illness. In this context, it is important to note that the depressive delusion topics have remained the same throughout time, as Krafft-Ebing teaches us in his 1874 book *Die Melancholie*. In schizophrenia, however, delusional ideas cover the most varied topics and are full of almost poetic symbols and thoughts. In fact, there have been great schizophrenic poets, such as Friedrich Hölderlin (1961). The appearance frequency of delusional ideas in depression ranges between 20% and 45% of the patients who have been hospitalized and who have suffered frank melancholy in the sense of the old endogenous depression, and between 10% and 15% among depressive patients in general, without distinguishing types or subtypes (Winokur, Scharfetter, Angst 1985; Tölle and Wefelmeyer 1987; Wolfersdorf, Steiner, and Keller 1987; Maj et al. 2007; Ostergaard et al. 2013).

The most common content is undoubtedly guilt, with its presence varying depending on sociocultural factors, but also on the type of depression. With respect to the first point, Kraepelin, 1904, had already observed the absence of guilt feelings in the depressive patients he studied in Java: "Guilt ideas were never manifested [by the patients]." He could also state that no severe depressive pictures were observed. Yap in Hong Kong (1965) and Pfeiffer (1969, 1971) in Indonesia found similar results. Yap summarized his findings with the following words: "Infrequent severe affective disorders, mild depressions with short duration and without guilt ideas, relative frequency of manic pictures, which are associated with confusion symptoms, and a very small proportion of suicide attempts" (Yap 1965: 105). In a study carried out in Concepción, Chile, on fifty-five depression patients who had required hospitalization, guilt ideas were found in only 11% of the patients (Doerr-Zegers et al. 1971), in comparison with a similar study carried out in Switzerland, where the frequency of guilt ideas reached 50% (Hoffet 1962). The second element, the relation between guilt ideas and the type of depression, has been emphasized by Stanghellini and collaborators (2006) in a study carried out in Italy on 116 patients who suffered from a major depressive episode. The authors divided these patients into two groups, those having the personality described by Tellenbach (1961, 1983) as *typus melancholicus* (eighty patients) and those who did not have that personality (thirty-six patients), and found clear differences in the way these two types of depression appear: the group with the typical Tellenbach's personality showed symptoms characterized by loss of vitality and guilt feelings, while in the other group, the one with personality features different to *typus melancholicus*, dysphoria and irritability predominated. Differences in other items, such as the presence of anxiety and of somatic symptoms, were not found. The Association for Methodology and Documentation in Psychiatry (AMDP) system was used for the measurement of psychopathological symptoms during the depressive episode. Among the several AMDP items, the authors selected only eight, one of these being "feelings of guilt." This AMDP system has been evaluated several times (Guy and Ban 1983; Baumann and Stieglitz 1983; 1989).

Following with the way in which guilt ideas in depression have been conceptualized, ICD-10 (1992) refers to the establishment of a sequence: ideas of self-depreciation, self-reproaches, and guilt ideas, being an indicator of the seriousness of the process. In mild or moderate depressive syndromes, both delusion and hallucinations constitute exclusion criteria. The DSMs (with very little differences between III and V, 1995, 2013), consider delusions as "specifiers" or seriousness criteria. Thus, they classify major depressive episodes in four groups: mild, moderate, severe without psychotic elements, and severe with psychotic elements; in this group the DSMs distinguish between those patients where psychotic elements are congruent with mood and those where this congruence is absent. All these systems define delusion as "a false belief based on incorrect inferences of reality." Different authors have questioned this definition of delusion, as in the case of Matussek 1963; Scharfetter 1985 and ourselves (Doerr-Zegers 1997). Thus, Matussek postulates that the non-correspondence between delusion and reality is not a mistake in the sense of a wrong logical conclusion, but rather the consequence of a much deeper disturbance, compromising the sphere of beliefs and of trust. In other words, the reality that would be at stake in delusion is not that of the objective world, but that reality opened to us both by the beliefs inhabiting us, as suggested by Ortega y Gasset (1974), and our capacity to trust. The delusional patient does not have too much faith by which he can excessively hold on to a determined idea. On the contrary, he is in need of it: "The delusional patient has very little capacity to believe and trust, and he substitutes this deficiency with supposedly objective knowledge" (Matussek, p. 64). Scharfetter, on the other hand, considers that the defining feature of delusion is not the content, but rather the fact that it implies a distorted relation with the world and with others. Finally, during the 1990s we carried out some studies on the relations between delusion and truth, coming to the conclusion that it is not a mistake in any case, but rather a deep truth (for the patient) that has lost its dialogical character, that is, its reference to other (Doerr-Zegers 1997).

PSYCHOPATHOLOGY OF DEPRESSIVE DELUSION

Throughout several studies on the topic, Wolfersdorf and collaborators (1987, 1989, and 1991) have provided a detailed characterization of depressive delusion which is worth noting. Here we will reproduce and comment on some of the most relevant features of the description provided by these authors:

1. "There is always a background of mood compromise." This coincides perfectly with our own findings. In our studies we have never seen depressive delusion without significant mood abnormalities and without the two other characteristic elements of depressive syndromes, which are the alteration of the biorhythms and the different forms of inhibition (Doerr-Zegers; 1971; 1979; 1993).

2. "The content of the delusion is congruent with the mood." This is a characteristic that has already been mentioned by classical authors (i.e. holothymic delusions, meaning that delusional ideas can be derived from mood) and it constitutes an important element for the differential diagnosis between psychotic symptoms of schizophrenic type and affective type. It is strange, however, that in the DSMs it is insistently stated that there is a sub-group of severe depressions "with psychotic elements" and "incongruent with the mood."

3. There is a "cognitive narrowing of the patient around the delusional topic." Strictly speaking, this is a characteristic also present in delusional disorders and has been studied in depth by W. Blankenburg, 1966. In this paper Blankenburg is able to describe step by step the way a given theme gradually invades the psychic life of a patient—like a tumor with metastasis—until it is finally transformed into a delusion.

4. "The impossibility of the content lies in the quantitative (there is no productive symptomatology, nor strange formulations)." In our opinion this is valid for the mild and moderate forms and not for very severe cases, nor for nihilist delusion. Thus, for example, there are patients who feel guilty for all the disasters of the world, something that is obviously impossible. Something similar occurs with the most serious cases of Cotard's syndrome, when delusional patients state that they are dead (Doerr-Zegers 2002).

5. "As in every delusion, it is a matter of *evidence* and not of a mere fear to becoming ill or being ruined." This statement highlights the difference between phobias and obsessions on one side, and delusions on the other.

6. "The paranoid ideas of self-reference and the hallucinations are congruent with the mood and are related to guilt." Both symptoms are relatively scarce and, as these authors state, they are indeed congruent with mood. In any case, we (Doerr-Zegers 1971) found a much lower frequency of guilt ideas (10.9%) than in Switzerland (around 50%) (Hoffet 1962), but a higher frequency of paranoid ideas. It should be noted that the ideas of harm and damage referring to relatives were more frequent than those referring to oneself. Our interpretation was focused on the respectively different predominant types of family in Chile and in Europe in that time: an extended family in the first case and a nuclear family in the second.

7. "The election of the (delusional) theme depends on the premorbid orientation to values and on socio-cultural factors." In fact, and as we discussed in the introduction and in the previous point, the frequency of appearance of guilt ideas, but also of paranoid ideas, has a clear relation to the type of society (Kraepelin 1904; Yap 1965; Pfeiffer 1969; Doerr-Zegers 1971).

8. "The remission is gradual" and "chronic delusional disorders are infrequent." This is also true, but we would add that within depression and delusion symptoms there

is a difference in terms of evolution. So, in patients who only show guilt, ruin, or illness ideas, the delusion disappears and there is an improvement in other depression
symptoms, while in those who present some form of Cotard's syndrome, remission can
take much longer.

An interesting clinical observation made by these authors refers to the fact that anxiety would
disappear when the delusion had been consolidated: the patient no longer feels fear about
being or becoming guilty anymore, but he *is* guilty and deserves punishment. The same is
valid for the ideas of economic ruin or suffering an incurable illness: the patient is already
ruined or ill, there is no way out any more, and the only possibility would be self-elimination.
On occasion, it is possible to distinguish between two forms of delusion, corresponding to
the different meaning of the German words *Schulden* and *Schuld*, debt in the sense of "being
in debt" and guilt as such. The first situation aims at remaining behind in respect to duties
and responsibilities, in the sense of the situation of "remanence" (i.e. lagging behind one's
own duties and commitments), described by Tellenbach (1961, 1980, 1983). In the second
situation the patient believes he is guilty of having already transgressed determined norms.
With respect to suicidal notions, Roose demonstrated in 1983 the relation existing between
it and guilt ideas, something that Metzger and Wolfersdorf (1988) confirmed later. However,
in a previous study (Wolfersdorf 1987), Wolfersdorf et al. (2007), had not found significant
differences in the number of suicides in a retrospective study in a delusional depression group
compared with another not delusional group. The explanation of these contradictory results
appears to lie in the more complete treatment received by the patients of the first investigation: antidepressants, antipsychotics, psychotherapy, post-discharge follow-up, etc.

   Another fact of interest and one that has to do both with the clinic and the epidemiology
of this illness is the increase in the frequency of delusional symptoms with age (Glatzel 1988;
Simkó 1983).

Nosological Considerations

The fundamental question stated with respect to this point is whether delusional depression is
a subtype of depression, in some way independent to it, or whether it is only a sign of severity.
Some North American authors have tended to consider it more as a different entity. Thus,
Charney and Nelson (1981). made a study of fifty-four delusional and sixty-six non-delusional
depressions, in which they compared the symptomatology, the evolution, the response to the
treatment, and the premorbid personality features, coming to the following conclusions: with
respect to the symptoms, in the group of delusional patients there were more states of agitation, rumination thoughts, and self-reproaches, while the group of non-delusional patients
showed a higher tendency toward inhibition, anxiety, and lack of energy. In all the other
symptoms, such as alteration of rhythms, loss of concentration, loss of interests, and suicidality, there were no significant differences. Regarding the progress of the illness, there were
no differences, with the exception of the fact that the patients with delusional depression
had also presented delusions in 80% of the previous episodes, while in the non-delusional
group this had occurred only in 12% of the cases. Regarding response to treatment, the difference was very clear: the patients with delusional depression did not react to treatment with

antidepressants only, but they did if antipsychotics and electroshock were added. The non-delusional patients, instead, had a good reaction to treatment with tricyclic antidepressants. Finally, these authors did not find differences in terms of personality features, since in both groups there was a clear predominance of obsessive and dependent features. The other types of abnormal personality features, such as the histrionic, narcissistic, paranoid, antisocial, or borderline, simply did not appear in the group of patients with delusional depression, while in the "non-delusional" group they did appear, but with low frequency: in 16% of the cases histrionic features are given, in 8% paranoid and narcissistic, and in only 4%, borderline. Antisocial features did not appear in either of the two groups. It is interesting to see the significant overlap between these findings and the description by Tellenbach (1961/1980) of *typus melancholicus* mentioned earlier, as the characteristic personality of unipolar depressions. The authors conclude that these findings—in particular the different reaction to treatment and the almost constant appearance of delusional depression with similar episodes in the past—allow us to suggest the hypothesis that they are two different nosological entities.

Another argument suggesting that delusional depression represents a different entity from unipolar depression is its clear bond with suicide. A study on this issue, carried out by Roose et al. (1983), and that spanned a period of twenty-five years, demonstrates that delusional depressive patients were five times more likely to commit suicide than non-delusional patients, and that the presence of delusion constitutes the most potent indicator of suicide in depressive patients.

Some European authors have questioned this idea of delusional depression as an independent nosological entity (Wolfersdorf 1987; Wolfersdorf et al. 1989). When applying the Diagnostic Interview Schedule (DIS) they did not find significant differences in depressive symptomatology, or in the presence of stressors that could have played a role in triggering the disease. They, as well as other authors (Roth 1988; Blankenburg 1991), consider delusional depression as a severe form of depression, in which the cognitive sphere is particularly compromised. However, this hypothesis is difficult to demonstrate, because it depends on what is understood by severity. If this is measured by the suffering accompanying the disease, it could be rather the contrary, since in general delusional patients suffer less that non-delusional patients, imprisoned as they are in their body and in their anxiety. Now, if severity is measured by suicidality, then this hypothesis would be correct, because the depressive-delusional patients are more likely to commit suicide. The other criterion that would support the thesis of severity is the resistance to treatment, since delusional symptoms are more difficult to treat and require antipsychotics in addition to antidepressants.

An interesting perspective, that would allow an understanding of why some depressive patients have delusions and others do not, is that given by Blankenburg (1991). This author argues that the answer could be found in the interaction between personality and biography. Blankenburg starts by accepting that Tellenbach's *typus melancholicus* (1961) is the characteristic personality of those who develop unipolar depression, and that it is characterized by a marked fixation with the different orders in which human existence is deployed: the order of inhabiting, of social life, of work, etc. *Typus melancholicus* are also people with a high self-demand, and because of that, very inclined toward feeling guilty. The existence of this personality, obtained by Tellenbach by means of phenomenological intuition, and called *typus melancholicus* by him, was demonstrated through numerous empirical studies by von Zerssen 1969; 1976; 1977; 1982; Zerssen et al. 1990; 1991) in Germany, by Anneliese Doerr-Álamos and Sandra Viani (1999) in Chile, and in Italy by Stanghellini (Stanghellini et al. 2006;

Stanghellini & Raballo 2007). This personality had also been described, though only partially, by the Japanese Shimoda in 1941. Alfred Kraus (1977; 1990) has added other elements to this type of personality that are worth considering: hypernomia (excessive attachment to norms) and intolerance to ambiguity. Blankenburg argues that perhaps the most determinant feature of this personality structure is not order, needs of proximity with the other, and solidity and conformity with social norms, but rather the way of being fixed to a determined project of life and/or of world and the type of identification with oneself characterizing it. This human "type" shows, as we mentioned previously, curious analogies with the results of studies by authors as varied and as distant in time as Abraham (1912/1971, p. 147) and Charney & Nelson (1981). Thus, both speak of "anancastic" and "depending" features in depressive patients, which corresponds fairly, although in different terminology, to Tellenbach's description of *typus melancholicus*. It is even more striking, in the same sense, that this author did not find antisocial features in his sample, and that histrionic and narcissistic features presented in minimal proportions, which does nothing but confirm the essential feature of *typus melancholicus*, which is the patient's preoccupation for the other, to the point of dependence on that person. Tellenbach could also demonstrate the way in which this personality type, with its specific way of interacting with the environment, generated situations he called "includence" and "remanence," from which the change toward melancholy arose.

But this would be valid for all the forms of melancholic depression, both non-delusional and delusional. And the question is why some patients suffer from delusions and others do not, when, as we saw, they are not independent diseases that should therefore have their own etio-pathogenesis, be it genetic, psychodynamic, or something else. Considering these backgrounds, we can approach Blankenburg's hypothesis: depressive patients who suffer from delusions are persons with all the characteristics of *typus melancholicus*, including orderliness, sensibility to guilt, hypernomia, etc., and who at some point in their lives—not necessarily before the beginning of the disease—have presented behaviors or have been involved in facts contradicting those personality features, for example, an infidelity, a sentimental rupture in which he was guilty, rivalries or negative feelings with respect to a beloved person, abandonments, etc. "They are in general isolated events that in a way are not integrated in the rest of the personality. And whether they are minor deviations of gross derailments, they remain as 'strange bodies' in the biography of these persons. It could be said that the pathogen in these cases is not *inauthenticity* (situation that uses to trigger anxious pictures), but *incompatibility* . . . " (Blankenburg 1991: 107).

Two examples from our casuistry:

1. Male of sixty-five years, admitted to the Psychiatric Hospital of Santiago with severe depression symptoms, agitation, guilt delusion, and suicidal thoughts. Working, responsible, and successful engineer both in Concepción—industrial city in the south of Chile—and later in Sao Paulo, where he later emigrated. He had four daughters from his first marriage, one of whom died at age sixteen from acute leukemia. This tragedy led—as is frequently the case—to the end of marriage, and the later development of a delusional disorder in his former wife. He abandoned the other three adolescent daughters, when he married for the second time and moved to Brazil. The daughters stayed with their mother for a time and then, when she became ill (a delusional disorder), they moved on and were very bonded with each other. The father set up a business in Brazil and his life carried on as normal with his new family, up to the day he had

the idea of stopping working. A short time later severe depressive symptoms appeared and his second wife called his daughters for them to collect him, because she was not willing to take care of this ill man. We found an emaciated man, with massive anxiety, almost at the extreme of agitation, delusional ideas of guilt, and of persecution.

2. Woman of seventy years, whom we examined in the Psychiatric University Clinic of Murcia, Spain, when the author was teaching on a course there. She presented with very serious depression, with great corporeal compromise, guilt ideas, and an uncontrollable impulse to kill herself. Being hospitalized and thus unable to kill herself, she begged the treating physicians and then the author to give her a lethal injection, because she "did not deserve to live." We managed to calm her and engage in a dialogue with her, which allowed us to obtain the following information: she came from a family of farmers of very traditional habits and principles, she had married the man she loved, in the same socio-economical group as herself, with whom she had several children and was very happy for more than forty years of marriage. The described depression was triggered by the marriage and moving away of her daughter, and because of this severity hospitalization was necessary. We persuaded her to tell us many details of her life and herself, from which we concluded that she presented Tellenbach's typical hypernomic personality, with its forgetfulness of herself and its excessive dedication to the care of others. At the end of the interview we thought that there must be some shadow in this life so clear and transparent, and she did confess to us her secret: before marrying she had had an affair with the owner of the farm where her father worked, and she had never dared to confess this "slip" to her husband.

In both cases the same constellation is observed: a personality with all the features of *typus melancholicus* and a biographical event, occurring in the remote past and always denied or repressed, in which the patient had clearly transgressed the norms that were in some way imprinted on their way of being. In the first case it was having abandoned his daughters, even although they were already adolescents and that this incomprehensible behavior was a way of escaping from the pain caused by the death of his favorite daughter. In the second case it was not having confessed to her husband, when marrying, that she was not a virgin and that, even worse, she had experienced a great passion for the owner of the property where she and her family had lived and worked.

Blankenburg's hypothesis helps to solve the initial question: is delusional depression an independent nosological entity or only the expression of a worsening of the depressive disorder? The answer should be searched for in the biography of the patient, and more specifically, in the interaction and coherence existing between the type of personality and important decisions taken in life.

PHENOMENOLOGICAL ASPECTS OF DELUSIONAL DEPRESSION

As a contribution to the phenomenology of the delusional experience of depression, we will analyze a case of our casuistry suffering from Cotard's syndrome, the most extreme form of manifesting delusion in this illness. This patient was treated by me at the General Psychiatric Hospital of Santiago in the year 2001. With her consent, she was presented in the Clinical Meeting of the Hospital. She also consented that I analyzed (and published) her case from a phenomenological and psychodynamic perspective (Doerr-Zegers 2002).

The patient was forty years old, married, with three children, without a morbid background and described as being "excessively normal" up to the beginning of the illness, two months before being admitted to hospital. She was very dedicated to her husband and her children and had a very good relationship with her widowed mother and her brothers. Her illness began in relation to a dispute with her brothers for the inheritance that their mother, already eighty-five years old, wanted to distribute while she was still living. She began to suffer from severe insomnia, anxiety, lack of appetite, weight loss, and multiple physical pains. She was found trying to hang herself and brought urgently to the hospital. Here we will reproduce verbatim her words when being examined by us: "What happens is that I am completely dead; let us say that I am dead, that I am in vegetative state from my head to toes. I do not have touch, smell, or taste for food . . . My body is so light that it is as it did not exist. I do not get tired, I can walk kilometers and nothing happens to me . . . I would like to feel the weight of my eyes to be able to get asleep. How I am going to be able to rest if I do not feel my body? . . . And however, when I am touched, I feel something vague, but I do not feel it in my brain. Nothing scares me anymore; neither can I feel anger . . . I live a life of science fiction, the life of a dead person . . . When I take my children in the arms, I do not feel them . . . If my children knew that they love an artificial mom . . . I do not feel the direct contact with the things, neither with the others . . . When I was alive, I felt the things and was able to concentrate myself in what I did . . . Now, when I speak, the words get out of me, but those of the others do not enter my head . . . The only thing I want is to die, but I go on living because, seemingly, the heart beats, though I neither feel it . . . "

The patient showed all the symptoms consistent with a severe depression with psychotic phenomena and these have the particularity of going beyond the usual themes of guilt, poverty, and illness, up to stating that she is dead, though conscious. The premorbid personality corresponds to the *typus melancholicus*: very dedicated to others, working, responsible, "excessively normal." Her ordered life, her good relationship with her family also pointed to the same conclusion. The premorbid situation represents in a way the transgressions *sensu* Blankenburg, since she was very forthright with her mother and her brothers when defending her rights to her inheritance, even though the mother was still alive. And none of the members of her family were accustomed to see her reacting that way and must have showed surprise and sorrow, which contributed to her guilt feelings, which were imperceptibly transformed into a nihilistic delusion. In the following, we will study this patient's delusion in relation to the way she experiences her own body and then, in relation to her experience of the world and of others.

The fundamental experience of our patient is that her body has lost its weight, something that is, according to her, inherent in what it is to be alive. For this reason she does not get tired and "can roam indefinitely for miles and miles." Neither can she sleep, because she lacks "the weight of her eyes," and then she asks herself: "how am I going to rest if I don't get tired?" Now this ethereal lightness does not mean for her an expansion of her space or of her consciousness, but on the contrary, the confirmation of the greatest impediment possible: one's own death. The first paradox arises here, since common sense would normally associate death with the weight of material things, of inanimate objects, whilst life, on the other hand, implies (to a greater or lesser extent) elevation above the very weight that constitutes it: or, in other words, movement which opposes the force of gravity. Indeed, it could perhaps be argued that the upright position is the greatest triumph attained by life forms over this elemental force of gravity that reigns over the entire physical world. Nevertheless, the patient's lucid yet tormented consciousness identifies lack of weight with death. How can we understand this experience?

Even at those points of Husserl's work in which he develops the transcendent character of the pure consciousness with the greatest radicalism, a sort of thickness of the natural and spontaneous current of experience can be inferred from his descriptions, which directly connects us with corporeality (*Leiblichkeit*). Husserl attaches importance to the body with regard to the "original level of experience" (Husserl 1939/1999: section 6; Husserl 1999), and defines natural experience as a direct and immediate relationship with "the individual," which is established "through the body and its senses." Thus, in section 53, he affirms: "Only by virtue of its experienced relationship with the organism does consciousness become real human or brute consciousness, and only thereby does it acquire a place in the space belonging to nature and the time belonging to nature—the time which is physically measured." At another point, he speaks of a resistance to pure intentionality and that this resistance comes from the body, from the fact that we are an embodied consciousness. In summary, it is the body, the flesh, and its very materiality, which prevents consciousness from floating in the air, devoid of all content. Materiality is weight, and that is what this patient lacks. In a way, she has transformed herself into pure consciousness, separated from her body, which she regards as dead. Consciousness needs a heavy body, both to feel alive and in order to constitute intersubjectivity, as we will see later.

This extreme human experience, suffered in Cotard's syndrome, is a demonstration of the indissoluble bond between consciousness and body. Because one cannot think or feel from nowhere, without a body that has weight and needs, and gets tired and sleeps. With this context in mind, we should recall the nexus established by Levinas (1987) between the experience of *il y a* (there is) and insomnia. For him, basic experience occurs against an impersonal, anonymous background, where there is no subject, an experience of emptiness, of horror. "There is" is later broken by the emergence of the subject, who is able to take possession of him/herself and of the world and to say "I am." Now, in the realm of daily experience, this initial stage of subjectification corresponds to insomnia, to that "wakefulness that is completely devoid of objects . . . it is as anonymous as night itself. It is the night itself that stays awake" (Levinas 1987: 110, 111). It is interesting that insomnia is a key symptom of depressive illness and that our patient also has suffered, with particular intensity, from an inability to sleep. A characteristic feature of depressive insomniacs is that they are haunted by the feeling that no rest is possible, that their wakefulness will continue like this for all eternity. In them, the profound disturbance of temporality characteristic of this illness can already be glimpsed: "(Insomnia is a) wakefulness without purpose . . . time does not start here from any point, nor does it move or melt away. Only the external noises that can leave traces in insomnia introduce starting points in this situation without beginning or end, in this sort of immortality from which it is impossible to escape . . . " (Levinas 1993, p. 85).

With respect to her relationship with the world and with the others, the patient says that when she takes her children in her arms, she does not feel them. Nor does she feel direct contact with things or with others. Then she explains that she has no senses: "I have no sense of feeling or smell, nor taste for food." Specifying her relationship with others, and focusing it on dialogue, on verbal relations, she states: "Now, when I speak, the words (automatically) emerge from me, but those of other people don't enter my head." She also establishes an analogy between what happens to her and television images, which also "do not . . . enter into my head . . . " Finally, she refers to her total absence of feelings toward others, since "I can (not even) feel anger."

For Husserl (1950: section 53; Husserl 1982), the body is the link to one's insertion or being-in-the-world. Husserl writes: "We also recall that only by virtue of the connection joining a consciousness and an organism to make up an empirically intuited unity within Nature is any such thing as mutual understanding between animate beings pertaining to a world possible . . . " It is from the body that openness to intersubjectivity is produced. In the first place, because the body is the "zero point," the *Nullpunkt* (Husserl's original word in German to describe the body's position in its own perceptual field) from which the perceived world is organized. Everything or every quality is oriented in relation to my lived body (*Leib*). This is also the case for whatever is imagined or remembered, since whatever its characteristics, its qualities, or even its own spatiality, it can only be imagined or remembered in reference to my body. It is only then, starting from my own body and from the perception that I have of it, that I am able to constitute the world surrounding me, through which other bodies are spatialized. It is also in this way, from this center that is my body, that I am going to constitute the global world, the world of the Earth. From a phenomenological point of view, the Earth is at the center of the world and my body is at the center of the center, as a zero point.

Husserl (1936/1962: 203) also writes that "the spirit is in the space-temporality, wherever its *soma* (its material body) is" and later on he adds: " . . . which implies that it constantly has a privileged experience of its body and that, consequently, has consciousness of living and being capable of constantly acting in it, in the way of an Ego that suffers afflictions and at the same time acts." This is precisely what the patient has lost. By not having any sensation of her body, by feeling "dead," she cannot act, but she also does not experience "afflictions" be-cause, strictly speaking, one's embodied being, as Husserl argues in "Cartesian meditations" (Husserl 1960 section 24), does not originally appear to one as a spatial object, but is given to one immediately together with the appearance of something that is not one's body. When perceiving a thing in space, the subject "becomes aware of the pre-spatiality of his/her perceiving flesh; it is the appearance of the perceived thing that constitutes the opportunity for the pre-appearance of the flesh as an 'organ of perception' " (Bernet 1993). The depressed patient with Cotard's syndrome has returned to the space of horror and of insomnia, where nothingness and emptiness reign. By not perceiving, by not feeling "the other" ("I have no sense of smell, or of taste") or others ("when I take my children in my arms, I don't feel them"), she is not able to become aware of the "pre-spatiality of her perceiving flesh": conse-quently, the only possibility is that she feels her body to be "dead." When one ceases to be, in oneself, an embodied subject, the ego, that subject emerging from the primordial experience of "there is," is dissolved, since it only can exist when embodied. In the specific case of our patient, her incapacity to transcend, her inability to relate to "the other" reaches the point that she no longer understands words, since "they mean nothing to me . . . because my skull is dead . . . and words don't enter my head."

Now, according to Levinas, in the process of subjectification or hypostasis, the primordial experience of horror before the naked *il y a* ("there is") is followed by the emergence of "I am," of consciousness. The ego accesses language and, through it, to different intentionalities, coinciding in this point with the self-constitution of Husserl's ego. However, for Levinas, the process of subjectification is more complex and must always take the subjective experience of corporeality into account. What is more, this can take on different forms, which are not mutually exclusive. One form could be the mere appropriation of the world in function of its utility to me, of converting everything into what might be useful for me. This is going to be the road that will lead to technique. But the process can also be slow and retain the other as "another" through enjoyment. Otherness is deeply respected in enjoyment. The other is no longer merely an object to be manipulated, as in the case of appropriation, but is instead an enjoyable thing. The ego affirms itself by enjoying things, neutralizing their otherness, until it incorporates them into the immanence of its own subjectivity, which has arisen from enjoyment. "We live from a good soup, from the air, from the light, from shows, from work, from ideas, from dreams, etc. . . . here, it is not a question of objects or of representations. We (simply) live from them . . . (Neither) are they instruments or utensils, in Heidegger's sense of the term . . . they are always objects of enjoyment, which are offered to the taste already adorned and beautified" (Levinas 1969). That is to say, the transitiveness of feeding leads to the reflexive act: "living from . . . " converts the food into vital content; enjoyment of the food is transformed into enjoyment of oneself. Through his philosophy of sensibility, Levinas restores to the body its role in the emergence of subjectivity. "Enjoyment gives us the key to unveiling the original sense of the expression 'own body': in the transition from the famished body (dependent on the surrounding environment . . .) to the sovereign body (which . . . affirms its power against outside factors . . .), in that transition, the 'own body' is revealed to be embodied self-identification" (Sucasas 1998, p. 38). To summarize, in Levinas's own words, "life is love of life . . . it is satisfied sensibility" (Levinas 1969: 131).

However, the patient's inability to feel with her "dead body" is but the end of a process of loss of sensibility. This is a process that begins with that truly characteristic symptom of depression, anhedonia. Levinas has argued that the fundamental way in which the subject relates to the world is not through Heidegger's *Sorge* (or "care," 1927; 1962), but rather enjoyment. If we accept this premise, our patient's widely differing statements that her body is dead, whilst at the same time complaining that she does not taste her food, appear to us to be perfectly consistent. To experience or not the taste of food presupposes the act of eating and this, in turn, of being alive, which contradicts her statement that she is dead. It seems that she has lost the ability to enjoy things and that this occurred to her—according to our knowledge of her history—shortly before suffering the onset of Cotard's nihilistic delusion. The inability to experience enjoyment is, in a way, a synonym for death, because, for Levinas, "life is satisfied sensibility."

The most perfect way of having a relationship with the world and with "otherness" is attained through our fellow human beings. In this relationship, Levinas stresses two things: the face and the caress. The face of "the other" is transcendence personalized and, through it, through the face of the loved one, humanity in its entirety is revealed to me in its helplessness. It is for this reason that the relationship with "the other" is fundamentally ethical, because when the ego discovers the fragility of all humanity in the face of a loved one, it feels inclined to say: "Here I am; I am taking charge of you." Now, the most special and personal way of accessing "the other" is the caress: "The caress is, like contact, sensibility; but the caress transcends sensitivity . . . The caress consists in not imprisoning anything . . . (It) searches, it seeks out. It is not with the intentionality of unveiling, but of searching: it marches toward the invisible. In a certain sense it *expresses* love, but suffers because of its

inability to say it" (Levinas 1969, p. 267). We are unable to provide here a more detailed explanation of the caress but we would like to point out the fact that, if we accept that these two
elements of sensibility—the face of "the other" and the caress by means of which I get close
to him/her—are key to the building of intersubjectivity, we must acknowledge that both are
practically absent in cases of deep depression. For our patient "the others," rather than faces,
are masks and she herself feels like one when she wonders how her children can love an "artificial" mother. The others are not faces for her, and neither is she a face for others (that is,
in terms of Levinas's definition of the face).The entire mystery of the face has disappeared
and both she and her children have been transformed into inanimate beings, into "artifices."
And, if she cannot acknowledge their faces, all the more reason for her not to feel able to caress them, an issue to which she expressly refers when she stresses, time and time again, her
inability to "feel them" as (living) persons when she takes them in her arms.

Depression would thus be the loss of the very insertion of a human being-in-the-world and,
consequently, of any possibility of transcendence. What we have discovered through our analysis of the experiences of a patient with Cotard's syndrome corresponds exactly with what we
found decades ago in a phenomenological analysis of a depressive stupor (Doerr-Zegers and
Tellenbach 1980): the reification and chrematization of the body as a core feature of depression.

We have undertaken a phenomenological analysis of an extreme form of depressive delusion, which appears in Cotard's syndrome. The analysis has allowed us to confirm that depressive delusional experiences are not a mere judgment ("I am a prophet"; "I am persecuted
by the mafia"), but the expression in words of a global change of corporality. The patient does
not only claim to be dead, but she describes a series of bodily sensations from which she
concludes her condition of being dead: "I do not have touch smell nor taste for food . . . " or
"Nothing scares me anymore; nothing makes me angry . . . " or "I do not feel the contact with
objects or people . . . ," etc. From that bodily experience, she comes to the conclusion that she
is dead.

Exactly the opposite happens in schizophrenic delusion, where it is a matter of cognition, of knowledge externalized in a judgment, of deep evidence arising in a rough or
gradual form in the patient and breaking the community sense of truth as identical to reality. Schizophrenic delusions are not a mistake, but a deep truth that has lost its dialogic
character: the other does not participate in the constitution of truth experience (Doerr-
Zegers 1984). Gadamer fully agreed with that in a personal conversation (1985): I asked him
what he thinks about the essence of this strange psychopathological phenomenon and he
answered: "delusion is a lonely truth." And this is what we always observe in schizophrenic
delusions: they emerge either from an endogenous background in the sense of Karl Jaspers's
"primary delusion" (1963), or its appearance is the consequence of a hallucinatory experience ("the voices told me that . . . ") which, given its perceptual character, is not questionably
by the patient. In both cases the other is absent. Instead, in depressive patients, the delusional
statement emerges from a determined way of feeling oneself in the body, which is inserted in
a world whose ontological level is not modified as it occurs in schizophrenic delusions. The
fundamental structures of reality such as identity, space, and time are the same we all share.
Following a distinction posed by Pelegrina 2006, we could say that in depressive delusions,
what is altered is not the "sense" but the "meaning" of things. For the depressive patient as for
the healthy person, things "mean" the same, but their "sense," that is, the way they affect us
for the fulfillment of our lives, is disturbed.

BIBLIOGRAPHY

Abraham K. (1912). "Ansätze zur psychoanalytischen Erforschung und Behandlung manisch-depressiven Irreseins und verwandter Zustände. In J. Cremerius (ed.), *Psychoanalytische Studien zur Charakterbildung. Bd. II. Conditio humana.* Frankfurt: S. Fischer, p. 30.

American Psychiatric Association. (1995). *Diagnostic and Statistical Manual of mental Disorders*, 4th edn, International Version. Washington, DC: American Psychiatric Association.

American Psychiatric Association. (2013). *Diagnostic and Statistical Manual of Mental Disorders*, 5th edn. Arlington, VA: American Psychiatric Association.

Baumann U. and Stieglitz R.D. (1983). *Testmanual zum AMDP-System. Empirische Befunde zur Psychopathologie.* Berlin: Springer.

Baumann U. and Stieglitz R.D. (1989). "Evaluation des AMDP-Systems anhand der neueren Literatur (1983–1987)." *Fortschritte für Neurologie und Psychiatrie.* 57: 357–739.

Bernet R (1993). ¿Una intencionalidad sin sujeto ni objeto? En: De Lerner P (ed.). *El Pensamiento de Husserl en la Reflexión Filosófica Contemporànea.* Ediciones Pontificia Universidad Católica del Perú, pp. 151–180. Lima.

Blankenburg W. (1966). "Die Verselbständigung eines Themas zum Wahn." *Jahrbuch für Psychologie, Psychotherapie und Medizinische Anthropologie* 13: 137.

Blankenburg W. (1991). "Der melancholische Wahn." In *Depressions-Konzepte Heute: Psychopathologie oder Pathopsychologie?* Ch Mund, P Fiedler, H Lang, A Kraus (eds), pp. 95–114. Berlin, Heidelberg, New York, London, Paris, Tokyo, Hong Kong, Barcelona: Springer Verlag.

Charney D. S. and Nelson J. C. (1981). "Delusional and Non-delusional Unipolar Depression: Further Evidence for Distinct Subtypes." *American Jornal of Psychiatry* 338(3): 328–333.

Doerr-Álamos A. and Viani S. (1999). "Personalidad premórbida en los distintos cuadros afectivos." *Acta Psiquiátrica Psicológica de. América Latina.* (Buenos Aires) 45: 41–50.

Doerr-Zegers O. (1979). "Análisis fenomenológico de la depresividad en la melancolía y en la epilepsia." *Actas Luso Españolas de Neurología, Psiquiatría y Ciencias Afines* 7 (2ª Etapa): 291–304.

Doerr-Zegers O. (1984). "Verdad y delirio." *Revista Chilena de Neuropsiquiatría* 22: 193–199.

Doerr-Zegers O. (1993). "Fenomenología de la corporalidad depresiva." *Salud Mental* (México) 16(3): 22–30.

Doerr-Zegers O. (2002). "Fenomenología de la corporalidad en la depresión delirante." *Salud Mental* (México) 25(4): 1–9.

Doerr-Zegers O, et al. (1971). "Del análisis clínico-estadístico del síndrome depresivo a una comprensión del fenómeno de la depresividad en su contexto etio-patogénico." *Rev. Chil. Neuropsiquiat* 10: 17–39.

Doerr-Zegers O. and Tellenbach H. (1980). Differentialphänomenologie des depressiven Syndroms. *Der Nervenarzt* 51: 113–118.

Gadamer, H. G. (1985). Personal communication.

Glatzel J. (1988). "Melancholie und Wahn." In M. Spitzer, F. A. Uehlein, and G. Oepen (eds.), *Psychopathology and Philosophy.* Berlin, Heidelberg, New York, London, Paris, Tokyo: Springer.

Guy W. and Ban T. A. (1983). "The AMDP and NCDEU/BLIPS Systems: Similarities and Differences." *Modern. Problems of Pharmacopsychiatry* 20: 185–192.

Heidegger M. (1927/1963). *Sein und Zeit.* Tübingen: Max Niemeyer Verlag.

Heidegger M. (1962). *Being and Time*. New York, London, Toronto, Sydney, New Delhi, Auckland: Harperperennial Modern Thought.

Hoffet H. (1962). Typologische Gliederung depressiver Syndrome und somatotherapeutische Indikationsstellungen, pp. 5–17. Basel, New York: Karger Verlag.

Hölderlin F. (1961). *Sämtliche Werke*. Frankfurt am Main: Insel Verlag.

Husserl E. (1939/1999). *Erfahrung und Urteil*, Paragraph 6. Hamburg: Felix Meiner Verlag. Translation in English (1975). *Experience and Judgement*. Evanston: Northwestern University Press

Husserl E. (1960). *Cartesian Meditations: An Introduction to Phenomenology*, trans. Dorian Cairns. The Haag: Martinus Nijhoff.

Husserl E. (1962). *Die Krisis der europäischen Wissenschaften und die transzendentale Phänomenologie* (ergänzende Texte). Husserliana VI, Paragraph 303. Den Haag: Martinus Nijhoff. Translation in English (1970). *The Crisis of European Science and the Transcendental Phenomenology*. Evanston: Northwestern University Press.

Husserl E. (1982). "Ideas Pertaining to a Pure Phenomenology and to a Phenomenological Philosophy." *Third book: Phenomenology and the Foundation of the Science*, trans. Kersten F., paragraphs 39 and 53. Dordrecht: Kluwer Academic Publishers.

Husserl E. (1999). *The Essential Husserl. Basic Writings in Transcendental Phenomenology*. Bloomington and Indianapolis: Indiana University Press.

Kraepelin E. (1904). "Vergleichende Psychiatrie." *Zentralblatt für Nervenheilkunde und Psychiatrie* 27: 433–437.

Kraft-Ebbing R. (1874). *Die Melancholie*. Erlangen: Enke Verlag.

Kraus A. (1977). *Sozialverhalten und Psychose Manisch-Depressiver*. Stuttgart: Ferdinand Enke Verlag.

Kraus A. (1990). "Der melancholische Wahn in identitäts-theoretischer Sicht." In *Wahn und Perspektivität*, pp. 66–78. W Blankenburg (ed.). Stuttgart: Ferdinand Enke Verlag.

Levinas E. (1969). *Totality and Infinity. An Essay on Externality*, trans. A. Lingis. Pittsburgh: Duquesne University Press.

Levinas E. (1987). *Time and the Other*, trans. R. A. Cohen. Pittsburgh: Duquesne University Press.

Levinas E. (1993). *El tiempo y el Otro. Barcelona – Buenos Aires—* México: Ediciones Paidós, p. 85.

Ma M., Pirozzi R., Magliano L., Fiorillo A., and Bartoli L. (2007). "Phenomenology and Prognostic Significance of Delusions in Major Depressive Disorder: A 10-Year Prospective Follow-Up Study." *The Journal of Clinical Psychiatry* 68(9): 1411–1417.

Matussek P. (1963). "Psychopathologie II: Wahrnehmung, Halluzination und Wahn." In *Psychiatrie der Gegenwart*. Band I/II. Berlin, Göttingen, Heidelberg: Springer Verlag.

Metzger R. and Wolfersdorf M. (1988). "Suicides Among Patients Treated in a Ward Specializing in Affective Disorders." In H. J. Möller, A. Schmidtke, and R. Welz (eds.), *Current Issues of Suicidology*, pp. 101–108. Berlin, Heidelberg: Springer Verlag.

Ortega y Gasset J. (1974). "Ideas y creencias." In *Obras Completas, Tomo V. Madrid: Revista de Occidente*, 6th edn, pp. 379–405.

Ostergaard S. D., Bertelsen A., Nielsen J., Mors O., and Petrides G. (2013). "The Association Between Psychotic Mania, Psychotic Depression and Mixed Affective Episodes Among 14,529 Patients with Bipolar Disorder." *Journal of Affective Disorders* May, 147(1–3): 44–50.

Pelegrina H. (2006). *Fundamentos antropológicos de la psicopatología*. Madrid: Editorial Polifemo.

Pfeiffer W. M. (1969). "Die Symptomatik der Depression in transkultureller Sicht." In H. Hippius und H. Selbach (eds.), *Das depressive Syndrom*, pp. 151–167. München, Berlin, Wien: Urban & Schwarzenberg.

Pfeiffer W. M. (1971). *Transkulturelle Psychiatrie: Ergebnisse und Probleme*. Stuttgart: Georg Thieme Verlag.

Roose P. R., et al. (1983). "Depression, Delusions, and Suicide." Amercian Journal of Psychiatry 140(9): 1159–1162.

Roth W. (1988). *Die wahnhafte Depression: ein Kontrollgrupenvergleich bei stationären depressiven Patienten*. Medizinische Disssertation. Universität Ulm.

Scharfetter Ch. (1985). *Allgemeine Psychopathologie. 2. überarbeitete Auflage*. Stuttgart, New York: Thieme Verlag.

Shimoda K. (1941) siehe: Shinfuku N. and Ihda S. (1969). "Über den prämorbiden Charakter der endogenen Depression—Immodithymie (später: Immobilithymie) von Shimoda." *Fortschrittr für Neurologie und Psychiatrie* 37: 545–552.

Simkó A. (1983). "Neue Beiträge zur Psychopathologie der Schuld-Wahndepression." *Fortschritte Neurologie und Psychiatrie* 51: 249–253.

Stanghellini, G., et al. (2006). "Typus Melancholicus: Personality Structure and the Characteristics of Major Unipolar Depressive Episodes." *Journal of Affective Disorders* 93: 159–167.

Stanghellini G. and Raballo A. (2007). "Exploring the Margins of the Bipolar Spectrum: Temperamental Features of the Typus Melancholicus." *Journal of Affective Disorders* 93: 159–167.

Sucasas JA (1998). La subjetivación. Hipóstasis y gozo, Anthropos (Barcelona) 176: 38–43.

Tellenbach H. (1961). *Melancholie*. Berlin, Göttingen, Heidelberg: Springer Verlag, 1. Auflage. Translation into English *Melancholy*. (1980) Pittsburgh: Duquesne University Press.

Tellenbach H. (1983). *Melancholie*. Berlin, Heidelberg, New York, Tokyo: Springer Verlag, 4. erweiterte Auflage

Tölle R. und Wefelmeyer T. (1987). "Wahn bei Melancholie." In H. Olbrich (Hrsg.), *Halluzinationen und Wahn*. Berlin, Göttingen, Heidelberg: Springer Verlag.

Winokur G., Scharfetter C., and Angst J. (1985). "A Family Study of Psychotic Symptomatology in Schizophrenia, Schizoaffective Disorder, Unipolar Depression and Bipolar Disorder." *European Archives for Psychiatry and Neurological Sciences* 134: 295–298.

Wolfersdorf M. (1987). "Depressiver Wahn, Todesangst und Suizid." *Suizidprophylaxe* 14: 260–282.

Wolfersdorf M., Steiner B., and Keller F. (1987). "Die wahnhafte Depression: Zur Diagnose und Therapie." *Neuropsychiatrie* 2: 193–203.

Wolfersdorf M., Keller F., and Steiner B. (1989). "Wahnhaft Depressive in der psychiatrischen Klinik: Unterscheiden sich wahnhafte von nicht wahnhaften Depressiven?" *Krankenhausarzt* 62: 722–726.

Wolfersdorf M., Roth W., Steiner B., Keller F., Straub R., and Hole G. (1991). "Psychopathologie und Therapie der wahnhaften Depression." In *Depressions-Konzepte Heute: Psychopathologie oder Pathopsychologie?* Ch Mundt, P Fiedler, H Lang, A Kraus (eds) pp. 115–132. Berlin, Heidelberg, New York, London, Paris, Tokyo, Hong Kong, Barcelona: Springer Verlag.

Wolfersdorf M., et al. (2007). "Delusional Depression and Suicide." *Acta Psychiatrica Scandinavica* 76(4).

World Health Organization. (1992). *The ICD-10. Classification of Mental and Behavioural Disorders*. Geneva: World Health Organization.

Yap P. M. (1965). "Phenomenology of Affective Disorders in Chinese and Other Cultures." In von A. V. S. de Revek and R. Porter (eds.), xxx, pp. 84–105. Ciba Foundation Symposion. London: A. Churchill Ltd.

Zerssen D. v., unter Mitarbeit von Koeller D-M, and Rey E.-R. (1969). "Objektivierende Untersuchungen zur prämorbiden Persönlichkeit endogen Depressiver: Methodik und vorläufige Ergebnisse." In H. Hiipius and H. Selbach (Hrsg.), *Das depressive Syndrom*, pp. 183–205. München, Berlin, Wien: Urban & Schwarzenberg.

Zerssen D. v. (1976). "Der 'Typus melancholicus' in psychometrischer Sicht." *Zeitschrift für Klinische Psychologie und Psychotherapie* 24: 200–220, 305–316.

Zerssen D. v. (1977). "Premorbid Personality and Affective Psychoses." In G. D. Burrows (ed.), *Handbook of Studies on Depression*, pp 79–103. Amsterdam, London, New York: Excerpta Medica.

Zerssen D. v. (1982). "Personality and Affective Disorders." In E. S. Paykel (ed.), *Handbook of Affective Disorders*, pp. 212–228. Edinburgh, London, Melbourne, New York: Churchill, Livingstone.

Zerssen D. v. (1991). "Zur prämorbiden Persönlichkeit des Melancholikers." In Ch. Mundt, P. Fiedler, H. Lang, and A. Kraus (eds.), *Depressionskonzepte Heute: Psychopathologie oder Pathopsychologie?* pp. 76–94. Berlin, Heidelberg, New York, London, Paris, Tokyo, Hong Kong, Barcelona: Springer Verlag.

Zerssen D. v. and Pössl J. (1990). "The Premorbid Personality of Patients with Different Subtypes of an Affective Illness: Statistical Analysis of Blind Assignment of Case History Data to Clinical Diagnoses." *Journal of Affective Disorders* 18: 39–50.

CHAPTER 75

··

PARANOIA

··

PAOLO SCUDELLARI

CLINICAL INVESTIGATION RAISES QUESTIONS ABOUT ANTHROPO-PHENOMENOLOGY

THE theme of "complexity" of scientific "object" has been summarized in the concept of "challenge of complexity" by E. Morin (1985). This concept represents a constant challenge to find the more global and the least mutilating possible meaning in front of multiform observable segments of the world. This concept does not belong to a particular theory or to a particular discipline, but is, rather, a general discourse regarding all of science.

The notion of complexity, in this sense, is not the answer to a problem, but is instead "the *re-awakening towards a problem*: the eruption of an irreducible uncertainty in our knowledge, and the fall of myths of completeness, exhaustiveness, omniscience which, for centuries, like comets, indicated the road of modern science" (Bocchi 1985).

But the positive aspects of the complexity are equally important. These include the growth of a "multidimensional thought" (Morin 1985), which can be described as the awareness that various disciplinary categories are but many aspects of the same reality. These aspects must be distinct but, above all, must be rendered as communicating.

In the face of the perpetual temptation to enclose the world in a pre-established structure, E. Morin, the great expert of epistemological problems, suggests a new approach to knowledge which he calls the "method of complexity." "The method of complexity [as E. Morin clarifies] asks us to think without ever closing the concepts, without ever breaking the closed spheres, in order to re-establish the articulations between that which is disjointed, forcing ourselves to understand the multidimensionality . . . " (Morin 1985: 59).

Unlike the traditional model of scientific knowledge—a neutral and omnipotent model of thought which claims to represent reality as it is—Morin suggests a new profile of knowledge. His model is aware of its own limitations and its temporariness and this new attitude facilitates the discovery of new possibilities and new ways of reading the world.

Psychopathology ought to be located today in the domain of complex science including its specific "challenge of complexity." Psychopathology is in need of exactly that which E. Morin calls "multidimensional thought" which is an interdisciplinary, methodological attitude, or rather, a transdisciplinary attitude.

Within this "complex" perspective, the hermeneutic approach (*comprehensive-interpretative*)—which was originally suggested to psychiatry by Jaspers (1913)—is the only one able to give again freshness and specific originality to psychopathology, after many years of extreme poverty in which the phenomenological approach seemed to have exhausted its task.

At this point, it is important to note that between hermeneutic and phenomenological approaches there is no discontinuity of horizons. In fact, phenomenological philosophy, as a descriptive doctrine of the phenomena of consciousness—phenomena consisting of events *sui generis* that are "experiences of meanings"—is unavoidable inserted in a hermeneutic horizon (Husserl 1913). "Consciousness," according to phenomenology, is steeped with meanings and interprets incessantly, because of its vision of the world, all of the things it encounters. Thus as for hermeneutic thought also for phenomenology *to know is to interpret*.

Our interest is orientated toward the hermeneutic side of psychiatry, which deals with the individual specificity of every clinical history, with the continuity of sense, and with the intrinsic narrative intelligibility of every event, psychopathological or not.

This area of research belongs to a vast hermeneutic horizon and represents a point of intersection of the various points of view of the many other hermeneutic approaches. In such a complex context, psychopathology becomes a meeting area open to other, sometimes very different, methodological perspectives. Those perspectives should be open to narratological analysis as sequential analysis of a text and of its internal coherence, to psychoanalysis as symbolic re-reading and re-narration of a life, as well as to anthropology and phenomenology as an uninterrupted interrogation regarding variety, sense, and project of possible imaginary worlds of human being.

Paranoia and Surroundings: Examining Psychopathology through the Clinical Text

The merit of restoring full psychopathological dignity to the concept of paranoia goes to D. Cargnello (1984), who underlined the specific nature of paranoid delusions and the level of grandiosity that distinguishes them.

The concept of paranoid delusion today appears outdated and almost completely unused in clinical diagnosis, as demonstrated by the DSM-III-R (1987) which consigns to nosography the final, probably uncancelable nosographic residue of a psychopathological notion of such complex history and problematic articulation. The DSM-III-R replaces the term "paranoia" (still present in the DSM-III of 1980) with the term "delusional disorder," characterized by the absence of bizarre aspects. Only in relation to querulous delusion is reference made to the old term "querulous paranoia."

The DSM-IV (1994) completely eradicates the lexical term paranoia for reasons no more clearly motivated than "being theoretically compromised."

The DSM-5 (2014) reinstates the "delusional disorder," attempting to describe it using specifiers: erotomanic type, grandiose type, jealous type, persecution type, somatic type, mixed type, unspecified type.

The nosographic specifiers distinguish between paranoid personality disorder and delusional disorder with paranoid features. A personality disorder is defined as a mental disorder manifested in maladapted thoughts and behaviors expressed pervasively, inflexibly, and permanently, involving the cognitive, affective, and interpersonal spheres of an individual's personality. A delusional disorder is instead delineated by the presence of a delusion for at least a month in the absence of marked compromise in the individual's functioning, with the exception of the impact of the delusion itself and its ramifications. It thus appears to underline a qualitative and quantitative difference: qualitative in that the personological architecture is not considered in subjects with a delusional disorder, while instead the personological architecture pervasively and stably constitutes personality disorders. Quantitative in difference of intensity, which appears to stop at a suspicious and diffident interpretative attitude toward others in paranoid personality disorder, while in delusional disorder it reaches its maximum expression in the creation of erroneous convictions not subject to critical judgment, leading to the altered conception of reality of delusion.

Perhaps under pressure from the need to facilitate diagnosis in order to establish therapies and prognoses, this system often appears to lose the narrative continuity of the individual, explaining any discontinuities in the symptom groupings with the concept of "co-morbidity." These generic "treatment" categories are not intended to substitute "sense" based categories of indicators, and they should coexist in clinical practice. In this way it is possible to identify the paranoid dimension, previously an indistinct continuum from normal to pathological, while also avoiding the risk of being led astray by the patient's own predominant ideas, which in the paranoiac are very striking at first impression and appear to sum up the entire disease, encouraging practitioners to overlook the contexts in which they arise and of which they represent only a superficial manifestation.

Based on the psychopathological ideas of D. Cargnello, who made an extraordinary psychopathological analysis of paranoid delusion ("The Ernst Wagner case," 1984), we understand that the concept of paranoia represents an absolutely indispensable concept in certain psychoses marked by cold grandiosity and a coherent defensive structuring of the delusional Ego.

We also consider this concept to be of great heuristic value, if we bear in mind that paranoid delusions appear to define an area of transition between common thought and delusional thought, in contrast with truly schizophrenic forms in which the disintegration of the personality, the structural disorders of thought, and autistic apragmatism indicate an almost complete detachment from socially accepted thoughts and behavior.

In its various editions the DSM once again reveals a lack of coherent organization of psychopathological thought, marking the current moment of crisis in psychopathology, after reaching the highest expression of its potential around the 1930s. Tracing the history of the concept of "paranoia" means going back to the origins of psychopathological thought, perceiving it once again in its most vital and essential sense.[1]

---

[1] For a detailed critical review of the concept of paranoia and the problems that it raises see Lanteri-Laura, Del Pistoia, and Bel Habib (1985).

A BRIEF HISTORY OF THE CONCEPT
OF PARANOIA

In the VI edition of his treatise (1899), Kraepelin defined paranoid delusion as: "The slow development, due to internal causes, of a lasting and unyielding delusional system, which acts while the lucidity and order of thought, of thinking and acting, remain perfectly intact." It is underlined that the personological structure is always conserved.

French language psychiatry transferred the substance of the Kraepelinian definition into the concept of "chronic systematized delusion," a cornerstone of French psychiatric culture (De Clérambault 1921; Claude and Montassut 1926; Ey and Pujol 1955; Nacht and Racamier 1958; Racamier 1966). The "chronic systematized delusion" was contrasted against the "paranoid" degeneratively evolving forms of schizophrenia.

In the analysis of the forms of "chronic systematized delusion" by the French school there was a failure, in the view of the present author, to adequately underline the aspect that most typifies paranoia: cold narcissistic grandiosity, which had originally been immediately identified, both in France (Dupré 1919, cited by Ferrio 1970) and in Italy (Tanzi 1923).

Returning to the historical vicissitudes of the concept of "paranoia," it should be remembered that over the years it referenced semantic areas of psychopathology of variable extension, which are briefly summarized here, all of them having in common the attempt to describe a personological structure.

From the early 1900s some authors in the French and German schools identified as a basis for paranoid delusions a particular personality structure variously labeled as: "abortive paranoia" (Gaupp 1910), "paranoiac character or structure" (Sauget 1955; Schultz 1955; Kranz 1958), "paranoiac constitution" (Dupré 1919; Delmas 1932), "minor paranoia" (Genil-Perrin 1926), and "paranoiac psychopathology" (Kehrer 1951).

All these labels can be unified under a number of character traits summarized as follows: psycho-rigidity, diffidence, excitability and irritability, extreme susceptibility to criticism, aggression and threats, tendency to overestimate personal talents and qualities, propensity toward feelings of envy and jealousy, tendency toward denigration and dissimulation, and fanatical enthusiasm for pure ideologies as long as these provide a totalizing means for interpreting the world.

Duprè (1919), for example, succinctly summarized the paranoiac constitution in three points: 1) hypertrophy of the Ego, pride, feeling of superiority; 2) moody and diffident temperament with a tendency for hostile misinterpretation of the environment and malevolent interpretation of the deeds of others; 3) error of judgment with permanent and implacable dialectical stance toward unilateral, egotistical, biased judgments.

The classic authors who made a decisive contribution to this issue include Kretschmer (1950). He rendered the concept of "paranoiac character" dynamic by establishing relationships between key life-events, and unified through the concept of "paranoiac development," personality, biography, and delusion.

"At the root of paranoid development," states Kretschmer, "lies a complex of defeat and a tormented sense of guilt which, over decades of evolution of the personality, leads to the establishment, by way of hypercompensation, of a dense system of thoughts of grandeur, hate, and revenge, an unbounded overestimation of the self paired with a sthenic aggressive conception of life."[2]

This now classic approach was recently taken up again with great originality by Kohut (1971, 1978) in terms of "narcissistic pathology."

It is noteworthy that both Kretschmer and Kohut dedicate time to explicating their model using a character from German Romantic literature (inspired by a real historical figure), Michael Kohlhaas, from a story by Kleist dating back to 1826 and seen as an emblematic example of paranoid litigiousness.

The short story provides an amusing description of the insatiable thirst for revenge of the protagonist, the victim of an unusual narcissistic offense.

Kretschmer sees the behavior of the protagonist as a perfect example of the development of delusions of grandeur. Kohut, in turn, sees in Kleist's story the best representation in German literature of the theme of narcissistic anger and implacable litigiousness. His article "Thoughts on Narcissism and Narcissistic Anger" (1978: 125) describes it as follows: "Kleist's novella recounts the destiny of a man who, like Captain Ahab, is trapped in an implacable narcissistic rage. It is the greatest representation in German literature of the motive of revenge, a theme that plays an important part in the national destiny of Germany, whose thirst for revenge after the defeat in 1918 almost arrived at the destruction of the entire western civilization."

By indicating Kleist as one of the authors who (together with Melville in "Moby Dick") best represented the most prominent features of narcissistic pathology, Kohut repeatedly underlines the theme of paranoid grandiosity, interpreting it as a specific defensive strategy that he defines as "chronic defensive grandiosity" or "defensive narcissism."

The present authors in turn also underline how the sphere of paranoid personalities hinges on the counterphobic attitude of systematic opposition and anticipatory vengefulness, all powered by an inexhaustible megalomaniacal drive.

Indeed, ever since the time of Kraepelin, there was a perception of the diagnostic problem of differentiating between paranoid delusions and paraphrenic delusions, in which the fabulatory-megalomaniacal core always emerges centerstage. Kraepelin himself appears to have repeatedly considered the possibility of positioning them very close to the fantastic paraphrenias, sensing the latent megalomaniacal nucleus, often inaccessible to observation, present in this pathology. As will be seen, this issue is not irrelevant from the psychopathological and phenomenological perspective, considering how scarcely the paranoiac imagination has been investigated. In order to discern the paranoiac imagination and its temporality from paraphrenic delusions, Callieri and Maci (2008), who underline particular operative modalities of memory, characterized the paranoiac with temporarily displaced reconstructions, and frequent omissions that impede the natural chaining together of events, despite the evocations of individual elements appearing largely precise and accurate. This probably derives from a wider operation of selective attention that strives for a unitary

---

[2] Hypersensitivity to offenses (the so-called "asthenic pole") is the common trait, according to Kretschmer, of these personological structures, and this very particular susceptibility stimulates pathologically aggressive reactions (the "sthenic pole"), with diverse clinical expressions (querulous delusion, delusional jealousy, erotomanic delusion). The combination in different proportions of these typological characteristics leads to "delusional sensitivity developments" (self-referential delusions of a persecutory nature) or "grandiose developments" (including the classic querulous delusion).

and exhaustive knowledge of the world, often repetitive but never fleeting. In paraphrenia in this sense a larger role appears to be played by interpretation, with the construction of more ephemeral and fleeting meanings that take different directions from one moment to another.

In summary, in the sphere of chronic psychoses, paranoid delusions appear to lie entirely outside of the schizophrenic range, almost defining a form of transition between common thought and deluded thought. For this reason above all, paranoia represents a crucial node not so much for clinical practice but rather for psychopathological reflection and psychiatric epistemology, lying as it does between common thought and delusion, between personality structure and symptom.

Paranoia between Personality Structure and Symptom

All the authors that have dealt with the issue of paranoia agree in identifying the aspects of tenacious and fanatical combativeness that characterize the personological structure of the paranoiac, to the extent that it has even been called "delusional action" (Serieux and Capgras 1902). Its psychological identikit is defined with great precision by Tanzi (Tanzi and Lugaro 1923). This author, considered by the present author to be undervalued, makes the paranoiac into a sort of champion of idealism, identifying the characteristics of narcissistic grandiosity that locate him, taking into account the necessary historical perspective, within the psychopathological area that today is defined as typical of the "narcissistic personality disorders."

Tanzi's identikit is as follows:

Wild independence of character, misanthropy, pride, dogmatism, fanaticism "both in religion and irreligiousness" ... The delusions of paranoiacs are not rooted in a defect in intelligence, but rather in the singularity of a character which has essential elements that include marked selfishness, an extremely high opinion of the self, a diffident attitude towards others, an expansive and militant sense of mysticism, a chivalrous spirit of active protection or passive devotion to an amorous ideal, a sensitive intolerance of injustice even when imaginary ... and above all a rare tenacity and constancy of driving sentiments that give direction to a tirelessly combative behaviour.

The sensitive aspects that permeate the character of the paranoiac and that trigger his fanatical litigiousness are summed up by Tanzi as:

By reconstructing his past the paranoiac finds traces of continuous, widespread, insuperable insidiousness even in the smallest childhood conflicts, an unjust castigation, a toy that broke as soon as it was purchased, an excessively hot drink, favouritism in the marks awarded at school, in the omission of an invitation ... But over the long term the persecuted becomes in turn the active and obdurate persecutor. He makes unfounded accusations, appeals to courts of law with petitions and denunciations, not obtaining satisfaction he disdains from referring further to the courts that are seen as weak, partial, or corrupted by his persecutors; finally he decides to take justice into his own hands.

(Tanzi and Lugaro 1923: 738, 749, 750).

The characteristic imprint of paranoiac action is that it is essentially social action. Underlying the paranoid delusional experience Tatossian recognizes "the calling into question of the identity of the social role" and tellingly notes that the persecuted paranoiac essentially calls more for the confession of the aggressor rather than the interruption of the aggression, the jealous paranoiac requests more the acknowledgment of guilt by the other rather than his love, and the querulous paranoiac calls for a *just* sentence rather than financial compensation.

The area of narcissistic pathology was mentioned in relation to the paranoid personality. It is no accident that Kohut himself identifies in "narcissistic rage" the driving element of these vindictive paranoid inclinations. In an article in 1978 Kohut writes:

> The most horrific human destructiveness [is found] under the form of ordering and organizing activities in which the destructiveness of the actors is amalgamated with the absolute conviction of their greatness . . . The need for revenge, to settle an insult, to compensate a damage by any means, and an implacable constriction to pursue all these ends . . . are the characteristics of narcissistic rage. In narcissistic personalities and paranoiacs, extreme sadism, the adoption of a policy of pre-emptive attack, the need for revenge and the desire to transform a passive experience into an active one are the remedies by which an individual, inclined towards shame, responds to situations that could potentially provoke shame.

(Kohut 1978: 145, 146)

The same author identifies more precisely the problem of narcissistic pathology as an oscillation between shame and rage, and when analyzing the concept of "chronic narcissistic rage," touches on the issue of transition between paranoid personality structure and delusional symptomology. The shame/rage oscillation closely resembles the oscillation between the two asthenic/sthenic poles, within which, according to Kretschmer, the whole range of paranoid delusional developments are arrayed.

B. Callieri and M. Maci confirm the role of shame as the greatest injury within narcissistic vulnerability, and to the narcissistic ideal. Shame, in all its gradations, can be caused by interaction with the other, with his gaze, which may be perceived as directed to the most hidden and least tolerated psychic world, experienced as a sometimes unbearable attack on the individual. Well aware of this experience, Nietzsche wrote "Who is evil? He who wants to shame me" (122).

The theme of shame thus runs through various existential dimensions of paranoia, and can develop through interactions with the other, developing under his gaze; an invasive, intrusive gaze that easily introduces persecutory feelings. As Callieri and De Vincentis showed, the meaning of life and the dynamics of the gaze present spatial peculiarities: through the gaze *the other* expands, coming to be where it falls, lending the capacity to grasp and violate the most profoundly private sphere. On the other hand, shame can be experienced in the most exclusive relationship with the ideal of the Ego, starting from emotions or thoughts that do not fit easily with the image that we would like to present to ourselves, and be recognized as by others.

As Rossi Monti (2009) underlined with reference to Meissner's idea, *shame*, compared to the more circumscribed *guilt*, assumes a global nature, because it is addressed toward a global image of self, exposed to self-judgment: "From this experience of shame the paranoiac emerges with its inversion into dysphoric anger, in marked irritability and haughty suspiciousness . . ."

According to Kohut, "chronic narcissistic rage" is the expression of the insistence of exercising total and omnipotent control over the subject, in response to an episode of shame, experienced as an uncancelable stain that spoils and undermines a reality experienced narcissistically, in the pure reflection of the self.

Someone who has suffered a narcissistic injury of this type "has no rest until he cancels the offence of the one who dared to oppose, disagree, or even simply outshine the subject." Narcissistic rage, when it expands and becomes chronic, tends to lead to loss of the limitations inherent to the power of self, which will tend to increasingly attribute its own failings and weaknesses to the malevolence and corruption of external "objects" that do not collaborate. This sets up a self-feeding persecutory cycle that encourages the rage and narcissistic omnipotence. Chronic narcissistic rage is defined by Kohut as "one of the worst torments of the human psyche, both in the initial endogenous and preliminary form of protest and spitefulness, and in the exteriorized form of isolated vengeful acts or carefully planned vendettas."

To better clarify the words of Kohut it can be added that the argumentative tactic, embraced within "chronic rage," is constantly at work to anticipate and counterphobically defer the ever looming persecutory anxiety. So much confrontational effort, centered on vengeful action, is much more easily observable compared to the submerged world of the paranoid imagination, which is consequently insufficiently investigated. This explains the reductive (even if appropriate) label of "delusion in action" (Serieux and Capgras 1902).

Sooner or later this type of anticipatory defense will fail in its attempt to maintain sufficient distance between the phobogenic and persecutory figures that he is trying to defend against. It is for this reason that the counterphobic strategy of chronic rage, tirelessly striving to destroy the phobic ghosts that assail the paranoiac world, is in any case always imbued with anxiety and implies a regime of instability between two diametrically opposite poles: megalomaniacal defense and persecutory risk.

For Cargnello the persecutory urgency and megalomaniac urgency are two poles between which the psychopathology of paranoia oscillates. "Persecution and grandiosity usually appear together. They are like a sound and its echo, like an object and its reflected image, like the backwards and forwards of a pendulum . . . " (from the play *Wahn* by E. Wagner, in Cargnello 1984).

This unstable system is implicit in incurable paranoiac vengefulness, an oscillating self-reflecting movement which endlessly presents the two opposite and specular faces of the paranoiac world.

For Callieri and Maci, the megalomaniacal core of the paranoiac, with his quest for ever higher ideals of justice, the pursuit of ambitious and distant political projects, religious faith experienced to its maximum, offers the paranoiac not only the possibility of hiding his experiences of shame, but also of seeking out a social role that compensates him for experiences of inferiority and limitation. The paranoiac's battle assumes an ever more epic value, against human limitations and the crumbling of his identity if faced with the multitude.

These authors thus consider it no accident to see the manifestation of a delusional drift around forty to forty-five years, a period of life according to Del Pistoia (1985): "In terms of experience of the world, this age brings awareness of a change in horizon after completing 'life's journey' . . . But it is also above all the age in which future time loses the unending uncertainty it had at twenty years . . . " It is an age of taking stock, which can result in narcissistic injuries or in simpler anxieties of finiteness, including that of mortality which the advancing years present.

Delle Luche (cited by Callieri and Maci) notes: "In the world of the paranoiac there is no place for grey normality, for habit, the common, the anonymous, in final analysis for accepting the human condition of finiteness. He inhabits the totipotent dimension of the un-limited, literally, accepting to position himself outside the world and outside of time, in the universe of fetishistic constructions simultaneously real and imaginary."

PARANOIA BETWEEN PASSION AND REASON

Referring to the contradistinction between passion and reason in the paranoiac world, Callieri and Maci deny the possibility of an Aut-Aut logic instead, with these interweaving and interfacing in a constant co-presence of ideo-affective aspects. A strong emotional charge is recognized as the *primum movens* in the history of the development of paranoia. It is followed by a phase in which delusional ideas of explanation or correction are hypothetical in nature, and the delusion appears barely structured, often accompanied by experiences of anxious self-referentiality. A possible evolution thus appears that of structured delusional ideation, in which "everything is explained." During this transition there is an ever increasing gap between the affective aspect, not acknowledged but suffered and the source of a search for acknowledgment, and the rational aspect, comprising an excessively simple logic in its *blinding luminosity* while unknowingly always remaining too emotionally polarized.

The contribution of Rossi Monti (2009) on the genesis of the evolutionary stages of para-noiac delusion underline how, after the establishment of the delusion, there can be a main-tenance stage of the same, which will become ingrained as a fundamental protective shield around a "secret and timeless emotional strongbox" containing painful and unacknowl-edged affective elements.

A root of pathos is thus identified in pre-reflective consciousness, which Callieri and Maci, following in the footsteps of Rossi Monti, describe: "It is the sensation of the zone of shadow that surrounds any noetic orientation in the world; and it is from this zone and this time that the proto-nucleus of delusion takes form, which "through interactions" with the external world and with cognitive/intellectual elements, will become the true nucleus of the delusion." But the noetics of the paranoiac world is unusual: elements of similarity can be identified between the noetics of a scientist and that of a paranoiac, in that "neither looks freely at the world, but instead the facts that come to their knowledge are already perceived in a certain way, and are thus *ideational*."

This lens through which knowledge is filtered, limiting the field to certain elements, comprises selective attention and inattention, differentiating the scientist and the paranoiac from the common man. However, the paranoiac, unlike the scientist, has a disowned affec-tive pole, which bends and distorts the observed reality to its need for control and totalitari-anism, lending it omnipotent and inhuman features.

The metaphoric area of this regime of antithesis and defensive opposition appears to be effectively described in the words dedicated by Durand (1963) to the so-called "Diurnal Regime of the Imagination" and to its typical "Schizomorphic structures": "Here the imagination appears marked by a pre-occupation for the recovery of lost power, of a fitness degraded by a fall . . . Ascension is imagined *against* falling and light *against* shadows . . . Light has the tendency to become a lightning bolt or sword and ascension to trample the defeated adversary."

Many aspects of the paranoiac imagination and its delusional transformations appears to draw on this register of confrontation and struggle, of fanatical combativeness and absolute and totalizing idealism (Muscatello et al. 1985a).

ON THE PARANOIAC "IMAGINARY WORLD"

Paranoid delusions, in their thematic multiplicity and their stark and undeniable formal homology, pose a major phenomenological problem. Even the most acute analysts and psychopathologists all appear to align themselves with an approach that could be defined essentially as behavioral, when they delineate the imaginary world of paranoiacs. The authors concentrate mainly on the tenacious and fanatical combativeness of the paranoiac, underlining above all the typical behaviors of querulous mania, implacable intolerance, antagonistic grandiosity, a particular aggressiveness that frequently culminates in unpredictable "escalation to action." As already seen, the paranoiac has also been convincingly defined by Serieux and Capgras (1902) as "delusion in action." More recently Racamier (1966) spoke of paranoiacs in terms of "ghostly silence."

What we do know is that paranoid delusions are those that undergo the longest and most complex incubation. Tanzi states: "As regards the internal elaboration of their delusions, paranoiacs do not usually recount these to anyone, because pride in their beliefs makes them unwilling to reveal their shadows."

Paranoiacs, in terms of both pathological personality and delusional phenomenology, appears to be distinguished by the unusual aridity of their imaginary world. Is this aridity genuine? Or a dissimilation that draws a curtain of reticence around the imaginary world?

In the face of this enigma there are numerous questions that phenomenologists can and must ask themselves, and there are many paths that they need to follow in order to seek answers. For example, an effort might be made to establish what fantasy is hidden behind the apparent aridity of a querulous manic behavior. It appears likely that there would be a highly articulated imaginary world around the issue of justice, a unique phantom of justice, a particularly radical form of idealization of the law. And one might query: what ascetic and chivalrous dream lies behind an erotomanic delusion? Or what dazzling mythologizing complexity is hidden in the core of a genealogical delusion? And so on . . .

A phenomenology of inner life should be able to grasp the anthropological aspect of a delusional development with all its latent narrative and communicative possibilities.

However, neither traditional psychiatry nor psychoanalysis have provided answers to any of these questions, though fundamental from a psychopathological phenomenological perspective.

In reality, only an interpretation of the imaginary world and some if its recurrent metaphors could illuminate certain paranoid behaviors (querulous manic and others, including those with "escalation to action"), which so often appear unpredictable and inexplicable.

Cargnello adopts this approach in the analysis of the case of Ernst Wagner, "the paranoiac exterminator," and manages to open a crack into his megalomaniac imaginary world through an analysis of his drama *Wahn* (Delusion), which remained unpublished in Italy for many years, only emerging in 1984 as an appendix to Cargnello's essay. The second act of *Wahn* in particular allows us to uncover the secret nucleus of the paranoid nature of the author.

As Cargnello specifies, the epiphany of unconfined grandiosity and unlimited power appears when the protagonist of the play, the paranoiac Ludwig, identifies himself with the grandiose historical figure of Nebuchadnezzar and his megalomaniac fantasies of dominion and "Gulliverization" of the world.

Cargnello's phenomenological analysis insightfully recalls the considerations of E. Canetti (1960) on the relationship between paranoia and power, and focuses very revealingly on the paranoiac imagination of E. Wagner, which provides some access to the background to his exterminatory gesture (Muscatello et al. 1985b).

THE ERNST WAGNER CASE

On the eve of the First World War an obscure primary school teacher, Ernst Wagner, committed a double atrocity: he stabbed his wife and four young children to death in their sleep, and then went into the town where he had taught a long time previously, Muhlhausen. Here he set a large number of houses on fire and killed nine inhabitants with his pistol while wounding various others more or less seriously.

This massacre was not the result of a sudden madness, but instead the conclusion of a plan for revenge that had gradually been developing over a period of more than ten years. He was convinced that a sin he committed (libidinous deeds with animals) was written on his face and that everybody was aware of his secret unnatural habits. Soon the suspicion of being persecuted, first by some and then by all the inhabitants of the town transformed into certainty and ultimately in fanatical, intransigent conviction. He decided to avenge himself for this.

Quickly recognized as mentally ill and committed for life to a mental asylum, he became the subject of incessant study by a great clinical therapist of the times, Robert Gaupp (1910), who defined him as paranoiac, dedicating much of his research work to the case. Ever since, this famous case has been widely discussed in central European psychiatric treatises, even the most recent.

Ernst Wagner was well-educated and highly intelligent. Above all he had a very high conception of self: a writer since his early years, little by little he ended up proclaiming himself the greatest living German playwright. In his final years there emerged a typical querulous manic delusion, focused on the writer F. Werfel, who he accused of having plagiarized important parts of his work. The dispute even had judicial developments.

Among his works certainly the most outstanding is the play *Wahn* (Delusion), composed in 1921, but published in a scientific monograph only in 1968. With obvious identification between the author and the main protagonist, the plot traces out the affairs of King Ludwig II of Bavaria, who committed suicide by drowning. It is an extraordinary example of literary "staging" of madness, and the play is a unique document in psychiatric case studies through the ages: it had never previously happened that a person affected by a delusion of persecution and grandeur described, with undeniable precision and depth, another case of delusional persecution and grandeur.

As Cargnello writes, "there is no question that in Ernst Wagner's work delusion becomes "drama" or rather "tragedy": no longer merely a clinical manifestation, but an oppressive or even tragic expression of how essentially deficient or distorted interpersonal relations are expressed. . . . Only exceptionally authentic documents, like those provided by the diary annotations of Strindberg, or the play *Wahan* by Ernst Wagner give us an idea of what the experience of a *delusional existence* really means."

In his essay dedicated to this play, D. Cargnello, in addition to providing an unsurpassable profile of the paranoiac world that we in turn are trying to track down, he also believed he had revealed this passionate interweaving of madness and literature.

The essay can be read and interpreted on at least three levels:

1) The play *Wahn* (Delusion), unknown to the public and known only to a narrow circle of specialists and refined experts on the great German tradition of psychopathology, including among others Danilo Cargnello.
2) The biography of E. Wagner, the paranoid playwright and author of this extraordinary text, which offers a dramatically personal interpretation of the delusional experience of the author reflected in the protagonist of the play, the paranoiac and suicidal Ludwig of Bavaria. The story of E. Wagner is also closely interwoven with the history of psychopathology and in particular with the definition of the concept of "paranoia," to the point that the term "Gaupp's Paranoia" is used with reference to Gaupp, a psychiatrist and expert on Wagner, whose case he studied throughout his life.
3) The third and most important level is D. Cargnello's illuminating commentary, which attempts to reconstruct, through rare period documents and enthusiastic analyses of the text of the play, a phenomenological profile of paranoia.

There are numerous possible connections between these levels of interpretation, with the text containing multiple metalevels, but certainly the most important is the possibility of seeing the drama of the madness of Ludwig of Bavaria through the eyes and interpretation of the paranoiac Wagner, who serves as a sort of reflecting conscience for the protagonist of the play, the paranoiac Ludwig.

E. Wagner described his work as follows (cited by Cargnello 1984):

> The play *Delusion* could only have been written by me. One who has seen all infernos and horrors. . . . I too have been to hell, *in the centre of the hottest of the fiery pits*. For this reason in the play I talk of one who, even if seated high on a throne, is nevertheless a companion in suffering. He lived in equal torment and damnation! *Drama of lived experienced*? Yes. *Drama of destiny*? Yes. . . . I did not write lightly but with seriousness, with bleeding seriousness. Anyone who reads me must know this.

This extraordinary overlap between the author's world and the world of his character induces Cargnello to speak of a "human document unique in its kind. In it a victim of delusional persecution-grandeur speaks of another victim of persecution-grandeur. A paranoiac describing somebody he considers to be paranoiac!"

The Wagner/Ludwig reflection represents the prototype for all the reflections and symmetries that emerge within the play. Fundamental among the proliferation of Ludwig's "doubles" are the specular transpositions of Ludwig/Frederick of Prussia and Ludwig/ Nebuchadnezzar, delusional incarnations of two extreme poles, between which the psychological structure of paranoia oscillates: persecutory phase and megalomaniacal phase. "Persecutory delusion and delusion of grandeur," says a character in the play, "they usually appear together. They are like the sound and its echo, like the object and its reflected image, like the backwards and forwards of a pendulum . . . "

Wagner also adds, through the figure of the psychiatrist in his appearance in the third act, that "the delusion of persecution is the face and the *essence/* the delusion of grandeur is the mask and the *appearance*" (III, 2). Here the author's phenomenological analysis reveals the modality of the dialectic between persecutory phase and megalomaniacal phase, the hinge of which, binding and keeping the two poles together, according to Cargnello is a profound modification that occurred in the existential structure of the With-Being (*Mit-Daisen*).

Picking up on Binswanger's observations described in *Schizophrenie* (1957), Cargnello sustains that when the world of peers (*Mit-Welt*), represented in the play by the King of Prussia, becomes oppositional, humiliating, and distressing, then the Being attempts to abandon this world to take refuge in its "own" world (*Eigen-Welt*) which, in contrast to the lowness of humiliation, rises up to the heights of megalomaniacal grandiosity.

Nevertheless, the attempt to abandon the world of peers is always a failure since, as Heidegger (1927) teaches, the With-Being is an inescapable structure of Being: hiding in a personal world, in terms of both physical isolation and in terms of increasing delusional rigidity and consequent break down of dialogical communication with the Other, is always a case of coexistence, defective as it may be, and it can never be an existence outside of coexistence. Otherwise stated, isolation only exists in reference to those from whom isolation is desired and, precisely on the strength of this relation, the others are in all cases present within the isolation in the defective manner of being at a distance. So, Ludwig/ Nebuchadnezzar is such only as a grandiose and solipsistic mask, contrasting with the persecutory dialectic Ludwig/Frederick of Prussia. The grandiose identification only exists in reference to the persecutory anxiety and right from the start this thwarts the aim of the megalomaniacal narcissistic identification of Ludwig with Nebuchadnezzar. It is precisely because Ludwig/Nebuchadnezzar cannot exist without Ludwig/Frederick of Prussia that the persecutory phase and megalomaniacal phase are intrinsically tied to each other, the second as echo and response to the existential intention of the first.

Structured as symmetrical and unstable counterpositions, that dramatize the counterpositions between Ludwig's two main "doubles," the persecutory and the megalomaniacal, the text concludes with the suicide of the protagonist, a suicide that expresses the final resolution of the two antagonistic forces in play. This appears to occur at the moment in which megalomania and persecution merge into a single gesture, that of suicide, the only gesture of defeat that can be transformed by megalomaniacal idealization.

As Balzac wrote in "Lost Illusions," "suicide is the effect of a feeling that might be called, if you like, self esteem in order not to confuse it with the word honour. The day in which a man disdains of himself, the moment in which the reality of life contrasts with his hopes he kills himself, thus rendering homage to the society in the face of which he does not want to remain stripped of his virtues and splendour."

At an extreme point in his development the defensive position of paranoia, hinged on narcissistic grandeur, can implode into psychosis, through the uncovering of an irremediable loss of self esteem, in the encounter with one's own Ego irremediably injured in honor, impoverished, and stripped of every illusion. And the moment of the specular encounter with the self is the mortal confrontation with one's own incurable imperfection. Now the mirror remains the final object. The final medium that reflects a shame and imperfection that can no longer be avoided. *So the figure reflected back from the surface of the mirror presents itself as a double or twin that we do not like and do not love and which, symmetrically does not love us.* Here appears the image of the twin "enemy" (Girard 1972), and the mirror becomes the medium for a relationship with one's own Ego charged with violence and death, like the theatre of an implacable duel with our own lookalike-enemy. In this case the specular double inevitably transforms into a "persecutory double." The poet George Trakl (1919) expressed the latent persecutory nature of the "specular double" and the twin enemy as: "From the illusory void of a mirror, / slow and uncertain, / from darkness and horror / emerges a face: Cain! / Imperceptible rustle of the curtain, / from the window the Moon looks into a void / I remain alone with my assassin."

This is also the psychotic theme analyzed by Otto Rank (1914) in literature and folklore: the autonomization of the specular alter ego. The recurrent theme analyzed by Rank is that of the appearance of a double which can equally be a specular image or shadow, which suddenly becomes autonomous and persecutes the protagonist, establishing a total and unchallenged dominion over him. The story can end in a duel in which protagonist kills the double and finds himself mortally wounded. Or it might happen that the double, as in the novel of the same name by Dostoyevsky, takes over the identity of the protagonist driving him mad, behaving, in the author's own words, "like a burning mirror." Or, as in the play *Delusion*, it happens that the lookalike-enemy, identifiable in the portrait-mirror of the Prince of Prussia that looms in persecution over every scene, drives the protagonist Ludwig to suicide.

The relationship of reflection/identification between Ludwig and Frederick of Prussia, always present on the scene as a large portrait with which Ludwig constantly dialogues, thus presents itself as an implacable struggle between duelling/lookalikes which concludes, as in the mythology of the double, in the suicide of the protagonist. The grandiose paranoiac shell worn like armor by the character Ludwig, expressed in ambitious fantasies of ascension (refuge in his high castles) and of omnipotent control over the world (the delusional transformation into the figure of Nebuchadnezzar, autocrat and warrior), should be considered as the extreme refuge from persecutory dread, the extreme megalomaniacal effort to escape the symmetrical violence of one's own double.

The operation is delusional and governed by the principle of the instability of the roles, and so does not succeed. It is thrown back hyperbolically amplified onto the protagonist who ends up subjected to the law of "an eye for an eye" advanced and triggered by his own megalomaniacal violence. He becomes, so to speak, the sacrificial victim.

E. Wagner's play appears to stage the tragic contest of paranoia in the most direct way: that of the unstable reversibility of roles. Ludwig's encounter with the portrait-mirror of the Prince of Prussia puts into motion an oscillating movement of persecutory dread and megalomaniacal retaliation that culminates in a grandiose fantasy of revenge and destruction of his eternal enemy/persecutor, the Prussian Prince.

The megalomaniacal apex is reached in the delusional creation of another mirror image of the protagonist, that of Nebuchadnezzar, and in the hallucinatory fantasy of dominion over a world governed from above, "Gulliverized" and magically manipulable. As Cargnello writes, "the epiphany of unconfined grandiosity and unlimited power appears when Nebuchadnezzar comes onto the scene (or rather Ludwig disguised as Nebuchadnezzar), transformed by his illusions of grandeur."[3]

However, the unstable oscillating game of the two figures of the paranoia, a game of endlessly rising stakes, contains within it, within its definition, a possible exit from its hyperbolic track: the final challenge, the final victory, and the final megalomaniacal disguise to face the persecutory challenge appears to be suicide. We can try asking ourselves why.

Suicide appears to be a sort of short-circuit between the two poles of the reflection: persecuted and persecutor end up reciprocally catching each other, merging into a single entity, that of the suicidal figure, thus repeating the path defined in the mythology of the "double." As already seen, in the duel with his lookalike the protagonist always finds himself mortally wounded.

In the mythology of the "double" we find a prefiguration of one of the latent psychopathological expressions of paranoia, its suicidal expression.

THE METAPHOR OF THE COURT OF LAW IN A CASE OF QUERULOUS MANIA

In a case of querulous mania-type paranoia that came under our observation, it was possible to identify the two antagonistic and specular figures of the paranoid world: persecution and grandeur. This patient gave us insight into the surprising imaginary background to a behavior typical of querulous mania (linked to themes of entitlement in the division of a hypothetical inheritance). Only through extended observation was it possible to identify an extensive multifocal delusion of which the querulous mania represented the culminating manifestation.

This case appeared to answer an exquisitely phenomenological question that we had already asked ourselves: what singular phantom of justice is hidden behind the apparent aridity of querulous manic behavior?

The world of patient S. appeared to be organized around a grandiose scenic "metaphor" that shone a beam of light into his internal world and on his structures of meaning. One *topos* of his imaginary world was the Court of Law.

During one interview the patient S. provided a distressing and visionary image of the court and the rituals celebrated there, depicting a place more metaphysical than real, a context that evoked simultaneously the altar and the gallows. The following is an extract from the transcription of S. referring to the picture he had invented of the court and the trial.

> The most important event that can be staged in a courtroom is a trial. In this case the mundane routine work that distinguishes much of the court's activity is elevated and becomes a rite. It

---

[3] The world of Nebuchadnezzar appears to condense in particular scenic metaphors of power and control. These are: the statue of Fame, which grips a bunch of glittering threads that radiate out over the world; a megaphone that amplifies and spreads the sovereign's commands everywhere; a movable mirror that like the lens of a telescope allows visual inspection of every corner of the world. The extreme control exercised by these instruments coincides with a sort of miniaturization of the world which renders gigantic the sovereign power of the one who controls it. This is the "Gulliverization" effect implicit in certain visual fantasies of dominion.

is a rite of roles and opposing strategies: on one side is the counsel for the prosecution, on the other the counsel for the defence.

The scene is awe-inspiring. In the centre of the predella is the court judge, who can transform when required into executioner. Seated to his right are the barristers nominated by the court, dressed in capes and military style headwear. To his left is the court disposed in balconies. Before him, sometimes shielded with a grid, are the accused. There is frequent altercation: the opposite parties spy on each other, study each other's moves, offend each other. This makes the trial a tense struggle requiring a large room with numerous bolt holes represented by the surrounding rooms and passages. The trial is distinct from other rituals of public life because there is always a guilty party who for justice or destiny, is also always condemned.

What we see is a grandiose counterphobic fantasy, used by S. to subtract himself from the persecutory risk of identification with the guilty party ("who for justice or destiny, is also always condemned"). The patient identified the court as the ideal place for the transfer of both his grandiose vengefulness and his latent persecutory anxiety.

His scenographic reconstruction, which resembles an altarpiece, is dominated by a symmetrical pyramidal structure, the vertex of which is represented by the solemn figure of a judge, "who can transform when required into executioner. Seated to his right are the barristers elected by the court, dressed in capes and military style headwear. To his left is the court disposed in balconies. Before him, sometimes shielded with a grid, are the accused."

This petrified paranoid scenography is imbued with signs of anxiety and suspicion that compromise its rigorous symmetry. In this room, says S., there are "numerous bolt holes represented by the surrounding rooms and passages." These passages and escape routes, are the scenographic rendering of the persecutory anxiety of S.[4]

In reality, in the trial celebrated in this courtroom, *de re tua agitur*.

The subtle persecutory atmosphere perceived in the courtroom scenography is emblematically summed up in S.'s final words. "The judge can transform when required into executioner" and "the accused, for justice or destiny, is also always condemned."

The Chance and Destiny evoked by S. as factors that loom indecipherably over the outcome of the trial, also represent the ultimate and most uncontrollable risk to which the two protagonists in the trial are exposed, the judge and the accused. The pair of opposites, by *Chance*, or *Destiny* can always invert in polarity: the judge can become the accused, the executioner can transform into the executed. This is the source of the sinister unease that circulates in the court during the enigmatic trial.

There is a symmetrical and reversible relationship between punisher and punished. In reality Chance and Destiny pair the two opposing figures of the courtroom in a sort of "malign symmetry" that implies the possible reversibility of the roles. The two figures that represent the persecutory and megalomaniacal aspects of the paranoid world are fatally bonded together. They are "like a sound and its echo, like an object and its reflected image, like the backwards and forwards of a pendulum . . .," to repeat the words cited by Danilo Cargnello

---

[4] Following Kafka ("The Trial," 1935) the trial has also become a literary topos. In one of the chasms of the court building in which the protagonist is to be tried is the studio of the painter Titorelli, specialized in portraits of judges. Here in the eyes of the protagonist Josef K., the Goddess of Justice depicted in a large canvas undergoes a slow metamorphosis, transforming into the Goddess of the Hunt. The trial is thus the place where the Goddess of Justice is deformed by the wildest and most persecutory arbitrariness that transforms her into an enigmatic Goddess of the Hunt.

(1984) regarding the Wagner case. Looking closely, the opposing and specular figures of the judge and the accused present the psychopathological theme of the "double" as persecutory lookalike. Within the logic of the "double," the judge has always also been the accused, and the punisher has always been destined to be punished.

This inescapable truth, beyond any illusionistic play on opposites, is revealed down to the smallest details in a short story by Kafka ("In the Penal Colony" (1919)), which can almost be considered the model parable for paranoiac existence. This story tells of a torture instrument which is also a capital punishment machine. It is designed like a hoeing device and with countless needles it carves the reason for the condemnation into the body of the condemned, before stabbing him to death. The accused only learns toward the end of his torment, like a revelation, the commandment that he has infringed.

At the end of the story the official and custodian of the machine, who is also judge and executioner, condemns himself to its judgment in order to illustrate its exemplary operation. The commandment that the executioner has carved into his back is: "Be just!"

The conclusion of the Kafkian parable lies in the final description of the lifeless body of the official: "He remained as he had been in life; there was not the minimal sign of the promised redemption; what all the others had found in the machine, the official had not found . . ."

Every expectation of redemption and catharsis that the official, like a paranoiac, invested in the justice system, here finds its definitive failure, a failure that we would define as ontological. As Cargnello underlines, in delusion "the presence no longer develops, it can only turn in and torment itself . . . without a true tomorrow, without a true future, reduced as it is to an eternal, sterile, and, above all, *inauthentic repetition.*"

PARANOIA: PROGNOSIS OR DESTINY?

The crucial question we posed is as follows: can the paranoid style of existence, in its repetitiveness, its faithfulness to delusional "truth," converge with the concept of "destiny"? And how distant (or close) is this word from the lexical meaning of prognostic inevitability?

Anthropo-analytic psychopathology cuts dazzlingly right across all the clinical-nosographic tradition of Kraepelinian memory, the latter fixated on the iron hard and reductive concept of "prognostic destiny," but in its way paying homage to "destiny" as such, paying its debt to "destiny," through the key concepts of "anthropological disproportion" (Binswanger), of "disanimating omnipotence" (Racamier 1966), of "failed existence" (Binswanger 1959), as markers of a specific anthropological style.

The Danish philosopher S. Kierkegaard (1844, 1849) anticipated and clarified in an incredible conceptual synthesis the two key concepts underlined above, "disanimating omnipotence" and "anthropological disproportion." In two extraordinary essays ("The Concept of Anxiety" (1844) and "The Mortal Illness" (1849)), he analyzed the risks faced by a subjectivity enclosed within an abstract omnipotence, in a project of self that provides neither conditioning nor limits. This anthropological disproportion (as Binswanger would put it, 1923) frustrates the Ego, which disappears into the enforced repetition of its own implacable certainties.

Kierkegaard (1849: 244) calls this rigid model of existence, so fixed in its certainties, the "*mortal illness*":

> The Ego desperately wants to enjoy the satisfaction of being its own self creator, of developing itself, of being itself, it wants to have the glory of this plan . . . of the sovereign project according to which it has defined itself . . . and this is precisely the final moment at which a fully intact individual becomes a mirage.

Retracing Kierkegaard's thesis in his own way, Binswanger states that paranoid existence is one that "holds on anxiously to its singularity," pursuing it beyond any possible relationship with the other. Striving to live for its own singularity, the existence necessarily fails, or as he writes, "the existence eliminates the ground that gives it substance."

The risk that these existences lose their way along certain hazardous passages of their anthropological journey in some cases reaches the high probability of a clinical prognosis, and in the view of the authors this determines the unfortunate destiny of paranoia and justifies our hopes for the predictive resources of phenomenological psychopathology.

ACKNOWLEDGMENTS

A special thanks to the psychiatry residents of the School of Bologna, F. Cerrato, R. Emiliani, L. Gammino, P. Lupoli, S.Valente, and E. Volta, who have built, around the theme of paranoia, a passionate "laboratory" of psychopathological thought.

BIBLIOGRAPHY

American Psychiatric Association. (1980). *Diagnostic and Statistical Manual of Mental Disorders, DSM-III*. Washington D.C.: APA.

American Psychiatric Association. (1987). *Diagnostic and Statistical Manual of Mental Disorders, DSM-III—R*. Washington D.C.: APA.

American Psychiatric Association. (1994). *Diagnostic and Statistical Manual of Mental Disorders, DSM-IV*. Washington D.C.: APA.

American Psychiatric Association. (2013), *Diagnostic and Statistical Manual of Mental Disorders, DSM-V*. Washington D.C.: APA.

Ballerini A. and Rossi Monti M. (1990). *La vergogna e il delirio: un modello delle sindromi paranoidee*. Torino: Bollati Boringhieri.

Balzac H. (1986). *Illusioni perdute*. Milano: Garzanti.

Binswanger L. (1959). *Drei Formen Missglückten Daseins*. Tübingen: Max Nieneyer, Verlag.

Binswanger L.(1982). "Uber Phanomenologie. Ztschr." *Ges. Neur. Psychiatr* 82,10, 1923. Trad. It.: Sulla fenomenologia in: Per un'Antropologia Fenomenologica, Feltrinelli, Milano, 1982

Bocchi G. and Cerruti M. (a cura di) (1985). *La sfida della complessità*. Milano: Feltrinelli.

Callieri B. and Maci C. (2008). *Paranoia—passione e ragione*. Roma: Anicia.

Canetti E. (1972). *Masse und Macht*. Hamburg: Claassen Verlag, 1960. Trans. *Massa e potere*. Milano: Rizzoli.

Cargnello D. (1984). *Il caso Ernst Wagner*. Milano: Feltrinelli.

Claude H. and Montassut M. (1926). "Delimitation de la paranoia legitime." *Encephale* 1(57): 63.

Clerambault (De) G. (1921). "Delires passionels: erotomanie, revendication, jalousie" *Bull. Soc. Clin. Med. Ment.* 61, 71.

Delmas F. A. (1932). "Le role et l'importance des constitutions en psychopathologie" *Congrès Alién. Neurol.*, Limoges.

Dilthey W. (1974). "Einleitung In Die Geisteswissenschaften." In *Gesammelte Schriften*. Vol. I. Leipzig: Teubner. Trans. *Introduzione alle scienze dello spirito*. Firenze: La Nuova Italia.

Durand G. (1963). *Les structures anthropologiques de l'Imaginaire* Paris: Presses Universitaires de France. Trans. *Le strutture antropologiche dell'Immaginario*. Bari: Dedalo, 1972.

Eidelberg L. (1954). *An Outline of a Comparative Pathology of the Neuroses. Trans. Patologia comparata delle nevrosi*. Firenze: Einaudi, 1959.

Ey H. and Pujol R. (1955). "Groupe des Délires chroniques." *Encycl. Méd.Chir., Psychiatrie*, 37299 D 10, 10, Paris.

Ferrio C. (1970). *Trattato di Psichiatria Clinica e Forense*. Torino: UTET.

Gadamer H. G. (1960). *Wahrheit und Methode. Grundzüge einer philosophischen Hermeneutik*. Tübingen: Mohr. Trans. *Verità e metodo. Lineamenti di un'ermeneutica filosofica*. Milano: Bompiani, 1983.

Gaupp R. (1910). "Zur Lehre von der Paranoia" *Nervenartz* XVIII: 167.

Genil-Perrin G. (1926). *Les paranoiaques*. Paris: Maloine.

Girard R. (1972). *La Violence et le Sacré*. Paris: Editions Bernard Grassé. Trans. *La violenza e il sacro*. Milano: Adelphi, 1980.

Heidegger M. (1927). *Sein und Zeit*. Tübingen: Max Niemejer. Trans. *Essere e Tempo*. Torino: UTET, 1969.

Husserl H. (1913). *Ideen zu einer reinen Phänomenologie und phänomenologischen. Philosophie. Erstes Buch: Allgemeine Einführung in die reine Phänomenologie. Trans. Idee per una fenomenologia pura e per una filosofia fenomenologica*. Torino: Einaudi, 1976.

Jaspers K. (1913). *Allgemeine Psychopathologie*. Berlin, Gottingen, Heidelberg: Springer-Verlag. *Trans. Psicopatologia Generale*. Roma: Il Pensiero Scientifico, 1964.

Kafka F. (1919). "*In der Strafkolonie*" Lipsia: Wolff. Trans. "*Nella colonia penale.*" In *Racconti*. Torino: Frassinelli, 1949.

Kafka F. (1935): "*Der Prozess.*" Berlin: Schocken Verlag. Trans. "*Il processo.*" Torino: Frassinelli, 1963.

Kehrer F. A. (1951). "Kristische Bemerkungen zum Paranoia-Problem." *Nervenartz* 22: 121.

Kierkegaard S. (1844). *Begrebet Angest. En simpel psychologisk-paapegende Overveielse i Retning af det dogmatiske Problem om Arvesynden*. Trans. *Il concetto dell'angoscia*. Milano: SE, 2007.

Kierkegaard S. (1849). *Sygdommen til Døden*.

Kleist (Von) H. (1975). *Michael Kohlaas*. Milano: Rizzoli.

Kohut H. (1971). *The Analysis of the Self*. London: Hogarth Press. *Trans. Narcisismo e Analisi del Sé*. Torino: Boringhieri, 1976.

Kohut H. (1978). *The Search for the Self*. New York: International Universities Press. *Trans. La Ricerca del Sé*. Torino: Boringhieri, 1982.

Koyrè A. (1968). *Newtonian Studies*. Chicago: The University of Chicago Press.

Kraepelin E. (1899). *Leherbuch der Psychiatrie*. Leipzig: Joh. Ambros. Barth.

Kranz H. (1958). "Die schizoide Fehlhaltung." In Frankl, von Gebsattel, and Schultz (eds.), *Handbuch der Neurosenlehre und Psychotherapie*. Munchen: Urban-Schwarzenberg.

Kretschmer E. (1950). *Medizinische Psychologie*. Stuttgart: Thieme. Trans. *Manuale teorico pratico di Psicologia Medica*. Firenze; Sansoni, 1952.

Lanteri-Laura G., Del Pistoia L., and Bel Habib H. (1985). "Paranoia." *Encycl. Méd.Chir., Psychiatrie*, 37299 D 10, 10, Paris, 1985.

Morin E. (1985). "Le vie della complessità." In *La sfida della complessità*, pp. 49–60. A cura di G. Bocchi e M. Cerruti. Milano: Feltrinelli.

Muscatello C. F. (1984). "Percorsi psicopatologici del narcisismo." *Riv. Sper. Freniat.*, 108: 1299.

Muscatello C. F., Scudellari P., Inglese S., Ravani C., and Pardi G. "Note per una fenomenologia delle personalità paranoicali—I parte." *Riv. Sper. Fren.*, 104: 841.

Muscatello C. F., Scudellari P., Ravani C., and Pardi G. (1985). "La paranoia fra struttura di personalità e sintomo." *Atti del XXXVI Congresso della S.I.P.*, Milano.

Muscatello C. F., Scudellari P., Ravani C., and Bologna M. (1985a). "Figure del Regime Diurno dell'immaginario: L'immaginario paranoicale." *Atti del XXXVI Congresso della S.I.P.*, Milano.

Muscatello C. F., Scudellari P., Ravani C., and Bologna M. (1985b). "Considerazioni sulla paranoia in margine al dramma 'Wahn' di E. Wagner." *Atti del XXXVI Congresso della S.I.P.*, Milano.

Muscatello C. F., Scudellari P., Ravani C., and Bologna M. (1987). "Note per una fenomenologia delle personalità paranoicali. Aspetti dell'immaginario paranoicale—II parte." *Riv. Sper. Fren.* CXI: 48.

Muscatello C. F. and Scudellari P. (1993). *Figure del narcisismo. La metafora del fiore e le sue metamorfosi grafiche in un caso di anoressia mentale*. Castrovillari: TEDA Editrice.

Muscatello C. F. and Scudellari P. (1998). "Prognosi e destino. Comprensione narrativa e predittività degli eventi psicopatologici." *Comprendere* 8: 115–124.

Nacht S. and Racamier P. C. (1958). "La Théorie psychanalytique du délire." *Rev. Franc. Pschoan.*, XXV (Juill.–Octobre): 4–5.

Racamier P. (1966). "Esquisse d'une clinique psychanalytique de la paranoia." *Rev. Franc. Psychoan.* 30: 125.

Rank O. (1914). "*Der Doppelgänger.*" Imago, Leipzig, Wien.

Ricoeur P. (1969). *Le conflict des l'interprètation*. Paris: Editions du Seuil. *Trans. La sfida semeiologica*. Roma: Armando, 1974.

Ricoeur P. (1986). *Du texte à l'action*. Paris: Editions du Seuil. *Trans. Dal testo all'azione*. Milano: Jaca Book, 1989.

Rossi Monti M. (2009). *La conoscenza totale, Paranoia, Scienza e Pseudo-scienza*. Roma: Fioriti.

Sauget H. (1955). "Névroses de caractère. Caractères névrotiques." *Encycl. Méd. Chir., Psychiatrie*, 37320 A 10, Io, Paris.

Schultz J. H. (1955). *Grundfragen der Neurosenlehre*. Stuttgart: Thieme.

Serieux P. and Capgras K. (mai-juin I902). "Les psychoses à base d'interpretations delirantes." *Ann. Méd. Psychol.*

Tanzi E. and Lugaro E. (1923). *Trattato delle malattie mentali*, 2nd edn. Milano: Società Editrice Libraria.

Tatossian A. (1979). *La phénoménologie des psychoses*. Paris: Masson. *Trans. La fenomenologia delle psicosi*. Roma: Fioriti, 2003.

Trakl G. (1919). "Die Dichtungen."

CHAPTER 76

AUDITORY VERBAL HALLUCINATIONS AND THEIR PHENOMENOLOGICAL CONTEXT

MATTHEW RATCLIFFE

INTRODUCTION

AUDITORY verbal hallucinations (hereafter, AVHs) are frequently associated with schizophrenia diagnoses but also occur in several other psychiatric conditions, as well as in the non-clinical population. In order to investigate how they are caused and how they might be treated (if they require treatment), it is essential to get the phenomenology right. Otherwise, there is a risk of failing to distinguish different experiences that need to be explained in different ways or even seeking to explain the wrong thing entirely, a point that applies equally to treatment. This is not to suggest that we need rely *exclusively* on phenomenological research in order to pin down the nature of AVHs. We can also draw on non-phenomenological findings in order to corroborate, clarify, or challenge phenomenological claims. For example, suppose it is assumed that AVHs are much like veridical auditory experiences, but it then turns out that patterns of brain activity associated with audition are entirely absent. In such a scenario, non-phenomenological findings would prompt us to reconsider the phenomenology.

However, where AVHs are concerned, one might think that the required phenomenological work is easily done. The term "auditory verbal hallucination" already says it all: a *hallucination* is an experience that resembles perception in one or another sensory modality, but which occurs in the absence of an appropriate external stimulus. By implication, an *auditory verbal hallucination* is an experience of hearing someone speak, which occurs in the absence of a speaker. Such definitions are commonplace in the literature. For example:

> Voices are defined as a sensory perception that has a compelling sense of reality, but which occurs without external stimulation of the sensory organ.
>
> (Hayward, Berry, and Ashton 2011: 1314)

> Auditory hallucinations (AHs) are auditory experiences that occur in the absence of a corresponding external stimulation and which resemble a veridical perception.
>
> (Waters et al. 2012: 683)

> Auditory verbal hallucinations (AVHs) are a sensory experience that takes place in the absence of any external stimulation whilst in a fully conscious state.
>
> (de Leede-Smith and Barkus 2013: 1)

This understanding is consistent with the (remarkably cursory) description of AVHs supplied by DSM-5: "Auditory hallucinations are usually experienced as voices, whether familiar or unfamiliar, that are perceived as distinct from the individual's own thoughts" (American Psychiatric Association 2013: 87). The only further qualification offered here is that cases where someone is falling asleep or waking up should be excluded. But again, it might seem that the relevant experiences are easy enough to comprehend: they are just like hearing someone speak. If that is right, then cursory definitions and descriptions are unproblematic. It is obvious what the relevant phenomenology consists of and so the phenomenological preliminaries can be dispensed with quickly.

This article will show that matters are considerably more complicated. The kinds of experience routinely labeled as "AVHs" are diverse, and many of them are not at all like hearing someone speak. Furthermore, in the context of severe psychiatric illness, AVHs are generally not circumscribed perceptual anomalies. They are embedded in much wider-ranging phenomenological disturbances, of a kind that are difficult to describe. It is debatable whether and to what extent these disturbances correspond to established diagnostic categories. Hence, if AVH experiences are to be adequately characterized and differentiated, in-depth phenomenological research is needed, of a kind that is able to acknowledge, describe, and distinguish profound disturbances in the overall structure or *form* of experience. Current phenomenological psychopathology acknowledges that AVHs are often unlike mundane perceptual experience and that they arise within the context of more encompassing experiential changes. Nevertheless, it offers what is at best an incomplete account, one that is questionable in several respects.

INTERPRETING VOICES

Talk of "hearing a voice" can mean different things in different circumstances, as exemplified by utterances such as "okay, I hear what you're saying," "I hear you loud and clear," and "I hear you," which can convey understanding, endorsement, or both, rather than merely registering the receipt of a verbal communication. Potentially different connotations should also be kept in mind when interpreting first-person reports of "voice-hearing" in psychiatric illness. The need for interpretive caution is recognized by Sarbin (1967: 363), who takes it as given that the relevant experiences are "imaginings" of one kind or another, but does not assume that they resemble veridical perceptual experiences. It is the clinician, and perhaps not the patient, who construes them as such:

> What are the antecedent and concurrent conditions that lead a person publicly to report his imaginings in such a way as to lead a psychologist, psychiatrist, or other professional to designate the described imagining as an hallucination?
>
> (Sarbin 1967: 363)[1]

A clinician's interpretation may be influenced by factors that have no bearing on the nature of the experience. For instance, whether a person says "I hear a voice" or "it is *as if* I hear a voice" is determined, in part, by age, linguistic ability, and whether or not she is a native language speaker. Drawing on J. L. Austin (1962), Sarbin adds that talk of things seeming "real" also poses considerable interpretive challenges. Hence, even where someone explicitly refers to "hearing" one or more "voices," it should not simply be assumed that she has an auditory experience of speech when nobody is present.

What is at least clear from first-person reports is that the various experiences labeled as AVHs are diverse. As Jaspers remarks in *General Psychopathology*:

> [W]e often find "voices" as well, the "invisible" people who shout all kinds of things at the patient, ask him questions and abuse him or order him about. As to content, this may consist of single words or whole sentences; there may be a single voice or a whole jumble of voices; it may be an orderly conversation between the voices themselves or between them and the patient. They may be women's, children's or men's voices, the voices of acquaintances or unknown people, or quite undefinable human voices. Curses may be uttered, actions of the patient may be commented on or there may be meaningless words, empty repetitions. Sometimes the patient hears his own thoughts spoken aloud.
>
> (Jaspers 1963: 73).

More recent studies have identified several dimensions of variation, including whether the voice addresses the subject in the second person or refers to her in the third person, whether its experienced origin is internal or external to the subject, the number of voices heard, the degree to which voices are personified, the thematic content of utterances, how elaborate the content is, whether or not there are hallucinations in other modalities, degree of control over voices, and degree of distress caused (e.g. Nayani and David 1996). Nevertheless, it remains unclear which differences are superficial and which more profound. In fact, it is not even clear which criteria should be employed to distinguish degrees of profundity or to classify AVHs into subtypes for one or another purpose. One thing that does become apparent, however, is that many so-called "AVHs," most likely the majority, are quite unlike hearing someone speak. Nayani and David (1996) report that 49% of their subjects heard voices "through their ears as external stimuli," while 38% experienced them as occurring in "in internal space," and 12% experienced both, while Leudar et al. (1997: 888–889) state that 71% of their subjects heard only internal voices, 18% heard voices "through their ears," and 11% heard both. Internal voices are often described as lacking some or all auditory characteristics. This is perhaps best exemplified by the reports of congenitally deaf "voice-hearers," who often express bemusement when

---

[1] Over time, it may be that the patient adopts some of the language that health-care professionals employ to describe her condition. Hence a clear distinction can no longer be drawn between her own narrative and one that labels her experiences as "hallucinations." This makes interpretation even more challenging.

asked whether their voices have one or another auditory property (Atkinson 2006). But many others similarly report voices that originate in an internal location, often "in the head," and that lack some or all auditory qualities. These experiences may also be described in terms of receiving a communication from elsewhere, reading in the absence of a text, having a perception-like experience of something that remains somehow thought-like, or as *like* telepathy. That they differ substantially from other AVHs, which are experienced as audition-like and as originating in an external location, is clear from the testimonies of those who experience both types and contrast them, sometimes explicitly stating that they use the term "voice" to refer to two different kinds of experience (Ratcliffe and Wilkinson 2015; Ratcliffe 2017).

Phenomenologically inspired approaches to AVHs recognize that the relevant experience is often quite unlike hearing someone speak. For instance, Henriksen, Raballo, and Parnas (2015: 167) take it to be more a "sort of direct inner intuition" than a "sensory experience." In support of that interpretation, they quote first-person accounts such as the following:

> "... often, I cannot tell if I have a thought, if it's the voice, or if it's a feeling I have."

> "... the voice seems partly real, but at the same time distorted. It can also appear as a face or a text. I cannot really describe the sound."
>
> (quoted by Henriksen, Raballo, and Parnas 2015: 167)

Such experiences are not usually mistaken for veridical auditory communications, and are instead distinguished from them with ease (although this is not to deny that confusion can occur). As noted by J. H. van den Berg (1982: 105), psychiatric patients often know "full well the difference in nature between their hallucinations and their perceptions." They may even give their voices a "special name," to indicate that they have a "recognizable character of their own which distinguishes them from *perception* and also from *imagination*." So a person might refer to *hearing voices* and insist that she *really does hear voices*, while at the same time speaking and acting in a way that implies recognition of their distinctness from mundane auditory perceptions. This is consistent with the wider phenomenon of double-bookkeeping, where a person's words and actions indicate an equivocal attitude toward delusions and perceptions; they are perception- and belief-like in certain respects but at the same time set apart from mundane perceptions and beliefs (e.g. Sass 1994). Phenomenological approaches have tended to focus on AVH experiences of this kind, and have sought to develop accounts of more enveloping phenomenological disturbances that they depend upon.

AVHs as Symptoms of Self-Disorder

A consistent theme in phenomenological psychopathology is that AVHs are largely attributable to global changes in the *form* of experience—not *what* is experienced but *how*. So they are not isolated "hallucinations," which occur against a backdrop of otherwise unproblematic experience. The emphasis of discussion has been on AVHs in schizophrenia. The earliest descriptions of dementia praecox/schizophrenia, by Emil Kraepelin and Eugen Bleuler, identify profound disturbances in the experience of *self*, involving pervasive changes in perception, emotion, thought, and agency. Kraepelin (1919: 3) writes that there is a "peculiar destruction of the internal connections of the psychic personality," while Bleuler (1950: 9) refers to a "splitting of the psychic functions," where "the personality loses its unity." The theme of *self-disturbance* or *self-disorder* in schizophrenia has been further developed by subsequent phenomenological psychopathology. Several recent discussions have adopted the term "minimal self."[2] As described in detail by Zahavi (2014), minimal self is not an *object* of reflective or pre-reflective experience; it is not an isolable *quale* or *feeling* of any kind; it is not a transcendental condition for the possibility of experience that lies *behind* the relevant experiences; and it is not a mere abstraction from experience. Rather, it is an indispensable structural condition for experience, which is integral to all experiences. As such, it is an inextricable aspect of experience, as opposed to an isolable component. Zahavi (2014: 22) thus refers to it as a sense of "mineness" that is inseparable from the "distinct manner, or *how*, of experiencing."

The concept of minimal self has been applied, in slightly different ways, to the phenomenology of schizophrenia by Thomas Fuchs, Josef Parnas, Louis Sass, and others. It is proposed that AVHs presuppose wider-ranging phenomenological disturbances, which arise before the onset of specific symptoms such as hallucinations and delusions. These disturbances centrally implicate the most basic experience of selfhood, the minimal self. For example, Sass (2014: 5–6) states that schizophrenia involves a "disturbance of minimal- or core-self experience" or "ipseity," the "sense of existing as a vital and self-identical *subject* of experience or *agent* of action." Parnas et al. (2005: 244) refer to the erosion of a "basic self-awareness (ipseity)," something that more usually operates as a "*medium* or a *mode* in which specific intentional experiences, such as perception, thinking, or imagination, articulate themselves" (244). Fuchs (2013: 248) likewise emphasizes the disruption of a "first-person perspective" that "inhabits all modes of intentionality and imbues them with a sense of mineness."

Disturbances of minimal self envelop all aspects of the structure of experience—the sense of being immersed in a world, how one experiences and relates to other people in general, the sense of time, bodily experience, and experiences of agency, perception, thought, and emotion. Although the emphasis of discussion varies somewhat, it is consistently maintained that a profound alteration in the overall *structure* or *form* of experience takes hold in the prodromal stages of schizophrenia, and precedes more specific symptoms (Parnas and Sass 2001). It is further claimed that seemingly localized symptoms, including AVHs, are only *intelligible* in the context of a subtle and hard-to-describe alteration in the global structure of experience. Hence they are not "atomistic, self-sufficient, thing-like symptoms." Rather, they are "meaningfully interrelated facets of a more comprehensive and characteristic gestalt change in the patient's experience (field of consciousness) and existence" (Larøi, de Haan, Jones, and Raballo 2010: 235).

More specific, and largely complementary, accounts have also been offered of *how* changes in the sense of self (and, by implication, in the overall structure of experience) give rise to AVHs. The common theme is that one becomes estranged from one's own thought processes, which are experienced as increasingly alien, as somehow object-like. Sass (e.g. 1992, 1994, 2003, 2007, 2014) offers an influential account, which emphasizes what he calls "hyperreflexivity": a largely involuntary attentiveness to aspects of experience that are more usually unproblematic and inconspicuous. In his words, it is "a condition in which phenomena that would normally be inhabited, and in this sense experienced as part of the self, come instead to be objects of focal or objectifying awareness" (Sass 2003: 153). AVHs and other kinds of anomalous experience are thus attributable, at least in part, to a kind of

---

[2] For references to complementary themes in earlier phenomenological writings see e.g. Sass (2001) and Fuchs (2012).

alienating self-awareness (e.g. Sass 1992: 226–235). Thoughts are no longer integral to a medium *through which* one engages with the world and instead appear curiously conspicuous and alien. Along with this, there is a more general sense of practical disengagement from the world as a whole and from other people, as well as a pervasive detachment from one's thoughts, perceptions, and activities.

Others similarly suggest that AVHs involve thought becoming somehow object-like. Henriksen, Raballo, and Parnas (2015: 172) refer to the "morbid objectification of inner speech" as an "essential" precursor to the formation of AVHs, whereby a medium of awareness, *through* which one experiences and engages with one's surroundings, gradually becomes an object of awareness. There is, they say, a kind of "dissociation" between the "sense of self" or "ipseity" and the "flow of consciousness." This is presupposed by the intelligibility of AVHs; such experiences involve a quasi-perceptual sense of alienation from one's own thoughts, of a kind that could not arise against the backdrop of a more mundane experience of the self and its surroundings.[3]

Proponents of this view tend to maintain that the phenomenological "gestalt" within which AVHs crystallize is specific to schizophrenia: self-disturbance in schizophrenia is uniquely pronounced, and also qualitatively distinctive from other kinds of self-disorder. It has been further proposed that self-disorder is detectable before the onset of clinically significant levels of disturbance (Cermolacce, Naudin, and Parnas 2007; Raballo and Parnas 2011: 1018). This raises the possibility of employing phenomenologically inspired methods for the purposes of early detection and thus early intervention. To this end, Parnas and colleagues have developed the Examination of Anomalous Self-Experience (EASE), a detailed checklist for a semi-structured, phenomenological interview, the principal aim of which is to reliably detect disorders of minimal self-awareness that are specific to the schizophrenia spectrum (Parnas et al. 2005). So, to summarize, the overall picture is that AVHs, or at least certain kinds of AVH, are preceded by and depend upon a distinctive disturbance of the overall structure of experience, of a kind that is specific to schizophrenia. This disturbance alienates the subject from her own thoughts (or, more specifically, inner speech), to such an extent that she eventually comes to experience some of them in a quasi-perceptual, object-like way.

AN INCOMPLETE STORY

It is plausible to insist that many AVHs are not like hearing a voice, and also that such experiences tend to arise against a backdrop of wider-ranging phenomenological disturbances. Even so, the explanatory power of the self-disorder account is currently rather limited. Furthermore, certain aspects of the account are unclear, and others questionable.

[3] On one interpretation, AVHs of this type are indistinguishable from experiences of thought insertion (TI). If TI is taken to involve an experience of alienation from thought *content*, rather than from the *process* of thinking, then it could equally be described as a perception-like experience of thought content, which is exactly how Henriksen et al. (2015) conceive of AVHs. For a more detailed defense of the view that TI is to be identified with (a certain kind of) AVH, see Ratcliffe and Wilkinson (2015); Ratcliffe (2017). For an attempt to retain the AVH/TI distinction in such cases, see Humpston and Broome (2016).

For one thing, why AVHs are experienced only episodically remains unexplained. If there is an all-enveloping phenomenological change that renders thought somehow perception-like, then surely all thoughts, or at least all thoughts of a certain type (for instance, those that take the form of inner speech) would be experienced in this way. One might respond that the relevant change is temporally inconsistent, and therefore disrupts some thoughts to a greater extent than others. While this might accommodate the sporadic nature of the experiences, it leaves their content-specificity unaccounted for. AVHs in severe psychiatric illness tend to have consistent and often quite specific thematic contents. For instance, voices are often abusive; over 50% of those voice-hearers with psychiatric illness diagnoses report critical, hostile, abusive voices (Nayani and David 1996; Leudar et al. 1997). Until the self-disorder approach can show why global changes in the structure of experience lead to sporadic, content-specific experiences, it remains importantly incomplete.

In addition, the claim that self-disturbance culminates in an *object-like* experience of thought is not wholly clear, and may involve a degree of equivocation over the term "object." On one reading, "object" refers to an *object of experience*. In other words, it pertains to *whatever it is that we experience*, as distinct from any qualities attached to the *act of experiencing*. So one could say that, while our thoughts ordinarily have objects, they are not themselves objects. Nevertheless, even if it is accepted that thoughts are not ordinary objects of experience, it seems plausible to maintain that we can be reflectively (and perhaps unreflectively) aware of our own thoughts in this way without feeling alienated from them. And the claim that thought becomes object-like is intended to convey something more specific than this. Thoughts become somehow akin to a type of object of perception: an inanimate entity that is external to the self. But in what respect? Sometimes, it seems as though the answer is that they acquire sensory properties that are ordinarily attributed to certain entities and occurrences in the external environment but not to thoughts. Consistent with this, Parnas et al. (2005: 241) refer to a "perceptualization of inner speech or thought," stating that inner speech takes on "*acoustic* and in more severe states *auditory* qualities." There are also descriptions of inner speech becoming "more pronounced" before the onset of voices, with "subtle pre-psychotic distortions of the stream of consciousness—such as abnormal sonorization of inner dialogue and/or perceptualization of thought" (Raballo and Larøi 2011: 163). With this, thought ceases to be part of the medium *through which* we experience and engage with our surroundings and instead becomes something separate from ourselves, something we confront. However, the appeal to sensory properties is in tension with the admission that AVHs are quite unlike auditory perceptual experiences. Furthermore, much the same contrast between alienated and non-alienated experiential contents arguably applies to perception as well. For example, in *Autobiography of a Schizophrenic Girl*, Renee describes her experiences of previously familiar objects as follows:

> Objects are stage trappings, placed here and there, geometric cubes without meaning.... When, for example, I looked at a chair or a jug, I thought not of their use or function—a jug not as something to hold water and milk, a chair not as something to sit in—but as having lost their names, their functions and meanings; they became "things" and began to take on life, to exist.
>
> (Sechehaye 1970: 44, 55–56)

In the case of an AVH, the claim is not that inner speech is experienced as akin to a mundane auditory perception. A more appropriate comparison would be with the kind of alienated perceptual experience described by Renee. However, that being the case, it is inaccurate to say that thought becomes perception-like, given that thought is experienced as *alien* in a way that can equally be contrasted with mundane, non-alienated perceptual experiences of "objects." The relevant sense of alienation should therefore be distinguished from the adoption of perceptual characteristics. It does not require such characteristics and, even if they are present, they do not account for it. Talk of "objectification" thus refers to a sense of alienation that requires further clarification, something that differs from both ordinary thought and ordinary perception.

But perhaps the most substantial problem with the minimal self account of AVHs is the widespread insistence that self-disorder, of the relevant kind, is schizophrenia-specific. That position is explicit in the writings of Parnas and some of his collaborators, although others are less committal.[4] Current applications of the label "schizophrenia" most likely accommodate a far wider range of experiences. So the self-disorder proposal is presumably intended to be revisionary, at least to some extent. By identifying schizophrenia with a certain type of self-disorder, the intention is to apply the diagnosis in a more principled, discerning, and restrictive way. Let us accept, for the sake of argument, that the self-disorder account of schizophrenia is right. The problem we then face is that schizophrenia-specific self-disorder does not seem to be necessary for AVHs, including those AVHs that involve perception-like experiences of alienated thought content. It is widely acknowledged that AVHs can occur in non-clinical, healthy subjects as well, although their frequency in the non-clinical population is debated (e.g. Aleman and Larøi 2008: chapter 3; Watkins 2008; McCarthy-Jones 2012: chapter 7). Some further maintain that the AVH experiences of healthy and clinical subjects are much the same. For instance, Romme and Escher (e.g. 2006) suggest that what distinguishes the two populations is not their experiences per se but how they react to those experiences. In clinical subjects, voices and the like are a source of considerable distress, nurturing a pervasive feeling of disempowerment and helplessness.

One response on behalf of the self-disorder view is to reject the claim that the experiences are relevantly similar. It might initially seem that they are, but only because of a failure to explore the comparative phenomenology in sufficient depth. Stanghellini et al. (2012) note that the relevant studies are seldom sufficiently receptive to potential phenomenological differences, and argue that detailed first-person descriptions in fact point to quite different experiences. Henriksen, Raballo, and Parnas (2015) also emphasize various differences between AVHs in schizophrenia and in healthy subjects. Hence distinguishing between AVHs in healthy subjects and in those with schizophrenia diagnoses may not be so much of a problem. Nevertheless, the same cannot be said of AVHs in schizophrenia and in other types of psychiatric illness. AVHs are associated with several other conditions, including posttraumatic stress disorder, psychotic depression, bipolar disorder, and borderline personality disorder. For example, Upthegrove et al. (2016) quote frequencies of 70% in schizophrenia, 23% in bipolar disorder, and 46% in borderline personality disorder. First-person accounts of abusive, insulting, or threatening voices in these populations have much in common. Now, it could be that certain experiences are more common in schizophrenia than elsewhere, such as "running commentary or arguing voices" (Henriksen, Raballo, and Parnas 2015: 178). But

---

[4] For instance, Sass (2014: 5) is more generally cautious about the schizophrenia construct. He suggests that, although flawed, it does at least appear seem to suggest "some subtle but underlying factor at the core of a psychiatric condition that is perhaps best conceived of as a syndrome (and probably represents a final common pathway with diverse etiological origins)."

even Romme and Escher (2006: 167) are happy to concede that voices commenting in the third person are more common in those with schizophrenia diagnoses. What remains the case is that all sorts of other AVH experiences do not seem to be schizophrenia-specific, and are common to several diagnostic categories. Claims for the schizophrenia-specificity of a certain type of AVH tend to contrast AVHs in schizophrenia with AVHs in non-clinical populations (e.g. Henriksen, Raballo, and Parnas 2015). However, not enough work has been done to support the claim that they are equally distinguishable from AVHs in other clinical populations. And, in the absence of any evidence to the contrary, the default assumption should be that these experiences have much in common.

A related problem for the self-disorder account is that not all AVHs in severe psychiatric illness are quite so different from veridical auditory experiences. While some involve encountering thought or inner speech in a perception-like way (the nature of which needs to be spelled out more clearly), others are more like hearing someone speak. Wu (2012) thus proposes that many AVHs are exactly as the term would suggest: non-veridical auditory perceptual experiences of voices. In a clinical context, Dodgson and Gordon (2009) make a more specific case for what they call "hypervigilance hallucinations," which are to be distinguished from inner speech AVHs. The former arise due to pervasive anxious anticipation, of a kind that is commonplace in psychiatric illness and diagnostically non-specific. Because the subject is always on the alert, anticipating self-directed communications with negative thematic contents, there is an increased disposition toward false positives, where ambiguous sensory information is interpreted (and also *experienced*) in terms of voices. Even without recourse to a principled taxonomy of AVH-subtypes, it is clear that an anomalous experience of inner speech is very different from an over-interpretation of perceptual stimuli, and it is equally clear that the two experiences come about in different ways.[5] Both kinds of experience are associated with schizophrenia diagnoses. And, if they are both to be explained in terms of self-disorder, the relevant explanation needs to distinguish the ways in which a common, underlying self-disorder gives rise to two very different types of experience.

Given these various concerns, it is clear that the self-disorder account of AVHs requires further refinement. As things stand, phenomenological approaches are not even close to showing that the majority of AVHs occurring in schizophrenia are diagnostically specific. Of course, it could be that schizophrenic self-disorder is one of many different phenomenological contexts in which these experiences can arise. But, if that is so, we would have to concede that, although self-disorder might be sufficient to bring about AVHs, it is not necessary for them. And this would involve abandoning strong claims about AVHs *only being intelligible* in the context of a distinctive phenomenological "gestalt," thus substantially weakening the position. Worse still, it would open up the possibility that self-disorder is not even sufficient for AVHs. If one accepts that it is not necessary, then one cannot simply assume that it has a role to play when it is present. Perhaps it is just an accompaniment, an associated symptom. Or, to really complicate matters, perhaps schizophrenia-specific self-disorder is necessary and sufficient for some types of AVHs, necessary but not sufficient for others, sufficient but not necessary for others, and neither necessary nor sufficient for others. All four possibilities remain open. An alternative option would be to concede that the degree and

---

[5] The possibility remains that the difference between other kinds of external, audition-like AVH and internal, thought-like experiences is more a matter of degrees, that there is a spectrum of experiences (Humpston and Broome 2016).

type of self-disorder required for AVHs of one or another type is not, after all, schizophrenia-specific. Whatever the case, the claim that AVHs are only intelligible in relation to a certain kind of profound phenomenological disturbance needs more work. The types of AVH in question need to be specified more clearly, as does the kind of "objectification" they involve. And the alleged specificity to schizophrenia needs to be reconciled with the much wider range of most, if not all, types of AVH experience.

Trauma and Psychosis

To conclude, I want to briefly contrast the self-disorder view with another, currently popular, way of thinking about AVHs. This alternative maintains that AVHs are not symptoms of schizophrenia. They are instead attributable to traumatic experiences and to an associated sense of alienation from other people, neither of which are consistently associated with one or another psychiatric diagnosis. Two prominent advocates of the view are Marius Romme and Sandra Escher, who insist that "voices" originate in unresolved trauma and are essentially relational in nature. They propose that we reconceptualize "psychosis" as an "emotional crisis," of a kind that is essentially interpersonal in nature and also embedded in a wider sociocultural context. "Voices," they maintain, should not be regarded as illness symptoms that are to be eliminated through treatment. Rather, we should seek to make sense of them, to grasp their emotional meanings and their relationships to life-history. So the aim is not so much to get rid of them as to help the person come to terms with them and, in so doing, to reduce the distress they cause (e.g. Romme et al. 2009; Romme and Escher 2012).

Setting aside the specifics of Romme and Escher's approach, the view that AVHs are closely associated with trauma is a plausible one. There is a substantial literature pointing to strong correlations between childhood abuse, as well as other traumatic events at various life stages, and the later onset of psychosis. There are also correlations between types of abuse and specific symptoms. For instance, childhood sexual abuse is particularly strongly associated with AVHs. Some symptoms are most reliably associated with combinations of childhood and adulthood trauma, and there are also dose-response relationships. In the majority of cases, there is every reason to believe that first-person reports are accurate (e.g. Larkin and Morrison 2006). An emphasis on the relational nature of AVH experiences and on their interpersonal causes is in tension with claims made by Parnas and colleagues. While acknowledging that self-disorder inevitably implies profound changes in the interpersonal sphere, they insist that self-disorder comes first, both phenomenologically and causally. Instead of emphasizing the interpersonal and social, they seek to identify genetic causes. Raballo, Sæbye, and Parnas (2009: 348) go so far as to state that the "primary relevance" of work on self-disorder in schizophrenia is to "etiological research into the genetic architecture of schizophrenia."[6]

---

[6] See also Raballo and Parnas (2011). However, not all advocates of a self-disorder approach place so much emphasis on genetic causes. Borda and Sass (2015) and Sass and Borda (2015) acknowledge potential roles for various different biological and non-biological causes at different life-stages. They also emphasize the heterogeneity of schizophrenia and propose a broad distinction between two kinds of scenario. In one of these, onset is early, negative symptoms predominate, and self-disorder is a prominent cause. In the other, onset is acute, positive symptoms are more salient, and "secondary factors" may have a greater role to play than "primary" self-disorder.

The association with interpersonal trauma does at least serve to account for the content-specificity of AVHs, as well as the frequent negativity of content. It also accommodates varying degrees of personification. A voice, and the personality that comes to be associated with it, could resemble—to varying degrees and in different ways—a particular person, such as an abuser or perhaps a protector. That said, there is a lack of clarity here too. It is sometimes unclear whether the position is that AVHs are often incorrectly taken to be symptoms of schizophrenia or, alternatively, that the schizophrenia construct should be dismissed altogether. For instance, Longden, Madill, and Waterman (2012) maintain that voices are attributable to dissociation rather than psychosis but at the same time reject the distinction between them (rejecting, by implication, a distinction between schizophrenia and affective disorders). But you can't have it both ways. It is also unclear which types of AVH are associated with trauma and which are not, or whether the relational contexts in which post-traumatic AVHs arise also amount to pervasive alterations in the overall form of experience, along the lines of what phenomenological psychopathology has sought to describe.

Regardless of the many gray areas, it at least appears that these two positions are opposed to each other. One of them attributes AVHs to self-disorders, which are responsible for disturbances of interpersonal relatedness, have a largely genetic origin, and are specific to schizophrenia. The other takes AVHs to be essentially interpersonal, relational phenomena, does not recognize the existence of pre-intersubjective self-disorder, insists that AVHs have an interpersonal origin (in most cases), and rejects the association with schizophrenia. The contrast is an intriguing one, given that both positions are developed in detail, supported by substantial bodies of evidence, and in many respects plausible. As is evident from a brief scan of the sources they tend to cite, the two have, to date, proceeded in near-complete isolation from each other. Nevertheless, there is at least one author in the phenomenological tradition who comes close to combining them. Wolfgang Blankenburg (1969/2001, 1971/2012) describes altered experience of self, body, world, and other people, of the kind associated with schizophrenia, in terms of a pervasive loss of habitual, bodily, *commonsense*, or a loss of *natural self-evidence* (*Verlust der natürlichen Selbstverständlichkeit*). With this, a previously taken-for-granted, unthinking confidence is gone and everything seems strangely unfamiliar. Thus, as Sass similarly emphasizes, what once operated as an unthinking background to thought, experience, and activity is now oddly conspicuous. Blankenburg adds that this "commonsense" is inextricable from how a person relates to others. It is, he says, "primarily related to an intersubjective world (*mitweltbezogen*)." To be more specific, it consists of a confidence that is inextricable from the ability to sustain a kind of habitual, pre-reflective "trust" other people (*Vertrauenkönnen*). Furthermore, adverse events that occur during interpersonal development can either fail to nurture or derail the "basic trust" upon which a wider commonsense depends (1969/2001: 307, 310).

What we have here is an account that combines an emphasis on profound and wide-ranging phenomenological changes (involving a sense of alienation from the world, one's activities, one's body, and even one's own thoughts) with an acknowledgment of their inextricability from the interpersonal sphere and from patterns of interpersonal development. This points to various potential ways of bringing the two together.[7] Perhaps Blankenburg's loss of commonsense is to be identified with self-disorder, in which case the "minimal self"

---

[7] For an attempt to develop such an approach in detail, see Ratcliffe (2017).

would have to be conceived of as a "relational self" too, something that depends for its integrity on a primitive sense of trust in others. Alternatively, it could be that loss of commonsense is sometimes or always preceded by a more fundamental disturbance of minimal self.[8] And, if a more primitive form of self-disturbance is sufficient for loss of commonsense but not necessary for it, we are then faced with the question of whether disruption of commonsense (of whatever degree) can fuel the development of one or another kind of AVH, even in the absence of underlying self-disorder. Last but not least, there is the issue of whether any types of AVHs, or any of the wider-ranging experiential disturbances that they depend upon, reliably track the diagnostic category "schizophrenia," rather than severe psychiatric illness more generally. Perhaps they do but, as things stand, the jury is still out.

ACKNOWLEDGMENTS

Thanks to Matthew Broome and Louis Sass for commenting on an earlier version of this article. Thanks also to Sam Wilkinson for many helpful conversations concerning this topic.

BIBLIOGRAPHY

Aleman A. and Larøi F. (2008). *Hallucinations: The Science of Idiosyncratic Perception.* Washington: American Psychological Association.

American Psychiatric Association. (2013). *Diagnostic and Statistical Manual of Mental Disorders,* 5th edn. Arlington: American Psychiatric Association.

Atkinson J. R. (2006). "The Perceptual Characteristics of Voice-Hallucinations in Deaf People: Insights into the nature of Subvocal Thought and Sensory Feedback Loops." *Schizophrenia Bulletin* 32: 701–708.

Austin J. L. (1962). *Sense and Sensibilia.* Oxford: Clarendon Press.

Berg J. H. van den. (1982). "On Hallucinating: Critical-historical Overview and Guidelines for Further Study." In A. J. J. de Koning and F. A. Jenner (eds.) (1982). *Phenomenology and Psychiatry,* pp. 97–110. London: Academic Press.

Blankenburg W. (1969/2001). "First Steps Towards a Psychopathology of 'Common Sense,'" trans. A. L. Mishara. *Philosophy, Psychiatry & Psychology* 8: 303–315.

Blankenburg W. (1971/2012). *Der Verlust der natürlichen Selbstverständlichkeit: Ein Bertrag zur Psychopathologie symptomarmer Schizophrenien.* Berlin: Parodos Verlag.

Bleuler E. 1950. *Dementia Praecox or the Group of Schizophrenias,* trans. J. Zinkin. New York: International Universities Press.

Borda J. P. and Sass L. A. (2015). "Phenomenology and Neurobiology of Self Disorder in Schizophrenia: Primary Factors." *Schizophrenia Research* 169: 464–473.

Cermolacce M., Naudin J., and Parnas J. (2007). "The 'Minimal Self' in Psychopathology: Re-examining the Self-disorders in the Schizophrenia Spectrum." *Consciousness and Cognition* 16: 703–714.

---

[8] Fuchs (2015) acknowledges and discusses in detail the kind of phenomenological change Blankenburg describes. He also recognizes its inextricability from interpersonal dynamics. Nevertheless, he continues to maintain that alteration of a "pre-reflective, embodied self" has priority and necessitates disruption of social relations.

de Leede-Smith S. and Barkus E. (2013). "A Comprehensive Review of Auditory Verbal Hallucinations: Lifetime Prevalence, Correlates and Mechanisms in Healthy and Clinical Individuals." *Frontiers in Human Neuroscience* 7(Article 367): 1–25.

Dodgson G. and Gordon S. (2009). "Avoiding False Negatives: Are Some Auditory Hallucinations an Evolved Design Flaw?" *Behavoural and Cognitive Psychotherapy* 37: 325–334.

Fuchs T. (2012). "Selbst und Schizophrenie." *Deutsche Zeitschrift für Philosophie* 60: 887–901.

Fuchs T. (2013). "The Self in Schizophrenia: Jaspers, Schneider and Beyond." In G. Stanghellini and T. Fuchs (eds.), *One Century of Karl Jaspers' General Psychopathology*, pp. 245–257. Oxford: Oxford University Press.

Fuchs T. (2015). "Pathologies of Intersubjectivity in Autism and Schizophrenia." *Journal of Consciousness Studies* 22(1–2): 191–214.

Hayward M., Berry K., and Ashton A. (2011). "Applying Interpersonal Theories to the Understanding of and Therapy for Auditory Hallucinations: A Review of the Literature and Directions for Further Research." *Clinical Psychology Review* 31: 1313–1323.

Henriksen M. G., Raballo A., and Parnas J. (2015). "The Pathogenesis of Auditory Verbal Hallucinations in Schizophrenia: a Clinical-Phenomenological Account." *Philosophy, Psychiatry & Psychology* 22: 165–181.

Humpston C. S. and Broome M. R. (2016). "The Spectra of Soundless Voices and Audible Thoughts: Towards an Integrative Model of Auditory Verbal Hallucinations and Thought Insertion." *Review of Philosophy and Psychology* 7: 611–629.

Jaspers K. (1963). *General Psychopathology*, trans. from the German 7th edn. (1959) J. Hoenig and M. W. Hamilton. Manchester: Manchester: University Press.

Kraepelin E. (1919). *Dementia Praecox and Paraphrenia*, trans. R. M. Barclay. Edinburgh: E. & S. Livingstone.

Larkin W. and Morrison A. P. (eds.) (2006). *Trauma and Psychosis: New directions for Theory and Therapy*. London: Routledge.

Larøi F., de Haan S., Jones S., and Raballo A. (2010). "Auditory Verbal Hallucinations: Dialoguing between the Cognitive Sciences and Phenomenology." *Phenomenology and the Cognitive Sciences* 9: 225–240.

Leudar I., Thomas P., McNally D., and Glinski A. (1997). "What Voices can do with Words: Pragmatics of Verbal Hallucinations." *Psychological Medicine* 27: 885–898.

Longden E., Madill A., and Waterman M. G. (2012). "Dissociation, Trauma, and the Role of Lived Experience: Toward a New Conceptualization of Voice Hearing." *Psychological Bulletin* 138: 28–76.

McCarthy-Jones S. (2012). *Hearing Voices: The Histories, Causes and Meanings of Auditory Verbal Hallucinations*. Cambridge: Cambridge University Press.

Nayani T. H. and David A. S. (1996). "The Auditory Hallucination: a Phenomenological Survey." *Psychological Medicine* 26: 177–189.

Parnas J. and Sass L. A. (2001). "Self, Solipsism and Schizophrenic Delusions." *Philosophy, Psychiatry & Psychology* 8: 101–120.

Parnas J., Møller P., Kircher T., Thalbitzer J., Jansson L., Handest P., and Zahavi D. (2005). "EASE: Examination of Anomalous Self-Experience." *Psychopathology* 38: 236–258.

Raballo A., Sæbye D., and Parnas J. (2009). "Looking at the Schizophrenia Spectrum Through the Prism of Self-disorders: An Empirical Study." *Schizophrenia Bulletin* 37: 344–351.

Raballo A. and Larøi F. (2011). "Murmurs of Thought: Phenomenology of Hallucinating Consciousness in Impending Psychosis." *Psychosis* 3: 163–166.

Raballo A. and Parnas J. (2011). "The Silent Side of the Spectrum: Schizotypy and the Schizotaxic Self." *Schizophrenia Bulletin* 37: 1017–1026.

Ratcliffe M. (2017). *Real Hallucinations: Psychiatric Illness, Intentionality, and the Interpersonal World*. Cambridge MA: MIT Press.

Ratcliffe M. and Wilkinson S. (2015). "Thought Insertion Clarified." *Journal of Consciousness Studies* 22(11–12): 246–269.

Romme M. and Escher S. (2006). "Trauma and Hearing Voices." In W. Larkin and A. P. Morrison (eds.) (2006). *Trauma and Psychosis: New Directions for Theory and Therapy*, pp. 162–191. London: Routledge.

Romme M., Escher S., Dillon J., Corstens D., and Morris, M. (2009). *Living with Voices: 50 Stories of Recovery*. Ross-on-Wye: PCCS Books.

Romme M. and Escher S. (eds.) (2012). *Psychosis as a Personal Crisis: An Experience-Based Approach*. London: Routledge.

Sarbin T. R. (1967). "The Concept of Hallucination." *Journal of Personality* 35: 359–380.

Sass L. A. (1992). *Madness and Modernism: Insanity in the Light of Modern Art, Literature, and Thought*. New York: Basic Books.

Sass L. A. (1994). *The Paradoxes of Delusion: Wittgenstein, Schreber, and the Schizophrenic Mind*. Ithaca: Cornell University Press.

Sass L. A. (2001). "Self and World in Schizophrenia: Three Classic Approaches." *Philosophy, Psychiatry & Psychology* 8: 251–270.

Sass L. A. (2003). "'Negative Symptoms,' Schizophrenia, and the Self." *International Journal of Psychology and Psychological Therapy* 3: 153–180.

Sass L. A. (2007). "Contradictions of Emotion in Schizophrenia." *Cognition & Emotion* 21: 351–390.

Sass L. A. (2014). "Self-disturbance and Schizophrenia: Structure, Specificity, Pathogenesis." *Schizophrenia Research* 152: 5–11.

Sass L. A. and Borda J. P. (2015). "Phenomenology and Neurobiology of Self Disorder in Schizophrenia: Secondary Factors." *Schizophrenia Research* 169: 474–482.

Sechehaye M. (1970). *Autobiography of a Schizophrenic Girl*. New York: Signet.

Stanghellini G., Langer A. I., Ambrosini A., and Cangas, A. J. (2012). "Quality of Hallucinatory Experiences: Differences between a Clinical and a Non-clinical Sample." *World Psychiatry* 11: 110–113.

Stein E. (1917/1989). *On the Problem of Empathy*, trans. W. Stein. Washington: ICS Publications.

Upthegrove R., Broome M. R., Caldwell K., Ives J., Oyebode F., and Wood S. J. (2016). "Understanding Auditory Verbal Hallucinations: a Systematic Review of Current Evidence." *Acta Psychiatrica Scandinavica* 133: 352–367.

Waters F., Allen P., Aleman A., Fernyhough C., Woodward T. S., Badcock J. C., Barkus E., Johns L., Varese F., Menon M., Vercammen A., and Larøi F. (2012). "Auditory Hallucinations in Schizophrenia and Nonschizophrenia Populations: A Review and Integrated Model of Cognitive Mechanisms." *Schizophrenia Bulletin* 38: 683–692.

Watkins J. (2008). *Hearing Voices: A Common Human Experience*. South Yarra: Michelle Anderson.

Wu W. (2012). "Explaining Schizophrenia: Auditory Verbal Hallucination and Self-Monitoring." *Mind & Language* 27: 86–107.

Zahavi D. (2014). *Self and Other: Exploring Subjectivity, Empathy, and Shame*. Oxford: Oxford University Press.

CHAPTER 77

....

AFFECTIVE TEMPERAMENTS

....

ANDREA RABALLO AND LORENZO PELIZZA

TEMPERAMENTS: THE HIPPOCRATIC ARCHAEOLOGY OF A CONCEPT

....

THE concepts of temperament and character are probably among the most ancient, tentative conceptualization of the constituents of mental states. For example, the notion that different kinds of temperament are constitutionally based affective-behavioral dispositions can be traced back to Hippocratic medicine with the theory of the four humors (Akiskal 1996). Such theory—based on analogic coherence—attempted to bridge the constituents of the macro-cosmos (i.e. the four basic elements of the Universe) with the bio-psychological constitution of the individual (i.e. fluids, secreting organs, and temperamental features) (see Table 77.1).

According to Hippocratic medicine the harmonic balance ("eucrasia") among the four humors was a prerequisite for somatic and physical health. The pathophysiology of disease states was therefore explained as a consequence of the "*dyscrasia*" (i.e. a dis-proportion of the humors) and the relative proportions of bodily humors was expected to influence and predict individual character types.

Since then, the notion of temperament has been broadly used to denote the temporally stable biological core of personality (i.e. an individual's activity level, as reflected in his biorhythms, moods, and related cognitions as well as their variability) as opposed to the set of more malleable, acquired dispositions and interpersonal styles, that constitute the characterological determinants of personality (Bouchard 1994). In this sense, despite a complex conceptual history, temperament has remained a sort of "bridge between the psychology and biology of affective disorders" (Rihmer et al. 2010) and a canonic notion addressed by several leading authors since the last century.

Table 77.1 Synopsis of the Hippocratic humors, with related physical elements, organs, and temperamental features

Bodily Humor	Cosmologic Element	Reference Organ	Temperament	Character Attributes
Blood	Air	Heart	Sanguine	Courageous, hopeful, playful, care-free
Yellow bile	Fire	Liver	Choleric	Ambitious, leader-like, restless, easily angered
Black bile	Earth	Spleen	Melancholic	Despodent, quiet, analytical, serious
Phlegm	Water	Brain	Phlegmatic	Calm, thoughtful, patient, peaceful

KRAEPELIN: TEMPERAMENTS AS FUNDAMENTAL STATES

Almost a century ago, while consolidating the foundations of its nosography, Kraepelin (1921) separated temperamental variants from actual, clinically overt disease states. In particular, at the less severe margins of *"manic-depressive insanity,"* he identified four mild basic affective dispositions, termed depressive, manic, irritable, and cyclothymic. Such dispositions, which could frequently be found in the blood relatives of manic–depressive patients (Rihmer et al. 2010), were conceived as subclinical forms and potential precursors of major affective psychoses, which harbored their pathogenetic roots in adolescence and developmental years (Blaney and Millon 2009). In this respect, Kraepelin coined the notion of *"fundamental states"* as follows:

> . . . the real, the deeper cause of the malady [manic-depressive insanity] is to be sought in a permanent morbid state which must also continue to exist in the intervals between the attacks. . . .The permanent changes . . . essentially consist of *peculiarities in the emotional life* . . . [which] are observed with special frequency as simple personal peculiarities in the family of manic-depressive patients. . . . . We are, therefore, led to the conclusion that there are certain temperaments which may be regarded as *rudiments of manic-depressive insanity.* (1921: 117–118)

> Those were "the *depressive* temperament (constitutional moodiness), the *manic* temperament (constitutional excitement), and the *irritable* temperament" plus the *cyclothymic* temperament, "in which moodiness and excitement frequently and abruptly alternate with each other." (1921: 118)

These fundamental states (see appendix) might emerge as peculiar forms of psychic personality without further development or may became the starting point of a morbid process with multiple manic-depressive episodes.

KRETSCHMER: TEMPERAMENT AND ENDOGENOUS PSYCHOSES

In the same years, Kretschmer (1925) exploring the transition between normal variants, specific temperamental accentuations, and endogenous psychoses (Harnic et al. 2011), conceptualized temperament as an "affectivity behavior" linking physical constitution and psychological features. He proposed that human emotions were to be differentiated along two dimensional axes: mood and sensitivity. The mood dimension was represented on a spectrum from joy to sadness, usually combined in each individual in "*diathetic proportion*"; whereas the sensitivity dimension ranged from sensitive to dull, typically balanced in the "*psychesthetic proportion*" of the person. Based on the relative contribution of one or another axes (i.e. mood and sensitivity), Kretschmer distinguished two basic types of personality: "*cyclothymic*" and "*schizothymic*." Within the mood dimension, the continuum ranged from cyclothymia (variant of norm) to cycloid personality disorder ("*cycloid temperament*") to manic-depressive illness (Glezerman and Balkoski 2002), while along the sensitivity dimension, the continuum included schizothymia (variant of norm), schizoid personality disorder ("*schizoid temperament*"), and schizophrenia. According to such an overarching view Kretschmer explicitly claimed:

> We shall no longer look on certain types of personality as psychopathic abortive forms of certain psychoses, but vice versa, certain psychoses will figure as caricatures of certain normal types of personality. The psychoses are thus only rare exaggerated editions of large widespread groups of healthy constitutions. (1925: 207)

Crucially, in determining personality features, Kretschmer included emotional and psychomotor patterns, as well as psychic tempo (see Table 77.2).

Thus, if the prevalent personality trait of cyclothymia is the syntonic "capacity for living, feeling and suffering with his surroundings," the corresponding psychomotility is smooth and natural, whereas the psychic tempo oscillates from fast and mobile to slow (Glezerman and Balkoski 2002; Harnic et al. 2011). In schizothymia, the psychic tempo is characterized by abruptness and discontinuity, corresponding to a lack of psychomotor harmony between the emotional stimulus and the reaction, and to a broader attrition with the environment eliciting a general, excitable oversensitivity or distancing coldness (Kretschmer 1925). In this respect, Kretschmer's seminal investigations first offer an initial depiction of prototypical forms of human subjectivity that, through temperamental accentuations (i.e. schizoid and cycloid), might lead to overt psychotic states (i.e. schizophrenia and manic-depressive illness); and, second, suggest a shift of attention to the comprehensive phenomenological coherence among affective-emotional features, psychomotricity, and psychic tempo.

Table 77.2 Mood and sensitivity scale

	Cyclothymia	Schizothymia
Mood	Diathetic proportion: between elevated and depressed.	Psychesthetic proportion: between hypersensitive and anesthetic (cold).
Psychic tempo	Wavy temperamental curve: between mobile and comfortable.	Jerky temperamental curve: between unstable and tenacious.
Psychomotility	Adequate to stimulus, rounded, natural, smooth.	Often inadequate to stimulus, restrained, inhibited, stiff.

Data from Ernst Kretschmer (1925). *Physique and Character*. London: Kegan Paul, Trench, Trubner & Co.

TELLENBACH: *TYPUS MELANCHOLICUS* AND THE ANTHROPOLOGICAL VULNERABILITY TO AFFECTIVE DISORDERS

Partly inspired by Kretschmer, Tellenbach (1914–1994), extrapolated a set of distinctive features that inform the premorbid and inter-morbid personality structure liable to endogenous depression. Those characteristics (i.e. orderliness, conscientiousness) shape and inform a certain way of being-in-the-world that revolves around the possibility of developing major depression (melancholia) (Tellenbach 1980). In Tellenbach's view, the developmental pathways leading toward endogenous depression, are indeed promoted by the dialectic between a certain premorbid personality (broadly understood as an anthropological precondition), and critical existential events (Ambrosini et al. 2014). Those premorbid characteristics conferring existential vulnerability to major affective disorders, already transpire at the level of the personality structure through a stable and recognizable imprint. Such specific personality structure, termed *Typus Melancholicus* (TM), is better understood as a stable mode of relating to the world and oneself in a way that entails a potential for the development of affective episodes. TM is defined by a set of concomitant, stable characteristics that are rooted in the ethical–ontological level of value-formation and constitute the anthropological core of the individual orientation to the social world. Because of such axiological orientation, TM pre-structures a worldview that already entails a germ of potential decompensation (Stanghellini and Mundt 1997).

Core phenomenological features of the TM are orderliness (i.e. an accentuated seeking for order and harmony in the field of interpersonal relationships) and conscientiousness (i.e. an elevated self-expectation above the threshold of one's own possibilities), both fueled by the need to prevent feelings and attributions of guilt as well as to maintain the surrounding free of possible conflicts (Ambrosini et al. 2014). Because of the synergetic effect of orderliness and conscientiousness, TM is constantly engaged in fulfilling many obligations in a reliable and scrupulous way, in view of preserving a controllable and predictable negotiation with the potential requests from the surrounding world. Moved by a fundamental need to avert any potential feeling of guilt, TM's behavior is modeled on the perceived social expectation.

However, despite his efforts to preserve an ordered and controlled existential homeostasis, TM's radical refractoriness to being subject to the unforeseen in his/her existential field is unavoidably frustrated, inducing an important exposure to vulnerability (Stanghellini and Mundt 1997; Ambrosini et al. 2014).

Elaborating on Tellenbach, one of his scholars, Alfred Kraus identified two further features of the anthropological structure of the TM: hyper/heteronomy (i.e. an exaggerated norm adaptation and receptiveness toward external normative conventions) and intolerance of ambiguity (i.e. a cognitive and emotional-affective incapacity to accommodate opposite or conflicting characteristics concerning the same person or situation). Those core properties of TM have been condensed, operationalized, and field-tested in the "Criteria for Typus Melancholicus" (Stanghellini et al. 2006; Stanghellini and Raballo 2007). The typical way of being in the social world of the TM, is therefore based on a hyperthrophy of the "role identity" (the identity sovra-structure conferred to the person by her social function) at the expense of the "self-identity" (the self-determination of the personality beyond simple and straightforward identification with the agent of a social role), with a reduction of the vital dialectic between these two identities and, ultimately leading to an alienation of self-identity in the impersonal formalism of the role-identity (Kraus 1987).

From Premorbid Personality to Endogenous Depression: The Pathogenic Role of TM

The TM strives not to lag behind himself, he is always following his duties and perceived obligations related to the social role, and therefore, his entire life is stretched in an effort to pay his debts before contracting them. This precarious and effortful balance gets shattered in the pre-melancholic situation. The key feature of this situation is the emotion of despair that is the prodrome of melancholic breakdown. Crucially, Tellenbach emphasizes:

> What we call despair ("*Verzweiflung*") is remaining captured in doubt . . . To be precise, despair is not just hopelessness and desperation, not an ultimate or an arrival at an endpoint, but rather the movement backward and forward, an alternation, so that a definite decision ("*endgültige Entscheidung*") is no longer possible. (1980: 165)

The person is caught in a sort of decisional and agentic fibrillation, unable to resolve the ambivalence of being simultaneously moved toward two opposite directions. Rather than a loss of hope, the core of despair is an inexcruciable indecision, that cannot be solved by making a pragmatic choice, resulting in a profound alteration of temporality: "what previously came about in the mode of succession, now appears only in the necessity of simultaneity" (Tellenbach 1980: 167).

Similarly to the paralysis of lived time, despair also impacts lived space as the juxtaposition of alternative choices, in a sort of indecision cramp, jeopardizes the sequential order of actions, leading to a frenzied restlessness.

THE PRE-MELANCHOLIC PHASE AS SITUATION

In this context, the phenomenological concept of "situation" illuminates hidden aspects of the relationship between the person and the triggering interpersonal event that instantiates the transition to despair and ultimately to a melancholic episode. Indeed, the TM, with his inflexible value structure and hierarchic (although reliable and sacrificial) way of understanding life, invariably co-creates relational situations that gradually destabilize his vulnerability. Concretely, the TM is caught between the latent goal of complying in advance with the presumed expectations of the others and a high interpersonal sensitivity, constantly sharpened by his concern for orderliness and conscientiousness, intolerance of ambiguity and hyper/heteronomia. Therefore, in his permanent striving for social desirability (in the very impersonal and conventional sense of contextual social standards), he recursively approaches situations characterized by an unrestrained increase of the fixed tasks that gradually overwhelms his capacity to preserve predetermined order. Caught in such imbalance, the TM fails to strategically discriminate what can be momentarily prioritized or left aside. In phenomenological terms the pre-melancholic phase is catalyzed by two "situative constellations" (i.e. *includence* and *remanence*) that later induce the radical transformation of the self–world relation constituting the despair (Tellenbach 1980). Specifically, spatial *"includence"* indicates the self-contradiction of the TM actively attempting to meticulously maintain a homeostatic order while constantly expanding beyond his own limits and capabilities; whereas temporal *"remanence"* designates paradoxical tendency of canceling possible debts in advance, with the danger of remaining behind oneself with respect to personal expectations, emerging duties, as well as the irreducible unpredictability of the unforeseen. Both "includence" and "remanence" are to be understood as complementary and latent modes of being in the interpersonal world, actualized by the structural features of the TM. Despair intervenes at the confluence of the two situative constellations and experientially translates the pre-melancholic phase into the melancholic one (Tellenbach 1980; Stanghellini and Mundt 1997).

TEMPERAMENTS AND AFFECTIVE PHENOMENOLOGY

Since early hyppocratic conceptualizations, the status of temperaments within the broader sphere of mood phenomena has been central, although with phenomenologically elusive borders. Indeed, temperaments are not discernible just in terms of subjective mental states and in a clinical setting surface almost inferentially on the basis of both self-description and observational exploration, particularly of the reaction styles triggered by external stimuli as well as of behavioral expressions of the person. Concretely, if emotions are psychologically discernible, intentional states with relatively specific determinants (i.e. they are directed at particular objects, events, and situations) and circumscribed time frame, and moods are broader and less focused, atmospheric feeling-states that predetermine inchoate affective saliences (Aho 2017), temperaments are those background bio-psychic organizers that confer the rhythm and the affective attunement between the two. That is, they precondition the background orientation and mood coloring as well as the actualization of unfocused, global feeling-states into specific emotions.

Therefore, phenomenological investigations of abnormal human subjectivity while emphasizing a shift of attention from mere symptom aggregates (i.e. state-like indexes matching diagnostic polythetic criteria) to a broader range of phenomena (i.e. trait-like features of a given life-world that are coherent expressions of underlying vulnerability toward the potential development of a certain type of disorder), also encourage an in-depth dissection of affective phenomena and related anomalies. In this sense, for example, recognizing a personality structure such as the TM has important implications in understanding the clinical evolution of minor and major mood episodes, including the direction of the polarity and the symptom formation of acute mood episodes (Stanghellini et al. 2006; Stanghellini and Raballo 2007; Ambrosini et al. 2014).

Although the modern concept of affective temperaments has been operationalized mostly in a clinical descriptive framework (Akiskal 1996; Rihmer et al. 2010), primarily based on the works of Kraepelin and Kretschmer, important empirical and theoretical convergences with phenomenology suggest that TM's infrastructure is a potentially relevant modulator of intermorbid and long-term trajectory of mood disorders, constituting a trait-like vulnerability factor (Stanghellini et al. 2006; Stanghellini and Raballo 2007). However, whereas Tellenbach systematic work has been substantially re-annexed to contemporary research, essential phenomenological intuition from Kretschmer remains largely under-recognized. This is the case of the two kretschmerian axes—cycloid and schizoid—and their immanent articulation in psychic tempo, psychomotility, and mood proportion. This coincides with the phenomenological intuition of the interconnectedness between lived time, lived space and the coherent way of finding oneself in the world along the continuum of affective reactivity (anesthetic and hyperaesthetic) and mood orientation (from joy to sadness) (Kretschmer 1925; Aho 2017).

CONCLUSIONS

A phenomenological approach to affective temperaments is fundamentally aimed at improving the cross-sectional and prospective understanding the subjective nuances of affective states as well as their potential pathogenetic trajectories, through the lens of certain prototypical descriptors and organizers. Among those, the anthropological structure of the TM is an example of pre-pathologic, dispositional vulnerability to affective spectrum disorders, whereas the kretschmerian tripod (i.e. mood proportion, psychic tempo, and psychomotility) is an equally important clinical prism to discern the relative schizo- and cyclo-thymic axes. Finally, it is worth highlighting that an accurate clinical-psychopathological exploration of affective temperaments is essential for a clinically rational identification of qualitative thresholds along a continuum of severity from generic help-seeking to high-risk and overt affective syndromes.

BIBLIOGRAPHY

Aho K. (2017). "Affectivity and its Disorders." In G. Stanghellini, M. Broome, P. Fusar-Poli, A. Raballo, R. Rosfort, and A. Fernandez (eds.), *The Oxford Handbook of Phenomenological Psychopathology*, pp. 1–7. New York: Oxford University Press.

Akiskal H. S. (1996). "The Temperamental Foundations of Affective Disorders." In C. Mundt, K. Hahlweg, and P. Fiedler (eds.), *Interpersonal Factors in the Origin and Course of Affective Disorders*, pp. 3–30. London: Gaskell.

Ambrosini A., Stanghellini G., and Raballo A. (2014). "Temperament, Personality and the Vulnerability to Mood Disorders: The Case of the Melancholic Type of Personality." *Journal of Psychopathology* 393–403.

Blaney P. H. and Millon T. (2009). *Oxford Textbook of Psychopathology*, 2nd edn. New York: Oxford University Press.

Bouchard T. J. (1994). "Genes, Environment, and Personality." *Science* 264: 1700–1701.

Glezerman T. B. and Balkoski B. I. (2002). *Language, Thought and the Brain*. New York: Kluwer Academic Publisher.

Harnic D., Koukopoulos A., Mazza M., Janiri L., and Bria P. (2011). "Temperament as a Basic Element in Bipolar Spectrum and in Sub-Threshold Manifestations: A Brief Review of Psychiatric Literature." *Italian Journal of Psychopathology* 17: 213–224.

Kalachanis K. and Michailidis I. E. (2015). "The Hippocratic View on Humors and Human Temperament." European Journal of Social Behaviour 2: 1–5.

Kraepelin E. (1921). *Manic-Depressive Insanity and Paranoia*. Edinburgh: Churchill Livingstone.

Kraus A. (1982). "Identity and Psychosis of the Manic-Depressive." In A. de Koning and F. A. Jenner (eds.), *Phenomenology and Psychiatry*, pp. 201–216. London: Academic Press.

Kraus A. (1987). "Dinamique de role des maniaque-depressifs." *Psychologie Medicale* 19: 401–405.

Kretschmer E. (1925). *Physique and Character*. London: Kegan Paul, Trench, Trubner and Company, Ltd.

Rihmer Z., Akiskal K. K., Rihmer A., and Akiskal H. S. (2010). "Current Research on Affective Temperaments." *Current Opinion in Psychiatry* 23: 12–18.

Stanghellini G. and Mundt C. (1997). "Personality and Endogenous/Major Depression: An Empirical Approach to Typus Melancholicus—Theoretical Issues." *Psychopathology* 30: 119–129.

Stanghellini G., Bertelli M., and Raballo A. (2006). "Typus Melancholicus: Personality Structure and the Characteristics of Major Unipolar Depressive Episode." *Journal of Affective Disorders* 93(1–3): 159–167.

Stanghellini G. and Raballo A. (2007). "Exploring the Margins of the Bipolar Spectrum: Temperamental Features of the Typus Melancholicus." *Journal of Affective Disorders* 100(1–3): 13–21.

Tellenbach H. (1980). *Melancholy*. Pittsburgh: Duquesne University Press.

Appendix: Kraepelin's Fundamental States

Temperament	Main psychological features	Clinical expression
Depressive	• permanent gloomy emotional orientation infused in all life experiences • whole conduct influenced by anxiety, scrupulous conscientiousness, and lack of self-confidence	"Every moment of pleasure is embittered to them by the recollection of gloomy hours, by self-reproaches, and still more by glaringly portrayed fears for the future . . . life with its activity is a burden which they habitually bear with dutiful self-denial without being compensated by the pleasure of existence, the joy of work" (1921: 118).
Manic	• a permanently exalted mood associated with a sense of superiority that pervaded all interpersonal relationships • conduct and activities dominated by a unsteadiness and restlessness, possibly associated with inconstancy, aimless hyperactivity, talkativeness, interpersonal grumpiness, and distractibility	"Mood is permanently exalted, careless. . . . The patients have very marked self-confidence, put an extremely high value on their own capabilities and performances, boast with the most obvious exaggeration. . . . They show little sympathy with the sorrows of others; they enjoy deriding, teasing, and illusing those who, they think, are their inferiors. . . . They are usually ready for jokes, . . . for conversation and pastimes of all kinds" (1921: 125–128). "They are communicative, adapt themselves readily to new conditions, but soon they again long for change and variety. Without sufficient reason they change . . . position, are always beginning something new, make large plans and after a short time drop them again. . . . They speak readily and much . . . In conversation, the patients assume a free and easy tone, give . . . ironical answers, . . . sought-out allusions. . . . They make great claims and behave arrogantly. . . . they are extraordinarily distractible, and seek to escape in every way from the constraint of a systematic mental training . . . The train of thought is desultory, incoherent, aimless; judgment is hasty and shallow" (1921: 125–129).
Irritable	• mixture of manic and depressive features • Wavy mood coloring mainly dominated by irritability • conduct of life was subject to the most multifarious incidents	"In general, the patients are perhaps cheerful . . . but periods are interpolated in which they are irritable and ill-humoured, also perhaps sad, spiritless, anxious; they display from youth up extraordinarily great fluctuations in emotional equilibrium and are greatly moved by all experiences, frequently in an unpleasant way. . . . They are easily offended and hot-tempered; . . . and on the most trivial occasions fall into outbursts of boundless fury. . . . In the family also they are insufferable, capricious, . . . have attacks of jealousy. . . . Their power of imagination is usually very much influenced by moods and feelings. It, therefore, comes easily to delusional interpretations of the events of life" (1921: 130–131).
Cyclothymic	• frequent, more or less regular fluctuations of the psychic state to the manic or to the depressive side	"These are the people who constantly oscillate . . . between the two opposite poles of mood, sometimes 'rejoicing to the skies', sometimes 'sad as death'. To-day lively, sparkling, . . . full of the joy of life, the pleasure of enterprise, . . . after some time they meet us depressed. . . . ill-humoured, in need of rest. A patient . . . said that she was 'like a barometer, one time so, another time different'. . . . At first these deviations from the middle line are only occasionally perceptible once in a way and as rapidly passing attacks; but for the most part they have the tendency to return more frequently and to last always longer, indeed finally to fill up the whole life" (1921: 131–132).

....

CHAPTER 78

SCHIZOPHRENIC AUTISM

....

RICHARD GIPPS AND SANNEKE DE HAAN

INTRODUCING BLEULER'S *AUTISM*

....

THE concept of "autism" was introduced to psychiatry by Eugen Bleuler who also coined the term "schizophrenia." "Schizophrenia" arrived in 1908, "autism" in 1910; both were introduced to the wider world in Bleuler's 1911 monograph *Dementia Praecox oder Gruppe der Schizophrenien*.[1] Distinctly schizophrenic disturbances, he contended, were characterized at root by disturbances of the three "A"s of association, affectivity, and ambivalence; these underpinned further symptoms including the central disturbance in reality contact he called autism. What today often denotes a developmental *condition or disorder* ("early infantile autism," or "autistic spectrum disorder" (ASD)) started out as a descriptor for a pathognomonic *manner of being* met with in schizophrenia. Phenomenological psychiatry continues to deploy it in this sense. In fact, even in the early writings of the ASD forerunners Asperger (1944) and Kanner (1943), the term is primarily used adjectivally ("autistic") to describe the *character* of certain disturbances of affective contact in children. Yet whereas the children described by Kanner suffered a deficit in affective contact ab initio, the adult patients described by Bleuler had instead detached from a reality with which they had previously enjoyed emotional relations (Kanner 1973).

To understand the significance of the psychopathological question "what is schizophrenic autism?" it is important to start in the right place—which here means not simply assuming a positivist conception of nosology from the get-go. For, agree or not with its methods, classical psychopathology did not take itself to do well by proceeding positivistically, enumerating operationally defined signs and symptoms and merely collocating them into a construct designated "schizophrenia." Instead it took itself to be investigating the distinctive, intuitively recognizable, delusion-engendering alteration in self-state and world-relation underlying such signs and symptoms, even if—as Jaspers (1963: 96) wrote—"a clear presentation is hardly possible with so alien a happening." For the phenomenologist, reflective understanding of precisely what is distinctive about this state is not to be disposed of through lapsing instead into criterial checklists but, rather, to be pursued through the careful

---

[1] See Bleuler (1908); Bleuler (1910); and Bleuler (1911/1950). Bleuler's monograph was translated into English in 1950 and published as *Dementia Praecox or the Group of Schizophrenias*. Kuhn (2004) provides a helpful overview.

description of what intuitively were paradigmatic cases, which description does not shy away from deploying such metaphoric and philosophic concepts as are apt to and revelatory of its object (Minkowski 1927/1987: 190–191).

Schizophrenia, Bleuler tells us (1911/1950: 63–67),

> is characterised by a very peculiar alteration of the relation between the patient's inner life and the external world. The inner life assumes pathological predominance (autism). . . . The most severe schizophrenics, who have no more contact with the outside world, live in a world of their own. They have encased themselves with their desire and wishes (which they consider fulfilled) or occupy themselves with the trials and tribulations of their persecutory ideas; they have cut themselves off as much as possible from any contact with the external world. . . . This detachment from reality, together with the relative and absolute predominance of the inner life, we term autism. . . . In less severe cases . . . patients are still able to move about in the external world but . . . everything which is in contradiction to their complexes simply does not exist for their thinking or feeling. . . . The autistic world has as much reality for the patient as the true one, but his is a different kind of reality. . . . In milder cases the real and autistic worlds exist not only side by side, but often become entangled with one another in the most illogical manner. The doctor is at one moment not only the hospital-physician and at another the shoemaker, S., but he is both in the same thought-content of the patient. . . . Wishes and fears constitute the contents of autistic thinking. . . . The autistic thinking is the source of delusions, of the crude offences against logic and propriety, and all the other pathological symptoms.

Bleuler (1911/1950: 63 n. 19) explains to us that his coinage is nearly coterminous with Freud's *autoerotism* but that he chose a new term since Freud's greatly expanded sense of eros/libido can mislead. He also notes that, unlike Janet's quite *general* concept of "loss of the sense of reality" (i.e. diminished "fonction du réel"), he considers autism to characterize the patient's reality relation *only in the ambit of her unconscious emotional complexes*. Bleuler's "autism" meant a circumscribed withdrawal from reality—into what today we might call a "psychic retreat" (Steiner 1993) or "autistic enclave" (Tustin 1986)—prompted by unbearable emotional experiences.[2] According to Bleuler, it is this withdrawal which conditions the flourishing of delusional experience and thought—experience and thought which still express the trace of the unconscious complex that evoked them (Jung 1907/1936). Precisely what is the character of this retreat is our concern in this article.

The psychopathological significance of autism—that is, of this "very peculiar alteration" of the relation between inner life and external world—is that it is pathognomonic of schizophrenia. There is, undeniably, much diversity (of expression, course, and outcome) amongst the manifest symptoms of what Bleuler termed "the schizophrenias" (Boyle 2002). There are also, undeniably, other important pathognomic features of schizophrenic selfhood (especially radical disruptions in ego identity, coherence, demarcation, vitality, and agency (Scharfetter 2008)) which are not simply a function of autism. Nevertheless, it is autism in particular which is intuitively sensed in the clinician's "*praecox Gefühl*" (a distinctive resonance to schizophrenic disturbance which has been argued to be a reliable indicator of schizophrenia for phenomenologically skilled clinicians (Schwartz and Wiggins 1987; Grube 2006; Varga

---

[2] Bleuler's autism has to do with a *qualitative alteration* in the relation between the inner life and the world. The autism of today's ASD has instead to do with *deficits* in social relating and *restrictions* in patterns of interest (see DSM-5; DSM-III even offered schizophrenia as an exclusionary criterion for an autism diagnosis).

2013—although cf. Ungvari et al. 2010), and autism which marks what is distinctly psychotic or delusional about the patient's thinking. Lose the significance of such distinctive organizing *Gestalten* as autism and the self-disturbances, and we lose the rationale for a phenomenologically meaningful typification of psychopathological experience, and risk collapsing back into banal symptom checklists or objective psychological descriptions of altered cognition that do nothing to thematize the distinctiveness of schizophrenic existence.

Bleuler's (1911/1950) concept of "autism" covers a lot of ground; a standard criticism of it (Parnas and Bovet 1991; Dein 1966) has it that it covers too much. Thus we find within his concept all of:

1. an altered relation to reality,
2. a distinctive fantasy-involving form of thinking, and
3. a motivated retreat from the world.

Some clinicians who combine something of a phenomenological and psychoanalytical disposition (Laing 1960; Sechehaye 1956) follow Bleuler in preserving the gamut of (i)-(ii)-(iii). Phenomenologically, yet largely non-psychoanalytically, minded clinicians (e.g. Parnas and Bovet 1991; Sass 2001; Minkowski 1953; Stanghellini and Ballerini 2004; Blankenburg 1971) instead develop a restricted, yet phenomenologically deepened, conception of autism as (i)—that is, as a *defective pre-reflective vital attunement* with reality which ramifies through the forms of thought and experience, imbuing all the psychopathology that arises with a distinctively schizophrenic tonus. Non-phenomenological, yet psychoanalytically-inclined, clinicians (e.g. Segal 1977/1990; Freeman, Cameron, and McGhie 1958), by contrast, rather focus their attention on (ii)-(iii); thus Segal's distinction between symbolic equation and symbolism proper maps directly onto Bleuler's distinction between autistic and realistic thought. Clinicians who, whilst having neither inclination, yet remain attached to the concept (e.g. Dein 1966), restrict their attention to an under-theorized version of (i). Others (e.g. Von Domarus 1944; Ciompi 1988) appear to abandon autism, yet somehow hope to retain a coherent concept of "schizophrenia." Perhaps rather improbably they try to reconstruct what is pathognomic about it in terms of a disturbance of the form of thought (e.g. in atypical association or invalid logic). Indeed, Bleuler's own modestly psychoanalytic and latently phenomenological sensibilities sometimes gave way to a largely associationist schematism (Bleuler 1911/1950: Section X).

In the next section we consider the depth of understanding which a phenomenological approach has brought to the understanding of (i) the autistic unmooring of pre-reflective reality contact. That which follows considers (ii) the significance of fantasy, and in the final section we consider (iii) the essentially motivational aspect to an autistic retreat to omnipotent fantasy, thereby completing our deepened understanding of Bleuler's fundamental conceptualization of the autistic core of schizophrenic life.

ALTERED RELATION TO REALITY: PHENOMENOLOGICAL PERSPECTIVES

Both early (Minkowski 1927; Blankenburg 1971; Kimura 1982, 2001) and contemporary (Sass 2001; Parnas, Bovet, and Zahavi 2002; Mishara 2001; Urfer 2001) phenomenological theorists of schizophrenic autism stress disturbances in pre-reflective world-engagement as definitive of schizophrenic autism.

To situate the phenomenological psychiatrists' discussions of autistic selfhood it is important first to rehearse the phenomenological philosophers' conceptualization of selfhood as *being-in-the-world*. And to understand the phenomenological understanding of selfhood as being-in-the-world it is important first to grasp its motivation—which is to resist those dualistic conceptions of selfhood, widespread in our scientific and philosophical culture, which alienate us from our bodies, from one another, from our cultural resources, and from the physical environment.

The assumption of such dualistic conceptions is that we may understand what a self is independently of its relations to other selves, to its body, to language and other cultural practices, and to its proximal environment. Having accepted such assumptions the theorist's task then becomes explaining how an inner self makes contact with a separate, outer, other/ body/world.

By contrast, phenomenologists such as Heidegger (1927/1978) and Merleau-Ponty (1945/ 2002, 1964/1968) consider their task to be the unity-preserving description of an intrinsically embodied, cultural, and relational selfhood. As they understand it, we do not encounter one another as pre-individuated monads, but rather enjoy such determinate individuality as we possess in virtue of our recurrently-enacted differentiation from one another. Such differentiation not only individuates the self but places the self and other in intrinsically comprehending forms of moral and emotional relation (I am angry at her for stealing my book). The same goes for self and objects: we become distinguished as determinate acting, perceiving, and understanding selves as we develop comprehending intentional relations of perception and action to the objects with which we interact. These perceptual and active relations do not enjoy an intentionality derivative of that intrinsic to the philosophically concocted "inner representations" of a pre-individuated "inner mind." Rather they are replete with their own *sui generis* intentionality. Skills such as language use, and the more complex and determinate opportunities for understanding which it affords, are also not soldered on top of intrinsically non-linguistic corporeal foundations like a man on a horse or even like a centaur. Instead the best picture we have of the relation of linguistic and bodily sensibilities is simply that of the developing man himself: someone whose reality-relating motor performances in speech and writing because, with increasing enculturation, more and more complex and sensitive to the interactive situations of their performance. Finally, whilst we do engage in cognitive activity which is disengaged, deliberative, and abstract (e.g. in theoretical reasoning carried out in inner speech), this is a derivative refinement of, rather than a foundation for, our everyday interactive capabilities (e.g. the practical ability to engage in conversation).

The significance of a phenomenological conception for the understanding of schizophrenic autism is that it allows us to understand just how intimately connected are disturbances of everyday immersed relations to reality and disturbances of the integrity of selfhood. A dualistically conceived self is, one might say, already disconnected in its being from reality and from other selves—yet is not thought of as disturbed on that basis alone. An embodied interactive self, by contrast, is *constituted* by its participation with others and in its environmental situations. Disturb such participatory relations and the self itself falls apart since these relations constitute its being. Far from the sanity of outer world-relations being derivative of that of an inner self, the two can—once we drop the dualistic inner–outer picture—be seen as of a piece.

Minkowski (1927/1987)—himself more a Bergson aficionado, but whose thought (like Bergson's) is resonant with much in phenomenology—summarizes this self-destroying disconnect as a loss of "vital contact with reality." The kind of contact which concerns him is no mere ability to *abstractly represent* reality, but rather that which founds such representational capacities, namely our *lived ("vital") participatory indwelling* (Parnas, Bovet, and Zahavi 2002). As one of his patients famously described it: "I can reason quite well, but only in the absolute, because I have lost contact with life" (Minkowski 1927/1987: 210).

This contact, engagement, or resonance amounts to an ability to act appropriately without prior deliberation. A patient we once interviewed talked of realizing that his "humanity" had returned and his (schizophrenic) "illness" had left him the moment that, rightly judging his nieces to be in danger as they played too close to a ride at a funfair, he spontaneously emerged from his autistic state to rush over and scoop them up. We may also bring to mind those temporary respites from loss of reality contact in long-stay psychiatric patients who, faced with an emergency like a flood or a fire, come out of their catatonic stupor and provide help or make an orderly escape. A difficulty of maintaining such automatic, pre-reflective attunement to what matters is termed by Blankenburg a "crisis of common sense" or, following his patient Anne, a lack of "natural self-evidence" (Blankenburg 1971; Sass 2003): "What is it that I really lack? Something so small, so odd, but so important that you cannot live without it . . . What I lack really is the 'natural self-evidence' . . . It has simply to do with living, with living properly, that you are not so outside, outside of society, so expelled. . . . But I cannot find the right word for that which is lacking . . . I can never be properly present and participate. . . . It is simply, I don't know, not knowledge . . . Every child knows it! One usually just naturally picks it up. It is these simple things a human being needs to be able to live."

The schizophrenia sufferer may succumb to what Minkowski called "morbid rationalism": that is, suffer the replacing of, or actively compensate for, a disconnected know-how and instinct with abstract knowledge and involuntary or deliberative reflection (also called "hyperreflexivity") (Laing 1960; Sass 1992; Sass and Parnas 2003; de Haan and Fuchs 2010). Even though the morbid rationalist may be lost in excessively abstract reason rather than (as Bleuler allegedly has it) excessive imagination, the term "autism" still applies, Minkowski suggests, because the sufferer's *thinking* "no longer seeks to be integrated with reality." The sufferer *herself* may be attempting to safely compensate for destabilizing damage to participatory know-how through engaging with the world in a deliberative and reflective vein. However her disconnected *thinking* cannot, from this top-down vantage point, achieve its necessary footing in the unquestioned instinctive certainties of daily life (Wittgenstein 1975). Moreover, by reflecting on what is normally tacitly taken for granted, alienation from the world and others is increased rather than dissolved (Fuchs 2005).

It is important to note that this know-how is not best understood as task competence (e.g. knowing how to change a light bulb). Rather what matters is, on the whole, a capacity for ongoing, intuitively apt and flexible, synchronized attunement with the world (Van Duppen, 2017). The autistic individual no longer participates in the environment's particular rhythm of ambient becoming, but rather marches to the beat of her own drum. Or ultimately—since the beat of this drum is constituted through the self's relatedness—to an incoherent beat, or merely to a delusional semblance of a beat.

A disturbance in the rhythms of such background coordination and participation is particularly acute in interpersonal relations. Kimura (2001) highlights this with his notion of disturbances of the "in-between." People are who they are in their relations. On a dual-istic conception, conversations are possible because what meets are distinct pre-delimited selves who have things to tell each other. On a phenomenological conception, by contrast, the selves are what they are in and through such meetings; neither conversation nor self-hood enjoys ontological primacy—instead they are, to use Heidegger's term, equiprimordial. Interactions structure selfhood, so the self which withdraws from interaction risks impov-erishment and disintegration. On the other hand, the self which stays in such interactions as are marked by intrapersonal or interpersonal conflict risks breaking apart unless additional self-protective measures are deployed.

In summary, the phenomenological perspective aims to re-theorize what Bleuler in-tended by way of autistic disconnection from reality through its conception of a disloca-tion of pre-reflective participatory indwelling. The phenomenological psychopathologists understand autism as a dislocation from the world which may inspire and/or be fed by hyperreflexive, morbidly rationalistic, attempts to compensate with reason for what has been lost by way of instinct. Schizophrenic idiosyncrasy and delusion is seen as launching, and taking its distinctive form from, the bodily unmooring of the autistically disconnected subject.

Whilst this dislocation surely indexes a fundamental, pathognomic aspect of schizo-phrenic psychopathology, and one which Bleuler didn't have the conceptual resources to adequately interpret, it isn't clear that it yet captures enough of what is distinctive in schizophrenic autism. For what distinguishes Bleuler's autism is not merely that it signifies (i) the negatively characterizable condition of disconnection from reality, but that it also involves, as the other side of this coin, (ii) a positively characterizable condi-tion of preoccupation by an alternative domain which Bleuler hoped to characterize in terms of substitutive and unassailable fantasy (Bleuler 1911/1950: 373). This disconnected and dreamlike autistic world is part-constituted by wishes and fears, may coexist along-side reality-relations ("double-bookkeeping"), and—so the theory goes—provides the soil structure in which "delusions . . . and all the other pathological symptoms" grow. The following two sections aim to recapture what is further distinctive to autism in a way which yet respects the non-dualistic conception of selfhood offered by existential phenomenology.

AUTISTIC FANTASY VERSUS REALISTIC THOUGHT

While phenomenological psychiatry deepens our understanding of (i) disturbances of co-ordinated, immersed, self-structuring participation in the world, it does not deepen our understanding of, but instead simply rejects the significance of (ii) fantasy-ridden inward preoccupation. As Parnas, Bovet, and Zahavi (2002) comment, "the criterion 'withdrawal to fantasy life' is empirically false, if taken as a necessary one: there are seemingly extro-verted schizophrenics (e.g. certain disorganized patients) as well as patients who do not have a rich fantasy life." Yet criteria as such are not empirically true or false—instead they delineate the concepts which frame empirical judgments. And Bleuler already recognized what Parnas et al. note: the alternative autistic world of the schizophrenic patient may well be impoverished, and may coexist with, rather than displace, the extrovert schizophrenic's participation in reality (Bleuler 1911/1950: 65, 88). Given this we may legitimately wonder whether contemporary phenomenological psychiatrists have yet adequately grasped the significance of fantasy to autistic reality—and whether we can find an understanding of it that allows it to take its place at a conceptual table which the phenomenologist would recognize as properly set.

When justifying his coining of "autism" as distinct from Freud's reworking of Havelock Ellis's "autoeroti[ci]sm," Bleuler (1911/1950: 63 n. 19) mentions his wish to avoid what he saw as Freud's unusually broad conception of Eros. What he doesn't mention here is what in fact was his contention with Freud over whether an infant starts out life in an autistic domain of fantasy governed by the pleasure principle (hallucinatory wish-fulfillment), gradually making her way out to realistic thought governed by the reality principle, or whether the capacity for fantasy is rather a developmental achievement presupposing reality-contact. Freud and Piaget thought the former, Bleuler and Vygotsky the latter (Harris 2000). The debate is partly about developmental chronology, but more importantly about the very intelligibility of ascribing coherent fantasy either to an infant who has not yet learned to make relevant reality discriminations or to a psychotic adult whose reality function has become compromised.

The debate is one on which phenomenology has a bearing. If we start from that dualistic conception of intentional life which phenomenology disputes, a conception which sees mental life as self-standingly inner, it is easy to feel the attraction of Freud's and Piaget's standpoint. For on such a conception there seems nothing wrong in principle with suggesting that inner fantasy may precede or take over from outer reality contact. Yet if we take seriously the phenomenological conception of mind as structured in and by its world-relations, fantasy can hardly be given such a self-standing role. For reality contact now becomes not something abrogated by, but rather the condition of possibility of, genuine mental functions such as fantasy. But, one then might think, if reality contact is fantasy's condition of possibility, and reality contact is precisely what is disturbed in schizophrenia, then considerations of fantasy are irrelevant to the constitution of schizophrenic autism.

Yet to suppose this the end of the issue against (ii) the fantasy-invoking criterion ignores the possibility of a deeper phenomenological reinterpretation of Bleuler's criterion. Consider again the phenomenological conception of selfhood as equiprimordial with relation to non-self. A key contention of that conception is that self and other *co-arise*—that their *oppositional configuration is essential to their identity*. This, we propose, is also the structure of the relation between fantasy and reality perception. Essential to being a true imaginer or believer is being able to entertain a possibility in one's mind whilst knowing that this (in the case of belief) may not be, or perhaps (in the case of fantasy) is definitely not, a fact. If we turn now to Bleuler's (ii) fantasy criterion, the significance is not so much that one is "lost in a fantasy world" but that one is lost to *the* world in such a way that a distinction between fantasy and reality no longer finds instantiation in the form of one's thought.

A superficial, merely epistemic, gloss could be given to this, and it is indeed tempting to offer such a reading of the autist's situation—as if the problem were that, whilst there *is* yet a fact of the matter as to whether his thoughts are fantasies or genuine beliefs, he no longer knows what that fact of the matter is. Bleuler (1911/1950: 373–374) reports Pelletier saying that "above all, the patient does not differentiate anymore between reality and fantasy," yet of this Bleuler says that whilst it is "true in a certain sense" it still does "not get at the essence of" autism. The deeper suggestion he grasps for is that, in autistic states, there is an "inadequate or absent distinction between fantasy and reality" themselves (Bleuler 1911/1950: 374).

On this ontological, rather than epistemological, conception, becoming lost in autistic states involves becoming lost to states of mind in which imagination and reality-oriented thought are collapsed and so no longer constitute themselves as such in a mutual antagonism. The coin which has (i) an altered relation to reality as one of its faces has, we can now see, as its other (ii) an indistinction between reality and fearful (e.g. paranoid) or wishful (e.g. grandiose) fantasy. It is just what Freud (1919/1985: 367) called this "uncanny effect . . . produced by effacing the distinction between imagination and reality" which provides the disturbed soil from which grows the varieties of delusional thought and delusional experience. A healthy soil gives rise to a mind which can have both true and false beliefs, yet the autistic loss of "reality contact" runs deeper than any mere falsity of belief—to a state of mind-negating indistinction between the fantastic and the real.

Laing (1960) well describes the corrosive effects of autism on the meaningfulness of both realistic and fantastic thought in his account of the tragic patient who styled herself "the ghost of the weed garden":

> Reality did not cast its shadow or its light over any wish or fear. . . . Every wish met with instantaneous phantom fulfillment and every dread likewise instantaneously came to pass in a phantom way. Thus she could be anyone, anywhere, anytime. "I'm Rita Hayworth, I'm Joan Blondell. I'm a Royal Queen. My royal name is Julianne." "She's self-sufficient," she told me. "She's the self-possessed." But this self-possession was double-edged. It had also its dark side. She was a girl "possessed" by the phantom of her own being. Her self had no freedom, autonomy, or power in the real world. Since she was anyone she cared to mention, she was no one.

As Laing carefully articulates, the boons of the autistic state include a removal of the predicaments of the terrors of self-dissolution in the face of an unassimilable reality. Such terrors can be mitigated by delusionally reconfiguring them into thinkable fears of persecution or omnipotent wish fulfillments. Yet the costs of disturbing one's reality contact in this way are also considerable. For now the persecuting others are just as real—and just as unreal—as the reassuring therapist, and the autistic retreat becomes an autistic prison when there is no possibility of escaping from fear into what in its better moments can be a relatively reassuring, benign and nourishing reality.

The psychopathological significance of the Bleulerian criterion for autism of (ii) a withdrawal to fantasy life—or what with more phenomenological accuracy we may describe as withdrawal from a life in which fantasy and reality are distinct to a mode of being in which fantasy and reality are no longer distinct—is that it allows us to understand the unassailable *form* taken by schizophrenic delusion as a function of the autistic state. We turn now to Bleuler's conception of this withdrawal as (iii) motivated to see what light this may shed on delusional *content*.

MOTIVATED RETREAT: THE PSYCHODYNAMICS
OF AUTISTIC WITHDRAWAL

The conception of autism we now have on the conceptual table goes beyond the phenomenologists' (i) disturbed pre-reflective attunement to include as its transverse side (ii) the inward collapse of the living dialectic of imagination and reality-oriented thought. Part (iii) of Bleuler's conception of autism is that a retreat to this state is motivationally— i.e. psychodynamically—explicable. This has been rejected by phenomenologists from Minkowski (1927/1987) to Parnas and Bovet (1991) who instead lean toward a non-psychoanalytic, merely neurobiological, explanation of disturbed attunement. We contend that this rejection of (iii) risks further impoverishing our understanding of schizophrenic autism.

In what follows we take Minkowski's discussion as exemplary of a tendency in phenomenological psychiatry to presuppose an untenable dualism of matters psychodynamic and neurobiological. Due to this presupposition it fails to draw on the anti-dualistic resources of philosophical phenomenology, fails to pay careful phenomenological attention to what is manifest by way of unconscious motivation in its own case material, misconstrues unconscious motivation in terms of an implausible conscious intentionality, and deprives us of a clear vision of how delusional form and delusional content can be of a piece. We make no claim that this criterion (iii) is non-defeasible; there may be clinical cases in which there is reason to talk of autism in the absence of motivation. Our claim however is that affective motivation belongs properly and fundamentally to intentional life and reality contact, and that we should therefore need special reason to read its contribution out of, rather than reason to read it in to, the autistic situation.

According to Bleuler the retreat to autistic fantasy occurs in the ambit of the schizophrenic's complexes. The thought is simple and has been intuitively expressed by the poets: the schizophrenic, when it conflicts with his basic needs and threatens a shattering shame, "cannot bear very much of reality" (Eliot 1941). The retreat to the autistic state is akin to being lured to the devitalized world of the "faery folk" because "the world's more full of weeping than you can understand" (Yeats 1886/2011). The delusional thoughts and experiences with which he is now involved make spuriously intelligible, give an unreal appearance of manageability to, and symbolically undo, the shattering wounds he suffers. By reverse-engineering these manifest delusional thoughts and experiences we may discern the latent wounds.

Although Minkowski expresses some skepticism about Bleuler's psychodynamic conceptualization, his own case material appears to support it. Consider the case (Minkowski 1927/ 1987: 208) of a man who, when out walking, "was sometimes struck with the appearance of a woman. He would then return to his house, sit down on a chair, cross his arms and take up a position as symmetrical as possible to reflect on the event. He would try to solve the problem of why a woman's body made a particular impression on a man." Minkowski describes his morbid rationality beautifully, but gives no thought at all to what is here being sublimated in the bizarre attempts to solve a putatively intellectual problem—that is, the practical problem of how to get the desirable woman into his bed.

Or consider the case (Minkowski and Targowla 1885/2001) of Paul, a socially withdrawn 17-year-old schoolboy, whose morbid rationality and diminished vital contact with reality are again described beautifully. Just before his autism set in, Paul "seems to have been preoccupied with questions of a sexual nature; he would question his father and ask him for explanations, revealing a complete ignorance of the subject." At bedtime Paul would take more than an hour ensuring the handkerchief was placed perfectly under the bolster [*sic*]. He also spent hours in the bathroom, explaining this in terms of his preoccupation with the size of a feather duster in there, the exact time he entered, or the size of the crack at the door's base and whether he may be seen through it—which latter thought, Paul alleges, troubles him not at all. Again, it is hardly a great step to detect here a defensive retreat into autism from various sexual troubles. Minkowski and Targowla state that the "sexual curiosity that appears at the outset of the illness, which could be considered for that reason a point of departure, can only be a precursory sign of the interrogative attitude that takes a firm hold afterwards. In any case, it is this attitude that must be rectified before attending to anything else." Why it might not instead be that the sexual confusion continued to inspire the autistic retreat is just not considered.[3]

Consider, finally, the case (Minkowski 1927/1987: 210) of the schizophrenic woman who "in an advanced stage of her illness, passed the time making hats for herself. She had made 16 of them. One day, she lost two of them. As a form of retaliation against this she decided to break two of her mother's 16 cups." Once again we're not here going out on a limb if we risk a hypothesis about the symbolic resonance of the hats, cups, and breakages—for example, that the patient made hats to provide herself with her own version of that which she enviously felt her mother to cherish and withhold, so that, following her loss, she was driven to even the score by breaking two of her mother's cups.

Against the suggestion that the retreat to a split-off autistic state could be motivated, Minkowkisi (1953: 212–213) writes that "This loss—or, if we attribute it to the activity of the subject, this suppression—of tonality, can be but the result of an act of violence, of a punch as it were. It is here that the verb 'to split' achieves its full meaning, without . . . this in any sense referring to a deliberate and conscious action. The difference between this state of affairs and putting your head in the sand is here particularly clear." Later, in describing how the autistic state and the activity of self–world severance are the same phenomenon seen from different angles, he reasserts just "how cautious we must be in speaking here of 'activity'."[4] Yet as Laing (1963) notes, Minkowski also cites a patient who reported of himself that "I suppressed feeling as I suppressed all reality. I dug a moat around me." And as Laing also goes on to say, what we meet with here is the early twentieth-century phenomenological psychiatrist's bafflement at the concept of the dynamic unconscious (cf. Jaspers 1963).

Nobody could disagree with this, yet it speaks not at all against a psychodynamic conception of autism as motivationally intelligible world-withdrawal in the face of emotionally intolerable conflict. The key point is that activity may be emotionally motivated without being consciously willed and deliberative. Our question is whether, as Bleuler and Jung discern,

---

[3] The preoccupation with the handkerchief and bolster is curiously similar to the second case in lecture 17 of Freud's (1916–17/1991) Introductory Lectures, which the patient herself traced back to a psychosexual and Oedipal preoccupation.

[4] Our translation, with help from Manon Piette.

autistic unworlding and consequent delusion obtain principally in the ambit of the patient's active complexes, and so may be motivationally intelligible as a response to overwhelming conflict that reality contact presents for them, or whether it is *only* intelligible in neurobiological terms. With regard to Minkowski's patient who described himself as having "dug a moat around me": the fact that it's hard to imagine this as a series of individually intended conscious acts of suppression and "digging" in no way speaks against our taking it as an emotionally motivated activity, one which even the patient notices he has been undertaking.

Even though phenomenological attention to the above case studies of delusional experiences promotes a motivational understanding, phenomenological psychiatrists (e.g. Sass and Byrom 2015; Parnas, Bovet, and Zahavi 2002) typically refer to neurobiological causes rather than psychodynamically intelligible motivations when it comes to understanding the development of delusions. The question arises as to why these should be taken as exclusive, rather than the neurobiological factors providing part of the corporeal instantiation of the motivational ones.

One possibility is that a currently popular understanding of schizophrenia as a disturbance of a so-called "minimal self" (e.g. Nelson, Parnas, and Sass 2014; Sass, Parnas, and Zahavi 2011; Sass and Parnas 2003) obscures the psychodynamics of delusion development. Our thought here is that the more schizophrenia gets relayed at an ever more "basic" or "minimal" level, and accordingly explained in terms of "low-level" causes, the less room there appears to be for motivational factors—on the further assumption, that is, that motives are too "high-level" to be operative in this minimal self.

Against such a reconstructed conception we should like to reiterate that the motivational structure at stake in schizophrenic autism should not be misunderstood as conscious, deliberate reasoning. If one does think of psychodynamic processes as belonging to the domain of intentional contrivance, then there might well seem to be a gap between the disturbances of the self at a basic level and the domain of psychodynamic motivation. In this way it may start to seem as if deep disturbances of world-involvement must belong to neurobiology *rather than* to psychodynamic psychology. This points to a second concern: that it is hard to see how we may equate "basic" with "neurobiological" as opposed to "psychological" without opening up a problematic duality between neurobiological causes and psychological motivations. As phenomenologists we ought to be suspicious of any such dualism. The point is reinforced within psychoanalysis itself which introduced its concept of the "drive" precisely to overcome this dualism: physiological and psychological processes being united in the unitary phenomenon of the drive (Snelling 2001). From such a perspective a conflict between the imperatives of two or more neurologically supported drives constitutes the complexes that motivate autistic unworlding.

When riven with such a conflict and pulled in two directions I may possess enough ego capacity to mentally accommodate both sides of my ambivalence—or, even better, to achieve an integrative sublation (health). Failing that I may repress one half of the equation (neurosis)—or perhaps, if things go well, at least sublimate half the incompatible desires into more congenial forms. Or, if the above options are unavailable, I may detach from reality and enter the substitutive autistic domain (psychosis). Autistic withdrawal, on this model, is psychological and biological at the same time. Which, after all—given that we are bodily beings whose physiology and psychology cannot be seen apart from our striving, motivated, caring, being-in-the-world—is what we should expect.

CONCLUSIONS

If Bleuler's nascently phenomenological and more fully psychoanalytic vision is apt we ought to find autism obtaining in the ambit of the complexes. This is not to say that delusional thought in schizophrenia ought to only ever have conflicted matter as its topic. After all, once an autistic mode is triggered by activated complexes the subject in its grip may still think about and perceptually register a variety of unemotional matters, and some of this may obtain in a fully autistic rather than double book-keeping mode, perhaps providing the welcome distraction of an autistic lullaby. And perhaps, despite affective motivation toward or away from reality forming a proper and foundational part of reality contact itself, we will find reason to withhold reference to motivation in particular cases of autism. What Bleuler's encompassing concept of "autism" does entail, however, is: that delusional thought and experience develop consequent on the triggering of complexes; that enduring delusions will likely indirectly thematize the predicaments of the complexes; and that delusional thought and the underlying autism may be relinquished following the deactivation, strengthening of neurotic defenses against, and development of powerfully motivating interests which do not provoke, the complexes.

Whilst there is now a large amount of published case material that can be modeled in this manner, we do not have empirical studies confirming or disconfirming the model itself. In a article in a handbook on phenomenological psychiatry it's worth pausing at this point to ask what such an attempted confirmation ought to look like. For what's not at all obvious is that we should follow what the empiricist psychologist might suggest— namely develop separate indices of schizophrenia, schizophrenic autism, complex activation, complex intensity, drive activation, delusionality, etc. and see whether and how they correlate. For that to seem plausible we should need to suppose that the concept of "autism" after all works *not* to deepen our very understanding of what it means to be schizophrenic, nor of what it means for thought and experience to take delusional forms, but instead references a separable phenomenon which has these as its mere upshot. Yet such a conception was never set on the table for us by Bleuler, and has no place within a phenomenologically-oriented psychiatry. The concept of autism is precisely that: a concept, not a judgment or hypothesis. It offers us an ontological vision, or a fundamental organizing understanding, of schizophrenic life—and what would it even mean to try to evidence a vision? (Gipps 2019).

What a phenomenological approach can help achieve is the recovery of a conception of autism as an organizing *gestalt*, one that deepens our reflective understanding of what we already intuitively grasp when we meet with schizophrenic delusionality. Until now phenomenological approaches have typically ditched Bleuler's positive markers of autism (the (iii) motivated retreat to (ii) a "wish-fulfilling" domain) to focus merely on his negative marker (the (i) loss of vital contact with reality). This article has suggested a phenomenologically inspired re-theorization of the (ii) wishful element of autistic thought: not as a retreat to imagination but as a retreat to a psychological mode which no longer instantiates a distinction between the imaginary and the real. It also suggested that the phenomenologist's suspicions regarding (iii) the psychoanalytically inspired criterion, motivated either by prior non-phenomenological commitment to a neurobiological model, or by antipathy to versions of unconscious motivation misconstrued along the lines of conscious choice, could be mitigated by recovering the unity of matters biological and motivational in the concepts of the drive and the complex. It is then perhaps not by negating, but by deepening, our reflective grasp of the character of such positive elements of Bleuler's "autism" that phenomenological approaches can truly show their worth: by revealing the essential unity not only of the two faces (lost reality, and reality-fantasy indistinction) of the autistic coin, but also of the delusional etchings on these faces, etchings revealing the shattering terror and devitalizing compromises of the schizophrenic predicament.

BIBLIOGRAPHY

Asperger H. (1944). "Die autistischen Psychopathen im Kindesalter." *Archiv für Psychiatrie und Nervenkrankheiten* 117: 76–136.

Blankenburg W. (1971). *Der Verlust der natürlichen Selbstverständlichkeit. Ein Beitrag zur Psychopathologie symptomarmer Schizophrenien*. Vol. 21, *Beiträge aus der allgemeinen Medizin*. Stuttgart: Enke.

Bleuler E. (1908). "Die Prognose der Dementia praecox (Schizophreniegruppe)." *Allgemeine Zeitschrift für Psychiatrie und psychischgerichtliche Medizin* 65: 436–464.

Bleuler E. (1910–1911). "Zur Theorie des schizophrenen Negativismus." *Psychiatrisch-Neurologische Wochenschrift* 12(18–21): 171–176, 184–187, 189–191, 195–198.

Bleuler E. (1911/1950). *Dementia Praecox or the Group of Schizophrenias*, trans. J. Zinkin. New York: International Universities Press. Original edition, 1911.

Boyle M. (2002). *Schizophrenia: A Scientific Delusion?* 2nd edn. Hove: Routledge. Original edition, 1993.

Ciompi L. (1988). *The Psyche and Schizophrenia: The Bond Between Affect and Logic*, trans. D. L. Schneider. Cambridge MA: Harvard University Press.

de Haan S. and Fuchs T. (2010). "The Ghost in the Machine: Disembodiment in Schizophrenia—Two Case Studies." *Psychopathology* 43(5): 327–333.

Dein E. (1966). "On the Concept of Autism." *Acta Psychiatrica Scandinavica* 41 (S191): 124–135.

Eliot T. S. (1941). *Burnt Norton*. London: Faber & Faber.

Freeman T., Cameron J., and McGhie A. (1958). *Chronic Schizophrenia*. London: Tavistock Publications Limited.

Freud, S. (1916–17/1991). Introductory Lectures on Psychoanalysis. *Penguin Freud Library*, vol 1, trans. James Strachey, ed. Albert Dickson. Harmondsworth: Penguin.

Freud, S. (1919/1985). "The 'Uncanny'." *The Pelican Freud Library*, vol. 14, trans. James Strachey, ed. Albert Dickson. Harmondsworth: Penguin, 335–376.

Fuchs T. (2005). "Corporealized and Disembodied Minds: A Phenomenological View of the Body in Melancholia and Schizophrenia." *Philosophy, Psychiatry, and Psychology* 12(2): 95–107.

Gipps R. G. T. (2019). "A New Kind of Song: Psychoanalysis as Revelation." In R. G. T. Gipps and M. Lacewing (eds.), *The Oxford Handbook of Philosophy and Psychoanalysis*, pp. 443–456. Oxford: Oxford University Press.

Grube M. (2006). "Towards an Empirically Based Validation of Intuitive Diagnostic: Rümke's 'Praecox Feeling' Across the Schizophrenia Spectrum: Preliminary Results." *Psychopathology* 39: 209–217.

Harris P. L. (2000). *The Work of the Imagination*. Malden: Blackwell Publishing.

Heidegger M. (1927/1978). *Being and Time*. Malden: Blackwell Publishing.

Jaspers K. (1963). *General Psychopathology*, trans. J. Hoenig and M. W. Hamilton. Manchester: Manchester University Press. Original edition, 1913/1923.

Jung C. G. (1907/1936). *The Psychology of Dementia Praecox*, trans. A. A. Brill. Vol. 3, *Nervous and Mental Disease Monograph Series*. New York & Washington: Nervous and Mental Disease Publishing Company.

Kanner L. (1943). "Autistic Disturbances of Affective Contact." *Nervous Child* 2: 217-250.

Kanner L. (1973). *Childhood Psychoses: Initial Studies and New Insights*. Washington: V. H. Winston.

Kimura B. (1982). "The Phenomenology of the Between: On the Problem of the Basic Disturbance in Schizophrenia." In A. J. J. De Koning and F. A. Jenner (eds.), *Phenomenology and Psychiatry*, pp. 173-185. New York: Grune & Stratton.

Kimura B. (2001). "Cogito and I: A bio-logical Approach." *Philosophy, Psychiatry, & Psychology* 8(4): 331-336.

Kuhn R. (2004). "Eugen Bleuler's Concepts of Psychopathology." *History of Psychiatry* 15: 361-366.

Laing R. D. (1960). *The Divided Elf*. London: Tavistock Publications.

Laing R. D. (1963). "Minkowski and Schizophrenia." *Review of Existential Psychology & Psychiatry* 3: 195-207.

Merleau-Ponty M. (1945/2002). *Phenomenology of Perception*, trans. C. Smith. London: Routledge. Original edition, 1945.

Merleau-Ponty M. (1964/1968). *The Visible and the Invisible. Followed by Working Notes*, trans. A. Lingis. *Northwestern University Studies in Phenomenology & Existential Philosophy*. Evanston: Northwestern University Press. Original edition, 1964.

Minkowski E. (1927). *La schizophrénie. Psychopathologie des schizoides et des schizophrènes*. Paris: Payot.

Minkowski E. (1927/1987). "The Essential Disorder Underlying Schizophrenia and Schizophrenic Thought." In J. Cutting and M. Shepherd (eds.), *The Clinical Roots of the Schizophrenic Concept*, pp. 188-212. Cambridge: Cambridge University Press. Original edition, 1927.

Minkowski E. (1953). *La schizophrénie. Psychopathologie des schizoides et des schizophrènes*. Revised edition. Paris: Desclée de Brouwer.

Minkowski E. and Targowla R. (1885/2001). "A Contribution to the Study of Autism: The Interrogative Attitude." *Philosophy, Psychiatry, & Psychology* 8(4): 271-278.

Mishara A. L. (2001). "On Wolfgang Blankenburg, Common Sense, and Schizophrenia." *Philosophy, Psychiatry, & Psychology* 8(4): 317-322.

Nelson B., Parnas, J. & Sass L. A. (2014). "Disturbance of minimal self (ipseity) in schizophrenia: clarification and current status." *Schizophrenia Bulletin* 40(3): 479-482.

Parnas J. and Bovet P. (1991). "Autism in Schizophrenia Revisited." *Comprehensive Psychiatry* 32(1): 7-21.

Parnas J., Bovet P., and Zahavi D. (2002). "Schizophrenic Autism: Clinical Phenomenology and Pathogenetic Implications." *World Psychiatry* 1(3): 131-136.

Sass L. A. (1992). *Madness and Modernism. Insanity in the Light of Modern Art, Literature and Thought*. New York: BasicBooks.

Sass L. A. (2001). "Self and World in Schizophrenia: Three Classic Approaches." *Philosophy, Psychiatry, & Psychology* 8(4): 251-270.

Sass L. A. (2003). "'Negative Symptoms', Schizophrenia, and the Self." *International Journal of Psychology and Psychological Therapy* 3(2): 153–180.

Sass L. A. and Parnas J. (2003). "Schizophrenia, Consciousness, and the Self." *Schizophrenia Bulletin* 29(3): 427–444.

Sass L. A., Parnas J., and Zahavi D. (2011). "Phenomenological Psychopathology and Schizophrenia: Contemporary Approaches and Misunderstandings." *Philosophy, Psychiatry, & Psychology* 18(1): 1–23.

Sass, L. A. and Byrom G. (2015). "Phenomenological and neurocognitive perspectives on delusions: A critical overview." *World Psychiatry* 14(2): 164–173.

Scharfetter C. (2008). "Ego-Fragmentation in Schizophrenia: A Severe Dissociation of Self-Experience." In A. Moskowitz, I. Schäfer, and M. J. Dorahy (eds.), *Psychosis, Trauma and Dissociation: Emerging Perspectives on Severe Psychopathology*, pp. 51–64. Chichester: John Wiley & Sons, Ltd.

Schwartz M. A. and Wiggins O. P. (1987). "Typifications. The First Step for Clinical Diagnosis in Psychiatry." *Journal of Nervous and Mental Disease* 175(2): 65–77.

Sechehaye M. (1956). *A New Psychotherapy in Schizophrenia*, trans. G. Rubin-Rabson. New York: Grune & Stratton.

Segal H. (1977/1990). *The Work of Hanna Segal: A Kleinian Approach to Clinical Practice*. Northvale: Jason Aronson Inc.

Snelling, D. (2001). *Philosophy, Psychoanalysis, and the Origins of Meaning*. Basingstoke: Ashgate.

Stanghellini G. and Ballerini M. (2004). "Autism: Disembodied Existence." *Philosophy, Psychiatry, and Psychology* 11: 259–268.

Steiner J. (1993). *Psychic Retreats: Pathological Organizations in Psychotic, Neurotic and Borderline Patients*. London: Routledge.

Tustin F. (1986). *Autistic Barriers in Neurotic Patients*. London: Karnac.

Ungvari G. S., Xiang Y.-T., Hong Y., Leung H. C. M, and Chiu, H. F. K. (2010). "Diagnosis of Schizophrenia: Reliability of an Operationalized Approach to 'Praecox-Feeling.'" *Psychopathology* 43: 292–299.

Urfer A. (2001). "Phenomenology and Psychopathology of Schizophrenia: The Views of Eugene Minkowski." *Philosophy, Psychiatry, & Psychology* 8(4): 279–289.

Van Duppen Z. (2017). "The Intersubjective Dimension of Schizophrenia." *Philosophy, Psychiatry, & Psychology* 24: 399–418.

Varga S. (2013). "Vulnerability to Psychosis, I-thou Intersubjectivity and the Praecox-Feeling." *Phenomenology and the Cognitive Sciences* 12(1): 131–143.

Von Domarus E. (1944). "The Specific Laws of Logic in Schizophrenia." In J. S. Kasanin (ed.), *Language and Thought in Schizophrenia*, pp. 104–114. Berkeley: University of California Press.

Wittgenstein L. (1975). *On Certainty*. Oxford: Blackwell.

Yeats W. B. (1886/2011). "The Stolen Child." In M. L. Rosenthal (ed.), *Selected Poems and Four Plays*, pp. 2–4. New York: Simon and Schuster.

CHAPTER 79

DYSPHORIA IN BORDERLINE PERSONS

MARIO ROSSI MONTI
AND ALESSANDRA D'AGOSTINO

LIVING ON THE EDGE: THE BORDERLINE INSTABILITY

BORDERLINE personality disorder (BPD) is one of the most enigmatic disorders in the contemporary psychopathological scenario. On the one hand, it represents the most diagnosed condition in the area of personality disorders; it is also the main object of both theoretical and clinical reflection. On the other hand, it is far behind other major psychiatric disorders in awareness and research, due to its complexity and multiple possibilities of expression, but also due to the serious difficulties experienced by mental health professionals in dealing with it. Particularly, one of the main problems of borderline personality disorder is that its clinical constellation is highly variegated, so that it might be better pictured as an area rather than a line. This area is very difficult to describe. Several authors have tried to do that during the last fifty years (Zanarini 1993; Linehan 1993; Bradley et al. 2005; Lenzenweger et al. 2008). Among them, M. Schmideberg (1959) has proposed the most representative "portrait" of borderline personality disorder, describing it as being essentially stable in its instability.

First, instability affects the way in which BPD has been theorized. Borderline personality disorder is primarily an entity suspended among other clinical entities: in general, between neurosis and psychosis. Besides, it is an entity suspended among syndrome, nosographic category, and structural organization. Moreover, it is an entity suspended among symptoms, due to the wide range of possible combinations of disturbances legitimizing the BPD diagnosis and making the borderline patient capable of moving among very different mental functioning levels so that sometimes he finds the resources to live his life in a less self-destructive manner.

Secondly, instability affects the BPD identity component. The borderline patient is unable to develop a stable and consistent image of himself as a person and is dominated by an inner sense of emptiness resulting in basic uncertainties that occur in all fields of life (the "syndrome of identity diffusion" described by Kernberg 1975). For this reason, the border-line identity has been defined as "liquid" (Acquarini 2006), but not in the sense that it tends to adapt to the shape of a container, rather in the sense of a fluidity continuously in search of a container (Stanghellini 2008). The container, however, invariably turns out to be disap-pointing, opening the way to the series of relational short circuits to which the borderline patient is dramatically accustomed.

Thirdly, instability affects the BPD emotional level, which is rapidly changing and highly variable. The borderline patient is a very sensitive "barometer" reacting to minimal vari-ations of the environmental pressure and being overwhelmed by a mixture of violent emotions, such as depression tinged with irritation (dysphoria), anger, emptiness, boredom, excitement, and omnipotence. As these violent emotions appear, just as quickly they disap-pear, thus leaving behind the rubble of the continuity of the self, as well as more or less disas-trous effects in relationships.

Fourthly, instability affects the BPD impulsivity area. The borderline impulsivity is in continuous oscillation between the extroversion of the impulses (i.e. risky behaviors, chal-lenging behaviors, and sometimes really suicidal equivalents) and the introversion of the impulses (i.e. self-harming and suicidal behaviors). From this point of view, the borderline patient is torn between acting his impulsivity outward, thus exporting his interior drama in the reality, and acting it inward, thus making the wound a means for regulating intolerable emotions.

Finally, instability affects the BPD relationship with reality. In the borderline psychopathology—it is said—reality testing is preserved. This is true at a phenomenological-descriptive level. Indeed, the DSM-5 diagnostic criteria for borderline personality disorder refer to transient impairments of reality testing and the appearance of reversible para-noid breaks. Literature and clinical observations have highlighted how these psychotic experiences emerging in borderline patients are not real psychotic experiences but inter-mediate experiences: quasi-psychotic experiences, quasi-delusions, quasi-hallucinations (Zanarini et al. 1990). In sum, it is as if the borderline patient is neither able to be depressed (because his depression is described as "atypical") nor delusional and hallucinatory in a full sense. He is always on the edge, trapped in his "stable instability."

For all these reasons, the borderline patient can be seen as a real *migrant* of psychopa-thology (Rossi Monti and D'Agostino 2009), as there is no possibility of fixing him at a cer-tain point of his pathway. So, what is it possible to say about him? In order to understand what it feels like for a borderline to be a borderline, a shift is needed from the description of psychiatric symptoms to the dimension of lived experience.

Pathways of Dysphoria

Over the past years, psychiatric literature has emphasized the fact that the infinite facets of the borderline psychopathology might be just the superficial manifestation—in the context of relationships—of an unstable emotional core functioning as the true BPD *driving force* (Glenn and Klonsky 2009; Cole et al. 2009). But what does emotional instability exactly mean? First of all, several terms are used in literature to describe the same or related phe-nomena, including affective instability, emotional dysregulation, mood swings, emotional impulsiveness, and affective lability (Broome et al. 2015). According to a recent systematic review, emotional instability consists of "rapid oscillations of intense affect, with a difficulty in regulating these oscillations or their behavioural consequences" (Marwaha et al. 2014: 1805).

In the specific context of BPD, several authors have focused on the oscillation between dysphoria and anger—an oscillation that is particularly sensitive to interpersonal variables (Goodman et al. 2009; Stanghellini and Rosfort 2013a, 2013b; Rossi Monti and D'Agostino 2014), thus making emotional instability in BPD different from that (if present) in mood disorders, where it is less dependent on the context and more related to the polarities of depression/euphoria, euthymia/depression, and euthymia/euphoria (Henry et al. 2001).

To what extent does dysphoria differ from anxiety, depression, and anger? And, most importantly, what is dysphoria? The word "dysphoria" derives from the ancient Greek *dysphoros*, formed from *dis-*, "difficult," and *phero*, "to bear," meaning an oppressive and unbearable emotional condition. In psychiatric and clinical psychological literature, the term appears not only in the context of borderline personality disorder but even in that of mood or anxiety, being used as a synonym for sadness or subthreshold forms of depression and to describe a mixture of negative and unpleasant emotions lacking specificity (Voruganti and Awad 2004; Cella et al. 2008). So, things are not clear and a deeper understanding of dysphoria is needed. In order to allow it and follow the line of research opened almost thirty years ago by the so-called Vienna school (Berner et al. 1987; Gabriel 1987), it is essential to describe dysphoria as a "psychopathological organizer" (Rossi Monti and Stanghellini 1996), that is, a framework conferring a unitary meaningfulness to heterogeneous declinations of pathological phenomena. In this sense, dysphoria can be seen as a process which structures the BPD experience in multiple, psychopathological pathways moving from basic lived experience to symptomatic disturbances (and vice versa), through here-and-now lived experience.

A first pathway can be traced back to a "background dysphoria" dominating the basic lived experience of BPD. This is an unpleasant, uncomfortable, negative, and oppressive condition, characterized by a mixture of tension, irritability, discontent, and unhappiness (Starcevic 2007) with all the features of mood: it is enduring, devoid of an intentional object, unmotivated, rigid, difficult to articulate, encompassing the whole horizon of the subject and affecting his relationship with the world, others, and himself (Rossi Monti 2012; Rossi Monti and D'Agostino 2014). In other words, "it is the long-lasting and profound emotional tonality . . . in which the borderline person is enmeshed" (Stanghellini and Rosfort 2013b: 266). In this sense, it represents the persistent, tormenting experience of BPD.

Background dysphoria, however, does not exist *in vacuo*. Rather, it has a relational nature. This means that the pathway of background dysphoria intersects with another factor characterizing BPD functioning: a "negative interpersonal disposition." This is a sort of vulnerability to interpersonal dysfunction constituted by three subdimensions: a) hostile distrust, that is, the cognitive component of hostility consisting of negative beliefs of others seen as threating antagonists (Barefoot 1992); b) interpersonal sensitivity, that is, a relational reactivity combining abandonment fears, rejection sensitivity, and intolerance of aloneness (Gunderson and Lyons-Ruth 2008); c) impaired empathy, that is, a difficulty in the multidimensional (including both cognitive and affective components) capacity to apprehend another person's state of mind (Davis 1983).

In particular context-dependent circumstances, background dysphoria and negative interpersonal disposition compact together into a second pathway ending up in a specific condition: "situational dysphoria," which pervades the here-and-now lived experience of BPD. This is a contingent state of pressure, urge (to act), and quasi-explosion, which is very dependent on the environmental, relational, and interpersonal context. It is a kind of impatience and intolerance developing into a drive to violent action (not necessarily in the sense of physical violence, but rather of a great intensity of the emotions involved). It is like feeling "on the edge," together with a tendency to anxiety, apprehension, and intensification of reactivity and vigilance in a state of dysphoric alertness. In this sense, it represents the cyclic, temporary experience of BPD.

Taken together, background dysphoria, negative interpersonal disposition, and situational dysphoria constitute, so to speak, the "interpersonal-affective specialty" of BPD. The variety of symptomatic disturbances can be located in this perspective as the external side of this interpersonal-affective specialty or, said another way, as the end of all the pathways of dysphoria. At this point, situational dysphoria plays a key role. Loaded with background dysphoria and negative interpersonal disposition, and solicited by contingent stressful events, situational dysphoria needs an escape route. This is found by following two other pathways: one disorganizing and another organizing, each ending up in different, acute phenomena. A single paragraph will be dedicated to the description of each of these pathways.

EMPTINESS OR THE DISSOLVED SELF

The first pathway (disorganizing) of situational dysphoria ends up in a state of disorganization and confusion with respect to personal identity. Tension, irritability, and urge (to act) cannot break down the dysphoric mood in order to orient it toward a specific object. Rather, dysphoria shows all its "centrifugal" drive, dispersing the various aspects of the self instead of aggregating them in some form of recognizable identity. As a result, the vagueness of the self contributes to the vagueness of the other, and vice versa.

Such a state of disorganization affects not only the patient, but also the clinician in the therapeutic relationship, who might be forced to try to "organize" the dysphoric pathway. This organizational attempt often results in acts that are symmetrical to those of the patient, just leading to the breakdown of the relationship. However, these oscillations of one's own sense of identity occurring during the sessions can be also seen as a sort of clinical organ of perception useful to understand what is happening in the therapeutic relationship in that moment (Searles 1994).

Besides, on a more intimate level of the self (Meares et al. 2011), the identity diffusion corresponds to a series of painful experiences of emptiness, insubstantiality, and inauthenticity—the lived side of identity diffusion (Rossi Monti 2016). But what is "emptiness"? A patient calls it the "syndrome of the empty mirror" (Ruggiero 2012), meaning that, when he tries to imagine a mental image of himself, he sees just a black hole that makes the reality of his physical existence questionable. However, this emptiness is not a synonym of loss or lack of something. In fact, while in the experience of lack the person suffers from the disappearance of the object, in the experience of emptiness the person suffers from a painful incoherence, that is, a subjective sense of lack of coherence (Wilkinson-Ryan and Westen 2000).

Moreover, emptiness has many ways of manifesting itself. First of all, emptiness can manifest itself through the feeling of being inhabited by something dead, which leads the person to live a sense of hopeless desolation. This emptiness is different from the previous one because the person identifies aspects of himself as dead or lifeless (i.e. the experience of the "alien self," as described by Fonagy et al. 2002), and those make him close to finding an intentional object with which to converse. Secondly, emptiness can manifest itself as a result of a worn-out relationship, when exhausting proximity blurs each other's boundaries. In this sense, the experience of emptiness makes thought disappear and the feeling of the self dissolving (Lolli 2012).

Finally, emptiness can manifest itself in a more dramatic way when it characterizes not only the patient's inner world but even his outside world. In this case, the risk of suicide is particularly high, because of the disconnection of dysphoric irritability from the world. More frequently, however, the disorganizing dysphoria-emptiness pathway can divert to impulsive actions. When the experience of emptiness is equivalent to the experience of painful incoherence, impulsive actions give greater cohesion and coherence to the self, restoring a sense of vitality (a "desperate vitality," as described by Stanghellini and Rosfort 2013a) and regaining hope. Instead, when the experience of emptiness corresponds to the experience of excessive proximity, impulsive actions strongly re-establish the borders of the self.

ANGER AND THE ORGANIZATION OF PAIN

The second pathway (organizing) of situational dysphoria ends up in anger. In its Latin and Greek roots (*angor, ancho*), *anger* refers to strangling, meaning an emotion normally conceived as involving a personal offence or somehow having been wronged by another person (Stanghellini and Rosfort 2013a). In this sense, anger has several functions: a) to cancel a source of irritation or pain; b) to remove an obstacle to gratification; c) to restore a sense of autonomy in the face of very frustrating situations (Kernberg 1992, 1994). In the first two cases, anger identifies an object as "source" of pain or "obstacle" to gratification. In the third case, instead, anger has an effect on the self.

In light of this premise and in order to better describe the role of anger in BPD, it is important to introduce a phenomenological distinction between affects and moods. While affects are responses to a phenomenon perceived as their motivation and typically involve an explicit intentional object that directs and informs the affect itself, moods are normally not directed or informed by any particular object but rather introduce an ambiguous and highly frustrating emotional vacuum (Rosfort and Stanghellini 2009). Anger and dysphoria can be inserted into this dialectic. In fact, if anger can be considered as an affect, dysphoria can be described as a mood. What does it mean? We will try to explain it now, focusing on four main areas: object, hope, self, and authenticity (Rossi Monti and D'Agostino 2014).

First of all, anger is the means through which the borderline patient reacts to every minimal breaking in empathy: anger emerges when the patient feels that the other will not assume the function he desperately needs. In fact, anger makes the object clearly visible, strongly characterized, and stand out very distinctively. It allows the BPD patient to switch from the state of vagueness typical of dysphoric mood (where the object is blurred, nebulous, and ambiguous) to a condition in which the object is crisp and clear. In this sense, anger has a "centripetal" role, coagulating the emotional dispersion by identifying each time an object/interlocutor (Rossi Monti and D'Agostino 2014).

Secondly, the expression of anger implies the existence of hope. This means that anger makes the patient believe that the object, the environment, or reality itself will react to the violence of the stimulus, thus assuming the role it had never played or had lost. Anger, in fact, is different from resignation; it is a desperate vital reaction that presupposes the possibility of a response by an interlocutor. At the same time, anger defends from the pain of separation and loss: a mind kept busy by angry fantasies somehow is still clinging to what it has lost (Rossi Monti and D'Agostino 2014).

Thirdly, anger gives consistency to the self. As anger mounts, the object becomes the real reason for pain, thus allowing the person to assume a clear and consistent accusatory role toward it. This gives him the possibility of perceiving his own self as cohesive and powerful. In other words, anger unravels the fog organizing an undefined and therefore intolerable psychic pain: in this state, the patient believes he sees things clearly and knows why he is suffering.

Lastly, anger tests the authenticity of the object. Borderline anger brings the object out of the shadow, opens it like a can opener, and forcibly extracts its true nature (Rossi Monti and D'Agostino 2014). This is a sort of load test helpful for evaluating how the object reacts to pressure and stress. The objective is to verify the soundness of the other, but also to discover its true features, as if only by seeing people bleeding in a traumatic situation the borderline patient could see how they really are.

THE BODY AS A BLOWHOLE

Alongside anger, the second pathway of situational dysphoria can also *organize* itself into a concrete self-oriented behavior, ending up in non-suicidal self-injury (NSSI) (i.e. the act of deliberately producing bodily injury, such as cutting or burning). Research shows that 70–75% of borderline patients enact self-injurious behaviors (Clarkin et al. 1983; Zisook et al. 1994; Kerr et al. 2010). The most common form of NSSI is cutting (80%), but bruising (24%), burning (20%), head banging (15%), and biting (7%) also seem to be frequent (Gunderson and Ridolfi 2001). So, NSSI could be defined as a real "behavioral specialty of the patient with BPD" (Gunderson 1984). Why? And what relationship do these behaviors have with dysphoria?

Undoubtedly, NSSI has the "advantage" of positioning negative emotions in a behavioral circuit that leads to a state of lowered tension. It is a momentary oasis of peace, a sort of discharge to the ground. In other words, cutting the flesh represents an attempt to modulate or staunch a negative and oppressive mood condition, precipitating it in a place that has a name and is objectifiable, delimited, and so also "curable." It is as if the body (in its surface) could be a concrete and visible blowhole from which to let compressed and overwhelming emotions spill out. Which emotions? What must be evacuated? We have tried to clarify this point, proposing six "meaning-organizers" (Rossi Monti and D'Agostino 2009) as synthesizing schemes of comprehension connecting different pathological experiences into unitary cores of meaningfulness (Rossi Monti and Stanghellini 1996).

Concretizing

The wounds function as a means to transform a mental pain into a physical one, to control intolerable feelings through the body. It might be an attempt to give shape to an invisible, wandering, and boundless mental pain by localizing it in the body, or to fill a distressing inner emptiness with a bodily sensation. At the moment of cutting, time stops and everything is concretely focussed on the physical pain (always lower than the psychological pain) and on bleeding.

Punishing–Eradicating–Purifying

The wounds function as a means to punish/eradicate some inner "evil" in order to detoxify/purify oneself. It is a way to punish a bad self, to assail one's thoughts, feelings, and memories, or even to unconsciously repeat an emotional sequence connected to a history of childhood abuse: repetition here replaces recollection, functioning as a shield against bad memories. This way, cutting the skin creates an open window through which the inner tension can be released, and all the bad and the alien can wriggle out from the interior of the body (Pestalozzi 2003).

Regulating Dysphoria

The wounds function as a tool to modulate the dysphoric mood typical of the borderline existence. NSSI becomes a way to get at least temporary relief from distressing tension, to transform chaos into calm, and to control the mixture of negative emotions made by tension, irritability, discontent, and confusion, which is the chronic, painful background to the borderline experience. Besides, self-injury can also be helpful in interrupting the depersonalization/derealization cycle, searching for lively and stimulating experiences in physical pain to feel not empty or dead but alive.

Communicating Without Words

The wounds function as a language to convey something inexpressible through words, but also as a way to control others' behavior and emotions by eliciting caregiving responses from them. Just to be precise, this is not a form of *manipulation* since this term means a mode of thought and behavior requiring complex and sophisticated mental functions which in most BPD cases is gravely compromised (Stanghellini 2014). Rather, in borderline psychopathology there is mostly an inability to freely treat the other as an autonomous and independent object and the necessity instead to treat him or her as a "subjective object" (Winnicott 1969).

Building a Memory of Oneself

The wounds function as a way to secure a memory of oneself. The skin is a surface on which to carve and mark certain circumstances, events, and emotions that correspond to significant turning points. A patient calls his self-inflicted wounds "my notches." In this sense, self-cutting becomes a way to make sure that certain events have left a concrete and visible trace—a trace one can immediately locate on one's skin. Another patient speaks of her wounds as a way to mark on her skin the evil she felt inside.

Turning Active

The wounds function as a way to transform passively endured or externally imposed experiences into active ones. This way, an intrinsically traumatic sense of helplessness is transformed into a more reassuringly self-inflicted "trauma." However, self-cutting is also an attempt to *shed skin* instead of changing oneself. There is also a social dimension to the "wounds": they can take on the characteristics of a ritual through which one's need to feel in control of one's body is acted out (Lemma 2005). The wounds, in this sense, become brands to exhibit as truly distinguishing features.

These six meaning-organizers may interweave themselves, representing from time to time the core organizer of the behavior, meaning that self-injuring causes a temporary relief from negative symptoms (i.e. anxiety, depersonalization, or desperation) but also refers to experiences of salvation, healing, and protection of one's own structure (Favazza 1996). Far from being a deconstructive passage to the act, it assumes the valence of a self-constructive "act of passage," that is, a mean for crossing and conjuring the flood of suffering (Le Breton 2003, 2007).

WHAT ABOUT SHAME?

Summarizing the main concepts expressed so far, dysphoria appears to be a predominant feature in BPD, saturating the emotional scenario with its multiple pathways. This is true, but it is not all. The emotional storm that the borderline patient experiences tends to overshadow other emotions that are often difficult to catch but still relevant in the "economy" of his lived experience. This is the case with shame. Despite clinical evidence, in fact, the role of shame in borderline psychopathology has always been poorly studied. This is strange because shame is a central feature in most BPD experiences: traumatic childhood events, anger, and acting-outs, above all. Besides, shame is a sensitive marker in BPD of all those moments in which the relational distance is reduced and the shadow of the other (and the dependence on him) appears; in those moments the patient experiences a painful unveiling of his powerlessness. So, shame seems to be a *core emotion* of the borderline psychopathology (Rossi Monti and Princigalli 2009).

More specifically, the position that shame has in BPD can be described at three levels: a) shame as a part of the core generating the borderline psychopathology; b) the relationship between shame and anger; c) shame as a developmental progression marker (Rossi Monti and Princigalli 2009). Regarding the first level, shame must be considered in strict relationship with trauma/abuse. In fact, although the traumatic vulnerability factors cannot be thought as a direct cause of BPD, there is no doubt that early traumatic experiences amplify the risk for developing psychopathology (in general) and the risk for developing borderline psychopathology (in particular). In this complex core generating BPD, shame has a central position, belonging to the area of traumatic emotions. The disorganizing function of the traumatic events exposes the powerlessness of the subject, giving rise to shame, which is responsible, in turn, for a further disorganizing process.

Regarding the second level, shame must be considered in a sort of recursive relationship with anger. The oscillation between "humiliating shame" and "implacable anger" or "narcissistic anger" theorized by Kohut (1971) resumes, in a more dynamic way, the oscillation between "sthenic" and "asthenic" dispositions in paranoid syndromes, described by Kretschmer (1918). Kretschmer arrived at the conclusion that even in the area of paranoia, which is most typically made up of combative and fanatical personalities, one can trace an "asthenic thorn," a vulnerable point, a "hidden focus of very old feelings of insufficiency" (Ballerini and Rossi Monti 1990). So, a "shame–anger spiral" (Scheff 1987) takes place from the intolerance of this shameful feeling of insufficiency, which is therefore transformed into an angry feeling against the others seen as persecutors because they are witnesses and responsible for the powerlessness of the patient. Similarly, an opposite anger–shame spiral can take place. In this second case, however, shame is considered as a by-product (together with anxiety and guilt) of the conflict between intense destructive/aggressive impulses and relative powerlessness of the Ego structures in dealing with them.

Regarding the third and final level, shame must be considered as having different dimensions or as a "stack" (Zilkha 2004) with both disorganizing and organizing areas: if the dimension of shame-ignominy belongs to the first area, the dimension of shame-modesty belongs to the second area. In the latter meaning, the emergence of shame reveals a differentiation process, in which something new—shameful—starts coming up to the surface. During a psychotherapeutic treatment, for example, the moment of the shame may coincide with the discovery of one's real dependence on others, with the unveiling of one's most fragile and vulnerable aspects which can no longer be hidden behind the crust of the background dysphoria or the barrage of angry impulsive breaks.

The ability to recognize this moment as a first developmental step, together with the ability to tolerate the burden of shame, in the personality structure of the patient and in the therapeutic relation, opens to a further evolution in the therapeutic process, which, according to Adler (1981), corresponds to a transition from borderline to narcissistic level of functioning, seen as along a continuum. As Bromberg states (2001), in fact, the therapeutic relation must be able to gradually sustain the patient in his attempts to experience his structure as stable and strong enough to resist the intervention from the subjectivity of the other without this threat to overwhelm his sense of self unleashing a wave of shame and fear associated with the irreparable trauma of early life.

In conclusion, our clinical experience suggested to us the need to reconsider borderline personality disorder as having an essential interpersonal-affective psychopathological core. In this sense, we proposed dysphoria as the marker of different levels of the borderline subjective experience, thus organizing both its basic lived experience (together with a negative interpersonal disposition) and its here-and-now lived experience. Working on dysphoria at these levels from a therapeutic point of view could be helpful in preventing the development of symptomatic disturbances.

BIBLIOGRAPHY

Acquarini E. (2006). "Identità liquida nel Borderline. Una ricerca condotta con l'Identity Disturbance Questionnaire (IDQ)." *Psichiatria di Comunità* 1: 48–56.

Adler G. (1981). "The Borderline-Narcissistic Personality Disorder Continuum." *American Journal of Psychiatry* 138: 46–50.

Ballerini A. and Rossi Monti M. (1990). "Shame and Delusion." *Comprendre* 5: 13–26.

Barefoot J. C. (1992). "Developments in the Measurement of Hostility." In H.S. Friedman (ed.), *Hostility, Coping & Health*, pp. 13–31. Washington: American Psychological Association.

Berner P., et al. (1987). "Psychopathological Concepts of Dysphoria." *Psychopathology* 20: 93–100.

Bradley R., et al. (2005). "The Borderline Personality Diagnosis in Adolescents: Gender Differences and Subtypes." *Journal of Child Psychology and Psychiatry* 46: 1006–1019.

Bromberg P. M. (2001). *Standing in the Spaces: Essays on Clinical Process, Trauma, and Dissociation*. Hillsdale: The Analytic Press.

Broome M. R., et al. (2015). "Mood Instability: Significance, Definition and Measurement." *The British Journal of Psychiatry* 207: 283–285.

Cella M., et al. (2008). "The Relationship Between Dysphoria and Proneness to Hallucination and Delusions Among Young Adults." *Comprehensive Psychiatry* 49: 544–550.

Clarkin J. F., et al. (1983). "Prototypic Typology and the Borderline Personality Disorder." *Journal of Abnormal Psychology* 92: 263–275.

Clarkin J. F., et al. (1993). "Factor Structure of Borderline Personality Disorder Criteria." *Journal of Personality Disorders* 7: 137–143.

Cole P. M., et al. (2009). "Emotional Instability, Poor Emotional Awareness, and the Development of Borderline Personality." *Development and Psychopathology* 21: 1293–1310.

Davis M. H. (1983). "Measuring Individual Differences in Empathy: Evidence for a Multidimensional Approach." *Journal of Personality and Social Psychology* 44: 113–126.

Favazza A. (1996). *Bodies Under Siege. Self-mutilation and Body Modification in Culture and Psychiatry*. Baltimore: The John Hopkins University Press.

Fonagy P., et al. (2002). *Affect Regulation, Mentalization and the Development of the Self*. London: Other Press.

Gabriel E. (1987). "Dysphoric Mood in Paranoid Psychoses." *Psychopathology* 20: 101–106.

Glenn C. R. and Klonsky E. D. (2009). "Emotion Dysregulation as a Core Feature of Borderline Personality Disorder." *Journal of Personality Disorders* 23: 20–28.

Goodman M., et al. (2009). "Quieting the Affective Storm of Borderline Personality Disorder." *American Journal of Psychiatry* 166: 522–528.

Gunderson J. G. (1984). *Borderline Personality Disorder*. Washington: American Psychiatric Press.

Gunderson J. G. and Ridolfi E. (2001). "Borderline Personality Disorder. Suicidality and Self-mutilation." *Annals of the New York Academy of Sciences* 932: 61–73.

Gunderson J. G. and Lyons-Ruth K. (2008). "BPD's Interpersonal Hypersensitivity Phenotype: A Gene-Environment-Developmental Model." *Journal of Personality Disorders* 22(1): 22–41.

Henry C., et al. (2001). "Affective Instability and Impulsivity in Borderline Personality and Bipolar II Disorders: Similarities and Differences." *Journal of Psychiatric Research* 35: 307–312.

Kernberg O. (1992). *Aggression in Personality Disorders and Perversion.* New Haven and London: Yale University Press.

Kernberg O. (1994). "Aggression, Trauma and Hatred in the Treatment of Borderline Patients." *Psychiatric Clinics of North America* 17: 701–714.

Kernberg O. F. (1975). *Borderline Conditions and Pathological Narcissism.* New York: Aronson.

Kerr P. L., et al. (2010). "Nonsuicidal Self-Injury: A Review of Current Research for Family Medicine and Primary Care Physicians." *Journal of the American Board of Family Medicine.* 23: 240–259.

Kohut H. (1971). *The Analysis of the Self.* New York: International Universities Press.

Kretschmer E. (1918). *Der sensitive Beziehungswahn.* Berlin: Springer.

Le Breton D. (2003). *La peau et la trace. Sur les blessures de soi.* Paris: Métailié.

Le Breton D. (2007). *En souffrance. Adolescence et entrée dans la vie.* Paris: Métailié.

Lemma A. (2005). *Under the Skin. A Psychoanalytic Study of Body Modification.* London: Routledge.

Lenzenweger M., et al. (2008). "Refining the Borderline Personality Disorder Phenotype through Finite Mixture Modelling: Implications for Classification." *Journal of Personality Disorders* 22: 313–331.

Linehan M. (1993). *Cognitive-Behavioral Treatment of Borderline Personality Disorder.* New York: Guilford Press.

Lolli F. (2012). *L'epoca dell'inconscio.* Milano, IT: Mimesis.

Marwaha S., et al. (2014). "How is Affective Instability Defined and Measured? A Systematic Review." *Psychological Medicine* 44(9): 1793–1808.

Meares R., et al. (2011). "Is Self-disturbance the Core of Borderline Personality Disorder? An Outcome Study of Borderline Personality Factors." *Australian and New Zealand Journal of Psychiatry* 45: 214–222.

Pestalozzi J. (2003). "The Symbolic and Concrete: Psychotic Adolescents in Psychoanalytic Psychotherapy." *International Journal of Psychoanalysis* 84: 733–753.

Rosfort R. and Stanghellini G. (2009). "The Feeling of Being a Person." *Philosophy, Psychiatry, and Psychology* 16(3): 283–288.

Rossi Monti M. (2012). "Borderline: il dramma della disforia." In M. Rossi Monti, *Psicopatologia del presente. Crisi della nosografia e nuove forme della clinica,* pp. 15–63. Milano, IT: FrancoAngeli.

Rossi Monti M. (2016). "The Window and the Wound: Dysphoria and Anger in Borderline Disorders." In G. Stanghellini and M. Aragona (eds.), *An Experiential Approach to Psychopathology. Phenomenology of Psychotic Experiences,* pp. 61–77. Cham, ZG: Springer.

Rossi Monti M. and Stanghellini G. (1996). "Psychopathology: An Edgeless Razor?" *Comprehensive Psychiatry* 37: 196–204.

Rossi Monti M. and Princigalli V. (2009). "Psicopatologia borderline: il posto della vergogna." *Psichiatria di Comunità* 8(3): 129–141.

Rossi Monti M. and D'Agostino A. (2009). *L'autolesionismo.* Roma, IT: Carocci.

Rossi Monti M. and D'Agostino A. (2014). "BPD from a Psychopathological-Dynamic Perspective." *Journal of Psychopathology* 20: 451–460.

Ruggiero I. (2012). "The Unreachable Object? Difficulties and Paradoxes in the Analytical Relationship with Borderline Patients." *International Journal of Psychoanalysis* 93: 585–606.

Scheff T. J. (1987). "The Shame–Rage Spiral: A Case Study of an Interminable Quarrel." In H. Block Lewis (ed.), *The Role of Shame in Symptom Formation*, pp. 109–149. Hillsdale: Lawrence Erlbaum.

Schmideberg M. (1959). "The Borderline Patient." In S. Arieti (ed.), *American Handbook of Psychiatry*, pp. 398–416. New York: Basic Books.

Searles H. (1994). *My Work with Borderline Patients*. New York: Aronson.

Stanghellini G. (2008). *Psicopatologia del senso comune*. Milano, IT: Raffaello Cortina.

Stanghellini G. (2014). "De-Stigmatising Manipulation: An Exercise in Second-Order Empathic Understanding." *South African Journal of Psychiatry* 20: 11–14.

Stanghellini G. and Rosfort R. (2013a). "Borderline Depression: A Desperate Vitality." *Journal of Consciousness Studies* 20(7–8): 153–177.

Stanghellini G. and Rosfort R. (2013b). "Borderland." In *Emotion and Personhood. Exploring Fragility—Making Sense of Vulnerability*, pp. 261–295. Oxford: Oxford University Press.

Starcevic V. (2007). "Dysphoric about Dysphoria: Towards a Greater Conceptual Clarity of the Term." *Australasian Psychiatry* 15(1): 9–13.

Stone M. H. (1990). "Treatment of Borderline Patients: A Pragmatic Approach." *Psychiatric Clinics of North America* 13: 265–285.

Voruganti L. and Awad A. G. (2004). "Neurolepetic Dysphoria: Towards a New Synthesis." *Psychopharmacology* 171: 121–132.

Wilkinson-Ryan T. and Westen D. (2000). "Identity Disturbance in Borderline Personality Disorder: An Empirical Investigation." *American Journal of Psychiatry* 157: 528–541.

Winnicott D. W. (1969). "The Use of an Object and Relating through Identifications." In D. W. Winnicott, *Playing and Reality*, pp. 115–127. London: Tavistock.

Zanarini M. C. (1993). "BPD as an Impulse Spectrum Disorder." In J. Paris (ed.), *Borderline Personality Disorder: Etiology and Treatment*, pp. 67–85. Washington: American Psychiatric Press.

Zanarini M. C., et al. (1990). "Discriminating Borderline Personality Disorder from Other Axis II Disorders." *American Journal of Psychiatry* 127: 161–167.

Zanarini M. C., et al. (2008). "The Ten-Year Course of Physically Self-Destructive Acts Reported by Borderline Patients and Axis II Comparison Subjects." *Acta Psychiatrica Scandinavica* 117. doi:10.1111/j.1600-0447.2008.01155.x

Zilkha N. (2004). "Honte." *Adolescence* 439: 245–256.

Zisook S., et al. (1994). "Reported Suicidal Behavior and Current Suicidal Ideation in a Psychiatric Outpatient Clinic." *Annals of Clinical Psychiatry* 6: 27–31.

CHAPTER 80

PSYCHOSIS HIGH-RISK STATES

LUÍS MADEIRA, ILARIA BONOLDI, AND BARNABY NELSON

INTRODUCTION

PSYCHOTIC episodes are archetypes of severe psychiatric syndromes and of a profound disruption of psychosocial development with great personal strain and social and economical burden. More significantly, they can mark the beginning of severe psychiatric conditions such as schizophrenia and bipolar and depressive disorders. Despite numerous advances in treatment of these disorders, morbidity and mortality and overall burden are one of the greatest found in clinical medicine (Murray 1996; Rössler et al. 2005). The rise of clinical "High-Risk states" pinpoints such measurable risk and has allowed primary prevention (along with early detection and intervention) before the onset of a mature syndrome. This is a novel approach to severe mental disorders which attempts to change their natural history. Research has shown that only a "uniquely evidence-informed, evidence-building and cost-effective reform provides a blueprint and launch pad to radically change the wider landscape of mental health care and dissolve many of the barriers that have constrained progress for so long" (McGorry 2015: 310). This development has allowed nosological and phenomenological enquires in clinical High-Risk states, highlighting a range of categories and phenomena these patients go through and allowing the trial of assorted potential preventive interventions.

There are various seminal inputs for "early symptoms" of mental disorders such as Griesinger (1867) and Kraepelin (Kraepelin and Lange 1927) and, particularly for schizophrenia, in Bumke (1936). However, before reporting on the range of "early" symptoms in clinical High-Risk states, some conceptual clarifications are necessary since the terms "initial/early," "precursor," "prodromal," and "basic" symptoms cannot be used interchangeably. The concept of early symptoms is credited to Bleuler portraying the symptoms of early schizophrenia (Bleuler 1950). They characterize predelusional states as including unspecific and seldom recognizable (1) affective symptoms, such as indifference and apathy, (2) obsessive and compulsive ideation and (3) "hysteric and neurasthenic" fluctuant symptoms. The concept of "prodromal" symptoms is attributed to Mayer-Gross and these include change in activity, psychasthenic complaints and the lack of affective resonance, depersonalization phenomena, compulsive symptoms without anxiety, hypochondriac symptoms, compulsive symptoms, and whirlwind thought processes (manic tonality) (Mayer-Gross 1932). Further analysis of the early stages of schizophrenia by Huber and Gross allowed for the use of the terms "precursor" and "prodromal" symptoms (Huber 1985; Gross and Huber 1985; Huber and Gross 1989; Gross et al. 1987). The "precursor" symptoms represented symptoms that precede (months) the prodromal phase and psychosis and are of limited duration—hours/days (rarely months/years)—completely remitting before psychosis. The term "prodromal" symptoms considered those that preceding psychosis would not remit on during the state and that would show a fluctuating course. The concept of basic symptoms was laid by Huber (Huber and Gross 1989) to describe the subjective experiences lived and depicted by patients in the initial phases of schizophrenia and in post-psychotic states. These included fluctuating cognitive, motivational (fatigability, reduction of energy and resistance, reduction in activity, indecision/ambivalence), and emotional experiences and the reduction in coping capacity (to changes), the will to be with others and patience (experience of irritability and discomfort). They also included perceptual disturbances ranging from sight, noise, taste and smell, or cenesthetic experiences. These symptoms were not specific to schizophrenia, but present in organic brain syndromes and in melancholic depression too. These studies considered symptoms defined retrospectively (after the diagnosis of psychosis), an approach that was later abandoned to in favour of the use of these terms in prospective analysis. However, a subset of these symptoms—taken as "basic" symptoms—were found to be predictive of subsequent development of psychosis, particularly schizophrenia. These include nine cognitive disturbances (Cognitive Disturbances scale: COGDIS), such as subjective disturbances of thought process (interference, blockages, pressure), as well as inability to divide attention, disturbances of expressive and receptive speech, unstable ideas of reference, and captivation of attention by details of visual field.

Also, and notably for the study of the early symptoms of psychosis, seminal literature has focused on the predelusional state of mind, evoking good representations of what today would characterize a prodromal state ("the augury of something or happening" (Fava et al. 2008)). Important depictions include those of Jaspers (1963) and particularly of Conrad (1997, translated in Broome et al. 2013). The latter depicts the initial phase of psychosis ("trema") as a change in the atmosphere where the all-together perceptual field becomes imbued with subtle changes of uncertainty and threat. Patients report experiencing an increased tension "as if there was something in the air" and a reduction of their capacity to act upon reality (they felt they could not move or make decisions as before) (Conrad 1997).

However, most empirical research is traced only to the 1960s in both European psychiatry, with Huber's concept of basic symptoms (Schultze-Lutter, Ruhrmann et al. 2012) (see later), and in American-Australian psychiatry and data that, two decades later, would serve as the basis for retrospective early detection studies proposing that 73% of all patients with psychosis had a five-year prodromal phase (Häfner et al. 1992; Häfner et al. 1998). Basic symptoms are subjective disturbances in drive, affect, thinking, speech, perception, motor action, central vegetative functions, and stress tolerance occurring in psychosis. For example, the basic symptom, "thought pressure," a self-reported "chaos" of unrelated thoughts, can be described as follows: "If I am stressed out my mind gets chaotic and I have great problems thinking straight. Too many thoughts come up at once" (Schultze-Lutter 2009:7). Unlike positive psychotic symptoms, basic symptoms are not associated with abnormal thought content and reality testing and insight is preserved (Gross 1989; Huber and Gross 1989). Longitudinal studies on basic symptoms in putatively prodromal patients by Klosterkotter (Klosterkötter et al. 2001) supported their very high sensitivity (96%) and high specificity (70%) for transition to schizophrenia.

In the 1990s in Australia, the criteria for a Ultra-High-Risk (UHR) group were developed by Jackson, McGorry, and Yung (Yung et al. 1996; Jackson et al. 1994) and the first clinical service for subjects at risk for developing psychosis was created by Yung et al. (1996). UHR criteria include three cohorts of persons as High-Risk: the attenuated psychotic symptoms (APS) group, including subjects with subthreshold (for intensity of frequency) psychotic symptoms; the brief limited intermittent psychotic episode (BLIP) group which refers to phenomena that are frankly psychotic, but occurring for short periods of time; genetic risk and deterioration syndrome (GRD) group which expresses vulnerability defined through family history of psychosis or diagnosis of schizotypal personality disorder in the individual, coupled with decline in functioning.

Various points are relevant for the discussion (1) that the clinical High-Risk states are biased to the schizophrenia spectrum, (2) that criteria are heterogeneous, and (3) numerous instruments exist to detect these disorders.

The first point refers to the fact that many of the sources of the criteria identify features of the schizophrenic spectrum (including language disturbances, isolation, and blunting of affect). Indeed, and despite the fact that criteria are meant to identify risk for psychosis, research has shown that they are strongly biased toward detection of schizophrenic psychosis. A meta-analysis of twenty-three studies on subjects at risk for psychosis has shown that criteria for psychosis risk are biased toward an identification of early phases of schizophrenia spectrum rather than affective psychosis: 73% of subjects who transitioned to psychosis met schizophrenic spectrum criteria, while only 11% met criteria for affective psychosis (Fusar-Poli et al. 2008). Recent interest in studying the bipolar at-risk state has allowed new instruments being developed to detect subjects at risk such as the Bipolar Prodrome Symptom Interview and Scale–Prospective (BPSS-P) (Correll et al. 2014). However, these are not currently routinely included in UHR assessment.

Secondly, the criteria for clinical High-Risk states identify distinct features leading to a significant heterogeneity in samples. Some of the criteria are epistemological rules—for instance, having a family history of schizophrenia as in the genetic risk and deterioration syndrome (GRD), while others comprise phenomenological features—such as the basic symptoms (BS) and the attenuated psychotic symptoms (APS) group of UHR (Olsen and Rosenbaum 2006). Despite this, these states now have a comprehensive volume of research to sustain their clinical relevance and their consistency and validity (Yung et al. 2006; Carr et al. 2000; Ruhrmann et al. 2010; Broome et al. 2005). These include (1) evidence from neurocognitive studies (for metanalysis see (Fusar-Poli, Deste et al. 2012; Woodberry et al. 2008; Giuliano et al. 2012); (2) genetic and imaging studies (for meta-analysis see: Smieskova et al. 2010; Fusar-Poli, Radua et al. 2012; Fusar-Poli et al. 2011), (3) functional (Fusar-Poli et al. 2007); and (4) neurochemical imaging studies (Fusar-Poli and Meyer-Lindenberg 2013a; Fusar-Poli and Meyer-Lindenberg 2013b; Howes et al. 2007; Stone 2009). This chapter focuses specifically on the phenomenological criteria (APS and BS) and considers other candidates for relevant phenomena in the clinical High-Risk states including the Examination of Anomalous Self-Experience (Parnas et al. 2005), Truman symptoms

(Fusar-Poli et al. 2008), and abnormal bodily phenomena (Stanghellini et al. 2012). Both the APS and BS select subjects with sub-threshold phenomena for a psychotic episode, which portray subtle changes in their experiencing of themselves (including their thoughts) and the world. Despite their similarities APS and BS segregate different subjects, APS detecting later and clinically more relevant phases while BS aim to identify earlier phases which could also be the target of intervention (Keshavan et al. 2011; Klosterkötter et al. 2013). Some have suggested that their simultaneous use would allow higher significance for transition (Fusar-Poli, Borgwardt et al. 2008).

The third point refers to the complexity range of measures and instruments used in the depiction of clinical High-Risk states as well as those that select BS symptoms. The first include the Comprehensive Assessment of At-Risk Mental State (CAARMS) (created in Melbourne in the Personal Assessment and Crisis Evaluation (Yung et al. 2005)); the Structured Interview for Prodromal Symptoms (SIPS) and the companion Scale of Prodromal Symptoms (SOPS) (Miller et al. 2003); the Early Recognition Inventory for the Retrospective Assessment of the Onset of Schizophrenia (ERIraos) (Häfner et al. 2013); the Basel Screening Instrument for Psychosis (BSIP) (Riecher-Rössler et al. 2007; Riecher-Rössler et al. 2008), or even a self-rating prodromal scale (Loewy et al. 2005). The CAARMS in Australia and SIPS/SOPS in the United States are equivalent of those with disseminated use including those used in Europe. The ERIraos is used in Germany and Italy to assess schizophrenia onset retrospectively and BSIP is a Basel scale developed in an Early Detection of Psychosis Clinic. For the BS the Bonn Scale for the Assessment of Basic Symptoms (BSABS) (Gross et al. 1987) was the original scale and comprehensively addressed these symptoms. These cognitive and perceptual experiential features can be assessed by the Schizophrenia Proneness Instrument, Adult version SPI-A (Schultze-Lutter, Addington et al. 2007) and its child and youth version SPI-CY (Schultze-Lutter, Marshall et al. 2012). Other instruments focus on particular subsets of phenomena which are candidates for clinical relevance in clinical High-Risk states including the anomalous self-experiences which are encompassed in the EASE (Examination of Anomalous Self-Experience (Parnas et al. 2005)) and abnormal bodily phenomena as the ABPq (Abnormal Bodily Phenomena questionnaire (Stanghellini et al. 2014)).

ATTENUATED PSYCHOTIC SYMPTOMS AND BASIC SYMPTOMS

This section assembles and details the phenomena that have been considered both in the APS and BS as providing early detection of risk of developing psychosis. Despite the amount of research on the presence and reliability of these symptoms, we recommend some phenomenological a priori premises that should be borne in mind when analyzing the available literature. First, many of the phenomena that are studied in the High-Risk states are transposed from full-blown functional psychosis (particularly schizophrenic psychosis) and were therefore depicted in established psychiatric disorders and not in adolescence or early adulthood. Before taking at face value the narration of experiences in schizophrenic and affective psychosis one must take in consideration the impact of the coexistent thought and language disturbances—together these might produce a second level of changes in experiences and symbols being used by patients (not the normal narration of disturbed experiences but the disturbed narration of normal experiences). This leads us to the second suggestion—that the "intact insight and reality testing" considered in the High-Risk states is key to the psycho-pathological import of derealization and depersonalization experiences. The derealization and depersonalization that are deeply imbued in the construct of psychosis rely highly on the fact that the person has lost contact with reality (e.g. delusions and hallucinations), as other forms of these experiences are fairly common in non-psychotic situations such as in anxiety and adaptive reactions. So for them to remain valuable in the assessment of High-Risk states great care and detail should be taken in the analysis of the phenomena these persons portray. And this hints at the last problem: that the concept of psychosis stands for a radical change in subjectivity which includes a loss of contact with reality and a heterogeneous range of phenomena where thought processes, and new bodily and world meanings occur and lead to subjective arousal. The phenomena in High-Risk states, by their inceptive nature, are conceptually apart from the drastic change of a psychotic state. All three reasons make the phenomenological enquiry of these states as stimulating as it is ambitious and we present the state-of-the-art position with regard to their study across objective and subjective phenomena.

Objective Phenomena

The identification of the objective phenomena occurring in High-Risk states can come from the clinician but also from family and friends who identify various behavioral changes which are present in a third-person perspective. Most of them involve changes in social and occupational functioning. Some of these symptoms are identified as negative symptoms including being socially withdrawn and presenting autistic features. In addition to (and often preceding) attenuated positive symptoms of psychosis, social isolation, impaired occupational functioning, and difficulties in interpersonal relationships, as well as other negative symptoms, are among the main presenting complaints of subjects seeking help and meeting criteria for psychosis risk. In fact, impairment in psychosocial functioning is a characteristic feature of the psychosis risk state (Velthorst et al. 2010), associated with poor longitudinal outcome (Fusar-Poli et al. 2010).

Moreover, High-Risk subjects usually present with comorbid diagnoses, such as anxiety, depression, and substance use disorders (Fusar-Poli et al. 2014; Fusar-Poli et al. 2013; Lencz et al. 2004). Multicenter studies on large High-Risk samples showed that the most common positive symptoms are unusual thought content and perceptual abnormalities. Regarding negative symptoms, half of High-Risk subjects experience poor functioning and a significant proportion presents decreased ideational richness, while disorganization symptoms are less frequently noted (Addington et al. 2015). Trouble with focus and attention is usually the most common disorganized symptom, whereas dysphoric mood is the general symptom more often portrayed (Alderman et al. 2015). Some studies reported more severe negative symptoms at presentation, followed by positive, general, and disorganization symptoms (Ruhrmann et al. 2010; Comparelli et al. 2014; Fulford et al. 2014; Lee et al. 2014; Velthorst et al. 2009). Amongst negative symptoms, social anhedonia is the most common. Suicidal ideation is also present in a significant proportion of subjects at risk for psychosis.

More than half of High-Risk patients have at least mild suicidal ideation, while almost half of them have attempted suicide before engaging with an early intervention service (Hutton et al. 2011).

Subjective Phenomena

Many, if not the larger part, of the phenomena that constitute APS and BS are subjective in nature—self-reported changes in experiencing (Yung and McGorry 1996; Klosterkötter et al. 2013). Some are broad-spectrum and encompassed in descriptive psychopathology textbooks including neurotic-like symptoms such as changes in concentration and attention, diminution of initiative and motivation, general anxious and depressive moods, and social isolation. Others have been conceptualized in more detail and include a disturbance in the understanding of reality (e.g. perplexity and other derealization and depersonalization phenomena), disturbance in thought process experienced as hyperreflexivity, diminished sense of presence and increased distance to the world, and a change in stance—existence as "singular." Also some specific sets of phenomena have now been operationalized in the clinical High-Risk states, including Truman symptoms (Fusar-Poli, Howes et al. 2008), anomalous subjective self-experiences (Parnas et al. 2005), and abnormal bodily phenomena (Stanghellini et al. 2014). This section discusses the former changes and presents the state-of-the art position of the latter phenomena.

Disturbed Grip on Reality: Perplexity, Derealization, and Depersonalization Phenomena

Early psychiatric literature portrays the features of impending psychosis as arrangements of perplexity, depersonalization, and derealization experiences which are included in the ideas of delusional atmosphere/mood (Jaspers 1963; Schneider 1939; Binswanger 1957; Broome et al. 2013; Matussek 1987a). Such states are depicted as a "psychologically irreducible...subtle, pervasive, and strangely uncertain light—intolerable but vague content (sensations, mood)" (Jaspers 1963: 98). Such a perplexed subject is depicted as enduring "the oppressive awareness of one's inability to cope with a given internal and external situation, this awareness being experienced as something that cannot be explained, something that has to do with one's own self" (Storring 1940: 79). This subject also suffers a decrease in their empathic capacity and/or a decline in psychic and motor activity and/or a detachment from the world (see more in Störring 1987). The relation of perplexity with early psychosis is inscribed in seminal contributions from (1) Conrad's depiction of *trema*, described as a state of hyper-awareness similar to that experienced by an actor just before going on stage where reality is saturated with hidden/mysterious qualities not in the foreground, "rather all what constitutes the background, all the surrounding space from which trees and bushes, whisper and ululate arise: they are precisely the very obscurity and background" (Conrad 1966: 41); (2) to Binswanger and Matussek's portrayal of subjects being "at-mercy" as if "hooked to the perceptual elements" of being enslaved to the world they perceive (Matussek 1987a) (see more in Mishara 2010). This has been expressed by Sass more recently expressed: "Every detail and event takes on an excruciating distinctness, specialness, and peculiarity—some meaning that always lies just out of reach, however, where it eludes all attempts to grasp or specify it" (Sass 1992: 52).

Such a disturbed "grip" or "hold" on the world as that appearing in clinical High-Risk states (Sass and Parnas 2003; Borda and Sass 2015) appears to involve deficits in context processing and abnormal discrimination between familiar and strange stimuli leading to perceptual disorganization and disintegration (Martin and Pacherie 2013; Sass 2004). A composite loss of "perceptual organization" constitutes a failure to structure stimuli (Uhlhaas and Silverstein 2005) and the lack "perceptual integration" characterize a disturbance of their intermodal synthesis (Postmes et al. 2014). These have been found in schizophrenia samples and ground various deficits in these subjects (Uhlhaas and Silverstein 2005; Phillips and Silverstein 2003; Postmes et al. 2014) who have lost the ability to evaluate context, and particularly in differentiating external and internal stimuli which together constitute their unstable reality (that lacks clarity) and their disturbed feeling of presence (Nelson et al. 2014b; Nelson et al. 2014a), and later in the chapter).

These subjects also endure another form of disturbance of "grip" conceptualized as the incapacity to coherently deal with the foreground stimuli. Such impediment leads to a disturbed focus and to a rigid attention where relevant and non-relevant stimuli both become salient. This was coined as "the abnormal salience hypothesis" (Kapur et al. 2005; Kapur 2014), a term designating how stimuli usually in the background come forward and interfere with those in the foreground. It constitutes a form of disturbance of attention where the subject is unable to focus or becomes abnormally focused on specific stimuli (Fletcher and Frith 2008; Kapur et al. 2005; Kapur 2014; Nelson et al. 2014a; Matussek 1987b; Postmes et al. 2014). Such changes occur early on in HR states where the subject complains of losing his ability to focus and his affordances (Gibson 2014)—meaning the things that were previously important in the subject's experiential world. The HR subject finds it difficult to navigate a world deprived of personal meanings (Sass and Pienkos 2015) and easily forms strange perspectives on the world (Sass and Byrom 2015) he inhabits.

However, some reservations remain regarding the unrestricted use of such depersonalization and derealization phenomena as markers of the risk of psychosis. First, these experiences have phenomenological complexity allowing for different portrayals of a phenomenon and similar portrayals of different phenomena (Simeon et al. 2008; Simeon and Abugel 2008). Indeed, attempts to break through this phenomenological complexity could be helpful in the distinction of schizophrenic forms from other forms (Simeon et al. 2008). Second, "depersonalization and derealization" are the third most common psychopathological symptoms (after anxiety and depressive mood) occurring in non-schizophrenic pathologies, in normal adaptive reactions and in anxiety-provoking situations or even as voluntary responses (e.g. in introspection or meditation (Sass et al. 2013)). It would then be possible for anxiety disorders, depressive disorders (Brauer et al. 1970), and depersonalization disorder (Simeon et al. 1997) to have their own constitutive forms (Renard et al. 2017). It is possible to postulate particular forms of depersonalization including (1) a "melancholiform" form constituting a *state* of reduced vitality where sensations or emotions are less vivid and (2) a "schizophreniform" form that would be *traitlike,* an internal distance to oneself since childhood, leading to the self becoming externally observed (one's own body, mind, thoughts, emotions, actions), reflected upon (hyperreflexivity), and therefore felt with a sensation of alienation.

Yet it is also possible to conceive that for the latter forms (considered of schizophrenic bearing) there could be *secondary* forms (Sass 2014; Borda and Sass 2015; Sass and Borda 2015; Hunt 1976; Sass, Pienkos, Nelson et al. 2013; Sass and Pienkos 2013). At an epistemic level, these secondary or consequential forms would arise as defensive factors that occur *in* but are not distinctive *of* schizophrenia. Phenomenologically they would be akin to the primary forms yet they would occur in the above disorders even having volitional (or quasi-volitional) counterparts that would take place in introspection or meditation. Indeed, and beyond theoretical consideration, recent studies (Sass et al. 2013a; Sass et al. 2013b) have explored specific *patterns* that would in term allow the clarification of schizophreniform, non-schizophrenic forms (Sass et al. 2013b) or even non-pathological forms (Sass et al. 2013a) and a study in clinical High-Risk states has particularly focused on this detail (Madeira et al. 2017).

These disturbances in understanding reality are intimately related with three other experiences in High-Risk states that are detailed next—an increased preoccupation and cognitive introspection (hyperreflexivity), a change in the feeling of "presence," and the experience of singularity of existence.

Hyperreflexivity: (In)Voluntary Rumination and Inward Attitudinal Stance

This concept refers to the subjective complaint of an increasing tendency (volitional and non-volitional) to attend to internal processes and to phenomena previously tacitly dealt and to which the subject was not self-conscious (Sass 1992; Sass et al. 2011). The first (and rather obvious) explanation for High-Risk subjects' self-absorption derives from the alienation that their states involve—solitude as ground for thinking. Yet, and hinting a possible primary involvement in High-Risk states, that similar self-absorbed configuration of experience is a primary feature of Conrad's depiction of delusion formation—"the subject turns inward, reflecting and introspecting upon the most trivial things" (Broome et al. 2013: 181). Further examination into the latter arrangement has conceptualized this as a psychopathological symptom with two forms—primary (operative) and secondary (compensatory)—a division which appears to be supported by the latest translational studies.

Automatic or "Operative Hyperreflexivity" is related to the previously described "salience hypothesis" (Kapur 2014; Roiser et al. 2013)—elements previously in the background of the perceptual field become salient and in need of reflection. The subject's sense of self is disturbed as such—the normal sense of self—requires that consciousness is at least partially turned *off*. It has been described as the "subtle but pervasive replacement of natural engagement in the world with introspective ruminations" (Sass et al. 2011) or as a transformation from "retrospective introspection" to a "simultaneous introspection" (Parnas et al. 2016). Such form of *"overthinking"* is intimately linked with the feeling of being a spectator of one's own experiences—no longer *living* (being-in-the-world) and rather *thinking* (musing on the world). This has been neurobiologically explained as disturbed perceptual intermodal integration and also, and particularly, the inability to "triangulate" all sensory inputs (afferent/body ownership) from his self in action (efferent/body agency) (Gamma et al. 2014;

Jeannerod 2003; Parnas et al. 1996; Schwabe and Blanke 2007; Tsakiris et al. 2007; Tsakiris 2010; van den Bos and Jeannerod 2002; Wylie and Tregellas 2010).

A reflective (or secondary) hyperreflexivity refers to an ancillary form of overthinking—aiming attention to what would normally be experienced as part of oneself or yet—moving focus from the explicit world to the implicit dimensions of experience (these include cenesthetic and proprioceptive experiences). Seminally, this subordinate upsurge in cognitive rumination was conceptualized by (Blankenburg 1971) as a consequence of *Verlust der natürlichen Selbstverständlichkeit*—the loss of the natural self-evidential nature of anything. Such loss of natural evidence is another link between forms of hyperreflexivity and the previously described disturbed grip on reality and the feeling of perplexity that imbues High-Risk states. Neurobiologically this could constitute the (over)activation of Default-Mode Network involved in "self-referential" tasks (Nelson et al. 2014b; Murray et al. 2012; Northoff et al. 2006; Qin and Northoff 2011; van der Meer et al. 2010), part of the "neural circuitry of self" (Brent et al. 2014) and an altered salience of perceptions (Nelson et al. 2014a).

This is closely related to the diminution in the feeling of being present in the world (see the following section) as in all three forms of hyperreflexivity (isolation, primary, and secondary) as "thoughts" are experienced unsuitable alternatives to previous experiential features and understanding of the world—and a painful distance to the world takes hold.

Diminished Self-Presence: Experiential Distance

Another key feature of High-Risk states is the sense of decline in one's presence in the world, together with the feeling that experience is no longer unique to the subject (Sass and Parnas 2003)—shorn of its *Meinhaftigkeit* or *moiété* [myness] and could now become the experience of everyone else. Again as with hyperreflexivity, the loss of self-presence is conceptualized as both primary and secondary. Primary diminished self-presence (diminished self-affection) refers to the loss of being present as living and being a unified subject of awareness or agent of action. It is an expression of the distortions of first-person perspective resulting from the loss of ipseity, which will be discussed later in this chapter. At first it can be seen in close relation to the previous experiences: (1) the subject can no longer take for granted his selfhood and (2) many tacit experiences become salient and explicit. Yet such reduction involves more than the loss of ownership and agency, and entails also the failure to distinguish oneself from others (Herrera et al. 2006; Lallart et al. 2009; Riva et al. 2014; Zahorik and Jenison 1998). Neurobiological evidence for disturbance of body ownership points to disturbance of bottom-up multisensory integration and areas such as right temporo-parietal junction (TPJ) and posterior parietal cortex (Ehrsson et al. 2005; Tsakiris et al. 2008). These areas, together with the somatosensory cortex and the insula, are responsible for the neuronal representations of a bodily self (see more in Borda and Sass 2015).

Another form of experiencing diminished self-presence could refer to intentional or defensive processes of withdrawing from the world and reducing the sense of existing or of being an agent of action. Many of the previous experiences involve variable degrees of (usually high) stress levels that, together with the persistent sense of not being able to cope with reality, result in an appalling experience. It is not surprising if the High-Risk subject attempts to remove himself from such reality and to aim increasingly for self-objectification (to increase clarity on his reality). Indeed this could also explain some of the depersonalization phenomena occurring in post-trauma which would motivate such secondary form of removal. These processes appear to involve the same brain correlates—hyperactivation of the Default-Mode Network and the hypoactivation of Central Executive Network of the salience network (Moran et al. 2013; Nekovarova et al. 2014; Nygård et al. 2012; Sass and Borda 2015).

Special Sets of Phenomena

The following phenomena are selective sets that group the previous phenomena into meaningful clusters of symptoms, which acquire particular importance in the High-Risk research.

Truman Symptoms

One of the special forms of derealization and perplexity recognized in High-Risk states (Madeira et al. 2016a) was symbolized by the construct—"Truman symptoms" (TS) (Fusar-Poli et al. 2008). The idea refers to the 1998 Peter Weir movie, in which the protagonist (Truman) is first unaware of being in a television show and gradually becomes suspicious that his world is one of constructed reality (Fusar-Poli et al. 2008). TS represent a profound change of the subjective experience and of self-awareness, resulting in an unstable first-person perspective with varieties of derealization, disturbed sense of ownership, fluidity of the basic sense of identity, distortions of the stream of consciousness, and experiences of disembodiment (Fusar-Poli et al. 2008). They involve rumination on altered subjective phenomena and an increasing self-awareness. Keeping the "as if" component (not a delusion), he might reach a "Truman explanation" that explains what, how, and why he experiences that.

TS are particularly relevant to the psychopathology of UHR group as a form of attenuated psychotic symptom (Fusar-Poli et al. 2008) and because they describe the cultural expression of a psychopathological phenomena in a group familiar with the information technologies (such as the internet and virtual reality).

Anomalous Subjective Self-Experiences

The disturbances of the self (Sass 2017; Kircher and David 2009; Parnas et al. 1998; Sass and Parnas 2003; Zahavi 2008) contain many of the previous descriptions of subjective symptoms and are currently central topics of psychopathological research in High-Risk subjects (Brent et al. 2014; Nelson et al. 2008; Nelson et al. 2012). Disturbances of the "basic"/ "core"/"minimal" self are considered the primary disturbance—mainly representing a disruption of ipseity. Such loss of ipseity would then forefront the distortions of the first-person perspective (diminished self-presence and self-affection, changes in process of thought and perception (disturbed grip on the cognitive-perceptual world) including the loss of "natural evidence" and increased reflexivity and also derealization and depersonalization experiences (see earlier in the chapter). Disturbances of basic self have strong neurobiological translational research accounts (Borda and Sass 2015; Sass and Borda 2015) of delusion formation in prodromal and early phases of psychosis that point to a neurobiological underlying alteration in salience processing of stimulus (Mishara and Fusar-Poli 2013; Roiser et al. 2013; Winton-Brown et al. 2014). The range of experiences resulting from the disturbance of ipseity have been operationalized in the EASE (Parnas et al. 2005) and EAWE interview (Sass et al. 2017) (Examination of Anomalous Self-Experience and Examination of Anomalous World Experience, respectively). This interview selects phenomena which involve "subjectively experiencing" a (1) disturbed way of thinking, (2) being-in-the-world, (3) one's own body, (3) interpersonal relations, and (5) principles and attitudes on the world one lives in. It has also shown a good internal and external validity and its use in subjects at high risk of psychosis (Nelson et al. 2012; Nelson, Thompson, Chanen et al. 2013; Nelson et al. 2009; Nelson et al. 2013) and in prodromal phases of schizophrenia (Parnas 2005; Nelson et al. 2012) has suggested it could be used as an early marker. It should not be understated that a crucial feature of this model is the fact that it is should be assumed as an "overall," "holistic," or "gestalt-like" disturbance and not indexed to a single (quantitative) measure (Parnas et al. 2005; Parnas et al. 2014).

Abnormal Bodily Phenomena

A similar research track has now explored the prevalence and relevance of abnormal bodily phenomena (ABP) in patients with a first psychotic episode and, in particular, in subjects who have been diagnosed with schizophrenia (Stanghellini et al. 2012; Stanghellini et al. 2014).

ABP have been considered in patients with psychosis and particularly schizophrenia even in their seminal representations (Jaspers 1963). The notion of ABP is related to the ideas of disturbed coenesthesia (Röhricht and Priebe 2002), assortments of uncanny bodily feelings with or without delusional interpretation, kinesthetic hallucinations (Ey 1973; Uhlhaas and Mishara 2007), and disruptions of body structure and boundaries (see more in Stanghellini et al. 2014). As a group, ABP are subjective phenomena that were taken as quasi-ineffable in nature and lacking sensible, specific, and reliable tools to assess them and therefore, until recently, they have been absent from our diagnostic textbooks.

The "Abnormal Bodily Phenomena Questionnaire" (ABPq) (Stanghellini et al. 2014; Stanghellini et al. 2012) allows a systematized enquiry of these experiences. Studies using ABPq have shown an assortment of bodily phenomena occurring in schizophrenia (Stanghellini et al. 2014) in the first episode psychosis (Stanghellini et al. 2012). These include uncanny feelings of numbness, loss of body vitality, the sense of disappearance of body parts, change in form (such as shrinking or enlargement), dimension (as unusual heaviness or lightness), or even "movement of internal parts" of the body (Stanghellini, Ballerini, Blasi et al. 2014; Ey 1973; Dupré 1925).

Various studies suggest that ABP occur as trait features before the first psychotic episode in patients with schizophrenia (Hemsley 1998; Klosterkötter et al. 2001; Röhricht and Priebe 2002; Stanghellini 2009; Gallese and Ferri 2013; Schultze-Lutter, Ruhrmann et al. 2007). The Comprehensive Assessment of At-Risk Mental State scale (CAARMS) already selects disturbances of bodily phenomena as relevant to the High-Risk profile. A recent study (Madeira et al. 2016b) explored the prevalence and implications of Abnormal Bodily

Phenomena in subjects considered at high risk of psychosis and found they were highly prevalent (while absent from matched healthy controls) raising the possibility that ABP could be a phenotypic component of High-Risk psychopathology. Some of the assorted ABP experiences reported by the High-Risk subjects included: the experience of violation "when he stretched his hand I felt an energy entering my body. That energy was pounding my right side until it break in"; experience of externalization "I felt that my body had become as a boiling soup and I was no longer in control of my energy that flows around me. Then my body became an ingredient in the soup parts of me are the vapors and rest of the soup"; morbid objectivization "I felt my brain freezing. Then thoughts were moving so slowly I could feel them drive from ear to ear," and devitalization "The loss of the animal part in me, I lost it! I feel that I act as I was programmed, even eating and I feel like a robot, even my arms feel artificially attached to me" (among others, see Madeira et al. 2016b).

CONCLUDING REMARKS

The relevance of this contemporary field of research comprises ontological (considering the possibility of prevention and early intervention in psychiatry) and epistemological (merging of assorted neurobiological, philosophical, and epidemiological contributions) novelties. To handle and keep expanding such breadth of knowledge, researchers and clinicians should consider enough conceptual and phenomenological detail on the experiences that occur in High-Risk states. Such knowledge is vital in contemporary predictive and translational research which will ultimately guide the integration of phenomenological data with the neurocognitive and neurobiological models. This chapter has reviewed the assortment of phenomena portrayed by subjects in High-Risk states of psychosis and focused on subjective symptoms. In this sense, High-Risk states not only bear the anticipation of a new scenario in the identification and treatment of psychiatry disorders but also they have been, and must continue being, an archetype of a phenomenologically informed psychopathology.

BIBLIOGRAPHY

Addington J., et al. (2015). "North American Prodrome Longitudinal Study (NAPLS 2): The Prodromal Symptoms." *The Journal of Nervous and Mental Disease* 203(5): 328–335.

Alderman T., et al. (2015). "Negative Symptoms and Impaired Social Functioning Predict Later Psychosis in Latino Youth at Clinical High Risk in the North American Prodromal Longitudinal Studies Consortium." *Early Intervention in Psychiatry* 9(6): 467–475.

Binswanger L. (1957). *Schizophrenie*. Neske: Pfullingen.

Blankenburg W. (1971). *La perte de l'évidence naturelle, contribution à la psychopathologie des schizophrénies pauvres en symptômes*, trans. Jean-Michel Azorin et Tatoyan. Presses Universitaires de France, Psychiatrie Ouverte.

Bleuler E. (1950). *Dementia praecox; or, The Group of Schizophrenias*. New York: International Universities Press.

Borda J. P. and Sass L. A. (2015). "Phenomenology and Neurobiology of Self Disorder in Schizophrenia: Primary Factors." *Schizophrenia Research* 169(1–3): 464–473.

Brauer R., Harrow M., and Tucker, G. J. (1970). "Depersonalization Phenomena in Psychiatric Patients." *The British Journal of Psychiatry: The Journal of Mental Science* 117(540): 509–515.

Brent B. K., et al. (2014). "Self-disturbances as a Possible Premorbid Indicator of Schizophrenia Risk: A Neurodevelopmental Perspective." *Schizophrenia Research* 152(1): 73–80.

Broome M. R., et al. (2005). "Outreach and Support in South London (OASIS): Implementation of a Clinical Service for Prodromal Psychosis and the at Risk Mental State." *European Psychiatry: The Journal of the Association of European Psychiatrists* 20(5–6): 372–378.

Broome M. R., Harland R., and Owen G. S. (2013). *The Maudsley Reader in Phenomenological Psychiatry*. Cambridge: Cambridge University Press.

Bumke O. (1936). *Lehrbuch der Geisteskrankheiten*, 4th edn. München: J. F. Bergmann-Verlag.

Carr V., et al. (2000). "A Risk Factor Screening and Assessment Protocol for Schizophrenia and Related Psychosis." *The Australian and New Zealand Journal of Psychiatry* 34(Suppl.): S170–S180.

Comparelli A., et al. (2014). "Basic Symptoms and Psychotic Symptoms: Their Relationships in the at Risk Mental States, First Episode and Multi-episode Schizophrenia." *Comprehensive Psychiatry* 55(4): 785–791.

Conrad K. (1966). *Die beginnende Schizophrenie*. Stuttgard: Thieme.

Conrad K. (1997). *La Esquizofrenia incipiente* (transl. 1958 German 1st edition). Madrid: Fundacion Archivos de Neurobiologia.

Correll C. U., et al. (2014). "The Bipolar Prodrome Symptom Interview and Scale-Prospective (BPSS-P): Description and Validation in a Psychiatric Sample and Healthy Controls." *Bipolar Disorders* 16(5): 505–522.

Dupré E. P. (1925). *Pathologie de l'imagination et de l'émotivité*. Payot, Paris: Bibliotèque Scientifique.

Ehrsson H. H., Holmes N. P., and Passingham R. E. (2005). "Touching a Rubber Hand: Feeling of Body Ownership is Associated with Activity in Multisensory Brain Areas." *The Journal of Neuroscience: The Official Journal of the Society for Neuroscience* 25(45): 10564–10573.

Ey H. (1973). *Traite des Hallucinations* (2 Vols.) Paris: Masson.

Fava G., et al. (2008). "Prodromal Symptoms and Intermittent Drug Medication in Mood Disorders." *Pharmacopsychiatry* 24(01): 28–30.

Fletcher P. C. and Frith C. D. (2008). "Perceiving is Believing: A Bayesian Approach to Explaining the Positive Symptoms of Schizophrenia." *Nature Reviews Neuroscience* 10(1): 48–58.

Fulford D., et al. (2014). "Symptom Assessment in Early Psychosis: The Use of Well-Established Rating Scales in Clinical High-Risk and Recent-Onset Populations." *Psychiatry Research* 220(3): 1077–1083.

Fusar-Poli P., et al. (2007). "Neurofunctional Correlates of Vulnerability To Psychosis: A Systematic Review and Meta-Analysis." *Neuroscience and Biobehavioral Reviews* 31(4): 465–484.

Fusar-Poli P., Borgwardt S., and Valmaggia L. (2008). "Heterogeneity in the Assessment of the At-Risk Mental State for Psychosis." *Psychiatric Services* 59(7): 813.

Fusar-Poli P., Howes O., et al. (2008). "'Truman' Signs and Vulnerability to Psychosis." *The British Journal of Psychiatry* 193(2): 168.

Fusar-Poli P., et al. (2010). "Social Dysfunction Predicts Two Years Clinical Outcome in People at Ultra High Risk for Psychosis." *Journal of Psychiatric Research* 44(5): 294–301.

Fusar-Poli P., et al. (2011). "Neuroanatomy of Vulnerability To Psychosis: A Voxel-Based Meta-Analysis." *Neuroscience and Biobehavioral Reviews* 35(5): 1175–1185.

Fusar-Poli P., Deste G., et al. (2012). "Cognitive Functioning in Prodromal Psychosis." *Archives of General Psychiatry* 69(6): 562–571.

Fusar-Poli P., Radua J., et al. (2012). "Neuroanatomical Maps of Psychosis Onset: Voxel-Wise Meta-Analysis Of Antipsychotic-Naive VBM Studies." *Schizophrenia Bulletin* 38(6): 1297–1307.

Fusar-Poli P., et al. (2013). "Outreach and Support in South London (OASIS), 2001–2011: Ten Years of Early Diagnosis and Treatment for Young Individuals at High Clinical Risk for Psychosis." *European Psychiatry: The Journal of the Association of European Psychiatrists* 28(5): 315–326.

Fusar-Poli P. and Meyer-Lindenberg A. (2013a). "Striatal Presynaptic Dopamine in Schizophrenia, Part I: Meta-Analysis of Dopamine Active Transporter (DAT) Density." *Schizophrenia Bulletin* 39(1): 22–32.

Fusar-Poli P. and Meyer-Lindenberg A. (2013b). "Striatal Presynaptic Dopamine in Schizophrenia, Part II: Meta-Analysis of [(18)F/(11)C]-DOPA PET Studies." *Schizophrenia Bulletin* 39(1): 33–42.

Fusar-Poli P., et al. (2014). "Comorbid Depressive and Anxiety Disorders in 509 Individuals with an At-Risk Mental State: Impact on Psychopathology and Transition to Psychosis." *Schizophrenia Bulletin* 40(1): 120–131.

Gallese V. and Ferri F. (2013). "Jaspers, The Body, and Schizophrenia: The Bodily Self." *Psychopathology* 46(5): 330–336.

Gamma F., et al. (2014). "Early Intermodal Integration in Offspring of Parents with Psychosis." *Schizophrenia Bulletin* 40(5): 992–1000.

Gibson J. J. (2014). *The Ecological Approach to Visual Perception*. New York: Psychology Press Classic Editions.

Griesinger W. (1867). *Mental Pathology and Therapeutics*, translated from german by C Lockhart Robertson and James Rutherford. The new Sydenham Society, London.

Gross G. (1989). "The 'Basic' Symptoms of Schizophrenia." *The British Journal of Psychiatry. Supplement* (7): 21–25, 37–40.

Gross G. and Huber G. (1985). "Psychopathology of Basic Stages of Schizophrenia in View of Formal Thought Disturbances." *Psychopathology* 18(2–3): 115–125.

Gross G., Huber G., and Klosterkötter J. (1987). *Bonner Skala für die Beurteilung von Basissymptomen*. Berlin, Heidelberg, New York: Springer-Verlag.

Giuliano A. J., et al. (2012). "Neurocognition in the Psychosis Risk Syndrome: A Quantitative and Qualitative Review." *Current Pharmaceutical Design* 18(4): 399–415.

Häfner H., et al. (1992). "IRAOS: An Instrument for the Assessment of Onset and Early Course of Schizophrenia." *Schizophrenia Research* 6(3): 209–223.

Häfner H., et al. (1998). "The ABC Schizophrenia Study: A Preliminary Overview of the Results." *Social Psychiatry and Psychiatric Epidemiology* 33(8): 380–386.

Häfner H., Maurer K., and an der Heiden W. (2013). "ABC Schizophrenia Study: An Overview of Results Since 1996." *Social Psychiatry and Psychiatric Epidemiology* 48(7): 1021–1031.

Hemsley D. R. (1998). "The Disruption of the "Sense of Self" in Schizophrenia: Potential Links with Disturbances of Information Processing." *The British Journal of Medical Psychology* 71(Pt 2): 115–124.

Herrera G., Jordan R., and Vera L. (2006). "Agency and Presence: A Common Dependence on Subjectivity?" *Presence: Teleoperators and Virtual Environments* 15(5): 539–552.

Howes O. D., et al. (2007). "Molecular Imaging Studies of the Striatal Dopaminergic System in Psychosis and Predictions for the Prodromal Phase of Psychosis." *The British Journal of Psychiatry. Supplement* 51(51): s13–s18.

Huber G. (1985). *Negative or Basic Symptoms in Schizophrenia and Affective Illness.* 4th World Congress of Biological Psychiatry, Philadelphia.

Huber G. and Gross G. (1989). "The Concept of Basic Symptoms in Schizophrenic and Schizoaffective Psychoses." *Recenti progressi in medicina* 80(12): 646–652.

Hunt H. T. (1976). "A Test of the Psychedelic Model of Altered States of Consciousness." *Archives of General Psychiatry* 33(7): 867–876.

Hutton P., et al. (2011). "Prevalence of Violence Risk Factors in People at Ultra-High Risk of Developing Psychosis: A Service Audit." *Early Intervention in Psychiatry* 6(1): 91–96.

Jackson H. J., McGorry P. D., and McKenzie D. (1994). "The Reliability of DSM-III Prodromal Symptoms in First-Episode Psychotic Patients." *Acta Psychiatrica Scandinavica* 90(5): 375–378.

Jaspers K. (1963). *General Psychopathology*, 7th edn. Manchester: Manchester University Press.

Jeannerod M. (2003). "The Mechanism of Self-Recognition in Humans." *Behavioural Brain Research* 142(1–2): 1–15.

Kapur S. (2014). "Psychosis as a State of Aberrant Salience: A Framework Linking Biology, Phenomenology, and Pharmacology in Schizophrenia." *American Journal of Psychiatry* 160(1): 13–23.

Kapur S., Mizrahi R., and Li M. (2005). "From Dopamine to Salience to Psychosis—Linking Biology, Pharmacology and Phenomenology of Psychosis." *Schizophrenia Research* 79(1): 59–68.

Keshavan M. S., DeLisi L. E., and Seidman L. J. (2011). "Early and Broadly Defined Psychosis Risk Mental States." *Schizophrenia Research* 126(1–3): 1–10.

Kircher T. and David A. S. (2009). "Self-Consciousness: An Integrative Approach from Philosophy, Psychopathology and the Neurosciences." In T. Kircher and A. David (eds.), *The Self in Neuroscience and Psychiatry*, pp. 445–474. Cambridge: Cambridge University Press.

Klosterkötter J., et al. (2001). "Diagnosing Schizophrenia in the Initial Prodromal Phase." *Archives of General Psychiatry* 58(2): 158–164.

Klosterkötter J., et al. (2013). "Prediction and Prevention of Schizophrenia: What Has Been Achieved and Where To Go Next?" *World Psychiatry: Official Journal of the World Psychiatric Association (WPA)* 10(3): 165–174.

Kraepelin E. and Lange J. (1927). *Psychiatrie*, 9th edn. Leipzig: J A Barth.

Lallart E., Lallart X., and Jouvent R. (2009). "Agency, the Sense of Presence, and Schizophrenia." *Cyberpsychology & Behavior: The Impact of the Internet, Multimedia and Virtual Reality on Behavior and Society* 12(2): 139–145.

Lee T. Y., et al. (2014). "Symptomatic and Functional Remission of Subjects at Clinical High Risk for Psychosis: A 2-Year Naturalistic Observational Study." *Schizophrenia Research* 156(2–3): 266–271.

Lencz T., et al. (2004). "Nonspecific and Attenuated Negative Symptoms in Patients at Clinical High-Risk for Schizophrenia." *Schizophrenia Research* 68(1): 37–48.

Loewy R. L., et al. (2005). "The Prodromal Questionnaire (PQ): Preliminary Validation of a Self-Report Screening Measure for Prodromal and Psychotic Syndromes." *Schizophrenia Research* 79(1): 117–125.

Madeira L., Bonoldi I., Rocchetti M., Brandizzi M., et al. (2016a). "Prevalence and Implications of Truman Symptoms in Subjects at Ultra High Risk for Psychosis." *Psychiatry Research* 238: 270–276.

Madeira L., Bonoldi I., Rocchetti M., Samson C., et al. (2016b). "An Initial Investigation of Abnormal Bodily Phenomena in Subjects at Ultra High Risk for Psychosis: Their Prevalence and Clinical Implications." *Comprehensive Psychiatry* 66: 39–45.

Madeira L., et al. (2017). "Basic Self-Disturbances beyond Schizophrenia: Discrepancies and Affinities in Panic Disorder—An Empirical Clinical Study." *Psychopathology* 50(2): 157–168.

Martin J.-R. and Pacherie E. (2013). "Out of Nowhere: Thought Insertion, Ownership and Context-Integration." *Consciousness and Cognition* 22(1): 111–122.

Matussek P. (1987a). "Studies in Delusional Perception (Translated and Condensed) Originally published in 1952." In *The Clinical Roots of the Schizophrenia Concept*, pp. 87–103. Cambridge: Cambridge University Press.

Matussek P. (1987b). "Studies in Delusional Perception." In *The Clinical Roots of the Schizophrenia Concept*. CUP Archive.

Mayer-Gross W. (1932). "Die Klinik der Schizophrenie." In *Handbuch der Geisteskrankheiten Vol IX*. Berlin, Germany.

McGorry P. D. (2015). "Early Intervention in Psychosis." *The Journal of Nervous and Mental Disease* 203(5): 310–318.

Miller T. J., et al. (2003). "Prodromal Assessment with the Structured Interview for Prodromal Syndromes and the Scale of Prodromal Symptoms: Predictive Validity, Interrater Reliability, and Training to Reliability." *Schizophrenia Bulletin* 29(4): 703–715.

Mishara A. L. (2010). Klaus Conrad (1905–1961): Delusional Mood, Psychosis, and Beginning Schizophrenia. *Schizophrenia Bulletin* 36(1): 9–13.

Mishara A. L. and Fusar-Poli P. (2013). "The Phenomenology and Neurobiology of Delusion Formation During Psychosis Onset: Jaspers, Truman Symptoms, and Aberrant Salience." *Schizophrenia Bulletin* 39(2): 278–286.

Moran L. V., et al. (2013). "Disruption of Anterior Insula Modulation of Large-Scale Brain Networks in Schizophrenia." *Biological Psychiatry* 74(6): 467–474.

Murray C. J. L. (1996). "The Global Burden of Disease: A Comprehensive Assessment of Mortality and Disability from Diseases, Injuries and Risk Factors in 1990 and Projected to 2020." Edited by A. D. Lopez and C. J. L. Murray, p. 43. Harvard School of Public Health.

Murray R. J., Schaer M., and Debbané M. (2012). "Degrees of Separation: A Quantitative Neuroimaging Meta-Analysis Investigating Self-Specificity and Shared Neural Activation between Self- and Other-Reflection." *Neuroscience and Biobehavioral Reviews* 36(3): 1043–1059.

Nekovarova T., et al. (2014). "Bridging Disparate Symptoms of Schizophrenia: A Triple Network Dysfunction Theory." *Frontiers in Behavioral Neuroscience* 8: 19.

Nelson B., et al. (2008). "The Phenomenological Critique and Self-Disturbance: Implications for Ultra-High Risk ("Prodrome") Research." *Schizophrenia Bulletin* 34(2): 381–392.

Nelson B., et al. (2009). "A Disturbed Sense of Self in the Psychosis Prodrome: Linking Phenomenology and Neurobiology." *Neuroscience and Biobehavioral Reviews* 33(6): 807–817.

Nelson B., Thompson A., and Yung A. R. (2012). "Basic Self-Disturbance Predicts Psychosis Onset in the Ultra High Risk for Psychosis "Prodromal" Population." *Schizophrenia Bulletin* 38(6): 1277–1287.

Nelson B., Thompson A., Chanen A. M., et al. (2013). "Is Basic Self-Disturbance in Ultra-High Risk for Psychosis ("Prodromal") Patients Associated with Borderline Personality Pathology? *Early Intervention in Psychiatry* 7(3): 306–310.

Nelson B., Thompson A., and Yung A. R. (2013). "Not All First-Episode Psychosis is the Same: Preliminary Evidence of Greater Basic Self-Disturbance in Schizophrenia Spectrum Cases." *Early Intervention in Psychiatry* 7(2): 200–204.

Nelson B., Whitford T. J., Lavoie S., and Sass L. A. (2014a). "What are the Neurocognitive Correlates of Basic Self-Disturbance in Schizophrenia? Integrating Phenomenology and Neurocognition: Part 2 (Aberrant Salience)." *Schizophrenia Research* 152(1): 20–27.

Nelson B., Whitford T. J., Lavoie S., and Sass L. A. (2014b.) "What are the Neurocognitive Correlates of Basic Self-Disturbance in Schizophrenia?: Integrating Phenomenology and Neurocognition. Part 1 (Source Monitoring Deficits)." *Schizophrenia Research* 152(1): 12–19.

Northoff G., et al. (2006). "Self-Referential Processing in Our Brain—A Meta-Analysis of Imaging Studies on the Self." *NeuroImage* 31(1): 440–457.

Nygård M., et al. (2012). "Patients with Schizophrenia Fail to Up-Regulate Task-Positive and Down-Regulate Task-Negative Brain Networks: An fMRI Study Using an ICA Analysis Approach." *Frontiers in Human Neuroscience* 6: 149.

Olsen K. A. and Rosenbaum B. (2006). "Prospective Investigations of the Prodromal State of Schizophrenia: Review of Studies." *Acta Psychiatrica Scandinavica* 113(4): 247–272.

Parnas J. (2005). "Clinical Detection of Schizophrenia-Prone Individuals: Critical Appraisal." *The British Journal of Psychiatry. Supplement* 48(48): s111–s112.

Parnas J., Innocenti G. M., and Bovet P. (1996). "Schizophrenic Trait Features, Binding, and Cortico-Cortical Connectivity: A Neurodevelopmental Pathogenetic Hypothesis." *Neurol Psychiatry Brain Res* 4(4): 185–196.

Parnas J., et al. (1998). "Self-Experience in the Prodromal Phases of Schizophrenia: A Pilot Study of First-Admissions." *Neurol Psychiatry Brain Res* 6(2): 97–106.

Parnas J., et al. (2005). "EASE: Examination of Anomalous Self-Experience." *Psychopathology* 38(5): 236–258.

Parnas J., Carter J., and Nordgaard J. (2014). "Premorbid Self-Disorders and Lifetime Diagnosis in the Schizophrenia Spectrum: A Prospective High-Risk Study." *Early Intervention in Psychiatry* 10(1): 45–53.

Parnas J., et al. (2016). "The 'Schizophrenic' in the Self-Consciousness of Schizophrenic Patients, by Mari Nagai (1990)." *History of Psychiatry* 27(4): 493–503.

Phillips W. A. and Silverstein S. M. (2003). "Convergence of Biological and Psychological Perspectives on Cognitive Coordination in Schizophrenia." *Behavioral and Brain Sciences* 26(01): 65–82.

Postmes L., et al. (2014). "Schizophrenia as a Self-Disorder Due to Perceptual Incoherence." *Schizophrenia Research* 152(1): 41–50.

Qin P. and Northoff G. (2011). "How is Our Self Related to Midline Regions and the Default-Mode Network?" *NeuroImage* 57(3): 1221–1233.

Renard S. B., et al. (2017). "Unique and Overlapping Symptoms in Schizophrenia Spectrum and Dissociative Disorders in Relation to Models of Psychopathology: A Systematic Review." *Schizophrenia Bulletin* 43(1): 108–121.

Riecher-Rössler A., et al. (2007). "The Basel Early-Detection-Of-Psychosis (FEPSY)-Study? Design and Preliminary Results." *Acta Psychiatrica Scandinavica* 115(2): 114–125.

Riecher-Rössler A., et al. (2008). "Das Basel Screening Instrument für Psychosen (BSIP): Entwicklung, Aufbau, Reliabilität und Validität." *Fortschritte der Neurologie Psychiatrie* 76(4): 207–216.

Riva G., Waterworth J., and Murray D. (2014). *Interacting with Presence*. Walter de Gruyter GmbH & Co KG, Warsaw/Berlin.

Röhricht F. and Priebe S. (2002). "Do Cenesthesias and Body Image Aberration Characterize a Subgroup in Schizophrenia?" *Acta Psychiatrica Scandinavica* 105(4): 276–282.

Roiser J. P., et al. (2013). "Neural and Behavioral Correlates of Aberrant Salience in Individuals at Risk for Psychosis." *Schizophrenia Bulletin* 39(6): 1328–1336.

Rössler W., et al. (2005). "Size of Burden of Schizophrenia and Psychotic Disorders." *European Neuropsychopharmacology: The Journal of the European College of Neuropsychopharmacology* 15(4): 399–409.

Ruhrmann S., et al. (2010). "Prediction of Psychosis in Adolescents and Young Adults at High Risk." *Archives of General Psychiatry* 67(3): 241–251.

Sass L. A. (1992). *Madness and Modernism*. Basic Books: New York.

Sass L. A. (2004). "Schizophrenia: A Disturbance of the Thematic Field." In Embree L, ed. *Gurwitsch's Relevancy for Cognitive Science*, pp. 59–78. Dordrecht, Holland: Springer Netherlands.

Sass L. A. (2014). "Self-Disturbance and Schizophrenia: Structure, Specificity, Pathogenesis (Current issues, New directions). *Schizophrenia Research* 152(1): 5–11.

Sass L. A. (2017). *Madness and Modernism: Insanity in the Light of Modern Art, Literature, and Thought*, rev edn. Oxford: Oxford University Press (orig 1992: NY: Basic Books).

Sass L. A. and Parnas J. (2003). "Schizophrenia, Consciousness, and the Self." *Schizophrenia Bulletin* 29(3): 427–444.

Sass L., Parnas J., and Zahavi D. (2011). "Phenomenological Psychopathology and Schizophrenia: Contemporary Approaches and Misunderstandings." *Philosophy, Psychiatry, & Psychology* 18(1): 1–23.

Sass L. and Pienkos E. (2013). "Varieties of Self-Experience: A Comparative Phenomenology of Melancholia, Mania, and Schizophrenia, Part I." *Journal of Consciousness Studies* 20(7–8): 103–130.

Sass L., Pienkos E., and Nelson B. (2013a). "Introspection and Schizophrenia: A Comparative Investigation of Anomalous Self Experiences." *Consciousness and Cognition* 22(3): 853–867.

Sass L., Pienkos E., Nelson B., et al. (2013b). "Anomalous Self-Experience in Depersonalization and Schizophrenia: A Comparative Investigation." *Consciousness and Cognition* 22(2): 430–441.

Sass L. A. and Borda J. P. (2015). "Phenomenology and Neurobiology of Self Disorder in Schizophrenia: Secondary Factors." *Schizophrenia Research* 169(1–3): 474–482.

Sass L. and Byrom G. (2015). "Phenomenological and Neurocognitive Perspectives on Delusions: A Critical Overview." *World Psychiatry: Official Journal of the World Psychiatric Association (WPA)* 14(2): 164–173.

Sass L. and Pienkos E. (2015). "Faces of Intersubjectivity." *Journal of Phenomenological Psychology* 46(1): 1–32.

Sass L., et al. (2017). "EAWE: Examination of Anomalous World Experience." *Psychopathology* 50(1): 10–54.

Schneider K. (1939). *Psychischer Befund und Psychiatrische Diagnose; (later editions renamed Klinische Psychopathologie)*, English translation: Clinical Psychopathology (1959) from 5th edn, New York: Grune & Stratton.

Schultze-Lutter F., Addington J., et al. (2007). *Schizophrenia Proneness Instrument, Adult Version (SPI-A)*. Rome: Giovanni Fiorito Editore.

Schultze-Lutter F., Ruhrmann S., et al. (2007). "The Initial Prodrome of Schizophrenia: Different Duration, Different Underlying Deficits?" *Comprehensive Psychiatry* 48(5): 479–488.

Schultze-Lutter F. (2009). "Subjective Symptoms of Schizophrenia in Research and the Clinic: The Basic Symptom Concept." *Schizophrenia Bulletin* 35(1): 5–8.

Schultze-Lutter F., Marshall M., and Koch E. (2012). *Schizophrenia Proneness Instrument Child and Youth (SPI-CY)*, Giovanni Fioriti, Geneva.

Schultze-Lutter F., Ruhrmann S., et al. (2012). "Basic Symptoms and the Prediction of First-Episode Psychosis." *Current Pharmaceutical Design* 18(4): 351–357.

Schwabe L. and Blanke O. (2007). "Cognitive Neuroscience of Ownership and Agency." *Consciousness and Cognition* 16(3): 661–666.

Simeon D., et al. (1997). "Feeling Unreal: 30 Cases of DSM-III-R Depersonalization Disorder." *American Journal of Psychiatry* 154(8): 1107–1113.

Simeon D. and Abugel J. (2008). *Feeling Unreal: Depersonalization Disorder and the Loss of the Self*. Oxford: Oxford University Press.

Simeon D., et al. (2008). "De-constructing Depersonalization: Further Evidence for Symptom Clusters." *Psychiatry Research* 157(1–3): 303–306.

Smieskova R., et al. (2010). "Neuroimaging Predictors of Transition to Psychosis—A Systematic Review and Meta-Analysis." *Neuroscience and Biobehavioral Reviews* 34(8): 1207–1222.

Stanghellini G. (2009). *Psicopatologia del senso comune*. Milano: Oxford University Press.

Stanghellini G., et al. (2012). "Abnormal Bodily Experiences May Be a Marker of Early Schizophrenia?" *Current Pharmaceutical Design* 18(4): 392–398.

Stanghellini G., Ballerini M., Blasi S., et al. (2014). "The Bodily Self: A Qualitative Study of Abnormal Bodily Phenomena in Persons with Schizophrenia." *Comprehensive Psychiatry* 55(7): 1703–1711.

Stanghellini G., Ballerini M., and Cutting J. (2014). "Abnormal Bodily Phenomena Questionnaire." *Journal of Psychopathology* 20: 138–143.

Stone J. (2009). "Imaging the Glutamate System in Humans: Relevance to Drug Discovery for Schizophrenia." *Current Pharmaceutical Design* 15(22): 2594–2602.

Störring G. (1940). "Wesen und bedeutung des symptoms der ratlosigkeit bei psychischen erkrankungen." *The Journal of Nervous and Mental Disease* 90(6): 798.

Störring G. (1987). "Perplexity." In J. Cutting and M. Shepherd (eds.), *The Clinical Roots of the Schizophrenia Concept*, pp. 79–82. Cambridge: Cambridge University Press.

Tsakiris M. (2010). "My Body in the Brain: A Neurocognitive Model of Body-Ownership." *Neuropsychologia* 48(3): 703–712.

Tsakiris M., Schütz-Bosbach S., and Gallagher S. (2007). "On Agency and Body-Ownership: Phenomenological and Neurocognitive Reflections." *Consciousness and Cognition* 16(3): 645–660.

Tsakiris M., Costantini M., and Haggard P. (2008). "The Role of the Right Temporo-Parietal Junction in Maintaining a Coherent Sense of One's Body." *Neuropsychologia* 46(12): 3014–3018.

Uhlhaas P. J. and Silverstein S. M. (2005). "Perceptual Organization in Schizophrenia Spectrum Disorders: Empirical Research and Theoretical Implications." *Psychological Bulletin* 131(4): 618–632.

Uhlhaas P. J. and Mishara A. L. (2007). "Perceptual Anomalies in Schizophrenia: Integrating Phenomenology and Cognitive Neuroscience." *Schizophrenia Bulletin* 33(1): 142–156.

van den Bos E. and Jeannerod M. (2002). "Sense of Body and Sense of Action Both Contribute to Self-Recognition." *Cognition* 85(2): 177–187.

van der Meer L., et al. (2010). "Self-Reflection and the Brain: A Theoretical Review and Meta-Analysis of Neuroimaging Studies with Implications for Schizophrenia." *Neuroscience and Biobehavioral Reviews* 34(6): 935–946.

Velthorst E., et al. (2009). "Baseline Differences in Clinical Symptomatology Between Ultra High Risk Subjects with and without a Transition to Psychosis." *Schizophrenia Research* 109(1–3): 60–65.

Velthorst E., et al. (2010). "Disability in People Clinically at High Risk of Psychosis." *The British Journal of Psychiatry: The Journal of Mental Science* 197(4): 278–284.

Winton-Brown T. T., et al. (2014). "Dopaminergic Basis of Salience Dysregulation in Psychosis." *Trends in Neurosciences* 37(2): 85–94.

Woodberry K. A., Giuliano A. J., and Seidman L. J. (2008). "Premorbid IQ in Schizophrenia: A Meta-Analytic Review." *American Journal of Psychiatry* 165(5): 579–587.

Wylie K. P. and Tregellas J. R. (2010). "The Role of the Insula in Schizophrenia." *Schizophrenia Research* 123(2–3): 93–104.

Yung A. R. and McGorry P. D. (1996). "The Initial Prodrome in Psychosis: Descriptive and Qualitative Aspects." *The Australian and New Zealand Journal of Psychiatry* 30(5): 587–599.

Yung A. R., et al. (1996). "Monitoring and Care of Young People at Incipient Risk of Psychosis." *Schizophrenia Bulletin* 22(2): 283–303.

Yung A. R., et al. (2005). "Mapping the Onset of Psychosis: The Comprehensive Assessment of At-Risk Mental States." *The Australian and New Zealand Journal of Psychiatry* 39(11–12): 964–971.

Yung A. R., et al. (2006). "Testing the Ultra High Risk (Prodromal) Criteria for the Prediction of Psychosis in a Clinical Sample of Young People." *Schizophrenia Research* 84(1): 57–66.

Zahavi D. (2008). *Subjectivity and Selfhood*. Investigating the First-Person Perspective. Cambridge, Massachusetts: MIT Press.

Zahorik P. and Jenison R. L. (1998). "Presence as Being-in-the-World." *Presence: Teleoperators and Virtual Environments* 7(1): 78–89.

CHAPTER 81

···

PSYCHOPATHOLOGY
AND LAW

···

GARETH S. OWEN

INTRODUCTION

···

MIND is central to law and law shares the problem of mind's anomalies with psychiatry. But psychiatry and law approach psychopathology with very different systems of knowledge.

Psychiatry, as a branch of medicine, comes at psychopathology with categories of symptoms, diagnoses, biological dysfunction, and treatment. But it also makes use of psychological and sociological concepts. Psychology assumes a continuity of psychopathology with normal mental functioning and sociology assumes social determinants of psychopathology. This plural, or "biopsychosocial," body moves along. Its organs are professional organizations, service delivery, training programs, research activity, and exercises in self-critique (Bolton 2008; Ghaemi 2009). It creates the shared professional language of clinical psychopathology.

Law is concerned with justice and aims to respect the self-determination of adults whom it considers are in sound mind.[1] A core concept for human rights based law is personal autonomy and law operationalizes this with the components of valid consent (Jackson 2009). In recent decades, these categories have increasingly regulated, or have attempted to regulate, areas of health and social care where the language of clinical psychopathology is indigenous (Owen, Szmukler, Richardson, David, Raymont, Freyenhagen et al. 2013).

In the United Kingdom, and in several other jurisdictions, the psychiatric and legal approaches to psychopathology are increasingly mixing (Brown, Tulloch, Mackenzie, Owen, Szmukler, and Hotopf 2013) and this trend will probably continue (Select Committee on the Mental Capacity Act 2005 2014). Given the different origins and professional perspectives of clinical psychopathology and law this mixing is liable to create confusion but it also affords opportunities. Several commentators have criticized the current state of

---

[1] See e.g. Justice Benjamin Cardozo's classic statement of this principle in *Schloendorff v. Society of New York Hospital*, 105 N.E. 92 (N.Y. 1914). "Every human being of adult years and sound mind has a right to determine what shall be done with his own body." This has been repeated in various forms in superior courts since.

clinical psychopathology as narrowly based on symptoms (Andreasen 2007; Mullen 2007; Owen, Freyenhagen, Richardson, and Hotopf 2009; Cutting 2012; Parnas, Sass, and Zahavi 2013) and criticisms of mainstream theories of personal autonomy are also being expressed (Freyenhagen and O'Shea 2013; Series 2015; Tan, Stewart, and Hope 2009). These critiques emphasize the relational, social, and value-laden aspects of autonomy and complain that mainstream accounts are narrowly individualistic or formal.

When overlapping areas have become narrowed, or siloed, interdisciplinary research becomes important. Progress in both clinical psychopathology and legal understandings of personal autonomy may come from research strategies that include psychiatric, philosophical, and legal perspectives on psychopathology (Owen, Freyenhagen, Richardson, and Hotopf 2009).

Phenomenology

What about phenomenology? In psychiatry the word phenomenology strongly connotes Karl Jaspers's approach to psychopathology with his majestic textbook *General Psychopathology* as the primary source (Jaspers 1963). Ghaemi (2007) has persuasively argued that the core, and lasting, feature of Jaspers's approach was methodological pluralism—the introduction of the distinction between the methods of understanding (*Verstehen*) and explanation (*Erklären*) to psychiatry's self-consciousness. But phenomenology also has a specific meaning in philosophy (Smith 2013). I understand phenomenology in this philosophical sense as a qualitative discipline that interprets structures of subjectivity or the meanings and values structuring intentional mental life. It is both descriptive and analytical and engages with ethical and ontological matters. This philosophical sense of phenomenology has significant links with psychiatry (Broome, Harland, Owen, and Stringaris 2012) but much of it lies outside of Jaspers's approach.

On psychopathology and law Jaspers was remarkably silent. Before the 1930s he seems (by his own admission) to have taken the Imperial certainties of German mental health law rather too much for granted (Jaspers 1963: 793–795, 839–840) and, from the 1940s on, he seems to imply that little could be said about the relation of personal autonomy to psychopathology at all (Jaspers 1963: 755–756). That is perhaps understandable given his historical and cultural context. But the twenty-first century context is different and, as we shall see, we need to find balanced ways of thinking about psychopathology from an ethical and legal point of view.

Plan for this Chapter

Both Jaspers's methodological pluralism and an approach to psychopathology drawing upon phenomenology as a philosophical, qualitative discipline are used to inform the interdisciplinary approach taken in this chapter. It will start with a short introduction to the legal components of valid consent and then focus on decision-making capacity (DMC) and the clinical categories of frontal brain injury, schizophrenia, and depression. It will look at DMC using clinical epidemiological methods (in Jaspers's mode of *explanation*) and then clinical phenomenological methods (Jaspers's mode of *understanding*—though supplemented by phenomenology in the philosophical sense).

VALID CONSENT

Imagine you are deciding about a treatment, selecting a home, or purchasing a car. Now ask yourself, what makes these decisions valid?

This question concerns law because the decisions involve different parties in society (you, your doctor, your family, your bank, etc.) and law needs to work out whom to justifiably hold accountable should disputes arise. Law's approach is to posit three elements of valid consent (or valid decision): relevant information, DMC, and voluntariness (Jackson 2009).

RELEVANT INFORMATION

This element recognizes that a person cannot be held accountable for a decision unless they are in possession of, or could be in possession of, relevant and reasonable amounts of information about the nature and consequences of the decision. I might decide to take medication A but if I don't know that medication A is for psychosis or that it may have side effects then law will question valid consent.

DECISION-MAKING CAPACITY

Decision-making capacity (DMC) is the presumption that the psychological abilities upon which decision-making depends are present. The sort of decision-making abilities that are relevant here are ones that relate to self-determination, or, in other words, abilities to make decisions for oneself. Legislators and courts have the final word on what these abilities are. Grisso and Appelbaum (1998) have distilled much US case law on DMC into a four abilities model.

1. Ability to understand relevant information
2. Ability to appreciate that information
3. Abilitiy to reason with that information
4. Ability to express a choice

In English law "appreciation" and "reasoning" are replaced by "use" and "weigh" (the Mental Capacity Act 2005). Whatever the exact words used, the law is trying to capture abilities to absorb relevant information, deliberate with that information, and effect choice.

The abilities must relate to specific decisions when a decision has to be made (or was made), for example, a treatment decision, a residence decision, a financial decision.

This is the so-called functional test of DMC. It is not a diagnostic test or a test of "reasonable" decision. One can have DMC in the presence of symptoms and a psychiatric diagnosis and one can have it if making a choice that many would regard as unwise or unreasonable. If any of the four abilities are absent then DMC is lacking and valid consent (or refusal) cannot be given but to lack an ability it must be shown that it is due to psychopathology.[2]

Recent legal debate is addressing a gray area in between valid consent and lacking DMC called "supported decision-making." The idea is that if an individual with mental disability is at risk of lack of DMC then the provision of support may remove that risk and enable valid consent to be achieved (Series 2015). Debate focuses on what this support should look like and its scope and limits.

VOLUNTARINESS

Voluntariness is the requirement that choices are not valid if they are coerced. In the extreme case a gun to the head with the threat to pull the trigger unless X is decided rather than Y is not a valid consent to X even if all relevant information is disclosed to the person deciding and all decision-making abilities (see above) are present. In practice coercion comes in shades and the law gives recognition of a continuum of threat to voluntariness with the concept of "undue influence."

With this brief legal outline of valid consent in place we can see that the component where psychopathology most clearly becomes relevant is DMC. But we can also see that *clinical* psychopathology and DMC are not the same thing. To look at psychopathology through the perspective of DMC is to look at it differently.

EXPLAINING DMC IN TERMS OF CLINICAL PSYCHOPATHOLOGY

One way to *explain* (in Jaspers's sense) DMC in terms of clinical psychopathology is through the use of operationalized measures and the statistical methods of epidemiology. Random sampling from clinical settings using ICD-10 codes, symptom scales, and a validated tool for the assessment of DMC (the "MacCAT-T" (Grisso and Appelbaum 1998)) allows measurements of both clinical psychopathology and DMC and for associations between these variables to be tested statistically.

Here I will summarize a selection of studies from the literature that illustrate this approach at work and which contribute to knowledge in psychopathology and law.

---

[2] There is some debate about whether this "due to" requirement is superfluous but, if it is superfluous, it will be superfluous because the absence of the psychological abilities is a mental inability itself (i.e. a mental anomaly). So, either way, psychopathology and lacking DMC have a deep connection.

PSYCHIATRIC VERSUS MEDICAL

Much debate has concerned whether there is an essential difference between psychiatric disorders and medical disorders (Kendell 2001; Szasz 1996) but how does this debate relate to DMC? When acute psychiatric settings were compared with acute medical settings on prevalence of DMC for treatment there were in fact no significant differences (Lepping, Stanly, and Turner 2015). If one performs a subanalysis of the relevant decision-making abilities, then inability to appreciate was more salient than reasoning in the psychiatric setting and vice versa in the medical setting (Owen, Szmukler, Richardson, David, Raymont, Freyenhagen et al. 2013).

So a remarkable parity exists between psychiatry and the rest of medicine in terms of DMC; but the underlying decision-making inabilities in the two settings are different. Appreciation is a more evaluative ability than reasoning and because the fact/value dichotomy and relativistic attitudes toward values are so influential in contemporary culture (Putnam 2004) it is likely that the objectivity of DMC assessment will attract more skepticism in psychiatric contexts than medical ones. But reasoning is also an area of considerable debate in psychology and philosophy because of plentiful evidence of poor reasoning in the healthy population (Sutherland 1992) and so skepticism can be directed to the medical setting also (Kim 2013). This parity of skepticism simply points to the need for more in-depth study of what appreciation and reasoning, or "use or weigh" abilities mean.

FRONTAL BRAIN INJURY

In a sizable number of cases of damage to the human frontal lobe, neuropsychology has been unable to measure impairment (Crawford 1998) despite patients having marked problems with behavior and self-awareness post brain damage. The famous case of Phineas Gage (Harlow 1848) is a prototype here and in many similar cases DMC is at issue. In a study of patients with frontal brain injury using detailed neurocognitive tests and a legal standard for the appreciation ability, Dreer and colleagues (Dreer, Devivo, Novack, Krzywanski, and Marson 2008) reported that the problems meeting the appreciation standard were unexplained by extant neurocognitive measures. This clarifies an interesting conceptual problem: what kind of evidence is of use in assessments of DMC in frontal brain injury? In-depth clinical phenomenological studies may help us arrive at an answer.

SCHIZOPHRENIA

The symptom profile of schizophrenia is varied and complex and the validity of the diagnostic category remains disputed (Bentall, Jackson, and Pilgrim 1988). Which symptoms associate most strongly with DMC for treatment in people with schizophrenia? A study of inpatients with psychotic symptoms found that there is a rank order in the strength of association. Delusions and thought disorder associated most strongly and hallucinations and cognitive impairment associated least strongly (Owen, David, Richardson, Szmuker, Hayward, and Hotopf 2008). Also, the category of schizophrenia was associated with regaining DMC more slowly compared with other diagnoses (Owen, Ster, David, Szmukler, Hayward, Richardson et al. 2011).

So, looked at through the perspective of DMC for treatment, the symptoms of schizophrenia that are of greatest interest are delusions and thought disorder rather than hallucinations and cognitive impairments. And if one wants to know about time-frames for regaining DMC, then the diagnosis of schizophrenia is not without predictive validity. Many questions remain however about what is underpinning these associations between schizophrenia and DMC.

DEPRESSION

Depressive is extremely common and can be severe, recurrent, and disabling. The psychiatric literature on depression is vast and there is good evidence for effective treatments. But how does depression impact upon DMC for treatment? Systematic review of empirical evidence reveals a tiny literature in this area and DMC tools have measurement problems (Hindmarch, Hotopf, and Owen 2013). This may not be a practical problem if psychiatrists have other reliable ways of identifying DMC. One possibility is the clinical concept of insight. If a patient with severe depression is unable to decide for themselves about treatment then, so the thought may go, they will lack insight and be flagged up for professional attention that way. But studies of depression and insight show that insight lacks sensitivity for severe depression (Amador, Flaum, Andreasen, Strauss, Yale, Clark et al. 1994) and also lacks sensitivity as a test of DMC (Owen, David, Richardson, Szmuker, Hayward, and Hotopf 2008). In other words, patients with severe depression do not have characteristically low scores on insight and high scores on insight can be consistent with lacking DMC.

So we have another conceptual gap and a new question: what are the relevant variables for losing the ability to decide for oneself in depression? Again, in-depth clinical phenomenological studies may help.

UNDERSTANDING MENTAL CAPACITY IN TERMS OF CLINICAL PHENOMENOLOGY

We have seen that *explaining* DMC in terms of clinical psychopathology yields a kind of knowledge. It gives a pragmatic mapping and identifies gaps where more basic conceptual work is required. Where gaps are found the methods of *understanding* become indicated to illuminate the meaningful relations between states of mind and abilities to self-determine. Here sampling is purposeful rather than random and interpretation is in depth rather than statistical. A method of second-person phenomenology has been adapted for this purpose (Owen, Freyenhagen, and Martin 2015). In brief, this method uses first-person reports but probes and interprets them in the context of an open-structured interview in which the interviewer (and research team) aim to make sense of the reports and what they imply for self-determination. I will now report on some studies which, using this method, address some of the gaps identified above.

FRONTAL BRAIN INJURY

The gap between neurocognitive tests of human frontal brain function and inability to use and weigh information, discussed above, requires a bridge to be constructed. A recent study reviewed relevant neuropsychological research on awareness of deficit, meta-cognition, and somatic markers and conducted in-depth interviews with people with frontal brain injury (Owen, Freyenhagen, and Martin 2018). A key finding concerned *online awareness of disability*. Consider this excerpt from an interview with a research participant with injury to the frontal lobe:

> ABI4:   It was really weird because in the hospital, everyone else was really bad. Like they couldn't walk or talk, totally mute. . . . But I was fine, I was walking and talking, and I thought everything was fine. And when I went home, I was like gone. I couldn't walk, couldn't walk upstairs. I was stuck in bed, and I couldn't talk. . . . But when I was walking and talking I was fine. Every single day in the hospital I was asking if I could go home. "I want to go home, I want to go home. I'm fine, look at me. You can see I'm fine." So eventually they gave in and said "Go on then, go home." And once I was home it was just different, you know. Before that I'd felt like I was better, I was fine. . . .
>
> INTERVIEWER: So when you were in hospital you felt it was all ok, you were walking around, you could speak, think, express yourself . . .?
>
> ABI4:   I was feeling fine, . . . but once I got out of hospital I realized how bad I was.
>
> INTERVIEWER: Outside of hospital it didn't work out?
>
> ABI4:   No, that's when I realized how bad I was.

The excerpt shows that ABI4 does have awareness of his disability ("I realised how bad I was"). In the interview, and retrospectively, ABI4 shows awareness of his disability. But the excerpt also attests to an episode in which ABI4 lacked that awareness in a context when a decision had to be made.

A few minutes later in the interview:

> ABI4:   I want to get out, have a fresh start where no one knows me, and I don't know anybody, and start all over again. Start totally fresh, start a totally fresh life, a totally fresh life.
>
> INTERVIEWER: And when you think like that, do you want to do it by yourself, alone, or do you want help from others?
>
> ABI4:   Do it myself.
>
> INTERVIEWER: Do it yourself?
>
> ABI4:   Yeah. I mean my uncle, when he got out of the nick . . . 9 years or 10 years. . . . He's out now, he's living up north.... When I get out of hospital I could go and see him. . . .

> INTERVIEWER: So what you're saying is that what you prefer is to start again, without any help from others. That's very, very different to hospital, isn't it, where there's an enormous amount of help that you're getting.
>
> ABI4:   I don't need this bollocks [hospital care], I'm sick of it.

Recall that ABI4 has just been articulating his awareness of his disability and significant support needs. But as the conversation began to involve deliberation that implicates future support needs, he was unable to bring that awareness "online" to inform his decision-making. The consequences of such an inability can be seen in an excerpt from a different participant, in which the difference between offline and online awareness was exhibited rather dramatically.

> INTERVIEWER: I mean, for example, in the restaurant you had somebody kind of shout at you after you got irritated and you kind of got into an argument which had got a bit out of hand, and it sort of started because, whereas before you would have managed the situation, now you lose your temper?
>
> ABI3:   Yeah.
>
> INTERVIEWER: Can you think of examples like that?
>
> ABI3:   Yeah it does happen. It does happen. [*Noise from another patient in background.*] I'll go out there and punch her on the f***ing nose in a minute if she don't shut up!

Awareness of disability is an important variable for DMC in the population of patients with frontal brain injury. However, awareness of disability can take different forms (retrospective, concurrent, online) and psychiatry and law need to be able to recognize all of them. Practical consequences for assessment of DMC in frontal brain injury flow from this result (Owen, Freyenhagen, Martin, and David 2015; Owen and Martin 2016).

Schizophrenia

Jaspers thought that phenomenology was important in identifying schizophrenia as a valid category. In other words, he thought that when psychiatry takes an entirely third-personal approach to schizophrenia (e.g. an entirely biological approach) it was at risk of losing its object. But he thought phenomenology was important in a sort of negative sense. His view seemed to be that in trying to interpret certain core patient experiences we can experience a limit in the scope of *Verstehen* as a method of interpretation (this is what he meant by "un-understandability"). This limit, together with characteristic patient self-descriptions such as "passivity" experiences, denoted schizophrenic psychic life and demarcated it from affective psychic life (Jaspers 1963: 577–582). So the core phenomenology of schizophrenia for Jaspers seemed to be a conjunction of distinctive first-person experiences (e.g. passivity symptoms) and a distinctive second-person experience (the interviewer experiencing a fundamental limit in the interpretability of those experiences).

Assessment of DMC involves interpretation (typically centered on a face-to-face interview) so what might this Jasperian point mean in relation to DMC assessment?

To illustrate the challenges of interpretation being referred to here, take this speech act from a patient with a diagnosis of schizophrenia.

> I went to Samoa. This has been my life in total. I never went there. I was taken there again. We got on the plane that took off, we were supposed to be flying local, we thought, like in France or something. The plane ended up in Tahiti, but the islands were called something in Samoa, so I can't remember whether it was Tahiti or Samoa we were in. I think we were in Samoa, but my family, someone was saying it was Tahiti. We landed on an Island. In those times they never had airstrips. The plane that brought us down was a cargo plane because they never had passenger planes. My brother got hold of me and there was a great white shark in the water, off a fair bit—it looked like somebody was carrying a door on their back—it was that big the shark, its fin.
>
> (Owen 2016)

Clearly, understanding what is being meant in this communication is going to strain our common sense or folk psychological resources.

In the context of assessment of DMC, Banner and Szmukler (Banner and Szmukler 2013) have proposed interpretative approaches drawing upon the "radical interpretation" of philosopher Donald Davidson. The suggestion is that in DMC assessment we should aim to clarify the meaning of a decision-making process using the principle of charity. Davidson developed the principle of charity as a way to interpret any alien speaker from scratch (think of an anthropologist's task of interpreting the language of a tribe where no assumptions can be made about shared beliefs or words). According to Banner and Szmukler when, after good faith attempts, radical interpretation does not yield translation of meaning about a decision-making process—or a person's will— then one may be unable to attribute DMC. They draw a parallel with Jaspers's concept of un-understandability.

A different interpretative approach is to try to understand the phenomenological structure of the decision-making abilities and inabilities at play in schizophrenia. On this approach, lacking DMC in schizophrenia is not inherently to do with un-understandability but to do with distinct psychological threats to self-determination. When overt delusion or thought disorder is stripped back to its meaning with close textual interpretation of dialogue what kind of underpinning cognitive and emotional rigidity of decision-making can be identified? And how does this rigidity threaten the ability to use or weigh information in decision-making? This is work in progress.

DEPRESSION

Psychopathologists have often remarked on the understandable nature of depression. It is, for example, easy to empathize with feeling bad or hopeless in the wake of the negative life events that often accompany a depressive episode. But in relation to DMC for treatment this can be a catch. Appelbaum and Roth (1982) have put it well in the context of challenges in general medicine:

> Of all the psychopathological processes associated with refusal [of medical treatment], depression is the most difficult to recognize, because it masquerades as, "Just the way I would

think if it happened to me" . . . The depressed patient is frequently able to offer "rational" explanations for the choices that are made.

We have seen that there is work to do to specify decision-making abilities in depression. A key finding from a recent study aiming to do this (Owen, Freyenhagen, and Martin 2015) concerns temporal inability.

This excerpt illustrates what requires interpretation:

> INTERVIEWER: What's in your mind?
> D4: Well nothing
> INTERVIEWER: And in your feelings?
> D4: No, I ain't got no feelings . . .
> INTERVIEWER: Do you feel sad?
> D4: No I don't feel sad, I got no feelings at all, I don't think.
>   I'm anxious again. You know . . . everything's a distraction . . . to take me away from what's going to happen. You know I go back to my room and lie there ready, that's why I lie in my room.
> INTERVIEWER: Ready for what?
> D4: Ready for death.

In this case of someone with severe depression in good physical health, the future was being experienced in a characteristic way. The ability to experience the future as open was compromised (death was the dominating awareness) and there was inability to experience a present task of deliberation and choice about treatment as shaping the future. There was inability to project oneself into significant normative differences and also inability to imagine different future treatment scenarios in some degree of detail when needed. Taken together this cluster of temporal inabilities can call into question self-determination in relation to treatment. How can there be using or weighing about X when the future has become normatively flattened in relation to X?

In the cases of mild–moderate depression studied, these temporal abilities were preserved (Owen, Freyenhagen, and Martin 2015) and here the concept of supporting decision-making to enable valid consent (see above) is likely to be more relevant than DMC assessment.

With an understanding of the relevant abilities and inabilities, we are in a better position to try to implement better strategies for the assessment of DMC in depression.

CONCLUSION

Psychiatry and the law share mind as a problem. Once we step back and reflect that psychopathology concerns the human being then the shared nature of the problem is not surprising. Clinicians are concerned with promoting human health and quality of life; law is concerned with ensuring that the human being's fundamental rights are respected. One point of specific overlap concerns DMC.

This chapter has summarized an interdisciplinary research approach to DMC. Some classic concepts from the clinical psychopathological stable—brain injury, schizophrenia, delusion, insight, and depression—have been looked at through the perspective of DMC and using the methodological pluralism of Jaspers. Starting with the perspective (or lens) of "*Erklären*," measurement of DMC patterns in selected clinical populations has been presented and this has also clarified some questions that are unsolved such as "how does frontal brain injury or depression impact on abilities to self-determine?" These questions have then been addressed using the perspective of *Verstehen* and this has generated new hypotheses about decision-making abilities (i.e. opportunities for the perspective of *Erklären* to grow) but also new illuminations of self-determination to aid those who must assess DMC in individuals. Ultimately, the assessment and navigation of DMC relates to a single human being and, as Jaspers taught us, a human being will elude the *single* perspective of either *Erklären* or *Verstehen*.

Much work is still to be done in this area of psychopathology and law and the field of research is comparatively new. But there are grounds to think the interdisciplinary approach outlined here contributes to a balanced and objective understanding of the normative dimensions of psychopathology.

Acknowledgments

The Wellcome Trust supported this work.

Bibliography

Amador X. F., Flaum M., Andreasen N. C., Strauss D. H., Yale S. A., Clark S. C., et al. (1994). "Awareness of Illness in Schizophrenia and Schizoaffective and Mood Disorders." *Archives of General Psychiatry* 51(10): 826–836.

Andreasen N. C. (2007). "DSM and the Death of Phenomenology in America: An Example of Unintended Consequences." *Schizophrenia Bulletin* 33(1): 108–112.

Appelbaum P. S. and Roth L. H. (1982). *Treatment Refusal in Medical Hospitals, in Report of the President's Commission for the Study of Ethical Problems in Medicine and Biomedical and Behavioral Research*, p. 434. Washington: US Government Printing Office.

Banner N. F. and Szmukler G. (2013). "'Radical Interpretation' and the Assessment of Decision-making Capacity." *Journal of Applied Philosophy* 30(4): 379–394.

Bentall R. P., Jackson H. F., and Pilgrim D. (1988). "Abandoning the Concept of 'Schizophrenia': Some Implications of Validity Arguments for Psychological Research into Psychotic Phenomena." *British Journal of Clinical Psychology* 27: 303–324.

Bolton D. (2008). *What is Mental Disorder?* Oxford: Oxford University Press.

Broome M., Harland R., Owen G. S., and Stringaris A. (eds.) (2012). *The Maudsley Reader in Phenomenological Psychiatry*. Cambridge: Cambridge University Press.

Brown P., Tulloch A., Mackenzie C., Owen G., Szmukler G., and Hotopf M. (2013). "Assessments of Mental Capacity in Psychiatric Inpatients: A Retrospective Cohort Study." *BMC Psychiatry* 13(1): 115.

Crawford J. R. (1998). "Introduction to the Assessment of Attention and Executive Functioning." *Neuropsychological Rehabilitation* 8: 209–211.

Cutting J. (2012). *A Critique of Psychopatholgy*. Berlin: Parados Verlag.

Dreer L. E., Devivo M. J., Novack T. A., Krzywanski S., and Marson D. C. (2008). "Cognitive Predictors of Medical Decision-Making Capacity in Traumatic Brain Injury." *Rehabilitation Psychology* 53(4): 486–497.

Freyenhagen F. and O'Shea T. (2013). "Hidden Substance: Mental Disorder as a Challenge to Normatively Neutral Accounts of Autonomy." *International Journal of Law in Context* 9(1): 53–70.

Ghaemi S. N. (2007). "Pluralism in Psychiatry: Karl Jaspers on Science." *Philosophy, Psychiatry and Psychology* 14(1): 57–66.

Ghaemi S. N. (2009). *The Rise and Fall of the Biopsychosocial Model.* Baltimore: Johns Hopkins University Press.

Grisso T. and Appelbaum P. S. (1998). *Assessing Competence to Consent to Treatment: A Guide for Physicians and Other Health Professionals.* New York: Oxford University Press.

Harlow J. M. (1848). "Passage of an Iron Rod Through the Head." *Boston Medical and Surgical Journal* 39(20): 5.

Hindmarch T., Hotopf M., and Owen G. (2013). "Depression and Decision-making Capacity for Treatment or Research: A Systematic Review." *BMC Medical Ethics* 14(1): 54.

Jackson E. (2009). *Medical Law,* 2nd edn. Oxford: Oxford University Press.

Jaspers K. (1963). *General Psychopathology.* Manchester: Manchester University Press.

Kendell R. E. (2001). "The Distinction Between Mental and Physical Illness." *British Journal of Psychiatry* 178: 490–493.

Kim S. Y. (2013). "Varieties of Decisional Incapacity: Theory and Practice." *British Journal of Psychiatry* 203(6): 403–405.

Lepping P., Stanly T., and Turner J. (2015). "Systematic Review on the Prevalence of Lack of Capacity in Medical and Psychiatric Settings." *Clinical Medicine (London)* 15(4): 337–343.

Mental Capacity Act (2005).

Mullen P. E. (2007). "A Modest Proposal for Another Phenomenological Approach to Psychopathology." *Schizophrenia Bulletin* 33(1): 113–121.

Owen G. S. (2016). "An Approach to the Patient with Bizzarreness." In M. Aragona and G. Stanghellini (eds.), pp. 221–229. Switzerland, Springer.

Owen G. S., David A. S., Richardson G., Szmuker G., Hayward P., and Hotopf M. (2008). "Mental Capacity, Diagnosis and Insight." *Psychological Medicine* 22: 1–22.

Owen G. S., Freyenhagen F., Richardson G., and Hotopf M. (2009). "Mental Capacity and Decisional Autonomy: An Interdisciplinary Challenge." *Inquiry* 52(1): 79–107.

Owen G. S., Ster I. C., David A. S., Szmukler G., Hayward P., Richardson G., et al. (2011). "Regaining Mental Capacity for Treatment Decisions Following Psychiatric Admission: A Clinico-ethical Study." *Psychological Medicine* 41(1): 119–128.

Owen G. S., Szmukler G., Richardson G., David A. S., Raymont V., Freyenhagen F., et al. (2013). "Decision-making Capacity for Treatment in Psychiatric and Medical In-patients: Cross-sectional, Comparative Study." *British Journal of Psychiatry* 203(6):461–467.

Owen G. S., Freyenhagen F., and Martin W. (2015). "Temporal Inabilities and Decision-making Capacity in Depression." *Phenomenology and the Cognitive Sciences* 14(1): 163–182.

Owen G. S., Freyenhagen F., Martin W., and David A. S. (2015). "Clinical Assessment of Decision-making Capacity in Acquired Brain Injury with Personality Change." *Neuropsychological Rehabilitation* 19: 1–16.

Owen G. S. and Martin W. (2016). "Brain Injury, Mental Capacity and Unwise Decisions." *Elder Law Journal* 6: 83–87.

Owen G. S., Freyenhagen F., and Martin W. (2018). "Assessing Decision-making Capacity After Brain Injury: A Phenomenological Approach [with Commentaries]." *Philosophy, Psychiatry & Psychology* 25(1): 1–19.

Parnas J., Sass L. A., and Zahavi D. (2013). "Rediscovering Psychopathology: The Epistemology and Phenomenology of the Psychiatric Object." *Schizophrenia Bulletin* 39(2): 270–277.

Putnam H. (2004). *Collapse of the Fact Fact/Value Dichotomy and Other Essays*. Cambridge, MA: Harvard University Press.

Select Committee on the Mental Capacity Act 2005. (2014). "Mental Capacity Act 2005: Post-legislative Scrutiny." House of Lords.

Series L. (2015). "Relationships, Autonomy and Legal Capacity: Mental Capacity and Support Paradigms." *International Journal of Law and Psychiatry* 40: 80–91.

Smith D. W. (2013). *Phenomenology. The Stanford Encyclopedia of Philosophy* (Winter 2013 Edition). Available from: http://plato.stanford.edu/archives/win2013/entries/phenomenology/

Sutherland S. (1992). *Irrationality*. London: Penguin.

Szasz T. S. (1996). "The Myth of Mental Illness." *American Psychologist* 15: 113–118.

Tan J. O. A., Stewart A., and Hope T. (2009) "Decision-making as a Broader Concept. *Philosophy, Psychiatry, & Psychology* 16(4): 345–349.

CHAPTER 82

ATMOSPHERES AND THE CLINICAL ENCOUNTER

CRISTINA COSTA, SERGIO CARMENATES, LUÍS MADEIRA, AND GIOVANNI STANGHELLINI

INTRODUCTION

MOST of present research in psychiatry focuses on objective phenomena that are measurable both by self-reported scales and semi-structured interview schedules. Yet some question the assumption of improved reliability and accuracy of clinical diagnoses (Norgaard et al. 2012; Regier et al. 2013) and we've witnessed a viral proliferation of the so-called *co-morbidity* (Kessler et al. 2005a; Kessler et al. 2005b). Yet comorbidity is problematic as "in psychiatry, cases of *true co-morbidity* are relatively rare since, for most disorders, we do not know enough about the underlying pathophysiology to be able to determine whether the disorders are truly clinically distinct" (First 2005). Some consider that there has been no etiological, pathogenic, or therapeutic breakthrough and that our awe is mainly due to technology-driven developments. One concern is the possibility of the strengthening of academic *anti-psychiatry*, another is the increasingly worrying credibility of psychiatry as a profession (Oyebode and Humphreys 2011). The specific pressures of clinical and academic career profiles have made researchers who are lacking clinical skills and clinicians who may not find the time or skills to carry out research. We see simple questions such as "What is characteristic of Schizophrenia?" keep eluding clinicians and scientists in our field, and their answers are unsatisfying to both. Most relevant to the present moment is the possibility of multidisciplinary teams that could encompass clinical and mathematical skills and also other skills such as those from cognitive science, neuroscience, and humanities.

Some of the present contributions to respond to these denigrations include reappraising the nature of psychiatric phenomena and, in particular, identifying the role of subjectivity and intersubjectivity. Schizophrenia is a particularly good example of these phenomena where seminal descriptions include "a *peculiar transformation* of feeling, thinking and perceiving, found nowhere else in this particular fashion" (Bleuler 1950) or "we have intuitions of a whole which we call schizophrenia but we do not grasp it. Instead we enumerate a vast number of particulars . . . while each of us only comprehends the whole from his own new experience of actual contact with such patients" (Jaspers 1997: 581–582). This has been considered under the premise of a disturbance of subjectivity by some European psychopathologists. They consider that it is inherent to a disturbance of a prototypical core self whose properties were not fluctuating surface psychotic symptoms but trait enduring features that have been present since early life. More recently, others consider that changes in the intersubjective taking place in the encounters with patients also seem to be implicated in the early detection of schizophrenia (Pallagrosi et al. 2016). The appraisal of what these elements represent place the reader in the field that this chapter focuses on—atmospheres and their disturbances.

These elements, ineffable and unarticulated in our psychopathological textbooks, are therefore dismissed from the psychiatric interview (Stanghellini and Mancini 2017). Clinicians are forced (1) to identify and describe the assortment of phenomena that are selected in classical psychopathological textbooks and (2) to a process of distancing themselves to a third-person perspective and a conceited scientific attitude that restricts the possibilities of the encounter. Both of these are a product of operational definitions and of the creation of diagnostic criteria, whose utility is unarguably linked to the contemporary effort to systematize psychiatry. Endorsed by our current nosography, this method has been adulated and applied significantly to the clinical encounter. It has hampered a generation of psychiatrists from identifying intersubjective phenomena, here appraised as a fair part of the clinical encounter bearing psychopathological meaning and also ground for the core of scientific knowledge of psychiatry (Stanghellini 2007).

Assessing and appraising atmospheres requires that we question two scientific premises: (1) an aseptic and static observation of phenomena in a third-person perspective allows their full disclosure (the position where mental symptoms present themselves) and (2) the dualistic intuition that encompasses our scientific minds suits the exploration of these phenomena. With this in mind, the experience of atmospheres is grounded on the suspension of two prejudices. The first one refers to the idea that the active participation in the encounter compromises the objectivity of the encounter. The second one concerns the intuitive reduction of phenomena to polarized qualities that are expected to define them.

ONTOLOGY OF ATMOSPHERES

> Atmospheres are indeterminate above all as regards their ontological status. We are not sure whether we should attribute them to the objects or environments from which they proceed or to the subjects who experience them. We are also unsure where they are. They seem to fill the space with a certain tone of feeling like a haze.
>
> (Böhme 1993: 114)

Is the Nature of Atmospheres Subjective or Objective?

As phenomena, atmospheres are ineffable and therefore their nature eludes most descriptions. They could be considered emotions, perceptions, or *emotional saliences*, emotional aspects of a situation that are immediately noticed prior to cognitive determination (Griffero 2014). Their distinctive feature is that they arise in the space between a person (or a sentient being) and a setting (person, thing, or situation) and are not traceable to them (Costa et al. 2014). So they are unlike ordinary emotions in the fact that they have no directedness—subject to an object—and they are felt as emerging from the outside of the subject's body. This description is similar to the depiction of emotions by the pre-Socratic philosophers or by Homer as external forces hitting the subject who feels them (Costa et al. 2014). Keeping an indeterminate location and direction, they have an ontologically intermediate status, which allows them to inform the subject about himself (subjectively) and about the world (objectively) (Costa et al. 2014).

In order to understand the experience of atmospheres one must avoid sustaining an introjectionist conception of feelings and attributing them directly to the subject. These are intuitive conceptions, brought to us by our cultural embedding, yet not suitable to our object of study. Instead consider the existence of bodily experiences as anterior to abstractions as such or that simply do not fit them. In this sense, Schmitz's work toward the absolute desubjectivization of emotions, including atmospheric ones, goes to the extreme of considering them as autonomous objects, entirely independent from the subject and the other elements in space (Schmitz 1969). Boehme does not go as far, considering the atmosphere the product of *Ekstases*, affective qualities radiating from objects, a place, or a person, tincturing the space between (Böhme 1993). Groundbreaking as they are, these conceptions do not divert from the ontological dualism that impedes the understanding of the atmospheric phenomenon. Griffero gives us a more consistent look, depicting it as "an in-between made possible by the co-presence of subject and object," safeguarding however, that "the in-between is not reified to the point of counting as a third element which, as a membrane, is interposed between the two margins" (Griffero 2014: 121). Instead, atmospheres are to be regarded as fragile phenomena, whose existence depends on the participation of the subjects who perceive them and whose objectivity depends on the possibilities of feeling of participants, for they are ever-changing "constantly seek(ing) renewed completion" (Grant 2013: 23; Costa et al. 2014).

Are Atmospheres Interior or Exterior Phenomena?

Pictorialists, artists that belong to the aesthetic movement that dominated photography during the later nineteenth and early twentieth centuries, aim at eliciting atmospheres by the use of vague shapes and blurred contour lines in their pictures (Nordström 2008). Their focus in the photo is quite literally on the air itself rather than the concrete objects photographed, which they find, is accountable for the general feeling conveys. Hence a key aspect of the atmospheric perception: atmospheres refer to the elusive and almost indefinable air that imbues and envelops a given situation (Costa et al. 2014). As intermediate phenomena that blur the objective–subjective dichotomy, their spatiality dwells in the loosened lines between interiority and exteriority, "filling the space between, not as a material object which fills another espousing the shape the other imposes" (Minkowski 1936: 86) "but rather as a vibration in which the perceived and the perceiver meet and merge" (Griffero 2014: 6). They are spatially diffuse feelings that convey basic emotional tones to the lived space, which resemble Stern's *vitality affects* and their dynamic qualities (Stern 2010). These include for instance "calming," "relaxing," "comforting," "tense," "heavy," or "light" tones that animate or dampen the background sense of life. For instance, in the sentence "the ambience in the room was tense," one is referring both to a private interior and a collective exterior phenomenon (Costa et al. 2014).

PHENOMENOLOGY OF ATMOSPHERES

Perception of an In-between

As intermediate phenomena atmospheres are not traceable to either of the individual participants. This is a very important point since it differentiates them from *auras*, the concept introduced by Benjamin (2009), to portray an objective property that emanates and therefore belongs to a person, or a thing, or a place, as part of their identity or essence. As an example, in ballet the spectator is not expected to experience the *aura* of the dancers (Costa et al. 2014; Böhme 2013). The object of contemplation is the atmosphere itself which arises while they are performing, "a quasi-thing, not less autonomous in relation to things than a melody is in relation to simple noise" (Griffero 2014: 18). The perception of atmospheres relies on the acknowledgment of an anti-dualistic autonomy to this in-between that is easily seen in less egocentric societies to the present day. In Japan for instance, there is a vast lexicon to designate the dynamics of intermediate phenomena: the *ma* designates the void or the gap between things, and simultaneously expresses the objective place and the subjective feeling it imparts; the interpersonal *aida*, a *being between* or the original common place that founds both everyday sociality and the individual self, the latter both in its external and internal composition and orientation (Griffero 2014; Cutting 2001).

Synaesthesia

Atmospheres belong to the pre-reflective realm of experience. They are lodged in the pathic moment of perception (Straus 1963), where the distinction between subject and object is fuzzy and no experience is monosensorial. Rather, one sense mode automatically elicits other sensorial modalities in a synaesthetic continuum. Their synesthetic nature is perfectly illustrated by Merleau Ponty, when referring to the haptic foundations of atmospheric sounds: "there is an objective sound which reverberates outside me in the instrument, an atmospheric sound which is between the object and my body, a sound which vibrates in me as if I had become the flute or the clock" (Merleau-Ponty 2005: 264). Marcel Duchamp's *musical sculpture* for instance, entails more than an acoustic experience, a visual-tactual one (Costa et al. 2014).

Significance

To perceive an atmosphere implies, other than receiving or apprehending sensorial data, the involvement in a situation and the participation in the global awareness of that situation. Situations encompass an atmospherically perceived significance that precedes any cognitive attribution, which means that they are not grounded in sign-referent semiotics, but in the effect produced in the lived body (Griffero 2014). Nevertheless, the attempts to reproduce them in the various forms of art—by choreographers, directors, painters, perfumers, etc.— proves their accessibility to reflective exercise. This reflective potentiality leads us to its relevance in the clinical encounter, which we will expose in the following section.

Phenomenological Assessment

In order to experience an atmosphere one must be predisposed to receiving it. According to Schmitz this predisposition is what allows the distanced influence of atmospheres (Böhme 1993). The potential inclusiveness of an aesthetic attitude in the phenomenological method used in the psychiatric interview resides in two features that are common to the aesthetic object and to the phenomenological object, which are (1) the aesthetic properties of an object can only appear if one allows the object's detachment from one's intention, just as the phenomenon appears when one is detached from any preconceptions; (2) the aesthetic properties only arise when the object is stripped of its ordinary meaning, likewise, the phenomenon appears when our pre-reflective natural attitude is suspended (Fenner 2008; Costa et al. 2014). Duchamp's ready-mades, whose aesthetic appraisal requires us to suspend common sense, are an example of this intersection.

ATMOSPHERES AS OBJECTS OF PSYCHIATRY

How are such fragile and unstable phenomena capable of psychopathologic meaning? The relevance of atmospheres in psychiatry is not without precedence. In his book *La Schizophrénie*, Minkowski claims that a psychiatrist should do more than enumerate symptoms "observing like a passive spectator, like when we are observing a microscopic slide, listing and classifying psychotic symptoms to achieve a so-called 'scientific' diagnosis is not going to be enough." The psychiatrist should aim at that which is essential and not available for exterior observation "we will feel with the patient and this will be an important element of our psychiatric judgement," thereby coining the term *diagnostique par pénétration* (Minkowski 2002: 94). Rümke, in the controversial report, stated that the psychiatric diagnosis is first formulated without the awareness of the psychiatrist relying on elements that are different from the ones that he will later use to justify it (Rümke 1941). For Rümke the psychiatric diagnosis is based on non-observable data. He went as far as saying that the determination of symptoms and the diagnosis of schizophrenia was to be made through the *Praecox Gefühl*, a specific feeling experienced by the clinician when encountering a patient with schizophrenia (Broome et al. 2012). More recently it has been revisited by Grube who established the percentage of correct diagnosis relying on the *Praecox Gefühl* of 86.6 based on the ICD-10 and 83.6 according to the DSM-IV (Grube 2006; Varga 2010). Doerr-Zegers introduced the term *Melancholie Gefühl*, a feeling that affects the clinician when meeting a melancholic patient (Doerr-Zegers 2015). Tellenbach developed the concept of *atmospheric diagnosis* (Tellenbach 1968). His conception of atmosphere is not along what is here presented, but the fact is that, similarly to his predecessors, he considered that during the encounter with a patient, the clinician is led to feel so-called atmospheric qualities perceptible in a bodily-sensuous way that permeate the process of diagnosing. In the therapeutic realm, Musalek has imported social aesthetics into the clinical encounter with the concept of *healing atmospheres*, which he conceives as spaces of possibilities (Musalek 2010). The same author, in conjunction with Schlimme, also introduced the term *paranoid atmospheres*, when referring to the atmospheres emerging in a deluded patient in their everyday interactions, which sustains the persistence and maintenance of the delusions (Schlimme 2009).

These are examples of atmospheres and their portrayals in psychiatry as accessible phenomena capable of disclosing psychopathologic meaning. Permeating the interaction with the patient they aid in the diagnostic process and have therapeutic implications (Musalek 2010). We will focus on the first two in the next sections.

Atmospheric Affordances

Some of the best-accomplished descriptions of atmospheres are found in psychiatric literature. Conrad, when referring to delusional mood, depicts it as something "in the air" and compares it to the atmospheric experience of walking alone in the woods. "The intermediate space between the invisible and what lies behind . . . has lost its neutrality. It is not the tree, nor the bush we see, the rustle of the tree tops or the cry of the owl we hear, but rather everything that is hidden, the space from which the tree, the bush, the rustle and the cry stand out: the very darkness and what is hidden as such" (Conrad 1963: 98; Mishara 2010). Jaspers depicts the delusional atmosphere as follows: "the environment is somehow different—not to a gross degree—perception is unaltered in itself but there is some change which envelops everything with a subtle, pervasive and strangely uncertain light . . . with this delusional atmosphere we always find an objective something there, even though quite vague, a something which lays the seed of objective validity and meaning" (Jaspers 1997: 98). In both descriptions, the atmosphere is disturbingly vague yet spatially present to the point of restricting our movements and ultimately our freedom. The fact that Conrad chose the example of the woods to illustrate part of the delusional mood demonstrates the openness of atmospheres to reflexive exercise and above all, its interpersonal objectivity. The experience of walking alone in the woods at night and the salience of that particular intermediate space set off feelings of disquiet and of being watched while walking, which are intersubjectively understood. Hence, the perception of atmospheres demands a special objectivity. We could therefore assume that situations, like walking in the woods, have certain *atmospheric affordances*—"ecological invites or meanings that are ontologically rooted in things or quasi-things" (Griffero 2014: 51), which are relatively inter-observable and prone to repetition (Griffero 2014). This is the core of the relevance of atmospheres as significant psychiatric objects.

Diagnostic Atmospheres

In the clinical encounter the most undefined bodily expressiveness of the patient, like a specific posture or a subtle fading of the prosody, are experienced in the lived space as atmospheres, in a precise and concrete fashion, before acquiring any intentional stance. For instance, when the depersonalized melancholic patient explains, "there is only emptiness around me" (von Gebsattel 1954: 25), the emptiness is immediately and evidently perceived by the clinician not as an absence but as an emptiness that is present in a quasi-concrete way. Recently, Doerr-Zegers and Stanghellini described their experience when meeting a schizophrenic patient as "a feeling of surmounting him. My lived body expands . . . I become bigger and feel that I invade David [the patient] . . . But his not wanting to look plus his standing bent and walking backwards does not produce in me that light sensation of nausea and repulsion we have in front of a stuporous depressive" (Otto Doerr-Zegers 2015: 4). Atmospheres are bodily resonant qualities of the lived space, manifest as *affordances* that build on the multimodal sensorial continuum of experience and guide our intuitive grasping of reality.

Schmitz structured the experience of space in three levels. The first level is the space of location (*ortsraum*), a geometric, measurable space. The second is the space of lived body directedness (*richtungsraum*) grounded in the motor suggestions of the surrounding space. The third level is the space of vastness (*weiteraum*), a non-measurable, non-directional absolute space centered in the lived body, the unnoticed background space that escorts our optokinetic movements (Schmitz 1969; Griffero 2014). When direction begins to narrow the lived body's vastness, the former two types of space arise. Atmospheres drift in the space of vastness. They are mostly elicited by the expressive attributes of a situation as well as intermodal motion and rhythmic configurations with its harmonies and dissonances that shape the space of vastness whilst being bodily experienced. Concerning the latter, Ligeti depicts them as "static, self-contained (music) without either development or traditional rhythmic configuration." In his music, atmospheres arise through the use of different rhythms in simultaneity, which create a volumetric sound structure that retains the melody. Giacometti's bronze sculptures *L'Homme qui marche* and *L'Homme du doigt* or Rui Chafes's iron sculptures like *During Sleep* illustrate the role of the expressive qualities in atmospheric perception. They are made of heavy raw materials, yet they immediately elicit the experience of lightness. It is the atmosphere that makes this determination possible. Hence, atmospheres are present in the genesis of our global awareness of situations. Just as in the theatre "the first scenes directly instill in us a certain emotion, which orients our entire comprehension," also in the clinical encounter it is not enough to identify symptoms, it is rather necessary that there be ascertained "a certain world-quality within which the problem or intrigue takes on meaning" (Dufrenne 1973: 188).

Fragile Understanding

Tarkovsky's discontinuities as the eroded images of abandoned places, the irregularity of surfaces, the erratic presence of water and the loosened narrative, elicit all senses and engage the viewer in a construction of meaning that is grounded in direct experience. We propose a similar engagement in the clinical encounter. Pallasmaa developed the concept of *fragile architecture*, which advocates a shift from the visual to the haptic understanding of architecture, relying on the whole sensorial experience (Pallasmaa 2005; 1999). Through this new understanding he intends to replace "the feeling of external control and visual effect by a heightened sense of interiority and tactile intimacy" (MacLeod 2013: 29). We suggest an analogous shift when assessing psychopathological phenomena, grounded on the clinician's own pathic pre-reflective experiences, thereby coining the term *fragile understanding*.

In the *Ellen West* case, her mode of existence is described as alternating between flying or floating over the clouds in relation with periods of hope and crawling like a worm in phases of desperation (Binswanger 2016). In *The Waves* by Virginia Wolf the author writes "I am rooted but I flow . . . I stream like a plant in the river, flowing this way, flowing that way, but rooted" (Woolf 2015: 59). These are examples of the relevance of the pre-reflective realm, particularly the lived body and space, in organizing experience (Figueira and Madeira 2011).

As a means of organizing our fragile understanding of atmospheres we suggest that clinicians rely mainly on the pre-reflective experiential realms, such as lived body and space, through which the expressive qualities in atmospheric perception, could for instance be described as expanding, retracting, being light or heavy, empty or full, floating, undulating or flat, etc. The phenomenological descriptions of these domains of experience carry the seed for interpersonal objectivity and the awareness of prototypic atmospheres to be disclosed. Hopefully, the intimate experience of atmospheres will also add empathic qualities to the encounter, having further implications in the therapeutic realm, like the strengthening and the unveiling of possibilities in the doctor-patient relationship (Musalek 2010; Picardi et al. 2017).

CONCLUSION

In this chapter we have attempted to clarify the intermediate ontological status of atmospheres. We have acknowledged them as immediately and directly perceived phenomena, which precede any cognitive attribution, whilst guiding our intuitive grasping of reality. In the particular setting of the clinical interview we have noticed their presence as phenomena, from which the encounter, and also the process of diagnosis, take on meaning. Although they certainly belong to the pre-reflective realm of experience, their openness to reflective exercise is manifest in the vast lexicon used to describe them. This has led us to recognize their inter-observability and proneness to repetition. Our final assertion is that these particular features account for an understanding that engages the clinician as an active participant in the delicate process of meaning making, which we coined *fragile understanding*, relying essentially on two distinctive domains of the pre-reflexive experience—lived space and lived body. Hopefully, the training of psychiatrists in this kind of understanding may have implications in the diagnostic realm, and in the therapeutic realm, namely by reinforcing the patient-doctor empathic relationship.

BIBLIOGRAPHY

Böhme G. (1993). "Atmosphere as the Fundamental Concept of a New Aesthetics." *Thesis Eleven* 36: 113–126.
Böhme G. (2013). "The Art of the Stage Set as a Paradigm for an Aesthetics of Atmospheres." *Ambiances*. https://journals.openedition.org/ambiances/315
Benjamin W. (2009). *The Work of Art in the Age of Mechanical Reproduction*. New York: Classic Books America.

Binswanger L. (2016). *Le Cas Ellen West. Schizophrénie. Deuxième étude*. Gallimard: Collection Bibliothèque de Philosophie.

Bleuler E. (1950). *Dementia Praecox or the Group of Schizophrenias*. New York: International Universities Press.

Broome M. R., Harland R., Owen G. S., and Stringaris A. (2012). *The Maudsley Reader in Phenomenological Psychiatry*. Cambridge: Cambridge University Press.

Conrad K. (1963). *La Esquizofrenia incipiente. Intento de un analisis de la forma del delirio*. Madrid: Alhambra.

Costa C., Carmenates S., Madeira L., and Stanghellini G. (2014). "Phenomenology of Atmospheres. The Felt Meanings of Clinical Encounters." *Journal of Psychopathology* 20: 351–357.

Cutting J. (2001). "On Kimura's Ecrits de psychopathologie phenomenologique." *Philosophy, Psychiatry, & Psychology* 8(4): 337–338.

Doerr-Zegers O. (2015). "Hermeneutics, Dialectics and Psychiatry." *Philosophical Anthropology* 1(1): 37–49.

Dufrenne M. (1973). *The Phenomenology of Aesthetic Experience*. Evanston: Northwestern University Press.

Fenner D. (2008). *Art In Context: Understanding Aesthetic Value*. Athens, Ohio: Swallow Press/ Ohio University Press.

Figueira M. L. and Madeira L. (2011). "Time and Space in Manic Episodes." *Dialogues in Philosophy, Mental and Neuro Sciences* 4(2): 22–26.

First M. B. (2005). "Mutually Exclusive versus Co-Occurring Diagnostic Categories: The Challenge of Diagnostic Comorbidity." *Psychopathology* 38: 206–210.

Grant S. (2013). "Performing an Aesthetics of Atmospheres." *Aesthetics* 23(1): 12–32.

Griffero T. (2014). *Atmospheres: Aesthetics of Emotional Spaces*. Farnham, Surrey ; Burlington, VT: Ashgate.

Grube M. (2006). "Towards an Empirically Based Validation of Intuitive Diagnostic: Rümke's 'Praecox Feeling' Across the Schizophrenia Spectrum: Preliminary Results." *Psychopathology* 39(5): 209–217.

Jaspers K. (1997a). *General Psychopathology*. Baltimore and London: Johns Hopkins University Press, vol I.

Jaspers K. (1997b). *General Psychopathology*. Baltimore and London: Johns Hopkins University Press, vol II.

Kessler R. C., Berglund P., Demler O., Jin R., Merikangas K. R., and Walters E. E. (2005a). "Lifetime Prevalence and Age-of-Onset Distributions of DSM-IV Disorders in the National Comorbidity Survey Replication." *Archives of General Psychiatry* 62(6): 593–602.

Kessler R. C., Chiu W. T., Demler O., and Walters E. E. (2005b). "Prevalence, Severity, and Comorbidity of 12-Month DSM-IV Disorders in the National Comorbidity Survey Replication." *Archives of General Psychiatry* 62(6): 617–627.

MacLeod S. (2013). *Museum Architecture: A New Biography*. Oxon and New York: Routledge.

Merleau-Ponty M. (2005). *Phenomenology of Perception*. Taylor and Francis e-Library.

Minkowski E. (1936). *Vers une cosmologie. Fragments Philosophiques*. Paris: Aubier.

Minkowski E. (2002). *La Schizophrénie*. Paris; Petite Bibliothèque Payot.

Mishara A. L. (2010). "Klaus Conrad (1905–1961): Delusional Mood, Psychosis, and Beginning Schizophrenia." *Schizophrenia Bulletin* 36(1): 9–13.

Musalek M. (2010). "Social Aesthetics and the Management of Addiction." *Current Opinion in Psychiatry* 23: 530–535.

Nordström A. (2008). *True Beauty: Pictorialism and the Photograph as Art, 1845–1945.* Vancouver Art Gallery. Vancouver/Toronto/Berkeley: Douglas & McIntyre.

Norgaard J., Revsbech R., Sæbye D., and Parnas J. (2012). "Assessing the Diagnostic Validity of a Structured Psychiatric Interview in a First-Admission Hospital Sample." *World Psychiatry* 11: 181–185.

Otto Doerr-Zegers G. S. (2015). "Phenomenology of Corporeality. A Paradigmatic Case Study in Schizophrenia." *Actas Españolas de Psiquiatría* 43(1): 1–7.

Oyebode F. and Humphreys M. (2011). "The Future of Psychiatry." *The British Journal of Psychiatry* 199(6): 439–440.

Pallagrosi M., Fonzi L., Picardi A., and Biondi M. (2016). "Association between Clinician's Subjective Experience during Patient Evaluation and Psychiatric Diagnosis" *Psychopathology* 49: 83–94.

Pallasmaa J. (1999). "Hapticity and Time—Notes on Fragile Architecture." *RIBA Discourse Lecture*, London, 78–84.

Pallasmaa J. (2005). *The Eyes of the Skin: Architecture and the Senses.* Chichester, West Sussex: Wiley-Academy.

Picardi A., Pallagrosi M., Fonzi L., and Biondi M. (2017). "Psychopathological Dimensions and the Clinician's Subjective Experience." *Psychiatry Research* 258: 407–414.

Regier D. A., Narrow W. E., Clarke D. E., Kraemer H. C., Kuramoto S. J., Kuhl E. A., and Kupfer D. J. (2013). "DSM-5 Field Trials in the United States and Canada, Part II: Test-Retest Reliability of Selected Categorical Diagnosis." *American Journal of Psychiatry* 170: 59–70.

Rümke H. C. (1941). "Das Kernsymptom der Schizophrenie und das 'Praecox Gefühl'." *Zeitschrift für die gesamte Neurologie und Psychiatrie* 102: 168–175.

Schlimme J. E. (2009). "Paranoid Atmospheres: Psychiatric Knowledge and Delusional Realities." *Philosophy, Ethics, and Humanities in Medicine* 4(14): 1–8.

Schmitz H. (1969). *System der philosophie. Der Gefuehlsraum.* Bonn: Bouvier.

Stanghellini G. (2007). "The Grammar of the Psychiatric Interview." *Psychopathology* 40(2): 69–74.

Stanghellini G. and Mancini M. (2017). *The Therapeutic Interview.* Cambridge: Cambridge University Press.

Stern D. N. (2010). *Forms of Vitality: Exploring Dynamic Experience in Psychology, the Arts, Psychotherapy and Development.* New York: Oxford University Press.

Straus E. (1963). *The Primary World of Senses: A Vindication of Sensory Experience.* New York: Free Press of Glencoe.

Tellenbach H. (1968). *Geschmack und Atmosphäre.* Salzburg: O. Müller.

Varga S. (2010). "Vulnerability to Psychosis, I-thou Intersubjectivity and the Praecox-feeling." *Phenomenology and the Cognitive Sciences* 12(1): 131–143.

von Gebsattel V. E. (1954). *Prolegomena einer medizinischen Anthropologie.* Berlin: Springer.

Woolf V. (2015). *The Waves.* Oxford: Oxford University Press.

CHAPTER 83

THE PSYCHOPATHOLOGY OF PSYCHOPATHS

JÉRÔME ENGLEBERT

INTRODUCTION

THE objective of this article is to present a holistic conception of psychopathy inspired by phenomenological psychopathology and to compare it with the mainstream nosographic diagnosis. First, two major theoretical works dedicated to this nosographic entity are discussed. One is German: Schneider's *Psychopathic Personalities* (Schneider 1923). The other is American: Cleckley's *The Mask of Sanity* (Cleckley 1941). The well-known work of Hare (Hare 2003) is then summarized, including the so-called *Hare Psychopathy Checklist* (PCL-R), as well as the critique by Cooke et al. (Cooke and Michie 2001; Cooke et al. 2004, 2007, 2012).

Next, I illustrate how a structural-phenomenological approach enhances the psychopathological investigation of psychopathy. I first compare Binswanger's conception of mania with psychopathic functioning. Patients' behavior is similar but the difference relates to the dialectic between the ego and the alter ego. A patient with mania is affected by a fundamental crisis of the ego, which a psychopath does not have. A second dimension relates to emotions and the adaptive dimension of psychopathy. An epistemological discussion of the concept of emotions reveals that psychopaths are competent at managing emotional stimuli, which bestows a psychological advantage upon them. Finally, a reflection enlightened by the contributions of phenomenological philosophy (Stein 1989; Scheler 2008; Zahavi 2005, 2011) on empathy and sympathy clarifies the presentation of "psychopathic *being-in-the-world*." Starting with the tension between clinical practice and criticism of the dominant diagnostic scales, we consider the "essential characteristics" of the psychopathic disorder to be: reification of the alter ego without an ego-related disorder, emotional coldness as it provides adaptive benefits, and empathic skills without sympathy.

PHENOMENOLOGICAL PSYCHOPATHOLOGY
OF PSYCHOPATHY?

As a discipline, the purpose of phenomenological psychopathology is to identify the logical structure of psychological functioning; it favors an approach based on understanding over interpretation or explanation (Stanghellini 2009; Cutting 2012; Englebert 2013). One of its aims is to identify the specific psychological features inherent to nosographic entities (the dimension of eidetic phenomenology which focuses on the study of essences and identification of the basic components of phenomena—in the specific field of phenomenological psychopathology, we speak about specific *being-in-the-world*). This method partly derives from Minkowski's legacy (1927, 1966), who suggested engaging in a "psychology of the pathological" rather than a "pathology of the psychological," that is, seeking a structural understanding of psychological organization. This approach to psychopathology is intrinsically clinical; the fundamentals of its research topics—phenomena—emerge from clinical practice (Stanghellini 2009; Nordgaard et al. 2013). This theoretical essay is informed by clinical situations involving psychopaths who were interviewed in prison or in forensic centers.

If phenomenological psychopathology is interested, largely, in psychotic issues, many studies do analyze other psychopathological disorders and psychopathological manifestations (Broome et al. 2013). Work on the consideration of psychopathy in a phenomenological paradigm, as far as it is concerned, is recent. These studies are particularly interested in the subject's experiential dimension of time and show deficits in the imagination of the future and massive deficits with respect to *mental time travel* (McIlwain 2010; Levy 2014; Berninger 2017). Let's also mention the amazing approach of philosopher Glover (2014) at Broadmoor high-security psychiatric hospital, in England, which analyzes the moral and ethical dilemmas of the psychopathic subjects he went to meet (along with other diagnoses). If they observe cognitive and moral bias in their speech, Glover's hypothesis is precisely to consider that such biases are in parallel to those seen in many people considered normal (Glover 2014). Finally, let's notice that the work of phenomenological psychopathology centered on psychopathy also discusses the emotional dimension of this disorder (Beringer 2016; Englebert 2013b, 2015).

Strictly speaking, psychopathy or "psychopathic personality" is not a medical/psychiatric diagnosis. As we shall see, the psychopath is in fact absent from domineering nosography as in the DSM or ICD. However, this diagnosis is of considerable importance in many contemporary debates on psychopathology because of its many clinical and societal issues. Important links are identified between the psychopathic trait and other disorders such as antisocial personality disorder (Hare 2003; Hare et al. 1991), borderline personality (González et al. 2016), and schizophrenia (Abu-Akel et al. 2015). From a developmental point of view, many studies underline connections between certain psychological disorders of childhood and adolescence (including Callous-unemotional line) and the development of psychopathic characteristics into adulthood (Bird and Viding 2014; Frick et al. 2014; Henry et al.

2016; Muratori et al. 2016). Finally, a clarification of psychopathy is very important for the forensic field and for the psychopathological reflection on criminal matters (Kiehl and Sinnott-Armstrong 2013; Englebert 2013).

Historical and Contemporary Nosographies

Historical Background

Psychopathy was described in the early nineteenth century by Pinel. He observed that some subjects presented a state of *"manie sans délire"* [insanity without delusion][1] (Pinel 1800: 151). This early description is very important as it will enable us to explain the problem inherent to modern conceptions of psychopathy. The work of Schneider and Cleckley gradually led to a common and still current definition of psychopathy: a serious disorder or imbalance of the character or personality that does not include psychosis or significant mental deficiency (Schneider 1923; Cleckley 1941).

In contemporary nosographic work, psychopathy occupies an ambiguous position. This uncertainty is reflected in its absence from the DSM-IV and DSM-5 and from the ICD-10 and future ICD-11.

According to Schneider (1923), psychopaths present antisocial manifestations and character disorders such as instability, irritability, inability to adapt, increased tendency to commit crimes and consume drugs and alcohol, etc. In addition, psychopathy is said to be characterized by a firm opposition to social rules and norms (see Table 82.1). Cleckley (1941) identifies sixteen key signs that tend to describe a typical psychopath. This is an individual who is characterized by *superficial charm and high intelligence,* who does not suffer from *delusions or irrational thinking,* but also does not present signs of *neurosis, guilt or shame. Lacking in insight* and presenting *emotional reactions* described as *poor,* a psychopath is also *unable to behave appropriately in interpersonal relations. Hypocritical and untruthful, egocentric and incapable of love,* this is *a person who cannot be counted on,* is *unable to learn from experience,* or *follow a life plan.* Finally, in addition to *engaging in inadequately motivated antisocial behavior,* a psychopath *demonstrates fantastic and objectionable behavior under the influence of alcohol,* has an *impersonal and trivial sex life,* and *is unlikely to attempt suicide* (see Table 82.1).

The Hare Psychopathy Checklist—Revised

Despite the lack of a definition in the international classifications, an important movement in the literature attempted to formulate a pragmatic definition of psychopathy, based on

---

[1] The traditional English translation is certainly not the best since it translates the word *"manie"* [mania] with "insanity" as in French we mean by the word *"folie."* For our purposes we will retain the notion of mania to be able to dialogue with the theses of Binswanger on the manic state and to refine our critique of the scale of Hare (see section on "Mad?: The Dialectics of Ego and Alter Ego in Psychopaths and Manic Subjects").

the work of Hare (2003). *The Hare Psychopathy Checklist—Revised* (PCL-R) presents a set of behavioral, interpersonal, and affective characteristics, including egocentricity; manipulation; insensitivity to others; irresponsibility; unstable relationships; impulsivity; lack of empathy, remorse or guilt; and poor behavioral control. All of the PCL-R items is presented in a summary table below (see Table 83.1). These signs are most likely to manifest in antisocial behavior (Hare 2003; Cooke et al. 2004). These antisocial characteristics are part of the clinical picture, but they are not sufficient to diagnose psychopathy: a psychopathic subject necessarily has an antisocial personality, but the opposite is not necessarily true (Hare 2003; Hare et al. 1991; Cooke et al. 2004). According to this conception, one might consider psychopathic personality to be a way of adapting to the world through affective and interpersonal experiences (Cooke et al. 2004), whereas the antisocial dimension is primarily a set of behaviors involving transgressions against social laws and standards (Hare 2003; Hare et al. 1991).

This work adds a specific set of items to the diagnosis of antisocial personality disorder in order to isolate psychopathy as a specific nosographic entity. These items mainly concern the interpersonal sphere and the affective dimension.

Table 83.1 Summary of criteria for psychopathy

Schneider's criteria	Cleckley's criteria	Hare's criteria
Antisocial manifestations	Superficial charm and high intelligence	Glibness and/or superficial charm
Instability		Grandiose sense of self-worth
Irritability	Does not suffer from delusions or irrational thinking	Need for stimulation and/or proneness to boredom
Inability to adapt		
Tendency to commit crimes	Does not present signs of neurosis, guilt, or shame	Pathological lying
		Conning and/or manipulative
Drugs and alcohol consumption	Lacking in insight	Lack of remorse or guilt
	Emotional reactions described as poor	Shallow affect
Characterized by a firm opposition to social rules and norms		Callous and/or lack of empathy
	Unable to behave appropriately in interpersonal relations	Parasitic lifestyle
		Poor behavioral controls
	Hypocritical and untruthful	Promiscuous sexual behavior
	Egocentric and incapable of love	Early behavior problems
	This is a person who cannot be counted on	Lack of realistic, long-term goals
		Impulsivity
	Unable to learn from experience or follow a life plan	Irresponsibility
	Engaging in inadequately motivated antisocial behavior	Failure to accept responsibility for own actions
	Demonstrates objectionable behavior under the influence of alcohol	Many short-term marital relationships
		Juvenile delinquency
	Has an impersonal and trivial sex life	Revocation of conditional release
		Criminal versatility
	Is unlikely to attempt suicide	

Other Instruments

I should make it clear that my goal is not to present a comprehensive examination of all contemporary models of psychopathy. I will only include the presentation of three other instruments: the *Psychopathic Personality Inventory* (Lilienfeld and Widows 2005; Uzieblo et al. 2010; Skeem et al. 2011), the *Triarchic Psychopathy Model* (Patrick et al. 2009) and the *Self-Report of Psychopathy–Short Form* (Paulhus et al. 2015). The former was revised in 2005 to become the PPI-R and now comprises 154 items organized into eight subscales (Lilienfeld and Widows 2005). The items are grouped into two overarching and largely separate factors (Factor 1—Fearless dominance: Social influence, Fearlessness, Stress immunity; Factor 2—Impulsive antisociality: Machiavellian egocentricity, Rebellious nonconformity, Blame externalization, Carefree nonplanfulness), plus a third factor that is mainly dependent on scores on the other two (Cold-heartedness).

Meanwhile, the *Triarchic model* (Patrick et al. 2009) suggests that different conceptions of psychopathy emphasize three observable characteristics to varying degrees: boldness (low fear including stress-tolerance, toleration of unfamiliarity and danger, and high self-confidence and social assertiveness), disinhibition (poor impulse control, including problems with planning and foresight, lacking affect and urge control, demand for immediate gratification, and poor behavioral restraints), and meanness (Lacking empathy and close attachments with others, disdain of close attachments, use of cruelty to gain empowerment, exploitative tendencies, defiance of authority, and destructive excitement seeking).

Finally, the *Self-Report of Psychopathy–Short Form* (SRP-SF) (Neumann and Pardini 2014; Paulhus et al. 2015). Derived from and shown to correlate highly with the PCL (2003), the SRP was developed for use in nonforensic populations as a practical and brief method to assess psychopathic traits. The latest version of this scale contains twenty-nine items and may provide an efficient method of measuring psychopathic traits among larger samples. The items are grouped into four dimensions of psychopathy: affective callousness, interpersonal manipulation, antisociality, and erratic lifestyle.

Despite the interest of these tools, I formulate my critical discussion on the basis of the PCL-R alone, as it remains the reference tool in criminological and psychopathological assessments in the field of forensics. I also specify that none of these tools falls within the scope of psychopathological phenomenology. Let's now discuss Cooke et al.'s criticism of the PCL-R's factor structure, and particularly the presence of antisocial characteristics in the diagnosis of psychopathy (this critique is also not made from a phenomenological point of view).

Critique of the Presence of an Antisocial Dimension

Cooke et al.'s work (Cooke and Michie 2001; Cooke et al. 2004, 2007, 2012) stimulated a lively debate on whether antisocial behaviors are or are not necessary in characterizing a subject as a psychopath (Patrick 2006; Vitacco 2007). This ambiguity already existed in the work of Schneider (1923) and Cleckley (1941). However, Cleckley was the researcher who most clearly considered the possibility of a diagnosis of psychopathy without the presence of antisocial or illegal behavior (Cleckley 1941; Patrick 2006).

The *Comprehensive Assessment of Psychopathic Personality* (CAPP) (Cooke and Michie 2001; Cooke et al. 2004, 2007, 2012) supports a different premise for defining the psychopathic entity. This conception, which has also been strongly influenced by Cleckley's work, is a multidimensional model of personality that consists in six dimensions and includes each of the dysfunctional traits observed in psychopathic personality disorder, except for the antisocial factor (and those related to sexual promiscuity and short-term cohabitation relationships in the PCL-R). These authors consider the antisocial factor as "secondary symptoms," which follow from the psychopathic lifestyle. Thus, the model excludes the elements related to the subject's behavioral and criminal history. According to this criticism, the interpersonal and affective facets are the "central constituents" of the psychopathic personality.

These developments are very important and allow one to go one step further in understanding the psychopathic individual's psychology, but they still seem to stop short of one crucial step: carrying out an in-depth psychopathological study of psychopathy. I formulate my critical discussion on the basis of the PCL-R alone, as it remains the reference tool in criminological and psychopathological assessments in the field of forensics.

FOR A PSYCHOPATHOLOGICAL APPROACH OF PSYCHOPATHY

My objective is to seek out the meaning structure and the signification that links different signs of the disorder. According to Jaspers's proposal (Jaspers 1913), the purpose in psychopathology is to *understand* the puzzle that is presented, observe the phenomena, and seek to obtain a significant overall picture. The starting point I suggest, paradoxically, is to examine *manic being-in-the-world*.

Mad? The Dialectics of Ego and Alter Ego in Psychopaths and Manic Subjects

Ludwig Binswanger (1960) conducted a systematic analysis of the "reification of the alter ego" in manic subjects. One of the fundamental characteristics of mania, in this author's view, is seeing other people as "interchangeable" and "utilitarian." Although Binswanger does not address this question, we can make an analogy with psychopathic functioning, which also presents this tendency to reify others. Psychopathic patients may say, for example: "The others are objects I use when I need them; in my eyes, they are no more"; "What counts for me is the pleasure I get from what I'm doing; the role of other people isn't very important"; "I wanted to carry out a successful robbery and no one was going to stop me. To succeed, I had to kill him. He didn't represent anything more than an obstacle to me" [Source: own clinical experience].

Clearly, though, from a clinical perspective, mania and psychopathy are very different phenomena. In what ways? When Pinel describes psychopathic behavior as "*manie sans délire*," it is important to define what is meant by "madness." The work of Binswanger suggests "the constitution of the alter ego" and "the ego" as a basis for discussing the dysfunctions of manic *being-in-the-world* (Binswanger 1960).[2] His thesis is that, in manic subjects, a disorder affecting the constitution of the alter ego coexists with a disorder of the constitution of the ego, or I:

> If in mania the alter ego is not completely constituted, and thus remains largely a stranger, or even a strange thing—a mere object taken, pushed aside and rejected, used and consumed by something—then the causes are naturally not in the alter ego but in the ego.
>
> (Binswanger 1960: 93; my translation)

This observation is critical since it presents mania as a subclass of psychosis, which Binswanger considers, based on Husserl's work, as a failure of "appresentation" [Appräsentation]. When two people meet, "what is present to us is different but is accompanied by the same appresentation" (Binswanger 1960: 75). These two people share a set of common representations that allow them to consider each other as an *alter ego* and to share a common world. Thus, in Binswanger's understanding of the term, appresentation is an intersubjective, intuitive, and pre-cognitive phenomenon that enables one to form relationships and that must necessarily be shared by the various partners. This a priori is crucial for the sharing of common meaning and natural self-evidence in social exchanges. It is precisely this faculty that is said to be deficient in psychotic pathologies (including mania).

Binswanger cites the example of one of his manic patients, Elsa Strauss, who entered a church and interrupted the ceremony to compliment the pianist and ask him for private lessons, offending the whole congregation. Words and actions, taken out of context, are not fundamentally incoherent or delirious, but they show a "failure of appresentation in mania and . . . the impossibility of constituting a common world" (Binswanger 1960: 78). The essence of psychosis in Binswanger's view is to escape this implicit common appresentation. This thesis can be superimposed on modern concepts of psychosis according to phenomenological psychopathology (Parnas et al. 2002; Stanghellini 2004; Sass 2014). For Binswanger, the manic reification of the other and the problem affecting the alter ego can be situated in a disorder affecting a psychotic ego. The determining factor in discriminating between manic and psychopathic subjects is at this level: the former have a disorder of the constitution of the alter ego explained by a disorder of the ego, while the latter have the same disorder but with an intact ego.

The Core Characteristic of Psychopathy: Reification of Others Without an Ego-Related Disorder

The major difference between manic and psychopathic reification of the other is clearly identifiable by clinicians. For manic patients, other people are just a casual means of implementing their own projects, of enjoying themselves or their grandiosity. Their instrumentalization of others is direct, clearly pre-reflexive, even "naïve."

They do not even try to imagine what goes on in other people's minds, because this does not play a role in their projects. Their empathetic awareness of other people is non-existent

---

[2] For an overview of the concept of *being-in-the-world*, refer to selected papers of Ludwig Binswanger (1963) and for a presentation of the manic mode of *being-in-the-world*, see Broome et al. (2013: 197–203).

(however, they can also be exquisitely sensitive to the emotions of others and can feel responsible—in a grandiose way—for all of their suffering). In contrast, for psychopaths, other people are a means of gaining power and pursuing their goals in a cold, insidious way. Their instrumentalization of others has a reflective, well-thought-out component, which is somewhat "Machiavellian." They may well use imagination and "theory of mind" in order to deceive, lie, and misuse others to achieve their own ends.

Thanks to Binswanger's analysis of the crisis of the ego and the alter ego, we can refine this description. The radical and fundamental difference between manic and psychopathic subjects is that the latter do not present problems with the ego or I; to put it more simply, they do not have psychotic symptoms. A psychopath presents a disorder affecting the alter ego, via the reification of others (a symptom shared with manic subjects) but without presenting an ego-related disorder (a symptom not shared with manic subjects). Unlike a manic subject, a psychopath is able to maintain a stable ego and a coherent identity while still reifying others. For the psychopath, the alter ego problem is not secondary to a problem with the ego in its function as an appresentative structure.

Now let us reconsider the twenty items of the PCL-R. Based on the recommendations of the CAPP (Cooke and Michie 2001; Cooke et al. 2004, 2007, 2012), I eliminate the so-called secondary items, which are less relevant to a psychopathological approach. The remaining thirteen items are as follows: 1. *Glibness and/or superficial charm*; 2. *Grandiose sense of self-worth*; 3. *Need for stimulation and/or proneness to boredom*; 4. *Pathological lying*; 5. *Conning and/or manipulative*; 6. *Lack of remorse or guilt*; 7. *Shallow affect*; 8. *Callous and/or lack of empathy*; 9. *Parasitic lifestyle*; 13. *Lack of realistic, long-term goals*; 14. *Impulsivity*; 15. *Irresponsibility*; 16. *Failure to accept responsibility for own actions*.

The semiological picture presented above describes manic subjects just as well as psychopaths. Needless to say, I don't think these two diagnostic entities are the same. Because it limits its analyses to a survey of interpersonal and affective dimensions considered as isolable signs, and does not provide a structural and psychopathological synthesis, this model is unable to explain the difference between mania and psychopathy.

Still, in the light of Pinel's proposal to consider psychopathy as "insanity without delusion" ["*manie sans délire*"], we should not be surprised by this finding. The overview of Binswanger's work highlighted that the difference between mania and psychopathy is located not really at the level of strictly behavioral signs but at the psychopathological level, based on the essential dialectic between the alter ego and the ego. Hence the decisive affiliation of mania with psychosis and not that of psychopathy. The latter should be considered a personality disorder. This allows us to remember that, of course, these two disorders are fundamentally and essentially different from a psychopathological point of view and with regard to their respective mode of *being-in-the-world*.

Adapted? Is Psychopathy a Generalized Maladaptation?

One of the problems in understanding psychopathy may be to immediately consider it as a disorder (Cutting 2012; Englebert 2013), without further thought, and thus viewing it a priori as a maladaptation. For evolutionary psychopathology (De Block and Adriaens 2011; Brüne 2008; McGuire and Troisi 1998; Stevens and Price 2000; Demaret 2014), many behaviors considered to be pathological must have an adaptive value in the original environment in which the morphology and psychology of our species were shaped. A change in time (a behavior in another era) or space (a behavior in another context, or social, cultural. or economic situation) may make a symptom appear adaptive (e.g. anorexia nervosa in times of famine). Regarding psychopathy, one might suggest that:

> The social function of psychopaths depends on conditions in the environment. In times of peace, we lock them up; in times of war, we count on them and cover them with medals.
>
> (Demaret 2014: 29; my translation)

Classically (Schneider 1923; Cleckley 1941; Hare 2003), psychopathy is associated with a general or specific emotional deficit, affecting the processing and production of emotion. Basic research tends to partially disconfirm this hypothesis (Poythress and Hall 2011; Brook et al. 2013; Casey et al. 2013; Maes and Brazil 2013; Bird and Viding 2014). Although the emotional dimension is considered to be the basis for the process of adaptation and social interaction and is assumed to have a regulating function (Sartre 1939; Fuchs 2013; Englebert 2013), the hypothesis that psychopaths have an emotional deficit is contradictory. I suggest instead that psychopaths are able to understand and manage emotional phenomena. This conception is in opposition to the "poor," "narrow," and "immature" emotional life attributed to psychopaths (Schneider 1923; Cleckley 1941; Hare 2003). It corresponds to the adaptive conception considered by Demaret (2014). In times of war, the psychopath does not suddenly regain the emotional competence he had lost in times of peace.

Emotional Coldness

"Emotional coldness" must be distinguished from "emotional deficit." Emotional coldness, if we can agree on a definition, is clearly one of the fundamental clinical signs of psychopathy. Hare (2003) defines emotional coldness as one of the four facets of psychopathy (and thus an essential trait). I agree with this claim. He then defines it with four items: *Lack of remorse or guilt* (item 6), *Shallow affect* (item 7), *Callous and/or lack of empathy* (item 8) and *Failure to accept responsibility for own actions* (item 16). This second point is not satisfactory because Hare's definition does not perfectly delimit the concept. Emotional coldness should instead be considered a way of managing emotional manifestations calmly and coolly, without precipitation. (This is difficult to relate to item 14 of the PCL-R, "impulsivity," which describes antisocial subjects but not true psychopaths, strictly speaking.) Emotional coldness is a preferred method of managing emotion calmly and keeping some distance, as well as a tendency to take the time to analyze emotional experiences triggered in oneself or in others. This tendency should not be considered as being more or less adaptive, effective, or pathological than a "warm" emotion management style (tendency to react faster, by trial and error, "naturally," or "romantically"). It is probably more profitable to have a preferred method (a style) of emotion management than to manage emotion in a more random, less coherent way. Depending on an individual's social, relational, or professional situation, it may be more adaptive to manage emotions either "coldly" (political leader, emergency physician, etc.) or "warmly" (group facilitator, performing artist, etc.). This means that the emotional coldness generally attributed to psychopaths may be considered partly as an adaptive advantage, which can also be found in numerous people who have no personality disorders or social or emotional deficits.

Bad? Empathy or Sympathy Disorder?

Psychopaths are generally said to have an empathy deficit (Hare 1999; Decety et al. 2013). Once again, it is necessary to define this concept. If we examine the definition more closely, we can see that a psychopath does not actually have an empathy disorder but a sympathy disorder. This difference is crucial as it enables us to distinguish between psychopathy (sympathy disorder) and schizophrenia (empathy disorder).

The concept of empathy is evoked so often that researchers often forget to define and analyze it. Some researchers with philosophical background point out that empathy is actually a phenomenon that is very difficult to delimit, and when closely examined, complicated to define (Stein 1989; Scheler 2008; Zahavi 2005, 2011). The most widely accepted definition can be summarized in this way: it is the psychological mechanism whereby an individual manages to intuitively represent another person's emotional experience or suffering. In this definition, the concept of empathy does not consider the subject's response to this representation. It is therefore a "representational ability" that allows for "understanding of others." It can be differentiated from sympathy, the object of which is other people's well-being (Scheler 2008; De Waal 2008; van der Weele 2011). Empathy is related to intuitive, implicit understanding and knowledge. Sympathy involves compassion and attention to others' well-being.

Empathetic knowledge is not "intellectual." Rather, it is a kind of intuitive, implicit knowledge that arises immediately when we meet another person. This is a primary form of intersubjectivity based on bodily expression and intercorporeality. This "implicit empathy" underlies social exchanges (Stanghellini 2004; Englebert 2013). In addition to this *pre-reflexive* tendency, psychopathologists develop a method of understanding other people's experiences. This "conative empathy" is a *reflexive* and *explicit* practice used to promote the development of intersubjectivity between the clinician and the patient. We can distinguish between two "kinds" of empathy: the clinician's (conative and explicit) and the patient's (implicit).

The investigation of implicit empathy needs to go into more depth in the case of psychopathy. A disorder affecting empathy (considered as the faculty of representing other people's experiences at the emotional, sentimental, or cognitive level) leads to a diagnosis of schizophrenia, rather than psychopathy. From this point of view, we must formally reconsider the hypothesis that psychopaths are affected by an empathy deficiency. On the other hand, it seems very possible that they have a "sympathy disorder." A psychopath has no difficulty identifying other people's feelings and experiences (unlike a person with schizophrenia), but he finds them completely irrelevant, as is other people's well-being. The analysis of other people and their experiences is strictly utilitarian and is unrelated to concern for or attention to their well-being. For example, a psychopath can describe his victims' suffering (showing evidence of empathy) but can coldly explain that they are of no importance to him (he feels no sympathy). Generally, psychopaths know that other people are bundles of emotions but they never "lose themselves" in this affective experience. A psychopathic rapist said about his victims: "What do you want me to say? That won't change anything for them. Maybe it did hurt them, but how do you expect that to change things for me? . . . What I think now won't change anything about their situations or mine"; "I can well understand when other people want to express their feelings but it's got nothing to do with me. What other people feel isn't important to me" [Source: own clinical experience]. This sympathy disorder, which takes the form of being able to imagine other people's emotional experiences without being affected by them, may obviously overlap with the emotional coldness discussed above.

This new way of considering psychopathic affectivity has an impact on clinical practice but also on the field of research (Englebert 2015). The relationship the psychopath has with emotions should not be considered a mere deficit but, from a certain point of view, an individualistic adaptive advantage. Discrimination between empathy (psychopathic competence) and sympathy (not a psychopathic skill) points out some weaknesses in diagnostic tools such as scale Hare (Hare 2003), but also, for example, allows to reconsider an expanding field of study such as the dimensions of Callous-unemotional traits in individuals at risk of developing a psychopathic personality, especially among adolescents (Bird and Viding 2014; Frick et al. 2014; Henry et al. 2016; Muratori et al. 2016). The proposals developed in this article may suggest that the unemotional intrinsic dimension should be discussed again through a complex consideration and take into account the discrimination between emotional understanding of others (empathy) and emotional response to them (sympathy).

Conclusion

The purpose of this article was to examine psychopathy and the classical approaches to evaluating it through the lens of phenomenological psychopathology. Despite some behavioral similarities, the psychopathological analysis allowed us to distinguish between mania and psychopathy, to restore to psychopathy the emotional competence it had been considered not to have, and to differentiate between empathy and sympathy. The adaptive qualities that have been preserved, consistently with the mastery of empathy, do not preclude a moral disorder via the loss of sympathy for other people. Finally, this phenomenological study enabled us to identify a fundamental structural characteristic of psychopathy, namely the ability to reify other people and to keep one's own ego intact.

The tools of phenomenological psychopathology gave us the means to identify the structuring and characteristic elements of psychopathic functioning and to point out the shortcomings of contemporary nosographies and theories related to this specific entity. Resorting to structural-phenomenological methods proved essential for not reducing this condition to a mere maladaptation or to an (emotional) deficit, and to try to understand the *being-in-the-world* of these particular patients.

Bibliography

Abu-Akel A., Heinke D., Gillespie S. M., Mitchell I. J., and Bo S. (2015). "Metacognitive Impairments in Schizophrenia are Arrested at Extreme Levels of Psychopathy: The Cut-off Effect." *Journal of Abnormal Psychology* 124(4): 1102–1109.

Berninger A. (2017). "Temporal Experience, Emotions and Decision Making in Psychopathy." *Phenomenology and the Cognitive Sciences* 16(4): 661–677.

Binswanger L. (1960). *Melancholie und manie. Phänomenologische studien*. Pfullingen: Günther Neske.

Binswanger L. (1963). *Being-in-the-World*. New York: Basic Books.

Bird G. and Viding E. (2014). "The Self to Other Model of Empathy: Providing a New Framework for Understanding Empathy Impairments in Psychopathy, Autism, and Alexithymia." *Neuroscience & Biobehavioral Reviews* 47: 520–532.

Brook M., Brieman C. L., and Kosson D. S. (2013). "Emotion Processing in Psychopathy Checklist—Assessed Psychopathy: A Review of the Literature." *Clinical Psychology Review* 33(8): 979–995.

Broome M. R., Harland R., and Owen G. S. (2013). *The Maudsley Reader in Phenomenological Psychiatry*. Cambridge: Cambridge University Press.

Brüne M. (2008). *Textbook of Evolutionary Psychiatry: The Origins of Psychopathology*. Oxford: Oxford University Press.

Casey H., Rogers R. D., Burns T., and Yiend J. (2013). "Emotion Regulation in Psychopathy." *Biological Psychology* 92(3): 541–548.

Cleckley H. (1941). *The Mask of Sanity*. St. Louis: Mosby.

Cooke D. J. and Michie C. (2001). "Refining the Construct of Psychopathy: Towards a Hierarchical Model." *Psychological assessment* 13(2): 171–188.

Cooke D. J., Michie C., Hart S. D., and Clark D. (2004). "Reconstructing Psychopathy: Clarifying the Significance of Antisocial and Socially Deviant Behavior in the Diagnosis of Psychopathic Personality Disorder." *Journal of Personality Disorders* 18(4): 337–357.

Cooke D. J., Michie C., and Skeem J. (2007). "Understanding the Structure of the PCL-R: An Exploration of Methodological Confusion." *British Journal of Psychiatry* 49(s): 39–50.

Cooke D. J., Hart S. D., Logan C., and Michie C. (2012). "Explicating the Construct of Psychopathy: Development and Validation of a Conceptual Model, the Comprehensive Assessment of Psychopathic Personality (CAPP). *International Journal of Forensic Mental Health* 11(4): 242–252.

Cutting J. (2012). *A Critique of Psychopathology*. Berlin: Parados.

De Block A. and Adriaens P. R. (2011). "Why Philosophers of Psychiatry Should Care about Evolutionary Theory." In P. R. Adriaens and A. De Block (eds.), *Maladapting Minds: Philosophy, Psychiatry, and Evolutionary Theory*, pp. 1–32. Oxford: Oxford University Press.

De Waal F. B. (2008). "Putting the Altruism Back into Altruism: The Evolution of Empathy. *Annual Review of Psychology* 59: 279–300.

Decety J., Chen C., Harenski C., and Kiehl K. A. (2013). "An fMRI Study of Affective Perspective Taking in Individuals with Psychopathy: Imagining Another in Pain Does Not Evoke Empathy." *Frontiers in Human Neuroscience* 7(489): 1–12.

Demaret A. (2014). *Éthologie et psychiatrie*. J. Englebert and V. Follet (eds.) 2nd edn., pp. 1–164. Bruxelles, Belgium: Mardaga.

Englebert J. (2013). *Psychopathologie de l'homme en situation*. Paris: Hermann.

Englebert J. (2013b). "Some Evidence for a Psychopathological Consideration on Psychopathy." *Annales Médico-Psychologiques* 171(3): 141–153.

Englebert J. (2015). "A New Understanding of Psychopathy: The Contribution of Phenomenological Psychopathology." *Psychopathology* 48(6): 368–375.

Frick P. J., Ray J. V., Thornton L. C., and Kahn, R. E. (2014). "Can Callous-unemotional Traits Enhance the Understanding, Diagnosis, and Treatment of Serious Conduct Problems in Children and Adolescents? A Comprehensive Review. *Psychological Bulletin* 140(1): 1–57.

Fuchs T. (2013). "The Phenomenology of Affectivity." In K. W. M. Fulford, M. Davies, R. G. T. Gipps, G. Graham, J. Z. Sadler, G. Stanghellini, and T. Thornton (eds.), *The Oxford Handbook of Philosophy and Psychiatry*, pp. 612–631. Oxford: Oxford University Press.

Glover J. (2014). *Alien Landscapes?: Interpreting Disordered Minds*. Harvard: Harvard University Press.

González R. A., Igoumenou A., Kallis C., and Coid J. W. (2016). "Borderline Personality Disorder and Violence in the UK Population: Categorical and Dimensional Trait Assessment." *BMC Psychiatry* 16: 180.

Hare R. D. (1999). *Without Conscience: The Disturbing World of the Psychopaths among Us*. Guilford Press.

Hare R. D. (2003). *The Hare Psychopathy Checklist—Revised Manual*, 2nd edn. Toronto: Multi-Health Systems.

Hare R. D., Hart S. D., and Harpur, T. J. (1991). "Psychopathy and the DSM-IV Criteria for Antisocial Personality Disorder." *Journal of Abnormal Psychology* 100(3): 391–398.

Henry J., Pingault J. B., Boivin M., Rijsdijk F., and Viding E. (2016). "Genetic and Environmental Aetiology of the Dimensions of Callous-Unemotional Traits." *Psychological Medicine* 46(2): 405–414.

Husserl E. [1931] (1960). *Cartesian Meditations*. London: Martinus Nijhoff Publishers.

Jaspers K. (1913). *General Psychopathology*, 7th edn. Baltimore: Johns Hopkins University Press.

Kiehl K. A. and Sinnott-Armstrong W. P. (2013). *Handbook on Psychopathy and Law*. Oxford: Oxford University Press.

Levy N. (2014). "Psychopaths and Blame: The Argument from Content." *Philosophical Psychology* 27(3): 351–367.

Lilienfeld S. O. and Widows M. R. (2005). *PPI-R: Psychopathic Personality Inventory Revised: Professional Manual*. Lutz, FL: Psychological Assessment Resources, Incorporated.

Maes J. H. R. and Brazil I. A. (2013). "No Clear Evidence for a Positive Association between the Interpersonal-affective Aspects of Psychopathy and Executive Functioning." *Psychiatry Research* 210(3): 1265–1274.

McGuire M. T. and Troisi A. (1998). *Darwinian Psychiatry*. Oxford: Oxford University Press.

McIlwain D. (2010). "Living Strangely in Time: Emotions, Masks and Morals in Psychopathically Inclined People." *European Journal of Analytic Philosophy* 6(1): 75–94.

Minkowski E. [1927] (2002). *La schizophrénie*. Paris: Payot.

Minkowski E. [1966] (1999). *Traité de psychopathologie*. Paris: Les empêcheurs de penser en rond.

Muratori P., Lochman J. E., Manfredi A., Milone A., Nocentini A., Pisano S., and Masi G. (2016). "Callous Unemotional Traits in Children with Disruptive Behavior Disorder: Predictors of Developmental Trajectories and Adolescent Outcomes." *Psychiatry Research* 236: 35–41.

Neumann C. S. and Pardini D. (2014). "Factor Structure and Construct Validity of the Self-Report Psychopathy (SRP) Scale and the Youth Psychopathic Inventory (YPI) in Young Men." *Journal of Personality Disorders* 28(3): 419–433.

Nordgaard J., Sass L. A., and Parnas J. (2013). "The Psychiatric Interview: Validity, Structure, and Subjectivity." *European Archives of Psychiatry and Clinical Neuroscience* 263(4): 353–364.

Parnas J., Bovet P., and Zahavi D. (2002). "Schizophrenic Autism: Clinical Phenomenology and Pathogenetic Implications." *World Psychiatry* 1(3): 131–136.

Patrick C. J. (2006). "Back to the Future: Cleckley as a Guide to the Next Generation of Psychopathy Research." In C. J. Patrick (ed.), *Handbook of Psychopathy*, pp. 605–617. New York: Guilford.

Patrick C. J., Fowles D. C., and Krueger R. F. (2009). "Triarchic Conceptualization of Psychopathy: Developmental Origins of Disinhibition, Boldness, and Meanness." *Development and Psychopathology* 21(3): 913–938.

Paulhus D. L., Neumann C. S., and Hare R. D. (2015). *Manual for the Self-Report Psychopathy Scale*, 4th edn. Toronto: Multi-Health Systems.

Pinel P. (1800). *Traité médico-philosophique sur l'aliénation mentale ou la manie*. Paris: Caille et Ravier.

Poythress N. G. and Hall J. R. (2011). "Psychopathy and Impulsivity Reconsidered." *Aggression and Violent Behavior* 16(2): 120–134.

Sartre J.-P. (1939). *Esquisse d'une théorie des émotions*. Paris: Hermann.

Sass L. A. (2014). "Self-disturbance and Schizophrenia: Structure, Specificity, Pathogenesis." (Current issues, New directions). *Schizophrenia Research* 152(1): 5–11.

Scheler M. (2008). *The Nature of Sympathy*. New Jersey: Transaction Publishers.

Schneider K. [1923] (1950). *Psychopathic Personalities*. London: Cassell.

Skeem J. L., Polaschek D. L. L., Patrick C. J., and Lilienfeld S. O. (2011). Psychopathic Personality: Bridging the Gap between Scientific Evidence and Public Policy." *Psychological Science in the Public Interest* 12(3): 95–162.

Stanghellini G. (2004). *Disembodied Spirits and Deanimated Bodies: The Psychopathology of Common Sense*. Oxford: Oxford University Press.

Stanghellini G. (2009). "The Meanings of Psychopathology." *Current Opinion in Psychiatry* 22(6): 559–564.

Stein E. (1989). *On the Problem of Empathy*, Vol. 3. Washington: ICS Publications.

Stevens A. and Price J. (2000). *Evolutionary Psychiatry: A New Beginning*, 2nd edn. London: Routledge.

Szilasi W. (1959). *Einfuhrung in die Phaenomenologie Edmund Husserls*. Tubingen: Niemeyer.

Uzieblo K., Verschuere B., Van den Bussche E., and Crombez G. (2010). "The Validity of the Psychopathic Personality Inventory—Revised in a Community Sample." *Assessment* 17(3): 334–346.

van der Weele C. (2011). "Empathy's Purity, Sympathy's Complexities: De Waal, Darwin and Adam Smith." *Biology & philosophy* 26(4): 583–593.

Vitacco M. J. (2007). "Psychopathy." *British Journal of Psychiatry* 191(s): 357–358.

Zahavi D. (2005). *Subjectivity and Selfhood: Investigating the First-person Perspective*. London: MIT Press.

Zahavi D. (2011). "Empathy and Direct Social Perception: A Phenomenological Proposal." *Review of Philosophy and Psychology* 2(3): 541–558.

....

CHAPTER 84

A PHENOMENOLOGICAL-CONTEXTUAL, EXISTENTIAL, AND ETHICAL PERSPECTIVE ON EMOTIONAL TRAUMA

ROBERT D. STOLOROW

PHENOMENOLOGICAL CONTEXTUALISM

BEFORE I turn to trauma proper, I offer a very brief overview of the theoretical lens through which I have sought to grasp its essential features over the course of some three decades. Intersubjective-systems theory, the name of my collaborators' and my (Stolorow, Atwood, and Orange 2002) psychoanalytic perspective, is a phenomenological contextualism. It is phenomenological in that it investigates and illuminates worlds of emotional experience and the structures that organize them. It is contextual in that it holds that such structures take form, both developmentally and in the therapeutic situation, in constitutive relational or intersubjective contexts. Recurring patterns of intersubjective transaction within the developmental system give rise to principles (thematic patterns, meaning-structures, cognitive-affective schemas) that unconsciously organize subsequent emotional and relational experiences. Such organizing principles are unconscious, not in the sense of being repressed, but in being pre-reflective; they ordinarily do not enter the domain of reflective self-awareness. These intersubjectively derived, pre-reflective organizing principles are the basic building blocks of personality development, and their totality constitutes one's character. Psychoanalytic therapy is a dialogical method for bringing this pre-reflective organizing activity into reflective self-awareness, particularly as it shows up within the therapeutic relationship.

TRAUMA'S CONTEXT-EMBEDDEDNESS

Early contexts of emotional trauma are a particularly important source of pre-reflective organizing principles. Nowhere is the context dependence of emotional life more vividly exemplified than in the phenomenon of emotional trauma. The explication of trauma's context dependence was foreshadowed in a sentence that my late wife Daphne (Dede) composed in our early joint article (Socarides and Stolorow 1984/1985): "The tendency for [painful] affective experiences to create a disorganized (i.e. traumatic) self-state is seen to originate from . . . faulty [affect] attunement, with a lack of mutual sharing and acceptance of affect states" (110). However, it was not until the aftermath of Dede's death in February 1991, when I experienced first-hand what I later came to call the unbearable embeddedness of being (Stolorow and Atwood 1992), that I turned my attention to trauma's context-embeddedness. The result was my chapter on emotional trauma in *Contexts of Being* (Stolorow and Atwood 1992), the book that George Atwood and I outlined the summer after Dede died.

I claimed in that chapter that emotional trauma is an experience of unendurable emotional pain and, further, that the unbearability of emotional suffering cannot be explained solely, or even primarily, on the basis of the intensity of the painful feelings evoked by an injurious event. Painful emotional states become unbearable when they cannot find a context of emotional understanding—what I came to call a relational home—in which they can be shared and held. Severe emotional pain that has to be experienced alone becomes lastingly traumatic and usually succumbs to some form of emotional numbing. In contrast, painful feelings that are held in a context of human understanding can gradually become more bearable.

Drawing on the work of Balint (1969), Ferenczi (1933), Kohut (1971), Krystal (1988), and Winnicott (1975), I contended that developmental trauma, in particular, must not be viewed as an instinctual flooding of an ill-equipped mental apparatus, as Freud (1926) would have it. Rather, developmental trauma was grasped as originating within a formative intersubjective context whose central feature is malattunement to painful affect—a breakdown of the child–caregiver inter-affective system, leading to the child's loss of affect-integrating capacity and thereby to an unbearable, overwhelmed, disorganized state. Painful or frightening affect becomes traumatic when the attunement that the child needs to assist in his or her tolerance and integration is profoundly absent. Such claims hold, pari passu, for adult-onset trauma as well (e.g. see Carr 2011). Finding a relational home for the pain of a traumatic loss may be particularly difficult. When Dede died, the person whom I would have longed to share in and hold my overwhelming grief was of course the very same person who was gone.

From the claim that developmental trauma is constituted in an intersubjective context wherein severe emotional pain cannot find a relational home in which it can be held, it follows that injurious childhood experiences in and of themselves need not be traumatic (or at least not lastingly so) or pathogenic, provided that they occur within a responsive milieu. Pain is not pathology. It is the absence of adequate attunement to the child's painful emotional reactions that renders them unendurable and thus a source of traumatic states and psychopathology. This conceptualization holds both for discrete, dramatic traumatic events and the more subtle "cumulative traumas" (Khan 1963) that occur continually throughout childhood.

One consequence of developmental trauma, relationally conceived, is that affect states take on enduring, crushing meanings (pre-reflective organizing activity). From recurring experiences of malattunement, the child acquires the unconscious conviction that unmet developmental yearnings and reactive painful feeling states are manifestations of a loathsome defect or of an inherent inner badness. A defensive self-ideal is often established, representing a self-image purified of the offending affect states that were perceived to be unwelcome or damaging to caregivers. Living up to this affectively purified ideal becomes a central requirement for maintaining harmonious ties to others and for upholding self-esteem. Thereafter, the emergence of prohibited affect is experienced as a failure to embody the required ideal, an exposure of the underlying essential defectiveness or badness, and is accompanied by feelings of isolation, shame, and self-loathing. In psychoanalytic therapy, qualities or activities of the therapist that lend themselves to being interpreted according to such unconscious meanings of affect confirm the patient's expectations that emerging feeling states will be met with disgust, disdain, disinterest, alarm, hostility, withdrawal, exploitation, and the like, or will damage the therapist and destroy the therapeutic bond. Such transference expectations, unwittingly confirmed by the therapist, are a powerful source of resistance to the experience and articulation of affect. Intractable repetitive transferences and resistances can be grasped, from this perspective, as rigidly stable states of the patient–therapist system, in which the meanings of the therapist's stance have become tightly coordinated with the patient's grim expectations and fears, thereby exposing the patient repeatedly to threats of retraumatization. The focus on affect and its meanings contextualizes both transference and resistance, and it is essential for the progress of therapy that such expectations and fears be carefully and repeatedly investigated.

A second consequence of developmental trauma is a severe constriction and narrowing of the horizons of emotional experiencing (Stolorow, Atwood, and Orange 2002: chapter 3), so as to exclude whatever feels unacceptable, intolerable, or too dangerous in particular intersubjective contexts. When a child's emotional experiences are consistently not responded to or are actively rejected, the child perceives that aspects of his or her affective life are intolerable to the caregiver. These regions of the child's emotional world must then be sacrificed in order to safeguard the needed tie. Repression was grasped here as a kind of negative organizing principle, always embedded in ongoing intersubjective contexts, determining which configurations of affective experience are not to be allowed to come into full being. For example, when the act of linguistically articulating an affective experience is perceived to threaten an indispensable tie, repression can be achieved by preventing the continuation of the process of encoding that experience in language. In such instances, repression keeps affect nameless.

Clinical Vignette

The following clinical vignette (a fictionalized composite) illustrates many of the ideas developed in this section.

A young woman who had been repeatedly sexually abused by her father when she was a child began therapy with a female trainee whom I was supervising. Early in the treatment, whenever the patient began to remember and describe the sexual abuse, or to recount analogously invasive experiences in her current life, she would display emotional reactions that consisted of two distinctive parts, both of which seemed entirely bodily. One was a trembling in her arms and upper torso, which sometimes escalated into violent shaking. The other was an intense flushing of her face. On these occasions, my supervisee was quite alarmed by her patient's shaking and was concerned to find some way to calm her.

I had a hunch that the shaking was a bodily manifestation of a traumatized state and that the flushing was a somatic form of the patient's shame about exposing this state to her therapist, and I suggested to my supervisee that she focus her inquiries on the flushing rather than the shaking. As a result of this shift in focus, the patient began to speak about how she believed her therapist viewed her when she was trembling or shaking: Surely her analyst must be regarding her with disdain, seeing her as a damaged mess of a human being. As this belief was repeatedly disconfirmed by her therapist's responding with attunement and understanding rather than contempt, both the flushing and the shaking diminished in intensity. The traumatized states actually underwent a process of transformation from being exclusively bodily states into ones in which the bodily sensations came to be united with words. Instead of only shaking, the patient began to speak about her terror of annihilating intrusion.

The one and only time the patient had attempted to speak to her mother about the sexual abuse, her mother shamed her severely, declaring her to be a wicked little girl for making up such lies about her father. Thereafter, the patient did not tell any other human being about her trauma until she revealed it to her therapist, and both the flushing of her face and the restriction of her experience of terror to its nameless bodily component were heir to her mother's shaming. Only with a shift in her perception of her therapist from one in which her therapist was potentially or secretly shaming to one in which she was accepting and understanding could the patient's emotional experience of her traumatized states shift from an exclusively bodily form to an experience that could be felt and named as terror. Through such naming within the therapeutic context, the painful states gradually became more bearable.

THE PHENOMENOLOGY OF TRAUMA

I turn now to a phenomenological description of traumatized states, as I myself have experienced them. When the book *Contexts of Being* (Stolorow and Atwood 1992) was first published, an initial batch of copies was sent "hot-off-the-press" to the display table at a conference where I was a panelist. I picked up a copy and looked around excitedly for my late wife, Dede, who would be so pleased and happy to see it. She was, of course, nowhere to be found, having died some twenty months earlier. I had awakened the morning of February 23, 1991, to find her lying dead across our bed, four weeks after her metastatic cancer had been diagnosed. Spinning around to show her my book and finding her gone instantly transported me back to that devastating moment in which I woke up and found her dead, and my world shattered. I was once again consumed with horror and sorrow.[1]

There was a dinner at that conference for all the panelists, many of whom were my old and good friends and close colleagues. Yet as I looked around the ballroom, they all seemed like strange and alien beings to me. Or more accurately, I seemed like a strange and alien being—not of this world. The others seemed so vitalized, engaged with one another in a lively manner. I, in contrast, felt deadened and broken, a shell of the man I had once been. An

---

[1] Borrowing a term from the Harry Potter book series (Rowling 2000), I call such experiences portkeys to trauma (Stolorow 2007, 2011), as discussed later in this article.

unbridgeable gulf seemed to open up, separating me forever from my friends and colleagues. They could never even begin to fathom my experience, I thought to myself, because we now lived in altogether different worlds.

Over the course of six years following that painful occasion, I tried to understand and conceptualize the dreadful sense of estrangement and isolation that seems to me to be inherent to the experience of emotional trauma. I became aware that this sense of alienation and aloneness appears as a common theme in the trauma literature (e.g. Herman 1992), and I was able to hear about it from many of my patients who had experienced severe traumatization. One such young man, who had suffered multiple losses of beloved family members during his childhood and adulthood, told me that the world was divided into two group: the normals and the traumatized ones. There was no possibility, he said, for a normal ever to grasp the experience of a traumatized one.

In 1998 I found an explanation for this estrangement in what I called the absolutisms of everyday life and presented my account in a brief article (Stolorow 1999): When a person says to a friend, "I'll see you later," or a parent says to a child at bedtime, "I'll see you in the morning," these are statements, like delusions, whose validity is not open for discussion. Such absolutisms are the basis for a kind of naive realism and optimism that allow one to function in the world, experienced as stable and predictable. It is in the essence of emotional trauma that it shatters these absolutisms, a catastrophic loss of innocence that permanently alters one's sense of being-in-the-world. Massive deconstruction of the absolutisms of everyday life exposes the inescapable contingency of existence on a universe that is random and unpredictable and in which no safety or continuity of being can be assured. Trauma thereby exposes "the unbearable embeddedness of being" (Stolorow and Atwood 1992: 22). As a result, the traumatized person cannot help but perceive aspects of existence that lie well outside the absolutized horizons of normal everydayness. It is in this sense that the worlds of traumatized persons are felt to be fundamentally incommensurable with those of others, the deep chasm in which an anguished sense of estrangement and solitude takes form (Stolorow and Atwood 1992: 467).

Trauma's Existential Significance

Once George Atwood and I, in the mid-1970s, had embarked upon our project of rethinking psychoanalysis as a form of phenomenological inquiry,[2] a focus on the mutually enriching interface of psychoanalysis and continental phenomenology became inescapable, and I began studying phenomenological philosophy, sometimes voraciously. In 2000, I formed a leaderless philosophical study group in which we devoted a year to a close reading of Heidegger's (1927) magnum opus, *Being and Time*. When I read the passages therein devoted to his existential analysis of Angst, I nearly fell off my chair! Both Heidegger's phenomenological description and ontological account of Angst bore a remarkable resemblance to what I had written about the phenomenology and meaning of emotional trauma two years earlier.

---

[2] An account of the historical evolution of this four-decades long collaborative project can be found in chapter 6 of *Structures of Subjectivity: Explorations in Psychoanalytic Phenomenology and Contextualism*, 2nd edn. (Atwood and Stolorow 2014).

Thus, Heidegger's existential philosophy—in particular, his existential analysis of Angst—provided me with extraordinary philosophical tools for grasping the existential significance of emotional trauma. It was this latter discovery that motivated me to begin doctoral studies in philosophy and to write a dissertation and two books (Stolorow 2007, 2011) on Heidegger, trauma, and what I came to call post-Cartesian psychoanalysis.

Like Freud (1926), Heidegger made a sharp distinction between fear and anxiety. Whereas, according to Heidegger (1927), that in the face of which one fears is a definite "entity within-the-world" (231), that in the face of which one is anxious is "completely indefinite" (231) and turns out to be "Being-in-the-world as such" (230). The indefiniteness of anxiety "tells us that entities within-the-world are not 'relevant' at all . . . [The world] collapses into itself [and] has the character of completely lacking significance" (231). Heidegger made clear that it is the significance of the average everyday world, the world as constituted by the public interpretedness of the "they" (*das Man*), whose collapse is disclosed in anxiety. Furthermore, insofar as the "utter insignificance" (231) of the everyday world is disclosed in anxiety, anxiety includes a feeling of uncanniness, in the sense of "not being-at-home" (233). In anxiety, the experience of "Being-at-home [in one's tranquilized] everyday familiarity" (233) with the publicly interpreted world collapses, and "Being-in enters into the existential 'mode' of . . . 'uncanniness'" (233).[3]

In Heidegger's (1927) ontological account of anxiety, the central features of its phenomenology—the collapse of everyday significance and the resulting feeling of uncanniness—are claimed to be grounded in what he called authentic (non-evasively owned) Being-toward-death. Existentially, death is not simply an event that has not yet occurred or that happens to others, as *das Man* would have it. Rather, it is a distinctive possibility that is constitutive of our existence—of our intelligibility to ourselves in our futurity and our finitude. It is "the possibility of the impossibility of any existence at all" (307), which, because it is both certain and indefinite as to its when, always impends as a constant threat, robbing us of the tranquilizing illusions that characterize our absorption in the everyday world, nullifying its significance for us. The appearance of anxiety indicates that the fundamental defensive purpose (fleeing) of average everydayness has failed and that authentic Being-toward-death has broken through the evasions that conceal it. Torn from the sheltering illusions of *das Man*, we feel uncanny—no longer safely at home.

I have contended that emotional trauma produces an affective state whose features bear a close similarity to the central elements in Heidegger's existential interpretation of anxiety and that it accomplishes this by plunging the traumatized person into a form of authentic Being-toward-death (Stolorow 2007, 2011). Trauma shatters the illusions of everyday life that evade and cover up the finitude, contingency, and embeddedness of our existence and the indefiniteness of its certain extinction. Such shattering exposes what had been heretofore concealed, thereby plunging the traumatized person into a form of authentic Being-toward-death and into the anxiety—the loss of significance, the uncanniness—through which authentic Being-toward-death is disclosed. Trauma, like death, individualizes us, in a manner that invariably manifests in an excruciating sense of singularity and solitude.

[3] Compare to the description of my traumatized state in the second paragraph of the preceding section, "The Phenomenology of Trauma."

The particular form of authentic Being-toward-death that crystallized in the wake of the trauma of Dede's death I characterize as a Being-toward-loss. Loss of loved ones constantly impends for me as a certain, indefinite, and ever-present possibility, in terms of which I now always understand myself and my world. My own experience of traumatic loss and its aftermath was a source of motivation for my efforts to relationalize Heidegger's conception of finitude by claiming that authentic Being-toward-death always entails owning up, not only to one's own finitude, but also to the finitude of all those we love. Hence, authentic Being-toward-death always includes Being-toward-loss as a central constituent. Just as, existentially, we are "always dying already" (Heidegger 1927: 298), so too are we always already grieving. Death and loss are existentially equiprimordial. Existential anxiety anticipates both death and loss.

Support for my claim about the equiprimordiality of death and loss can be found in the work of Derrida, who contended that every friendship is structured from its beginning, a priori, by the possibility that one of the two friends will die first and that the surviving friend will be left to mourn: "To have a friend, to look at him, to follow him with your eyes, . . . is to know in a more intense way, already injured, . . . that one of the two of you will inevitably see the other die" (Derrida 2001: 107). Finitude and the possibility of mourning are constitutive of every friendship.

DISSOCIATION, FINITUDE, AND TRAUMATIC TEMPORALITY

In the course of my investigations of the phenomenology and existential meaning of emotional trauma, I have conceptualized dissociation as the keeping apart of incommensurable emotional worlds, and I have rethought the phenomenon of dissociation in terms of the devastating impact of emotional trauma on our experience of temporality.[4] Dissociation, I contend, is traumatic temporality, and traumatic temporality is the condition for the possibility of the defensive use of dissociation.

A patient of mine (discussed in Stolorow 2007) with a long, painful history of traumatic violations, shocks, and losses arrived at her session in a profoundly fragmented state. Shortly before, she had seen her psychopharmacologist for a twenty-minute interview. In an apparent attempt to update her files, this psychiatrist had required the patient to recount her entire history of traumatization, with no attention given to the emotional impact of this recounting. The patient explained to me that with the retelling of each traumatic episode, a piece of herself broke off and relocated at the time and place of the original trauma. By the time she reached my office, she said, she was completely dispersed along the time dimension of her crushing life-history. Upon hearing this, I spoke just three words: "Trauma destroys time." The patient's eyes grew wide; she smiled and said, "I just came together again."

---

[4] By temporality I mean the lived experience of time.

I use the term portkey, which I borrowed from the Harry Potter book series (Rowling 2000), to capture the profound impact of emotional trauma on our experience of time. Harry was a severely traumatized little boy, nearly killed by his parents' murderer and left in the care of a family that mistreated him cruelly. He arose from the ashes of devastating trauma as a wizard in possession of wondrous magical powers, and yet never free from the original trauma, always under threat by his parents' murderer. As a wizard, he encountered portkeys—objects that transported him instantly to other places, obliterating the duration ordinarily required for travel from one location to another.[5] Portkeys to trauma return one again and again to an experience of traumatization.[6] As shown dramatically in the foregoing paragraph, the experience of such portkeys fractures, and can even obliterate, one's sense of unitary selfhood, of being-in-time.

Trauma devastatingly disrupts the ordinary, average-everyday linearity and "ecstatical unity of temporality" (Heidegger 1927: 416), the sense of "stretching-along" (426) from the past to an open future. Experiences of emotional trauma become freeze-framed into an eternal present in which one remains forever trapped, or to which one is condemned to be perpetually returned through the portkeys supplied by life's slings and arrows. In the region of trauma all duration or stretching along collapses, past becomes present, and future loses all meaning other than endless repetition. In this sense it is trauma, not, as Freud (1915) would have it, the unconscious that is timeless.

Because trauma so profoundly modifies the universal or shared structure of temporality, the traumatized person quite literally lives in another kind of reality, an experiential world felt to be incommensurable with those of others. This felt incommensurability, in turn, contributes to the sense of alienation and estrangement from other human beings that typically haunts the traumatized person. Torn from the communal fabric of being-in-time, trauma remains insulated from human dialogue.

The endless recurrence of emotional trauma is ensured by the finitude of our existence and the finitude of all those with whom we are deeply connected. Authentic temporality, insofar as it owns up to human finitude, is traumatic temporality. "Trauma recovery" is an oxymoron—human finitude with its traumatizing impact is not an illness from which one can recover. "Recovery" is a misnomer for the constitution of an expanded emotional world that coexists alongside the absence of the one that has been shattered by trauma. The expanded world and the absent shattered world may be more or less integrated or dissociated, depending on the degree to which the unbearable emotional pain evoked by the traumatic shattering has become integrated or remains dissociated defensively, which depends in turn on the extent to which such pain found a relational home[7] in which it could be held. This is the essential fracturing at the heart of traumatic temporality. Dissociation just is traumatic temporality.

---

[5] My wife, Dr. Julia Schwartz, first brought this imagery of portkeys to my attention as a metaphor that captures the impact of trauma on the experience of temporality.

[6] See the first paragraph of the section, "The Phenomenology of Trauma" for a vivid personal example of such a portkey.

[7] In authentic existing, such a relational home is also itself recognized as finite.

Therapeutic Implications: Emotional Dwelling

How can a therapeutic relationship be constituted wherein the therapist can serve as a relational home for unbearable emotional pain and existential vulnerability? Recently (Stolorow 2014), I have been moving toward a more active, relationally engaged form of therapeutic comportment that I call emotional dwelling. In dwelling, one does not merely seek empathically to understand the other's emotional pain from the other's perspective. One does that, but much more. In dwelling, one leans into the other's emotional pain and participates in it, perhaps with aid of one's own analogous experiences of pain. I have found that this active, engaged, participatory comportment is especially important in the therapeutic approach to emotional trauma. The language that one uses to address another's experience of emotional trauma meets the trauma head-on, articulating the unbearable and the unendurable, saying the unsayable, unmitigated by any efforts to soothe, comfort, encourage, or reassure—such efforts invariably being experienced by the other as a shunning or turning away from his or her traumatized state.

Let me give an example of emotional dwelling and the sort of language it employs from my own personal life. In the immediate aftermath of my late wife Dede's death, my soul brother, George Atwood, was the only person among my friends and family members who was capable of dwelling with me in the magnitude of my emotional devastation. He said, in his inimitable way, "You are a destroyed human being. You are on a train to nowhere." George lost his mother when he was eight years old, and I think his dwelling in and integrating his own experience of traumatic loss enabled him to be an understanding home for mine. He knew that offering me encouraging platitudes would be a form of emotional distancing that would just create a wall between us.

If we are to be an understanding relational home for a traumatized person, we must tolerate, even draw upon, our own existential vulnerabilities so that we can dwell unflinchingly with his or her unbearable and recurring emotional pain. When we dwell with others' unendurable pain, their shattered emotional worlds are enabled to shine with a kind of sacredness that calls forth an understanding and caring engagement within which traumatized states can be gradually transformed into bearable and nameable painful feelings.

Concluding Remarks: Toward an Ethics of Finitude

What is it in our existential structure that makes the offering and the finding of a relational home for emotional trauma possible? I have contended (Stolorow 2007, 2011) that just as finitude and vulnerability to death and loss are fundamental to our existential constitution, so too is it constitutive of our existence that we meet each other as "brothers and sisters in the same dark night" (Vogel 1994: 97), deeply connected with one another in virtue of our common finitude. Thus, although the possibility of emotional trauma is ever present, so too is the possibility of forming bonds of deep emotional attunement within which devastating emotional pain can be held, rendered more tolerable, and, hopefully, eventually integrated. Our existential kinship-in-the-same-darkness is the condition for the possibility both of the profound contextuality of emotional trauma and of the mutative power of human understanding.

I suggest, as does Vogel (1994), that owning up to our existential kinship-in-finitude has significant ethical implications insofar as it motivates us, or even obligates us, to care about and for our brothers' and sisters' existential vulnerability and emotional pain. Imagine a society in which the obligation to provide a relational home for the emotional pain that is inherent to the traumatizing impact of our finitude has become a shared ethical principle. In such a society, human beings would be much more capable of living in their existential vulnerability, anxiety, and grief, rather than having to revert to the defensive, destructive evasions of them so lamentably characteristic of human history. In such a societal context, a new form of identity would become possible, based on owning rather than covering up our existential vulnerability. Vulnerability that finds a hospitable relational home could be seamlessly and constitutively integrated into whom we experience ourselves as being. A new form of human solidarity would also become possible, rooted not in shared grandiose and destructive ideological illusion, but in shared recognition and respect for our common human finitude. If we can help one another bear the darkness rather than evade it, perhaps one day we will be able to see the light—as finite human beings, finitely bonded to one another.

ACKNOWLEDGMENTS

This article was originally published as "A Phenomenological-Contextual, Existential, and Ethical Perspective on Emotional Trauma" by Robert D. Stolorow in *The Psychoanalytic Review* 102(1): 123–138, https://doi.org/10.1521/prev.2015.102.1.123
Copyright © 2015, Guilford Press.

BIBLIOGRAPHY

Atwood G. E. and Stolorow R. D. (2014). *Structures of Subjectivity: Explorations in Psychoanalytic Phenomenology and Contextualism*, 2nd edn. London: Routledge.

Balint, M. (1969). "Trauma and Object Relationship." *International Journal of Psycho-Analysis* 50: 429–435.

Carr R. B. (2011). "Combat and Human Existence: Toward an Intersubjective Approach to Combat Related PTSD." *Psychoanalytic Psychology* 28: 471–496.

Derrida J. (2001). *The Work of Mourning* P.-A. Brault and M. Naas (eds.) Chicago: University of Chicago Press.

Ferenczi S. (1933). "Confusion of Tongues between Adults and the Child." In *Final Contributions to the Problems and Methods of Psycho-analysis*, pp. 156–167. London: Hogarth Press.

Freud S. [1915] (1953–74). "The Unconscious." In J. Strachey (ed. and trans.), *The Standard Edition of the Complete Psychological Works of Sigmund Freud*, 24 vols, 14: 159–204. London: Hogarth Press.

Freud S. (1926). "Inhibitions, Symptoms and Anxiety." Standard ed., 20: 77–175.

Heidegger M. [1927] (1962). *Being and Time*, trans. J. Macquarrie and E. Robinson. New York: Harper & Row.

Herman J. (1992). *Trauma and Recovery*. New York: Basic Books.

Khan M. M. R. [1963] (1974). "The Concept of Cumulative Trauma." In *The Privacy of the Self*, pp. 42–58. Madison: International Universities Press.

Kohut H. (1971). *The Analysis of the Self*. Madison: International Universities Press.

Krystal H. (1988). *Integration and Self-healing: Affect, Trauma, Alexithymia*. Hillsdale: Analytic Press.

Rowling J. K. (2000). *Harry Potter and the Goblet of Fire*. New York: Scholastic Press.

Socarides D. D. and Stolorow R. D. (1984/1985). "Affects and Self Objects." *The Annual of Psychoanalysis* 12/13: 105–119.

Stolorow R. D. (1999). "The Phenomenology of Trauma and the Absolutisms of Everyday Life: A Personal Journey." *Psychoanalytic Psychology* 16: 464–468.

Stolorow R. D. (2007). *Trauma and Human Existence: Autobiographical, Psychoanalytic, and Philosophical Reflections*. New York: Routledge.

Stolorow R. D. (2011). *World, Affectivity, Trauma: Heidegger and Post-Cartesian Psychoanalysis*. New York: Routledge.

Stolorow R. D. (2014). "Undergoing the Situation: Emotional Dwelling is More Than Empathic Understanding." *International Journal of Psychoanalytic Self Psychology* 9(1): 80–83.

Stolorow R. D. and Atwood G. E. (1992). *Contexts of Being: The Intersubjective Foundations of Psychological Life*. Hillsdale: Analytic Press.

Stolorow R. D., Atwood G. E., and Orange D. M. (2002). *Worlds of Experience: Interweaving Philosophical and Clinical Dimensions in Psychoanalysis*. New York: Basic Books.

Vogel L. (1994). *The Fragile "We": Ethical Implications of Heidegger's Being and Time*. Evanston: Northwestern University Press.

Winnicott D. W. (1975). *Through Paediatrics to Psychoanalysis*. New York: Basic Books.

SECTION SEVEN

PHENOMENOLOGICAL PSYCHOPATHOLOGY

SECTION EDITORS: MATTHEW R. BROOME
AND PAOLO FUSAR-POLI

....

CHAPTER 85

PHENOMENOLOGICAL PSYCHOPATHOLOGY AND NEUROSCIENCE

....

GEORG NORTHOFF

Neither the 'brainless' psychiatry of the middle of the 20th century, nor the "mindless" variety of the past 30 years should be taken to represent the most we can achieve. The future should yield a synthesis.

(Panksepp 2004: 17)

INTRODUCTION

....

Methodological Gap between Experience and Brain

Psychopathology concerns the empirical and theoretical framework in which symptoms, behavior, and experiences in psychiatric patients can be described, categorized, and classified (Parnas, Sass, and Zahavi 2008; Parnas, Sass, and Zahavi 2013; Stanghellini 2009a; 2009b; Stanghellini and Broome 2014). Different empirical and theoretical frameworks have been suggested in past and present approaches to psychopathology, including cognitive psychopathology (David and Halligan 2000; Halligan and David 2001), affective psychopathology (Panksepp 2004), phenomenological psychopathology (Fuchs 2007; 2013; G. Northoff 2015b; Parnas et al. 2008; Parnas et al. 2013; Stanghellini 2009a; 2009b; Stanghellini and Broome 2014), clinical psychopathology (current classification systems like DSM-5 and ICD-10), and the recent Research Domain Operational Classification (RDoC) classification that entails behavioral and computational psychopathology (Cuthbert and Insel 2013).

Despite their virtues for single functions (like affective, cognitive, etc.), all these approaches suffer from a methodological gap between the brain, on the one hand, and experience and symptoms on the other. Neither approach shows why or how the symptoms and their experience are related to and based on the brain. This is not a problem specific to psychiatry though but holds for current neuroscience in general. We currently do not know how and why the neuronal activity of the brain generates or yields mental features like self and consciousness. This lack of knowledge reverberates particularly in psychiatry where the various psychopathological symptoms are essentially mental symptoms.

The different psychopathological approaches take either side of the gap, that is, mental or neuronal, as a starting point. For instance, phenomenological psychiatry takes experience or consciousness itself as starting point and focuses on exploring first-person experiences in detail (Parnas et al. 2008; Parnas, Sass, and Zahavi 2012; Stanghellini 2009a; 2009b). Specifically, the focus is on the first-person experience of time and space as well as body, self, and world. The brain, in contrast, nowhere surfaces in experience in particular, and phenomenology in general, since it cannot be accessed in experience in first-person perspective but only in observation as in third-person perspective. The brain is thus excluded in experience of the own self, body, and world including time and space in particular and phenomenology in general. Such exclusion of the brain in experience or consciousness occurs by default, for example, on methodological grounds, since the brain cannot be accessed in experience in first-person perspective.

The exclusion of the brain in experience raises the question for phenomenological psychopathology of how experience can be linked to the brain. This question becomes even more crucial given the fact that recent brain imaging shows the relationship of psychopathological symptoms to neural alterations in the brain. That leaves open though how the experience of those psychopathological symptoms and of self, world, and body including time and space can be related to the brain and its neural changes. In other words, phenomenological psychopathology needs to establish a bridge or link to the brain and thus from phenomenal to neural activity. How is that possible? One way is to search for a "common currency" that is shared by both, experience and brain, and, at the same time, underlies our experience of self, body, and world as well as our observation of neural activity changes in the brain. I suggest in this chapter that such "common currency" shared between experience and brain consists in time and space. Alterations in time and space may then be manifest in both abnormal experience of self, body, and world as well as abnormal neural activity changes in the brain. Psychopathological symptoms may then ultimately be traced to alterations in time and space hence my suggestions of what I describe as "spatiotemporal psychopathology." Considered in this way, spatiotemporal psychopathology can be considered an extension of phenomenological psychopathology from experience to the brain.

Very much like phenomenological psychopathology, biological psychiatry too is confronted with a gap, although this occurs from the opposite side. Biological psychiatry investigates the brain's neuronal states in all their molecular, genetic, cellular, regional, and network levels as they can methodologically be approached in third-person perspective. However, this leaves out experience and its first-person perspective. Experience is thus excluded on methodological grounds in biological psychiatry in the same way and as much as the brain is often (though not always) excluded in phenomenological psychiatry. The methodological gap between experience and brain is thus mutual, being fostered from both sides, brain and experience, for example, biological and phenomenological psychiatry.

How now can we bridge the gap from biological psychiatry to phenomenological psychopathology? For that we need to go back to what potentially underlies the observed neural activity changes in the brain which, as I will demonstrate below, can be found in the temporal and spatial organization of the brain's neural activity. There is recent empirical evidence that such temporal and spatial changes do indeed feature psychiatric disorders like depression and schizophrenia (see below). These alterations in time and space underlying the observed brain's neural activity may then provide the bridge to the abnormal experience of time and space that underlie the abnormal experience of self, body, and world as investigated in phenomenological psychopathology. Spatiotemporal psychopathology can consecutively be considered an extension of biological psychiatry from the brain toward experience in more or less the same way (though reversed direction) as it is an extension of phenomenological psychopathology from experience to the brain. In the following, I shall specify the exact positioning and characterization of spatiotemporal psychopathology as extension of both phenomenological psychopathology and biological psychiatry in methodological regards which will be followed by illustrating such approach by specific examples.

"Common Currency" Between Experience and Brain

How can we close the gap between experience and brain? Closing this gap is central for psychiatry since we need to understand the processes that transform abnormal neuronal into phenomenal states which psychiatric patients experience in first-person perspective. How can we apprehend these transformative processes, for example, neuronal-phenomenal transformation? For that we may want to search for a shared overlap or "common currency" between neuronal and phenomenal states that drives the transformation of the former into the latter.

The shared overlap or common currency between neuronal and phenomenal states, for example, brain and experience, may consist in spatiotemporal features. On the side of the brain, it is the spontaneous activity (rather than its stimulus-induced or task-evoked activity that may be central in providing or constituting such spatiotemporal structure (see below for details). The brain's spontaneous activity shows certain spatiotemporal features, a particular spatial and temporal structure in its neural activity that surfaces in and is transformed into phenomenal state, for example, experience (see (Northoff 2014a) for many examples). One would consequently expect a common, similar, or analogous spatiotemporal structure between the brain's spontaneous activity and the phenomenal features of experience.

Such common, similar, or analogous spatiotemporal structure between brain and experience amounts to what I describe as "spatiotemporal correspondence." The concept of spatiotemporal correspondence means that the brain's spontaneous activity and the phenomenal features of experience show corresponding or analogous spatial and temporal features: the spatial and temporal configuration or structure of the neural activity in the brain's spontaneous activity surface in the spatial and temporal features within which the contents of experience (like specific objects or events including body, self, and world) are integrated and thus structured and organized. For instance, a recent study of ours demonstrated that private

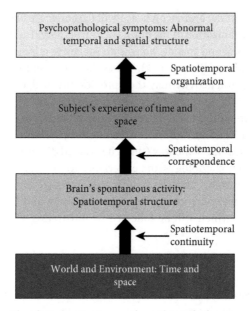

FIGURE 85.1 Different levels in spatiotemporal psychopathology.

self-consciousness is directly related to the temporal patterns of spontaneous or resting state activity across different frequency ranges (as indexed by what is described as "power law") (Huang, Obara, Davis IV, Pokorny, and Northoff 2016). This suggests that mental features like self may be rooted in spatiotemporal features of the brain's spontaneous activity. The self as mental feature may then be characterized in spatiotemporal terms, that is, by specific spatiotemporal schemata or structure rather than by cognition of particular contents (see Figure 85.1).

Unlike biological psychiatry that focuses on the brain itself independent of its respective ecological context, phenomenological psychiatry emphasizes the integration of experience including the subject of experience within the ecological context of the world. There is continuity between experience and world with such continuity often assumed to be mediated by the body, for example, experience of the body as lived body (see for instance Northoff and Stanghellini (2016)). Such continuity between subject and world is deemed central for making experience including the first-person perspective itself first and foremost possible.

Spatiotemporal Psychopathology

What exactly is the "common currency" that allows for continuity between experience and brain? The continuity between experience and brain may ultimately be traced to the continuity between world and brain. Let us give an empirical example. Duncan et al. (2015) recently demonstrated that early childhood traumatic experience is manifest in adulthood in the spatiotemporal patterns of the brain's spontaneous activity (as indexed by entropy) which, in turn, impacts subsequent stimulus-induced activity in relation to aversive stimuli. The continuity between experience and brain can thus be traced to continuity between world and brain as it is manifest in the spatiotemporal pattern of the latter's spontaneous activity. One may consequently want to speak of "spatiotemporal continuity" between world and brain. The concept of "spatiotemporal continuity" refers to the fact that certain spatial and temporal features are continuous from world to brain as for instance when certain temporal differences in the environment (as between specific stimuli) resurface in the temporal difference of the brain's spontaneous activity.

I postulate that the two features as introduced here, spatiotemporal correspondence and spatiotemporal continuity, are hallmark features of what can be described as "spatiotemporal psychopathology" (Northoff 2015a; 2015b; 2015c; 2015d). The concept of "spatiotemporal psychopathology" refers to the fact that psychopathological symptoms are conceived primarily in spatiotemporal terms rather than in cognitive (as in cognitive psychopathology), phenomenological (as in phenomenological psychopathology), affective (as in affective psychopathology), or neuronal terms (as in biological psychopathology).

How does such spatiotemporal psychopathology stand in relation to the other forms of psychopathology? One central distinguishing feature concerns the contents of our experience. Biological psychiatry, in contrast, focuses on contents in that it aims to reveal the neural underpinnings of the cognitive, affective, sensorimotor, and social contents. This is different in spatiotemporal psychopathology. Here the focus is not on contents at all but rather on how these contents can be characterized in spatial and temporal terms including their respective spatiotemporal context which, phenomenologically, can be traced to the life-world, for example, the world as experienced. The focus is thus not on contents themselves but on the spatiotemporal structure within which the contents are organized. Psychopathological symptoms are consequently characterized by structure-based alterations of temporal and spatial structure rather than content-based changes. This puts spatiotemporal psychopathology in close relation to phenomenological psychopathology that also considers the contents of experience in the wider context of self, body, and world. However, spatiotemporal psychopathology is even more radical than phenomenological psychopathology in that the central phenomenological constituents like self, body, and world are also conceived in spatiotemporal terms and thus within the context of time and space.

The aim of this chapter is to introduce spatiotemporal psychopathology and the way it may complement and extent phenomenological psychopathology by bridging the methodological gap between brain and experience. In the first section I will provide examples for spatiotemporal correspondence between neuronal and psychopathological features. Specifically, I will discuss how spatial changes in the brain's spontaneous activity translate into abnormal experience of the self in major depressive disorder (MDD). This is followed by the second section where I will focus on spatiotemporal continuity. Specifically, the second section highlights the special relevance of temporal changes in spontaneous activity and its relation to the world and how that translates into hallucinations in schizophrenia. Finally, in the third section, I will briefly discuss the method of such spatiotemporal psychopathology and distinguish it from the methods relied on in other forms of psychopathology with a special focus on showing the continuity between spatiotemporal and phenomenological psychopathology.

Spatiotemporal Correspondence: Spontaneous Activity's Spatial Structure and Self in Depression

As an example of the approach of spatiotemporal psychopathology, we can examine major depressive disorder (MDD). In a recent meta-analysis Alcaro (Alcaro, Panksepp, Witczak, Hayes, and Northoff 2010) looked at the brain's resting state activity, that is, the neural activity that can be observed in different regions and networks during the absence of specific stimuli or tasks (Logothetis et al. 2009). This yielded hyperactive regions in medial prefrontal cortex like perigenual anterior cingulate cortex (PACC) and ventromedial prefrontal cortex (VMPFC) (as well as subcortical midline regions as thalamic regions like the dorsomedial thalamus and the pulvinar, pallidum/putamen and midbrain regions like ventral tegmental area (VTA), Substantia nigra (SN), the Tectum, and the periaqueductal gray (PAG). In contrast, resting state activity was hypoactive in lateral prefrontal cortex regions being reduced in the dorsolateral prefrontal cortex (DLPFC) (and other regions like the posterior cingulate cortex (PCC) and adjacent precuneus/cuneus (Alcaro, Panksepp, Witczak, Hayes, and Northoff 2010) (see also (Kuhn and Gallinat 2013) for similar results). Especially the medial prefrontal resting state hyperactivity changes in PACC and VMPFC seems to be somehow specific for depression since in schizophrenia there is rather hypoactivity (see (Kuhn and Gallinat 2013; Zhu et al. 2012) (see Figure 85.2).

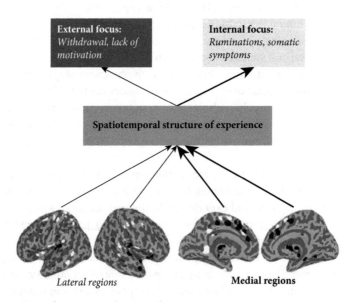

FIGURE 85.2 Spatial correspondence in depression.

The medial prefrontal regions like PACC and VMPFC are core regions of the default-mode network (DMN) while lateral prefrontal regions like DLPFC are part of the central executive network (CEN). A recent meta-analysis of resting state functional connectivity observed the following abnormal changes in these networks that seem to be (more or less) specific to MDD as distinguished from other psychiatric disorders (Kaiser, Andrews-Hanna, Wager, and Pizzagalli 2015). The DMN shows functional hyperconnectivity among its regions and especially between anterior and posterior midline regions. In contrast to the regions within the DMN, regions within the CEN show functional hypoconnectivity and are also less connected to parietal regions implicated in attention toward the external environment. This suggests spatial imbalance between the two networks with an abnormal spatial shift toward the DMN and away from the CEN with the former also enslaving the latter (as suggested by abnormally negative functional hyperconnectivity between DMN and CEN (Kaiser et al. 2015). These findings are specific to MDD as in BD such a pattern cannot be observed (Martino et al. 2016) while in schizophrenia functional connectivity between DMN and CEN is positive (rather than abnormally negative as in MDD) (Carhart-Harris et al. 2013).

In sum, the data provide evidence for abnormal resting state hyperactivity in medial prefrontal regions as part of the DMN in MDD while there is resting state hypoactivity in lateral prefrontal regions as part of the CEN. This suggests abnormal reciprocal modulation between medial and lateral prefrontal cortex with resting state activity being abnormally increased in the former and decreased in the latter. Abnormal opposite or reciprocal modulation between medial and lateral prefrontal cortical resting state activity in MDD is further supported by analogous functional connectivity: increased functional connectivity in PACC-VMPFC and thus within DMN is accompanied by decreased functional connectivity in lateral prefrontal cortex and the CEN (Hasler and Northoff 2011; Northoff 2014a; Northoff and Synille 2014; Zhu et al. 2012). One can thus speak of abnormal reciprocal modulation between medial/DMN and lateral/CEN prefrontal cortex with their spatial balance tilting abnormally toward the former at the expense of the latter.

The question then is how is the abnormal spatial balance between medial and lateral prefrontal cortex related to the psychopathological symptoms in MDD? This spatial imbalance on the level of the brain's spontaneous activity is well reflected on the phenomenal level: MDD patients' experiences are characterized by an increased focus on their own internal contents as consisting in either thoughts, as in ruminations with increased self-focus, or/and the body leading to the various unspecific somatic symptoms, for example, increased body-focus. In contrast, these patients' experience is no longer focused on the external environment at all, for example, decreased environment-focus, which psychopathologically is manifest in social withdrawal and lack of motivation. Consequently, one can say that the abnormal spatial structure in the brain's spontaneous activity translates and surfaces in the spatial structure of experience, for example, the spatial organization of contents with regard to body, self, and environment, which in turn leads to the various kinds of psychopathological symptoms.

SPATIOTEMPORAL CONTINUITY: SPONTANEOUS ACTIVITY'S TEMPORAL STRUCTURE AND HALLUCINATION IN SCHIZOPHRENIA

Lakatos, Schroeder, Leitman, and Javitt (2013) conducted an EEG study in schizophrenic patients whom they presented a stream of auditory stimuli (i.e. tones) with regular, that is, rhythmic interstimulus intervals (1500ms). They presented the stream of auditory stimuli with some deviant stimuli (20%) that were distinguished in their frequency. Subjects had to either passively listen (passive task), detect the easily detectable deviant stimuli (easy task), or detect the more difficult (variation by frequency) detectable stimuli (difficult task).

They observed that the phase coherence (i.e. the intertrial coherence/ITC) in different frequency ranges like delta (1-4Hz that mediates basic processes of the brain's attunement to its respective environmental context; Northoff (2014a; 2014b)) (in central electrodes that can be traced back to neural activity in auditory cortex) increased from the passive over the easy to the difficult condition with the latter showing the highest degree of ITC at stimulus onset in the delta range. However, this was only the case in healthy subjects whereas such task-related increase in delta ITC was not observed in schizophrenic patients. These patients were not able to properly align or shift their auditory cortical phase onsets in the delta range (that corresponded to the stimulation frequency with the ITI of the presented tones) to the onset of the tones and thus to properly adapt their neural activity to the task. This suggests decreased phase alignment or entrainment to external auditory stimuli.

Interestingly, in the intertrial interval (1500ms) task-dependent amplitude in the delta range could be observed with the highest amplitude in the difficult task. This again was observed only in the healthy subjects whereas schizophrenic subjects did not show such delta amplitude in the ITI. In contrast to the phase, that is, ITC, power in delta did not increase during any of the conditions in either healthy or schizophrenic patients. There was, however, a power increase in other frequency ranges, that is, theta (5-7HZ as related to memory processes) and beta (12-30HZ as related to sensorimotor processing) /gamma (30-40HZ as related to sensory processing) range from passive over easy to difficult tasks in healthy subjects. Schizophrenic patients showed an abnormally strong 7hz increase while the beta/gamma power was decreased especially during the difficult condition. Finally, reduced delta ITC correlated with both the behavioral measure, for example, the detection rate of the deviant tones, and the electrophysiological index, the P300 (in response to deviant tones), in schizophrenic subjects. Importantly, reduced delta ITC also predicted the severity of psychopathological symptoms (as measured with BPRS) and especially the positive symptoms (including hallucinations, delusions, and excitement).

Abnormal, that is, reduced entrainment of phase onsets to external stimuli have also been observed in other studies in schizophrenia as for instance in response to 40hz auditory stimuli (Hamm et al. 2015; Hamm, Gilmore, Picchetti, Sponheim, and Clementz 2011). Other studies also observed major abnormalities in phase resetting in delta (1-4Hz) and theta (5-8Hz) ranges in schizophrenia (Doege, Jansen, Mallikarjun, Liddle, and Liddle 2010a; Doege et al. 2010b) during an auditory oddball task, which, even more interestingly, predicted the degree of positive symptoms in schizophrenia, for example, disorganization (see also Hamm et al. (2011)). Unfortunately, there are no clear findings as yet about cross-frequency coupling between reduced delta phase reset and the phase/power (or amplitude) of higher frequencies in the beta or gamma range. Based on the findings described here, one would predict that decreased delta phase reset is closely linked to reduced cross-frequency coupling to beta and gamma as it is supported indirectly by the findings (and the impact of delta phase ITC on ERP like P300) (see above).

Taken together, these findings suggest that schizophrenic patients remain unable properly to link their internal auditory cortical neural activity, as indexed by phase onsets in delta, to a stream of external auditory stimuli. Lakatos et al. (2013) speak of deficits in active predictive sensing by phase resetting that does not allow schizophrenic patients to increase their cortical excitability at stimulus onset for the subsequent processing of external stimuli. Given the evidence described above, one may indeed assume severe deficits in phase entrainment (or alignment) to external stimuli, that is, internal–external alignment in schizophrenia.

More generally put, phase resetting allows for internal–external stimulus' (or, more generally, rest/brain–environment) alignment and thus for what Schroeder and Lakatos (2009a; 2009b; Schroeder, Lakatos, Kajikawa, Partan, and Puce 2008; Schroeder, Wilson, Radman, Scharfman, and Lakatos 2010) describe as "rhythmic mode" of brain function. The rhythmic mode of brain function can be characterized by good phase alignment of the brain's low frequency fluctuations (like delta) to the statistical frequency distributions of the external stimuli; this entails also that the high frequencies (like beta and gamma) show decreased power. In contrast, the brain may also operate in a "continuous mode" where the low frequencies are no longer phase-aligned to the external stimuli while the higher frequencies are now decoupled (i.e. low cross-frequency coupling) from the lower ones and show stronger power than in the rhythmic mode (Schroeder and Lakatos 2009a, 2009b; Northoff, 2014b).

Given the findings in auditory cortex with decreased delta ITC, increased resting state gamma, decreased task-evoked gamma (see above) and, to some degree, also decreased cross-frequency coupling, one would assume the auditory cortex in schizophrenia would operate in a continuous rather than rhythmic mode in relation to its respective environmental context. These temporal alterations mean that the schizophrenic patients' auditory cortical resting state activity can no longer align and adapt itself to its respective auditory environment, that is, external stimuli and remains quasi "decoupled" or "dissociated" from the external environment. One may consequently want to speak of "sensory decoupling" that describes the reduced entrainment or phase alignment to external sensory stimuli. Instead, as indicated by Lakatos et al. (2013), auditory cortical activity may rather align or entrain itself to internal stimuli or events (like thoughts). Instead of suppressing internal activity during entrainment to external stimuli, auditory cortical activity may instead phase align and entrain itself to internal stimuli of the ongoing resting state while, at the same time, suppressing its alignment to external stimuli (see Figure 85.3).

Specifically, periods of high cortical excitability as provided by the long phase durations of delta oscillations, may now be shifted or reset in orientation on the temporal timing of internal stimuli (like self-generated thoughts) rather than external stimuli (like tones), for example, reversed entrainment or phase alignment. However, that is a hypothesis at this point which needs to be investigated in the future. Such "reversed entrainment or phase alignment" to internal (rather than external) stimuli entails that there is spatiotemporal discontinuity (rather than spatiotemporal continuity) between world/environment and brain in the

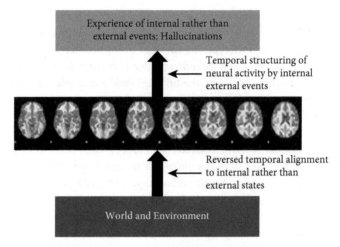

FIGURE 85.3 Spatiotemporal (dis)continuity in schizophrenia.

spontaneous activity. This is phenomenally reflected in the decoupling of experience from the ecological context, for example, the world and results psychopathologically in auditory hallucinations (and probably delusions).

Rather than focusing on outward contents originating within the world, experience turns inwards to internal contents such as delusions and hallucinations. The abnormal temporal structure of the brain's spontaneous activity, that is, its phase onsets including their temporal detachment from the temporal structure of the tones' onsets, manifests itself in the shift from external tones to internal contents like hallucinations. The abnormal temporal structure of the brain's spontaneous activity with its lacking phase shift during the tones thus translates into hallucinations as abnormal contents in experience. Rather than originating in the cognitive contents of cognitive function, hallucinations may then be traced to the abnormal temporal structure of the brain's spontaneous activity and its detachment from the temporal structure of the tones in the world.

SPATIOTEMPORAL PSYCHOPATHOLOGY VERSUS PHENOMENOLOGICAL PSYCHOPATHOLOGY

Direct Link with "Common Currency" between Brain and Experience

How can we characterize the methodology of spatiotemporal psychopathology and how does it compare to other forms of psychopathology? First and foremost, spatiotemporal psychopathology views and approaches psychopathological symptoms in terms of spatial and temporal features rather than contents themselves: psychopathological symptoms are traced to abnormal spatial and temporal structuring of cognitive, affective, social, and sensorimotor contents. For instance, one may hypothesize that the internal thought contents are processed in depression in a spatial context that puts abnormal emphasis on them at the expense of external contents leading to ruminations and increased self-focus. The internal contents, for example, the thoughts are thus structured and integrated spatially in an abnormal way. The same applies to schizophrenia where the spontaneous activity can no longer structure and organize its own temporal features, that is, its phase onsets, in order to align and link them to the auditory tones. Psychopathological symptoms are thus traced to abnormal spatial and temporal structuring of sensorimotor, cognitive, affective, and social contents in perceptions, emotions, and cognitions.

Such spatiotemporal approach distinguishes spatiotemporal psychopathology from other forms of psychopathology that view psychopathological symptoms in either cognitive, affective, behavioral, or phenomenal ways (See Table 85.1).

Spatiotemporal psychopathology aims to establish direct links between neuronal and phenomenal states by focusing on the spatiotemporal features as shared overlap or "common currency" between the brain's spontaneous activity and experience. The spatiotemporal features allow the transformation from neuronal into phenomenal activity thus establishing a direct link between brain and experience; the temporal and spatial features as constructed by the brain's spontaneous activity allow for extending and transforming neuronal into phenomenal activity. At the phenomenal level those very same spatial and temporal features are experienced in first-person perspective as for instance described in the concept of "phenomenal time" (Northoff and Stanghellini 2016) and the "stream of consciousness" (James 1890). The experience of time and space, in turn, underlies our experience of self, body, and world as main focus of phenomenological psychopathology. Spatiotemporal psychopathology can therefore be considered as much as an extension of the brain/biological psychiatry to experience/phenomenological psychopathology as it can be regarded as extension from the later to the former. Metaphorically speaking, spatiotemporal psychopathology provides the bridge

Table 85.1 Comparison between different forms of psychopathology

	Spatiotemporal Psychopathology	Affective Psychopathology	Cognitive Psychopathology	Phenomenological Psychopathology	Descriptive Psychopathology
Psychopathological symptoms	Spatiotemporal features	Affective features	Cognitive features	Phenomenal features	Operational features
Link neuronal and mental	Direct and spatiotemporal	Indirect through affect	Indirect through cognition	none	none
Neural activity	Spontaneous activity	Task-evoked activity	Task-evoked activity	none	none
Role of experience	Methodological starting point	Emotional feeling	none	Starting and end point	none
Self, body, and world	Secondary constructs	Body as basis of emotions	Cognitive constructs	Lived body as primary	Operational constructs
Time and space	Primary pre-phenomenal constructions	No special role	Cognition of time and space	Phenomenal features: Inner time/space consciousness	No special role

between experience and brain and like any bridge in reality, it allows for direct access from both sides, namely, phenomenal and neural.

This is different in the other forms of psychopathology where there is a rather indirect link between brain and experience with regard to symptoms: the psychopathological symptoms are here conceived to be mediated by the cognitive, affective, or behavioral functions of the brain (or the phenomenal features of experience). Such an indirect link ultimately opens a gap between brain and symptoms as described above.

Spatiotemporal psychopathology focuses mainly on the brain's spontaneous activity rather than the task-evoked or stimulus-induced activity. This is different in the other forms of psychopathology that target cognitive, affective, and/or behavioral functions as related to stimulus-induced or task-evoked activity in the brain.

Spatiotemporal Psychopathology Versus Phenomenological Psychopathology

Spatiotemporal psychopathology shares with phenomenological psychopathology the assumption of a central role of experience. Both take very seriously experience as the subjective account of what objectively is described as psychopathological symptoms. In that sense spatiotemporal psychopathology can be considered as phenomenological as phenomenological psychopathology. In other words, spatiotemporal psychopathology in this sense can be considered an extension of phenomenological psychopathology that shifts the focus from self, body, and world to their underlying temporal and spatial features in experience. Taken in this sense, spatiotemporal psychopathology may be considered a subset of phenomenological psychopathology specifically with regard to the experience of time and space and how that is related to the experience of self, body, and world.

However, unlike phenomenological psychopathology, spatiotemporal psychopathology does not remain within the boundaries of experience itself. It goes beyond experience in that it aims to link experience to the brain and its neural activity. That raises the question for the "common currency" between experience and brain which, per spatiotemporal psychopathology, can be found in temporal and spatial features: both the brain's neural activity especially its spontaneous activity and experience share the spatial and temporal structuring and organizing of contents—spatiotemporal features are the "common currency" between experience and brain.

Methodologically, this amounts to what can be described as "double access" in spatiotemporal psychopathology. The symptoms can be accessed in terms of the brain and its neural activity and, at the same time, in terms of their experience by the respective subject. Both the brain's neural activity and the subjects' experience are conceived in primarily spatiotemporal terms—the brain's neural activity changes may then be conceived in the spatiotemporal features of the subject's experience and vice versa. One can for instance investigate whether the degree of shift between self- and environment-focus, that is, the spatial shift between internal and external contents corresponds to the spatial shift between medial/DMN and lateral/CEN prefrontal cortical regions (see above). Analogous correspondence between neuronal and mental features can be observed in the temporal domain. The degree of temporal detachment of the brain's phase onsets from the environment's tones may correspond to the degree to which the subject's experiences are determined by internal (rather than external) contents like delusions and hallucinations. In short, spatiotemporal psychopathology supposes spatiotemporal correspondence and continuity between neural and experiential activity.

The role of self, body, and world are different in spatiotemporal psychopathology. Phenomenological psychopathology takes subjective experience of time and space as well as of self, body, and world as the central and most basic features of psychopathology. Spatiotemporal psychopathology, in contrast, focuses mainly on time and space, for example, the subjective experience of time and space, as the most basic and fundamental experiential dimensions as they underlie our experience of self, body, and world. Self, body, and world are not neglected but, unlike in phenomenological psychopathology, they are no longer considered as independent constituents of experience. Instead, they are traced to spatial and temporal features. As mentioned above, a recent study shows that self-consciousness can be linked with the overall temporal structure of the spontaneous activity (Huang et al. 2016). The same holds analogously for the body, that is, the lived body, that can be traced to the spatial structure of the brain's spontaneous activity (Northoff and Stanghellini 2016). These data lent support to the view that self, body, and world may by themselves be conceived in the spatiotemporal terms of the brain's spontaneous activity.

Why does spatiotemporal psychopathology conceive self, body, and world in spatiotemporal terms rather than as basic phenomenal constituents by themselves? This makes it possible for spatiotemporal psychopathology to transgress the boundaries of experience and to link it with the brain. Time and space are considered as the bridge or "common currency" between experience and brain since, as I suggest, they allow for transforming merely neuronal activity (as we can observe it in the brain) into phenomenal features (as we can experience them). Spatiotemporal psychopathology thus complements phenomenological psychopathology by extending it beyond its own phenomenal boundaries that is, the border of experience, to the brain and its spontaneous activity. At the same time, spatiotemporal psychopathology extends the borders of neuroscience beyond the brain itself to experience. In the case of both transitions from experience to brain and brain to experience, spatiotemporal features serve as guiding thread and "common currency" underlying both our experience of self, body, and world as well as our observation of neural activity changes in the brain. Accordingly, as already pointed out above, spatiotemporal psychopathology can be regarded as extension of both phenomenological psychopathology and biological psychiatry though from reversed directions.

Finally, it should be pointed out that, due to its functional role as bridge between experience and brain, spatiotemporal psychopathology is somewhat intrinsically hybrid. It is phenomenal in that it relies and draws on experience of time and space. At the same time spatiotemporal psychopathology is neuronal in that it searches for how time and space are constructed and realized by the brain and its spontaneous activity. Taken in this sense, spatiotemporal psychopathology can be considered truly neurophenomenal (rather than being either purely neuronal or phenomenal) (Northoff 2014a; 2014b).

Finally, taken in a more philosophical context, spatiotemporal psychopathology can be considered a methodological or epistemological framework for investigation of psychopathology in particular and mental features like self and consciousness in general. Finally, spatiotemporal psychopathology also carries an ontological dimension in that it targets time and space, for example, the construction of time and space by the brain in its relation to body and world, as they actually exist and are real in the world. The rather complex reality of psychiatric disorders as basic disturbances of self, body, and world as thematized so well in phenomenological psychopathology is thus well reflected in the hybrid nature of spatiotemporal psychopathology.

CONCLUSION

I have in this chapter suggested a novel approach to psychopathology, namely, to conceive psychopathological symptoms in terms of their underlying spatiotemporal features. Spatiotemporal psychopathology assumes correspondence and continuity between the spatial and temporal features of the brain's spontaneous activity on the one hand and the spatial and temporal structure underlying psychopathological symptoms. Such spatiotemporal correspondence was exemplified by ruminations in depression. Moreover, spatiotemporal psychopathology assumes continuity between the spatial and temporal features of the world and those of the brain entailing spatiotemporal continuity. For instance, such spatiotemporal continuity is disrupted in schizophrenia which may be central in constituting hallucinations and delusions.

Spatiotemporal psychopathology aims to complement and extend phenomenological psychopathology beyond the phenomenal boundaries of experience reaching out to the brain. Specifically, spatial and temporal features shared by both experience and brain are sought to correspond with each other; the changes in the spatiotemporal structure of the brain's spontaneous activity are assumed to surface and translate into abnormal spatiotemporal structuring on the phenomenal level of experience resulting in the various kinds of psychopathological symptoms. Methodologically, this requires double access: the spatiotemporal psychopathologist needs access to subjects' experience like a phenomenological psychopathologist while, at the same time, he requires access to the brain's spontaneous activity just as the spatiotemporal neuroscientist. This will ultimately enable spatiotemporal psychopathology to bridge the gap by providing time and space as "common currency" between experience and brain, for example, by their shared spatiotemporal features.

BIBLIOGRAPHY

Alcaro A., Panksepp J., Witczak J., Hayes D. J., and Northoff G. (2010). "Is Subcortical-Cortical Midline Activity in Depression Mediated by Glutamate and GABA? A Cross-Species Translational Approach." *Neuroscience & Biobehavioral Reviews* 34(4): 592–605.

Carhart-Harris R. L., Brugger S., Nutt D. J., Stone J. M. (2013). "Psychiatry's Next Top Model: Cause for a Re-think on Drug Models of Psychosis and other Psychiatric Disorders." *Journal of Psychopharmacology* 27(9): 771–778. doi: 10.1177/0269881113494107

Cuthbert B. N. and Insel T. R. (2013). "Toward the Future of Psychiatric Diagnosis: The Seven Pillars of RDoC." BiomedCentral (BMC) *BMC Medicine* 11: 126. doi: 10.1186/1741-7015-11-126

David A. S. and Halligan P. W. (2000). "Cognitive Neuropsychiatry: Potential for Progress." *J Neuropsychiatry Clinical Neuroscience* 12(4): 506.

Doege K., Jansen M., Mallikarjun P., Liddle E. B., and Liddle P. F. (2010a). "How Much Does Phase Resetting Contribute to Event-related EEG Abnormalities in Schizophrenia?" *Neuroscience Letters* 481(1): 1–5.

Doege K., Kumar M., Bates A. T., Das D., Boks M. P. M., and Liddle P. F. (2010b). "Time and Frequency Domain Event-related Electrical Activity Associated with Response Control in Schizophrenia." *Clinical Neurophysiology* 121(10): 1760–1771.

Duncan N. W., Hayes D. J., Wiebking C., Brice T., Pietruska K., Chen D., and Northoff G. (2015). "Negative Childhood Experiences Alter a Prefrontal-Insular-Motor Cortical Network in Healthy Adults: A Multimodal rsfMRI-fMRI-MRS-dMRI Study." *Human Brain Mapping* 36(11): 4622–4637. doi: 10.1002/hbm.22941

Fuchs T. (2007). "The Temporal Structure of Intentionality and Its Disturbance in Schizophrenia." *Psychopathology* 40(4): 229–235.

Fuchs T. (2013). "Temporality and Psychopathology." *Phenomenology and the Cognitive Sciences* 12(1): 75–104.

Halligan P. W. and David A. S. (2001). "Cognitive neuropsychiatry: Towards a Scientific Psychopathology." *Nature Reviews Neuroscience* 2(3): 209–215.

Hamm J. P., Gilmore C. S., Picchetti N. A., Sponheim S. R., and Clementz B. A. (2011). "Abnormalities of Neuronal Oscillations and Temporal Integration to Low- and High-Frequency Auditory Stimulation in Schizophrenia." *Biologicll Psychiatry* 69(10): 989–996. doi: 10.1016/j.biopsych.2010.11.021

Hamm J. P., Bobilev A. M., Hayrynen L. K., Hudgens-Haney M. E., Oliver W. T., Parker D. A., and Clementz B. A. (2015). "Stimulus Train Duration But Not Attention Moderates γ-Band Entrainment Abnormalities in Schizophrenia." *Schizophrenia Research* 165(1): 97–102. doi: 10.1016/j.schres.2015.02.016

Hasler G., and Northoff G. (2011). "Discovering Imaging Endophenotypes for Major Depression." *Molecular.Psychiatry* 16(6): 604–619.

Huang Z., Obara N., Davis H. H. IV, Pokorny J., and Northoff G. (2016). "The Temporal Structure of Resting-State Brain Activity in the Medial Prefrontal Cortex Predicts Self-Consciousness." *Neuropsychologia* 82: 161–170. doi: 10.1016/j.neuropsychologia

James W. (1890). *Principles of Psychology*. Cambridge, Mass: Harvard University Press.

Kaiser R. H., Andrews-Hanna J. R., Wager T. D., and Pizzagalli D. A. (2015). "Large-Scale Network Dysfunction in Major Depressive Disorder: A Meta-analysis of Resting-State Functional Connectivity." *JAMA psychiatry* 72(6): 603–611. doi: 10.1001/jamapsychiatry.2015.0071

Kuhn S. and Gallinat J. (2013). "Resting-State Brain Activity in Schizophrenia and Major Depression: A Quantitative Meta-analysis." *Schizophrenia Bulletin* 39(2): 358–365.

Lakatos P., Schroeder C. E., Leitman D. I., and Javitt D. C. (2013). "Predictive Suppression of Cortical Excitability and Its Deficit in Schizophrenia." *The Journal of Neuroscience* 33(28): 11692–11702.

Logothetis N. K., Murayama Y., Augath M., Steffen T., Werner J., and Oeltermann A. (2009). "How Not to Study Spontaneous Activity." *Neuroimage* 45(4): 1080–1089. doi: 10.1016/j.neuroimage.2009.01.010

Martino M., Magioncalda P., Huang Z., Conio B., Piaggio N., Duncan N. W., Rocchi G., Escelsior A., Marozzi V., Wolff A., Inglese M., Amore M., and Northoff G. 2016. "Contrasting Variability Patterns in the Default Mode and Sensorimotor Networks Balance in Bipolar Depression and Mania." *Proceedings of the National Academy of Sciences of the United States of America* 113(17): 4824–4829. doi: 10.1073/pnas.1517558113

Northoff G. (2014a). *Unlocking the Brain: Volume 1: Coding*. Oxford: Oxford University Press.

Northoff G. (2014b). *Unlocking the Brain. Volume II: Consciousness*. Oxford: Oxford University Press.

Northoff G. (2015a). "Spatiotemporal Psychopathology I: Is Depression a Spatiotemporal Disorder of the Brain's Resting State?" *Journal of Affective Disorder*. 190: 854–866. doi: 10.1016/j.jad.2015.05.007

Northoff G. (2015b). "Spatiotemporal Psychopathology II: What Does a Psychopathology of the Brain's Resting State Look Like?" *Journal of Affective Disorder* 190: 867–879. doi: 10.1016/j.jad.2015.05.008

Northoff G. (2015c). "Is Schizophrenia a Spatiotemporal Disorder of the Brain's Resting State?" *World Psychiatry* 14(1): 34–35.

Northoff G. (2015d). "Resting State Activity and the "Stream of Consciousness" in Schizophrenia-Neurophenomenal Hypotheses." *Schizophrenia Bulletin* 41(1): 280–290. doi: 10.1093/schbul/sbu116

Northoff G. and Synille E. (2014). "Depression and GABA-A Cross-Level Translational Hypothesis." *Molecular Psychiatry* 19(9): 966–977. doi: 10.1038/mp.2014.68

Northoff G. and Stanghellini G. (2016). "How to Link Brain and Experience? Spatiotemporal Psychopathology of the Lived Body." *Frontiers Human Neuroscience* 10: 172.

Panksepp J. (2004). *Textbook of Biological Psychiatry*. Wiley Online Library.

Parnas J., Sass L. A., and Zahavi D. (2008). "Recent Developments in Philosophy of Psychopathology." *Current Opinion in Psychiatry* 21(6): 578–584.

Parnas J., Sass L. A., and Zahavi D. (2012). "Rediscovering Psychopathology: The Epistemology and Phenomenology of the Psychiatric Object." *Schizophrenia Bulletin* 39(2): 270–277. doi: 10.1093/schbul/sbs153.

Parnas J., Sass L. A., and Zahavi D. (2013). "Rediscovering Psychopathology: The Epistemology and Phenomenology of the Psychiatric Object." *Schizophrenia Bulletin* 39(2): 270–277. doi: 10.1093/schbul/sbs153

Schroeder C. E., Lakatos P., Kajikawa Y., Partan S., and Puce A. (2008). "Neuronal Oscillations and Visual Amplification of Speech." *Trends in Cognitive Science* 12(3): 106–113. doi: 10.1016/j.tics.2008.01.002

Schroeder C. E. and Lakatos P. (2009a). "Low-Frequency Neuronal Oscillations as Instruments of Sensory Selection." *Trends in Neuroscience* 32(1): 9–18. doi: 10.1016/j.tins.2008.09.012

Schroeder C. E. and Lakatos P. (2009b). "The Gamma Oscillation: Master or Slave?" *Brain Topography* 22(1): 24–26. doi: 10.1007/s10548-009-0080-y

Schroeder C. E., Wilson D. A., Radman T., Scharfman H., and Lakatos P. (2010). "Dynamics of Active Sensing and Perceptual Selection." *Current Opioni in Neurobiology* 20(2): 172–176. doi: 10.1016/j.conb.2010.02.010

Stanghellini G. (2009a). "A Hermeneutic Framework for Psychopathology." *Psychopathology* 43(5): 319–326.

Stanghellini G. (2009b). "The Meanings of Psychopathology." *Current Opinion in Psychiatry* 22(6): 559–564.

Stanghellini G. and Broome M. R. (2014). "Psychopathology as the Basic Science of Psychiatry." *The British Journal of Psychiatry* 205(3): 169–170.

Zhu X., Wang X., Xiao J., Liao J., Zhong M., Wang W., and Yao S. (2012). "Evidence of a Dissociation Pattern in Resting-State Default Mode Network Connectivity in First-Episode, Treatment-Naive Major Depression Patients." *Biological Psychiatry* 71(7): 611–617.

CHAPTER 86

PHENOMENOLOGICAL PSYCHOPATHOLOGY AND QUALITATIVE RESEARCH

MASSIMO BALLERINI

WHAT IS QUALITATIVE RESEARCH

CAN qualitative research (QR) be considered as a set of empirical studies the findings of which are simply delivered without any numerical (statistical) procedures (Fossey et al. 2002)?

Such a concept is largely unsatisfactory as QR has a further, distinctive value (Razafsha et al. 2012). QR is an empirical investigation "into meaning" (Shank 2002) which sets about "to make sense of, or to interpret, phenomena in terms of the meanings people bring to them" (Denzin and Lincoln 2000).

A plurality of qualitative methodologies (QMs) are available to researchers: they diverge in the modality of data collection (Palinkas 2014). In psychiatry, the most commonly employed are *field observations* (direct observations of the investigated phenomena where they take place), *focus groups* (peer groups that discuss personal experience), and *in-depth interviews* (extensive investigations of subjective experiences).

The Standards of Qualitative Research

Looked at globally, QMs display a set of common principles:

a) *Meanings as results*

QR involves an interpretative approach to experimental data, with findings reflecting the personal perspective (subjective meanings, attitudes, and beliefs) toward the topic under inquiry (Razafsha et al. 2012).

b) *Conceptualizations as an inductive process*

Data conceptualization is the outcome of research, rooted in the "unfolding" of the empirical data.

Using interpretative procedures, the collected data gradually produces overall meanings, generating categories with specific properties. This approach has been referred as "Grounded Theory" (Pidgeon and Henwood 1996). In contrast, quantitative research necessitates a priori defined paradigms, provided with hypotheses to challenge, the supposed intervening variables and their assessment measures (Glaser 2002).

c) *Naturalistic real-world approach*

QR is not confined to laboratory paradigms, but rather looks at the "contextualized" real-world relevance of the topics under investigation. In this sense, QR has been defined as "naturalistic" while the quantitative research—based on laboratory paradigms—is referred to as "experimental" (Denzin and Lincoln 2000).

d) *Active role of researchers*

Researchers must be actively engaged in the research setting in order to facilitate the production of empirical data (Glesne and Peshkin 1992). In this sense, QR promotes the role of clinical settings as the place where is possible to integrate treatment with research procedures (Stanghellini and Ballerini 2008).

Why a Phenomenological Psychopathology Background for Qualitative Research?

A hermeneutical approach to *anomalous subjectivity* is the core feature of phenomenological psychopathology. Phenomenological psychopathology is addressed to investigate *anomalous experiences* in order to disclose their overall meaning, their value, and the existential arrangement they emerge from (Stanghellini 2004; Nordgaard et al. 2013); it promotes "high resolution" understanding of patients' anomalous subjectivity, avoiding the "tunnel vision" of many mainstream rating scales (Stanghellini and Ballerini 2008). It is useful in refining psychiatric phenotypes, thus improving the differential typology of mental disorders. Also, the findings have proved to be very useful in developing specific rating scales (Parnas et al. 2005).

Phenomenological psychopathology represents an excellent theoretical background for QR—particularly for in-depth interview—by promoting "systematic but flexible" investigation of patients' apparently unstructured experiences (clinical phenomena). Psychiatric disorders are not simple checklists of independent symptoms or mere collections of isolated fragments, rather they constitute salient unities, meaningful wholes, or coherent structures (Stanghellini 2004; Nordgaard et al. 2013), that are grounded on the disturbances of the fundamental, unitary relationship of self–others–world.

A structure is a web of interconnected signs and symptoms that reveals a proper, coherent order—paradoxical in severe mental illness—a unitary meaning, and a global value.

On the other hand, psychiatric disorders, articulated in manifolds of morbid experiences, are peculiar existential stances (Binswanger 1956). Despite all the patients' biographical details and personal variations, they display a typical invariant structure residing in specific (anomalous) arrangements of patients' structures of subjectivity (see below).

To capture the overall meaning of pathological *salient unities* or *structures* one must study in depth the specific modes of anomalous subjectivity.

Classical phenomenological psychopathology produced outstanding documentations of severe elusive mental disorders, but it has been criticized for not fulfilling the modern standards of empirical research (Stanghellini and Ballerini 2011a). Phenomenological psychopathology-oriented research needs to be "disciplined" in a comprehensible, transmissible, and reliable methodology, so I will examine the essentials of phenomenology, to improve comprehension of the methodology and summarize its key points.

THE ESSENTIALS OF PHENOMENOLOGY

Phenomenology has become a major stream of philosophical investigation (see Heidegger 1927; Sartre 1943; Merleau-Ponty 1945; Husserl 1971a, b, 2000). In recent decades, phenomenology has shared its research agenda with the cognitive sciences as well as looking for a useful integrative approach with neuroscience (Varela 1996).

What is Phenomenology?

Phenomenology studies how the world—intended in the widest sense—is experienced (or assumed) in each person's consciousness. It is not a mere description of the appearances the world; phenomenology points out the very structure of our experiential world (how the experiences structure themselves within an individual's consciousness) and which are their condition of possibility).

Consciousness, Intentionality, and Subjectivity

Consciousness is not merely an object of the world but it is our "access" to the world, the "where" the world is structured and actualized (Gallagher and Zahavi 2012); the objects of the world are constituted within consciousness, that is, they are experienced disclosing their meanings by the means of the structure of consciousness (Husserl 1971a, 1971b). The fundamental properties of consciousness are at issue (see Lutz and Thompson 2003; Van Gulick 2014).

In the phenomenological perspective, two main features of consciousness have to be underpinned—intentionality and subjectivity.

Intentionality (Husserl 2000) means that our consciousness is ever directed about something: thinking, imaging, dreaming, feeling, etc., are diverse forms of intentionality. Intentionality shapes the form of our experience (i.e. thinking or hearing). Discriminating different forms of intentionality is an immediate and automatic process in healthy subjects (i.e. each one is able to feel immediately if he or she is thinking or hearing).

However, every mental state presupposes a subject. Subjectivity is our being-in-the-world (Merleau-Ponty 1945). Consciousness is subjective since whatever experience I have or I do, this is—from the beginning and without any reflective stance—my experience (Gallagher and Zahavi 2012). Subjectivity is not a label over-imposed on experience (Sass and Parnas 2003): the first-person perspective is the way experience structures itself within consciousness (Henry 1990).

There is no experience without consciousness and no consciousness without a subject. Finally, phenomenology is not a form of mere subjectivism, but it endorses a first-person subjective approach in order to reconstruct the objectivity of the world.

How to Grasp the Overall Meaning of Experience: The Phenomenological Methodology

Phenomenology provides a disciplined methodology (see Husserl 1971a, 1971b), to depict the typical invariant features of a given experience, brilliantly summarized by Gallagher and Zahavi (2012) as "the phenomenological toolkit." What does it contain?

The suspension of all common sense attributions regarding a given phenomenon is the first step to evidence the modes through which an experience is given or structured. Its complementary aspect is the phenomenological reduction; this is a "correlational inter-dependence between specific structures of subjectivity and specific modes of appearance or given-ness" (Gallagher and Zahavi 2012) of an experience.

The removal of natural attitude and the phenomenological reduction liberate us from a naturalistic dogmatism—they act to comprehend the cognitive or "constitutive" mode (Husserl 2000) by which we organize the meanings of experience—to appreciate how subjectivity manifests itself in the experiences we live.

Now we have to grasp the ideally necessary features, that is, the typical invariant characteristics of such an experience, or its essential (*eidetic*) *feature*.

We have to abandon our reliance on the specific (particular, circumstantial, incidental) features of the considered phenomenon and concentrate on the invariant properties (or qualities) that define this phenomenon; we can imagine intuitively a lot of variation of the considered phenomenon but there is something necessary and invariant that, as Husserl says, "holds up" along the variations we can perform. Some characteristics remain constant, or re-sist, this form of eidetic (or essential features) variation. You may imagine a gallery of cars or a set of guilt experiences: which is the core set of properties (or qualities) that properly define an object such as *a car* or *a certain* lived experience as a *guilt experience*? Some characteristics remain constant or resist this form of eidetic (or essential features) variation. You can modify these features in your imagination to determine when the concept loses its essence. This core set of properties represents the essence or the essential feature of the experience.

To discover if such an exercise is a peculiar or idiosyncratic account, a final step is necessary. We have to corroborate our finding by way of an interpersonal validation (Gallagher and Zahavi 2012). To be valid, this set of essential properties has to be shared by the others (intersubjective validation or interpersonal corroboration). This is crucial as it may extend the validity criteria from classical phenomenological paradigm to a naturalized *form of validity* as required by modern empirical sciences (Roy et al. 1999).

Naturalizing Phenomenology

The phenomenological method may fit the standards of empirical research, including neurosciences (Varela 1996), but how can we combine the subjective, first-person perspective, including its eidetic/transcendental criteria of validity with the objective, third-person perspective whose validity resides in complex, sub-personal (or pre-phenomenal) mechanisms and/or in mathematical procedures?

We have to avoid any correlative approach (Gallagher and Varela 2003) where the phenomenal (the experiential level) and the trans-phenomenal or transcendental level (the condition of possibility of experience) are reduced to mere correlates of sub-personal mechanisms. Here, the risk is to transform phenomenal and trans-phenomenal to a mere epiphenomenal approach.

To bridge the gap, we have to employ two methodological strategies. First, we have to look for "common properties" between the account of phenomena furnished by phenomenology and that provided by neuroscience (Gallagher and Zahavi 2012); in other words, *common properties* strategy means that we have to grasp the specular or mirroring unfolding of the properties as depicted by the two perspectives.

Second, we must impose a *reciprocal constraints* strategy to each discipline with careful attention to the findings evidenced by the other one in the same topic of research; these findings have to be carefully considered in the formulation of theoretical models as they are cogent points of reference (Gallagher and Varela 2003). For example, empirical science criteria of validity require findings to be generalizable according to standardized numerical procedures. Thus, to be valid, phenomenological psychopathology findings have to be translated in transpersonal constructs applicable not only to paradigmatic cases but to a class of individuals, that is, people suffering schizophrenia. Next, they have to be confirmed by standard psychometric procedure (Roy et al. 1999).

Naturalized phenomenological psychopathology, rooted in the standards of empirical research, may contribute to a better definition of phenotypes, improving the differential typology and readdressing many neurobiological investigations.

The Phenomenological Psychopathology Toolkit

How can we translate the phenomenological method in the study of anomalous subjectivity? Here, first-person subjective experiences articulated in personal narratives are converted in transpersonal constructs, valid for a class of individuals—that is, people suffering from schizophrenia (Stanghellini and Ballerini 2008).

I will summarize the theoretical key points of phenomenological psychopathology-oriented QM: this set of principles may be termed "the Phenomenological Psychopathology Toolkit" since it is strictly related to the "phenomenological toolkit" above.

Structures of Subjectivity and Their Morbid Distortions

The systematic investigation of anomalous subjectivity is the main focus of phenomeno-logical psychopathology. To look at the purpose of phenomenological psychopathology-oriented QM, it is useful to stretch some essential features of subjectivity. Through the work of Merleau-Ponty (1945) embodiment is recognized as playing a foundational role, and has become a key topic in neuroscience (Varela et al. 1991), including cognitive science (Gallese and Sinigaglia 2011). Embodiment means that the lived body is the constitutive element of our being-the-world (Merleau-Ponty 1945), since:

1) it is fundamental to the primordial—experiential—sense of self, named *ipseity* (Sartre 1943; Henry 1990) or core self (Damasio 2000) or basic or minimal self (Zavahi 2005; Gallagher 2013a); the basic self is pure, absolute subjectivity, the first person perspective, the way in which every kind of experiences takes form. Here, the term basic—adopted by phenomenology in the recent years (see Fuchs 2010)—echoes the classic term transcendental

According to the Husserlian lesson (Husserl 1991), Gallagher (2005) outlined transcendental temporality as the milestone of basic subjectivity. Transcendental temporality consents to the automatic fluid integration, moment by moment, of the present (primal impression), the past (retention), and future (protention), organizing any experiential object or action.

However, basic (or transcendental) temporality is the constitutive mode of conscious-ness (Husserl 1991) since it allows the fluid flow of the stream of experiences. Temporal infrastructures (retention and protention) substantiate the sense of myness of experience and the sense of agency.

2) the lived body structures the self/other demarcation
3) it represents the departure point and the frame of reference of our immersion in the world, organizing perception and our lived spatiality (Merleau-Ponty 1945)

Embodiment consents to our immediate apprehension of others—that is, the immediate (Gallagher 2013b), enactive (Hutto 2013) form of intersubjectivity.

The basic structures of subjectivity remain (Fuchs 2010) stable over time and are not dis-tinctive of specific individuals. They are implicit or automatic, pre-cognitive, pre-reflective, and pre-linguistic; normally transparent, they manifest themselves when distorted in pathology (Sass and Parnas 2003; Fuchs 2010).

Higher-order (Gallagher and Zahavi 2012) or propositional (linguistic) structures of subjectivity may be regarded as the modes in which a specific subjectivity (a specific in-dividual) is given: they are accessible to introspection, articulable in language and they evolve throughout the course of life; they enfold the extended (Damasio 2000) or narra-tive (Ricoeur 1984) self or personhood (Zavahi 2005; Gallagher 2013a) including the autobiographical—temporal—arrangement of memories; time and spatiality, as effectively lived by the subject; the system of values and the symbolization processes; finally, habits, attitudes, cognitive style, emotional reactivity, etc. The strategic, cognitively charged form of intersubjectivity might also be included.

This relationship between the basic/higher-order structures of subjectivity and neurocognitive abilities has been questioned (Fuster 2003; Nelson et al. 2014). Gallagher and Zahavi (2012) rejected a strict relationship between basic self or fundamental temporality and neurocognitive abilities; on the other hand, a correlation between episodic memory and narrative self is intuitive. Finally a link between symbolization processes and semantic memory has been proposed (Ballerini 2016a).

The structures of subjectivity are currently distorted in the course of psychiatric disorders. It may be argued that psychotic symptoms arise as a consequence of the morbid distortion of the basic structures of subjectivity, since the latter are the very condition of experience: in schizophrenia there are disturbances of basic self (Sass and Parnas 2003), fundamental temporality (Fuchs 2010; Stanghellini et al. 2016), and spatiality (Straus 1935).

Sometimes the patients directly experience their morbid arrangement; more frequently they manifest in overt psychotic (or pre-psychotic) symptomatology. Higher-order structures of subjectivity are interested by non-psychotic mental disorders (i.e. melancholic depression); psychosis too may involve them—i.e. the morbid arrangement of values (Stanghellini and Ballerini 2007) or the semantic attitude (Ballerini 2016a) over the course of schizophrenia.

The Lived Experience

In the phenomenological perspective, lived experiences are the single, interdependent, fragments or building blocks of our engagement in the world. Anomalous lived experiences or clinical phenomena are the object of phenomenological psychopathology since they reflect specific modes of abnormal subjectivity. Lived experiences possess four main features:

a) *A form*

This is the way experience is given, the mode it presents itself within subjectivity. Different types of experiences (i.e. thinking, hearing, feeling) reflect different modes of intentionality (Parnas et al. 2013). The form an experience assumes (Jaspers 1913) plays a major diagnostic role (confronting a ruminative doubt with hearing an invisible voice). Note that some morbid experiences (e.g. thought broadcasting) overwhelm the embodied limits of experience.

b) *A content*

This is the informative side of experience—the information contained in the experience (Stanghellini and Ballerini 2008).

Every content is permeated by personal, biographical aspects and details. It reflects attitudes, habits, ways of acting, values, beliefs, thinking style, and emotional reactivity.

A specific content may be distinguished from its thematic disposition or arrangement—the existential category to which the specific content belongs.

Morbid conditions can vary in specific contents, but the thematic disposition may be the same.

c) *A position-taking*

Every experience conveys a position-taking or a personal value toward what is experienced. Content and personal value are often intertwined (Wyrsch 1949; Stanghellini 1997).

d) *An affective climate*

This is the what-it-is-like-to-be-in, the affective taint characterizing every experience (Nagel 1974). Some experiences are overwhelmed by the emotional climate. Sometimes an affective climate, such as psychotic anxiety, can deflagrate the form of experience (ruminative doubts of guilt may substantiate themselves in auditory verbal hallucinations).

Where is the Morbidity of Pathological Experiences?

What is not a normal experience is a complex question. The morbidity of an experience has not to be a mere normative judgment based on socio-political assumptions: psychiatry refuses to be centred on deviating social behavior. Morbid experiences impose themselves on a subject as a diktat. Patients experience the impossibility, or great difficulty, to transcend them.

Diktat experiences may:

A) impede the personal ability to resist, overwhelming the ability to cope and manage them (Stanghellini 1997). The threshold of pathological distress is inescapably subjective: patients frequently report suffering unmanageable or disabling distress, too intense or repetitive (Bolton 2013) to cope with. Even when morbid experiences are not ego-dystonic (i.e. manic euphoria), they are equally unmanageable

B) determine pain, withdrawal and solitude producing personal suffering, disability and impairment of expected, or willed, functions.(American Psychiatric Association 2013)

C) comport a rupture in the narrative continuity of life (Stanghellini 2013) or reveal, in the way they are given, the "corrosion" of basic structures of subjectivity (see above) originating psychotic or pre-psychotic symptoms. Interestingly in such as cases, the morbid experiences—in the way they take form—overpass the embodied limits imposed to the human species (i.e. thought broadcasting)

D) overwhelm the intersubjective validity of experiences that is their objective character, that is, the objectivity of perception (BInswanger 1957)

E) impose a loss of freedom, resulting in forms of derailment, corrosion, or alienation of the individuals' existential arrangement or presence in the world (Binswanger 1956)

In my opinion, one of these features is enough to depict an experience as pathological.

Patients lose the openness to the life-world, the possibility to project themselves in a common world with others, instead they experience a sense of "thrown-ness" as in a journey of no return.

Personal Narratives

We give sense to our experiences and that of others through language. Our native language represents a large stock of knowledge (Schutz 1962) we use to take account of our experiences and to communicate (Berger and Luckmann 1966). Narratives are linguistic meaningful reconstructions of life events (Stanghellini 2004).

In clinical or QR settings, we collect patients' experiences by means of their self-descriptions that depict what is moving within their consciousness.

Mental terms are highly polysemic: the same word (e.g. depression) may involve a manifold of experiences and meanings. In every case shared symbolism between researcher and patients has to be investigated.

Also, in describing mental states idiosyncratic metaphors that overpass any sociocultural boarder deserve the utmost attention.

Three main aspects of narratives have to be underpinned:

a) *Meaningfulness of narratives*

Man is an *animal symbolicum* (Cassirer 1923) and he is continuously engaged in conceptualizing reality. Facts, events, and objects are typified through linguistic meaningful constructs. Narratives are ever meaningful, even when they are poor or disconnected. They enact probabilistic connections between events, actions, moods, beliefs, values, etc. (Stanghellini 2004).

b) *Internal coherence of narratives*

This is the consistency of the linguistic structure, including syntactical arrangement, lexical articulation, temporal organization, and, finally, the absence of inexplicable contradictions (Lysaker et al. 2001).

c) *External coherence of narratives*

This is the sociocultural plausibility of the content as it matches social shared knowledge, symbolism, standards, values, and action (van Dijk 1980).

Every meaning displays a socially driven central core and a personal peripheral fringe. We are anchored to the social matrix of meanings but commonly reside also in the peripheral fringe (Schutz 1962). The cognitive style of everyday life world, also called natural attitude (Schutz 1962) and the standards of specific disciplines, draw the limits in which the sense of reality (objectivity) is preserved. Beyond these limits, meanings are immediately felt as original, strange, uncanny, and bizarre (Ballerini 2016a).

Transpersonal Constructs

Transpersonal constructs are the final aim of phenomenological psychopathology-oriented QR. They are synthetic schemes of comprehension; they outline the typical invariant features of anomalous experiences translating the first-person subjective perspective in third-person, objective descriptions (Stanghellini and Ballerini 2008). Transpersonal constructs reflect specific forms of patients' anomalous subjectivity—they describe efficaciously the existential arrangement of people affected by specific psychiatric disorders, contributing to the fine description of clinical phenotypes.

Transpersonal constructs may be considered the emergent prototypes, the central exemplars of a group of experiences that are similar in that they share a network of analogies (Wittgenstein 1953)

Prototypes are two-fold: they are the final results of the inquiry and the conceptual frameworks that help us to understand unstructured clinical reports.

There are first-order and second-order transpersonal constructs—the latter congregate in a single construct the meanings conveyed by the first. We may also distinguish *state*—and *trait-transpersonal constructs*, the latter being stable over time independently from clinical exacerbations. The very same transpersonal construct may appear to a lesser degree during the premorbid stage of a disorder, serving as a vulnerability marker, and it may heighten during the prodromal phase, becoming well-evident in the full-blown period.

THE BUILDING UP OF TRANSPERSONAL CONSTRUCTS

Transpersonal constructs are delineated by means of phenomenological "treatment" of patients' self-descriptions in order to advocate "the importance of the global grasping of a phenomenon as an organising and meaningful Gestalt" (Stanghellini and Ballerini 2008). This is the strategy to pursue.

a) *Suspension of the standard assumptions*

Collect patients' self-descriptions on the topic under investigation. For each one, suspend any common sense judgment; leave out any non-relevant (non-generalizable) personal biographical details; suspend assumptions on the mere formal description (i.e. specific form of symptomatology): Phenomenological psychopathology presumes general and clinical psychopathology but is primarily concerned to investigate how anomalous subjectivity reflects itself in patients' existential arrangement.

b) *Reduction and eidetic variation*

The overall meaning, that is, the essential feature of a given experience, emerges as "specific modes of appearance" (Gallagher and Zahavi 2012) of a structure of subjectivity within the experience itself (reduction). Sometimes a patient provides a declaration that appears to be a ready-to-hand, phenomenological treated, meaning structure. Such a description may serve as a proto-typical description.

Select similar experiences (sharing a common meaning organizer) using two method-ological strategies—denominated constant comparison and active sampling (Pidgeon and Henwood 1996).

a) *Constant Comparison*: collected data are compared, separated and finally grouped to-gether on the basis of their meaning resemblance. This is the way through which we can obtain significant categories.

b) *Active sampling*: as the process of investigation unfolds itself, new relevant cases are actively collected in order to deepen the researcher's emergent comprehension of phenomena.

Phenomenological psychopathology-oriented QM involves a dialectical relation between data collecting and interpretative procedure.

Ultimately, you will obtain a gallery of similar experiences: each one discloses an essen-tial feature that may be considered a variation of the very same core theme (*eidetic varia-tion*). Comparing this set of similar feature, you can grasp the essential core, the meaning organizer subtending all of these. This is a transpersonal construct and must reflect the morbid arrangement of a structure of subjectivity.

Define clearly the basic properties characterizing each and provide reliable operational definition and organize the hierarchic structure of emergent transpersonal constructs dis-tinguishing categories and sub-categories.

c) *Interpersonal corroboration*

Consensual qualitative research (CQR) is a well-established methodology (Hill et al. 2005) to promote interpersonal corroboration of QR findings, ensuring them a "first-level" objectivity.

A clear-cut procedure is available, making CQR methodology understandable, appli-cable, and reliable. The fundamental characteristic is "consensus" between researchers: the emergent findings require to be approved by independent judges. Consensus involves the whole process: the number and the type of transpersonal constructs, their denomination, and finally their operational definitions. CQR invokes findings articulated in categories and sub-categories, that is, second- and first-order constructs. To be relevant or "typical" a transpersonal construct must to be displayed—at least—by more than half of the sample. Typicality is a very elementary form of representativeness. It must not to be confounded with standardized validation procedures (see below).

Finally, a control group is necessary to assess the disorder specificity of the findings.

THE VALIDITY OF TRANSPERSONAL CONSTRUCTS

The exhaustive validation of transpersonal constructs is a very complex issue since it involves both phenomenological and empirical science criteria of validity.

Phenomenological Psychopathology-Oriented Qualitative Methodology Criteria of Validity

In my opinion, within the context of QR, validation is tied to five criteria:

1) Phenomenal validity represents the adequate, satisfactory, and comprehensive description of the experiential level, and may be ensured by vividness and richness of details.
   When new cases cannot provide further information, the topic under investigation may be considered "saturated" or completed.
2) Eidetic or prototypical validity is the power to capture the essential (invariant) meaningful organizer of manifold morbid experiences (see above). This criterion (and the following) is fulfilled by means of "consensus" between researchers and auditors, as required by CQR methodology.
3) Phenomenological (*sensu stricto*) validity is the capacity to illustrate efficaciously how anomalous subjectivity manifests in peculiar forms of lived experiences.
4) *Typicality* is an initial form of objectivity (interpersonal-validity) provided by the means of CQR methodology.
5) *Disorder-related specificity* requires that specific transpersonal constructs should be able to discriminate between specific forms of mental disorders since the latter entail diverse existential arrangements. If specific transpersonal constructs do not satisfy this criterion, they reflect a form of morbid subjectivity that manifests itself in diverse anomalous existential arrangements.

Empirical Science Standards of Validity

Refined transpersonal constructs may be employed to draw rating scales that, in turn, must be validated according psychometric standards (i.e. explained variance, reliability, stability, sensibility, concurrent and divergent validity). This step is necessary to produce effectively generalizable (objective) data.

Exhaustively valid transpersonal constructs represent a form of naturalized phenomenology since they effectively convert the first-person perspective in third-person (transpersonal) objective constructs.

CONCLUSION: CAUTIONARY REMARKS ON QUALITATIVE RESEARCH

QR is useful for explorative studies of very complex, still uninvestigated topics, or to explore the real-world relevance of variables, usually investigated in laboratory paradigms. Hypothesis formulation is a major advantage of QR: findings may serve as the starting-point to formulate assessment tools to be further validated with standardized procedures (see Stanghellini, Ballerini, and Cutting 2014; Stanghellini, Ballerini, and Lysaker 2014). There are many excellent examples of phenomenological psychopathology-oriented QR—see studies concerning (in the context of schizophrenia) anomalies of self-experience (Sass and Parnas 2003), system of values (Stanghellini and Ballerini 2007), experience of social relationships (Stanghellini and Ballerini 2011b), the lived body (Stanghellini et al. 2014), and temporality (Stanghellini et al. 2016).

Recently I have discussed the notion of autism in schizophrenia analyzing—in a paradigmatic case—the distortions of the (basic and high order) structures of subjectivity (Ballerini 2016b).

QMs do not consent any form of correlation between findings or between findings and clinical or socio-demographical characteristics. QR is generally "cross-sectional" and it does not appear well conceived for longitudinal, long-term studies. A potential limitation of qualitative studies is that they may imply a selection bias excluding patients noncompliant to a dialogical approach. Finally, patients with high linguistic competence may be over-represented.

ACKNOWLEDGMENTS

For linguistic revision, Barbara Ciomei, European University Institute, Florence, Italy.

BIBLIOGRAPHY

American Psychiatric Association. (2013). *Diagnostic and Statistical Manual of Mental Disorders*, 5th edn. Washington DC.

Ballerini M. (2016a). "Semantic Processing and Semantic Experience in People with Schizophrenia: A Bridge between Phenomenological Psychopathology and Neuroscience?" *Journal of Psychopathology* 22: 94–105.

Ballerini M. (2016b). "Autism in Schizophrenia: A Phenomenological Study." In: G. Stanghellini and M. Aragona (eds), An Experiential Approach to Psychopathology What is it like to Suffer from Mental Disorders? pp. 281–300. New York: Springer.

Berger P. L. and Luckmann T. (1966). *The Social Construction of Reality*. New York: Doubleday.

Binswanger L. (1956). *Drei Formen Missglueckten Daseins*. Tubingen: Niemeyer.

Binswanger L. (1957). *Schizophrenie*. Pfullingen: Neske.

Bolton D. (2013). "What is Mental Illness?" In K. W. M. Fulford, M. Davies, R. G. T. Gipps, G. Graham, J. Z. Sadler, G. Stanghellini, et al. (eds.), *Handbook of Philosophy and Psychiatry*, pp. 434–450. Oxford: Oxford University Press.

Bolton D. (2013) and Damasio (2000): Cassirer E. (1923). *Philosophie der symbolischen Formen. Erster Teil. Die Sprache*. Berlin: B. Cassirer.

Damasio A. (2000). *What Happens: Body, Emotion and the Making of Consciousness*. London: Vintage.

Denzin N. K. and Lincoln Y. S. (2000). *Handbook of Qualitative Research*, 2nd edn. Thousand Oaks: Sage Publications.

Fossey E., Harve C., McDermott F., and Davidson L. (2002). "Understanding and Evaluating Qualitative Research." *Australian and New Zealand Journal of Psychiatry* 36: 717–732.

Fuchs T. (2010). "Phenomenology and Psychopathology." In D. Schmicking and S. Gallagher (eds.), *Handbook of Phenomenology and Cognitive Science*, pp. 547–573. Berlin, Heidelberg, New York: Springer.

Fuster J. M. (2003). *Cortex and Mind—Unifying Cognition*. Oxford: Oxford University Press.

Gallagher S. (2005). *How the Body Shapes the Mind*. Oxford: Oxford University Press.

Gallagher S. (2013a). "A Pattern Theory of Self." *Frontiers in Human Neuroscience* 7: 1–7.

Gallagher S. (2013b). "Intersubjectivity and Psychopathology." In K. W. M. Fulford, M. Davies, R.G.T. Gipps, G. Graham, J. Z. Sadler, G. Stanghellini, et al. (eds.), *Handbook of Philosophy and Psychiatry*, pp. 258–274. Oxford: Oxford University Press.

Gallagher S. and Varela F. J. (2003). "Re-Drawing the Map and Resetting the Time: Phenomenology and the Cognitive Sciences." *Canadian Journal of Philosophy* 29 (suppl): 93–132.

Gallagher S. and Zahavi D. (2012). *The Phenomenological Mind*, 2nd edn. London and New York: Routledge.

Gallese V. and Sinigaglia C. (2011). "What Is So Special About Embodied Simulation?" *Trends in Cognitive Sciences* 15(11): 512–519.

Glaser B. G. (2002). "Conceptualization: On Theory and Theorizing Using Grounded Theory." *International Journal of Qualitative Methods* 1.

Glesne C. and Peshkin A. (1992) *Becoming Qualitative Researchers: An Introduction*. White Plains, New York: Longman.

Heidegger M. (1927). *Sein und Zeit*. Halle: Niemeyer.

Henry M. (1990). *Phénoménologie Materielle*. Paris: Presses Universitaires de France.

Hill C. E., Knox S., Thompson, B. J, Williams E. N., Hess S. A., and Ladany N. (2005). "Consensual Qualitative Research: An Update." *Journal of Counseling Psychology* 52(2). doi:10.1037/0022-0167.52.2.196

Husserl E. (1971a). "Ideen zu einer reinen Phänomenologie und phänomenologischen Philosophie (*Erstes Buch: Allgemeine Einführung in die reine Phänomenologie*)," ed. K. Schumann, Husserliana III Nijoff the Hague; trans. F. Kersten, *Ideas Pertaining To A Pure Phenomenology And To A Phenomenological Philosophy* (1st book, 1980). The Hague: Nijoff.

Husserl E. (1971b). "Ideen zu einer reinen Phänomenologie und phänomenologischen Philosophie" (Drittes Buch: Die Phänomenologie und die Fundamente der Wissenschaften), ed. V. Marly Biemel Husserliana, trans. T. E. Klein, *Ideas Pertaining To A Pure Phenomenology And To A Phenomenological Philosophy* (3rd book). The Hague: Nijoff.

Husserl E. (1991). *On the Phenomenology of the Consciousness of Internal Time*, trans. and ed. J. B. Brough. Dordrecht and Boston: Kluwer Academic Publishers.

Husserl E. (2000). *Logical Investigations* (vol. 2). London: Routledge.

Hutto D. D. (2013). "Interpersonal Relating." In K. W. M. Fulford, M. Davies, R. G. T. Gipps, G. Graham, J. Z. Sadler, G. Stanghellini, et al. (eds.), *Handbook of Philosophy and Psychiatry*, pp. 249–257. Oxford: Oxford University Press.

Jaspers K. (1913). *Allgemeine Psychopathologie*. Berlin: Springer.

Lutz A. and Thompson E. (2003). "Neurophenomenology Integrating Subjective Experience and Brain Dynamics in the Neuroscience of Consciousness." *Journal of Consciousness Studies* 10(9–10): 31–52.

Lysaker P. H., Lysaker J. T. and Lysaker J.T. (2001). "Schizophrenia and the Collapse of the Dialogical Self: Recovery, Narrative and Psychotherapy." *Psychotherapy* 38: 252–261.

Merleau-Ponty M. (1945). *Phénoménologie De La Perception*. Paris: Gallimard.

Nagel T. (1974). "What is it Like to be a Bat?" *Philosophical Review* 83: 435–450.

Nelson B., Whitford T. J., Lavoie S., and Sass L. A. (2014). "What are the Neurocognitive Correlates of Basic Self-Disturbance in Schizophrenia? Integrating Phenomenology and

Neurocognition. Part 1 (Source Monitoring Deficits)." *Schizophrenia Research* January, 152(1): 12–19.

Nordgaard J., Sass L. A., and Parnas J. (2013). "The Psychiatric Interview: Validity, Structure, and Subjectivity." *European Archives of Psychiatry and Clinical Neuroscience*, June 263(4): 353–364.

Palinkas L. A. (2014). "Qualitative and Mixed Methods in Mental Health Services and Implementation Research." *Journal of Clinical Child Adolescent Psychology* 43(6): 851–861.

Parnas J., Møller P., Kircher T., et al. (2005). "EASE: Examination of Anomalous Self-Experience." *Psychopathology* 38: 236–258.

Parnas J., Sass L. A., and Zahavi D. (2013). "Rediscovering Psychopathology: The Epistemology and Phenomenology of the Psychiatric Object." *Schizophrenia Bulletin* March, 39(2): 270–277.

Pidgeon N. and Henwood K. (1996). "Grounded Theory: Practical Implementation." In J. T. Richardson (ed.), *Handbook of Qualitative Research Methods for Psychology and the Social Sciences*, pp. 86–101. Leicester: The British Psychological Society.

Razafsha M., Behforuzi H., Azari H., Zhang Z., Wang K. K., Kobeissy F.H., and Gold M. S. (2012). "Qualitative Versus Quantitative Methods." *Psychiatric Research Methods in Molecular Biology* 829: 49–62.

Ricoeur P. (1984). *Temps et récit. Tome II: La configuration dans le récit de fiction* Le Seuil.

Roy J. M., Petitot J., Pachoud B., and Varela F. J. (1999). "Beyond The Gap An Introduction To Naturalizing Phenomenology." In J. M. Roy, J. Petitot, B. Pachoud, and F. J. Varela (eds.), *Naturalizing Phenomenology*, pp. 1–53. Stanford: Stanford University Press.

Sartre J. P. (1943). *l'Être et le Nèant*. Paris: Gallimard.

Sass L. A. and Parnas J. (2003). "Schizophrenia, Consciousness, and the Self." *Schizophrenia Bulletin* 29(3): 427–444.

Schutz A. (1962). "Symbol, Reality and Society." In A. Schutz, *Collected Papers*, vol I. Den Haag: M. Nijhoff.

Shank G. (2002). *Qualitative Research. A Personal Skills Approach*. New Jersey: Merill Prentice Hall.

Stanghellini G. (1997). "For an Anthropology of Vulnerability." *Psychopathology* 30: 1–11.

Stanghellini G. (2004). "The Puzzle of the Psychiatric Interview." *Journal of Phenomenological Psychology* 35(2): 173–195.

Stanghellini G. (2013). "Philosophical Resources for the Psychiatric Interview." In K. W. M. Fulford, M. Davies, R. G. T. Gipps, G. Graham, J. Z. Sadler, G. Stanghellini, et al. (eds.), *Handbook of Philosophy and Psychiatry*, pp. 321–358. Oxford: Oxford University Press.

Stanghellini G. and Ballerini M. (2007). "Values in Persons With Schizophrenia." *Schizophrenia Bulletin* 33(1): 131–141.

Stanghellini G. and Ballerini M. (2008). "Qualitative Analysis: Its Use in Psychopathological Research." *Acta Psychiatrica Scandinavica* 117(3): 161–163.

Stanghellini G. and Ballerini M. (2011a). "What is it Like to be a Person with Schizophrenia in the Social World? A First-Person Perspective Study on Schizophrenic Dissociality—Part 1: State of the Art." *Psychopathology* 44(3): 172–182.

Stanghellini G. and Ballerini M. (2011b). "What is it Like to be a Person with Schizophrenia in the Social World? A First-Person Perspective Study on Schizophrenic Dissociality—Part 2: Methodological Issues and Empirical Findings." *Psychopathology* 44(3): 183–192.

Stanghellini G., Ballerini M., and Cutting J. (2014). "Abnormal Bodily Phenomena Questionnaire." *Journal of Psychopathology* 20: 138–143.

Stanghellini G., Ballerini M., and Lysaker P. H. (2014). "Autism Rating Scale." *Journal of Psychopathology* 20: 273–285.

Stanghellini G., Ballerini M., Blasi S., Mancini M., Presenza S., Raballo A., and Cutting J. (2014). "The Bodily Self: A Qualitative Study of Abnormal Bodily Phenomena in Persons With Schizophrenia." *Comprehensive Psychiatry* 55(7): 1703–1711.

Stanghellini G., Ballerini M., Presenza S., Mancini M., Raballo A., Blasi S., and Cutting J. (2016). "Psychopathology of Lived Time: Abnormal Time Experience in Persons With Schizophrenia." *Schizophrenia Bulletin* January, 42(1): 45–55.

Straus E. (1935). *Von Sinn der Sinne*. Berlin, Gottingen, Heidelberg: Springer.

van Dijk T. A. (1980) *Macrostructures: An Interdisciplinary Study of Global Structures in Discourse, Interaction, and Cognition*. Hillsdale: Erlbaum.

Van Gulick R. (2014). "Consciousness." In the *Stanford Encyclopedia of Philosophy*, ed. E. N. Zalta (first published Friday, June 18, substantive revision Tuesday, January 14. http://plato. stanford.edu/entries/consciousness/archives/

Varela F. J. (1996). "Neurophenomenology: A Methodological Remedy to the Hard Problem." *Journal of Consciousness Studies* 3: 330–350.

Varela F. J., Thompson E., and Rosch E. (1991). *The Embodied Mind: Cognitive Science And Human Experience*. Cambridge MA: MIT Press.

Wittgenestein L. (1953). *Philosophical Investigations*. New York: Macmillan.

Wyrsch J. (1949). *Die Person des Schizophrenen*. Studien zur Kilinik, Psychologie, Daseinsweise. Bern: Haupt.

Zahavi D. (2005). *Subjectivity and Selfhood: Investigating the First-Person Perspective*. Cambridge MA: MIT Press.

CHAPTER 87

PHENOMENOLOGICAL PSYCHOPATHOLOGY AND QUANTITATIVE RESEARCH

JULIE NORDGAARD AND MADS GRAM HENRIKSEN

INTRODUCTION

IN this article, we explore phenomenological psychopathology and discuss how this approach may be translated to quantitative research in psychiatry. Since phenomenological psychopathology is closely tied to the philosophical discipline of phenomenology, founded by Husserl and continued by philosophers such as Heidegger, Sartre, and Merleau-Ponty, an initial description of a few key features of phenomenology will be relevant. We then outline central characteristics of phenomenological psychopathology before examining, using the "EASE: Examination of Anomalous Self-Experience" scale (Parnas et al. 2005a) as an example, how this approach can, to some extent, be translated to quantitative-empirical research.

PHENOMENOLOGY

Phenomenology is usually defined as the study of phenomena.[1] In this context, phenomena designate that which appears in our subjective experience, for example, perceived or imagined objects or others. In the following, we briefly present three key features of phenomenology. First, phenomenology is characterized by a kind of essentialism (Merleau-Ponty 2002: vii), that is, phenomenology is not interested in mere description, however detailed and fine-grained, of empirical or mental objects, but in uncovering the essential, invariant

---

[1] For a detailed analysis of the concept of phenomenology, see para. 7 in Heidegger's *Being and Time* (Heidegger 2007: 49–63).

structures of its objects of inquiry.[2] Second, phenomenological inquiries do not start from a detached, theoretical stance but begin from factual existence, that is, from our already established relation to the world. The manner in which objects appear in our experiences (their *how-ness*) is considered to reveal something about their essence (their *what-ness* or *quidditas*). For example, spatial objects never appear in their totality but always in a partial way, from a certain perspective and distance. Given that objects always appear before an experiencing subject, the first-person perspective has a natural privilege in phenomenology, which also emphasizes that subjectivity always is embodied and embedded in a social, cultural, and historical context. Third, phenomenology is a form of transcendental philosophy, that is, it explores the conditions of possibility for experience and objectivity. Not only does phenomenology take its point of departure in factual existence, it radically strives to grasp our immediate, antepredicative, and pre-reflective contact with the world, which is always already there, prior to any philosophical reflection or scientific knowledge we may have of it. For example, phenomenology argues that consciousness essentially is characterized by intentionality (e.g. Husserl 2008; Sartre 2003), that is, *consciousness is consciousness of something* (e.g. the tree I perceive, remember, or imagine) *for someone* (i.e. the experiencing subject). Intentionality discloses simultaneously the world-directedness and self-manifestation of consciousness and therefore, from a phenomenological perspective, consciousness (as well as its disorders in psychopathology) cannot be satisfactorily studied as a mere object in the world, since it is fundamentally correlated to the experiencing subject.

PHENOMENOLOGICAL PSYCHOPATHOLOGY

Psychopathology is the study of distorted subjective experience (symptoms) and expressions (signs) and it forms the bedrock of psychiatry as a scientific and therapeutic discipline. Naturally, precise description of symptoms and signs is crucial to psychiatry. In mainstream psychiatry, the term "phenomenology" is often used synonymously with that of "descriptive psychopathology." It would, as we shall see, be a crude mistake to consider phenomenological psychopathology as a merely descriptive enterprise. In the following, simplified presentation of phenomenological psychopathology, we limit ourselves to three interconnected characteristics.[3]

---

[2] In other words, phenomenology aims at grasping necessary properties of the objects of investigation, i.e. properties that these objects cannot lack without ceasing to be these very objects. e.g. if we seek to uncover the essence of a sphere, we soon realize that properties such as mass and color are accidental properties—they are properties that may vary in different spheres. However, what cannot vary or lack, without a sphere ceasing to be a sphere, is the property that every point on its surface must be equidistant from its center—this is not an accidental but a necessary and sufficient property, articulating the very essence of the sphere. As a philosophical discipline, phenomenology has explored the essence of, e.g. perception or consciousness (e.g. Merleau-Ponty 2002; Husserl 2008) and existence (e.g. Heidegger 2007; Sartre 2003). From these works, it is also clear that phenomenology does not regard "essences" as somehow fixed entities, independent from historical development (e.g. Husserl 1984).

[3] We focus here only on the experiential dimension, leaving other important dimensions such as expression and behavior unaddressed (see instead Jansson and Nordgaard 2016). For an excellent anthology on the tradition of phenomenological psychopathology, see Broome et al. (2012).

First, phenomenological psychopathology tries to grasp patients' anomalous or abnormal experiences, for example, reflected in certain experiential *contents* such as the verbal content of a hallucinatory voice or the feeling of being depressed. More specifically, phenomenological psychopathology strives to "stay with" or "keep focus on" the patients' experiences, exploring "how" they are experienced by the patients themselves rather than inquiring into "why" the patients believe they are undergoing these experiences (which can of course often also be relevant for diagnostic or therapeutic purposes). For example, when asked about how she experienced her own body, a young female patient with schizophrenia reported, "I feel I have this void inside. I try to fill it with food but that isn't working well." When asked to clarify this vague complaint, she said, "I think the void is a feeling of inadequacy, loneliness, a feeling of not being sufficient, and lack of meaning. I really don't know who I am, what I'm supposed to do, and what I'm here for." This description casts a different light on the initial complaint, now indicating experiences of meaninglessness and a wavering sense of identity or self. In an effort to further clarify and grasp the nature of her experience, she was asked if the void has a spatial location. She replied, "Yes, I actually feel that it's right in the solar plexus. I feel it's gigantic, larger than my body. Like a big Pilates ball perhaps. There, I'm missing something. Some meaning is missing. I can physically feel the void. I have had it for many years. There is a space that is not filled out with anything. There's just a black void." The example illustrates how a phenomenological inquiry, keeping focus on the experience, may reveal psychopathological phenomena (in this case, somatic depersonalization and wavering sense of basic self) beneath an initially vague complaint.

Second, to grasp the patients' experiences, it is not sufficient to explore only their experiential content; the *form* of these experiences must also be examined (e.g. Henriksen 2013). For example, if a patient reports that she has the experience of "being looked at when walking in the street," it is critical to clarify the quality and form of her experience. For example, is this experience of self-reference on a delusional level or is it rather an "as-if" experience (i.e. with fairly intact reality judgment)? Moreover, is the experience of self-reference *secondary* to other mental states, exhibiting the thematic quality of these states—for example, is it an experience of others looking *reproachfully* at her (as often seen in depression) or of others looking *admiringly* at her (perhaps indicative of a hypo-manic state). Or is it a *primary*, athematic experience of being the center of others' attention *for no apparent reason* (indicative of a schizophrenia spectrum disorders) (Jansson and Nordgaard 2016: 142f.)? Moreover, certain psychotic experiences, for example, experiences of others having access to one's own thoughts or experiences of one's own movements being controlled by an external force, do not only involve abnormal experiential contents but seem also to involve a disturbance of certain basic structures of consciousness, for example, ego-boundaries (Schneider 1950; Nordgaard et al. 2008; Parnas and Henriksen 2016a). The importance of exploring the form of experience is hardly a new insight in psychiatry but rather an old and almost forgotten one—here in the words of Binet and Simon, "Some symptoms are characteristic, others are banal, or rather, in every symptom there is a banal part to be neglected and a characteristic part to remember. We must clarify the specific characteristics of each form of the symptoms studied, because *what matters most are not the symptoms but the mental state which conditions them*" (quoted in Jansson and Nordgaard 2016: 98; emphasis added). This brings us to our third characteristic.

Finally, subjective experiences, pathological or not, never appear in an atomistic, isolated, or free-floating fashion but are always embedded in an experiential, meaningful totality or gestalt—a web of mutually implicative relations that jointly facilitate a sense of meaning and coherence. Though it is often necessary to key in on and explore specific anomalous or abnormal experiences to clarify their precise content and form (vide supra), such a maneuver invariably entails an element of abstraction and this must always be kept in mind. In other words, an exclusive focus on singular symptoms and signs loses sight of the overarching experiential gestalt in which the subjective experiences are embedded and from which they receive their meaning, thereby basically distorting the reality of the patients' lived experiences. Unfortunately, this is more or less what occurred in the wake of the so-called "operational" revolution in psychiatry, which took place with the publication of DSM-III (APA 1980). The current edition, namely DSM-5 (APA 2013), focuses exclusively on discrete symptoms and signs, and diagnosing mental disorders consists simply in identifying and counting a sufficient number of symptoms or signs. After nearly four decades of operational psychiatry, psychiatry finds itself in state of crisis: we no longer see the forest (gestalt/syndrome) for the trees (symptoms and signs), psychopathological and differential-diagnostic knowledge is declining (Parnas 2015; 2017), nearly all features of psychopathology seem "dimensional" (Parnas and Henriksen 2016b), and psychiatric comorbidity is rapidly increasing (Maj 2005).

Phenomenological psychopathology offers resources to overcome this crisis, for example, by reasserting the importance of grasping the underlying psychopathological gestalt in diagnostic assessments. A gestalt is a characteristic phenomenological pattern, that is, a unifying structure of experiential, expressive, and behavioral phenomena, centered upon prototypical cases with a diminishing typicality toward the boundaries of the diagnostic category, where it may overlap other diagnostic categories (Jansson and Nordgaard 2016: 19f.; Nordgaard et al. 2013; Zandersen et al. in press). The relation between the gestalt and its manifestations (symptoms and signs) is reciprocal: the gestalt confers certain typicality on its concrete manifestations, while these manifestations simultaneously infuse the gestalt with its specific clinical rootedness (Parnas 2011; 2012). Crucially, different mental disorders have distinctive psychopathological gestalts, and a key point, repeatedly advocated by phenomenological psychopathology, is that this is the only valid way to grasp complex unities (e.g. the psyche). For example, Jaspers stressed, "In grasping particulars we make a mistake if we forget the comprehensive whole in which and through which they exist . . . the whole comes before its parts; the whole is not the sum of its parts, it is more than them; it is an independent and original source; it is form" (Jaspers 1997: 28–29). In other words, the specificity of mental disorders is not graspable at the level of singular symptoms and signs but only at the gestalt level. Since all symptoms and signs bear an imprint of the psychopathological gestalt they are a part of (e.g. vide supra on self-reference), identifying this imprint is central in any differential-diagnostic assessment. This identification, however, is not possible by non-clinicians, using a highly structured diagnostic interview schedule and where diagnosis are derived solely from (computer) algorithms, but requires substantial clinical experience, interviewing skills, education in psychopathology and differential-diagnosis, and supervision by experts.[4]

For example, according to both classical and recent phenomenologically oriented research on schizophrenia, the core of the schizophrenia gestalt is reflected in certain

---

[4] For details on the differential-diagnostic interview and insights into the core gestalt of different mental disorders, see Jansson and Nordgaard (2016).

specific, trait-like, non-psychotic features (e.g. fundamental symptoms (Bleuler 1950) and self-disorders (Parnas et al. 2005a)) and not in state-like or episodic features (e.g. positive symptoms). In other words, the basic, trait-like, non-psychotic features reflect the phenomenological essence of the disorder. Where Bleuler's fundamental symptoms largely were expressive features (signs), observable by the clinician, self-disorders are subjectively lived experiential anomalies (symptoms). In contemporary phenomenological psychopathology, self-disorders are best examined with the Examination of Anomalous Self-Experience (EASE) scale (Parnas et al. 2005a). The EASE offers a systematic exploration of the subjective, experiential dimension in schizophrenia spectrum disorders, allowing the clinician to identify some of the essential disturbances and thereby to grasp core aspects of the psychopathological gestalt of schizophrenia. To make these claims more tangible, we will in the following use the EASE scale as an example of how phenomenological psychopathology can be used to obtain detailed qualitative information about certain subjective disturbances and how this information then can be translated into quantitative data and analysis.

EASE AND QUANTITATIVE RESEARCH

The EASE scale offers a systematic, qualitative, and quantitative, semi-structured exploration of a variety of anomalous self-experiences (i.e. self-disorders), which, in different ways and on different levels, reflect a disordered or unstable experiential self.[5] The impetus that eventually led to the construction of the EASE scale arose from clinical work in a unit for young, first-admission patients, whom, it was suspected, were suffering from a schizophrenia spectrum disorder. Over a four-year period, Drs. Josef Parnas and Lennart Jansson interviewed approximately 100 patients with the purpose of exploring and grasping subjective, experiential aspects of schizophrenic autism (Parnas et al. 2005a: 237; Parnas and Bovet 1991). These comprehensive, in-depth, psychopathological interviews were phenomenologically oriented, open-ended, and tried to stimulate spontaneous self-reports about the patients' experiential life. A central finding was that many of these patients, in a relatively uniform way, reported an enduring lack of identity and feelings of self-transformation, and these experiences appeared to be at the very heart of the patients' suffering. These initial observations were later confirmed in two independent, systematic studies from Denmark (Parnas et al. 1998) and Norway (Møller and Husby 2000), respectively. In addition to the initial clinical interviews and the empirical data from the systematic studies, the EASE scale was inspired by classical descriptions of these subtle psychopathological phenomena primarily from the German and French tradition (found, e.g. in the works of Janet, Bleuler, Gruhle, Berze, Minkowski, and Blankenburg), by the work on "basic symptoms" by Huber,

---

[5] The notion of "self" refers here to the first-personal givenness of experience, which implies an immediate, pre-reflective sense of ipseity (Sass and Parnas 2003), for-me-ness (Zahavi 2014) or self-presence that transpires through the flux of time and changing modalities of consciousness and imbues all subjective experiences with a foundational, elusive, yet vital feeling of "I-me-myself." It is this minimal level of experiential selfhood that is disturbed in the schizophrenia spectrum disorders and often with consequences also at more complex, sophisticated levels of selfhood (see Parnas and Henriksen, "Selfhood and its Disorders," chapter 52 in this volume).

Gross, Klosterkötter, Schultze-Lutter, and their colleagues (e.g. Gross et al. 1987), and inputs from philosophy, especially Husserlian phenomenology (Parnas and Zahavi 2002; Sass and Parnas 2003). The EASE was created in collaboration between senior interdisciplinary scholars from three European countries, and it was finally published in 2005 (Parnas et al. 2005a). Today, it has been translated into fourteen languages (see www.easenet.dk for details).

The EASE scale comprises fifty-seven main items, aggregated into five domains: 1) Cognition and Stream of Consciousness; 2) Self-Awareness and Presence; 3) Bodily Experiences; 4) Demarcation/Transitivism; and 5) Existential Reorientation/Solipsism. Psychometric testing of the EASE scale has shown an excellent internal consistency—Nordgaard and Parnas (2014) reported a Chronbach's alpha coefficient $\alpha=0.90$ and Møller and colleagues (2011) reported $\alpha > 0.85$. A principal component analysis, using varimax rotation, of the five EASE domains yielded a one-factor solution, accounting for 59.8% of the total variance (Nordgaard and Parnas 2014). Good to excellent inter-rater reliability has been found among trained and experienced psychiatrists (Parnas et al. 2005b; Møller et al. 2011; Nordgaard and Parnas 2012). One study found an overall inter-rater reliability of the EASE total score above 0.80 (Spearman's coefficient, $p<0.001$) and a Cohen's kappa of 0.65 (Haug et al. 2012a). Another study reported nearly perfect agreement with a Cohen's kappa of 0.94 for the full EASE scale (Nordgaard and Parnas 2012), kappa values between 0.89–0.95 for the five EASE domains, and kappa values above 0.81 for all but two individual EASE items (Nordgaard and Parnas 2012). In other words, a high level of inter-rater reliability is achievable for the EASE scale. However, it must be noted that reliable scoring of EASE items requires extensive psychopathological knowledge, clinical experience, and training in the phenomenological use of the EASE scale. If the EASE scale is intended for research purposes, we strongly recommend following the certification program (see www.easenet.dk).

The EASE interview must always be performed in a semi-structured way, requiring that the interviewer is intimately familiar with the relevant psychopathology, specifically trained in how to inquire into the kind of experiences that are described in the EASE, and knowing precisely what is required to score EASE items as present or absent. All EASE items must be explored in the synchronic and diachronic context of other experiences, for example, does the relevant experience only occur in certain situations or it is situationally unbound? Does it have a state-like or trait-like character, that is, is it merely episodic or does it tend to articulate itself as a recurrent feature of the patient's conscious life (the latter must be the case)? To score an EASE item as present, the patient must always describe in detail and in his own words at least one concrete example of a relevant experience, and only by assessing this experience may the interviewer score the EASE item as present, if the experience fulfils the relevant item definition. In other words, a simple, affirmative answer ("yes") to a question about an EASE item is never enough to rate this item as present. Similarly, a simple, dissenting answer ("no") to a question about an EASE item is also not sufficient to rate this item as absent, if the patient, perhaps elsewhere the interview, offers a concrete example of the experience that addresses the EASE item in question. In both case, it is only the patient's concrete examples of her experiences that are assessed.[6] Crucially, many items in the EASE

---

[6] For details about how to conduct an EASE interview, see Parnas et al. (2005: 238f.) and Henriksen and Nordgaard (2016).

scale do not primarily target an anomalous experiential content but also the form of these experiences. For example, what is distinctive about "thought pressure" (EASE item 1.3) is not simply an experience of "having lots of thoughts" but the form of this experience. One patient with schizophrenia vividly described thought pressure in the following way: "My thoughts are like rockets, shooting in all directions at once. It's one big chaos" (Henriksen and Nordgaard 2014: 437). Thought pressure can be defined as rapid and/or parallel trains of thoughts that occur with a clear loss of meaning. In other words, it is the form of the experience rather than the specific contents of the different trains of thoughts that are essential when assessing the presence or absence of thought pressure. Patients with depression may also report "having lots of thoughts," but the form of their experiences is typically remarkably different. Usually, their thoughts are not disconnected but revolve around a common, dominant theme, for example, feelings of guilt or inferiority, and there is accordingly no similar loss of meaning. In this regard, the form of these experiences, which may come to light by exploring experiential contents, enables a distinction between thought pressure and ruminations. The task of the interviewer is to try to capture such essential features of the patients' anomalous self-experience.

The publication of the EASE scale has provoked huge interest, not only in the scale itself but also in phenomenological psychopathology and philosophical phenomenology more generally. Empirical EASE studies have been launched worldwide and, in the following, we list a few of the central results: i) self-disorders hyper-aggregate in schizophrenia spectrum disorders but not in other mental disorders (Parnas et al. 2005b; Raballo et al. 2011; Raballo and Parnas 2012; Haug et al. 2012a; Nordgaard and Parnas 2014); ii) the levels of self-disorders are similar among patients with schizophrenia and patients with the schizotypal disorder (Raballo and Parnas 2012; Nordgaard and Parnas 2014); iii) prospective studies indicate that self-disorders predict transition to psychosis in an ultra-high risk for psychosis sample (Nelson et al. 2012) and that high baseline scores of self-disorders predict later transition to a schizophrenia spectrum diagnosis (Parnas et al. 2011; 2016)—suggesting that self-disorders may be a unique candidate for early detection purposes (Nordgaard and Henriksen 2016); iv) self-disorders correlate with positive symptoms, negative symptoms, formal thought disorders, and perceptual disturbances, respectively (Nordgaard and Parnas 2014), but not with IQ or neurocognitive measures (Haug et al. 2012b; Nordgaard et al. 2015), except for impaired verbal memory (Haug et al. 2012b); and v) self-disorders are temporarily stable over a five-year period (Nordgaard et al. 2017, 2018)–for a review of the empirical studies, see Parnas and Henriksen (2014). Recently, there has been growing interest in trying to identify possible correlations between self-disorders and neurobiology (e.g. Borda and Sass 2015; Sass and Borda 2015; Mishara et al. 2016) and neurocognition (e.g. Sass, this volume; Nelson et al. 2014a; 2014b), respectively.

CONCLUSION

We have outlined core features of phenomenology and phenomenological psychopathology and used the EASE scale to exemplify how insights from the former disciplines can be translated into empirical and quantitative research in psychiatry. In brief, the EASE scale was initially developed through a series of comprehensive, phenomenologically oriented, open-ended psychopathological interviews conducted by senior research clinicians, striving to stimulate spontaneous self-reports about the patients' experiential life and eventually keying in on essential features of the patients' anomalies of self-experience (self-disorders). The scale was also informed by classical descriptions of subtle psychopathological phenomena, especially in the French and German tradition, by the work on "basic symptoms," and by philosophical insight from especially phenomenology. Not only was the scale informed by phenomenology, the EASE interviews themselves must also be conducted in a phenomenologically faithful way, that is, by conducting the interview in a semi-structured, conversational manner, by keeping focus on the patients' lived experiences (rather than possible explanations of their experiences), by identifying essential features of the patients' anomalies of self-experience, by exploring their state- or trait-like status, and by evaluating all self-disorders and other symptoms contextually. Finally, EASE ratings (items scored as present or absent) can then be subjected to quantitative, statistical data analysis. One of the most visible results of the impact of EASE research specifically and contemporary phenomenological psychopathology generally is the inclusion of "disturbances of self-experience" (i.e. self-disorders) as a defining feature of schizophrenia in the beta-version of the ICD-11. Whether or not this formulation will also be found in the published version remains to be seen. Finally, it should be noted that a new psychometric instrument, that is, the "EAWE: Examination of Anomalous World Experience" (Sass et al. 2017) has recently been published, allowing for further exploration and analysis of patients' experiences of the lived world.

Bibliography

American Psychiatric Association. (1980). *Diagnostic and Statistical Manual of Mental Disorders: DSM-III.* Washington: APA.

American Psychiatric Association. (2013). *Diagnostic and Statistical Manual of Mental Disorders: DSM-5.* Arlington: APA.

Bleuler E. (1950). *Dementia Praecox or the Group of Schizophrenias,* trans. J. Zinkin. New York: International University Press.

Borda J. P. and Sass L. A. (2015). "Phenomenology and Neurobiology of Self Disorder in Schizophrenia: Primary Factors." *Schizophrenia Research* 169: 464–473.

Broome M. R., Harland R., Owen G. S., and Stringaris A. (2012). *The Maudsley Reader in Phenomenological Psychiatry.* New York: Cambridge University Press.

Gross G., Huber G., Klosterkötter J., and Linz M. (1987). *Bonner Skala Für die Beurteilung von Basissymptomen.* Berlin, Heidelberg: Springer.

Haug E., Lien L., Raballo A., Bratlien U., Øie M., Andreassen O. A., et al. (2012a). "Selective Aggregation of Self-disorders in First-treatment DSM-IV Schizophrenia Spectrum Disorders." *Journal of Nervous and Mental Disease* 200: 632–636.

Haug E., Øie M., Melle I., Andreassen O. A., Raballo A., Bratlien U., et al. (2012b). "The Association Between Self-Disorders and Neurocognitive Dysfunction in Schizophrenia. *Schizophrenia Research* 135: 79–83.

Heidegger M. (2007). *Being and Time,* trans. J. Macquarrie and E. Robinson. Oxford: Blackwell.

Henriksen M. G. (2013). "On Incomprehensibility in Schizophrenia." *Phenomenology and the Cognitive Sciences* 12: 105–129.

Henriksen M. G. and Nordgaard J. (2014). "Schizophrenia as a Disorder of the Self." *Journal of Psychopathology* 20: 435–441.

Henriksen M. G. and Nordgaard J. (2016). "Self-disorders in Schizophrenia." In G. Stanghellini and M. Aragona (eds.), *An Experiential Approach to Psychopathology. What is it like to Suffer from Mental Disorders*, pp. 265–280. New York: Springer.

Husserl E. (1984). *The Crisis of European Sciences and Transcendental Phenomenology*, trans. D. Carr. Evanston: Northwestern University Press.

Husserl E. (2008). *Logical Investigations*, Vol. II, trans. J. N. Findlay. London: Routledge.

Jansson L. and Nordgaard J. (2016). *The Psychiatric Interview for Differential Diagnosis*. Switzerland: Springer.

Jaspers K. (1997). *General Psychopathology*, trans. J. Hoenig and M. W. Hamilton. London: Johns Hopkins University Press.

Maj M. (2005). " 'Psychiatric Comorbidity': An Artefact of Current Diagnostic Systems?" *British Journal of Psychiatry* 186: 182–184.

Merleau-Ponty M. (2002). *Phenomenology of Perception*, trans. C. Smith. London: Routledge.

Mishara A., Bonoldi I., Allen P., Rutigliano G., Perez J., Fusar-Poli P., and McGuire P. (2016). "Neurobiological Models of Self-Disorders in Early Schizophrenia." *Schizophrenia Bulletin* 42: 874–880.

Møller P. and Husby R. (2000). "The Initial Prodrome in Schizophrenia: Searching for Naturalistic Core Dimensions of Experience and Behavior." *Schizophrenia Bulletin* 26: 217–232.

Møller P., Haug E., Raballo A., Parnas J., and Melle I. (2011). "Examination of Anomalous Self-experience in First-episode Psychosis: Interrater Reliability." *Psychopathology* 44: 386–390.

Nelson B., Thompson A., and Yung A. R. (2012). "Basic Self-Disturbance Predicts Psychosis Onset In The Ultra High Risk For Psychosis 'Prodromal' Population." *Schizophrenia Bulletin* 38: 1277–1287.

Nelson B., Whitford T. J., Lavoie S., and Sass L. A. (2014a). "What are the Neurocognitive Correlates of Basic Self-Disturbance in Schizophrenia?: Integrating Phenomenology and Neurocognition. Part 1 (Source Monitoring Deficits)." *Schizophrenia Research* 152: 12–19.

Nelson B., Whitford T. J., Lavoie S., and Sass L. A. (2014b). "What are the Neurocognitive Correlates of Basic Self-Disturbance in Schizophrenia?: Integrating Phenomenology and Neurocognition. Part 2 (Aberrant Salience)." *Schizophrenia Research* 152: 20–27.

Nordgaard J., Arnfred S. M., Handest P., and Parnas J. (2008). "The Diagnostic Status of First-rank Symptoms." *Schizophrenia Bulletin* 34: 137–154.

Nordgaard J. and Parnas J. (2012). "A Semi-structured, Phenomenologically Oriented Psychiatric Interview: Descriptive Congruence in assessing Anomalous Subjective Experience and Mental Status." *Clinical Neuropsychiatry* 9: 123–128.

Nordgaard J., Sass L., and Parnas J. (2013). "The Psychiatric Interview: Validity, Structure and Subjectivity." *European Archives of Psychiatry and Psychology* 263: 353–364.

Nordgaard J. and Parnas, J. (2014). "Self-disorders and Schizophrenia-spectrum: A Study of 100 First Hospital Admissions." *Schizophrenia Bulletin* 40: 1300–1307.

Nordgaard J., Revsbech R., and Henriksen M. G. (2015). "Self-disorders, Neurocognition, and Rationality in Schizophrenia: A Preliminary Study." *Psychopathology* 48: 310–316.

Nordgaard J. and Henriksen M. G. (2016). "Self-disorders: A Promising Candidate for Early Detection." *Scandinavian Journal of Child and Adolescent Psychiatry and Psychology* 4: 12–13.

Nordgaard J., Handest P., Vollmer-Larsen A., Sæbye D., Thejlade Pedersen J., and Parnas J. (2017). "Temporal Persistence of Anomalous Self-experience: A 5 Years Follow-up." *Schizophrenia Research* 179: 36–40.

Nordgaard J., Nilsson L. S., Saebye D., and Parnas J. (2018). "Self-disorders in Schizophrenia-spectrum Disorders: A 5 Years Follow-up Study." *European Archives of Psychiatry and Clinical Neuroscience*, 268(7): 713–718.

Parnas J. (2011). "A Disappearing Heritage: The Clinical Core of Schizophrenia." *Schizophrenia Bulletin* 37: 1121–1130.

Parnas J. (2012). "The Core Gestalt of Schizophrenia." *World Psychiatry* 11(2): 67–69.

Parnas J. (2015). "Differential Diagnosis and Current Polythetic Classification." *World Psychiatry* 14: 284–287.

Parnas J. (2017). "Diagnostic Epidemics and Diagnostic Disarray: The Issue of Differential Diagnosis." In K. S. Kendler and J. Parnas (eds), *Philosophical Issues in Psychiatry IV: Classification of Psychiatric Illness*, pp. 143–145. Oxford: Oxford University Press.

Parnas J. and Bovet P. (1991). "Autism in Schizophrenia Revisited." *Comprehensive Psychiatry* 32: 1–15.

Parnas J., Jansson L., Sass L. A., and Handest P. (1998). "Self-experience in the Prodromal Phases of Schizophrenia: A Pilot Study of First Admissions." *Neurology, Psychiatry & Brain Research* 6: 107–116.

Parnas, J. and Zahavi, D. (2002). "The Role of Phenomenology in Psychiatric Classification and Diagnosis." In M. Maj, W. Gaebel, J. J. López-Ibor, and N. Sartorius (eds), *Psychiatric Diagnosis and Classification*, pp 137–162. World Psychiatric Association's Series on Evidence and Experience in Psychiatry. Chichester: Wiley.

Parnas J., Møller P., Kircher T., Thalbitzer J., Jansson L., Handest P., and Zahavi, D. (2005a). "EASE: Examination of Anomalous Self-experience." *Psychopathology* 38: 236–258.

Parnas J., Handest P., Jansson L., and Sæbye D. (2005b). "Anomalous Subjective Experience Among First-Admitted Schizophrenia Spectrum Patients: Empirical Investigation." *Psychopathology* 38: 259–267.

Parnas J., Raballo A., Handest P., Jansson L., Vollmer-Larsen A., and Sæbye D. (2011). "Self-experience in the Early Phases of Schizophrenia: 5-Year Follow-up of the Copenhagen Prodromal Study." *World Psychiatry* 10: 200–204.

Parnas J. and Henriksen M. G. (2014). "Disordered Self in the Schizophrenia Spectrum: A Clinical and Research Perspective." *Harvard Review of Psychiatry* 22(5): 251–265.

Parnas J., Carter J., and Nordgaard J. (2016). "Premorbid Self-disorders and Lifetime Diagnosis in the Schizophrenia Spectrum: A Prospective High-Risk Study." *Early Intervention in Psychiatry* 10: 45–53.

Parnas J. and Henriksen M. G. (2016a). "Mysticism and Schizophrenia: A Phenomenological Exploration of the Structure of Consciousness in the Schizophrenia Spectrum Disorders." *Consciousness and Cognition* 43: 75–88.

Parnas J. and Henriksen M. G. (2016b). "Epistemological Error and the Illusion of Phenomenological Continuity." *World Psychiatry* 15: 126–127.

Parnas J. and Henriksen M. G. (in press). "Selfhood and its Disorders." In: Stanghellini G., Broome M., Raballo A., Fernandez A., Fusar-Poli P., and Rosfort R. (eds)., *The Oxford Handbook of Phenomenological Psychopathology*. Oxford: Oxford University Press.

Raballo A., Sæbye D., and Parnas J. (2011). "Looking at the Schizophrenia Spectrum through the Prism of Self-disorders: An Empirical Study." *Schizophrenia Bulletin* 37: 344–351.

Raballo A. and Parnas J. (2012). "Examination of Anomalous Self-experience: Initial Study of the Structure of Self-disorders in Schizophrenia Spectrum." *Journal of Nervous and Mental Disease* 200: 577–583.

Sartre J.-P. (2003). *Being and Nothingness*, trans. H. E. Barnes. London: Routledge.

Sass L. A. (in press). "Schizophrenia as a Self-disorder." In: Stanghellini G., Broome M., Raballo A., Fernandez A., Fusar-Poli P., and Rosfort R., (eds.), *The Oxford Handbook of Phenomenological Psychopathology*. Oxford: Oxford University Press.

Sass L. A. and Parnas J. (2003). "Schizophrenia, Consciousness, and the Self." *Schizophrenia Bulletin* 29: 427–444.

Sass L. A. and Borda J. P. (2015). "Phenomenology and Neurobiology of Self Disorder in Schizophrenia: Secondary Factors." *Schizophrenia Research* 169: 474–482.

Sass L. A., Peinkos E., Skodlar B., Stanghellini G., Fuchs T., Parnas J., and Jones N. (2017). "EAWE: Examination of Anomalous World-Experience." *Psychopathology* 50: 10–54.

Schneider K. (1950). *Klinische Psychopathologie*. Stuttgart: Georg Thieme Verlag.

Zahavi D. (2014). *Self and Other: Exploring Subjectivity, Empathy, and Shame*. Oxford: Oxford University Press.

Zandersen M., Henriksen M. G., and Parnas J. (2018). "A Recurrent Question: What is Borderline?" *Journal of Personality Disorders*. Feb 22: 1–29. doi: 10.1521/pedi_2018_32_348 [Epub ahead of print].

CHAPTER 88

PHENOMENOLOGICAL PSYCHOPATHOLOGY AND PSYCHOTHERAPY

GIOVANNI STANGHELLINI

INTRODUCTION

PHENOMENOLOGICAL psychopathology is the discipline that provides clinicians with systematic knowledge about the abnormal phenomena that affect human existence and with a valid and reliable method to appraise them. Jaspers's *General Psychopathology* was the first systematic attempt to describe, define, and classify abnormal mental phenomena. Jaspers's project was deeply embedded in the intellectual atmosphere of the early twentieth century: to provide a language to talk about the concreteness of human existence, including its absurdity, anxiety, despair, and its invisible dimension. From different angles, this project was shared by phenomenology, existentialism, and psychoanalysis, and bears profound kinship and resonances with contemporary art and literature. This is the very meaning of the word "psychopathology": a discourse (*logos*) about the sufferings (*pathos*) of the human mind (*psyche*).

Jaspers declared that the main purpose of his project was not mere taxonomy, but also methodology. What we need, he argued, next to systematic and generalized knowledge, is the systematic awareness of the ways to gain such knowledge. Thus the basic purpose of psychopathology is to empower clinicians with a means to explore the patients' perspective. This issue was primarily inspired by phenomenology. Phenomenology is the method that stands at the basis of psychopathology. Phenomenological psychopathology is open to an unusual extent, in that it reveals aspects of experience that other approaches tend to overwrite or eclipse with their strong theoretical claims. Phenomenological psychopathology assumes that its primary object is the patients' personal being, thus putting all its efforts into focusing on the rich and varied forms and contents of their subjective experience as it is narrated by them. Phenomenological psychopathology and psychotherapy are spiritual allies in putting the person of the patient and her experience first, and in searching for a language to talk about this.

A SHARED TOOLBOX FOR PHENOMENOLOGICAL PSYCHOPATHOLOGY AND PSYCHOTHERAPY

This section links phenomenological psychopathology to understanding, and understanding to psychotherapeutic care. I briefly describe the main tools at use for establishing psychopathological knowledge as the basis for care. These include the *epoché*, empathic, eidetic, and dialectic understanding. The former is the practice of suspension of all prejudices necessary to bring to the foreground the patient's perspective. As such, it is the common root, the *conditio sine qua non* to develop personalized understanding, be it a kind of understanding based on immediate emotional resonance, or on the patient and tactful exploration and reconstruction of the world the patient lives in, or on the intuition of some core properties of his experiences and of the way they are interrelated in a meaningful *gestalt*. Both empathic and eidetic understanding are embedded in a dialectical framework: a patient's symptom is not the direct outcome of some dysfunction, rather the product of her need for self-interpretation with respect to her encounter with puzzling experiences.

Epoché

The word "*epoché*" means cessation. It involves suspending belief in something, or more exactly, not operating with some belief. In Husserl it is a way to bracket our habit of considering consciousness and the world based on common sense, as well as to put to one side the default natural science understanding of them, and making the transition to the properly phenomenological way of considering them (McKenna 1997). It includes a cessation of both our obvious/common sense and theoretical/scientific pre-knowledge. This cessation exhibits a respect for the evidence of experience and at the same time orients itself toward seeking the grounds of that evidence. Thus the *epoché* has a double orientation and paves the way to a double achievement. The first is that it allows to go "to the things themselves"—the acknowledgment of the evidence of experience, of the way things and events appear to consciousness, refraining from taking a position with respect to that evidence. The second is that it allows the grasping of the mental processes that make these "things" appear as they appear to consciousness—the world-constituting dimension of consciousness.

The concept of *epoché* is obviously one of the key methodological steps not only in philosophical phenomenology, but also in phenomenological psychopathology. Although Jaspers's (1913/1997) phenomenology differs from Husserl's eidetic and transcendental research since he focused mainly on the phenomenal level of experience, he was among the first to grasp the need of bracketing pre-knowledge in order to go to the psychopathological phenomena themselves. Jaspers's aim is to describe mental (abnormal) phenomena as they really are; with this he means as they are experienced and narrated by the patient. He uses the *epoché* as a way to establish empirically sound knowledge in the context of a hetero-phenomenology (phenomenology of the other person's experience), rejecting a priori theoretical doctrines in favor of an empirical approach focused on the direct analysis of the patient's lived experience. If and only if we bracket prejudices can we approach mental phenomena in order to study them as they really present to consciousness. Bracketing all theoretical biases is the quintessential methodological as well as ethical (i.e. maximum respect for the person as a subject of experience) prerequisite of psychopathological knowledge and care.

The concept of *epoché* differs from more recent naïve "atheoretical" stances because the latter do not bracket obvious pre-knowledge but implicitly assume it in the form of a covert neopositivist trust in the description of mental symptoms viewed as mere objects (Aragona 2013). On the contrary, the phenomenological *epoché* assumes that the objects of knowledge are not mere facts but are intentionally constituted in consciousness activity (Stanghellini and Aragona 2016).

Also, in order to preserve the *epoché* from a naïve objectivistic misunderstanding, we need to remember that the very nature of the praxis called *epoché* is not eliminating prejudices, rather it is to make them more evident. The epoché is a praxis whereby I can see my prejudices since it brings into view the world-constituting dimension of my acts of consciousness. The outcome of the *epoché* is *not* a *tabula rasa* that allows for a pure and unprejudiced impression of the real on my consciousness, but rather a wider and deeper awareness of my own prejudices.

A further caveat about the *epoché* is avoiding its presumed divinatory character since a further contribution of the *epoché* to field of mental health care is its link (established by some authors but not others) to recovering beyond mere appearances, a global and intuitive vision of essences. I will develop this theme in the paragraph on eidetic understanding.

Empathic Understanding

Understanding means grasping the "what-it-is-like" aspect of a given experience, and the meaning that given experience has for the person who lives it.

The late nineteenth century saw the emergence of an epistemological dispute concerning the most appropriate methods for the emerging human sciences (sociology, history, jurisprudence, economy, and the like), as well as the proper place of psychology and hence of psychopathology (is it a natural or a human science?). Psychopathology is not only a science of nature, but it is also a human science. In many instances, we are not satisfied to know that somebody acted as he did *because* some parts of his brain were activated, while others were inhibited. We also want to know *how* it feels to act in that given way. Also, if we want to know why he did so, we need to understand his reasons, his motivations, and his purposes. This is a different level that can be grasped only by means of a totally different method. This method is understanding (Jaspers's *Verstehen*); it consists in reproducing (*Nachbilden*) in ourselves what is actually taking place in the mind of that person. In Jaspers's psychopathology, such understanding was mainly an empathic understanding, basically a kind of emotional reliving (*Nacherleben*).

Jaspers proposes his method called "static understanding": although we do not observe directly the subjective experiences of our patients, we can make them present in our consciousness by means of a sort of transposition, of reviving in ourselves what the other is actually living. This is an empathic act that gives us the material for the appraisal of such subjective, private experiences. Such an empathic understanding requires a preliminary bracketing of our prejudices if we want to grasp the phenomenon as it presents itself from the patient's standpoint (see *epoché*).

Jaspers's concept of "understanding" has distinctive features that shall be briefly considered (Stanghellini and Aragona 2016).

(1) *Understanding is pathic* (that is, based on emotional experience). We understand when we grasp by empathy how certain thoughts and experiences are embedded in moods, wishes, or fears. Rational understanding is merely an aid to psychology, whereas pathic understanding brings us to very psyche of the person (Jaspers 1913/1997).

(2) *Understanding requires the right distance.* Empathic understanding is neither emotive fusion nor cold distance (Villareal and Aragona 2014). It is something in between, where the sympathetic tremulation of one psyche with the experiences of another coexists with the critical objectification of such experience (Jaspers 1913/1997). There is the need to modulate the distance between oneself and the patient and to continuously oscillate between objective categorization and the appreciation of individual existential subjectivity.

(3) *Genetic understanding is local* (does not lead to generalizations). Next to static understanding (reliving the other's experience), genetic understanding is what allows us to grasp the genesis of a phenomenon, that is, the motivations that led the person to perceive, feel, or act as he did. This knowledge is local in the sense that it cannot be subsumed under a general law. While in a given situation a person did something, in another situation the same person could also have done something else, so we can at best realize that a general tendency occurred, but we can never be sure that in similar circumstances the person in question will do the same again.

(4) *Understanding is limited.* We cannot always relive in ourselves what is happening in our interlocutor. We can understand phenomena that at least in principle we can or could re-experience ourselves, and this means that understanding is based on a common ground between human beings, a shared world of meanings that make it possible. Other phenomena are beyond the boundaries of ordinary empathic understanding. Famously, Jaspers's claim that schizophrenic primary delusions are ununderstandable raised several critiques. Jaspers's theorem of incomprehensibility was a stimulus to explore different ways to "understand" psychotic experiences. Jaspers himself mentions philosophical clarification as well as other forms of interpretation (not necessarily psychoanalytic) as other possible ways to transcend the limits of empathic understanding. If we see Jaspers's theorem of incomprehensibility from the angle of the ethics (rather than epistemology) it sets the agenda for a kind of clinical care based on approximation and coexistence, and as an exhortation to clinicians to navigate the space that separates them from their patients (Stanghellini 2013a).

(5) *The limits of understanding are changeable.* Understandability shall not be conceived as an intrinsic characteristic of a given psychopathological phenomena, but as an emerging relational property within the clinical encounter. The boundaries of our ability to understand depend on "consistency, deepness, and duration" of the therapeutic relationship (Ballerini 2003: 40), the characteristics of the clinical setting, the duration of the therapeutic relationship, and the personal characteristics of the patient and of the clinician (attention, patience, and imagination of the participants).

The analysis of the main features of Jaspers's concept of "understanding" raises several problems, the most important of which in the context of care is the limitations of spontaneous or first-order empathic understanding. Understanding is a much more complex task than simply putting oneself into the other's shoes. Sometimes, while performing this act of imaginative self-transposal we experience the radical otherness of the other. In some cases—maybe the most relevant in clinical practice—we do not feel immediately in touch with the other, we do not immediately grasp the reasons and meaning of his actions, although we purposively and knowingly attempt to put ourselves in his place. In the clinical setting we cannot simply rely on standard empathic capacities. Understanding requires a kind of training that goes beyond spontaneous and naïve empathic skills (Stanghellini 2016a; Stanghellini and Mancini 2017). The clinician's empathic capacities need some kind of education. I suggested (Stanghellini 2013b) naming *second-order empathy* the method required to grasp those experiences that are not understandable via simply transposing oneself into another person. To achieve second-order empathy is a complex process. First, I need to acknowledge that the life-world inhabited by the other person is not like my own. The supposition that the other lives in a world like my own—that is, that he lives time, space, his own body, others, the materiality of objects, etc. just like I do—is often the source of serious misunderstanding (see Section 6: Life-Worlds). In order to empathize with these persons I must acknowledge the ontological difference which separates me from the way of being-in-the-world that characterizes each of them. Any forgetting of this ontological difference will be an obstacle to understanding. Achieving second-order empathy thus requires bracketing my own pre-reflexive, natural attitude (in which my first-order empathic capacities are rooted), and approaching the other's world as I would do while exploring an unknown and alien country.

EIDETIC UNDERSTANDING

"*Eidos*" means essence. It is the core or defining property of a given phenomenon or set of phenomena. As is the case with empathic understanding, eidetic understanding also requires the bracketing of pre-given ordinary and theoretical knowledge to bring to the fore the phenomenon as it is given in consciousness. The process of eidetic understanding consists in progressively removing unessential properties and perspective views in order to grasp the essence of the thing itself. To achieve the *eidos* of a given set of phenomena one can adopt a method called *free fantasy variation*—a series of arbitrary variations although restricted to imagined instances of the phenomenon at issue. Roughly, if the phenomenon remains itself after progressively removing several features, but finally vanishes when a feature is eliminated, then that feature is its essence.

There is an *intuitional* and an *empirical* way to eidetic understanding (Stanghellini and Aragona 2016). Does the knowledge of the essence of a given phenomenon take place by abstraction or comparison of similar phenomena (as believed by the empiricists), or by a direct intuition of what is universal (as believed by the intuitionists)? This question explains interpretative fluctuations in the reception of Husserl's "rigorous method" (as Husserl himself used to call it) by clinicians. In phenomenological psychopathology, eidetic appraisal tends to fluctuate between scientific dissection of phenomenal appearances, at one side, and a more global and intuitive vision of essential themes on the other side.

Binswanger (1956), who imported Husserl's essences into the psychopathological debate, can be seen as an example of the intuitionist view. He claims that psychopathologists should advance, step by step, from the particular empirical and individual facts toward the meta-empirical, general pure essences described by Husserl. Binswanger appears well aware of the meaning Husserl had given to the word "essence" and to his eidetic research. Despite this fact, there are some significant differences in Binswanger's own way of conceiving essences. In fact, his essences are more akin to immediate artistic intuitions than Husserl's rigorous derivation from subsequent and systematic acts of eidetic variation. To Binswanger the grasping of the *eidos* is an act of seeing. Yet this *seeing* is not through the eyes, but is an immediate awareness that looks inside and may be more reliable than sensorial knowledge. Although this *intuitive* vision of essences in scientific phenomenology should not be confused with the artistic intuition, these two forms of intuition—he writes—have "undoubtful and strict relationships" which are beyond the contraposition between science and art.

An example of the interpretation of eidetic appraisal as a scientific dissection of phenomenal appearances can be found in the concept of "pheno-phenotype" (Stanghellini and Rossi 2014). In this view, mental symptoms are not accidental meaningless disturbances occurring to a patient. Rather they are the manifestation of some implicit quintessential "core" change in the fundamental structures of the patient's subjectivity. It is this fundamental global *core* of human subjectivity that transpires through the single symptoms and gives to the whole syndrome a specific and characteristic *gestalt* that many psychopathologists call "phenomenological essence." The *eidos* is the "kernel underlying the manifest symptoms in all their variety that keeps them meaningfully interconnected or united" (Urfer 2001). Indeed, all the symptoms of a syndrome can be seen as empirical variations of an essential property shared by all these symptoms. This eidetic property is the characteristic without which this set of symptoms will lose their identity (Husserl 1977).

To retrieve this core is basically an intellectual and rational enterprise that needs a rigorous method (not a "technique" in a strict sense), rather than an aesthetic performance. Or more exactly: it is not *only* an act of aesthetic intuition, exclusively based on the clinician's sensibility. The ability to recover the core or essence is an attitude and a kind of reasoning that can be taught, learnt, tested, and reproduced. Also, the attempt to find the *eidos* is not the idiosyncratic discovery that takes place in a private, inner space of a contemplative subject. Rather, it is the product of a process of confrontation. The description of this method, and its importance in the psychotherapeutic setting, will be described in the last section of this chapter.

Dialectic Understanding

The dialectic understanding of mental disorders assumes that mental symptoms are not the direct effects of a psychological or biological dysfunction (Stanghellini 2016b). Psychopathological symptoms are the outcome of a disproportion between the person and her disturbing experiences (Binswanger 1956)—namely estrangement from oneself and alienation from one's social environment. A person's symptom is the outcome of her need for self-interpretation with respect to her encounter with puzzling experiences (Jaspers 1913/1997). The person is engaged in trying to cope with and make sense of her puzzling experiences. Each patient, urged by the drive for the intelligible unity of her life-construction (Mayer-Gross 1920), plays an active role in interacting with these experiences and thus in shaping her symptoms and the course and outcome of her illness. The person's attitude is characterized by her attempt to achieve a self-interpretation of her disturbing and perplexing experiences, alongside a constant search for personal meaning (Stanghellini, Bolton, and Fulford 2013). The production of a symptom is the *extrema ratio* for alterity to become discernible (Stanghellini 2016a). Psychopathological symptoms are the outcome of miscarried attempts to give a meaning to distressing experiences, to explain and cope with them. The encounter with alterity may offer the vantage from which a person can see herself from another, often radically new, perspective. Thus, otherness kindles the progressive dialectics of personal identity. Narratives are the principal means to integrate alterity into autobiographical memory, providing temporal and goal structure, combining personal experiences into a coherent story related to the self.

The main difference between this person-centered understanding of mental disorders and an exclusively neurobiological model is that in the latter the patient is conceived as a passive victim of her symptoms, whereas the former attributes to the patient an active role in shaping her symptoms, course, and outcome. Each patient, as a "goal-directed being," plays an active role and stamps her autograph onto the raw material of her basic abnormal experiences. When a clinical syndrome emerges, the line of the pathogenic trajectory is the following: (1) a disproportion of alterity and the person's resources for understanding, of emotions and rationality, of *pathos* and *logos*, of otherness and selfhood bringing about a disturbing metamorphosis of self- and world-experience; (2) a miscarried auto-hermeneutics or self-interpretation of one's abnormal experiences and of the transformations of the life-world that they bring about; (3) the fixation in a psychopathological structure in which the dialectics between the person and alterity gets lost.

This person-centered, dialectic approach helps us to see the patient as meaning-making entity rather than passive individual. The patient "can see himself, judge himself, and mould himself" (Jaspers 1913/1997: 424). His attempts at self-understanding are not necessarily pathological and are potentially adaptive.

This approach contains a theoretical framework and practical resources for understanding the diversity of psychopathological structures, including symptom presentation, course, and outcome as a consequence of the different ways patients seek to make sense of and value the basic changes in self- and world-experiences. It also contains a framework for engaging with human fragility by means of a person-centered, dialectic therapy.

PHENOMENOLOGICAL PSYCHOTHERAPY AS A QUEST FOR MEANING

In endorsing the legacy of phenomenological psychopathology and its emphasis on the analysis of subjectivity by means of the first-person and second-person mode of understanding, phenomenologically oriented psychotherapy aims for a wide-range, fine-grained assessment of the patient's morbid subjectivity, not constrained in a priori fixed schemata such as specific techniques or structured question-and-answer procedures (Stanghellini and Mancini

2017). The phenomenological attitude in psychotherapy can be condensed in one single question: *What do we need to put ourselves* at the side *of the patient?* The first step is quite obvious: we need to perform a radical *epoché* with respect to all approaches that see mental disorders as failures of normative functioning, avoid the language reflecting deviance-laden and vice-laden conceptualizations of the patient's existential condition, and *give the word* to the patient himself in describing his perspective. In a formula: switch from negative to *positive pathography* (that is, a narrative of what is there, rather than on what is lacking, in the patient's life-world). The second step, also suggested by van den Berg (1955), is to switch from an introspective to an *extraspective pathography*. This means that if we want to know what-it-is-like to have a given experience we should not limit ourselves to explore the patient's subjective sensations, but to focus on the world as it appears to him.

This approach can provide the background for unfolding the phenomena of the patient's existence from the angle of the life-world inhabited by him, including all those details that resist standard semiological classification; and it can rescue the architectural nexus that lends coherence and continuity to them. Phenomenological psychopathology assumes that the manifold of phenomena of a given mental disorder has a meaningful coherence. Rather than being a mere aggregate of symptoms, they form a structured totality, that is, a meaningful whole. Also, the method of phenomenological psychopathology is a prerequisite for moving beyond pure static description of the life-world toward the illumination of the structures of subjectivity that allegedly generate and structure the phenomenal world.

In this section I describe the basic philosophical principles of the phenomenologically oriented framework for psychotherapeutic care. In this framework, psychotherapy can be defined as a quest for meaning based on the art of questioning. This includes five steps corresponding to five levels of meaningfulness (Stanghellini 2013b and 2016a).

Unfolding the Phenomena of the Life-World and Rescuing its Implicit Structure

The first step of phenomenological psychotherapy is unfolding the details of the patient's psychopathological world—its explication. Unfolding means to exposit, open up, or lay bare the pleats, creases, or corrugations of a text. The opposite of this is to garble, pervert, distort, or twist/ stretch/ strain the text itself. This operation can be seen as the necessary first step of all forms of understanding, consisting in an enlightenment or clarification of existence— *Existenzerhellung* in Jaspers's terms (Jaspers 1956).

The phenomenal world that comes into sight through the unfolding is seen as a *text* (Ricouer 1981). The product of unfolding is a text that reflects the phenomenal world, the world as it appears to the subject of experience, including all those details that resist standard semiological classification. In a given psychopathological text, there is much more than that which can be mapped using the catalogue of psychopathological symptoms (like phobias, formal thought disorders, or delusions). What becomes perspicuous is the texture that is immanent in the text itself, although it may remain invisible to or unnoticed by the author. Explication enriches understanding by providing further resources in addition to those that are immediately visible. The aim of this process is to rescue the *logos* of the phenomena in themselves, by "bringing unnoticed material into consciousness"—as Jaspers (1913/

1997: 307) would put it. The *logos* that is immanent in the intertwining of phenomena is called *sense*, that is, the internal coherence between the clinical (as well as subclinical and existential) phenomena found in a given condition of suffering (Ricouer 1981). Phenomenological psychopathology advocates the idea that the phenomena embedded in a given (normal or abnormal) form of existence are a meaningful whole. This has an important clinical implication. The standard understanding of the concept of "syndrome" is one which views it as a cluster of symptoms which happen to hang together not by any mutual phenomenological implication, but by their being otherwise unrelated effects of a common neurobiological cause. This alternative perspective holds that the manifold (abnormal) phenomena in a syndrome are meaningfully interconnected, that is, they form a structure. A psychopathological syndrome is not simply a casual association of (abnormal) phenomena. To have a phenomenological grasp on these phenomena is to grasp the structural nexus that lends coherence and continuity to them, because each phenomenon in a psychopathological structure carries traces of the underlying formal alterations of subjectivity.

Although this discourse is imbued with visual metaphors, it is important to note that this process of unfolding is profoundly rooted in hearing—or even better: listening and dialoguing—and in the power of the spoken word. The kind of seeing implied in this practice should be—to adopt Levin's (1993) terms—"multiple, aware of its context, inclusionary, horizontal and caring" (Jay 1994). Hearing contributes to an ethics based on reciprocity and belonging, as well as to establishing a kind of knowledge focused on subjective experiences and personal narratives.

Rescuing the Implicit Structures of the Self

The second stratum made visible by this process consists of the invisible conditions of possibility of the world disclosed in the first level. By rescuing the map of the world that is depicted in the text, we can approximate the architecture of the Self that constituted it. This is an exploration of the implicit structures of experience, or into the structures of the Self as the tacit and pre-reflexive conditions for the emergence of mental contents. It looks for the way consciousness must be structured to make phenomena appear as they appear to the experiencing Self. Looking for structural relationships consists in the unfolding of the basic structure(s) of subjectivity, that is, the way the Self appropriates phenomena.

The guidelines for reconstructing the life-world in which a person lives are the so-called *existentials*, the basic categories, or categorical characteristics, of the fundamental features of human existence, namely, lived time, space, body, otherness, materiality, and so on (Heidegger 1927/1962). In this way we can trace back this transformation of the life-world to a specific configuration of the embodied Self as the origin of a given mode of inhabiting the world, and perceiving, manipulating, and making sense of it. In order to grasp the transcendental framework of one's experience, one must turn one's gaze away from one's "mind" (and also from the "world" as it appears in straightforward cognition) and look for the world's spatiotemporal architecture which reflects it. The reconstruction of the patient's life-world, and of the transcendental structures of his Self, allows for the patient's behavior, expression, and experience to become understandable.

Narrating the Transcendental Origin of the Life-World

This kind of practice connecting a given experience (abnormal or not) with its transcendental condition of possibility may have pathogenetic implications, thus linking the research on meanings to that on causes of mental symptoms. The path to genetic understanding in psychopathology was opened by Jaspers, who described it as the "[i]nner, subjective, direct grasp of psychic connectedness" (Jaspers 1913/1997: 307). Genetic understanding, according to Jaspers, is a kind of knowledge that establishes meaningful connections between psychic phenomena. Jaspers argued that psychic events emerge out of each other in a way that we can immediately understand. For instance, we immediately understand that attacked people become angry and spring to defense, or a cheated person grows suspicious. The philosophical paragon inspiring Jaspers is Nietzsche's understanding of morality as connected to weakness: the awareness of one's weakness, wretchedness, and suffering gives rise to moral demands and religion, because in this roundabout way the psyche can gratify its will to power. Jaspers offers several examples of genetic understanding in psychopathology, among them psychic reactions and the development of passions. Jaspers insists on the character of immediateness and self-evidence in grasping meaningful connections in someone's life. To him, genetic understanding in psychopathology "is a precondition of the psychology of meaningful phenomena ... just as the reality of perception and of causality is the precondition of the natural sciences" (1913/1997: 303).

Husserl also developed, beyond static or descriptive phenomenology, another kind of genetic or constructive phenomenology that he called "explanatory" (Sass 2010). This is a kind of developmental or diachronic understanding studying the way complex modes of experience are constituted via the synthesis of more basic modes of lived experiences. The key dispositive of Husserl's explanatory phenomenology is motivational causality. It has been argued that "analyzing the basic constitution and explicating the implicit structure of experience, phenomenology offers another way of developmental understanding: it allows for a comprehension of the pre-reflective dimension of experience ... from which manifest symptoms arise" (Parnas and Sass 2008: 280). In this way, the dialogue moves beyond pure description and static understanding toward "an understanding of both the overall unity of that person's subjectivity and its development over time" (Parnas and Sass 2008: 264). This kind of narrative, based on the understanding of the basic architecture of the life-world, and on the structures of subjectivity which allegedly generate them, may allow us to both make sense of (rescue the personal meaning) and genetically understand (rescue the personal motivation of) a given symptom, be it an action or a belief.

Appropriation (by the Clinician) of the Patient's Life-World

The fourth level of meaningfulness made manifest by this exploration is the world that the text opens up in the patient when it is appropriated by the clinician. The clinician appropriates the sense of the patient's experience and suggests his view of it. To appropriate a text means to acknowledge the way the text belongs to the reader, the way the reader could inhabit it. It is an attempt at reducing the distance between the text and its reader. If the *interpretandum* were completely extraneous, the understanding enterprise would be condemned to a checkmate, and if it were completely familiar, there would be no sense in making an effort at interpretation. The clinician makes explicit his understanding as his own, that is, the vantage point from which he sees the patient's situation. This implies, in fact, a tension between extraneousness and familiarity. In this way, and only in this way, the clinician may become a "You" for his patient. The clinician appropriates the patient's world by means of his own imagination when he tries to reply to the question: "To make sense of the patient's otherwise absurd and otherwise meaningless behavior, I must imagine myself as if I were living in a world that has the following characteristics." This approximation to the patient's life-world is carried out by the clinician via as-if experiments that are metaphorically expressed.

Grasping the Importance of the Patient's Life-World

The meanings that we find in a text may exceed the intention of the author. This is the case with any kind of symptom. By unfolding the structures of a text, we can understand an author better than the author himself. Also, during this process of unfolding, the text lays in front of its author who can adopt a third-person stance over the text itself—and in the case of the symptom the patient can take a reflexive stance over the feel and the meaning of his experience, thus reinforcing his subjective and intersubjective sense of being a Self. The importance of a text reaches beyond this level of understanding and discloses the mode of being-in-the-world of that individual patient as a universal problem. It reveals the way his existence belongs to human existence as a whole, to the *condicio humana*. The text may display meanings that transcend the situation in which the text was produced. To grasp the importance of a text is to unfold "the revelatory power implicit in his discourse, beyond the limited horizon of his own existential situation" (Ricoeur 1981: 191). The importance of a text is what "goes 'beyond' its relevance to the initial situation" (Ricoeur 1981: 207). In virtue of its importance, a text acquires a universal (not merely contingent) meaning, and its author embodies a universal problem (he stops being a merely contingent sufferer).

THE PHD METHOD: PHENOMENOLOGY, HERMENEUTICS, AND PSYCHODYNAMICS

In the previous section, I explained the basic philosophical principles of phenomenological psychotherapy as a quest for meaning. In this section, I will provide the practical guidelines for performing it according to these principles.

The phenomenological method is based on the art of dialogue. The aim of dialogue is to obtain a sharper view of a given phenomenon through an exchange of views between two or more partners. It is literally and *inter-view* (Stanghellini and Mancini 2017). Emphasizing the dialogical nature of phenomenology, Ricoeur (1981) takes distance from the idea that phenomenology is about the idiosyncratic discovery of the *eidos* of a given phenomenon. The kind of phenomenology at issue here—namely hermeneutic phenomenology—is not (or is not *just*) an eidetic practice, rather it is an activity that takes place in an intersubjective space and its product is the outcome of a process of dialogical confrontation.

It should not come as a surprise that phenomenology, as the bedrock of care, is a dialogical practice. We, as human beings, are dialogue: of the person with herself, and with other persons. Mental disorder is the crisis of the dialogue of the person with the alterity that inhabits her, and with the alterity incarnated in the other persons. Human existence is a yearning for unity and identity. Yet, this attempt is unfulfilled in the encounter with alterity, that is, with all the powers of the involuntary. All this generates feelings of estrangement. Mental pathologies may be read as miscarried attempts to struggle for a sense of reconciliation, to heal the wounds of disunion. Care is an effort to reconstruct such a vulnerable dialogue of the soul with herself (Stanghellini 2016a).

The practice of care that derives from these assumptions is based on the integration of three basic dispositives, synthesized in the acronym PHD—bringing together phenomenology, hermeneutics, and psychodynamics (Stanghellini 2016a and 2016b).

Phenomenological Unfolding

As we have seen on the previous paragraph, the basic purpose of the unfolding is to empower clinician and patient with a systematic knowledge of the abnormal phenomena that affect the patient. "Unfolding" means to open up and lay bare the pleats of the patient's experiences. What comes into sight is the texture that is immanent in the patient's style of experience/action, although it may remain invisible to or unnoticed by him. Unfolding enriches understanding by providing further resources in addition to those that are immediately visible. The main aim of unfolding is to rescue the *logos* of the phenomena in themselves, that is, immanent in the intertwining of phenomena.

An outstanding example of phenomenological unfolding is given by Minkowski (Minkowski 1993; see in detail discussion in Stanghellini 2010). In a classic idiographic essay on the structure of depressive states, following an in-depth portrayal of the manifold abnormal experiences and sensations of a twenty-six-year-old man with a diagnosis of "ambivalent depression" (a subtype of major depression), mainly relying on this man's self-descriptions, Minkowski attempts to grasp the kernel underlying these symptoms. The patient reports his complaints and Minkowski carefully registers and systematically orders them. He documents cenesthopathic troubles ("I have the sensation of a stop of vegetative functions"), sensations of materialization ("I am nothing but a kind of animal function"), disorders of self-awareness ("I don't feel myself anymore. I don't exist anymore") and of intersubjectivity ("I resonate with people, I reflect their vibrations," "I have the impression to be rubbish thrown into life, so much I feel distant from the others"); he complains about disorders of action ("I have always the sensation of incompleteness"), and of temporalization ("I have been persuaded to be a person sick of time (*malade du temps*)," "I have the sensation that time passes very fast, faster than for the others, too fast," "I don't have the sensation of continuity anymore," "I have the obsession with the past").

So far, Minkowski's analysis is a scholarly example of phenomenal assessment: he records personal experiences, as idiosyncratic as they are, including those phenomena that are not categorized in ad hoc diagnostic checklists. To note, he is not simply interested in psychopathological symptoms in a traditional sense (indexes for diagnosis): he mentions neither disorders of ideation (delusions or other "false ideas") nor abnormal moods (sadness, anger, or anhedonia). Minkowski is concerned with reconstructing the patient's life-world, "the lived experience of the real world that surrounds him" (Lanteri-Laura 1993), more than counting his symptoms. To obtain this, he methodically brackets or suspends all the "ideo-affective" (cognitive and affective) contents of experience, and focuses on formal aspects or the spatiotemporal configurations that are implicit in the patient's experiences. The main guidelines for this are lived space and time, but the way the patient experiences his own body, self, and other persons are also included in Minkowski's inquiries. This patient's experiences, examined from this angle, depart from those one may find in the common-sense world in which we all live. Following this path, to a certain extent it is possible to feel or imagine what it is like to live in the patient's world. However, at this stage of reconstruction the life-world still lacks a core that keeps its parts meaningfully interconnected—the "underlying unity characteristic of particular types of abnormal lived world" (Sass 2001).

A psychopathological syndrome is the expression of a profound and characteristic modification of the human existence in its entirety. We need to grasp the intimate transformation of subjectivity underlying the manifold symptoms and conferring them their structural unity. In Minkowsky's own words (1993), "the way in which personality is situated, in normal as well as in pathological terms, in relation to lived time and lived space" (2), the "organized living unity" of abnormal psychic phenomena—"a *deeper symptom* compared to surface symptoms on which contemporary nosography is based" (Kendler 2008).

The procedure here credited to Minkowski can serve as a model to grasp the *eidos* that keeps the manifold of symptoms meaningfully interconnected. Indeed, all the symptoms presented by Minkowski's patient can be seen as empirical variations of an essential property shared by all these symptoms. In the case study illustrated by Minkowski, it is the patient himself that finds the right words to talk about the *eidos* of his sufferings: "*I am person sick of time.*" This seems to be the fundamental essential phenomenon that is always implicit and virtually present in all the manifest parts of his life-world (e.g. the sensation of a cessation of vegetative functions, the impression of being rubbish thrown into life, the sensation of incompleteness, the feeling that time passes very fast, the impression to lack temporal continuity and the obsession with the past).

The essential phenomenon is a disorder of the experience of time that gives the manifold abnormal phenomena affecting this patient its meaningful coherence. Minkowski writes that at the roots of our awareness of time there are two elements, distinct but intimately related: one dynamic in nature, preparing our "*élan*" toward the future, the other, more static, that can be called "the eternal" (*l'éternel*) (Minkowski 1993). Our normal experience of time results from its harmonious synthesis, so that time is neither experienced as a fugue nor as fixation. In pathological conditions, this synthesis falls apart. In major depressions, *l'élan* is overpowered by *l'éternel*. The core symptom is a disorder of conation or inhibition of becoming. This disorder of lived time transpires in all phenomena characterizing major depression, including the experience of a stagnation of endogenous vital processes, the experience of present and future dominated by the past, and the experience of the slackening of the flow of time (Stanghellini et al. 2016). All are supposedly the phenomenal manifestations of the pre-phenomenal disturbance of temporality called *conation*, that is, the basic energetic momentum (*élan*) of mental life that gives the sense of being alive and acting spontaneously, and which orientates one's life in the direction of the future. The disturbance of conation (time-sickness, *maladie du temps*) is the structural nexus that gives them unity and coherence; it allows for making sense of actions, thoughts, emotions, and experiences that would otherwise be inexplicable.

The unfolding thus helps to recover the implicit (not necessarily rejected), automatic (not censored), forgotten (not forbidden) sources that make phenomena appear as they appear to the patient, his drives, emotions, and habitus—the three emblematic components of the obscure and dissociated spontaneity that make up the involuntary dimension in human existence (Stanghellini 2016a).

Hermeneutic Analysis

The second moment of the PHD method is the analysis of the person's position-taking toward her experiences. This is called the hermeneutic moment (H) since it is focused on the way the patient interprets or makes sense of his own experiences. The central idea is that there is an active interplay between the person and her basic abnormal experiences (Stanghellini, Bolton and Fulford 2013). As self-interpreting animals, we continuously strive to make sense of what happens to us, or to make a *logos* out of *pathos*. The H moment of the PHD pays attention to the active role that the person has in taking a position and interacting with her abnormal and distressing experiences. The patient, with her unique strengths and resources as well as needs and difficulties, has an active role in shaping her symptoms, and the course and outcome of her disorder.

As the P moment unfolds the patient's life-world or world-experience, the H moment reveals the patients *worldview*. This concept refers to the person's philosophy of life, that is, the structure of values that orients her way to experience reality and her actions. Jaspers (Jaspers 1925) explains that a worldview consists of two parts: an "attitude," the pattern of mental existence by means of which the world is experienced, and a "world-picture," the whole of the mental content a person possess. Husserl further explains that a "world-view is thus essentially an individual accomplishment, a sort of personal religious faith; but it is distinguished from traditional faith, that of revealed religion, through the fact that it makes no claim to an unconditioned truth binding for all men" (Husserl 1936/1970: 389). A worldview is thus a mental framework or a *shelter* (*Gehause*) in which a person has her hold and seeks refuge from her dread of limit situations, those situations in which her existence can be put at jeopardy (Jaspers 1925).

Persons vulnerable to schizophrenia, for instance, may show an attitude of distrust toward conventional knowledge and attunement (Stanghellini and Ballerini 2007). Eccentric values in persons with schizophrenia are one aspect of an overall crisis of common sense and of these persons' difficulties in feeling attuned to the others and making sense of their behavior. The outcome of this has been designated as antagonomia (literally: striving against rules) and idionomia (the sentiment of the radical uniqueness and exceptionality of one's own internal law (*nomos*) with respect to common sense or the other human beings) (Stanghellini and Ballerini 2007). These quasi-philosophies are shelters or defensive housings (Jaspers 1925). In general, we enter into one of these shelters when common-sensical assumptions are jeopardized. When I enter into one of these protective casings, it becomes a structured and structuring organization for me. My worldview protects me from the moral pain produced by disturbing experiences, but endlessly produces other experiences of a similar kind.

It is extremely difficult to become aware of the shelter in which I live, of its precarious-ness, and of the way it structures my life-world and the relationships with other persons. My shelter is a disposition that generates practices, beliefs, perceptions, feelings, and so forth. Rescuing from the implicit the active role that values have in holding together a patient's shelter and in shaping his abnormal and distressing experiences is the *via regia* to help him to recalibrate his dysfunctional, miscarried position-taking and, finally, to recover his sense of responsibility and agency (Stanghellini 2016a).

An example of phenomenologically informed therapeutic values-based interviews may come from the case of anorexia (Fulford and Stanghellini, chapter 41). The psychopatho-logical core of the life-world of persons with anorexia nervosa is not feeling oneself in the first-person perspective, and in particular feeling extraneous from one's body and emotions (Stanghellini et al. 2012). This entails a fleeting feel of selfhood and an evanescent sense of identity (Stanghellini and Mancini in press). This vulnerable awareness of oneself is dis-turbing and generates the need to appraise oneself in alternative ways. One of the coping strategies or alternative means of self-recognition in these persons is feeling their body through the gaze of the others. The other has a key role in the life-world of persons with an-orexia since it is through being looked at by others that these persons can achieve a feeling of their own body and a sense of identity. Obviously, this coping strategy is not voluntarily adopted and remains largely unconscious. A second way to regain a sense of themselves is identifying oneself through one's passion for thinness as passions represent a rupture in the fleeting character of their emotional and bodily life. The ossification of this passion and of the related value is the expression of the need to compensate the disturbing, shameful, and anxiogenic fleeting sense of selfhood and identity.

The unfolding (P) of the life-world of persons with anorexia and the analysis of their value-structure and position-taking (H) is essential if we want to acknowledge that it's a mis-take to see these persons' values as merely imperfect cognition or as a kind of irrational or delusional belief about one's body or nutrition. Rather, their values are a kind of religion that goes beyond the rationality/irrationality divide. It is about the worth of life and the way to make one's life meaningful. Food for them has a moral value: it is a sin and a tempta-tion. Fatness and thinness—that is, one's bodily shape—have a moral value too. Fatness has a moral value as indicative of laziness, lack of self-care, and self-control. Thinness means the capacity to give a shape to oneself and is more valuable than anything else including health and life itself. Strict rules are needed not to do wrong and to be led astray. Starvation is the unique salvation practice.

Dynamic Analysis

The psychodynamic moment (D) of the PHD consists in tracing back the life-world (one's experiences and actions) and the worldview (one's values and position-taking) to the life-history in which they are embedded. To make sense of a given phenomenon is finally to posit it in a meaningful context, and this context includes the personal history of the patient.

With Binswanger (1928/1963) we call "personal life-history" the intimate interconnection of the contents of the person's experiences. Through histories (or narratives) we are able to articulate the reasons of our character and the meanings of the events that we encounter in our life. Narratives are patterns of meanings that contribute to make sense of my character and the *via regia* to work through the meaning of a given situation in my life. They moderate the ossification of the character and the traumatic potential of the event. They make our involuntary dispositions and the alterity contained in the event a dynamic part of our personal history. The psychodynamic analysis consists, first of all, in the analysis of the *pathogenic situation*, that is, of the life situation that kindles the existential crisis and the psychopathological decomposition. Contrary to the standard notion of "trauma" which sees the person passively undergoing a distressing event, the notion of "situation" shows both the active (the person actively concurs in creating the situation) and the passive roles (the persons does not consciously intends to create the situation) (Tellenbach 1961/1980). The pathogenic situation can be seen as a limit situation (Jaspers 1925) in which the vulnerable structure of the patient is made manifest. Limit situations may turn into a pathogenic situation when they impact a given existentially vulnerable person. Limit situations include vulnerability to guilt, inescapability of finitude, anxiety for freedom, fragility of one's body, loneliness of one's existence, etc.

The relation between pathogenic situations and existentially vulnerable personality is a *key-lock relation* (Kretschmer 1919) in the sense that each personality has its own specific limit situation. Fuchs offers some examples of such vulnerability: the hypochondriac's sensitivity to the perils of bodily existence, the anorexic's sensitivity to the dependency on a material body, the depressive's vulnerability in relation to freedom and guilt, and the narcissist's vulnerability to the limitation of possibilities (Fuchs 2013).

Existentially vulnerable persons establish themselves within the defensive walls of a housing to avoid the contents uncovered by their specific limit situation (Fuchs 2013). For instance, for obsessive structures, completeness and perfection are the basic assumption/housing that defends from contingency and unpredictability. For the melancholic type of personality (Tellenbach 1961/1980) orderliness and hypernomia defend from guilt feelings. For dependent personality, hanging on others is the way to avoid the anxiety of freedom. For narcissistic personality, continuously expanding one's status via success is a defense from finiteness, restriction, and imperfection.

The D moment of the PHD helps the patient to recognize her own limit situation and its implications, to accept it and to take a stance toward it. Limit situations thus uncover the basic conditions of existence, that is, its being at risk of failure, guilt, death, financial ruin, etc. Personality structures are housings or shelters meant to defend from these threats. Yet these housings are precarious, vulnerable. The analysis of the pathogenic situation thus leads to the analysis of the patient's *vulnerable structure*. This indicates a significant combination of stable characteristics that make up the ontological constitution around which the vulnerability of the person is organized. A person's vulnerable structure is the amalgamation of a certain set of values and beliefs that serve as a protection from this person's limit situation. For instance, *antagonomia* in persons with schizophrenia, that is, their claiming one's independence as the most important value, can be seen as a shelter or defensive structure against their feeling to be vulnerable to the influx coming from the external world since for them conventional (common sense) assumptions, social-shared knowledge, common ways of thinking and behaving, and immediate (empathic) relationships and emotional attunement are evaluated as dangerous sources of loss of individuation. The D moment of the PHD can lead a patient to understand one's own shelter, its basic assumptions or philosophy of life, as a fragile defense against one's own limit situation, and to the awareness of the failure of all attempts toward solution through housings.

The analyses of the pathogenic situation and of the vulnerable structure are part and parcel of psychodynamics as the basic presuppositions of psychodynamics are psychological (existential) continuity and psychological determinism (Brackel 2009). The former assumes that all events in a person's life (including those that look inconsistent) are lawful and potentially meaningful in a particular way for that person. The latter presumes that all events in a person's life have at least as one of their causes a psychological cause and can thereby be explained on a psychological basis. The PHD method endorses the first one, and only partially the second. The purpose of the D moment in the PHD method is not an archaeology, that is, the rescuing of a remote cause that is posited in the past (Stanghellini 2016a). The psychodynamic moment is not the search for a *big bang*. What is searched for is not a datum, an event that has taken place at the origin of a person's story. Rather, it is a phenomenon that allows the intelligibility of the other historical phenomena. It is something that belongs to a person's life-history that helps make intelligible a string of phenomena whose association might have passed unobserved. This "something" enforces the coherence and synchronic comprehensibility of the system (Agamben 2008: 93). Looking into a person's past has not the purpose of finding a remote traumatic event that causally explains (to explain technically means *scire per causas*) the following events that have taken place. Rather, the purpose is looking for the phenomenon—let's call it the *Urphänomen*—that can lend coherence to the person's life-history.

The *Urphänomen* is not chronologically original, but hermeneutically so. It may not be a traumatic event that has taken place in the remote past and gave origin to a given personal development. The *Urphänomen* is better understood as the best examplar of a class of phenomena that exhibits, shows, and points out the essential properties of that kind of phenomena. It is a single phenomenon in a person's life-history that, being very perspicuous in its singularity, can make intelligible an entire group of phenomena, whose semantic homogeneousness it has contributed to creating. If I discover the *Urphänomen* in a person's life-history, this will shed light on all other previously opaque phenomena by means of the analogy between itself and the other phenomena. The *Urphänomen* can transform a set of phenomena that, at face value, were unrelated into a *gestalt* of meaningfully related phenomena. It is not an aetio-pathogenic construct, but rather a hermeneutic one. It can generate pathogenic or aetiological hypotheses, but it should not be taken as an aetio-pathogenic construct per se. The task of reconstructing the "causes" of human behavior in all cases is based on and must therefore be preceded by—especially in a therapeutic context—that of reconstructing its meaning that motivates behavior. Thus, this task is first and foremost hermeneutical in nature.

Conclusion: A Decalogue for Phenomenological Psychotherapy

1) Suspending all common-sense as well as theoretical prejudices and focusing on the patient's subjective experience as they are narrated by him as the point of departure of any clinical encounter.

2) Encouraging the patient to unfold his experiences and make explicit his emotions and values as the core of his life-world and his personal horizon of meaning.

3) Helping the patient to reflect upon his experiences, express them in a narrative format, and identify a core meaning, or meaning-organizer, around which his narrative can become meaningful for him.

4) Supporting the patient in taking a position in front of the way he narrates and makes sense of his experiences.

5) The clinician's making explicit to the patient his own experiences elicited by the patient's narratives, and his own understanding of the patient's narrative (assumptions, personal experiences, beliefs) as if it were his own.

6) Through this process, the clinician also makes his own set of theoretical assumptions, personal experiences, values, and beliefs, explicit.

7) The clinician promotes a reciprocal exchange of perspectives with his patient.

8) Clinician and patient cooperate in the co-construction of a new meaningful narrative that includes and, if possible, integrates contributions from both the original perspectives.

9) The clinician tolerates diversity and potential conflicts of values and beliefs.

10) Finally, the clinician facilitates coexistence when it is not possible to establish consensus.

BIBLIOGRAPHY

Agamben G. (2008). *Signatura rerum. Sul metodo*. Torino: Bollati Boringhieri.

Aragona M. (2013). "Neopositivism and the DSM Psychiatric Classification. An Epistemological History. Part 2: Historical Pathways, Epistemological Developments and Present-day Needs." *History of Psychiatry* 24: 415–426.

Ballerini A. (2003). "La psicopatologia tra 'comprendere' e 'spiegare.'" In A. Garofalo and L. Del Pistoia (eds.), *Sul comprendere psicopatologico*, pp. 31–48. Pisa: Edizioni ETS.

Binswanger L. (1928/1963). *Being in the World. Selected Papers of Ludwig Binswanger*. New York: Basic Books.

Binswanger L. (1956). *Drei Formen missglueckten Daseins: Verstiegenheit, Verschrbenheit, Maniererertheit*. Tuebingen: Niemayer.

Brackel L. A. W. (2009). *Philosophy, Psychoanalysis, and the A-Rational Mind*. Oxford: Oxford University Press.

Fuchs T. (2013). "Existential Vulnerability: Toward a Psychopathology of Limit Situation." *Psychopathology* 46: 301–308.

Fulford K. W. M and Stanghellini G. "Values and Values-based Practise," Chapter 41, this volume.

Heidegger M. (1927/1962). *Being and Time*. Oxford: Blackwell/Harper and Row.

Husserl E. (1936/1970). *The Crisis of European Sciences and Transcendental Phenomenology: An Introduction to Phenomenological Philosophy*. Northwestern University Press.

Husserl E. (1977). "Seeing Essences as Genuine Method for Grasping the A Priori." In *Phenomenological Psychology*. The Hague: Martinus Nijhoff.

Jaspers K. (1913/1997). *General Psychopathology*, trans. J. Hoenig and M. W. Hamilton. Baltimore: The Johns Hopkins University Press.

Jaspers K. (1925). *Psychologie der Weltanschauungen*, dritte Auflage. Berlin: Springer.

Jaspers K. (1956) *Existenzerhellung*. Philosophie II. Berlin/Goettingen/Heidelberg: Springer.

Jay M. (1994). *Downcast Eyes. The Denigration of Vision in French Twentieth Century Thought.* Berkeley and Los Angeles: University of California Press.

Kendler K. S. (2008). "Introduction: Why Does Psychiatry Need Philosophy?" In K. S. Kendler and J. Parnas (eds.), *Philosophical Issues in Psychiatry. Explanation, Phenomenology, and Nosology*, pp. 1–16. Baltimore: Johns Hopkins University Press.

Kretschmer E. (1919). *Der sensitive Beziehungswahn. Ein Beitrag zur Paranoidefrage und zur psychiatrischen Charakterlehre.* Berlin/Goettingen/Heidelberg: Springer.

Lanteri-Laura G. (1993). "Introduction à l'oeuvre psychopathologique d'Eugène Minkowski (Postface)." In E. Minkowski (ed.), *Structure des depressions*, pp. 63–118. Paris: Nouvel Object.

Levin D. M. (1993). *Modernity and the Hegemony of Vision.* Berkeley and Los Angeles: University of California Press.

Mayer-Gross W. (1920). "*Uber die Stellungnahme zur abgelaufenen akuten Psychose: Eine Studie uber verstandliche Zusammenhange in der Schizophrenie* [Concerning the position-taking to past acute psychosis: A study of meaningful connections in schizophrenia]." *Zeitschrift fuer die Gesamte Neurologie und Psychiatrie* 60: 160–212.

McKenna W. R. (1997). "Epoché and Reduction." In L. Embree, et al. (eds.), *Encyclopaedia of Phenomenology*, pp. 177–180. Dordrecht/Boston/London: Kluwer.

Minkowski E. (1930/1993). "Etude sur la structure des états de depression (Les depressions ambivalentes)." In E. Minkowski (ed.), *Structure des depressions*, pp. 1–61. Paris, Nouvel Object.

Parnas J. and Sass L. A. (2008). "Varieties of 'Phenomenology': On Description, Understanding, and Explanation in Psychiatry." In K. S. Kendler and J. Parnas (eds.), *Philosophical Issues in Psychiatry: Explanation, Phenomenology, and Nosology*, pp. 239–278. Baltimore: Johns Hopkins University Press.

Ricoeur P. (1981). *Hermeneutics and the Human Sciences.* Cambridge: Cambridge University Press.

Sass L. A. (2001). "Self and World in Schizophrenia: Three Classic Approaches." *Philosophy, Psychiatry, & Psychology* 8: 251–270.

Sass L. A. (2010). "Phenomenology as Descriptions and as Explanation: The Case of Schizophrenia." In S. Gallagher and D. Schmicking (eds.), *Handbook of Phenomenology and the Cognitive Sciences*, pp. 635–654. Berlin: Springer.

Stanghellini G. (2010). "A Hermeneutic Framework for Psychopathology." *Psychopathology* 43: 319–326.

Stanghellini G. (2013a). "The Ethics of Incomprehensibility." In G. Stanghellini and T. Fuchs (eds.), *One Century of Karl Jaspers' General Psychopathology*, pp. 166–183. Oxford: Oxford University Press.

Stanghellini G. (2013b). "Philosophical Resources for the Psychiatric Interview." In K. W. M. Fulford, M. Davies, R. G. T. Gipps, et al. (eds.), *The Oxford Handbook of Philosophy and Psychiatry.* Oxford, Oxford University Press.

Stanghellini G. (2016a). *Lost in Dialogue. Anthropology, Psychopathology, and Care.* Oxford/New York: Oxford University Press.

Stanghellini G. (2016b). "Phenomenological Psychopathology and Care. From Person-Centered Dialectical Psychopathology to the PHD Method for Psychotherapy." In G. Stanghellini and M. Aragona (eds.), *An Experiential Approach to Psychopathology. What is it Like to Suffer from Mental Disorders.* Heidelberg/New York: Springer.

Stanghellini G. and Ballerini M. (2007). "Values in Persons with Schizophrenia." *Schizophrenia Bulletin* 33(1): 131–141.

Stanghellini G., Castellini G., Brogna P., Faravelli C., Ricca V. (2012). "Identity and Eating Disorders (IDEA): A Questionnaire Evaluating Identity and Embodiment in Eating Disorder Patients." *Psychopathology* 45: 147–158.

Stanghellini G., Bolton D., and Fulford K. W. M. (2013). "Person-centered Psychopathology of Schizophrenia: Building on Karl Jaspers' Understanding of Patient's Attitude toward his Illness." *Schizophrenia Bulletin* 39(2): 287–294.

Stanghellini G. and Rossi R. (2014). "Pheno-phenotypes: A Holistic Approach to the Psychopathology of Schizophrenia." *Current Opinion Psychiatry* 27(3): 236–241.

Stanghellini G. and Aragona M. (2016). "Phenomenological Psychopathology: Toward a Person-Centered Hermeneutic Approach in the Clinical Encounter." In G. Stanghellini and M. Aragona (eds.), *An Experiential Approach to Psychopathology. What is it Like to Suffer from Mental Disorders*, pp. 1–43. Heidelberg/New York: Springer.

Stanghellini G., Ballerini M., Presenza S., Mancini M., Northoff G., and Cutting J. (2016). "Abnormal Time Experiences in Major Depression: An Empirical Qualitative Study." *Psychopathology.* doi: 10.1159/000452892

Stanghellini G. and Mancini M. (2017). *The Therapeutic Interview. Emotions, Values and the Life-world.* Cambridge: Cambridge University Press.

Tellenbach H. (1961/1980). *Melancholy: History of the Problem, Endogeneity, Typology, Pathogenesis, Clinical Considerations.* Pittsburg: Duquesne University Press.

Urfer A. (2001). "Phenomenology and Psychopathology of Schizophrenia: The Views of Eugène Minkowski." *Philosophy, Psychiatry, & Psychology* 8: 279–289.

van den Berg J. H. (1955). *The Phenomenological Approach to Psychiatry. An Introduction to Recent Phenomenological Psychopathology.* Springfield: Thomas Publisher.

Villareal E. and Aragona M. (2014). "El concepto de 'comprensión' (Verstehen) en Karl Jaspers." *Vertex* 116: 262–265.

CHAPTER 89

PHENOMENOLOGICAL PSYCHOPATHOLOGY AND PSYCHIATRIC ETHICS

RENÉ ROSFORT

INTRODUCTION

ETHICS is a fundamental part of psychiatry, and also a constant challenge to psychiatry. As with other branches of medicine, care for vulnerable individuals is at the heart of psychiatry. Ethical principles and guidelines are established to secure recognition of the patient as a person. Since the humanitarian reforms of medical practice at the turn of the nineteenth century, the recognition that patients are persons has become an integrated part of medicine to the extent that is considered a fact on a par with our physiological and anatomical facts. Biological facts exist independently of human recognition, even though their existence is uncovered and corroborated by human beings. The fact that patients are persons is a different kind of fact. It is a normative fact. This means that it is a fact that cannot be discovered or ratified once and for all, but a fact that needs constant human recognition in order to exist. It is possible to understand and treat a patient as an impersonal human being in need of medical assistance. The patient is thus reduced to an object of our scientific curiosity or to a means to fulfil our professional ambition. Recognizing the patient as a person is to see, understand, and interact with the patient as an autonomous person with a particular history and with her own experience of and ideas about her life. While the cure of disease is the avowed goal of medicine, an ethical perspective is meant to make health professionals acknowledge—or remember—that all diseases are personal. A disease happens to a person who suffers in her or his own way. To put it concisely, one could argue that biomedical ethics is about securing care as a fundamental part of the medical cure. Care and the recognition of the patient as a person have become integral parts of contemporary medical practice, but how exactly to take care of the concrete person's suffering is still a challenge that health professionals are faced with daily. The complexity of health care stems from the fact that patients have their individual needs and ideas about themselves and their illness. Safeguarding the autonomy of the person is a principal ethical concern in caring for the patient, but the work to cure the patient also requires adopting an impersonal perspective on the suffering of the person. A medical approach has to adopt a stance capable of diagnosing and treating the impersonal and heteronomous factors at work in a person's illness, even when this course of treatment may go against the patient's understanding of her suffering. In no branch of medicine is this interplay of care and cure as intimately interwoven into the fabric of both theory and practice as is the case with psychiatry.

Psychiatric ethics is part of biomedical ethics, and as such it is concerned with mapping out and examining the ethical foundation, principles, theories, and methods concerning medical practice (Beauchamp and Childress 2013). Recent years have witnessed increasing attention to the distinctiveness of the ethical issues involved in psychiatry (Sadler, Van Staden, and Fulford 2015), and it has been argued that psychiatric practice involves many features (e.g. patient vulnerabilities, stigma, societal structures, controversy over the concept of mental disorder, consumer movements) that combine to make it a unique biomedical practice with ethical challenges that require different perspectives than can be provided with a traditional bioethical approach (Radden 2002; Bloch and Green 2006; Radden and Sadler 2009). Common to both bioethical approaches and the more recent approaches of psychiatric ethics is to treat ethical perspectives as relevant almost exclusively to the practice of psychiatry. In most approaches to mental illness, for example, biological and phenomenological approaches, ethics does not play an explanatory role in the theoretical work toward understanding a specific mental illness. The etiology and pathogenesis of a mental illness are considered to be unaffected by ethical questions, and norms and values come into the account either before the scientific investigations begin or after they have been concluded. Most psychiatrists would probably agree that the primary challenge for psychiatry is to connect anonymous biological explanations such as genetic and neurobiological functioning with the first-person experience of suffering. As Kenneth Kendler puts it: "We deal with symptoms of the mind. Stopping at third-person 'explanations' of disease mechanisms leaves our project unfinished. We also want, and our patients deserve, understanding in a first-person framework" (Kendler 2014: 936). One of the most long-standing debates in psychiatry concerns which of the two levels is the primary object of psychiatric research. Biologically oriented psychiatrists argue that the mental illnesses are to be assessed and explained primarily on a third-person, impersonal biological level (Insel and Cuthbert 2015). Phenomenologically oriented psychiatrists contend that mental illness is rooted in and developed through human experience, and that we therefore cannot explain any mental illness without taking into account the subjective aspects of that illness (Parnas, Sass, and Zahavi 2013). Common to both approaches, though, is the exclusion of ethics from the theoretical framework. In neither approach do ethical considerations figure as explanatory elements in the examination of mental illness. On these accounts, ethical issues such as the distinction between biological and experiential norms, between personal values and cultural norms, the sense of obligation, the demand of responsibility, the ideal of a good life, the question of justice, the challenge of identity concern psychiatry practice rather than psychiatric theory. Ethics in this way functions as a kind of "add-on" to the discipline of psychiatry, that is, as a normative perspective introduced from outside the discipline in order to secure patient rights or in other ways regulate the practice of psychiatry.

Ethics has never figured prominently in phenomenological psychopathology, so in this respect phenomenological psychopathology does not differ much from other psychiatric approaches. And yet, ethical considerations play a more critical role in phenomenological psychopathology than in most other approaches to mental illness. For the phenomenolog-ical psychiatrist mental illness not only involves disturbances of experience as the result of biological malfunctioning or environmental stressors. Mental illness is an illness *of* expe-rience, and we cannot hope to understand or treat a mental illness without examining the experiential disturbances involved in that illness. These disturbances affect our sense of identity, our self-awareness, and the way we experience time, world, and other people. The central role that experience, self-awareness, and sense of identity play in phenomenological psychopathology means that ethical considerations cannot but an integral part of the un-derstanding of mental illness. Human experience is value-laden, self-awareness is saturated with feelings, and our sense of identity is constituted by norms, conventions, and concerns. We are not able make sense of and deal with mental suffering without an examination of how norms and values inform and orient human existence. And perhaps even more importantly, understanding how to cure the mental suffering of a person involves a clarification of what the person cares about.

The argument of this chapter is that the interplay of cure and care is central to phenome-nological psychopathology, and that it is in the articulation of this interplay that we find the most significant contribution of phenomenological psychopathology to psychiatric ethics. In what follows, I will outline the relationship between ethics and phenomenological psy-chopathology by examining the perennial question of the good life, how to make sense of what we care about, the challenge of autonomy, and the problem of responsibility in relation to mental illness. I will use various philosophers to construct my argument, and primarily the works of two French phenomenologists from the twentieth century, Emmanuel Levinas and Paul Ricoeur. The work of these philosophers is concerned with showing that ethics is an integral part of human experience, and that we cannot understand what it means to be human without articulating the ethical core of what we care about. For Levinas and Ricoeur, phenomenological articulations of what we care about will bring out the personal character of ethical considerations. Ethics lurks in the simple question "what shall I do?" and, as the philosopher Volker Gerhardt argues:

> When one suddenly asks this question by oneself, then one has a consciousness of morality. Then responsibility lets itself know. Conscience is stirred and demands that one understands one's own duty.
>
> (Gerhardt 1999: 389; author's translation)

The phenomenological articulation of ethics as an integral part of human experience will support my argument that phenomenological psychopathology has a significant contribu-tion to make to psychiatric ethics. The phenomenological approach to psychopathology enables us to see that ethical considerations are not merely an external normative perspec-tive on psychiatry, but constitutive of the experience of mental illness and as such critical to the medical understanding of what a mental illness is.

Ethics and the Ambiguity of the Good Life

The good life has been a central topic in ethics since antiquity. In the *Republic*, Plato has Socrates discuss with the sophist Thrasymachus whether being just and honest contributes to a person's happiness or whether these virtues are merely foils covering more cynical power structures (Plato 1997: 981–998 [336b–354c]), and Aristotle opens the first systematic treatise on ethics, the *Nicomachean Ethics*, with the argument that every person wants to be happy, and that we all orient our lives around the idea of happiness (Aristotle 1984: 1729–1742 [1094a–1103a]). The problem is that the notions of the good life and happiness—as well as most other normative notions—are inherently vague and cause more confusion than clarity. Plato and Aristotle were of course aware of this, and the importance of their work, as is the case with subsequent moral philosophers, lies in the way they clarify and produce arguments for the norms and values that constitute our understanding of how to live a human life. Ethical examinations deal primarily with understanding our emotions, desires, and ideas in light of normative notions such as happiness and the good life. How to educate human beings so that they live peacefully and productively together in a society? How does a person become virtuous? How does a person learn to domesticate her desires and cravings in order to find a more permanent kind of happiness? In short, how can human beings live a good life?

The question of the good life dominated moral philosophy and ethical debates for millennia, but in the Enlightenment the philosophical priority of the good life was challenged by the idea of duty. Toward the end of the seventeenth century, the German philosopher Immanuel Kant revolutionized the philosophical debate about ethics and changed the cultural understanding of what it means to be a person. Inspired by the time-hallowed Christian tradition of neighborly love and contemporary Enlightenment ideas about autonomy and equality, Kant argued that the problem with orienting ethical considerations around the ideas of happiness and the good life is that human beings are inescapably selfish creatures who most of the time use their rational capacities to justify their own selfish interests. He writes: "[W]e like to flatter ourselves by falsely attributing to ourselves a nobler motive, whereas in fact we can never, even by the most strenuous self-examination, get entirely behind our covert incentives, since when moral worth is at issue, what counts are not actions, which one sees, but those inner principles of actions that one does not see" (Kant 1996a: 61–62). Our examinations of the good life and our understanding of virtue, character, and happiness cannot, on Kant's account, extricate themselves from our individual perspective, our ideas, our culture, our desires and inclinations, that is, our subjectivity. The idea of the good life is teleological and as such aimed at ideals of goodness and happiness. These ideals, however, cannot but be affected by the subjective values of the person or the intersubjective norms of the culture that constructs the ideals. The only way to escape the subjective particularity of our norms and values is to seek for a moral compass that leads to an understanding of goodness independent of our own interests and desires. Kant finds this compass to be an impersonal moral law capable of universalizing our particular human perspectives and thereby working toward securing equality, autonomy, and dignity for all human beings. In fact, Kant's radical argument is that we can only secure a life as autonomous human beings in and through our duty to respect the humanity that we share with other human beings. This humanity is secured by the moral law and consists in our rational capacity to liberate ourselves from our inclinations and desires. Only through this detachment from our natural inclination do we become free to choose our own life. To be human is thus to be an autonomous person, and to understand a human being as a person is to recognize a basic "freedom and independence from the mechanism of the whole nature" and to respect this freedom by never using a person "merely as a means," but only as "an end in itself" (Kant 1996b: 210).

The moral law with its impersonal imperatives of universality and humanity is therefore—paradoxically—that which secures our personal autonomy (Manganaro 1989: 41–65). One of Kant's most influential contributions to ethics is to be found in his argument for our duty to respect the humanity that makes every human being an autonomous person. Our individual human freedom is only possible through a respect for and a constant working for the freedom of the other person.

The good life and the respect for humanity are key topics in contemporary philosophical ethics, and both play a critical, although often tacit, role in mental health care. It is evident that mental health and the good life are entangled, that is, mental health is vital to a good life, and a good life is fundamental to our mental health. It is, however, not obvious how exactly mental health and the good life are related. There are of course many ways to approach this issue. Phenomenology offers an explanatory framework that allows us to examine how a person's ideas about the good life can both promote and disturb that person's mental health. This ambiguity of our ideas about a good life is connected with the norms and values that orient our existence. We experience our life through our ideas about how our life should be. Most of the time we do not explicitly articulate these ideas, but they still function as implicit points of orientation for our feelings, thoughts, and actions. The good life functions as a kind of horizon for our life, and we cannot, as Aristotle rightly points out, escape the desire for the good life. Ideas about a good life are in this sense constitutive of our experience of the world, other people, and ourselves. This also means that these ideas have significant impact on our mental health. Our hope for the good life can help us through disturbances of our mental health and alleviate our mental suffering. On the other hand, our inability to realize our ideas of a good life can make us despair and thus contribute to the disturbances of our mental health and intensify our metal suffering. Richard Bentall cogently captures this vital role of hope in mental health care: "Sometimes ordinary stories of triumph over adversity are inspiring. They remind us that hope is the fire that will guide us through darkness. Psychiatry's greatest sin has been to crush hope in those it has claimed to care for. Without hope the struggle for survival seems pointless. With hope, almost everything seems possible" (Bentall 2009: 288).

This ambiguity of the good life is closely connected with the duty to humanity. As we have seen, Kant introduced the duty to humanity in order to demonstrate the problematic character of our ideas of the good life. The duty to humanity concerns our recognition of human beings as autonomous persons. We have, according to Kant, a duty to recognize and respect our own autonomy and the autonomy of other people. These two basic aspects of autonomy—my autonomy as well as that of the other—present a constant challenge to our ideas about the good life. First of all, our ideas about the good life are never entirely our own, but significantly influenced by our upbringing, sociocultural, and biological factors, and as such the good life can be experienced as something that is imposed on us, and at times as an obstacle to our autonomy, to our sense of being an individual and unique self. Moreover, our ideas about what is good and meaningful change over time, and we might find ourselves alienated from the life that we have chosen to live. Our choices are, in other words, never truly transparent to ourselves, and who we want to be is often in tension with who we have become and what we actually do. Finally, ideas of the good life are inherently selfish and therefore risk making us blind to the fact that our life is lived through the coexistence with other people. Our ideas about the good life are in constant tension, if not outright conflict, with our duty to recognize and treat other human beings as autonomous persons who can never be used to further our own interests.

To be human is to be an autonomous person, and the challenges of autonomy to our ideas about the good life are fundamental to our mental health. To make sense of these challenges, we have to look at the experiential character of what we care about, and try to clarify the normative structure of our care and caring.

CARE AND CARING

The notion of care was introduced into phenomenology in 1927 by Martin Heidegger in his epochal work *Being and Time* (Heidegger 2010). The notion of care is central to Heidegger's endeavor to produce a theory of what it is to be human, an ontology, that is radically different from the traditional understanding in Western philosophy of human beings as primarily rational beings whose existence is and should be constituted by cognitively transparent norms and values secured by logic and reason. Heidegger does not deny that human beings are rational beings who orient themselves through cognitive norms and values. He does argue, though, that the idea of rationality has overshadowed the fact that human beings are also affective beings whose existence is saturated with feelings that they have not chosen and that they cannot make sense of (Heidegger 2010: 130). Human beings find themselves in the world and are engaged with the world before they try to understand the world and their place in it. We find ourselves in the world in a certain way. The world affects us and matters to us before we attempt to make reflective sense of what we care about. As Heidegger writes, in and through care a human being "is always already brought before itself, it has always already found itself, not as perceiving oneself to be there, but as one finds one's self in attunement" (Heidegger 2010: 132). We do not freely choose what we care about. We find ourselves affectively entangled with the world and other people to the extent that it is difficult to maintain a sense of identity. This means that we have to make sense of what we care about in order to understand who we are and how we actually want to live our life (Heidegger 2010: 307–309). Heidegger's analysis of care as the ontological structure of human existence brings out the normative character of human experience. Our existence matters to us, and we care about the world, other people, and ourselves. We cannot escape the normative structures of existence or the more or less articulate demands that those structures lay upon us. As Simon Blackburn cogently puts it, "*there is no getting behind ethics*. It comes unbidden. It comes with living" (Blackburn 1998: 2; emphasis in the original). Heidegger did not articulate the ethical implications of his understanding of care. His account of normativity remained impersonal and, as Karl Jaspers has pointed out, strangely solipsistic (Jaspers 1978: 33). One could argue that Heidegger's notion of care is a care without caring and that his account of normativity is a normativity without ethics. Nonetheless, his analysis of the normative complexity of care provided the foundation for several subsequent phenomenological investigations into the ethical character of human experience.

Among the most influential of these are the works of the French philosophers Emmanuel Levinas and Paul Ricoeur. Both philosophers are deeply indebted to Kant's notion of duty to humanity, and both are critical of what they understand to be Heidegger's impersonal understanding of normativity (Levinas 2001: 81–82; Ricoeur 2004: 9–10). Our lives are entangled the lives of other people, and an account of care without a duty to actually care about the concrete person in front of me is, for both philosophers, deeply problematic. We exist as persons together with other persons, and the interpersonal character of human existence makes ethics a fundamental part of what we care about. This fundamental role of ethics is inscribed in the normative structure of human experience. The phenomenology that we find in the work of Levinas and Ricoeur is oriented toward showing that the normative duty to humanity is not a demand arbitrarily or contingently imposed on human beings. That is to say, that the demand is not rooted in a specific cultural, social, or philosophical conception of human nature. It is constitutive of human experience. Seeing the other is experiencing the duty to take care of the other. It is an ethics that, so to say, grows out of experience. The other person matters to me whether I want to acknowledge it or not. In fact, I cannot escape the other. She is part of my life, and her simple presence is an ethical demand to me as a person.

This personal character of ethics, the experiential force of ethical obligations, comes out most vigorously in the philosophical poetry of Levinas:

> The face with which the Other turns to me is not reabsorbed in a representation of a face. To hear his destitution which cries out for justice is not to represent an image to oneself, but is to posit oneself as responsible, both as more and as less than the being that presents itself in the face. The being that presents himself in the face comes from a dimension of height, a dimension of transcendence whereby he can present himself as a stranger without opposing me as obstacle or enemy. More, for my position as *I* consists in being able to respond to the essential destitution of the other, finding resources for myself. The Other who dominates me in his transcendence is thus the stranger, the widow, and the orphan, to whom I am obligated.
>
> (Levinas 1969: 215)

The ethical obligation at the core of the duty to humanity—and the many ways this duty challenges my understanding of a good life—has rarely, if ever, been articulated more concretely or argued for more conspicuously than in the works of Levinas. The ethics of Levinas is radical in the sense that it explicitly argues for an asymmetric account of interpersonal relationship. We are infinitely responsible for the other, and we can never extricate ourselves from this responsibility. Our duty to the humanity of the concrete person in front of us should overshadow our care for living a good life. Levinas is not concerned with developing an ethics that combines the duty to humanity with our ideas about living a good life. On the contrary, Levinas argues against such attempts to accommodate our duty to the other with our care for ourselves. I have a duty to care for the other. My other cares and concerns must fade into the background in the encounter with the other person. The ethical approach of Levinas demands that I sacrifice my ideas of my good life for the other. I must "forget myself for my neighbor who looks at me" accepting that "[s]acrifice is the norm and criterion of the approach" (Levinas 1996: 76).

Levinas's radical phenomenological ethics constitutes an enduring contribution to psychiatric ethics. His phenomenological examinations of how the encounter with the other person challenges our ideas about what it means to be human making evident the conceptual shortcomings of our attempts to understand a concrete person. The medical environment can prefigure our vision, and our professional expertise can make us blind to the concrete individual who experiences and communicates his suffering. Levinas teaches us to see the person in the patient in front of us. Instead of understanding the other with our ideas and concepts, we have a responsibility for allowing the other to exist as a concrete person who we can never fully understand. We should, in other words, complement our heteronomous conceptual and symptomatic approach to the patient with an approach that allows for the autonomous suffering of this concrete person (Levinas 1998:148). In this sense, the ethics of Levinas is a constant and vital reminder to actually see the other person in the patient in front of us.

A phenomenological approach to psychopathology can contribute with more than an articulate and nuanced account of this vital demand to treat the patient as a person. The phenomenological approach also produces philosophical resources to make sense of how ethics plays into mental suffering in terms of the experienced tension between our ideas about the good life and the duty to humanity. To explore this question, we can turn to Paul Ricoeur in whose ethics we find an account of human identity that combines our ideas of the good life with the duty to humanity.

THE CHALLENGES OF AUTONOMY

Ricoeur constructs his ethics upon autonomy. To be human is to be autonomous, and a human life is the story of our effort to affirm our autonomy through the challenges of otherness. He develops this ethics of autonomy through phenomenological investigations of the tension between selfhood and otherness constitutive of human self-awareness. We become aware of being a self through the experience of otherness. This otherness is not different from or somehow distinct from me. It is an otherness that I am. I am an embodied, situated, and social being, and I experience myself through the encounter with the otherness of my body, the world, and other people.

This intimate otherness is implicitly manifest in bodily experience. I feel, think, and act through my body, and in this sense my body is an integral part of my pre-reflective awareness of being a self and constitutive of my sense of agency. I use my body to live my life thus making my body an organ of my autonomy. And yet my body is also a heteronomous organism among other biophysical organisms in nature, and as such subject to the anonymous functions and conditions of the natural world (Ricoeur 1992: 127). My body requires food, water, exercise, and sleep. My body ages, becomes sick, and eventually dies in spite of what I do. In and through my bodily experience I encounter an otherness that I am and yet that I may not want to be. This becomes obvious in the fact that I am not entirely in control of what I care about. My body has needs that may surprise, disgust, and even frighten me. And yet these needs are my needs although I do not identify with them. In Ricoeur's words, I have to live "with the otherness of the flesh that I am" (Ricoeur 1992: 326). This experiential tension between selfhood and otherness springs from our sense of autonomy, from our sense of agency and ownership, and the various challenges to this sense of autonomy are fundamental to our understanding of who we are. Otherness is constitutive of human identity. As seen with the experience of our own body, we experience who we are through the experience of passivity. This passivity constantly challenges our endeavor to become who we want to be, and through the experience of these challenges we discover that our identity is not entirely of our making, but constituted by that over which we have little or no control. In other words, we have to find ourselves through a passivity that is an inescapable part of our identity. The relation between selfhood and otherness in human identity is thus dialectical in the sense that we cannot understand selfhood without otherness or vice versa.

Our endeavors to understand ourselves are disturbed by the experience of not being who we want to be. The experiential fact that human self-understanding "hold together, side by side, the serene affirmation *I am* and the poignant doubt *Who am I?*" (Ricoeur 2004: 259) makes human identity constitutively fragile. To exist as a person, Ricoeur argues, is therefore to reappropriate oneself through the fragility of one's identity (Ricoeur 1970: 472). This reappropriation of our identity is not a choice, that is, it is not something that we can choose not to do. We can escape neither our fragility nor our autonomy. Ricoeur adopts Kant's duty to humanity, and he develops a phenomenological articulation of the notion of autonomy that is fundamental to Kant's understanding of humanity. Unlike Levinas and more in line with Kant, Ricoeur argues that the duty to humanity involves a respect for the autonomy of oneself as well as for the autonomy of the other: "Humanity is a way of treating human beings. This means neither you nor I. It is the practical ideal of 'the self' in you as well as me" (Ricoeur 1986: 72; translation slightly modified). We cannot construct a life through the sacrifice of our autonomy for the other. We have the duty to respect our own autonomy even through the most terrible experiences of suffering and loss. "The human being," Ricoeur states, "is the Joy of Yes in the sadness of the finite" (Ricoeur 1986: 140). He elaborates on this statement elsewhere:

> [A] meditation on unswerving necessity reaches its limit in the exultation of freedom, in the resumption of responsibility by means of which I exclaim: I am the one who moves this body which carries me and betrays me. I change this world which situates me and creates me according to the flesh. I give rise to being within and without myself through my choice.
>
> (Ricoeur 1966: 482–483; translation modified)

We experience the challenge of autonomy through the desire to create our own life or at least to find ourselves as ourselves in the life that we have been given. Every human being is a person, and yet to be a person is to care about being a certain kind of person. Our sense of autonomy is entangled with our dreams, hopes, and ideas about who we want to be, and we cannot escape this experience of being more than—or at least different from—what we are and what other people understand us to be. The paradox of autonomy is that our capacity to self-determine our life, to realize ourselves as the persons that we want to be, is also the very capacity that makes us feel at unease with ourselves. Our sense of autonomy makes our identity fragile because we are faced with the task of trying to hold our identity together through the encounter with otherness. We are responsible for our identity, and yet our identity is not of our own making. Nor can we understand who we are without understanding that our life is ineradicably interwoven with the life of other people.

The intimate otherness that we first experience through our own body makes itself known as the desire for the otherness of the other person in our thinking about the good life. In the desire for the other person, we find that otherness of the other person is as fundamentally constitutive of our identity as is the otherness of our body. And as is the case with my body, the other person is of course a challenge to my autonomy. He can say no to me, insult me, hurt me, or be a concrete obstacle to the realization of my ambition. I nevertheless need this person to recognize me as an autonomous person. My autonomy is in this sense entangled with the autonomy of the other person. The recognition of my autonomy is, according to Ricoeur, only possible through the recognition of the autonomy of the other person (Ricoeur 2005: 89–93). I need the other *to want* to see me as a person. This need for the other is entangled with an almost visceral sense of justice. I depend upon the recognition from the other, and my own recognition of the other as an autonomous person is, in turn, necessary for this recognition to actually satisfy my own need. In other words, I need the other to complete me:

> [T]he demand for justice is like hunger and like thirst. This means that the faculty of desiring is broader than organic concern. I am a lacuna and a lack of something other than bread and water . . . In the last analysis, it is the other who counts. We must always return to this. It is thus the good of the other which I lack. The "I" is empty with respect to the other "I." He completes me, just as food does. The being of the subject is not solipsistic; it is being-in-common. In this way the sphere of intersubjective relations can be the analog of the organic sphere, and the world of need can provide the fundamental metaphor of appetite: the other "I," like the "not-I"– as for example nourishment—comes to fill up my lack . . . The community is my good because it leads towards making me whole within the "we" where the lacuna of my being would be filled. In some moments of precious communion I sense tentatively that the isolated self is perhaps only a segment torn from such others who could have become a you for me.
>
> (Ricoeur 1966: 127–128; translation modified)

My identity is constituted by the otherness of the other person. I experience myself as a self through the other, and only through recognizing the otherness of the other can I become the person that I want to be. In this sense, Ricoeur uses phenomenology to articulate how our ideas of a good life depend upon a duty to humanity. This phenomenological work brings out the fragile character of human identity through the dialectics of selfhood and otherness. Our autonomy is challenged by an otherness that is part of who we are. We need this otherness to be the persons that we are, and yet this otherness can also disturb our sense of identity to the extent that we lose our sense of identity.

The ethics of Ricoeur brings out the fragility of human identity through the dialectics of selfhood and otherness. This dialectics is experienced in and through the challenge of human autonomy. The challenge of autonomy is not merely the experience of passivity in the encounter with the otherness of our body, the world, and other people. Autonomy is also experienced as a challenge through my desire to construct a good life for myself. I experience a need to make my life mine. The merit of Ricoeur's ethics consists in his phenomenological articulation of how this desire of autonomy can only be satisfied through the otherness that I am, that is, my body, the world, and most important the autonomy of the other person. Our recognition of autonomy—in ourselves and in the other—entails a demand of responsibility. We are responsible for reappropriating ourselves through our fragility. We experience ourselves to be, and other people expect us to be, responsible for how we live our life, and yet human responsibility is fragile. In the concluding section that follows, we will use Ricoeur's phenomenological articulation of what we could call the strength of fragility to argue that the notion of fragility is the conceptual link that allows us to see how ethics is not merely an external perspective on psychiatry but a necessary element of our attempt to understand mental illness.

THE STRENGTH OF FRAGILITY

The question of responsibility is central to psychiatry. Recognizing the patient as an autonomous person entails the problem of how to make sense of the demand of responsibility that is constitutive of the idea of autonomy. How do we treat the patient as an autonomous person without making him responsible for his illness? What are we to do with the problem of stigma, that is, how do we avoid producing feelings of shame and fear of blame in the patient when introducing talk about responsibility? These questions concerning how to approach the patient are rendered all the more urgent by the fact that experience of responsibility plays a central role in how the patient experiences her illness. The experience of autonomy and the ensuing problem of responsibility is one of the cornerstones of Karl Jaspers's formative account of psychopathology, particularly in his insistence on the importance of the patient's attitude to his illness:

> The will can *interfere* with the psyche which it may darken or illuminate, inhibit or yield to, inflate in some respect or repress in another. When the individual is ill, there are various possibilities open to him in so far as a state of illness is not an objective biological condition but a subjective state as well, in the form of an awareness of the illness. This latter is not merely something that happens alongside the illness, the mere reflection of its consciousness, but it is an effective factor which is an actual link in the morbid state itself.
>
> (Jaspers 1997: 424)

Ricoeur's account of the strength of fragility can clarify and make sense of the role of responsibility in mental illness. The dialectics of selfhood and otherness produce our identity, and it is this dialectics that makes our identity fragile. Understanding responsibility through the fragile character of human identity allows for a perspective on mental illness that avoids two dehumanizing approaches to mental illness: a biological approach that focuses exclusively on the impersonal otherness of mental illness and a moralizing approach that understands mental illness exclusively as a problem of the self. The dehumanizing effect in these approaches lies in their respective approach to autonomy and the consequent understanding of the role of responsibility in mental illness. The presentation of these approaches is not a description of actual psychiatric approaches, but a construction of two opposite extremes within which contemporary mental health care is conducted. The drawing up of these extremes serves as a way to bring out two attitudes of dehumanization that are present in mental health care in less extreme forms.

The first of these ways of dehumanizing the patient is to adopt a biological approach that explains mental illness exclusively in terms of an impersonal biological functionalism. This approach reduces the patient to a hapless victim of genetic or neuronal malfunctioning, and thereby eliminates or at least sidesteps the autonomy that we experience as fundamental to our humanity. The biological approach is often considered to be beneficial because of the hope that a medicalized approach can reduce the stigma that sadly still haunts people who suffer from a mental illness. A genetic or neurological biological explanation of mental illness relieves the patient of responsibility for her illness, and without talk about responsibility the patient will no longer have to endure blame, discrimination, or social exclusion because of her mental suffering (Illes et al. 2009; Austin and Honer 2007). There is no evidence, however, that decades of a near hegemony of biological explanations of mental illness has reduced the stigma of mental illness (Malla, Joober, and Garcia 2015; Schomerus et al. 2012; Kvaale, Gottdiener, and Haslam 2013). Biological explanations can actually increase the public fear of persons with mental illnesses because of the impersonal character of the illness, and they do not necessarily make patients themselves feel less guilty about their illness (Rüsch et al. 2010; Read et al. 2006). The problem with this argument for the biological dehumanization of mental illness is, as Jaspers points out in the quote above, that an impersonal biological explanation does not eliminate the subjective or experiential feature of a mental illness. Autonomy is constitutive of human experience. We experience the world, other people, and ourselves through a sense of selfhood, and the demand of responsibility comes, as we have seen, unbidden with our sense of being an autonomous person. It therefore seems impossible to eliminate the idea of responsibility, both on the part of the patient and in the eye of public. Persons who suffer from a mental illness cannot escape the feeling of responsibility, and people who interact with a mentally ill person are frightened by the conception of an anonymous and therefore completely irresponsible—in the etymological sense of not being answerable—conception of mental illness.

The other way of dehumanizing the patient is to approach mental illness as exclusively a problem of the self. This approach is not as easy to individuate or as theoretically clear-cut as the biological approach. While the biological approach to mental illness grows out of a consolidated biomedical model that openly—and some would say proudly—aims at removing from or at least significantly reducing the subjective factor in the account of mental illness, the moralizing approach is more promethean in character, and is perhaps more adequately characterized as an implicit cultural attitude rather than an acknowledged theoretical approach. This attitude dehumanizes the patient by making the patient more responsible for her illness or for her recovery than is actually humanly possible. This strong notion of responsibility is fostered by a problematic conflation of autonomy with the moral idea of freedom. The capacity to give laws unto oneself, to self-determine oneself, is not the same as being free to do whatever one wants to do. Human autonomy is not free in this sense. We have a sense of autonomy, and we experience ourselves as capable of and responsible for determining our own life, but this experience of being a self is rooted in what Ricoeur calls the otherness of our body, the world, and other people. Human freedom is experience of the difficulty of freedom, and such "human freedom is," as Ricoeur argues, "a dependent independence, a receptive initiative" (Ricoeur 2007: 228). As with the biological approach, this moralistic version of dehumanization rarely comes in a clear and undiluted form—although explicit moralistic accounts can be found in some religious approaches to mental illness, and in the public debate about eating disorders and addictive disorders (Scrutton 2015; Frank and Nagel 2017; Easter 2012). The moralizing attitude is, however, an always present danger for the patient, the public, and the therapist when thinking about or debating whether or not a concrete case qualifies as a mental illness. Once again we cannot but structure our experience and understanding of human beings around the notion of autonomy. The dehumanizing effect of the moralizing approach consists in transforming the experience of autonomy into a moral ideal of human freedom that disregards the concrete challenges of otherness that make our autonomy human.

The lesson that we can draw from these two ways of dehumanizing the patient is that the sense of autonomy that structures human experience means that we cannot avoid the notion of responsibility when trying to understand mental illness. The notion of responsibility is fundamental to our experience of what it means to be human, but the experience of responsibility never comes with the purity or clarity that we find in our conceptual construct of responsibility. The lived *experience* of responsibility is vital to our sense of being a self, and the normative *concept* of responsibility functions as an explicit point of orientation for our endeavor to make sense of who we are and how to live a good life. The experience of responsibility is inescapably subjective while the concept of responsibility becomes a norm by disregarding the individuality constitutive of the experience of responsibility. The challenge of thinking about responsibility consists in the fact that we cannot disregard either of these perspectives on responsibility. We understand our identity through our experience of being responsible, and at the same time we experience responsibility as a normative challenge. This obscure role that responsibility plays in our sense of identity brings out the importance of the notion of fragility that Ricoeur articulated through his phenomenological ethics.

The notion of fragility can function as a conceptual link between the (descriptive) understanding of mental illness and the (normative) practice of mental health care. Human identity is fragile because of the dialectics of selfhood and otherness constitutive of what humans care about. Mental illness is an illness of experience, and the notion of fragility allows us to articulate and make sense of the importance of care in mental suffering. We suffer through disturbances of what we care about, and our suffering is marked by what we care about. The recognition of this experiential fragility at the core of mental illness requires an acknowledgment and acceptance of an explanatory fragility in the sense that our various conceptual approaches to mental illness allow for the autonomy of suffering of the concrete person in front of us. Only by acknowledging the fragile character of our approach to the patient are we capable of recognizing that the vulnerability that makes the patient suffer is an expression of the fragility that makes her a person. One of the most important contributions of phenomenological psychopathology to psychiatric ethics is this notion of fragility. To be human is to be fragile. Fragility is not something to overcome or be rid of. It is both a phenomenon and a norm. Human experience is inescapably fragile, and only by recognizing this fragility—in ourselves and in the other person—can we hope for recovery.

BIBLIOGRAPHY

Aristotle (1984). "Nicomachean Ethics," trans. W.D. Ross and J.O. Urmson. In J. Barnes (ed.) *The Works of Aristotle, vol. 2*, pp. 1729–1867. Princeton: Princeton University Press.

Austin J. C. and Honer W. G. (2007). "The Genomic Era and Serious Mental Illness: A Potential Application for Psychiatric Genetic Counseling." *Psychiatric Services* 58: 254–261.

Beauchamp T. L. and Childress J. F. (2013). *Principles of Biomedical Ethics*, 7th edn. Oxford: Oxford University Press.

Bentall R. (2009). *Doctoring the Mind: Why Psychiatric Treatments Fail*. London: Allen Lane.

Blackburn S. (1998). *Ruling Passion. A Theory of Practical Reasoning*. Oxford: Oxford University Press.

Bloch S. and Green S. A. (2006). "An Ethical Framework for Psychiatry." *British Journal of Psychiatry* 188: 7–12.

Easter M. M. (2012). ""Not All My Fault": Genetics, Stigma, and Personal Responsibility for Women with Eating Disorders." *Social Science & Medicine* 75: 1408–1416.

Frank L. E. and Nagel S. K. (2017). "Addiction and Moralization: the Role of the Underlying Model of Addiction." *Neuroethics* 10: 129–139.

Gerhardt V. (1999). *Selbstbestimmung: Das Princip der Individualität*. Stuttgart: Reclam.

Heidegger M. (2010). *Being and Time*, trans. J. Stambaugh, revised by D.J. Schmidt. New York: State University of New York Press.

Illes J., Lombera S., Rosenberg J., and Arnow B. (2009). "In the Mind's Eye: Provider and patient Attitudes on Functional Brain Imaging." *Journal of Psychiatric Research* 43: 107–114.

Insel T. R. and Cuthbert B. N. (2015). "Brain Disorders? Precisely: Precision Medicine Comes to Psychiatry." *Science* 348: 499–500.

Jaspers K. (1978). *Notizen zu Martin Heidegger*, ed. H. Saner. München: R. Piper & Co. Verlag.

Jaspers K. (1997). *General Psychopathology*, trans. J. Hoenig and M. W. Hamilton. Baltimore: The Johns Hopkins University Press.

Kant I. (1996a). "Groundwork of the Metaphysics of Morals," trans. M. J. Gregor. In M. J. Gregor (ed.), *Immanuel Kant: Practical Philosophy*, pp. 37–108. Cambridge: Cambridge University Press.

Kant I. (1996b). "Critique of Practical Reason," trans. M. J. Gregor. In M. J. Gregor (ed.), *Immanuel Kant: Practical Philosophy*, pp. 132–271. Cambridge: Cambridge University Press.

Kendler K. S. (2014). "The Structure of Psychiatric Science." *The American Journal of Psychiatry* 171: 931–938.

Kvaale E. P., Gottdiener W. H., and Haslam N. (2013). "Biogenetic Explanations and Stigma: A Meta-Analytic Review of Associations Among Laypeople." *Social Science & Medicine* 96: 95–103.

Levinas E. (1969). *Totality and Infinity: An Essay on Exteriority*, trans. A. Lingis. Pittsburgh: Duquesne University Press.

Levinas E. (1996). "Enigma and Phenomenon." In A. T. Peperzak, S. Critchley, and R. Bernasconi (eds.), *Emmanuel Levinas: Basic Philosophical Writings*, pp. 65–78. Indianapolis: Indiana University Press.

Levinas E. (1998). *Otherwise than Being or Beyond Essence*, trans. A. Lingis. Pittsburgh: Duquesne University Press.

Levinas E. (2001). *Existence and Existents*, trans. A. Lingis. Pittsburgh: Duquesne University Press.

Malla A., Joober R, and Garcia A. (2015). "'Mental Illness is Like Any Other Medical Illness': A Critical Examination of the Statement and Its Impact on Patient Care and Society." *Journal of Psychiatry & Neuroscience* 40: 147–150.

Manganaro P. (1989). *Libertà sotto le leggi. La filosofia pratica di Kant*. Catania: C.U.E.C.M.

Parnas J., Sass L. A., and Zahavi D. (2013). "Rediscovering Psychopathology: The Epistemology and Phenomenology of the Psychiatric Object." *Schizophrenia Bulletin* 39: 270–277.

Plato (1997). "Republic," trans. G. M. A. Grube and C. D. C. Reeve. In J. M. Cooper and D. S. Hutchinson (eds.) *Platon: Complete Works*, pp. 971–1223. Indianapolis: Hackett Publishing Company.

Radden J. (2002). "Notes towards a Professional Ethics for Psychiatry." *Australian and New Zealand Journal of Psychiatry* 36: 52–59.

Radden J. and Sadler J. Z. (2009). *The Virtuous Psychiatrist: Character Ethics in Psychiatric Practice*. Oxford: Oxford University Press.

Read J., Haslam N., Sayce L., and Davies E. (2006). "Prejudice and Schizophrenia: A Review of the Mental Illness is an Illness Like Any Other Approach." *ActaPsychaitrica Scandinavica* 114: 303–318.

Ricoeur P. (1966). *Freedom and Nature: The Voluntary and the Involuntary*, trans. E. Kohak. Evanston: Northwestern University Press.

Ricoeur P. (1970). *Freud and Philosophy: An Essay on Interpretation*, trans. D. Savage. New Haven: Yale University Press.

Ricoeur P. (1986). *Fallible Man*, trans. C. A. Kelbley. New York: Fordham University Press.

Ricoeur P. (1992). *Oneself as Another*, trans. K. Blamey. Chicago: University of Chicago Press.

Ricoeur P. (2004). *The Conflict of Interpretations: Essays in Hermeneutics*, trans. W. Domingo, et al. London: Continuum.

Ricoeur P. (2005). *The Course of Recognition*, trans. D. Pellauer. Cambridge: Harvard University Press.

Ricoeur P. (2007). *Husserl: An Analysis of His Phenomenology*, trans. E. G. Ballard and L. E. Embree. Evanston: Northwestern University Press.

Rüsch N., Corrigan P.W., Todd A. R., and Bodenhausen G. V. (2010). "Implicit Self-Stigma in People With Mental Illness." *The Journal of Nervous and Mental Disease* 198: 150–153.

Sadler J. Z., van Staden W., and Fulford K. W. M. (eds.) (2015). *The Oxford Handbook of Psychiatric Ethics*. Oxford: Oxford University Press.

Schomerus G., Schwahn C., Holzinger A., Corrigan P. W., Grabe H. J., Carta M. G., and Angermeyer M. C. (2012). "Evolution of Public Attitudes about Mental Illness: A Systematic Review and Meta-Analysis." *Acta Psychaitrica Scandinavica* 125: 440–452.

Scrutton A. P. (2015). "Is Depression a Sin or a Disease? A Critique of Moralizing and Medicalizing Models of Mental Illness." *Journal of Disability & Religion* 19: 285–311.

CHAPTER 90

PHENOMENOLOGICAL PSYCHOPATHOLOGY AND AMERICA'S SOCIAL LIFE-WORLD

JAKE JACKSON

INTRODUCTION: THE CLUTTERED LIFE-WORLD OF MENTAL ILLNESS

WITHIN the United States, our societal understanding of mental illness is perpetually un-clear and insecure. An uncareful interpretation of contemporary social issues regarding psychopathology would state that we are in a crisis.[1] Any such "crisis" is not a recent one, but has presented as a perpetual crisis for at least the better part of the last century as the United States has had trouble reacting to the phenomenon of mental illness. My intent in these pages is to tease out some, but not all, of the different overlapping disciplinary attitudes toward mental illness.[2] I am not developing an overt phenomenology here, but rather rely on phenomenological method of pulling apart strands from the life-world of mental ill-ness discussions in the United States. By life-world I mean the Husserlian conception of the rich pre-reflective world of experience, where we find ourselves always already deployed, as "our most immediate and basic reality" (Parnas and Sass 2008: 255). This life-world is

---

[1] I use this term ironically, in the sense that discussions of crises in philosophy and other disciplines have been long cliché, even doubted in the beginning pages of Husserl's own *Crisis* text (Husserl, *The Crisis of European Sciences and Transcendental Phenomenology* 1954/1970). As I will cover in this article, the social crisis of mental illness is perpetual: both long-standing and constantly seen as an immediate threat requiring an even more immediate resolution.

[2] Three significant approaches to mental illness that I will not discuss are that of religion, psychoanalysis, and fiction, while each most certainly capture our cultural imagination with extremely complicated narratives. Religious narratives still cast mental illness as a sort of possession or spiritual battle. Such a viewpoint may have its merits, but often the connotation is that those with mental disorders have done something to deserve their suffering, which is a cruel practice. Psychoanalysis, while no longer as widespread in the academy as it was, still influences many public notions of mental health and disorder. Fiction, in any form, often presents the mentally ill in many negative ways often using indistinct depictions of madness as either comic relief, a force of evil, or a convenient plot twist.

inherently social, as our understanding of mental difference is inherently rooted in intersub-jective comparisons (Husserl 1954/1970). The life-world in this sense is rich with meaning, but it can at times be hard to discern meaning for oneself. Husserl describes the life-world as the background to our understanding of the world, more particularly our sciences or disciplines.[3] While different sciences/disciplines are taken up by particular scientists, the sciences quite clearly present themselves at a wider social level. Husserl writes in the *Formal and Transcendental Logic* that

> whether sciences and logic be genuine or spurious, we do have experience of them as *cultural formations* given to us beforehand and bearing within themselves their meaning, their 'sense': since they are formations produced indeed by the practice of the scientists and genera-tions of scientists who have been building them.
>
> (Husserl 1969: 8–9; emphasis mine)

Individuals encounter the logics of different disciplines and are free to make sense of both the reason and unreason of the surrounding world (Husserl 1954/1970: 6). To speak of a life-world of mental illness is to speak of an already-deployed fabric of disparate thoughts both from without and within mentally ill individuals, including through different disciplinary approaches to the question. Psychiatry and mental illness do not exist within a vacuum, but are constantly within a complicated world of conflicting social attitudes that are co-determined by these phenomena. I hope to show that there is a serious social need for phe-nomenological psychopathology where few other attitudes toward mental illness take lived experience seriously. Without a stronger emphasis on phenomenology and lived experience of patients, discussions of mental illness lose focus on what is important in terms of care and living together.

To approach the life-world of psychopathology in the US public is to approach a din of conflicting noises. The most blaring and self-conflicting noise is that of mainstream media, which both condemns the mentally ill for their potential of committing heinous crimes but at other times reprieves heinous acts as unavoidable. For example, when Dylann Roof massacred nine members of a historic black church in South Carolina in a deliberate hate crime attack, he was more readily identified by the FBI and press as mentally ill while they avoided discussing racism before the public even knew his name. Roof's racism was underreported and replaced by a media narrative that blamed mental illness for his attack (Butler 2015). The media narrative shifted away from blaming a white supremacist for being a white supremacist to blaming mental disorder.[4] While mental illness may be a factor in a mass shooter's actions, it is never the sole cause. It is far more statistically likely for a mentally

---

[3] In discussing the sciences, Husserl uses the word *Wissenschaften* which more widely applies not just to the natural sciences but to all disciplines in general. In this article I will discuss different "disciplinary" attitudes, but in a Husserlian sense, I could just as readily be using the word sciences.

[4] It is further important to note that when faced with the option to claim an "insanity defense" in order to seek leniency in his sentencing, Roof denied psychiatric evaluation. A handwritten manifesto found in his car reads "Also I want state [sic] that I am morally opposed to psychology. It is a Jewish invention, and does nothing but invent diseases and tell people they have problems when they dont [sic]" (quoted in Slack and Blinder 2017). Roof's refusal to be evaluated means that we cannot speculate on his mental state. Instead, we should directly evaluate his actions for the non-psychpathologizing answer; it was a racist and misogynist hate crime perpetrated out of Roof's premeditated ideological and violent plans.

ill individual to be the victim of violence than its perpetrator,[5] yet mental illness is blamed and quickly shirks responsibility from the perpetrator in such attacks.[6] The consequences of such media narratives shame mentally disordered individuals and often prevent them from seeking treatment either because they do not see such violent behavior in themselves, or for fear of being persecuted. Different disciplines are taken up and understood by individuals as evidence about the world. In this way, our understanding of mental illness is informed by different disciplinary practices and attitudes. General social attitudes, while not necessarily held by a mentally ill individual, still directly affect their day-to-day life in trying to navigate and understand their lives. The trouble that I want to outline is that the mentally ill have no clear recourse on how to treat or understand their respective conditions as well as their social status or responsibility within American society, especially as there are few disciplines that take lived experience seriously. Mentally ill individuals most often feel at odds with society at large. This sense of alienation and estrangement only worsens when the mentally ill person then faces social stigma. The position of the mentally ill individual trying to make sense of their condition in attempts to have a flourishing life is what I call being *epistemically adrift*. This is the phenomena of facing too many competing explanations as to what one should do that it becomes nearly impossible to discern what to do with oneself, even in regards to understanding whether one has a mental condition or if their anguish is their "choice." Epistemically adrift with nowhere safe to turn, many mentally disordered individuals turn to drastic actions as the only expected social roles for them are those of deviance and self-destruction.

Faced with a cacophony of different competing disciplinary approaches to mental health, those with mental disorders who try to navigate their own care and self-knowledge become epistemically adrift. This can be, in part, the end result of hermeneutical injustice, a form of epistemic injustice as outlined by Miranda Fricker (2007). Hermeneutical injustice is when an individual of a particular social identity is systematically denied access to knowledge that would be crucial to that individual's social flourishing (Fricker 2007). Yet, where Fricker examines cases of hermeneutical injustice a posteriori after a paradigm-shift in thinking, our general and scientific attitudes to mental illness are too conflicting for there to be a clear analysis of the full extent of hermeneutical injustice. In this case, there is no intended structure that blocks the mentally ill individual from access to knowledge about their condition, however I argue that it is due to the conflicted life-world of different interpretations of mental difference. The mentally ill experience a knowledge deficit for a multitude of reasons

---

[5] See Johnson et al. (2016) which discusses how mentally ill individuals are victims of violence at a higher rate than the general population. Additionally, see Fuller et al. (2015); Glied and Frank (2014); and Martinelli, Binney, and Kaye (2014) for discussions on how mental illness is not statistically a factor in violent crimes. Further, if mental disorder alone were the operative factor of violent behavior, the prevalence of mental disorders would lead to a higher rate of mass violence.

[6] There have additionally been attempts, both within psychiatric practices and from other disciplines, to pathologize racism as a mental illness or a symptom of mental illness. According to Thomas and Byrd (2016), such an attempt confuses widespread social problems with individual psychoanalysis and defers social responsibility against systemic racism. A fuller history of mental illness first being used as a way of explaining race and racism can be found in Gilman and Thomas's 2016 *Are Racists Crazy? How Prejudice, Racism, and Antisemitism Became Markers of Insanity.* This work studies how psychiatry of the nineteenth and twentieth centuries began with a justification of racist systems, only to change later to blaming racist behavior and ideology on mental illness when social attitudes had changed.

outside of their own mental health, including but not limited to stigma, socio-economic background, race, gender, or political climate. I will not be able to cover all of these possible identity politics problems within this essay, but will highlight a few examples along the way. The import of understanding mental illness socially is that there are many limited yet conflicting resources for the mentally ill to pursue, without any clear explanation of one's options. Within this essay, I will discuss several problems in three approaches to mental illness, through professional psychiatry, the anti-psychiatry movement, and the criminal justice system. However given the nature of my critique, I find it necessary to state one clear claim: mental disorder is a *real* phenomenon which affects countless individuals, both aware and unaware of their condition.[7] The ever-present debate on the existence of mental illness leaves individuals epistemically adrift and unable to determine how to live a flourishing life outside of being defiant in the face of stigmatizing norms.[8] Whatever the "truth" is to mental illness, it is epistemically covered over within interdisciplinary noise.

Troubles in Psychiatry

To open this section, I provide an anecdote that I believe exemplifies unreflective psychiatric attitudes and poor use of diagnostic tools in the public's cultural understanding. During the abnormal psychology unit of my high school Psychology 101 course, our class held a mock group therapy session. The teacher gave each student a role to play, a diagnostic name from the Diagnostic Statistical Manual (DSM) and a set of symptoms. We were then each to play our respective roles for the better part of the class period, then at the end guess who was what diagnosis. Some of us yelled, some ticked, and most laughed both with in and breaking character. I cannot remember the positive lessons of this exercise, but it is easy to extrapolate negative ones. The game suggests as many no doubt believe that mental disorder is easy to openly recognize, categorize, and dissect through a medical lens.[9] It presents mental disorder as merely reducible to a series of easily imitated quirks or behaviors. Further, it suggests that diagnostic tools such as the DSM have the capacity to read into any behavior that one presents, implying that those with neurodivergent traits or conditions are easy to spot or deconstruct from a distance, and reinforces mentally ill individuals' fear of stigma and being a spectacle for being abnormal. Additionally, the game suggests that there is a very typical social sick role that diagnoses play in social interaction, a limited set of possibilities for the mentally ill.

The profession and discipline of psychiatry is indispensable when it comes to explicating and understanding the wide array of mental disorder and divergence. Psychiatry, to put it broadly for the purposes of this essay, is the intersection of social and biological sciences devoted to categorizing and understanding mental health. However, psychiatry has several

---

[7] There is a live debate as to whether mental illness can truly be considered an illness, or disorder, or mere diversity across mental types. I will use mental illness and mental disorder interchangeably.

[8] For those who are epistemically adrift, I would argue along the lines of Nancy Nyquist Potter (2016), to say that being defiant/noncompliant in the face of stigmatizing practices is an ethical virtue in order to succeed in living a flourishing life.

[9] This game additionally showed that mental disorders were perhaps merely a joke or a spectacle.

compromising factors both external and internal that diminish its overall benefit. Externally, psychiatry is compromised by the general stigma of mental illness that pervades in our culture. This includes the problems caused by private health insurance companies that limit coverage for mental health treatment beyond prescription coverage for medications. Within the paradigm of private health insurance, lower-income US citizens generally have had difficulty accessing mental health treatment, both in regards to emergency care as well as preventive care due to cost of medical treatment out-of-pocket/not covered by insurance. Mental illness has been classified as a non-life-threatening condition by most private insurers before implementation of the Affordable Care Act (ACA, or crudely referred to as Obamacare). Without wider mental health insurance coverage, psychiatry has been effectively delegitimized as a medical field and seen more as a luxury service or emergency care. Before the ACA, mental health practitioners did not participate in the Medicaid program due to the low reimbursement rate, paying less than 53% of what private insurance companies paid for services (Olfson 2016: 986). It is unclear as to how beneficial the ACA will be in the long run for mental health amidst its contested history, but there is a clear increase in patients seeking mental health services since its implementation (Creedon and Lê Cook 2016; Weiss, Gross, and Moncrief 2016; Olfson 2016). The current Trump/Republican administration's plans to repeal the ACA without any clear plan for its replacement would only lead to increased numbers of adrift individuals, that is, they would lead to the destruction of the lifeline that mental health-care recipients require. The absence of affordable mental health care leaves many not only epistemically adrift, but in further grave danger. However the general trend set from poor insurance coverage is for mentally ill individuals not to seek therapy, but medications which are generally more likely to be covered and more cost-effective as they can be prescribed by a general practitioner instead of a specialty therapist. Limiting health insurance benefits toward mental health limits access to mental health services for those who are impoverished or otherwise also disadvantaged.

The APA's formation and subsequent editions of the DSM has been an attempt to categorize mental disorder into definitive kinds. However, due to conflicting notions of what mental illness is, the DSM-5 exists in the form of a long, general laundry list of conditions, disorders, and mental states.[10] There have been many due criticisms of this approach as the DSM has grown not only physically but in terms of its influence and use. One major problem is that the existence of the DSM has outweighed other forms of therapeutic engagement. Instead of engaging directly with patients themselves and their own given experience, practitioners are often more concerned with filling out checklists. Nancy Nyquist Potter writes that "the DSM works together with other epistemic practices that constrict many clinicians' access to knowing well. Thus clinicians shape themselves into, and are shaped into, a privileged way of knowing that elides many crucial factors that influence the experiences and needs of the person in front of them" (2016: 160). Relying upon the DSM without critical reflection on its limitations or the experiences of patients directly affects the patients' lives. When overreliance on the DSM continues in a clinical setting, clinicians commit hermeneutical injustices toward their patients. Nancy Andreasen argues that the unintended consequences of the DSM are dehumanizing, writing that "History taking—the central evaluation tool in

---

[10] A better description of the processes and motivations that go into the DSM's formation can be found in Cooper (2014) and Potter (2016).

psychiatry—has frequently been reduced to the use of *DSM* checklists. *DSM* discourages clinicians from getting to know the patient as an individual person because of its dryly empirical approach" (Andreasen 2006: 111). Andreasen describes this as the death of phenomenology in American psychiatry, which definitely seems to be the case when compared to Karl Jaspers's demand that psychiatrists must take on a phenomenological empathetic approach to patients. Jaspers writes that psychopathological "experience is best described by the person who has undergone it. Detached psychiatric observation with its own formulation of what the patient is suffering is not any substitute for this" (Jaspers 1959/1963: 55). The DSM's use implies that priority has been taken on pre-existing categorical definition over rich and ever-changing lived experience that it can never suitably cover.

The fault of not listening to the lived experience of patients would perhaps be better explained by bad tool use. The DSM presents not a totalized description of psychopathology, but rather focuses instead on bare minimum criteria as a diagnostic tool. As a result, the DSM has presented a very uniform and utilitarian description even for conditions that present themselves in unique ways. For example, the DSM-5 states that major depression is experiencing either a depressed mood or lack of interest or pleasure in activities and at least four of the following seven symptoms over a period of time spanning over two weeks: weight/diet changes, changes in sleep patterns, psychomotor problems, fatigue, feeling extreme guilt/worthlessness, problems thinking/concentrating, or continuous/obsessive thoughts of death/suicide (160–161). Depression appears in many different ways for individuals. Depression often *feels* different, where many sufferers remark upon their experiences in metaphors, yet the DSM's intention is to have a clear categorical definition that can be easily applied to a wide array of cases. Where an episode can be much shorter than the prescribed two weeks, psychiatrists insist on the duration for accurate results that cover a longer period of time rather than a fleeting episode. The DSM is a mere tool of categorization, but is often confused as a complete map of all possible mentally-divergent experiences. Some clinicians are too reliant upon the DSM and will rush to make the closest available, yet incorrect diagnosis, assuming that there is no psychopathological conceptual space that is unoccupied by the DSM.[11] In contrast, Rachel Cooper notes that "the rates with which diagnoses are made depend not only on the contents of the DSM, but also on the economic, cultural, and bureaucratic contexts within which diagnoses are made" (2014: 12). The dry language of the DSM presents a very objectivizing attempt at typifying subjective experience. A rush to diagnose based solely on preset diagnostic criteria is a possible case of hermeneutical injustice and leaves the patient epistemically adrift and conforming to the wrong treatment plan. The trouble is in confusing the DSM as the ultimate authority in clinical settings when a better understanding must go "back to the things themselves" and engage more directly with the patient's experience.[12]

Additionally in the case of the DSM, the tool shapes its own use by way of its own nosology and does not consult subjects regarding how it affects them socially. Most infamous is the inclusion of homosexuality as a diagnosis within early versions of the manual, which was only deleted from the DSM-II after extensive campaigning from gay rights activists against

---

[11] I am thankful to Matthew Broome for suggesting this point.

[12] "Back to the things themselves" (*zu Sachen selbst*) is one of Husserl's better-known catchphrases, arguing that our best understanding of the world must come from a direct engagement with phenomena as they appear.

such pathologizing in 1973 (Sadler 2005: 204–206). Psychiatrist John Sadler argues that this shows quite clearly that the diagnoses themselves clearly have a value beyond their claims to being "objective" categories (204). Later versions of the DSM included gender identity disorder, much to the dismay of transgender advocates as the term disorder implies that there is something bad or defective in their identity (206–210). The DSM-5 still includes "Gender Identity Disorders" as a general category that outlines "Gender Dysphoria" with criteria which amount to a describing the distressed experience that can result from social pressures but not fault the individual's gender identity (American Psychiatric Association 2013: 451-459). While the focus of this disorder's criteria has justly changed from the identity itself to the distress caused by external stigma, its continued inclusion presents rationaliza-tion for transphobia; claiming that those who identify with a different gender than assigned at birth are possibly mentally-disordered unfairly forces all trans-individuals within a psy-chiatric sick role and perpetuates the stigma around gender identity. The continued inclu-sion of Gender Dysphoria in the DSM still suggests that trans-individuals are aberrant and disordered, despite gender identity being irreducible along medical or psychiatric models. This still presents opportunity for psychiatric overreach, overdiagnosis, and transphobic stigma, as many trans-individuals do not feel distress over their identity, but nevertheless face continued stigma under a medicalized and dehumanizing lens.

Another dubious historical problem in nosology is highlighted by Jonathan Metzl's *The Protest Psychosis* where the very language used to describe schizophrenia changed between the DSM and the DSM-II. Metzl argues that the changes in diagnostic criteria language was implicitly racist as it more readily described and pathologized protest as mental illness, leading to a growth in diagnoses for African-American men in the late '60s and '70s (Metzl 2009: 98).[13] Based on events like Metzl describes, there have been many questions as to whether the terminology and history of schizophrenia is stigmatizing (Lasalvia et al. 2015). Schizophrenia as a concept has a sordid history where the term is completely misunderstood by the general public thanks to its changes as a diagnosis as well as pop-culture references. There have been many attempts to change or rename the condition altogether as Lasalvia et al. note, but one resounding fear is that changing the name will only cause for more confusion for those seeking or administering treatment (ibid.).

A final but less grievous example of the DSM instructing its own tool use is the removal of Asperger's syndrome from the DSM-5, lumping it instead within autism spectrum disorder (ASD). According to Miriam Solomon, this erasure has led to a loss of diagnostic meaning or identity for those previously diagnosed with Asperger's syndrome. She argues that since the DSM has no consideration for patient interests in creating or changing diagnostic categories, those who have found value in the Asperger's identity now suffer from hermeneutical in-justice, albeit Solomon is unsure whether this loss of diagnostic identity is an active harm against those who otherwise identify as having Asperger's (Solomon, 2017).[14] The DSM is a tool geared toward the purposes of diagnosis, which often leaves patients desolate and adrift of making any meaning for themselves.

---

[13] While the DSM has moved away from the psychoanalytic perspective that was in the DSM-II, this history of pathologizing protest still remains in cultural consciousness. Again, see Gilman and Thomas (2016).

[14] I am thankful to Miriam Solomon for sharing an early draft of this chapter.

Oftentimes mental illness stigma and poor psychiatric ethics appear in the political sphere, as we have seen again recently in the 2016 US presidential election and subsequent conversations about Donald Trump's policies, executive orders, and behavior as President. The grassroots social media call to #DiagnoseTrump over the summer of 2016 presented yet another betrayal of stigmatizing attitudes against mental illness from both outside and within the mental health field.[15] The call and pull of this particular movement became great enough that the APA's president, Maria Oquendo, had to step in to remind mental health professionals of the notorious Goldwater Rule: that it is a breach of ethics to diagnose a public figure from afar (Oquendo 2016). This rule was implemented in 1973 after a public outcry that Senator Barry Goldwater's 1964 candidacy for presidency had likely been ruined in part by a survey of psychiatric professionals who agreed that he was unfit, many of whom offering a wide array of unsolicited diagnoses. Oquendo's reminder came after multiple mental health professionals had already weighed in on Donald Trump's mental health and had given him armchair diagnoses of narcissistic personality disorder against APA ethics (Blake 2016). Since his electoral college win and inauguration, the resistance to Trump's presidency has only increased in references to his mental health, ramping up claims about narcissistic personality disorder as well as speculation that his erratic behavior can be blamed on his use of Propecia and the drug's "mental confusion" sideeffects (Brenoff 2017). The calls for diagnosing Trump even includes federal legislators, such as Congressman Ted Lieu from California, who for example, has tweeted "Last 24 hrs on Twitter, @realDonaldTrump went on rant about 'death & destruction,' 'FAKE NEWS,' & 'evil.' Should he get mental health exam?" (Lieu February 4, 2017 11:28AM EST). Lieu went on further to state to a reply to this tweet that "we are investigating" what grounds are possible to remove Trump over mental illness (ibid.).[16] Again as mentioned in the previous footnote, there are countless reasons to move to impeach or remove Trump from presidency, but the implication of medicalized reasons to remove him create a horrifying precedent for governmental overreach of biopolitics and patient privacy.[17]

But despite the increasing politicizing of Trump's mental health, there have been several within the psychiatric profession who actively resist the armchair reflections and bad medicalization inherent in trying to diagnose someone with mental disorder to declare them "unfit" to rule. Allen J Frances, the author of the DSM-5 criteria for narcissistic personality disorder himself, has come out to speak against the move to try to diagnose Trump from a distance. Frances states that despite many armchair psychologist diagnoses, Trump does not fit the criterion that narcissism causes "clinically significant distress or impairment" (Frances 2017). The question of "significant distress or impairment" points out yet another

---

[15] There are many reasons that one could object to Donald Trump's legitimacy as the President of the United States, let alone his candidacy to begin with, but none of these reasons (corruption, racism, complete disregard for the rule of law/constitution, etc.) are at bottom dependent upon his own psyche. I hold that a politician's mental health is irrelevant to their (in)eligibility to rule.

[16] Replies can be found listed under initial tweet: https://twitter.com/tedlieu/status/827916850973380608

[17] The same sort of unsettling policy has appeared in the gun control debate where politicians have argued for restricting not the sale of high-powered firearms at large, but preventing those with a history of mental illness from purchasing weapons. Such a preventative measure would require an invasively public database of individuals with mental disorder, furthering stigma and anguish while not likely curbing gun deaths in the United States.

issue with the DSM-5; it is designed to trace out disorder and suffering but finds no positive diagnostic value in contentment or flourishing. Nobody psychopathologizes the happy. Yet, I must question Frances's decision to weigh in against the armchair diagnosis debate by still hypocritically directly offering a diagnostic opinion in assessing Trump's sense of distress without consultation.

Frances then states that "Dismissing Trump as simply mad paradoxically reduces our ability to deal with his actions" (ibid.). Beyond the violation of ethics, the public's speculation and call for pathologizing Trump's behavior again shows an ugly attitude against the mentally ill and deflects our responsibility for handling his policies. This is rooted in the popular assumption that mentally ill individuals are inherently evil or at very least incompetent. These attempts to diagnose from the armchair show that everyday mental illness stigma has not left even those practicing psychiatry. No matter the state of a politician's mental health, to call on a public diagnosis in order to invalidate their candidacy or presidency is a disastrous overreach of ableist medicalizing attitudes. Claims about the "mental fitness" of the president do not seem to harm him personally or politically. The end result of the resistance to Trumpism has yet to come, but if it continues to pull mental health stigma to the forefront of its battle will only lead to further harm to mentally ill individuals within the United States.

ANTI-PSYCHIATRY

Anti-psychiatry, as the name implies, is a movement across multiple disciplines against the practices of psychiatry. In general, anti-psychiatrists cite ethical charges against the profession of psychiatry, which then often bleeds into metaphysical claims against the existence of mental disorder outside of obvious cognitive disability. Anti-psychiatric sentiments evolved, in part, out of public outcry following the publicized discovery of "back wards"—areas of mental asylums reserved for the most mentally disabled who were left within squalid conditions (Torrey 2014; Ferguson 2014). One of the leading figures of the anti-psychiatry movement was the psychoiatrist, Thomas Szasz, who argued that mental illness as conceived was a myth that perpetuated collectivist social control and infringed upon human freedom.[18] Szasz stresses the difference between more visibly physical diseases of the brain such as cognitive impairment with mental disturbances which he describes instead as "counterfeit illnesses" which in his view only resemble physical diseases in terms of unsound metaphors that do more damage than good (Szasz 1974). However, by accusing psychiatry as a whole as ideological propaganda and control, the anti-psychiatrists formed their own ideological contrarianism (e.g. Szasz co-founded the Citizens Commission on Human Rights (CCHR) with the Church of Scientology in a combined effort against psychiatric practices). The anti-psychiatry movement has sown irreparable doubt that has only further alienated mental difference and worsened the social status of the seriously mentally ill. Thomas Szasz's

---

[18] There are of course many other anti-psychiatrist thinkers, but I find Szasz to have had a relatively successful afterlife in US policy and understandings of mental illness. Some lump Michel Foucault in as an anti-psychiatrist, however I find that this label to be inaccurate. Foucault's work on mental illness is mainly a critique of the development of concepts, and does not make any definitive claim regarding the existence of phenomena behind these epistemic concepts (Foucault 1965).

intent to show that psychiatry is not a "legitimate" medicine relies upon a strong yet unexamined notion of medicine qua medicine. Delegitimizing psychiatry as an entire practice may have had the best intentions for some, but it nevertheless caused hermeneutical injustice toward the mentally ill in denying them access to self-knowledge through doubt. Szasz's polemical works argue tirelessly against the infringed freedoms of the "so-called" mentally ill, but does not account for what patients should do in seeking help. Despite anti-psychiatric criticisms and conjecture, there is no collectivized epistemic monopoly or conspiracy of psychiatric control to be found; as intimated in the previous section, systems of oppression and control seem more the result of ignorance and poor resources than willful or diabolical maleficence. Psychiatry is not a collectivist, let alone unified practice, no matter what anti-psychiatrists accuse it of being. Thomas Szasz's depiction of psychiatry is that of a lurking shadow conspiracy, further wedging the divide of distrust between society and medicine.

The relative success of the anti-psychiatry movement is clear today as psychiatry is still considered an entirely different field than medicine, implying and further reinforcing the belief in a rigid dualism between mind and body.[19] This success is also apparent within other social sciences, humanities, and popular press. The experience of being epistemically adrift that pervades in society due to psychiatric practices are not remedied, but compounded by anti-psychiatric attitudes. The cultural consciousness about mental illness becomes easily confused due to the existence of many self-described experts who claim different causes and "cures" for mental disturbance from diets to hobbies. Ann Cvetkovich's 2012 depression memoir/treatise entitled *Depression: A Public Feeling*, without citing "traditional" anti-psychiatrists, presents a strong contemporary embodiment of these attitudes. Beyond her own personal concerns regarding the psychiatric profession, Cvetkovich additionally casts doubt upon other depressives' experiences to the point of being "dissatisfied with more popular mainstream depression memoirs . . . all of which largely, if ambivalently, endorse pharmaceutical treatment . . ." (Cvetkovich 2012: 23).[20] Her work rests rather uncritically on the claim that depression is a spiritual affliction, rather than a psycho-physiological one, that is rooted within and caused by capitalism and racial oppression (by way of her own white guilt). While this may betray Cvetkovich's own anti-intersubjective thinking in the sense of denying the possibility of depression being rooted in other existential causes, she does still represent a contentious anti-psychiatric perspective about depression that presents itself as a typical epistemic authority. She inherits the overtly political posturings of the tradition concerned more readily with personal liberty than with the multiplicities of mental disorder.

CRIMINALIZED

Today, due to the decline of state hospitals and the growth of mass incarceration and police brutality, the seriously mentally ill have no safe haven. Slate and Johnson argue that prisons have become the de facto mental health system in the United States (2008: 59–61).

[19] I am thankful to Paolo Fusar-Poli for suggesting this point in manuscript comments.
[20] Cvetkovich does not state her reasons for distrusting anyone's recovery or relief through medication, but one can assume it has more readily to do with the pharmaceutical industry being a capitalist industry more than it has to do with medications' efficacy.

Currently, the largest inpatient mental health facility in the country is the Cook County Jail in Chicago with one third of its population suffering from mental illness, while nationally at least 400,000 mentally ill individuals are prison inmates (Ford 2015). This growth of "criminalized" mental illness has come about from the grand-scale deinstitutionalization movements following from the Kennedy administration in 1963 (Torrey 2014; Erickson and Erickson 2008; Slate and Johnson 2008; Rembis 2014). In psychiatrist and historian Fuller Torrey's account, it is clear that anti-psychiatric attitudes along with America's own obsession regarding personal freedoms led to deinstitutionalization while paradoxically throwing the mentally ill in jail by droves when they no longer had the societal recourses to better prevent criminal behavior.[21] This came as well with the advent of the growth of mass incarceration and the overcrowded prison industrial complex, where poor and minority individuals have been imprisoned indefinitely for only minor initial crimes (Alexander 2012; Davis 2003). With the decline of state mental hospitals, individuals with mental illness have no avenues for treatment, leading to a greater likelihood of deviant behavior, putting them at risk of arrest or police brutality.[22]

The industrial prison complex not only presents itself as a source of general anxiety for those under threat of incarceration, but its own machinations have created their own mental illness and social death for inmates. The implementation of solitary confinement has been proven to create its own distinctive mental disorder in inmates and has been deemed a method of torture and cruel and unusual punishment. The growing use of "special housing units" (SHU) in super-maximum prisons have created SHU syndrome, a unique condition that appears amongst solitary confinement prisoners that includes hyperresponsitivity to external stimuli, relatively idiosyncratic perceptual distortions, panic attacks, difficulty in concentration and memory, obsessional thoughts, and overt paranoia (Guenther 2013: 145). Solitary confinement, as it is a form of torture, *creates* mental illness and anguish. One of the few windows into the active practice of solitary confinement that we have had in the United States is the case of Chelsea Manning, the Army whistleblower. Manning faced further punishment within prison for a suicide attempt that resulted from previous solitary confinement and presumably her experience of gender dysphoria resulting from being kept in a male prison. She was found guilty of "conduct which threatens" for her suicide attempt "violating good behavior" and sentenced to an additional fourteen days of solitary confinement (Lennard 2016).[23] The logic of the current criminal justice system compounds the suffering of mental illness. Guenther argues that solitary confinement not only dehumanizes, but de*animalizes* inmates leading to them becoming completely unhinged through the process of becoming both legally and socially dead to the world (2013). To be legally and socially dead is an abject erasure of the mentally ill individual's lived experience.

[21] Torrey (2014) provides a rather full historical analysis of deinstitutionalization including its motivations and aftermath, which we are still seeing today.

[22] Again I want to point out Potter's (2016) argument for defiance as an epistemic and moral virtue in the face of conflicting motivations and interpretations of mental illness. While I agree with her that there must be an appropriate mean of defiance in the face of these mental health attitudes that I have discussed, the present threat of police and state violence makes for a harder case regarding judgment.

[23] Manning has since had her original sentence commuted by President Obama thanks to activists and large-scale petitions condemning her treatment and torture within solitary confinement. She was released in May 2017.

With the erosion of state hospitals and the growth of the industrial prison complex as well as the advent of militarized police forces, seriously mentally ill cases are de facto handled by police and the criminal justice system. Even worse, is that the criminal justice system, both at the level of the police and even at the level of the courts, is ill-prepared for considering mentally ill citizens' existence amongst society (Slate and Johnson 2008; Erickson and Erickson 2008).[24] Where many mentally ill individuals disappear almost entirely from the public view within prisons, countless examples of mentally ill individuals brutalized and killed by police pervade the public consciousness. In 2006, the Department of Justice estimated that persons with mental illness were four times as likely to be killed by police (Cordner 2006, cited in Slate and Johnson 2008: 83). One especially jarring case from 2016 is that of Charles Kinsey, an African-American *therapist* shot by Officer Jonathan Aledda in North Miami, Florida, while Kinsey was consoling one of his patients with severe autism who could not comply with the officer's demands. The local police union tried to alleviate outrage by admitting that the officer was not aiming for Kinsey, who was pleading that the officer did not shoot, but the patient that Kinsey was trying to protect (Helm 2016). Further, police shot and killed a mentally ill man named Alfred Olango in September 2016 in San Diego, California after his sister had called 911 in order to help him when he was having an episode (Al Jazeera 2016). In October 2016, NYPD officers shot and killed Deborah Danner, a schizophrenic African-American woman in the Bronx, in her own home when her neighbors had once again reported her erratic behavior. The police had in the past been called to Danner's apartment in order to aid her, but this time they entered, shot, and killed her as she defended herself with a baseball bat from their intrusion (Editorial Board 2016).[25] The examples of mentally ill citizens brutalized by police continue to grow, as "the risk of being killed during a police incident is 16 times greater for individuals with untreated mental illness than for other civilians approached or stopped by officers" (Fuller et al. 2015: 1). If police are the first line of treatment for mentally ill individuals, then they ought to be better trained to deal with mentally ill citizens, let alone supplied with less destructive means toward duty and service. The militarization of police only further ensures the destruction of seriously mentally ill individuals who do not have the ability to easily comply with police orders. With mentally ill deviant behavior being a direct concern for police and the increased public awareness of police brutalities and shootings, the mentally ill face a concrete fear without relief. Where the interaction between

[24] Where Slate and Johnson (2008) write on a wide array of mental health problems in the United States with hopeful and optimistic advice on where to turn, Erickson and Erickson (2008) describe the criminal justice system's utter inability to understand responsibility in the face of behavioral sciences and the so-called insanity defense. Erickson and Erickson show that incompetency to stand trial is a well-intentioned legal precedent that is both abused by defense lawyers and poorly understood by juries and judges alike, leading instead to a higher conviction rate for the mentally ill.

[25] More tragically, Danner had written an implicitly phenomenological account of her life with schizophrenia years before her fatal altercation with police. In this short essay she condemns the police for their poor training and practice with the severely ill and cites other instances of brutality. Danner's essay shows that her schizophrenia was not as bad as the stigma that she had faced for the condition which made her worry for her life and wellbeing (Danner 2012). Of course, race is a crucial factor in all three of these cases on top of mental disability. Any practical changes in combating mental illness stigma must also go hand in hand with anti-racist work in order to be fully effective in curbing socially manufactured anguish.

a police officer and citizen in the United States contains the chance of deadly force, the citizen always has reason for anxiety, which can only exacerbate atypical behavior.

THE NEED FOR OPEN LIVED EXPERIENCES AND PHENOMENOLOGICAL PSYCHOPATHOLOGY

In some closing remarks, I want to comment on the notion of normalcy. Perhaps prescient in the mock group therapy game I mentioned above, the most antagonistic and outspoken "character" was a classmate who had been assigned to play "normal."[26] This peer spent the entire session insecurely berating everyone around him, goading others in calling them all crazy and unstable.[27] In a life-world that pre-exists categorization and diagnostic criteria that are only designed to recognize that which is other or abnormal, what exactly is a mentally healthy individual in opposition to mental illness? It is crucial to note that the World Health Organization's definition of mental health is *not* that of mental "normalcy" or neurotypicality but instead "is defined as a state of well-being in which every individual realizes his or her own potential, can cope with the normal stresses of life, can work productively and fruitfully, and is able to make a contribution to her or his community" (World Health Organization 2014). This definition does *not* exclude ability for those who have mental illnesses or disorders to still nevertheless live within a relative state of mental health. That is, mental health is a condition of flourishing that is not precluded by having a different non-"normal" condition. What prevents those with mental disorders from being able to live flourishing lives of mental health is not necessarily the illness or condition, but the stigma and perpetuation of ignorance in society. Being epistemically adrift in a confusing and stigmatized society is more opposed to mental health than mental disorders are. The answer in the face of being epistemically adrift, I believe, is the virtue of defiance in the context of mental health settings as argued by Nancy Nyquist Potter (2016). Potter claims that in order to live a flourishing life, patients find themselves having to navigate being noncompliant with procedures and stigmatizing society. Being mentally ill in an epistemically adrift society requires self-advocating resistance in order to live well.

If we continue to consider mental illness as a bad and immoral thing, then neurotypical individuals are in an insecure and fragile position. Considering conditions such as posttraumatic stress disorder (PTSD) that arise out of a person's experience or environment, mental illness can develop and affect anyone at any time. Jaspers argues that ultimately, being mentally healthy is merely what appears along the majority or average while illness is that which is the minority or deviant (Jaspers 1959/1963: 779–780). Ultimately, normalcy is only possible to understand as the absence of deviance. Our understanding of mental illness is at bottom understood by its difference from the majority. But at no point can we confuse our disciplines as self-sufficient. Jaspers again states that "No outline of a human being as a whole

---

[26] I am personally hesitant to use the word normal in the context of mental health due to its stigmatizing implications, but this is what his card stated.

[27] I remarked after the game was over that if this peer accurately represented "normalcy," our society is doomed.

ever quite succeeds ... Every time we grasp at the whole it recedes and we are left with only a particular schema of the whole, one mode of complex unity among others" (1959/1963: 751). At best, different disciplinary attitudes can sketch out a partial understanding of human phenomena, but they cannot develop a full and lasting picture of human experience. To quote Bernhard Waldenfels, "for both the cultural and intercultural realms: *there are orders, but there is no one order*" (2006/2011: 82. Original emphasis). Each discipline provides a perspective of the world of mental phenomena, but we cannot reduce the phenomena to any one approach.

Without taking a serious phenomenological approach to mental illness—without a clear and open discussion which allows patients to share their experience of mental illness and to be treated with epistemically just practices—there is no hope for the mentally ill to find meaning in their condition. Conflicting narratives distract us from being able to get back "to the things themselves" regarding mental illness, and have allowed for horrendous criminal policies to appear instead of helpful treatment programs. Otherwise, "[m]erely fact-minded sciences make for merely fact-minded people" (Husserl 1954/1970: 6). Husserl argues that one can find individual meaning through the life-world itself, but a mentally ill individual who tries to make sense of their condition can easily find themselves epistemically adrift with no clear direction for life projects. Perhaps what we see in the United States today is a worst of both worlds scenario between psychiatric and anti-psychiatric models of mental health; the neurodivergent are both highly categorized and controlled by disciplinary methods, but they also face a societal doubt that mental illness is a real phenomenon that is unchosen. Society's attitudes, informed and misinformed by different disciplinary approaches, present mental illness as something *other*; mental illness is seen as a phenomenon that must always be kept at arm's length, ostracized, and condemned. The effect of this alienates the mentally ill even more than the conditions themselves. A society's widespread fear and discomfort with abnormality condemns and silences its abnormal inhabitants.

BIBLIOGRAPHY

Al Jazeera. (2016). "Alfred Olango: US police kill mentally ill black man." *Al Jazeera*. September 28. Accessed October 16, 2016. http://www.aljazeera.com/news/2016/09/alfred-olango-police-kill-mentally-ill-black-man-160928065635824.html

Alexander M. (2012). *The New Jim Crow: Mass Incarceration in the Age of Colorblindness*. Revised Edition. New York: The New Press.

American Psychiatric Association (APA). (2013). *Diagnostic and Statistical Manual of Mental Disorders. DSM-5*. Washington: American Psychiatric Publishing.

Andreasen N. C. (2006). "DSM and the Death of Phenomenology in America: An Example of Unintended Consequences." *Schizophrenia Bulletin* 33(1): 108–112.

Blake A. (2016). "The American Psychiatric Association Issues a Warning: No Psychoanalyzing Donald Trump." *The Washington Post*. August 7. Accessed September 27, 2016. https://www.washingtonpost.com/news/the-fix/wp/2016/08/07/the-american-psychiatric-association-reminds-its-doctors-no-psychoanalyzing-donald-trump/

Brenoff A. (2017). "Trump Takes Propecia, A Hair-Loss Drug Associated With Mental Confusion, Impotence." *Huffington Post*. February 2. Accessed February 4, 2017. http://www.huffingtonpost.com/entry/trump-propecia-haiir-loss_us_58936376e4b06f344e4058a6

Butler A. (2015). "Shooters of Color are Called 'Terrorists' and 'Thugs.' Why are White Shooters Called 'Mentally Ill'?" *The Washington Post.* June 18. Accessed September 27, 2016. https://www.washingtonpost.com/posteverything/wp/2015/06/18/call-the-charleston-church-shooting-what-it-is-terrorism/?utm_term=.d8263bef12d5

Cooper R. (2014). *Diagnosing the Diagnostic and Statistical Manual of Mental Disorders.* London: Karnac.

Cordner G. (2006). *People with Mental Illness.* Washington: Office of Community Oriented Policing Services, US Department of Justice.

Creedon T. B and Lê Cook B. (2016). "Access to Mental Health Care Increased but not for Substance Use, While Disparities Remain." *Health Affairs* 35(6): 1017–1021.

Cvetkovich A. (2012). *Depression: A Public Feeling.* Durham: Duke University Press.

Danner D. (2012). "Living with Schizophrenia." January 28. Accessed October 22, 2016. https://assets.documentcloud.org/documents/3146953/Living-With-Schizophrenia-by-Deborah-Danner.pdf

Davis A. Y. (2003). *Are Prisons Obsolete?* New York: Seven Stories Press.

Editorial Board. (2016). "The Death of Deborah Danner." *The New York Times.* October 20. Accessed October 22, 2016. http://www.nytimes.com/2016/10/21/opinion/the-death-of-deborah-danner.html?_r=0

Erickson P. E. and Erickson S. K. (2008). *Crime, Punishment, and Mental Illness: Law and Behavioral Sciences in Conflict.* New Brunswick: Rutgers University Press.

Ferguson P. M. (2014). "Creating the Back Ward: The Triumph of Custodialism and the Uses of Therapeutic Failure in Nineteenth-Century Idiot Asylums." In L. Ben-Moshe, C. Chapman, and A. C. Carey (eds.), *Disability Incarcerated: Imprisonment and Disability in the United States and Canada,* pp. 45–62. New York: Palgrave Macmillan.

Ford M. (2015). "America's Largest Mental Hospital Is a Jail." *The Atlantic.* June 8. Accessed September 28, 2016. http://www.theatlantic.com/politics/archive/2015/06/americas-largest-mental-hospital-is-a-jail/395012/

Foucault M. (1965). *Madness & Civilization: A History of Insanity in the Age of Reason,* trans. R. Howard. New York: Random House.

Frances A. J. (2017). "Trump Isn't Crazy." *Psychology Today.* January 31. Accessed February 4, 2017. https://www.psychologytoday.com/blog/saving-normal/201701/trump-isnt-crazy

Fricker M. (2007). *Epistemic Injustice: Power and the Ethics of Knowing.* Oxford: Oxford University Press.

Fuller D. A., Lamb L., Biasotti M., and Snook J. (2015). "Overlooked in the Undercounted: The Role of Mental Illness in Fatal Law Enforcement Encounters." *Treatment Advocacy Center.* Office of Research and Public Affairs. December. Accessed October 22, 2016. http://www.treatmentadvocacycenter.org/storage/documents/overlooked-in-the-undercounted.pdf

Gilman S. L. and Thomas J. M. (2016). *Are Racists Crazy? How Prejudice, Racism, and Antisemitism Became Markers of Insanity.* New York: New York University Press.

Glied S. and Frank R. G. (2014). "Mental Illness and Violence: Lessons from the Evidence." *American Journal of Public Health* 104(2): e5–e6.

Guenther L. (2013). *Solitary Confinement: Social Death and its Afterlives.* Minneapolis: University of Minnesota Press.

Helm A. B. (2016). "North Miami Police Officer Who Shot Therapist Identified; Sister of Autistic Man Gives Heartbreaking Statement." *The Root.* July 23. Accessed September 27, 2016. http://www.theroot.com/articles/news/2016/07/n-miami-police-officer-who-shot-therapist-identified-sister-of-autistic-patient-releases-heartbreaking-statement/

Husserl E. (1954/1970). *The Crisis of European Sciences and Transcendental Phenomenology*, trans. D. Carr. Evanston: Northwestern University Press.

Husserl E. (1969). *Formal and Transcendental Logic*, trans. D. Cairns. The Hague: Martinus Nijhoff.

Jaspers K. (1959/1963). *General Psychopathology: Volume I*, trans. J. Hoenig and M. W. Hamilton. Baltimore: Johns Hopkins University Press.

Jaspers K. (1959/1963). *General Psychopathology: Volume II*, trans. J. Hoenig and M. W. Hamilton. Baltimore: Johns Hopkins University Press.

Johnson K, Desmarais S. L., Grimm K. J., Tueller S. J., Swartz M. S., and Van Dorn R. A. (2016). "Proximal Risk Factors for Short-Term Community Violence Among Adults with Mental Illnesses." *Psychiatric Services* 67(7): 771–778.

Lasalvia A., Penta E., Sartorius N., and Henderson S. (2015). "Should the Label 'Schizophrenia' be Abandoned?" *Schizophrenia Research* 162: 276–284.

Lennard N. (2016). "The Military Logic of Punishing Chelsea Manning's Suicide Attempt." *The Nation*. September 28. Accessed October 16, 2016. https://www.thenation.com/article/the-military-logic-of-punishing-chelsea-mannings-suicide-attempt/

Lieu T. (2017). "Twitter Post." 11:28 AM EST, February 4. https://twitter.com/tedlieu/status/827916850973380608

Martinelli L. R., Binney J. S., and Kaye R. (2014). "Separating Myth from Fact: Unlinking Mental Illness and Violence and Implications for Gun Control Legislation and Public Policy." *New England Journal on Crime and Civil Confinement* 40(2): 359–378.

Metzl J. M. (2009). *The Protest Psychosis: How Schizophrenia Became a Black Disease*. Boston: Beacon Press.

Olfson M. (2016). "Building the Mental Health Workforce Capacity Needed to Treat Adults with Serious Mental Illnesses." *Health Affairs* 35(6): 983–990.

Oquendo M. A. (2016). "The Goldwater Rule: Why Breaking it is Unethical and Irresponsible." *American Psychiatric Association*. August 3. Accessed September 27, 2016. https://www.psychiatry.org/news-room/apa-blogs/apa-blog/2016/08/the-goldwater-rule

Parnas J. and Sass L. A. (2008). "Varieties of 'Phenomenology': On Description, Understanding, and Explanation in Psychiatry." In K. S. Kendler and J. Parnas (eds.), *Philosophical Issues in Psychiatry*, pp. 239–278. Baltimore: Johns Hopkins Press.

Potter N. N. (2016). *The Virtue of Defiance and Psychiatric Engagement*. Oxford: Oxford University Press.

Rembis M. (2014). "The New Asylums: Madness and Mass Incarceration in the Neoliberal Era." In L. Ben-Mosche, C. Chapman, and A. C. Carey (eds.), *Disability Incarcerated: Imprisonment and Disability in the United States and Canada*, pp. 139–159. New York: Palgrave Macmillan.

Sadler J. Z. (2005). *Values and Psychiatric Diagnosis*. Oxford: Oxford University Press.

Slack K. and Blinder A. (2017). "Dylann Roof Himself Rejects best Defense against Execution." *The New York Times*. January 1. Accessed February 4, 2017. https://www.nytimes.com/2017/01/01/us/dylann-roof-execution-defense-charleston-church-shooting.html?_r=0

Slate R. and Wesley Johnson W. (2008). *Criminalization of Mental Illness: Crisis and Opportunity for the Justice System*. Durham: Carolina Academic Press.

Solomon M. 2017. "On the Appearance and Disappearance of Asperger's Syndrome." In K. S. Kendler and J. Parnas (eds.), *Philosophical Issues in Psychiatry IV*, pp. 176–186. Oxford: Oxford University Press.

Szasz T. (1974). *The Myth of Mental Illness: Foundations of a Theory of Personal Conduct*. Revised Edition. New York: Harper & Row Publishers.

Thomas J. M. and Carson Byrd W. (2016). "THE 'SICK' RACIST: Racism and Psychopathology in the Colorblind Era." *Du Bois Review* 13(1): 181–203.

Torrey E. F. (2014). *American Psychosis: How the Federal Government Destroyed the Mental Illness Treatment System*. New York: Oxford University Press.

Waldenfels B. (2006/2011). *Phenomenology of the Alien*, trans. A. Kozin and T. Stähler. Evanston: Northwestern University Press.

Weiss E. L., Gross G. D., and Moncrief D. (2016). "Can Health Care Reform End Stigma toward Mental Illness?" *Journal of Progressive Human Services* 27(2): 95–110.

World Health Organization (WHO). (2014). "Mental Health: A State of Well Being." *World Health Organization*. August. Accessed February 5, 2017. http://www.who.int/features/factfiles/mental_health/en/

CHAPTER 91

PHENOMENOLOGICAL PSYCHOPATHOLOGY AND THE FORMATION OF CLINICIANS

GIOVANNI STANGHELLINI

INTRODUCTION

EDUCATION in mental health care is a long way from emphasizing adequate concepts and methods for exploring the patient's perspective. Since the publication of diagnostic manuals, many clinicians have confused operationalized criteria with handbooks of psychiatry and psychopathology, and diagnostic criteria with the whole picture of the illnesses. Consequently, a magnificent thesaurus of psychopathological knowledge, including in-depth descriptions of mental abnormal phenomena and syndromes, has simply been removed from educational programs. Moreover, educational programs make very little effort to bring to the fore the methodological problems that arise during the clinical interview, that is, how to get to know "what it is like" to experience a given symptom or abnormal phenomenon and why taking the other's perspective is relevant for clinical practice. The interview is not merely a clinical problem; rather, it may be considered an epistemological and ethical one. There is a need for a philosophically rich approach to the art of interviewing, especially for the task of exploring the patient's subjectivity. The risk is that mental health care as a discipline may lose its own identity if a rigorous assessment and attentive care to the patient's subjectivity is disregarded.

The need to go "back to fundamentals" has recently been argued for (Jablensky 2010; Stanghellini and Broome 2014). In this chapter I argue that psychopathology, as the discipline that assesses and makes sense of abnormal human subjectivity, should be at the heart of psychiatry and clinical psychology. It should be a basic educational prerequisite in the curriculum for mental health professionals and a key element of the shared intellectual identity of clinicians and researchers in this field. Yet how can young clinicians, who are so hungry for textbook knowledge, structured interviews, decision-making criteria, and therapeutic protocols be so patient as to endorse a kind of knowledge which is stubbornly aware of its limits, and resists all sorts of objectification and dogmatism? How can those who are looking for expert knowledge be satisfied with a kind of knowledge which conceives of itself as an "unlimited task" which takes place in the face-to-face, here-and-now encounter between two persons? How can they be happy with a mentor whose main teaching can be condensed into one sentence: "questions are more essential than answers, and every answer becomes a new question" (Jaspers 2003)?

Trainees' Unmet Needs in Learning Psychopathology

Given all that, it comes as a surprise that trainees and early career psychiatrists consider rediscovering psychopathology as one of the top priorities for their own future and for that of their patients (Fiorillo et al. 2013). According to the *Charter on Training of Medical Specialists in the EU: Requirements for the Specialty of Psychiatry* (UEMS 2005), educational programs during psychiatric residency should include structured training (with lectures, seminars, etc.) on psychopathology and other disciplines, which are held by students to represent the scientific bases of psychiatry (similar principles are reflected in the recommendation for undergraduate training; see Box 91.1).

Many studies (Lotz-Rambaldi et al. 2008; Oakley and Malik 2010; Muijen 2010; Rojnic Kuzman et al. 2012a, b; Kuzman et al. 2012) on the application of the UEMS recommendations in the different European countries showed great variability, in particular as regards training in psychopathology. The results of a survey (Fiorillo et al. 2016) exploring the current status of training on psychopathology in Europe to which forty-one representatives of early career psychiatrists of their national associations were invited to participate were the following:

- all respondents recognized psychopathology as a core component of training in psychiatry;
- a formal training course in psychopathology is available in twenty-nine out of the thirty-two surveyed countries and in most countries there is not a defined number of hours dedicated to psychopathology;
- teaching is mainly theoretical (96%) and discussion of clinical cases is routinely performed only in 24% of nations;
- structured training on psychometric tools is available in only ten countries (35%), and respondents from nineteen countries (73%) reported they used them routinely in clinical practice, even without formal training;
- trainees consider that the primary aims of studying psychopathology are (a) to assess psychiatric symptoms (47%), (b) to understand patients' abnormal experiences (33%), and (c) to make nosographical diagnosis (20%);

Box 91.1 Undergraduate teaching and training in psychiatry, core curriculum
          and assessment
Recommendations of the WPA co-sponsored meeting
Coventry March 18 and 19, 2013

The main recommendations from the meeting were:

1. Core curriculum and assessment guidelines and procedures need ongoing reviews especially in low income and developing countries.
2. When developing local policy for core curriculum and assessment guidelines, due consideration should be given to the different learning domains of knowledge, skills, and attitudes. Curriculum guidelines should include assessment procedures.
3. Course evaluation should be incorporated and made an integral component of formal teaching and of clinical placements.

The participants of the meeting proposed the following guiding principles for a core curriculum for undergraduate psychiatry to medical students. It is anticipated that adoption of these recommendations in different countries should ensure adherence to educational principles and promote high standards of mental health practice taking into account local contexts. (We use assessments to mean examination of what the students have learned and evaluation to examine if the teaching has delivered what it was supposed to do.)

CURRICULUM

Knowledge

By the end of medical school (or a locally specified time period) medical students should be able to:

1. Recognize common forms of psychopathology as well as the epidemiology, clinical manifestations, natural course, and response to treatment of common psychiatric disorders.
2. Familiarize themselves with common forms of pharmacological, psychotherapeutic, and psychosocial interventions and the evidence for these interventions.
3. Recognize local mental health problems including those related to natural disasters. war, migration, and indigenous populations.
4. Identify mental health promotion opportunities and interventions in the pathways to psychiatric care.
5. Highlight the impact of mental illness on the health economy and society and recognize the need for the inclusion of mental health promotion and treatment in public health policies.
6. Describe ethical, legal, and cultural influences/values on patient management.

Skills

1. Establish rapport with patients included those who have mental health problems and/or are acutely distressed and with their families as needed.
2. Take a full psychiatric history and assess the mental state (including a cognitive assessment).
3. Demonstrate clinical reasoning and present a diagnostic formulation (which includes being able to describe symptoms and mental state features, etiological factors, differential diagnoses, a plan of management and assessment of prognosis, and clinical ethical reasoning), which takes into account the biopsychosocial factors based on patients' wishes and best available evidence relevant to the local context.
4. Identify and apply those interventions for mental health promotion and common psychiatric conditions that can be provided by non-mental health specialists.

5. Recognize what constitutes a psychiatric emergency and when a referral is warranted and to whom.

Attitude

1. Evaluate societal attitudes toward mental illness and the values attached to mental health and illness.
2. Reflect on their own attitude to mental illness and their personal values and the impact these might have on the clinical care provided to patients.
3. Demonstrate compassion, empathy, dignity, and respect for patients and take into account the principles of autonomy, confidentiality, capacity, and consent as they relate to the local context.
4. Recognize the importance of developing professional relationships based on ethical standards, transparency, and probity.

Assessment

Psychiatry should be an important component of the examination process. Assessment could include the following components:

1. Attendance, participation, and successful completion of requirements of clinical placement as described in the local curriculum.
2. Clinical log books and/or cards that demonstrate evidence of clinical and reflective practice.
3. An observed assessment of their interviewing skills and ability to detect common psychiatric conditions (through a structured clinical exam or in a clinic).
4. Written exams to test clinical and theoretical psychiatric knowledge using MCQs, essays, patient management problems, or other written assessments techniques as per local needs and resources.
5. Viva or case-based discussion.

- the most frequently adopted psychopathological approach is the clinical one (65%) aimed at nosgraphical diagnosis, while the phenomenological approach is adopted in 22% of the countries and the descriptive approach in 18% of countries;
- Karl Jaspers, Emil Kraepelin, and Kurt Schneider are listed as the most influential psychopathologists, followed by Eugene Bleuler, Sigmund Freud, and Philippe Pinel;
- at the end of residency, 48% of respondents are not satisfied with the training they received in psychopathology, 21% believe that psychopathology "is not useful in clinical practice," 25% that it "is old-fashioned," and 50% that it "is of no interest for psychiatric practice." Six percent of respondents state that they have "no time to dedicate to the study of psychopathology";
- the most important unmet needs identified by residents in psychiatry are time dedicated to supervision (90%), time dedicated to studying psychopathology (73%), and opportunities to discuss patients' psychopathological phenomena in clinical practice (57%). Other unmet needs include lack of supervision, which is available in only eleven of the surveyed countries (35%), and lack of training in the use of psychometric tools scales, which should be a compulsory part of residency courses, according to 100% of respondents.

Five Reasons for Teaching
Phenomenological Psychopathology

The results of this survey demonstrate that the rediscovery of psychopathology is among the top priorities for training. Early career clinicians are not satisfied with the training they receive in psychopathology. They would like to see better educational opportunities in this field, requesting that theoretical knowledge be complemented by practical clinical skills. Yet famous recent editorials argue for the opposite (e.g. Ross, Travis, and Arbuckle 2015), that is, psychiatry training should be heavily focused on neuroscience. In this section I will explain why I disagree with them.

For past generations of residents in psychiatry (Maj 2013), Jaspers's *General Psychopathology* was recommended reading. Familiarity with that and other classics of psychopathology helped residents to see the DSMs as synopses of available knowledge and diagnostic algorithms to be used for clinical purposes—not as *handbooks* of psychiatry and psychopathology. This may not be the case for current residents, which may result in a high risk of misunderstanding and oversimplification. The main misunderstanding is, perhaps, that psychopathology is the name of an old-fashioned quasi-religious cult celebrating the dogma that psychiatry should be part of the medical humanities rather than a biomedical science. Actually, psychopathology brings into focus the primary—although not sole—"object" of psychiatry: the *psyche*, that is, the patient's abnormal experiences lived in the first-person perspective, embedded in anomalous forms of existence, and structured according to unusual meaning patterns. Psychopathology is a discourse (*logos*) about the sufferings (*pathos*) of the mind (*psyche*).

There are at least five reasons for psychopathology, and more exactly *phenomenological* psychopathology, to become once more a fundamental column of training in the field of mental health (Stanghellini and Fiorillo 2015):

- Phenomenological psychopathology provides clinicians with a method enabling them to capture the subtle nuances of patients' experience that constitute the essentials of the "psychiatric object" (Parnas 2013). The precise characterization of these nuances is, at present, the only secure basis for diagnosis and treatment, since experiential symptoms are by far more specific diagnostic indexes than any other kind of symptoms, including behavioral ones.
- Phenomenological psychopathology acknowledges that what patients manifest is not a series of mutually independent, isolated symptoms, but rather a certain structure of interwoven experiences, beliefs, and actions, all permeated by biographical details. What stands in front of the clinician is not an amorphous agglomerate of symptoms, but a person with a specific, meaningful, and (to a certain extent) coherent "form of life."
- Phenomenological psychopathology is a method for understanding a given phenomenon, that is, grasping the personal feel and meaning of an experience or set of experiences. Mental symptoms do not simply have subpersonal causes, but also a personal feel and meaning. Understanding is not the effect of a generalized knowledge, but is achieved by immersing ourselves in a particular situation. Thus, phenomenological

psychopathology preserves the individuality and uniqueness of the suffering person. It can operate in parallel with a traditional biomedical approach, since it does not exclude seeing abnormal phenomena as symptoms caused by a dysfunction to be treated, but additionally includes the exploration of personal meanings. Phenomenological psychopathology conceptualizes mental symptoms as the outcome of a mediation between the person and her abnormal phenomena (Stanghellini, Fulford, and Bolton 2013).

- Phenomenological psychopathology helps us not only to understand, but also to causally explain ("to explain" means *scire per causas*) a given abnormal phenomenon, or a set of abnormal phenomena, since it helps to characterize them. Any phenomenon, in order to be explained, must first of all be described in the greatest detail. Thus phenomenological psychopathology is a necessary prerequisite for linking clinical sciences to the neurosciences.

- The fifth reason is that the personal background, as a pre-reflective context of meaning and significance within which and against which persons construe the significance of their abnormal phenomena, should be part and parcel of a thorough clinical assessment. Thinness of phenotypes and simplification of clinical constructs are the consequences of a mainstream approach to psychopathological phenotypes that focuses on easy-to-assess operationalizable symptoms. Phenomenological investigations of abnormal human subjectivity suggest a shift of attention from mere symptoms (i.e. state-like indexes for nosographical diagnosis) to a broader range of phenomena that are trait-like features of a given life-world. Systematic explorations of anomalies in the patients' experience, for example, of time, space, body, self, and otherness, may provide a useful integration to the symptom-based approach. These abnormal phenomena can be used as pointers to the fundamental alterations of the structure of subjectivity characterizing each mental disorder (Stanghellini and Rossi 2014).

Psychopathology's Agenda

Psychopathology is a peculiar kind of discipline characterized by an "and-and" agenda bringing together generalized and individual knowledge, explaining and understanding, spontaneous and second-order empathy, technical education and human formation. All this should be acknowledged in establishing training curricula for clinicians.

Generalized and Individual Knowledge

While acknowledging the need for systematic knowledge, psychopathology also advocates the necessity for clinicians not to forget that each patient is an individual and not just the token of a given category. We expect generalized knowledge in science—and psychopathology is a science—but we also have to know that anything really meaningful tends to have a concrete form, and generalization destroys it (Jaspers 1997). Jaspers's *General Psychopathology* was the first systematic attempt to classify abnormal mental phenomena and became the most secure basis to establish a valid and reliable diagnosis. But Jaspers suggested that the knowledge thus established must not be used as the map of a continent but more like as an outline of possible ways to explore it (ibid.). Jaspers declared that the clinician's main preoccupation, next to taxonomy, should be methodology. Methodology, next to taxonomy, is the only way to avoid depersonalization and dehumanization of the "real" patient. What we need, next to systematic and generalized knowledge, is the systematic awareness of the ways to gain knowledge about an individual patient.

A reliable taxonomy did some good in psychiatry. We can remember the whimsical and idiosyncratic ways psychiatric diagnoses were given—or rejected, by the so-called anti-psychiatrists—in the 1970s and early 1980s. DSM and ICD, as well as structured and semi-structured interviews, contributed to changing this profoundly unscientific attitude toward systematic assessment and diagnosing. The technical biomedical turn of psychiatry in the 1970s was a reaction against this irrational attitude. To the technical approach, the scientific status of psychiatry is founded on reliable diagnosis. This is the right use of diagnostic manuals. Next to this, however, there is *abuse* of diagnostic manuals: the *reification* of diagnostic criteria. Diagnostic criteria are meant to index rather than thoroughly describe syndromes. We should not confuse our *DSM* diagnostic criteria with the disorders that they were designed to index (Kendler 2016). This is a conceptual error since diagnostic criteria are representations and not objects *in se*. Also, they are abstractions since mental disorders are not natural entities existing in themselves.

The effectiveness of the diagnostic process relies on two domains: diagnostic criteria and the interview method. Operational diagnostic criteria are instrumental in achieving high reliability in the domain of the diagnostic schema, primarily because of their reduction of criterion variance. Structured interview methods help to improve the reliability of diagnostic assignment by reducing information variance. These two domains are coupled in such a way that structured interviews are designed to explore only those symptoms that are relevant to establishing a diagnosis according to the diagnostic criteria themselves. The main goal is to discover whether a patient with a given set of signs/symptoms "meets criteria." Accordingly, interviewing is seen as a technique that should conform to the technical–rational paradigm of natural sciences in which psychiatry as a branch of biomedicine is positioned and the clinical encounter is thus conceived as a stimulus–response pattern.

Psychopathology teaches us to balance this attitude with attention to the individuality of the patient. To encourage true dialogue between interviewer and interviewee the interviewer should not presume to "know" a priori what is relevant to assess, and to possess the "whole picture" of the patient's illness, whilst the patient has just the "pieces" of the puzzle. "It is much more important to know what sort of a patient has a disease than what sort of a disease a patient has." This aphorism, attributed to Sir William Osler (one of the founders of modern medicine in the early twentieth century) (Osler 1921) reflects the importance of oscillating between generalized and individual knowledge when interviewing a patient.

Explaining and Understanding

As the science of human abnormal subjectivity, psychopathology brings into a clear epistemic focus the fact that mental health practice is based on two main, complementary methodological approaches: explaining and understanding. We causally explain a phenomenon when we find, by repeated experience, that that kind of phenomenon is regularly linked together with a number of other phenomena. Explanations are achieved by observation of events, by experiment and the collection of numerous examples (Jaspers 1997) which allow us to formulate general rules. This is the way we establish diagnostic categories and causal connections with subpersonal causes. Understanding, on the other hand, is achieved by immersing ourselves in a singular situation. It is not the effect of a generalized knowledge, rather fresh, personal intuition is needed on every occasion. An essential aspect of understanding is that it connects elements of the patient's conscious life and, by doing so, it makes visible to the clinician something that helps him to feel *what it is like* to be in the patient's mental state.

The attention to understanding other individuals is an essential virtue in the field of mental health care. Philosopher Martha Nussbaum (Nussbaum 2010) provides an unintentional portrait of the mental health clinician as a candidate prototype of a globally minded citizen (Stanghellini 2013a). The ideal citizen should have "the ability to think what it might be like to be in the shoes of a person different from oneself, to be an intelligent reader of that person's story; and to understand the emotions and wishes and desires that someone so placed might have" (Nussbaum 2010: 95–96). Also, she should possess the ability to have concern for the lives of others, to imagine a variety of complex issues affecting the story of a human life as it unfolds, and to understand human stories not just as aggregate data. This epitome should be able to see other persons, especially marginalized people, as fellows with equal rights and look at them with respect (25–26).

First- and Second-Order Empathy

Nussbaum's kind of understanding is, first and foremost, an ethical attitude that enables a person to put herself in someone else's shoes. In this vein, to understand empathically is to insist on and give radical attention to the irreducible and ultimate character of the givenness of the other's experience. For Jaspers too, the phenomenological attitude involved in his conception of empathic understanding allows him to see the other human being not as a clinical object or an isolated, physiological organism swirling around in a physical universe, but as a human being living a life similar, but never identical, to other human beings (Jaspers 1963).

Phenomenally, this kind of empathic experience is an experience of resonance between oneself and the other person. This basic form of empathy does not require any voluntary and explicit effort, but an attitude which is ethical in nature. Such an immediate understanding is only possible against a background of a similar life-world. We may call this type of empathy, which is at play from the very beginning of our life, nonconative—a kind of spontaneous and pre-reflective attunement between embodied selves through which we implicitly make sense of the other's behavior.

Yet understanding abnormal experiences (especially psychotic experiences like schizophrenic, melancholic, or manic ones) is based on a different kind of empathic attitude which departs from the ordinary concept of "empathy." To achieve this kind of empathy requires a kind of training that goes beyond nonconative empathic skills. Also, at the same time this other type of empathy avoids the pitfalls of conative empathy, that is, of the attempt to understand the other's experiences based on my own (the clinician's) personal experiences and on commonsense categories. This kind of empathic attitude can be named *second-order empathy* (Stanghellini 2013b; Stanghellini 2013c; Stanghellini 2016). To achieve second-order empathy is a complex process that should be taught in great detail to trainees. First of all one needs to acknowledge the autonomy of the other person, and consequently that the life-world of the other person is not like one's own. Second, one must learn to neutralize one's own natural attitude that would make one try to understand the other's experience as if it took place in a world like one's own. Third, one must try to reconstruct the existential structures of the world the other lives in. Fourth, one can finally attempt to understand the other's experience as meaningfully situated in a world that is indeed similar to one's own, but also constantly and indelibly marked by the other person's particular existence. The supposition that the other lives in a world just like my own—that is, he experiences time, space, his own body, others, the materiality of objects, etc. just as I do—is often the source of serious misunderstandings. Take the example of lived time: one day for a young man can be lived as growth and fulfillment, whereas an old man may live it as consumption and decline. An anxious person may be afflicted by a feeling that time vanishes, inexorably passes away, that the time that separates her from death is intolerably shortened. A patient in an early stage of schizophrenia may experience time as the dawn of a new reality. In order to empathize with these persons, I need to acknowledge the existential difference, the particular autonomy, which separates me from the way of being-in-the-world that characterizes each of them. Any forgetting of this difference will be an obstacle to empathic understanding since these people live in a life-world whose structure is (at least in part) different from my own. Achieving second-order empathy thus requires me to set aside my own pre-reflective, natural attitude (in which my first-order empathic capacities are rooted), and to approach the other's world as I would do if I was exploring an unknown and alien country (Stanghellini and Rosfort 2013).

Education and Formation

Thus psychopathology advocates a kind of curriculum for clinicians that complements professional educational aims (providing assessment and diagnostic skills) with personal formation (providing an epistemologically and ethically sound background for the encounter with patients). Clinicians need personal formation or cultivation alongside a thorough scientific education—restrictively understood as acquisition of technical knowledge and skill training. *Timeo hominem unius libris* ("I fear a man who has read only one book"). Besides other sources, training in this area will build on rich resources from classical philosophy and history of ideas (Fulford, Stanghellini, and Broome 2004). Since 2001, a full curriculum for philosophy of psychiatry was introduced in the Royal College of Psychiatrists' curriculum for higher psychiatric training, the "MRCPsych" (Royal College of Psychiatrists 2001). Students should be encouraged to read, as well as textbooks, not only essays, but also novels and poetry, as well as paying attention to everything that may help them develop their sensibility to what is *other* and their interest in making sense of otherness. Cultivating one's Self (*Bildung*) is a complement to memorizing pieces of professional equipment (Gadamer 2004). Psychopathology provides both educational resources (e.g. valid and reliable concepts and methods for establishing an accurate diagnosis) and that kind of sensitivity, namely the sensitivity to what is appropriate in dealing with others, for which knowledge of general principles does not suffice. Next to second-order empathy, *tact*, as the ability to feel an *atmosphere* and to attune with it in those situations that are not yet plainly and unambiguously defined, is an example of this. When evidence-based guidelines are still scarce (as is the case, for instance, with early psychoses), tact seems to be an indispensable resource for the clinician.

The clinical encounter is not only a cognitive-rationalistic performance but also an aesthetic experience (Costa et al. 2014). Tact is the sense that is present when one finds its limits in the limits of the other. Atmospheres are haptically experienced: the kind of understanding at play is a global awareness of the here-and-now and you-and-I situation, while the limits between oneself and the other are being defined and redefined. In order to grasp atmospheres, one must be predisposed to receive them. In 1907, Husserl wrote a letter to Hofmannsthal, comparing Hofmannsthal's theory of aesthetics to the phenomenological method which, as he wrote, "requires us to take a stance that is essentially deviating from the 'natural' stance towards all objectivity, which is closely related to that stance in which your art puts us as a purely aesthetical one with respect to the represented objects and the whole environment" (quoted in Costa et al. 2014). Husserl appears to be referring to the suspension of the natural attitude that would come to sustain the phenomenological method. The force of an aesthetic attitude in clinical practice resides in two features: (1) the aesthetic properties of an object can only appear if one allows the object's detachment from one's intention; (2) the aesthetic properties only arise when the object is stripped of its ordinary meaning. The former resembles the "disinterestedness" that especially psychodynamically-oriented clinicians endorse: to abandon the "desire" to simply eliminate the patient's symptoms. The second is much closer to the phenomenological epoché: the clinician has to learn how to avoid his intention of finding symptoms in order to allow the appearance of atmospheres.

The atmosphere's significance in the clinic encounter has long been recognized. Tellenbach considered that during the interaction with a patient, the clinician is led to feel certain atmospheric qualities that exceed the factual, but nevertheless permeate the process of understanding. This led him to develop the concept of "diagnostic atmosphere" (Tellenbach 1968). Minkowski used a similar term: *diagnostique par penetration* (Minkowski 1927) to refer to the importance of intuition (the non-cognitive grasping of the meaning of a phenomenon), particularly referring to the diagnosis of schizophrenia. These concepts are evidence to the fact that the two authors acknowledged the partaking of atmospheres in the understanding of phenomena.

Atmospheres belong to the pathic moment of experience, the moment when self and world are merged. The pathic transformations impressed by atmospheres are not directly accessible by ordinary language (not to mention to the technical language of general psychiatry). They can only be indirectly made sense of by a process that is metaphoric in nature. The leading role of metaphors in the process of understanding atmospheres reflects the pre-reflective nature of the experience (Costa et al. 2014). This process brings experience to the reflective realm, but will perpetually remain unfinished, as metaphors do not pin down atmospheres. On the contrary, they enhance atmospheres, amplifying them, and enchaining other metaphors.

The Personal Influence of the Teacher

Training institutions should finally recognize the importance of the influence of the teacher upon those who are being taught in the process of professional formation (Camac 1921).

This obviously implies that not only trainees, but also trainers need to be trained, selected, and supervised. In an age where technical skills are emphasized, teaching itself can be misunderstood as a technical performance rather than as a human encounter in which the teacher as a person is in the foreground.

This has long been considered a cornerstone in the field of arts, but scientific institutions seem to be tardy to acknowledge the importance—in the positive as well as in the negative— of the personal contact between mentor and pupil. From this personal encounter emanates an atmosphere which may inspire both. Within this inspiring atmosphere an institution may become a seat of learning, research, and knowledge, a place in which principles of thought and conduct can be established, instilled, and transmitted from generation to generation.

Bibliography

Camac C. N. B. (1921). "Introduction to the 1905 Edition of Osler W." In *Counsels and Ideals from the Writings of William Osler*. Boston/New York: Houghton Mifflin Company.

Costa C., Carmenates S., Madeira, L. and Stanghellini, G. (2014). "Phenomenology of Atmospheres. The Felt Meanings of Clinical Encounters." *Journal of Psychopathology* 20: 351–357.

Fiorillo A., Malik A., Luciano M., Del Vecchio V., Sampogna G., Del Gaudio L., et al. (2013). "Challenges for Trainees in Psychiatry and Early Career Psychiatrists." *International Review of Psychiatry* 25: 431–437.

Fiorillo A., Sampogna G., Del Vecchio V., et al. (2016). "Is Psychopathology Still the Basic Science of Psychiatric Education? Results from a European Survey." *Academic Psychiatry* 40: 242–248.

Fulford K. W. M., Stanghellini G., and Broome M. (2004). "What Can Philosophy Do for Psychiatry?" *World Psychiatry* 3: 130–135.

Gadamer H.-G. *Truth and Method* (2004), trans. J. Weinshemer and D. G. Marshall. New York: The Continuum Publishing Company.

Jablensky A. (2010). "Psychiatry in Crisis? Back to Fundamentals." *World Psychiatry* 9: 29.

Jaspers K. (1963). "Die phänomenologische Forschungsrichtung in der Psychopathologie." In K. Jaspers (ed.), *Gesammelte Schriften zur Psychopathologie*, pp. 314–328. Berlin: Springer-Verlag.

Jaspers K. (1997). *General Psychopathology*. Baltimore and London: The John Hopkins University Press.

Jaspers K. (2003). *Truth and Symbol*. Lanham: Rowman & Littlefield.

Kendler K. S. (2016). "Phenomenology of Schizophrenia and the Representativeness of Modern Diagnostic Criteria." *JAMA Psychiatry* 73(10):1082–1092.

Lotz-Rambaldi W., Schäfer I., Doesschate R., and Hohagen F. (2008). "Specialist Training in Psychiatry in Europe—Results of the UEMS-Survey." *European Psychiatry* 23: 157–168.

Maj, M. (2013). "Introduction: The Relevance of Karl Jaspers' General Psychopathology to Current Psychiatric Debate." In G. Stanghellini and T. Fuchs (eds.), *One Century of Karl Jaspers' General Psychopathology*, pp. xxiv–viii. Oxford: Oxford University Press.

Minkowski E. (1927). *La schizophrénie*. Paris: Editions Payot & Rivages.

Muijen M. (2010). "Training Psychiatrists in Europe: Fit for Purpose? Commentary on Psychiatric Training in Europe." *Psychiatry Bulletin* 34: 450–451.

Nussbaum M. (2010). *Not for Profit. Why Democracy Needs the Humanities*. Princeton and Oxford: Princeton University Press.

Oakley C. and Malik A. (2010). "Psychiatric Training in Europe." *Psychiatry Bulletin* 34: 447–450.

Osler W. (1921). *Counsels and Ideals from the Writings of William Osler*. Boston/New York: Houghton Mifflin Company.

Parnas J. (2013). "The Breivik Case and 'condition psychiatrica.'" *World Psychiatry* 12: 22–23.

Rojnic Kuzman M., Giacco D., Simmons M., Wuyts P., Bausch-Becker N., Favre G., et al. (2012a). "Psychiatry Training in Europe: Views from the Trenches." *Medical Teacher* 34: e708–e717.

Rojnic Kuzman M., Giacco D., Simmons M., Wuyts P., Bausch-Becker N., Favre G., et al. (2012b). "Are There Differences between Training Curricula on Paper and in Practice? Views of European Trainees." *World Psychiatry* 11: 135.

Ross D. A., Travis M. J., and Arbuckle M. R. (May 2015). "The Future of Psychiatry as Clinical Neuroscience: Why Not Now?" *JAMA Psychiatry* 72(5): 413–414.

Royal College of Psychiatrists. (2001). *Curriculum for Basic Specialist Training and the MRCPsych Examination*. London: Royal College of Psychiatrists.

Stanghellini, G. (2013a). "The Portrait of the Psychiatrist as a Globally Minded Citizen." *Current Opinion in Psychiatry* 26: 498–501.

Stanghellini G. (2013b). "The Ethics of Incomprehensibility." in G. Stanghellini and T. Fuchs (eds.), *One Century of Karl Jaspers' General Psychopathology*, pp. 166–181. Oxford: Oxford University Press.

Stanghellini G. (2013c). "Philosophical Resources for the Psychiatric Interview." In K. W. M. Fulford, et al. (eds.), *Oxford Handbook of Philosophy and Psychiatry*, pp. 321–356. Oxford: Oxford University Press.

Stanghellini G. (2016). *Lost in dialogue. Anthropology, Psychopathology and Care*. Oxford: Oxford University Press.

Stanghellini G., Fulford K. W. M., and Bolton D. (2013). "Person-centered Psychopathology of Schizophrenia. Building on Karl Jaspers' Understanding of the Patient's Attitude towards His Illness." *Schizophrenia Bulletin* 39: 287–294.

Stanghellini G. and Rosfort R. (2013). "Empathy as a Sense of Autonomy." *Psychopathology* 46(5): 337–344.

Stanghellini G. and Broome M. R. (2014). "Psychopathology as the Basic Science of Psychiatry." *British Journal of Psychiatry*. 205: 169–170.

Stanghellini G. and Rossi R. (2014). "Pheno-phenotypes: A Holistic Approach to the Psychopathology of Schizophrenia." *Current Opinions in Psychiatry* 27(3): 236–241.

Stanghellini G. and Fiorillo A. (2015). "Five Reasons for Teaching Psychopathology." *World Psychiatry* 14(1): 107–108.

Tellenbach H. (1968). *Geschmack und Atmosphäre*. Salzburg: Müller.

Union Européenne des Médecins Specialistes. (2005). "Report of the UEMS Section for Psychiatry, The Profile of a Psychiatrist." UEMS. http://www.uemspsychiatry.org/section/reports/2005Oct-PsychiatristProfile.pdf

CHAPTER 92

PHENOMENOLOGICAL PSYCHOPATHOLOGY AND PSYCHIATRIC CLASSIFICATION

ANTHONY VINCENT FERNANDEZ

INTRODUCTION

TODAY, the dominant systems of psychiatric classification are the fifth edition of the *Diagnostic and Statistical Manual of Mental Disorders* (DSM-5; APA, 2013) and the tenth edition of the *International Classification of Diseases* (ICD-10; WHO, 2004)—which, in its forthcoming eleventh edition, will largely converge with the DSM-5. Other systems include the *Psychodynamic Diagnostic Manual* (PDM-2; Lingiardi and McWilliams 2017), which is informed by psychoanalytic approaches, and the Research Domain Criteria (RDoC) initiative, a dimensional approach developed by the US National Institute of Mental Health (Cuthbert 2014; Cuthbert and Insel 2013). The goal of any psychiatric classification should be to provide a means of organizing and navigating the complex domain of mental disorders, thereby guiding both clinical practice and scientific research.

Most contemporary approaches aim for a biological classification. They assume that mental disorders are, at their basis, biological disease entities. The goal of classification is, therefore, to provide a set of categories that maps onto discrete biological diseases. However, in light of the DSM's failure to biologically validate its categories of disorder, psychiatrists are now looking to alternative approaches that might produce new classifications.

Some of these alternative approaches are grounded in phenomenology, a philosophical study of human experience and existence. Phenomenological psychopathologists describe not only "what it's like" or "what it feels like" to live with a mental disorder, but also how the structural features of human experience and existence—for example, intentionality, self-hood, temporality, and affectivity—alter in psychopathological cases. At this point, however, none of these classificatory *approaches* have culminated in a classification scheme like the ones we find in the DSM, ICD, or PDM. Here, I refer to a classificatory *approach* as a process or method of classifying phenomena. In the case of mental disorders, classificatory approaches might track, for instance, differences in experience, behavior, neurobiology, or treatment response. I refer to a classification *scheme* as the set of phenomena that an approach has grouped or delineated. In the case of the DSM, for instance, the scheme is the set of categories included in the manual. Therefore, to say that phenomenologists have developed only classificatory approaches means that they have methods for delineating the range of psychopathological conditions, but they have not actually produced their own scheme.

In addressing the topic of phenomenology and psychiatric classification, this chapter has two aims: First, it presents phenomenological critiques of the DSM/ICD approach to classification. Second, it delineates the various phenomenological approaches to classification. My intention is not to take a stand on the adequacy of any particular approach. Rather, my intention is to delineate the central features of these approaches side by side, and against the backdrop of the DSM/ICD, so that phenomenologists will be in a better position to debate these approaches and develop more effective systems of classification—for example, systems that more accurately align with neurobiological markers, predict course of illness, or guide targeted therapeutic interventions.

Phenomenological Critiques of Operationalism

Since the DSM-III (APA 1980), operationalism has been the dominant approach to classification and diagnosis. As employed in the DSM, an "operational approach" is one that categorizes and diagnoses disorders by reference to a set of easily observable symptoms, some number of which must be present for a predefined period of time.[1] Major depressive disorder (MDD), for example, is diagnosed when at least five of nine possible symptoms are present for at least two weeks. One of these symptoms must be either (1) depressed mood or (2) loss of interest or pleasure. The other symptoms include (3) significant weight loss or weight gain; (4) insomnia or hypersomnia; (5) psychomotor agitation or retardation; (6) fatigue or loss of energy; (7) feelings of worthlessness or excessive or inappropriate guilt; (8) diminished ability to think or concentrate; and (9) recurrent thoughts of death or suicidal ideation (APA 2013). Schizophrenia, by contrast, is diagnosed when at least two of five symptoms are present over a one-month period: (1) delusions; (2) hallucinations; (3) disorganized speech; (4) grossly disorganized or catatonic behavior; and (5) negative symptoms (in addition, at least one of the symptoms must be items 1, 2, or 3) (APA 2013).[2]

---

[1] In contemporary psychiatry, what goes under the label of "operationalism" is relatively superficial when compared with its early philosophical and scientific development in the work of Carl Hempel (1966), Edwin Boring (1945), and Percy Williams Bridgman (1938). While psychiatry's version of operationalism likely has its roots in this history, one should not assume that it takes over the fairly robust philosophical programs of these early figures. For a more detailed account of the history of operationalism in psychology and psychiatry, see Hasok Chang (2009) and Josef Parnas and Pierre Bovet (2015).

[2] Each diagnostic category includes additional criteria, such as significant impairment of one's ability to work, engage in self-care, or maintain social relations.

Notably, the DSM's major focus has been on enhancing inter-rater reliability—that is, increasing the likelihood that two or more clinicians will diagnose the same patient with the same condition. An operational approach, with its reliance on easily observable symptoms and structured diagnostic interviews, provides an effective means of enhancing reliability. But psychiatrists want more than reliability—they want validity. In most cases, this takes the form of an appeal to neurobiological underpinnings. However, as Assen Jablensky and Robert Kendell point out, there are numerous definitions of validity in psychiatry, with little agreement on which sense of validity should be privileged. A category might be considered valid if it

> (a) is based on a coherent, explicit set of defining features (construct validity); (b) has empirical referents, such as verifiable observations for establishing its presence (content validity); (c) can be corroborated by independent procedures such as biological or psychological tests (concurrent validity); and (d) predicts future course of illness or treatment response (predictive validity).
>
> (Jablensky and Kendell 2002: 10)

In light of this state of affairs, some psychiatrists—including Jablensky and Kendell—argue that we should appeal to a concept of utility instead of validity. Utility is achieved when a category or scheme "provides nontrivial information about prognosis and likely treatment outcomes, and/or testable propositions about biological and social correlates" (Kendell and Jablensky 2003: 9). Considering the DSM's shortcomings with respect to validity and utility, it has been the subject of widespread criticism from groups both inside and outside of mainstream psychiatry.

Phenomenological psychopathologists constitute one of these critical groups. Phenomenologists don't necessarily agree on how to approach the problem of validity or utility—some seem to endorse, for example, the view that phenomenology should assist in the process of distinguishing biological disease entities, whereas others defend a less naturalistic view. There are, however, three general criticisms of the DSM's operational approach that we find in the phenomenological literature:

1) It ignores how clinicians intuitively diagnose patients.
2) It neglects the organization among the various symptoms, treating them as disparate parts without a unified whole.
3) It allows categories to reify, inhibiting future refinement and revision of the classification scheme.[3] (Parnas and Bovet 2015; Schwartz and Wiggins 1987a, 1987b)

In general, phenomenological approaches to psychiatric classification claim to resolve all of these issues. In what follows, I outline four phenomenological approaches to classification, which I divide into two broad classes: type and dimension approaches. The first class includes ideal types, essential types, and prototypes. The second class includes a dimensional approach that I have recently proposed, which draws inspiration from the National Institute of Mental Health's Research Domain Criteria (RDoC) initiative.

---

[3] This situation is even more problematic when a diagnostic category encompasses a heterogeneity of conditions, as we find in the case of MDD (see e.g. Ratcliffe, Broome, Smith, and Bowden, 2013).

TYPIFICATION AND CLASSIFICATION

Before distinguishing the ideal type, essential type, and prototype approaches, it will be helpful to outline what they hold in common. All of these approaches aim to resolve the above shortcomings of the DSM's operational approach, and they do so in the following ways:

1) They take stock of how clinicians intuitively understand their patients—utilizing, rather than ignoring, this intuitive understanding.
2) They seek an organizing principle, a gestalt, or what Eugene Minkowski calls the *trouble générateur*, that makes sense of the total structure of the disorder.
3) They build in mechanisms for continued revision and refinement, treating current concepts as one step along the way to a better system of classification.

With respect to the first solution, all three approaches share the basic phenomenological insight that we perceive and make sense of our world through tacit types or categories. In everyday experience, these types are not explicitly defined and their boundaries are not always clear. Whenever we perceive something, we perceive it *as* some particular kind of thing; we never perceive a bare object. For example, if I walk through my garden and see that a rose has bloomed, I simply see it *as* a rose. In most cases, I don't list off explicit criteria to check whether it's a rose. I just know what a rose looks like.

But this doesn't mean that our typifications are never wrong. Perhaps I invite my friend, a botanist, over to show her my rose. Upon walking into the garden, she exclaims, "That's not a rose! It's a peony." Realizing that my initial typification was incorrect, I'm now open to being corrected by my friend. When she corrects me, she might teach me explicit criteria for distinguishing roses from peonies. And I might rely on these explicit criteria for some time. But, eventually, this too will become habitual and tacit. I'll develop my own expertise, immediately seeing a flower *as* a rose, a peony, or some other species.

Our typifications are, therefore, learned and refined in the course of everyday experience. I wasn't born knowing how to identify flowers; I learned what counted as a flower and how to distinguish among different kinds of flowers through everyday experience (and with a little guidance from my parents). And, even now, my ability to tacitly typify or categorize flowers remains relatively limited. The botanist is not only better at distinguishing peonies from roses; she can also distinguish among a wide variety of peonies and roses. And, as an expert, she can distinguish them intuitively, without appealing to explicit criteria. In this respect, to refer to the process of typification as *intuitive* simply means that it occurs tacitly or implicitly—not that it's based on an innate or unchanging base of knowledge.

Moreover, seeing *as* isn't simply a process of identifying and categorizing objects within the world. In addition to identifying and categorizing, I also have an immediate sense of how to take things up and put them to use. For example, when I see an object on my table *as* a mug, it immediately shows up to me as a vessel for holding tea, coffee, or hot chocolate. It also shows up to me as something I should wash in the kitchen sink or place in the dishwasher. In general, these actions aren't things that I have to explicitly reflect on or infer. To see an object *as* a mug just is to see it as something that can perform these functions and should be handled in these ways.

Phenomenologists argue that we employ tacit typifications not only in our experience of everyday objects, but also in our experience of other people. To navigate the social world, we typify people in a variety of ways and these typifications guide our initial interactions. When I walk into my classroom, I immediately perceive the people before me as my students and they perceive me as their professor. These tacit typifications shape how we engage each other, determining proper modes of address, expected behaviors, and so on. Such typifications can, of course, be pernicious: They might, for instance, become racial or gender stereotypes. However, phenomenologists argue that prejudices aren't inherently problematic (see e.g. Gadamer 1960/2013, 2008). We need presuppositions and assumptions in order to successfully navigate our environment (although we also need to be open to revising them in light of future experiences).

But what does everyday typification have to do with the practice of clinical psychology and psychiatry? Proponents of typification argue that clinicians have an intuitive understanding of their patients, and that this understanding often leads to an initial diagnosis (Schwartz and Wiggins 1987b). In the clinical encounter, the skilled clinician doesn't simply perceive a generic person who happens to exhibit an array of symptoms. Her perception often includes a tacit sense of her patient *as* depressed, *as* schizophrenic, *as* autistic, and so on. This initial perception can guide her process of questioning, helping her arrive at a final diagnosis. The operational, check-list diagnostic method of the DSM-5 ignores this skilled, intuitive mode of understanding and therefore fails to put it to use.

Over the past few decades, intuitive diagnosis has been overshadowed by the operational approach. However, there has been a recent renewal in studies of the effectiveness and accuracy of intuitive modes of diagnosis, focusing both on the diagnosis of schizophrenia (Gozé et al. 2018) and on the ability to identity those at risk of developing schizophrenia (Lindau et al. n.d.). These studies stress that the intuitive approach provides only a preliminary or tentative diagnosis. An expert psychiatrist should be guided by his typifications, but should not simply allow his initial intuition to determine the final diagnosis. Marcin Moskalewicz, Michael Schwartz, and Tudi Gozé (2018) argue that intuitive diagnosis, properly conducted, is not simply an immediate sense of the patient's condition. Rather, it is a temporally extended process in which the psychiatrist critically reflects upon his intuition or typification and seeks out disconfirming evidence. Moreover, they claim that this mode of diagnosis need not conflict with an operational approach. One might, for instance, be led to an initial diagnostic category through intuition, but confirm or disconfirm this intuition by employing operational criteria.

This practice of actively confirming or disconfirming an intuitive diagnosis is linked with the practice of revising and refining diagnostic categories themselves. This latter practice is as an attempt to make the diagnostic system more rigorous and scientific. We need to guarantee that our types accurately identify the conditions they're meant to diagnose and that these types don't reify into outdated and inaccurate categories. However, the three typification approaches do not necessarily agree on how we should make diagnosis scientific. Each proposes a slightly different method of harnessing everyday typifications, transforming them into scientific concepts and categories (Fernandez 2016).

These approaches are not, however, properly disambiguated in the literature. The essential type and prototype approaches, for instance, are sometimes presented as if they don't differ in any important respects from the ideal type approach. To head off potential confusions, I describe each approach below by focusing on their distinctive features, illustrating how each proposes a different way of making typifications scientific—and, ultimately, a different way of classifying mental disorders.

Ideal Types

The ideal type approach is championed by Schwartz and Osborne Wiggins. In the fields of psychology and psychiatry, this approach is rooted in Karl Jaspers's *General Psychopathology* (1913/1997). But Jaspers himself adapted it from Max Weber's initial proposal. Weber, the founder of modern sociology, argued that social phenomena could not be classified in the same manner as natural objects. The sociologist cannot create a classification akin to the periodic table of elements because social phenomena do not have hard boundaries—their manifestations are fluid and variable. To better capture the features of social phenomena, Weber developed the notion of an ideal type. As he defines it,

> An ideal type is formed by the one-sided *accentuation* of one or more points of view and by the synthesis of a great many diffuse, discrete, more or less present and occasionally absent *concrete individual* phenomena, which are arranged according to those one-sidedly emphasized viewpoints into a unified *analytical* construct (*Gedankenbild*). In its conceptual purity, this mental construct (*Gedankenbild*) cannot be found empirically anywhere in reality. It is a *utopia*.
>
> (Weber 1949: 90)

What is most important here—at least with respect to differentiating the phenomenological approaches to classification—is that the ideal type is not an empirical reality. It is ideal in the sense of being pure, uncontaminated by the messy details of the concrete world (Broome 2006).

But what makes ideal types scientific? As Schwartz and Wiggins explain, ideal types are heuristic devices. They provide the community of researchers and clinicians with a means of conceptually organizing their subject matter. As heuristic devices, ideal types aren't taken as "true"—that is, they aren't judged with respect to how accurately they represent some aspect of reality. Rather, by characterizing her concept as an ideal type, the researcher or clinician admits that no instance of the disorder in question will correspond exactly with her concept; the concrete manifestation might lack certain features included in the ideal type, or express additional features not included in the ideal type (Schwartz and Wiggins 1987a: 283). And, as Schwartz and Wiggins argue, this lack of perfect fit enhances the scientific value of ideal types; the precise ways in which the concrete instance of the disorder fails to correspond with the ideal type can guide the processes of both clinical diagnosis and scientific research.

The clinician's goal—as Schwartz and Wiggins present it—is to understand the patient in his particularity. Therefore, the ways in which the patient diverges from the ideal type can guide further inquiry into the unique nature of his individual condition. One of the researcher's goals, by contrast, is to produce a naturalistic or biological classification.[4] In this

---

[4] Among phenomenologists, it's by no means universally accepted that a biological classification should be our ultimate goal. However, in at least some of Schwartz and Wiggins's presentations of their program, the ideal type approach is characterized as a step along the way to a biological classification.

case, the ideal type provides a shared starting point for constructing hypotheses and carrying out experiments. As Schwartz and Wiggins explain,

> For psychiatric research, ideal types furnish the initial conceptual guidelines for the postulation of law-like regularities and the design of experiments to test such postulates. For clinical practice, ideal types predelineate the features of disorders so that clinicians know what to search for, focus on, and examine in particular patients.
>
> (Schwartz and Wiggins 1987a: 286)

Because ideal types are heuristic devices, their value is based entirely on their utility. If the community of researchers and clinicians finds that altering the ideal type (or replacing it altogether) better guides their research and clinical practice, then they are free to make such alterations or replacements. In this respect, the set of ideal types used to delineate the field of mental disorders is not taken as a definitive system of classification. It is one step along the way.[5]

Essential Types

The essential type approach was proposed by Josef Parnas and Dan Zahavi (2002) (although they do not call it by this name). Parnas and Zahavi ground their approach in Husserlian phenomenology: "a tradition specifically *aiming at grasping the essential structures of human experience and existence*" (2002: 143). However, there is an ambiguity in their adaptation of this approach to the study of mental disorders. They initially characterize their phenomenological approach to psychiatric diagnosis and classification as if it is identical with Schwartz and Wiggins's approach:

> A concept of "ideal type" or "essence" plays here an important role. Ideal type exemplifies the *ideal and necessary* connections between its composing features. Ideal type transcends what is given in experience: e.g. all my possible drawings of a straight line will be somehow deficient (for instance if examined through a microscope) compared to the very (ideal) concept of a straight line.
>
> (Parnas and Zahavi 2002: 157)

Here, Parnas and Zahavi appeal directly to Schwartz and Wiggins's (1987a) ideal types. But their further characterizations seem to present a substantially different project; as Matthew Broome has pointed out, Parnas and Zahavi seem to conflate Weberian ideal types with Husserlian essences (Broome 2006: 311).

If we look further into how Parnas and Zahavi characterize their approach, we find a key distinction between ideal types and essential types, which hinges on their relation to necessity. According to Parnas and Zahavi, the "[p]henomenological approach to anomalous experience is precisely concerned with bringing forth the typical, and *ideally necessary* features of such experience" (2002: 157; my emphasis). As they explain, their approach identifies essential features of categories of mental disorder, rather than just essential features of human

---

[5] This characterization is, notably, in contrast with Weber's use of ideal types. Weber's goal was not to use ideal types as a step toward a naturalistic conceptualization of social phenomena. Rather, he thought that social phenomena were best classified through ideal types.

experience as such. In order to discover these essential features, they suggest that that we employ Husserl's eidetic reduction, which involves a process of imaginative variation:

> This process of imaginative variation will lead us to certain borders that cannot be varied, i.e. changed and transgressed, without making the phenomenon cease to be the kind of phenomenon it is. The variation consequently allows us to distinguish between the accidental properties, i.e. the properties that *could* have been different, and the essential properties, i.e. the invariant structures that make the phenomenon be of the type it is.
>
> (Parnas and Zahavi 2002: 157)

On this approach, a condition that fails to display an essential feature simply won't count as the disorder in question. Parnas and Zahavi's emphasis on essential features will, therefore, produce more rigid categories than Schwartz and Wiggins's ideal types because ideal types do not identify necessary features of disorders; they are heuristic devices with no truth value. But this is not to suggest that Parnas and Zahavi's categories will not be amenable to revision and refinement. As they explain, to claim that something is an essential feature of a disorder is not to claim that this has been proved once and for all. It's possible that one was mistaken in labeling a feature "essential." Future phenomenological analyses might provide reason to believe that the feature is contingent or accidental (even if common or typical) (Parnas and Zahavi 2002: 157).

Prototypes

The prototype approach, like ideal type and essential type approaches, is intended to make the everyday process of typification scientific. Parnas and Shaun Gallagher (2015) propose prototypes as an alternative to operational classification and diagnosis. According to Parnas and Gallagher, "A prototype is a *central example* of a category in question (a sparrow is more characteristic of the category 'bird' than is a penguin or an ostrich), with a graded dilution of typicality toward the borders of the category, where it eventually overlaps exemplars from neighboring categories" (2015: 73; my emphasis). As they characterize it here, a prototype is neither a utopic *ideal* nor a clearly defined *essence*. Unlike an ideal type, a prototype is a concrete exemplar of the disorder, which necessarily implies that such an exemplar actually exists. And, unlike an essential type, a prototype does not establish a set of necessary and essential features of the condition in question. Rather, the prototype is itself a concrete instance of the condition. Other conditions are categorized based on how closely they match this particular instance.

Moreover, Parnas and Gallagher characterize their particular version of prototypes as a "prototype-gestalt," which highlights the unity and organization of symptoms. However, an apparent contradiction arises in their characterization of the gestalt. They say, "A gestalt instantiates a certain *generality of type*. Yet, this type-generality is always deformed, because it inheres in a particular, concrete and situated individual. The particular token always attenuates the ideal clarity and pregnancy of type" (2015: 75). By suggesting that there is no perfect, concrete instance of the condition, Parnas and Gallagher characterize their approach as if it's akin to Schwartz and Wiggins's ideal types—and they refer directly to Schwartz and Wiggins's work on the topic (1987a, 1987b). This seems to contradict their initial characterization: They initially argued that—on their prototype approach—categories are defined, or anchored, by appealing to a concrete exemplar. But if the prototype or exemplar is an *imperfect* instantiation of its category—as they suggest in their second characterization—then it can't be what's anchoring the category; the prototype does not stand, as it were, in the center of the category. Parnas and Gallagher seem to appeal to an ideal type with respect to which the prototype itself is judged as adequate or inadequate.

I don't mean to suggest that this apparent contradiction is necessarily unresolvable. There might be some manner of reconciling these two approaches: For example, the prototype might be a useful diagnostic or teaching tool, while the ideal type is what the psychiatrist ultimately appeals to when revising his classificatory scheme. However, Parnas and Gallagher don't seem to acknowledge the apparent contradiction in the first place, and therefore offer no resolution of their own.[6]

In addition to this ambiguity, another confusion arises when we consider Schwartz, Wiggins, and Michael Norko's (1989, 1995) early work on the relationship between ideal types and prototypes. However, I believe this confusion can be avoided once we understand that their critique of prototypes does not apply to the version presented by Parnas and Gallagher. Schwartz, Wiggins, and Norko suggest that prototypes have two major shortcomings: First, prototypes consist of a set of attributes without conceptual unity; Jaspers, for example, says that a prototype is "a disjointed enumeration" of features (Schwartz et al. 1989: 6). Second, prototypes cannot produce novel concepts because they are constructed by surveying psychiatrists about how they diagnose and understand their patients—prototypes merely reflect the current understanding of mental disorders (1989: 6). However, from the above account, it should be clear that neither of these critiques apply to Parnas and Gallagher's prototype approach. Despite the ambiguities in their approach, they clearly posit a gestalt organization among the prototype's features and they do not believe that prototypes are constructed by merely surveying and averaging typical ways of understanding mental disorders.

DIMENSIONS

Until recently, all phenomenological approaches to classification and diagnosis have been type approaches. However, I have proposed a phenomenological-dimensional approach to psychiatric research and classification (Fernandez, 2019).[7] The primary motivation behind this approach is psychiatry's recent shift from categorial approaches to dimensional approaches.

---

[6] These ambiguities are compounded by Parnas and Gallagher's apparent use of "prototype" and "exemplar" as synonyms. In their initial characterization of their prototype approach, they appeal to Edouard Machery's work on concept formation. But Machery clearly distinguishes between "prototype" and "exemplar" approaches to concept formation. As he describes it, "a prototype of a class is a body of statistical knowledge about the properties deemed to be possessed by members of this class" (Machery 2009: 83). An exemplar, by contrast, "is a body of knowledge about the properties believed to be possessed by a particular member of a class" (Machery 2009: 93). In light of this, it seems that Parnas and Gallagher's proposal is akin to an "exemplar" approach, which therefore diverges substantially from what's often called a "prototype" approach.

[7] Thomas Fuchs and Mauro Pallagrosi have also proposed the use of a dimensional approach for the study of psychopathological temporality (Fuchs and Pallagrosi 2018).

By "dimensional," I do not refer to the DSM-5's construction of new, graded categories, such as autism spectrum disorder. Rather, I refer to approaches that dispense with categories altogether, beginning, instead, from basic aspects of human experience or behavior. If psychiatry continues in this direction—which seems likely—then the gulf between phenomenology's categorial approach and mainstream psychiatry will only widen. In light of this, I've suggested that phenomenologists embrace a broadly dimensional approach, thereby reducing barriers to interdisciplinary collaboration between phenomenologists and psychiatrists.

Psychiatry's major dimensional approach is the Research Domain Criteria (RDoC) initiative developed by the US National Institute of Mental Health. The RDoC aims to produce a new *research* classification (i.e. one not currently intended for use in clinical practice) based on dimensions or constructs (the terms are used interchangeably) of human experience and behavior. Constructs are clustered into broad domains, such as Cognitive Systems or Social Processes. The Social Processes domain includes, for example, the constructs of Affiliation and Attachment, Social Communication, Perception and Understanding of Self, and Perception and Understanding of Others. Some of these constructs are then divided into subconstructs. For example, Perception and Understanding of Self includes the subconstructs of Agency and Self-Knowledge. By orienting research through this matrix, researchers achieve two ends: First, they can investigate psychopathological conditions without framing their investigations through the lens of invalid DSM categories. Second, they can study how this dimension manifests across both normal and abnormal conditions; they might study, for instance, how agency is compromised across subjects who would typically be diagnosed with depression, bipolar disorder, and schizophrenia.

How can we develop a dimensional approach for use in phenomenology? While a broadly dimensional approach might draw inspiration from the RDoC, it need not conform with the RDoC matrix (i.e. its set of domains, constructs, and subconstructs). I have argued that a phenomenological matrix of domains and dimensions can be drawn from what Heidegger calls "existentials," and other phenomenologists refer to as "transcendental," "essential," or "ontological" structures (Fernandez 2017, 2019). Each existential is a basic feature of human existence, such as intentionality, selfhood, affectivity, or temporality. These existentials constitute the basic domains of phenomenological psychopathology, with each existential further distinguished into its various structural moments, or features, which constitute its dimensions. The domain (or existential) of Selfhood, for instance, can include the dimensions of Core Self and Narrative Self, with each dimension further subdivided or specified as required. The Core Self might include features such as (1) Cognition and Stream of Consciousness; (2) Self-Awareness and Presence; (3) Bodily Experience; and (4) Demarcation/Transitivism of the self–world boundary (see Parnas et al. 2005).[8] We can then investigate each of these domains, constructs, and subconstructs across the full range of normal and abnormal experience, moving beyond current diagnostic categories.[9]

---

[8] These items are adapted from the Examination of Anomalous Self Experience (EASE) (Parnas et al. 2005). As I've argued elsewhere, the EASE does not translate directly into the kind of dimensional approach I am proposing, but some of its items can be appropriated for dimensional analysis (Fernandez, 2019).

[9] For a more complete account of a phenomenological-dimensional approach, including illustrative examples, see Fernandez (2019).

My phenomenological-dimensional approach is—at this time—only a proposal. However, some phenomenologists have already conducted studies with a broadly dimensional outlook. I briefly outline two of these studies here with the intention of providing some insight into what a phenomenological-dimensional approach might look like in practice. First, I outline Louis Sass and Elizabeth Pienkos's comparative study of selfhood across melancholia, bipolar mania, and schizophrenia. Second, I outline Matthew Ratcliffe's study of temporal disturbances in depressive disorders. While these authors don't explicitly characterize their work as dimensional in the sense I've described here, these studies investigate how basic existential structures alter across psychopathological conditions; they're framed through what I've called the basic domains and dimensions of human existence, rather than through current diagnostic categories.

Sass and Pienkos study how one dimension of experience—the core self—alters across three categories of disorder. One feature of the core self that they explore is the experience of the self–world boundary, or the way in which I experience myself and my identity in relation with my environment. As they argue, in melancholia the boundary between self and world is enhanced or increased; the world feels distant or unreachable. In mania, by contrast, the boundary between self and world is significantly diminished, sometimes culminating in an experience of mystic union (Sass and Pienkos 2013: 124). We might assume that this manic experience is akin to schizophrenia, which also involves a diminished self–world boundary. However, Sass and Pienkos argue that this apparent similarity is superficial. If we carefully attend to the way this dimension of experience can change, we'll find that there are important differences in the experience of the self–world boundary between mania and schizophrenia. The experiences differ in two key respects: First, in mania the diminished self–world boundary is typically accompanied by a positive or neutral mood, whereas in schizophrenia it is typically accompanied by feelings of anxiety in which the subject feels invaded by the external world. Second, in mania there is often a sense of oneness with the world, whereas schizophrenia can include a sense of solipsism (the world is produced by my mind and has no independent reality).

While Sass and Pienkos's study still refers to current diagnostic categories, the categories don't frame their investigation. Rather, their investigation is framed through the dimension of selfhood, which allows them to test and further articulate categorial boundaries. Such an investigation would be impossible if a study were confined to a particular category or had to assume the validity of current diagnostic categories from the start. Moreover, this suggests that dimensional and categorial approaches need not be mutually exclusive. A dimensional approach might help us refine clinical diagnostic categories.

Another broadly dimensional approach is employed in Matthew Ratcliffe's study of temporal disturbances in depressive disorders. Instead of comparing different diagnostic categories, Ratcliffe uses a dimensional analysis to assess the alleged homogeneity of depressive disorders. By showing that people diagnosed with depression report a variety of temporal disturbances, he casts doubt on the belief that we've identified a single, unified condition, and motivates the project of reclassifying depressive disorders.

Many people with depression report changes in their temporal experience, such as the sense of time slowing down or stretching out (similar to the temporal experience of boredom). Ratcliffe, however, argues that if we attend more carefully to descriptions of temporal experience in depressive episodes, we'll find a wide variety of temporal disturbances expressed across these reports. Ratcliffe clusters these disturbances into three groups: loss of significance, loss of conative drive, and loss of life projects (Ratcliffe 2012). First, some people report that future possibilities are not enticing or worth pursuing. Among this group, some report that future possibilities are insignificant as such—that is, future possibilities are experienced as having no significance for anyone. Others report that possibilities are insignificant for themselves but understand that others might experience them as significant. Second, some people report that future possibilities are significant and worth pursuing, yet they lack any drive or motivation to pursue them. Third, some people report that future possibilities don't show up at all; they have no sense of who they might be in the future. This is often accompanied by a sense that one will never escape their depression (Ratcliffe 2012: 121; see also Aho 2013; Fernandez 2014; Maiese 2018). Any of these disturbances might be experienced independently of the others, but there are also cases in which multiple disturbances occur simultaneously.

Ratcliffe concludes that the diversity of temporal disturbances across people diagnosed with depressive disorders—specifically, with major depressive disorder—suggests that we might not be dealing with one homogeneous condition. There might be a heterogeneity of conditions that, due to imprecise diagnostic criteria, are classed as a single category of disorder. As Ratcliffe says,

> I have suggested that "depression" and more specific subcategories of depression such as "major depression" encompass a range of subtly different changes in the structure of temporal experience. I have not attempted to provide a comprehensive taxonomy here. However, I have offered the beginnings of an interpretive framework for doing so and explored at least some of the variety.
>
> (Ratcliffe 2012: 134)

While Ratcliffe doesn't provide a new classification scheme of depressive disorders, he does provide some tools that might help us construct a new scheme. These examples suggest that a dimensional approach can undermine the validity of current diagnostic categories, motivate the need for a new classification, and provide new conceptual distinctions that can be used to reclassify psychopathological conditions.

While I believe there are good reasons for phenomenologists to move toward a dimensional approach, I want to suggest that this new approach might be compatible with type approaches. Type approaches seek the basic organizing principle of the disorder in question—the *trouble générateur* or core gestalt (Parnas 2012). They aim not only to understand the relationship between parts and whole, but also to identify the core disturbance from which the various symptoms arise. In the case of schizophrenia, for instance, many phenomenologists have argued that the variety of symptoms can be tied to a core disturbance in the structure of selfhood; once we understand how selfhood has altered in schizophrenia, we can make sense of a variety of experiences, such as hallucinations as well as delusions of thought insertion and alien control. These experiences arise because of a breakdown in the sense of agency and ownership of one's thoughts, feelings, and perceptions. A dimensional approach, with its focus on identifying and articulating alterations in specific domains and dimensions of human existence, provides a method of identifying these core disturbances. If such an approach is viable, then phenomenology's type and dimension approaches will not only coexist, but can be mutually complementary (Fernandez, 2019).

Conclusion

In this chapter I have provided an overview of phenomenological approaches to psychiatric classification. First, I articulated phenomenological critiques of the operational approach: (1) It ignores how clinicians intuitively diagnose patients, (2) it neglects the organization among various symptoms, and (3) it allows categories to reify. Second, I described three different type or typification approaches to psychiatric classification—ideal types, essential types, and prototypes—and showed how these approaches differ (despite their occasional conflation in the contemporary literature). Third, I outlined a phenomenological-dimensional approach to psychiatric classification, which starts from existentials, or basic domains of human existence, rather than current diagnostic categories.

My intention, however, was not to argue for the superiority of the dimensional approach over type approaches. Rather, the primary aim of this chapter is to encourage and facilitate philosophical debate over the best ways to classify psychiatric disorders. Phenomenology has the potential to make substantial contributions to the project of psychiatric classification. But its internal ambiguities and inconsistencies will need to be resolved before phenomenologists can move forward with a classification scheme of their own. This overview of the field should provide a useful starting point for future dialogue and debate.

Bibliography

Aho K. (2013). "Depression and Embodiment: Phenomenological Reflections on Motility, Affectivity, and Transcendence." *Medicine, Health Care and Philosophy* 16(4): 751–759.

American Psychiatric Association. (1980). *Diagnostic and Statistical Manual of Mental Disorders*, 3rd edn. Washington, D.C.: The American Psychiatric Association.

American Psychiatric Association. (2013). *Diagnostic and Statistical Manual of Mental Disorders*, 5th edn: DSM-5. Washington, D.C.: American Psychiatric Publishing.

Boring E. G. (1945). "The Use of Operational Definitions in Science." *Psychological Review* 52(5): 243–245.

Bridgman P. W. (1938). "Operational Analysis." *Philosophy of Science* 5(2): 114–131.

Broome M. (2006). "Taxonomy and Ontology in Psychiatry: A Survey of Recent Literature." *Philosophy, Psychiatry, & Psychology* 13(4): 303–319.

Chang H. (2009). "Operationalism." In E. N. Zalta (ed.), *The Stanford Encyclopedia of Philosophy* (Fall 2009). Metaphysics Research Lab, Stanford University. Retrieved from https://plato.stanford.edu/archives/fall2009/entries/operationalism/

Cuthbert B. N. (2014). "The RDoC Framework: Facilitating Transition from ICD/DSM to Dimensional Approaches that Integrate Neuroscience and Psychopathology." *World Psychiatry* 13(1): 28–35.

Cuthbert B. N. and Insel T. R. (2013). "Toward the Future of Psychiatric Diagnosis: The Seven Pillars of RDoC." *BMC Medicine* 11(1): 126.

Fernandez A. V. (2014). "Depression as Existential Feeling or De-Situatedness? Distinguishing Structure from Mode in Psychopathology." *Phenomenology and the Cognitive Sciences* 13(4): 595–612.

Fernandez A. V. (2016). "Phenomenology, Typification, and Ideal Types in Psychiatric Diagnosis and Classification." In R. Bluhm (ed.), *Knowing and Acting in Medicine*, pp. 39–58. Lanham: Rowman and Littlefield International.

Fernandez A. V. (2017). "The Subject Matter of Phenomenological Research: Existentials, Modes, and Prejudices." *Synthese* 194(9): 3543–3562.

Fernandez A. V. (2019). "Phenomenology and Dimensional Approaches to Psychiatric Research and Classification." *Philosophy, Psychiatry, & Psychology.*

Fuchs T. and Pallagrosi M. (2018). "Phenomenology of Temporality and Dimensional Psychopathology." In M. Biondi, M. Pasquini, and A. Picardi (eds.), *Dimensional Psychopathology*, pp. 287–300. Cham: Springer International Publishing.

Gadamer H.-G. (2008). *Philosophical Hermeneutics*, ed. D. E. Linge. Berkeley: University of California Press.

Gadamer H.-G. (2013). *Truth and Method*, revised 2nd edn. London; New York: Bloomsbury Academic. (Original work published 1960)

Gozé T., Moskalewicz M., Schwartz M. A., Naudin J., Micoulaud-Franchi J.-A., and Cermolacce M. (2018). "Is 'Praecox Feeling' a Phenomenological Fossil? A Preliminary Study on Diagnostic Decision Making in Schizophrenia." *Schizophrenia Research.* doi.org/10.1016/j.schres.2018.07.041

Hempel C. (1966). *Philosophy of Natural Science.* Upper Saddle River: Prentice Hall.

Jablensky A. and Kendell R. E. (2002). "Criteria for Assessing a Classification in Psychiatry." In M. Maj, W. Gaebel, J. J. López-Ibor, and N. Sartorius (eds.), *Psychiatric Diagnosis and Classification*, 1–24. New York: John Wiley & Sons.

Jaspers K. (1997). *General Psychopathology*, trans. J. Hoenig and M. W. Hamilton. Baltimore: Johns Hopkins University Press. (Original work published 1913)

Kendell R. and Jablensky A. (2003). "Distinguishing between the Validity and Utility of Psychiatric Diagnoses." *American Journal of Psychiatry* 160(1): 4–12.

Lindau J. F., Broome M., Cipriani A., Brandizzi M., Masillo A., Catone G., . . . Nastro P. F. (Unpublished Manuscript). *Clinical Impression Assessment of the Pre-psychotic Phase of Schizophrenia (CIAPPS): A Screening Questionnaire.*

Lingiardi V. and McWilliams N. (eds.). (2017). *Psychodynamic Diagnostic Manual, 2nd edn: PDM-2.* New York: The Guilford Press.

Machery E. (2009). *Doing Without Concepts.* Oxford: Oxford University Press.

Maiese M. (2018). "Getting Stuck: Temporal Desituatedness in Depression." *Phenomenology and the Cognitive Sciences* 17(4): 701–718.

Moskalewicz M., Schwartz M. A., and Gozé T. (2018). "Phenomenology of Intuitive Judgment: Praecox-Feeling in the Diagnosis of Schizophrenia." *AVANT. Trends in Interdisciplinary Studies* 9(2): 63–74.

Parnas J. (2012). "The Core Gestalt of Schizophrenia." *World Psychiatry* 11(2): 67–69.

Parnas J. and Zahavi D. (2002). "The Role of Phenomenology in Psychiatric Diagnosis and Classification." In M. Maj, W. Gaebel, J. J. López-Ibor, and N. Sartorius (eds.), *Psychiatric Diagnosis and Classification*, pp. 137–162. New York: John Wiley & Sons.

Parnas J., Møller P., Kircher T., Thalbitzer J., Jansson L., Handest P., and Zahavi D. (2005). "EASE: Examination of Anomalous Self-Experience." *Psychopathology* 38(5): 236–258.

Parnas J. and Bovet P. (2015). "Psychiatry Made Easy: Operation(al)ism and Some of Its Consequences." In K. Kendler and J. Parnas (eds.), *Philosophical Issues in Psychiatry III: The Nature and Sources of Historical Change*, pp. 190–212. Oxford: Oxford University Press.

Parnas J. and Gallagher S. (2015). "Phenomenology and the Interpretation of Psychopathological Experience." In L. J. Kirmayer, R. Lemelson, and C. A. Cummings (eds.), *Re-visioning Psychiatry: Cultural Phenomenology, Critical Neuroscience, and Global Mental Health*, pp. 65–80. New York: Cambridge University Press.

Ratcliffe M. (2012). "Varieties of Temporal Experience in Depression." *Journal of Medicine and Philosophy* 37(2): 114–138.

Ratcliffe M., Broome M., Smith B., and Bowden H. (2013). "A Bad Case of the Flu? The Comparative Phenomenology of Depression and Somatic Illness." *Journal of Consciousness Studies* 20(7–8): 198–218.

Sass L. and Pienkos E. (2013). "Varieties of Self-Experience: A Comparative Phenomenology of Melancholia, Mania, and Schizophrenia, Part I." *Journal of Consciousness Studies* 20(7–8): 103–130.

Schwartz M. A. and Wiggins O. P. (1987a). "Diagnosis and Ideal Types: A Contribution to Psychiatric Classification." *Comprehensive Psychiatry* 28(4): 277–291.

Schwartz M. A. and Wiggins O. P. (1987b). "Typifications: The First Step for Clinical Diagnosis in Psychiatry." *The Journal of Nervous and Mental Disease* 175(2): 65–77.

Schwartz M. A., Wiggins O. P., and Norko M. A. (1989). "Prototypes, Ideal Types, and Personality Disorders: The Return to Classical Psychiatry." *Journal of Personality Disorders* 3(1): 1–9.

Schwartz M. A., Wiggins O. P., and Norko M. A. (1995). "Prototypes, Ideal Types, and Personality Disorders: The Return to Classical Phenomenology." In W. J. Livesley (ed.), *The DSM-IV Personality Disorders*, pp. 417–432. New York: Guilford Press.

Weber M. (1949). *Methodology of Social Sciences*, ed. H. A. Finch and E. A. Shils. Glencoe, IL: The Free Press.

World Health Organization. (2004). *International Statistical Classification of Diseases and Related Health Problems: 10th Revision*. Geneva: World Health Organization.

CHAPTER 93

PHENOMENOLOGICAL PSYCHOPATHOLOGY AND CLINICAL DECISION-MAKING

EDUARDO IACOPONI AND HARVEY WICKHAM

The Father, speaking to the Director: "I say that to reverse the ordinary process may well be considered a madness: that is, to create credible situations, in order that they may appear true. But permit me to observe that if this be madness, it is the sole raison d'être of your profession, gentlemen."

(from *Six Characters in Search of an Author*, Pirandello 1921: 7)

INTRODUCTION

CLINICAL decision-making in medicine and psychiatry is a complex and multi-layered process that is influenced by a variety of factors (Montgomery 2006). There has been increasing interest in a more precise understanding of why clinicians choose one diagnosis or intervention over another, in the hope that such an understanding might reduce errors. Concepts about decision-making, borrowed from non-clinical fields such as business theory and economic analysis, have been employed in various clinical settings (Groopman 2007). The awareness that heuristic biases often carry the risk of systematic cognitive errors has also contributed to the thinking about decision-making in clinical practice (Tversky and Kahneman 1974; Kahneman 2011). More recently, thanks to developments in technology and informatics, there has been considerable interest in using operational clinical guidelines to develop algorithmic computer programs that supposedly will eventually replace fallible clinicians (Caspar, Berger, and Frei 2016).

In the practice of psychiatry, factors related to the psychiatrist, the patient, and to their clinical encounter, are known to influence clinical decision-making (Mayou 1978; Crumlish and Kelly 2009). One of the main factors is the information obtained during the interaction between patient and clinician (Bhugra et al. 2011). Magnavita (2016), in a recent review, proposed that effective clinical decision-making in mental health practice is sustained by five pillars: (a) access to high-quality empirical evidence, such as clinical trials and other data about outcomes of clinical interventions; (b) building of clinical expertise, which is the gradual accumulation of objective and tacit knowledge over years of apprenticeship and clinical practice; (c) use of sound theoretical constructs, stemming from biomedical or psychological and social models; (d) use of ethical considerations; and (e) knowledge of decision theory. Within the second pillar lies, possibly, the contribution of the clinician's expertise in the application of phenomenological psychopathology.

THE PHENOMENOLOGICAL APPROACH

It is, to the authors' minds, somewhat puzzling that the phenomenological approach to psychopathology does not appear to have greater recognition in the psychiatric clinical decision-making literature. Since its inception last century (Jaspers 1913/1968; Jaspers 1913/1997; Wiggins and Schwartz 2013), it has been hailed as key to the detailed description and understanding of the problems presented by our patients. In bringing the phenomenological method into clinical practice, it is not necessary to utilize the strict outlook of bracketing or "*epoché*," with its radical suspension of all preconceptions and judgment when listening to our patients. Ratcliffe (2009) described what he calls a modest approach as:

> A phenomenological stance . . . is a methodological shift, whereby one comes to appreciate that there are certain questions which cannot be satisfactorily addressed from the standpoint of empirical science or from any other standpoint that takes a sense of reality for granted. This stance does not demand the total removal of all existential commitment from one's methodological orientation. What is required is the *acknowledgement* that there is an experientially constituted sense of reality and belonging, coupled with a commitment to study and attempt to describe this and other aspects of experience, using whatever means are at our disposal.
>
> (Ratcliffe 2009: 227)

This constitutes a unique opportunity to enter the realm of our patients. In Sass and Volpe's (2013) words:

> . . . subjective symptoms . . . are emotions, inner processes, and sensory manifestations like fear, grief or cheerfulness [that] cannot be perceived by sensory organs but only by putting ourselves into another's soul, by empathy—the only clinical method which allows depicting as clearly as possible the various inner psychological conditions as they are experienced by the patients.
>
> (Sass and Volpe 2013: 187)

By enabling access to patients' inner lives, obtaining evidence during clinical encounters, and bringing the opportunity for patients to relive and reflect on their experiences, the phenomenological method makes an unquestionably significant contribution to clinical decision-making in psychiatry.

COMPETING FORCES IN CLINICAL
DECISION-MAKING IN PSYCHIATRY

The phenomenological approach, despite all its praised advantages, has always had to compete for space with other models and theories of psychopathology. When it came into existence a century ago, it placed itself outside the forces of neurobiology and psychoanalysis, almost as an attempt to solve what was already then an intractable impasse between these dominant models. Psychiatrists at the time, unconvinced by any overarching explanation for their patients' plight, opted to make regular use of this new approach.

But the past decades have seen fewer psychiatrists reliably engaging with the phenomenological approach. At least, this is the impression that we have from practicing psychiatry in inner city London. Our patients, like Pirandello's characters, have to wait a long time before their stories are sensibly embraced, and before a meaningful understanding of their problems can begin. This delay will be illustrated in the clinical encounters described later in this chapter. The barriers that our patients face in their search for a clinician to make their stories real are many and diverse. Several reasons have been considered to explain such shrinking in the influence of phenomenological psychopathology.

Widespread Use of Diagnostic Manuals

Andreasen (2007) associated the decline of phenomenology with the increase in importance of diagnostic classifications in psychiatry such as the *Diagnostic and Statistical Manual*, 3rd edition (American Psychiatric Association 1980), suggesting that phenomenology was sacrificed in the search of the golden fleece of reliability in psychiatric diagnosis (Fulford and Sartorius 2009). Although in many ways an advance in the understanding of and communication about psychiatric disorders (Haslam 2013), the reliance on diagnostic manuals rendered psychiatry a hostage to symptoms checklists. By feeding the illusion of objectivity, the diagnostic manuals, even in their latest versions (*Diagnostic and Statistical Manual*, 5th edition, American Psychiatric Association 2013) have marginalized other valid ways—such as phenomenology—of confronting the inevitable uncertainty of our patients' complex presentations (Pearce 2014; Callard 2014).

Shape of Mental Health Services

Other reasons for the supposed decline of phenomenological psychopathology have also been considered. In England, for instance, some of the changes in the delivery of public mental health services resulted in a shift of attention from psychopathology to behavior during increasingly reduced periods of inpatient care, with patients being discharged from hospital wards as soon as their behavior is settled, allowing minimal time for in-depth exploration of their psychopathology (Smith et al. 2015; Green and Griffiths 2014). Moreover, the changes in the delivery of services have markedly reduced the time that clinicians are allowed to spend with patients, practically eroding their ability to explore symptoms and bringing phenomenological clinical practice to a point of near total marginalization.

Once under the care of community teams, our patients, now in contact with a completely different group of clinicians, are encouraged, under the predominant "Recovery Approach" (Slade 2009; Tondora et al. 2014), to talk about their strengths rather than their symptoms, limiting the opportunity to further explore the nature of their psychopathology.

Getting Rid of Symptoms

Another reason proposed for the reduced emphasis in psychopathology is the growth over the past fifty years of the therapeutic interventions targeted at the amelioration and control of symptoms. Advances in psychopharmacology (Harrison et al. 2011; Anderson and McAllister-Williams 2016), and psychological therapies such as cognitive behavior therapy (Jolley et al. 2015) and acceptance and commitment therapy (Pots et al. 2016) have been made. These achievements, not available when asylum psychiatry was dominant, have understandably resulted in an intense pressure to use every interaction with patients for the evaluation and application of the new therapies.

In this therapeutic-oriented context, when clinicians meet their patients, it is implied that the aim of the encounter is to get rid of symptoms and not to explore them, therefore circumscribing even further the use of the phenomenological approach.

Dominance of Risk Assessment

Concurrently, in England, there has been a dramatic increase in the attention given to the risks associated with severe mental illness, particularly the risk of harm to others and the risk of suicide (Bolland and Bremner 2013; Care Quality Commission 2010). Only the foolhardy might argue that the assessment of risk is an unimportant aspect of psychiatric care. Indeed, the authors contend that a phenomenology-oriented approach is possibly the best way to obtain a meaningful understanding of risk.

But this is not what is observed in current clinical practice. Instead, the already limited time spent with patients is being used to complete standardized risk assessment forms—required for financial indemnity rather than clinical purposes (see Department of Health 2007)—that have limited, if any, predictive value. Beyond the pointlessness of such forms is the upsetting fact that our patients clearly become withdrawn when they notice that, during the clinical interaction, we are more concerned about ourselves (worries about inquiries, media exposure, peer criticism, job loss) than about their plight. It then takes a good clinician, and the development of a trustful relationship, for our patients to re-engage in an empathic interview and allow a more relevant exploration of their thinking.

Training to Become a Psychiatrist: Physical or Mental Health Care

Psychiatrists, like other clinicians, learn how to practice mainly through observing others in action during several years of apprenticeship. During this period they also develop mechanisms of defense that will protect them from the considerable and relentless suffering they are exposed to. If, in their training, junior psychiatrists don't see their seniors engaged into the phenomenological approach to psychopathology, they are less likely to overcome their own fears of empathizing with severely disturbed patients, and less likely to find themselves in situations and settings that promote a closer contact and a better understanding of the clinical problems.

In addition to the lack of opportunity to observe phenomenological interviews, trainee psychiatrists in England now have to comply with the recent national call to improve the quality of our patients' physical health care. Here again, no one would dispute the importance of measures aimed at reducing the unacceptably high levels of physical morbidity and mortality our patients face (Thornicroft 2011). But, in practice, these measures came to depend considerably on the general medical knowledge of trainee psychiatrists, who have ended up being responsible for performing physical examinations and investigations and for referrals to cardiologists or endocrine physicians, and a host of other tasks. And this means less and less time for trainees to become involved with the assessment and management of complex clinical presentations, as is the *métier* of psychiatrists.

And these general medicine knowledge and skills are surely measured in end-of-training examinations, particularly in standardized assessments with role players (Malik et al. 2011), which mandatorily include physical examination stations. The format of these stations, each of which lasts seven to ten minutes, basically bans the assessment of the skills needed for a phenomenological interview, and it drives psychiatric trainees not only to the practice of very brief and fragmented interactions with patients, but also to the belief that mechanized interviewing is the gold standard of psychiatric practice.

CLINICAL ENCOUNTERS

Given all these barriers, it is somewhat surprising that phenomenological psychiatry can still contribute to sound clinical decision-making. In a dialectical manner, perhaps there is a limit beyond which we cannot crush any further the search for meaningful connections lingering behind the symptoms.

The following clinical encounters will illustrate this point. They are pointedly more detailed than the short and context-less descriptions commonly found in the psychiatric literature. While based on patients we've met over the years, they do not portray any individual in particular. We trust that there is no way that anyone can recognize himself or herself from the following accounts. While these clinical encounters are fairly typical of our practice, and while they do reflect our main clinical approach, they are by no means representative of all the encounters we have we our patients.

The Case of Amil

Amil was taken by his friend to an emergency department on Good Friday after he had been found wandering the streets of London naked in a confused state. One of his friends reported that for the fortnight before, he had been abusing drugs, behaving strangely, and expressing odd ideas about witches. When interviewed by a junior doctor Amil calmly explained that he had stepped outside his front door after waking from sleep, that the door shut suddenly behind him, and he had been walking around to find a way back inside his home. When questioned regarding his beliefs about witches he explained that he could not tell much more as nobody would understand him. He added that he was about to be married to somebody who was unknown to him, but didn't elaborate further on this subject either. The junior doctor recorded that although Amil had some strange beliefs, they did not appear to hold delusional intensity. He was discharged from the emergency department with a plan for a follow-up appointment with the local community mental health services. No diagnosis was made on this occasion.

He never attended any appointment with the community team. Three months later he was admitted to hospital involuntarily due to disturbed behavior that included stripping off his clothes, urinating on the floor, standing motionless with his face pressed against an internal window, and giving bizarre answers to questions. Amil was unable to explain why he was in hospital, stating that he hadn't done anything wrong or disruptive, wasn't loud, or displaying inappropriate behavior. He then became guarded, stating he was a very important person, had several security guards and servants at home, and hence could not give further information due to the "privacy of his social status." It was recorded by the on-call trainee psychiatrist that Amil was experiencing psychotic symptoms. When reviewed the following day by the ward trainee psychiatrist, the impression was that Amil had returned to his usual "jovial" self and could be discharged from hospital. A diagnosis of acute stress reaction in the context of a mixed personality was made. Later that day Amil was briefly reviewed by the senior psychiatrist, who did not probe for psychotic symptoms but cemented the plan for Amil to be discharged from hospital and to be re-referred to the local community mental health team.

Three days later Amil was arrested for arson, having lit rubbish he had amassed outside a neighbor's front door. He was subsequently convicted and sentenced to prison for eighteen months. His next contact with mental health professionals occurred a few months after his release from prison, when he was arrested after he was found again piling rubbish against his neighbor's door and attempting to light it. Back in hospital, it became clear to all involved that it would not be possible to care for Amil without an adequate comprehension of what was going on in his mind.

"Why do you think you are you here Amil?" was the first question that the senior psychiatrist asked him. But this time the question was asked in the context of a desire to understand, through accurate empathy, active listening, questioning, clarification, confrontation, exploration, interpretation, reframing, reflection, and silence. Amil's trust eventually evolved and, in turn, his story unfolded. He told of a kernel of unease developing into a pervasive feeling of persecution, and crystallizing into a realization of Christian maleficence being practiced against him by a neighbor. Driven by what he believed to be the neighbors' intolerance of his sexuality, Amil became convinced that his own conversion to Judaism through marriage would be a proselytistic act of such significance that all Christians would be prevented from practicing their faith, and this would in turn release him from his suffering. Their sorcery, however, foiled this divine plan, and so Amil set about burning the witches, a method of execution employed by many societies for activities considered criminal, such as witchcraft and homosexuality. He felt safe from his Christian neighbors when he was in prison, but as soon as he returned home their persecution of him continued. This time, with his story properly told, Amil was successfully treated in hospital, with all his symptoms resolving and his insight completely regained. Unfortunately, a combination of legal injunctions and eviction meant that he was unable to return to his home of twenty years. The missed opportunity for practicing phenomenological psychopathology earlier had a real and significant impact on Amil and on those around him.

The Case of Fredrik

When Fredrik was in the second year of his sociology degree, he experienced something completely new: a sense of being observed all the time, of being connected to a global network of people who, like him, cared about the future of planet Earth. It wasn't unpleasant, and it didn't worry him much, but it was unusual. He was twenty-one years old at the time. He frequently smoked cannabis with friends, but not more or less often than he had done before going to University. He'd been quite happy since leaving his parents' home in London, and kept regular contact with them on social media.

About a year later, and a few months before his final exams, the experiences became more intense. He had the impression that he was under constant surveillance and started thinking he had done something wrong, although he wasn't sure what. His friends had noticed some changes in his behavior, but only felt the need to take him to the emergency department when he stopped talking, eating, and sleeping. Fredrik agreed to be admitted to the local psychiatric ward.

Helped by sedative medication, Fredrik slept solidly for a few days and, when he was ready to be interviewed, he told the hospital psychiatrist, in a polite but vague manner, that he was now fine and all he'd needed was a few good nights' good sleep. He didn't elaborate in any of his answers. Since he was more alert and interactive on the ward, and there wasn't anything in his behavior that suggested the presence of a psychotic or affective illness, Fredrik was told that he would be discharged from hospital.

Then, unexpectedly, on the planned day of his discharge, Fredrik cut both his wrists with a penknife, causing deep cuts that required stitching. From then on, his behavior changed considerably: he became demanding and verbally abusive, telling nurses that nobody cared about him, and that he would try to kill himself if they insisted on discharging him. It was another two months before he left the hospital. Despite this longer than expected admission, the psychiatric team couldn't reach a clear diagnosis, as most of the interviews with Fredrik were consumed by the management of his behavior on the ward. There were suggestions that he had suffered a drug-induced psychotic episode, and also a view, held mainly by the nursing team, that he had borderline personality disorder traits.

The transition to living with his parents again wasn't easy at first, but there were no major behavioral upheavals either. When things were reasonably settled, Fredrik and the community psychiatrist arranged to meet for a prolonged exploratory session, with the aim of clarifying his psychiatric diagnosis. Fredrik himself had been demanding to know his diagnosis. Aware of the diagnostic challenges (i.e. psychosis versus personality disorder), the community psychiatrist chose to use the phenomenological approach by attempting to be free of bias, to assume a genuine stance of "presuppositionlessness," to imagine what it was for Fredrik to be himself at that point in time, and to fully empathize with his current existence.

The session started well, with Fredrik able to talk about some of those unusual experiences and beliefs he had before being admitted to hospital. As the clinical interaction progressed, the psychiatrist became gradually aware of a certain emotional shallowness in the way Fredrik interacted, and also his inability to bring any depth to his account of events. Such shallowness and poverty in the content of speech reminded the psychiatrist of patients who suffered from long-standing psychotic illness, but this couldn't possibly be the case with Fredrik, who only recently had been performing well academically at University. Then, when he was talking about his plans for the future, Fredrik unexpectedly became very tense and started saying "I'm good for nothing . . . I'm a waste of space . . . I hate my current existence . . . I despise this person I have become . . . please have the compassion to allow me to die." From this point on, while getting increasingly distressed, all Fredrik could do was to repeat the same sentences many times, looking fixedly at the floor, rocking his upper body back and forward, punching his head hard with his fists, not responding to any of verbal interventions, as if in a tunnel, detached from the world. After unsuccessfully trying to use supportive interventions, the psychiatrist chose to be silent and waited until Fredrik's distress gradually dimmed.

On the basis of this assessment, the psychiatrist, together with her team, decided that it would be unproductive, and even cruel, to further attempt exploratory sessions with Fredrik. No final diagnosis had been reached. In fact, in addition to the initial hypotheses of psychosis and personality disorder, possible negative syndrome symptoms, dissociative symptoms, and even autism spectrum disorder symptoms were considered. As a consequence of this assessment, the awareness of the complexity of Fredrik's presentation increased. Most importantly, it became clear that Fredrik himself had only partial awareness of what was going on with him, and whatever awareness he had was the cause of considerable suffering.

The community clinical team very much appreciated the use of the phenomenological approach. They also decided that, while they would have to wait for firm psychiatric diagnoses, all clinical effort should be, at least temporarily, directed at caring rather than curing interventions.

CONCLUSION

The views and cases described above are based on our experience as psychiatrists working in busy inner city mental health services in London and therefore hardly representative of what goes on in other parts of the world, where phenomenological psychopathology is hopefully more assiduously used to aid clinical decision-making. But it is still clear that it is very difficult to dislodge the inevitable alliance between time-restricted patient contact and symptom checklists. In busy wards and recovery-orientated community clinics, the use of phenomenology-based interviews will not be at the forefront of decision-making, and will not be learned by junior psychiatrists.

Would it help if phenomenological psychopathology became "manualized," or if its usefulness were tested empirically against other competing approaches to clinical decision-making? Certainly not. This would go completely against the whole point of the phenomenological approach, in its passionate defense of the need to keep in contact with a dimension of being human that all other approaches in medicine and psychiatry appear to have lost sight of. But can any approach satisfactorily embrace this human dimension? Pirandello's character, *the Father*, sharing the same world as Jaspers's, quite miserably concluded that:

> But don't you see that the whole trouble lies here. In words, words. Each one of us has within him a whole world of things, each one of us his own special world. And how can we ever come to an understanding if I put in the words I utter the sense and value of things as I see them; while you who listen to me must inevitably translate them according to the conception of things each one of you has within yourself. We think we understand each other but we never really do!
>
> (Pirandello 1921: 14)

In fact, paradoxically, it is perhaps exactly this stubborn insistence that we can and indeed must keep listening to and understanding our patients that will keep phenomenological psychopathology alive and perhaps even more and more essential for clinical decision-making in the future.

BIBLIOGRAPHY

American Psychiatric Association (1980). *Diagnostic and Statistical Manual of Mental Disorders*, 3rd edn (DSM-III). Washington DC: American Psychiatric Publishing.

American Psychiatric Association (2013). *Diagnostic and Statistical Manual of Mental Disorders*, 5th edn (DSM-5). Washington DC: American Psychiatric Publishing.

Anderson I. and McAllister-Williams R. (eds.) (2016). *Fundamentals of Clinical Psychopharmacology*, 4th edn. Boca Raton: CRC Press.

Andreasen N. (2007). "DSM and the Death of Phenomenology in America: An Example of Unintended Consequences." *Schizophrenia Bulletin* 33: 108–112.

Bhugra D., Easter A., Mallaris Y., and Gupta S. (2011). "Clinical Decision Making in Psychiatry by Psychiatrists." *Acta Psychiatrica Scandinavica* 124: 403–411.

Bolland B. and Bremner S. (2013). "Squaring the Circle: Developing Clinical Risk Management Strategies in Mental Healthcare Organisations." *Advances in Psychiatric Treatment* 19: 153–159.

Callard F. (2014). "Psychiatric Diagnosis: The Indispensability of Ambivalence." *Journal of Medical Ethics* 40: 526–30.

Care Quality Commission. (2010). *Guidance about Compliance: Essential Standards of Quality and Safety*. London: CQC.

Caspar F., Berger T., and Frei L. (2016). "Using Technology to Enhance Decision Making." In J. Magnavita (ed.), *Clinical Decision Making in Mental Health Practice*, pp. 3–21. Washington DC: American Psychological Association.

Crumlish N. and Kelly B. (2009). "How Psychiatrists Think." *Advances in Psychiatric Treatment* 15: 72–79.

Department of Health. (2007). *The National Health Service Litigation Authority*. Norwich: HMSO.

Fulford K. W. M. and Sartorius N. (2009). "The Secret History of ICD and the Hidden Future of DSM." In M. Broome and L. Bortolotti (eds.), *Psychiatry as Cognitive Neuroscience: Philosophical Perspectives*, pp. 29–48. Oxford: Oxford University Press.

Green B. and Griffiths E. (2014). "Hospital Admission and Community Treatment of Mental Disorders in England from 1998 to 2012." *General Hospital Psychiatry* 36: 442–448.

Groopman J. (2007). *How Doctors Think*. New York: Houghton Mifflin Co.

Harrison P., Baldwin D., Barnes T., Burns T., Ebmeier K., Ferrier N., and Nutt D. (2011). "No Psychiatry Without Psychopharmacology." *British Journal of Psychiatry* 199: 263–265.

Haslam N. (2013). "Reliability, Validity, and the Mixed Blessings of Operationalism." In K. Fulford, M. Davies, R. Gipps, G. Graham, J. Sadler, G. Stanghellini, and T. Thornton (eds.), *The Oxford Handbook of Philosophy and Psychiatry*, pp. 987–1002. Oxford: Oxford University Press.

Jaspers K. (1913/1968). "The Phenomenological Approach in Psychopathology." *British Journal of Psychiatry* 114: 1313–1323.

Jaspers K. (1913/1997). *General Psychopathology*, 7th edn. Baltimore: Johns Hopkins University Press.

Jolley S., Garety P., Peters E., Fornell-Ambrojo E., Onwumere J., Harris V., Brabban A., and Johns L. (2015). "Opportunities and Challenges in Improving Access to Psychological Therapies for People with Severe Mental Illness (IAPT-SMI): Evaluating the First Operational Year of the South London and Maudsley (SLaM) Demonstration Site for Psychosis." *Behaviour Research and Therapy* 64: 24–30.

Kahneman D. (2011). *Thinking Fast and Slow*. London: Allen Lane.

Magnavita J. (2016). "Overview and Challenges of Clinical Decision Making in Mental Health Practice." In J. Magnavita (ed.), *Clinical Decision Making in Mental Health Practice*, pp. 3–21. Washington DC: American Psychological Association.

Malik A., Bhugra D., and Brittlebank A. (eds.) (2011). *Workplace-based Assessments in Psychiatry*, 2nd edn. London: RCPsych Publications.

Mayou R. (1978). "Psychiatric Decision Making." *British Journal of Psychiatry* 130: 374–376.

Montgomery K. (2006). *How Doctors Think: Clinical Judgment and the Practice of Medicine*. New York: Oxford University Press.

Pearce S. (2014). "DSM-5 and the Rise of the Diagnostic Checklist." *Journal of Medical Ethics* 40: 515–516.

Pirandello L. (1921/2014). *Six Authors in Search of a Character*. London: CreateSpace.

Pots W., Fledderus M., Meulenbeek P., ten Klooster P., Schreurs K., and Bohlmeijer E. (2016). "Acceptance and Commitment Therapy as a Web-Based Intervention for Depressive Symptoms: Randomised Controlled Trial." *British Journal of Psychiatry* 208: 69–77.

Ratcliffe M. (2009). "Understanding Existential Changes in Psychiatric Illness: The Indispensability if Phenomenology." In M. Broome and L. Bortolotti (eds.), *Psychiatry as Cognitive Neuroscience: Philosophical Perspectives*, pp. 223–244. Oxford: Oxford University Press.

Sass H. and Volpe H. (2013). "Karl Jaspers' Hierarchical Principle and Current Psychiatric Classification." In G. Stanghellini and T. Fuchs (eds.), *One Century of Karl Jaspers' General Psychopathology*, pp. 185–207. Oxford: Oxford University Press.

Slade M. (2009). *Personal Recovery and Mental Illness: A Guide for Mental Health Professionals*. Cambridge: Cambridge University Press.

Smith G., Nicholson K., Fitch C., and Mynors-Wallis L. (2015). *Background Briefing Paper by the Commission to review the provision of acute inpatient psychiatric care for adults* in Englands, Wales and Northern Ireland. https://www.rethink.org/media/1290275/CAAPC%20Background%20Briefing%20Paper.pdf

Thornicroft G. (2011). "Physical Health Disparities and Mental Illness: The Scandal of Premature Mortality." *British Journal of Psychiatry* 199: 441–442.

Tondora J., Miller R., Slade M., and Davidson L. (2014). *Partnering for Recovery in Mental Health: A Practical Guide to Person-centered Planning.* Chichester: Wiley Blackwell.

Tversky A. and Kahneman D. (1974). "Judgment Under Uncertainty: Heuristics and Biases." *Science* 185: 1124–1131.

Wiggins O. and Schwartz M. (2013). "Phenomenology and psychopathology: in search of a method." In G. Stanghellini and T. Fuchs (eds.), One century of Karl Jaspers' General Psychopathology, pp 16--26. Oxford: Oxford University Press.

CHAPTER 94

PHENOMENOLOGICAL PSYCHOPATHOLOGY AND PSYCHOANALYSIS

FEDERICO LEONI

THE TWINS OF THE CRISIS

AT the dawn of the twentieth century, the state of psychiatry as a science looked fragile and gloomy: the literature was growing, broad nosographic classifications were being developed, but psychiatry was still an imperfect neurology and a failed science. Research on the histo-pathological correlates of mental illness had not led to the desired results. As a consequence, in the absence of a reliable biological foundation for their discipline, psychiatrists remained at the margins of medical science. From a biological perspective—the only one psychiatry considered reliable—the possibility of curing mental illness appeared a distant and unlikely hope. This therapeutic impotence seemed to leave open only two possibilities: 1) a more or less coercive internment of patients in hospitals and asylums; 2) an accumulation of clinical descriptions that were, however, bound to remain abstract and sterile, and disconnected from therapeutic interventions, unless further interpreted.

The twentieth century began, in psychiatry, with two grand experiments, both of which aimed at breaking through the impasse described above by questioning the jurisdiction of the natural sciences, or at least the idea of science promoted by the natural sciences of the time. These two experiments were psychoanalysis and phenomenological psychopathology. The beginnings of psychoanalysis can be traced either to Freud and Breuer's *Studies on Hysteria* (1895) or to Freud's *Interpretation of Dreams* (1900) and *Psychopathology of Everyday Life* (1901), while those of phenomenology and phenomenological psychopathology can be traced to Husserl's *Logical Investigations* (1900), or Jaspers's *General Psychopathology* (1913). What emerged from these works was a particular cultural climate, a common atmosphere, in which different paths and trends converged and sometimes intertwined, thereby shaping a new landscape. Wittgenstein would have detected some "family resemblances" between psychoanalysis and phenomenological psychopathology; indeed, both shared a number of characteristic features, and some minor and major themes resonated from one side of the field to the other. Similarities were as numerous as differences, and there were as many common battles as internal conflicts. Psychoanalysis and phenomenological psychopathology appeared united in their dissatisfaction for their common background, but their path diverged as soon as it came down to their main goals. However, the way they constructed and interpreted the clinical descriptions of their most famous cases was profoundly different: while psychoanalytic narration focused on the unconscious, the psychopathological narration concentrated on consciousness.

THE DISCOVERY OF THE UNCONSCIOUS

With his *Interpretation of Dreams*, Freud had opened a window on the unconscious as it manifested itself in dreams and in the darkness and secrecy of night. However, it was his *Psychopathology of Everyday Life* that carried the most disturbing message: in this work, the darkness of night had also engulfed daylight. According to Freud, there was another kind of life that continually eluded and directed our waking life, sometimes overthrowing it. This could be seen in those fleeting and baffling experiences that Freud called "slips" or "faulty actions." According to Freud, our consciousness is dominated—or continually nourished, if you will—by a meaning that has originated elsewhere. We are inhabited by a drive that is ours without being ours, by a knowledge that is in us without our knowing anything about it. All this unconscious content emerges through the gaps, the slips, and the intermittences of our consciousness. Husserl's perspective, instead, was completely different. Phenomenology officially began with his *Logical Investigations*, in two volumes, which emphasized how the operations of consciousness lay at the core of the logical procedures and the validity of the objects studied by logicians. A few years earlier, in his *Philosophy of Arithmetic*, Husserl had explored the territory of arithmetic, arguing that even in this case the mathematician's "spiritual operations"—as he called them—lay at the basis of those mathematical entities we tend to regard as existing independently, irrespective of the fact that someone contemplates them or not. According to Husserl, it is not because of the already-existing numbers that the mathematician can perform his or her operations; rather, it is because of the mathematician's operations and specific acts of consciousness that something like a number or a certain relationship between numbers can acquire its existence and objectivity.

On the one hand, therefore, psychoanalysis claimed that the unconscious was the cause of and the engine behind our seemingly autonomous conscious life. On the other, phenomenology presented consciousness as a relentless and inescapable meaning-generating mechanism. In the overall, psychoanalysis declared that our conscious life, literally, does not know what it does. In this sense, what we actually do and think would always be different—or other—from what we think we are doing and thinking. For this reason, Jacques Lacan defined the unconscious as the "discourse of the Other."

THE DISCOVERY OF CONSCIOUSNESS

Husserl's phenomenology as a whole can be seen as a constantly modified and updated illustration of the effectiveness of the operations of consciousness, of their imperceptible and tenacious capacity to shape meanings and to generate subjective experiential contents, interpersonal and cultural expressions, and even the most impersonal scientific objects. This way, phenomenology seems to ban the unconscious from its visual field as an unnecessary hypothesis; however, this exclusion is only a partial one. In fact, if every content of experience, every subjectively experienced emotion, and every scientific object is the result of the constitutive activity of consciousness, then phenomenology becomes a kind of archaeology: an archaeology of the underground operations of consciousness as a necessary premise of what appears on the surface of experience. Consciousness must be other from the contents it generates: if everything we experience is constituted by consciousness, then consciousness itself must by definition elude our experiential grasp. The act of consciousness, in other words, must be unconscious. Roughly, these were the same arguments advanced by the young Sartre in his *Transcendence of the Ego* (1934). According to Sartre, the act of consciousness, which brings everything to consciousness, could not be fully grasped and bring itself to consciousness: it could only replicate itself in the form of an unperceived mental act accompanying every object of reflection. However, there was more to the story. What the early Husserl had called consciousness and described as an act or set of acts, had been by the late Husserl gradually and increasingly investigated in its depth, in its perceptual roots and in its continuity with bodily expressiveness and mobility. As a result, what for the early Husserl or Sartre was as an almost disembodied act, in the subsequent history of phenomenology gradually took on flesh and bones and was characterized also in terms of desire. This is particularly evident in Merleau-Ponty's *Phenomenology of Perception* (1945) and even more in his *The Visible and the Invisible* (1964), where he explicitly connected his "phenomenology of carnality"—as he defined it to emphasize its progress with respect to Husserl's phenomenology of the body—with the Freudian perspective and the question of the unconscious. The guiding idea was still that of a constantly active, actual, and desiring unconscious always on the verge of breaking through the smooth and unsuspecting surface of consciousness. However, the texture of such act was no longer that of early phenomenology—vaguely Fichtean, abstract, and asexual—but rather a "fleshy" one made of gestures and expressions, sexuality, and creation.

UNCONSCIOUS AS CAUSE, CONSCIOUSNESS AS SURFACE

Yet the psychoanalytic unconscious was something else. Psychoanalysis was itself something like an archaeology: it also aimed to interpret the emerged land of conscious life through the exploration of a submerged and boundless continent. It was immediately structured as an art of listening to a patient, as a more or less wandering hermeneutics that gradually identified the traces of something else, of a latent but decisive and insistent meaning. Psychoanalysis, however, interpreted this meaning as a trauma and as the main cause. It was a complex interplay between, on the one side, a procedure typical of the "sciences of the spirit" (as they were called at the time), based on interpretation, deciphering, and the hermeneutics of suspicion, and, on the other, a method typical of the natural sciences, grounded on the search for a materially conceived cause.

Such cause was inscribed within a complex theory of trauma and temporality of the trauma, which can be traced primarily to Freud's famous *Clinical Case of the Wolf-Man* (1914). This man presumably had witnessed a traumatic event in his infancy, when, however, such an event could not have acquired a properly traumatizing meaning. The trauma, according to Freud, was therefore deposited in the child's memory without taking on a precise significance. Only at a later time, when the child had developed a broader knowledge of life, that insignificant event, so far dormant in the man's permanently active integral and uncensored memory, was redefined as traumatic, censored by the rules of conscious life and thrown in the unconscious as a scene suppressed because unacceptable. In the Freudian and, more generally, psychoanalytic perspective, the causal role of the unconscious remained central, whether the cause was to be identified with the event itself or with its re-signification by means of a subsequent knowledge; in this sense, Lacan argued that what is properly traumatic is only language, symbols, or the culture at large. Such an idea of causality based on the notion of the unconscious had no place in phenomenology.

Karl Jaspers wrote his *General Psychopathology* when he was a young psychiatrist with a vast psychopathological knowledge and a stronger passion for hermeneutics than for phenomenology. Dilthey and Weber were his heroes. Only later did he discover Husserl's works and reframe his investigation first in phenomenological terms, and then according to an increasingly autonomous existentialism. With his *General Psychopathology* Jaspers wanted to rebuild psychopathology and rearrange its rich wealth of data in light of a theory of the understanding. Such theory was that of Dilthey's and, in general, that of the nineteenth- and twentieth-century "sciences of the spirit." At the center of this approach stood Dilthey's distinction between explanation (*Erklären*) and understanding (*Verstehen*), from which Jaspers was directly influenced.

According to this distinction, the natural sciences *explain* reality, and therefore understand it on the basis of causal connections. The sciences of the spirit, on the other hand, *understand* reality, and therefore explain it on the basis of motivational connections. It is true that Jaspers's psychopathology, just like Freudian psychoanalysis, abandoned the organicism typical of the psychiatry of the time; however, we should not forget that it did so by bluntly dismissing the causal way of explanation and investigation typical of the Freudian approach. The point for Jaspers was not to explain, but to explain *and* to understand, namely to identify, in the psychic life of a subject and in the words of a patient who spoke about his or her suffering, not a root cause of what was happening on the surface, but a set of reasons that were connected or intertwined on the surface of his or her conscious life. According to this view, there was nothing else outside the acts of consciousness and the overall actuality of our conscious life. This surface simply had no reverse side, no thickness, no depth, and no past. As Nietzsche (another favourite author of Jaspers, see his great *Nietzsche* book published in 1936) would say, this surface was all the depth and the mystery there was.

In the psychoanalytic perspective, the dialogical and interpretative moment was supposed to lead to an archaeology of traumatic causes. In Jaspers's psychopathology, instead, dialogue and interpretation culminated in a morphology of the acts of consciousness and in a reconstruction of the overall forms and modalities of organic relationship between the many contents of an experience or an existence, be it psychopathological or not. In Freud, the identification of the unconscious cause represented the turning point of the therapeutic treatment: ultimately, this could lead to the remission of the symptoms and to the patient's recovery, at least as long as a recovery could be reached in the Freudian perspective (cf. Freud, *Analysis Terminable and Interminable*, 1937).

In Jaspers, on the contrary, the goal of the therapeutic dialogue was the dialogue itself, which fostered the therapist's understanding of the psychopathological world of the patient and allowed him or her to share such understanding with the patient. Through this double movement, the dialogue opened the way for a recovery, to the extent that a similar term could be used within this perspective. On the one hand, the movement of understanding alleviated the experience of radical loneliness that went together with madness or, better, coincided with it. On the other hand, this understanding allowed the patient to take a stance toward an experience that was thought to be impossible to confront, this impossibility being another condition that, for Jaspers, went together with madness or, better, coincided with it.

Once again, these were conflicting approaches. This contrast, however, should be seen in light of the fact that psychoanalysis and phenomenology seemed to share similar perspectives: the relationship between the conscious and the unconscious, the opposition between explanation and understanding, and the idea of hermeneutics as archaeology or morphology. However, the routes and strategies along which they came to adopt such perspectives were very different. Psychoanalysis was born out of Freud's study of hysteria and developed through his constant focus on the world of neurosis: Anna O., Dora, Little Hans, the Rat Man, perhaps even the aforementioned Wolf Man, who actually showed signs that led others to hypothesize a more severe diagnosis. Phenomenological psychopathology, instead, was born in the context of psychiatry and immediately identified psychosis as its favorite object of study. The very first cases studied by Jaspers clearly belong to this area. A number of young women who had moved to the city from the German countryside and had been hired by upper-class families as nannies had committed what he called "nostalgic murders." Soon after being hired, these women had developed a sense of rootlessness, of envy for the wealthy young mothers they were assisting, and of nostalgia for their own children whom they could not take care of. These feelings had gradually turned into hatred for the wealthy children, whom the nannies had eventually murdered. The great cases studied by Binswanger, such as those of Ellen West and Suzanne Urban (*Schizophrenia*, 1957), or by Wolfgang Blankenburg, such as that of Anne Rau (*The Loss of Natural Self-Evidence*, 1971), also belong to the area of psychosis.

THE VIRTUES OF COMPREHENSION AND THE VIRTUES OF THE INCOMPREHENSIBLE

Given the centrality that Jaspers assigned to the movement of understanding, his clear and resolute admission that primary delusions are un-understandable, that sooner or later the psychiatrist faced with a psychotic experience was bound to encounter something utterly incomprehensible might come as a shock. According to this view, in the mind of the patient there was an ideation, an affect, or a content, that had no place in the web of motivational connections that held his or her psychic life together. In short, the final message of Jaspers's *General Psychopathology* was that the truly psychotic core of psychosis eluded any form of psychopathological understanding. However, the idea that everything was understandable and could be brought down to a common measure and a common sense had been precisely the fundamental assumption behind Jaspers's method of understanding in the first place. The ethical implications of this assumption are easy to make out. Originally, the idea that everything was understandable implied that nothing would have been excluded from the human dimension, so that no patient would have been subjected to the purely nosographic gaze of organicist psychiatry, to the desolation of psychiatric institutions, and to the violence of the asylums. Not surprisingly, then, Jaspers's final admission appeared to many of his fervent followers as a premature and outrageous surrender. For the same reason, Ludwig Binswanger, from within the phenomenological movement, decided to reintroduce the idea of an integral comprehensibility of psychopathological experience, at the cost of a profound reformulation of Jaspers's theory of understanding. To understand, for Binswanger, meant to identify the structures of lived experience rather than to penetrate the contents of subjective experience and their overall connections. It meant in particular to isolate the forms of spatiality and temporality typical of the experience of the patient. What was to emerge from a similar analysis were the patient's characteristic modalities of organization of time or space, whose understanding, for Binswanger, depended on the identification of their genesis in a phenomenological sense—and genesis, in his view, meant *transcendental* genesis.

A phenomenology of time, according to Husserl, must conceive time as something "constituted": the temporality of experience, the meaning of temporality, the meaningfulness of experience, and the directionality of existence are shaped by the operations of our consciousness (see his *On the Phenomenology of Consciousness of Internal Time, 1893–1917*). While in the language of Husserl those operations were called "retention" and "protention," in that of Binswanger the transcendental genesis of a melancholic, manic, or schizophrenic temporality was linked to a "constitutional defect" (cf. *Melancholy and Mania*, 1960)—for example, to an excess of retention in the case of melancholic experience. In a sense, for a melancholic person, to experience a past that utterly swallows his or her sense of temporality is still a way to experience a certain temporality and still presupposes a temporal synthesis and a sense of time, although one perceived as senseless. The constitution of meaning tends to be reduced to zero, Binswanger seemed to say, without ever being able to reach that point.

Throughout his life, Binswanger exchanged letters with Freud: he considered himself a disciple of his, read his writings continuously and passionately, and adopted many of his clinical suggestions in his daily practice (Freud-Binswanger, *Briefwechsel 1908–1938*, 1992. However, there was one aspect that made Binswanger always distrustful of Freud and psychoanalysis: the question of the drive. In the eyes of Binswanger, psychoanalysis was affected by an irreparably naturalistic tendency. In the Freudian doctrine of the drive, with its all too openly hydraulic notion of psychic energy and its blatantly materialistic and sexual coloring, Binswanger saw the re-emergence of the specter of organicism. This was really too much for the adepts of the sciences of the spirit to take and incorporate in their own perspective. Binswanger's perspective certainly took inspiration from a phenomenology that placed the body (*Leib*) at the center of its inquiry, but its purpose was to make it an essentially perceptive and expressive body, not a body affected by sexual difference and dominated by the ungovernable force of pleasure.

Freudian materialism, one might say in a formula, was intolerable for Binswanger because it reintroduced the specter of meaninglessness as the driving force behind meaning: everything was pushed and moved by the drive, but the drive pushed simply because it pushed. As the proverbial rose, it bloomed simply because it bloomed. This idea marked a dividing line.

Incidentally, this explains the fact that often a "Christian" psychiatry has found in phenomenological psychopathology a way out of organicist materialism, a way that also prevented it from falling into the arms of psychoanalysis, especially in its Freudian or Lacanian version. It is true that, from a phenomenological perspective, one could still argue that even the synthesis, or the living presence, from which the genesis of meaning stems, does not have a meaning: the mechanism that generates meaning cannot be understood in terms of meaning. It is also true that, on the basis of Hcidegger's existential analytic, one could still argue that the openness of being-toward-death, which makes our very existence possible and posits the meaning of its constitutive openness, is itself senseless, because it derives from a resolute decision, as Heidegger calls it, a decision that does not draw on anything other than itself. This was precisely Heidegger's position as announced first in *Being and Time* (1927) and then openly embraced in his later works (*Time and Being*, 1963).

ANTI-HUMANIST BUT ANTI-NATURALIST

Influenced by these Heideggerian ideas, Jacques Lacan opted for what he called a "return to Freud," a decision that disconcerted many of Freud's followers. On the one hand, such a return was distrustful of Freud's naturalism and tried to rewrite Freudian psychoanalysis by freeing it from any organicist or positivist residue. It was a farewell to the Freudian model of psychic energy, to the hope that one day psychoanalytic discoveries could be re-translated in the language of psychobiology, and finally to the dream, if not a positivist at least an illusionistic one, that psychoanalytic treatment could finally reclaim the swamp lands of the unconscious and securely replace the darkness of the Id with the light of the Self.

On the other hand, Lacan's return to Freud was also distrustful of the phenomenological approach, since it regarded with suspicion those who planned to escape organicism and naturalism by embarking on a highly spiritualist journey. It was also a farewell to Husserl's operations of consciousness, to the idea that the constitution of meaning was an inescapable threshold, and to the illusion that all meaning was understandable and all the apparent meaninglessness was still meaningful and therefore understandable. "We'd better leave this mushy notion of understanding," Lacan wrote, to "Jaspers and company" (*The Seminar of Jacques Lacan, Book III*, 1955–1956).

It is remarkable that Lacan's attack was directed at Jaspers, who in fact had conceded that the core of every psychosis could not be fully understood. However, incomprehensibility was for Jaspers a limit, a defeat, and not a major premise behind his method. On the contrary, to recognize this incomprehensibility and to establish a paradoxical relationship with this "elusive something" was for Lacan not a defeat, but an ethical gesture, perhaps an indispensable one for those wishing to follow the ethics of psychoanalysis, as he would later call it (*The Seminar of Jacques Lacan, Book VII*, 1959-1960). However, in order to understand Lacan's fundamental notion of incomprehensibility and the Heideggerian flavour of his return to Freud, it is necessary to take a short detour.

It is instructive that in the late aftermath of the Second World War Heidegger had to distance himself from the two most important interpretations of his work: that advanced by his devoted disciple Binswanger, and, secondly, that propounded by a more autonomous but no less indebted follower such as Sartre. In the case of Binswanger, Heidegger's accusation may sound cryptic (*Zollikon Seminars*): what for Heidegger was to be taken in an ontological sense, Binswanger had taken in an ontic sense. What for Heidegger was to be the subject of an ontology, in the hands of Binswanger had turned into an anthropology or a psychology. The radical nature of the investigation undertaken in *Being and Time* had been lost in the transition from the analytics of existence developed in *Being and Time* to the *Daseinsanalyse* developed in Binswanger's *Schizophrenia*. Binswanger took Heidegger's ontological vocabulary and directly applied it to his patients, thus contradicting one of the main efforts of Heidegger's philosophy which was precisely oriented to avoid every reference to the dimension of subject and subjectivity, the idea of subject being for Heidegger one of the major documents of the nihilism of Modernity.

The same accusation of misunderstanding was directed to Sartre. Immediately after the war, Sartre had published a famous pamphlet entitled *Existentialism is a Humanism* (1946). Heidegger had replied with his equally famous *Letter on Humanism* (1946). This time, he had articulated his case with more clarity, and his accusation was one of humanism. What for Sartre was a resource and a solution, for Heidegger was part of the problem or even the problem itself. And if the problem was nihilism, as Heidegger claimed, humanism was part of nihilism, not an antidote to it. Precisely the assumption that man had a privileged point of view on Being and that our subjective consciousness was the locus or the creator of meaning was not a convincing antidote to the problem of nihilism. In fact, this assumption was for Heidegger the embodiment of nihilism, since it claimed that meaning should come from above or emanate from the innermost of a privileged interiority, namely from an elsewhere that supposedly had the miraculous power to distill meaning, or, as the phenomenologists put it, to "constitute" it. It is in the wake of such fundamental anti-humanism that Lacan's notion of incomprehensibility and in general his—both Heideggerian and structuralist—return to Freud must be understood.

In the context of the human sciences, the theme of the "death of man," variously developed by the structuralists (Foucault, *The Order of Things*, 1966), expressed the same need that Heidegger had begun to voice in the field of philosophy at least since the 1930s. Meaning emerges by itself: experience does not need an underlying subject as its foundation, nor does it need a supervising consciousness or an unconscious that functions as another form of consciousness. If the unconscious plays a causal role, for Lacan, this causality should be seen as almost mechanical and blind in nature, as a law that generates certain effects not through a humanistic unconscious, but rather through a totally impersonal and mechanical one. Here lies the reason behind Lacan's constant appeal to Saussure's structural linguistics and Levi-Strauss's structural anthropology. All this allowed Lacan to reinterpret Freud by expunging from his perspective what still sounded too humanistic, psychological, romantic, or fictional.

For example, Freud roughly explained the Oedipus complex by saying that the child would like to be with his mother all the time so to enjoy her body and cuddles, but the father takes that magnificent toy away from him and forbids his essentially autoerotic satisfaction. As a result, the child gradually learns to postpone immediate gratification, and to desire a mediated and symbolized form of pleasure—that is, he learns to desire tout court. Lacan replaced these three characters—the child, the mother, and the father—with three pure functions. He called the mother the "thing," the indistinct object of the original enjoyment. The role of the father was taken by language. Rather than a man in flesh and blood, it is language that prevents the child (and in general the human animal) from remaining confined to his own environment and to a merely direct access to the world: thanks to the distance interposed by words, the child encounters the things of this world as filtered and transformed by language categories. As a consequence, the "thing" is never present, and the desire is a desire for what the language has nullified once and for all: the subject emerges as a mere "slippage," so to speak, an empty referent that language has interposed between the ghost of a forever lost object and the mirage of an object always propelled to the realm of other subjects and, more profoundly, to the desert land of language as *the* Other (*Seminar VII*).

Here was Lacan's Freudianism: not a psychological sequence of events, not a family romance, but a structure that revolved around itself, a machine that produced meaningful effects in a perfectly meaningless fashion. This way, the causal role of the unconscious was purified of both its organicist and spiritualistic overtones. Heidegger would perhaps have agreed, but would surely have been suspicious toward the mechanical and structural aspect of Lacanianism, since for him technology was an expression of nihilism as much as humanism was. To be more precise, technology was for Heidegger just the other side of the privilege over nature assigned by humanism to man, a nature that was in turn reduced to a usable and infinitely exploitable resource.

FIELD AND INTERPRETATION

It is worth recalling, however, that later on a less mechanical and desolate version of the post-Freudian unconscious was also elaborated, one equally committed to emphasize its subject-less, anonymous, and diffused character. In this case too, this version emerged at the intersection of the Freudian legacy and the debate surrounding the legacy of a now widely post-Husserlian phenomenology. Ideas of this sort were developed in the wake of French post-Kleinianism. There were multiple factors behind this process: the tremendous development of the Kleinian attention to the dynamics of transference and countertransference; the psychoanalytic development—pursued by analysts such as Andre Green and Pierre Fédida (cf. *L'absence*, 1978)—of certain phenomenological concepts such as "field" (Sartre) and, more importantly, "flesh" (Merleau-Ponty); a fruitful reinterpretation of the thought of the late Wilfred Bion (cf. Bion, *A Memoir of the Future*), which highlighted themes and concepts such as those of "becoming" and "O." One could argue that "O" becomes because it becomes, and that this ultimate root of being or doing, of ontology or ethics, is the target of both the theory and the practice of much of contemporary post-Freudian psychoanalytic thinking (cf. Ferro, *The bi-personal Field*).

Finally, mention should be made of Paul Ricoeur, who, combining his training in phenomenology with a profound Christian sensibility, devoted one of his most important works to Freud: *Freud and Philosophy: An Essay on Interpretation* (1965). The book, which was immensely influential, contained already what was to be Ricoeur's most mature theoretical proposal: an hermeneutics that saw in Freud *a* decisive model (but not *the* decisive one) and a stimulus to go beyond the psychoanalytic perspective. In fact, Ricoeur saw Freudian psychoanalysis as one of the most important expressions of what appeared to him as an overall tendency of contemporary thought, whose major representatives were Freud, Marx, and Nietzsche. With a formula destined to great fortune, Ricoeur baptized them "the three masters of suspicion." Whether it was about the economic structure governing a seemingly autonomous cultural superstructure (Marx), or the instinctual structure rooted in early infancy and still affecting adult psychic life (Freud), or, finally, the will to power ruling, from its dark depths, entire epochs, and cultural formations (Nietzsche)—whatever the specific case, for Ricoeur, an entire philosophical movement emerged as a form of generalized hermeneutics. More precisely, this movement developed as a practice of systematic deciphering of the surface in the direction of a hidden and decisive depth: in other words, as a hermeneutics of suspicion grounded on an archaeology.

Freud, however, represented for Ricoeur also an incentive to take a further step. Ricoeur wanted to combine such an archaeology, which lay at the core of Freud's whole enterprise, with what he called a teleology. Freud had shown that consciousness was not a master in its own mansion, but was driven and guided by what it did not know; Ricoeur, however, argued that consciousness itself was a powerful instance of re-signification, an original force that could be reduced to its archaeological roots. For Ricoeur, an existence was, therefore, something like a hermeneutics in action, both in the sense that it was a constant process of reinterpretation of a given content (archaeology), and a firm recovery and creation of such content—similarly to Jaspers's idea of freedom and responsibility, and also to a certain Lacanian sensibility for the logic of *après-coup* and re-signification (teleology).

CONCLUSION

Phenomenological psychiatry and psychoanalysis both descend from the crisis of nineteenth-century psychiatry. Psychopathological experiences are not meaningless dysfunctions. But on the meaning of their meaning, they immediately part ways. Phenomenology believes that sense is the transcendental constitution of objects and worlds, and that psychopathological experiences are the misadventures of the constitutive power of transcendental consciousness, down to its fading in the night of the world, down to psychotic fragmentation. Sense is sex, psychoanalysis thinks on the contrary, and if this definition may seem too brutal and outdated, we should recall that Lacan in his last years repeatedly insisted on this point. The fact is that other great psychoanalytic concepts belong to the reign of interpretation, therefore to the tradition of hermeneutic, which phenomenology itself rejoined after itsusserlian season. Drives on the contrary resist the hermeneutic, and exactly as they resist to interpretation, they push the subject within his constructions and within the discontents or the failures of his constructions. So phenomenology puts at the center man as the animal who constructs; psychoanalysis, man as the animal who desires.

BIBLIOGRAPHY

Binswanger L. (1957). *Schizophrenia*. Pfullingen: Neske.p
Binswanger L. (1960). *Melancholie und Manie*. Pfullingen: Neske.
Binswanger L. (1992). *Briefwechsel* (2000). Fischer: Frankfurt am Main.
Bion B. (1991). *A Memoir of the Future*. London: Karnac.
Blankenburg W. (1971), *Der Verlust der natürlichen Selbstverständlichkeit. Ein Beitrag zur Psychopathologie symptomarmer Schizophrenien*. Stuttgart: Enke Verlag.

Fédida P. (1978). *L'absence*. Paris: Gallimard.

Ferro A. (1999). *The Bi-personal Field. Experiences in Child-Analysis*. London: Routledge.

Foucault M. (1966). *The Order of Things. An Archaeology of the Human Sciences*. New York: Pantheon Books, 1994.

Freud S. (1900). Interpretation of Dreams, in *The Complete Psychological Works of Sigmund Freud*, vols 5 and 6. London: Hogarth Press, 1953–.

Freud S. (1901). Psychopathology of Everyday Life, in *The Complete Psychological Works of Sigmund Freud*, vol. 7. London: Hogarth Press, 1953–.

Freud S. (1914). Clinical Case of the Wolf-Man, in *The Complete Psychological Works of Sigmund Freud*, vol. 17. London: Hogarth Press, 1953–.

Freud S. (1937). Analysis Terminable and Interminable, in *The Complete Psychological Works of Sigmund Freud*, vol. 23. London: Hogarth Press, 1953–.

Heidegger M. (1927). *Being and Time*. Albany: SUNY Press, 2010.

Heidegger M. (1946). "Letter on Humanism." In M. Heidegger, *Basic Writings*. London: Routledge, 1977.

Heidegger M. (1963). *On Time and Being*. Chicago: University of Chicago Press, 2002.

Husserl E. (1891). *Philosophy of Arithmeti*. Dordrecht: Springer, 2003.

Husserl E. (1893–1917), *On the Phenomenology of Consciousness of Internal Time (1893–1917)*. Dordrecht/Boston: Kluwer, 1991.

Husserl E. (1900). *Logical Investigations*. London: Routledge and K. Paul, 1970.

Jaspers K. (1913). *General Psychopathology*. Chicago: University of Chicago Press, 1963.

Jaspers K. (1936). *Nietzsche. An Introduction to the Understanding of his Philosophical Activity*. Baltimore: Johns Hopkins University Press, 1997.

Lacan J. (1955–1956), *The Seminar of Jacques Lacan. Book III. The Psychoses*. New York: Norton & Co., 1997.

Lacan J. (1959–1960), *The Seminar of Jacques Lacan. Book VII. The Ethics of Psychoanalysis*. New York: Norton & Co., 1997.

Merleau-Ponty M. (1945). *Phenomenology of Perception*. London/ New York: Routledge, 2012.

Merleau-Ponty M. (1964). *The Visible and the Invisible*. Evanston: Northwestern University Press, 1968.

Ricoeur P. (1965), *Freud and Philosophy: An Essay on Interpretation*. New Haven: Yale University Press, 1970.

Sartre J.-P. (1934). *The Transcendence of the Ego. An Existentialist Theory of Knowledge*. New York: Hill&Wang, 1991.

Sartre J.-P. (1946). *Existentialism is a Humanism*. New Haven: Yale University Press, 2007.

CHAPTER 95

PHENOMENOLOGICAL PSYCHOPATHOLOGY AND AUTOBIOGRAPHY

ANNA BORTOLAN

INTRODUCTION

MEMOIRS and autobiographical accounts of mental illness have been widely utilized in phenomenological psychopathology and, in particular, in the investigation of depression (Fuchs 2013; Ratcliffe 2010; Ratcliffe 2015),[1] mania (Binswanger 1960; Bowden 2013), schizophrenia (Binswanger 1957; Parnas and Henriksen 2016; Sass 1994),[2] anorexia nervosa (Bowden 2012; Legrand 2010),[3] and borderline personality disorder (Stanghellini and Rosfort 2013). In this article I will provide a critical illustration of the different ways in which self-narratives[4] have been employed in this context and I will advance some suggestions as to how the use of life stories could further enhance the phenomenological understanding of mental illness and the therapeutic process.

---

[1] Some of the memoirs used in this context are, e.g. Brampton (2008), Plath (1966), Solomon (2001), Styron (2001), and Thompson (1995).

[2] e.g. Schreber (2000) and Saks (2007).   [3] e.g. Bruch (1978) and Bowman (2006).

[4] In this article I focus on autobiographical or life narratives, namely narratives which are about a real person's own story, as opposed to narratives which have as their subject historical or fictional characters. Autobiographical narratives themselves can have a literary character and be in the form of published or unpublished memoirs, but in this work I consider as falling within this category also the stories about oneself that are simply told, or, as put by Goldie, "just thought through in narrative thinking" (2012: 2). As such, the notion of autobiographical or life narrative employed here includes both memoirs and verbal and written reports of various kinds (e.g. the ones provided in structured or unstructured interviews, in response to questionnaires, and in personal communications). These accounts can cover more or less extended parts of one's life: some regard events which take place in just a few minutes or hours, while others span days, months, or even an entire lifetime.

THE USE OF MEMOIRS AND AUTOBIOGRAPHY IN PHENOMENOLOGICAL PSYCHOPATHOLOGY

The examination of first-person reports has long been a fundamental tool of phenomenological research and this is dependent in the first place on the distinctive aim and method of phenomenology as a discipline. At the core of this theoretical framework is the attempt to discover the fundamental structures of subjectivity, that is, to identify the conditions of possibility and essential features of experiences of different kinds (e.g. Husserl 1983, 1989). Classical and contemporary phenomenologists have investigated the nature of various forms of cognition and affectivity (e.g. Stein 2000), for example, trying to determine the characteristics which make states such as judgments, emotions, and desires the particular states they are. To do so, phenomenologists need to consider multiple instances of the phenomena at issue—for example, looking at different occurrences of what appears to be or is identified as an emotion—and single out the features which are invariant across them.[5] In this context, first-person testimonies are a very important resource, as they provide a wealth of examples of the subjective states in question, and it is by comparing and contrasting them that significant advancements toward the identification of their core structure can be made.

However, it is also for reasons specific to the nature of psychopathological experience that first-person narratives are central to the work of phenomenologists. By looking at the various ways in which experience is altered or disrupted in psychopathology, the structure of ordinary experience itself can indeed be more easily understood. As exemplified by the centrality of the analysis of neurological disorders in Merleau-Ponty's work (1945), the observation of the various ways in which everyday experience can be disrupted sheds light on aspects of that experience which may normally go unnoticed (Carel 2013). In addition, the understanding of first-person experience which is facilitated by the examination of illness narratives positively contributes to the ability of phenomenological psychopathology, and psychiatry more broadly, to provide a comprehensive and faithful account of the phenomena under consideration. Theoretical investigations of mental illness may be rooted in academic and clinical practices in which a distance exists between enquirers, health-care professionals, and sufferers, and the relationship between them can be influenced by a number of sociocultural and economic dynamics (e.g. Cooper 2004) which can contribute to the marginalization of the patients' experience. For example, at a time in which neurobiological models of mental illness enjoy great popularity, more authority may be attributed to clinicians and less attention and credit given to patients' reports. This might result in a more pronounced risk of misunderstanding the experiences that are investigated, potentially ignoring their specificity and the way in which they might diverge from dominant models of the illness.[6] In this

---

[5] Integral to the phenomenological method is the use of "free variation" (Husserl 1973), namely a procedure which consists in imagining possible ways in which a certain phenomenon could vary while remaining the same kind of phenomenon. As explained by Zahavi, "[s]ooner or later this imaginative variation will lead us to certain properties that cannot be varied, that is, changed and transgressed, without making the object cease to be the kind of object it is" (2003: 39). Through the use of this procedure the phenomenologist can then disentangle the object's contingent and essential features.

[6] The structured model of interview favored by biological psychiatry provides an example of this dynamic, since, due to its focus on determining the presence of particular symptoms, such model

context, the use of first-person narratives can help to prevent the development of partial and potentially distorting accounts, enhancing the degree of visibility and consideration which is given to the perspective of the patients and reducing the risk of them suffering various forms of "epistemic injustice" (Kidd and Carel 2017).

The use of autobiographical materials and memoirs in the investigation of mental illness can nevertheless also be problematic in various respects. In this regard, one of the issues to which attention has been drawn concerns the influence that social and cultural factors can have on both narrative form and content (Radden 2008; Radden and Varga 2013; Shapiro 2011: 69). Life stories are embedded in particular cultures (Bruner 2004) and tend to conform to certain communicative and literary conventions, and this is the case also for first-person accounts of mental illness. Due to the wide diffusion of autopathographies (Hawkins 1999), specific narrative rules and scripts are increasingly available to those who are willing to recount their psychiatric experience, and it is feared that this may negatively impact on the authenticity of these accounts.

In addition, specific concerns have been raised with regard to the reliability of autobiographical and, in particular, illness narratives (Shapiro 2011). First-person reports are often crafted after the events they describe have taken place, and such a temporal distance can be detrimental to the accuracy of what is reported. For example, Radden and Varga (2013) argue that, due to the various ways in which the position of the author of an autobiographical narrative might differ from that of the protagonist, the narrated contents are fundamentally "indeterminate." In particular, attention is drawn by Radden and Varga to the fact that, when the life-story is constructed, the author might be in possession of information which was unknown to him in the past, or might judge or feel about his previous experiences in a different way. According to them, the existence of these multiple gaps— "epistemic," "evaluative," and "emotional"—may interfere with the recollection process, so that what is recounted is not simply remembered but also "co-constructed" in the process (2013: 103).

Another criticism which can be moved against the use of first-person narratives in psychopathology has to do with the degree to which the experiences communicated in these narratives can be generalized. Galen Strawson (2004) has famously argued that not everybody is equally inclined to engage in narrative self-understanding, and that the lack of narrativization is not detrimental to the constitution and preservation of personal identity over time. As claimed by Woods, such a position is extremely relevant to research in the medical humanities, as it prompts questions regarding the universality and desirability of narrative practices related to the experience of illness (2011: 75–77). Due to a range of possible reasons, people may be "unwilling or unable" to report their experiences discursively (Broome 2006: 310), and this may provide a reason to question the usefulness and appropriateness of drawing on autobiographical accounts to identify universal structures of experience. Rather than being generalizable, these accounts could indeed just be representative of the experience of a particular group of individuals.

Criticisms regarding the authenticity, reliability, and generalizability of self-narratives would thus appear to challenge the claim that the examination of first-person accounts

constrains the amount and type of diagnostically relevant information that can be communicated to the clinician (Stanghellini 2013).

should play a fundamental role in phenomenological psychopathology. Such criticisms, however, can be responded to in various ways.

In the first place, and with reference specifically to the concerns about the influence that narrative conventions can have on the authenticity of patients' stories, it has been argued for instance that a self-narrative can faithfully describe one's own experience even if it does so by abiding to certain narrative conventions (Bowden 2013: 77; Shapiro 2011: 70). In addition, it may be the case that autobiographical stories can only exist as socially and culturally embedded. As observed by Bruner, "the tool kit of any culture is replete not only with a stock of canonical life narratives [. . .], but with combinable formal constituents from which its members can construct their own life narratives" (2004: 694), and this a fundamental resource for the person who is willing to engage in story-telling. In other words, the availability of specific narrative scripts through which to express one's own story, does not entail that the individual experiences which are related in accordance with those models are not genuine. On the contrary, the existence of specific narrative models may provide patients with the linguistic and conceptual scaffolding necessary to describe experiences which could otherwise be very difficult to report.

The criticisms concerning the reliability of autobiographical and in particular autopathographical narratives correctly identify factors and dynamics which have the potential to hinder the truthfulness of first-person accounts. However, there are various ways in which reliable and unreliable stories can be distinguished. In the first place, in order for it to be credible, a particular narrative needs to be not only internally consistent, but also coherent with other narratives and known facts about the narrator's life, the context, and the type of experience which is being described. Secondly, life narratives are rarely constructed or rehearsed in isolation,[7] thus meaning that narrators can be questioned by their audiences, and asked to clarify, refine, discard, or expand their accounts if need be. As such, it is arguable that a comprehensive assessment of narrative coherence and intersubjective validation can go a long way in reducing the indeterminacy of narrative contents highlighted by Radden and Varga (2013).

Finally, the concerns about the generalizability of illness narratives, and in particular Strawson's conception of autobiographical narrativity as just one among various possible forms of self-understanding (2004) can be responded to in different ways. On the one hand, it could be claimed that by making it possible to conceive of ourselves as unitary individuals who develop over time, narratives indeed support a fundamental form of self-consciousness. As such, rather than being an aspect of ordinary experience, disruptions of autobiographical narrativity would be integral to various forms of psychopathology.[8] On the other hand, even if Strawson is right in challenging the universality of narrative practices, it still needs to be acknowledged that autobiographical story-telling is for many people an important form of self-understanding. As such, the examination of life stories is still to be considered a valuable tool for the comprehension of a particular class of experiences, namely the ones undergone by people who construct and understand their identity through narrative means.

---

[7] For an account of the dialogical dimension of illness narratives see Frank (2000).

[8] This line of response to Strawson's position will not be developed further in this article. However, some of the insights presented in the second section of the text provide evidence in support of the idea that autobiographical story-telling is central to the development of non-pathological self-understanding.

DISRUPTIONS OF NARRATIVITY IN MENTAL ILLNESS: THE CASE OF DEPRESSION

In the first section of this article I have argued that, despite the various difficulties that this might raise, the use of memoirs and autobiographical narratives is of cardinal importance in phenomenological psychopathology. In this context, the relevance of first-person narratives depends also on the fact that various psychopathological disturbances consist in or are manifested through disruptions of narrative abilities. More specifically, a number of psychiatric illnesses have been argued to involve alterations of the "narrative self," namely a particular form of selfhood to the constitution of which autobiographical story-telling is considered to be central.

At the core of many conceptions of what such a self amounts to is the idea that autobiographical narratives make it possible for us to conceive of various parts of our life as joined together rather than as separate fragments. By establishing intelligible connections between different aspects of our experience, life stories portray our existence as characterized, at least to a certain extent, by order rather than chaos. Through story-telling, life can be conceived as having unity and a specific "architecture,"[9] namely as involving events which are causally and meaningfully interwoven.[10]

A very influential example of such a view, and one upon which contemporary phenomenological accounts significantly draw, is Paul Ricoeur's theory of narrative identity (1992). This theory is based on the distinction between two forms of identity—identity as sameness (*mêmeté*) and identity as selfhood (*ipséité*)—and on a specific conception of the relationship which exists between the two.

According to the notion of *mêmeté*, the identical is that which can be identified as the same over time because it undergoes little or no change. The notion of *ipséité*, on the contrary, indicates a form of identity which is kept through change: the identical, from this perspective, is that which remains the same while mutating. Ricoeur argues that narrativity is what makes it possible to mediate between these two forms of identity (1992: 148–149). In his opinion, the construction of an autobiographical narrative is indeed what enables the individual to create coherence and meaning across the variety of events and changes experienced in her life, a way to avoid dispersion and define a stable identity which is recognized as such by both the self and others.

In deep consonance with the insights put forward by Ricoeur, contemporary phenomenologists draw attention to the existence of a specific dimension of selfhood to the structure of which narrativity is fundamental. From this perspective, attention is drawn to the dynamic nature of the "narrative self," which is seen as something that evolves over time and is constituted through a plurality of reflective, social, and linguistic processes (Gallagher and Zahavi 2012; Stanghellini 2004; Zahavi 2005).[11]

---

[9] I borrow this notion from Pugmire (2005).

[10] The idea that, in order for something to count as a narrative, meaningful relations must hold between the events which are narrated is defended by Goldie (2000). However, also less robust accounts of what a narrative is have been put forward (e.g. Lamarque 2004).

[11] Phenomenological accounts argue in favor of the existence also of an experiential and pre-linguistic form of selfhood—the "minimal self" (e.g. Gallagher and Zahavi 2012; Zahavi 2005).

It is with disruptions of this form of selfhood that the core of depression is often identified. Englebert and Stanghellini, for example, argue that it is the creative aspect of narrative identity that is compromised in depression (2015: 698). According to them, while the ability to recount one's story remains intact in the illness, the capacity of the depressed persons to modify and innovate her self-understanding is impaired, thus making it very difficult to effect change even when it would be beneficial to do so given the circumstances of one's life.

The disturbances of narrative selfhood which characterize depression have also often been related to the specific alterations of affective experience which mark the illness. In depression the experience of pleasure and other positive emotions is radically diminished, and this appears to be an integral aspect of the disruptions of narrative identity undergone by the patients. For example, it has been maintained that due to the loss of emotional resonance, the life stories endorsed by the patients before the onset of the illness come to be experienced as inauthentic (Bortolan 2017a). In addition, Englebert and Stanghellini (2015) suggest that the loss of feeling hinders narrative self-understanding also because of the thwarting effect it has on motivation. Emotions are very powerful forces in driving our cognitive and practical activities and, in their opinion, it is because of the affective flattening they experience that depressed patients are not motivated to creatively reshape their self-conception (2015: 693).

Depression, however, is marked not only by the impoverishment or disappearance of certain emotions, but also by the emergence of affects which are rarely present in non-pathological experience and it has been claimed that this might lead to the crafting of narratives which possess specific characteristics with respect to both their form and content (Bortolan 2017a: 81–87).

At the origin of this idea is the acknowledgment that emotions are fundamental to the constitution and selection of narrative content. As remarked by Hardcastle (2003), it is because of their affective connotations that some experiences are included in the stories we tell about ourselves while others are excluded. Emotions, in other words, "tag" certain events as significant and these are the ones which "make it into our stories" (2003: 354). In addition, emotions can shape the contents of our narratives not only by marking certain events as significant or relevant for the purposes of our story-telling, but also by becoming narrative contents themselves.

Underlying the accounts of the narrative self discussed so far is the idea that integral to the processes through which we craft our life stories is the ability to take a position with regard to who we are and we want to be. Zahavi, for example, notices that a fundamental aspect of the development of narrative selfhood consists in the endorsement of specific values and beliefs, a process which shapes one's "personal character or personality" (Zahavi 2007: 193). In a similar vein, Rosfort and Stanghellini (2009: 254) claim that personhood is dependent on the ability to take an "evaluative stance" toward one's own experiences and to make decisions about what kind of person one aspires to be.

It seems that in depression, due to the presence of particular moods, such position-taking ability is disrupted, thus further contributing to the disturbances of narrative self-understanding. Radden (2013), for instance, has suggested that the moods experienced by the depressed person have distinct qualitative and quantitative features (2013: 97) which may hinder the patients' "epistemic agency," namely the ability to reflect on and submit their cognitive states to rational scrutiny. Radden acknowledges that moods have the power to shape our judgments and behaviors and that, in particular in the case of unipolar and bipolar disorders, they are very resistant to change. As such, when a depressed person is in the grip of a negative mood, it is very difficult for her to distance herself from the thoughts and evaluations, such as "disparaging self-assessments" (2013: 84), which are congruent with those moods, and, as a result, her ability to critically assess her mental states may be weakened.[12]

The affective alterations which mark depression can thus affect the patient's narrative self-understanding by impairing her ability to adequately evaluate herself, others, and features of the external world. As such, the alterations of affectivity and narrativity typical of the illness can also be ethically relevant, as they may significantly impact upon the person's moral knowledge and behavior.[13]

NARRATIVES AND THE RECOVERY PROCESS

As illustrated so far, the role played by narrative disturbances in mental illness has been a clear focus of research in phenomenological psychopathology. In particular, attention has been drawn to alterations of narrative selfhood and the various ways in which these are connected with disruptions of affective experience. Affectivity and narrativity, however, are also significantly involved in the treatment and recovery processes, and in the following I will provide an overview of some of the dynamics which are relevant in this context, suggesting some directions for further phenomenological investigation.

Narrativity contributes to emotional regulation in various ways and this is very relevant to the processes through which psychopathological disturbances can be managed and overcome. In the first place, engaging in story-telling activities can enhance the sense of being in control of one's own experience (Pennebaker and Seagal 1999). One reason why this is the case has to do with the fact that emotions are usually perceived as passive phenomena, something by which we are affected rather than states which we willfully trigger. Even when we actively pursue the experience of a particular emotion, its eventual emergence is experienced in itself as being independent of our voluntary control. Because of this, especially when emotions are particularly intense, we might feel unable to control them. Due to a sense of powerlessness we might engage in fewer attempts to regulate the emotions, which can then acquire greater intensity and, in a circular way, further increase our feelings of passivity. Story-telling can contrast these dynamics by virtue of its being an active process: thinking or narrating a story is an intentional act and, as such, it enhances our sense of having a degree of control over our experiences. This increased sense of control, in turn, inclines us to be more proactive in regulating our feelings, which results in less overwhelming emotions and in an increased sense of empowerment. This is particularly relevant to the experience of physical and mental illness, as these may be marked by the presence of intense and disruptive emotions. In this context, as observed by Charon, "to find the words to contain the disorder and its attendant worries gives shape to and control over the chaos of illness" (2001: 1898).

---

[12] Disruptions of narrative self-understanding involving alterations of position-taking abilities have been claimed to be present also in borderline personality disorder (Fuchs 2007) and bipolar disorder (Potter 2013).

[13] For a defence of this idea see Biegler (2011) and Bortolan (2017b).

Narrativity can contribute to emotional regulation also because it allows us to put distressing affects "in perspective." This is suggested, for example, by Angus and Greenberg (2011) in their conceptualization of "Emotion-Focused Therapy." Within this approach, attention is drawn to the fact that through story-telling emotions can be contextualized, that is, they can be situated in a particular space and time, and interpreted in light of specific personal and relational dynamics. As such, narrativity makes it possible to circumscribe emotional reactions whose boundaries at the experiential level might be blurred and to give the person the sense that distressing emotions are episodes that can eventually be overcome. As remarked by Angus and Greenberg (2011: 70), by attributing to an emotion a "clear beginning, middle, and end" and organizing the events along an "unfolding plotline," we can make the emotion itself not only more intelligible, but also more manageable.

In addition to the positive impact that it can have on emotional regulation, being involved in narrative activities inside and outside the therapeutic setting can contribute to the recovery process also in other ways. For example, being in contact with a plurality of real or fictional life stories may make it easier for the person to conceive of experiences which are precluded by the illness, and this in turn makes it more likely for these experiences to be undergone when the possibility arises. This dynamic reflects an aspect of the relationship between language and affectivity more broadly, and has been investigated by Colombetti (2009) with reference specifically to the impact that emotion labels and classifications can have on the structure of the affects themselves.

Colombetti (2009) observes that language gives us the possibility to "condense" complex experiences in relatively simple expressions. By being so labeled, she argues, certain affects are made "accessible" to people, who thus become more aware of the existence of particular experiential possibilities and more likely to undergo the relevant emotions. According to Colombetti, an example of this is provided by the Japanese expression "*mono no aware*," which designates the "awareness of the transient nature of all things" (2009: 19).[14] Colombetti notices that this particular experience appears to be referred to much more frequently in Japanese than, for example, in Italian poetry (where no single term exists for the word "aware"), and suggests that it is the existence of the word itself which determined the significance of the experience in Japanese culture (ibid.).

It is arguable that, similarly to what happens in the case of emotional labeling, by virtue of their being narrated, certain experiences and behaviors become more understandable and salient, and it is thus easier for those who engage with these narratives to conceive the events there represented as concrete possibilities.

These dynamics are particularly relevant to psychiatric experience, as it has been claimed that disruptions of one's sense of possibility are central to a number of psychopathological disturbances (Ratcliffe 2008). For example, Ratcliffe (2010) has shown that in depression the sense of what it is possible for one to achieve is deeply altered: for patients affected by severe forms of the illness recovery is seen as just unattainable and the person's distressing condition is perceived as insurmountable.

---

[14] Colombetti reports that the translation of "aware" is generally "pathos" or "sensitivity," while the meaning of the expression "mono no" is "of things" (2009: 19).

Given the power of narratives to shape the structure of emotions, modifying the stories with which patients identify can have a significant effect on their experience.[15] By being both passively and actively involved in story-telling, patients can imagine themselves in alternative roles, they can play parts which are different from the ones they usually embody, and, as result, become able to access emotions and behaviors which were precluded to them by the illness. These processes appear to reflect the dynamics around which also cognitive therapy revolves (e.g. Beck et al. 1979). According to this framework, it is through the modification of one's own beliefs and judgments that long-lasting affective and experiential changes can be triggered, and narratives seem to be a particularly effective tool for the generation of these cognitive shifts, as they provide the context in which the person's thoughts can be expressed, connected to each other, and negotiated.

CONCLUSION

This article has provided an illustration of various ways in which the use of memoirs and autobiographical narratives is central to phenomenological psychopathology. First-person accounts of mental illness are for the phenomenologist a fundamental source of information about the essential structure of the experiences she investigates. In addition, they play a significant role in the attempt to avoid the construction of one-sided and potentially distorting psychiatric models. However, the debate still seems to be open with regards to what would be the best way to structure, collect, and use first-person reports in a clinical context, and this is an issue to which further research should be devoted.[16] Furthermore, as shown in the second section of the article, alterations or the breakdown of narrative structures are often integral to psychopathological disturbances, and, as such, their consideration is something from which phenomenological accounts of psychiatric experience cannot prescind. In the existing literature and in this article, attention has been devoted in particular to the narrative disruptions which mark depression, but the body of phenomenological research in this area could be fruitfully extended by examining autobiographical narrativity in other forms of psychiatric and neurological illness. Finally, as highlighted in the last section, autobiographical story-telling is central also to the dynamics which are in play in therapeutic and recovery processes and further inquiry into this area appears to be a promising avenue for future research in phenomenology.

---

[15] It must be noted that the fact that engaging in autobiographical story-telling can have positive psychological effects does not guarantee that the narratives are accurate or that the person will be willing to uphold them indefinitely. Due to the constructive nature of memory and narrativity, the life stories we tell may be questioned by others, or come to be doubted by ourselves at a later stage.

[16] An important question in this regard has to do with the degree to which both clinicians and patients should be trained in phenomenology and asked to apply the phenomenological method when soliciting, examining, and providing first-person testimonies. On this point, see e.g. Gallagher and Brøsted Sørensen (2006).

ACKNOWLEDGMENTS

Some of the research presented above was conducted in my position as an Irish Research Council Government of Ireland Postdoctoral Fellow, as an integral part of the project "The Phenomenology of Self-Esteem" [GOIPD/2016/555]. I thus wish to thank the Irish Research Council for its support, as well as Matthew Broome and Paolo Fusar-Poli for very helpful comments on a previous version of the text.

BIBLIOGRAPHY

American Psychiatric Association (APA). (2013). *Diagnostic and Statistical Manual of Mental Disorders*. DSM-5, 5th edn. Arlington: American Psychiatric Association.

Angus L. E. and Greenberg L. S. (2011). *Working with Narrative in Emotion-Focused Therapy. Changing Stories, Healing Lives*. Washington: American Psychological Association.

Beck A. T., Rush A. J., Shaw B. F., and Emery G. (1979). *Cognitive Therapy of Depression*. New York: The Guilford Press.

Biegler P. (2011). *The Ethical Treatment of Depression. Autonomy through Psychotherapy*. Cambridge, MA: MIT Press.

Binswanger L. (1957). *Schizophrenie*. Pfullingen: Neske.

Binswanger L. (1960). *Melancholie und Manie. Phänomenologische Studien*. Pfullingen: Neske.

Bortolan A. (2017a.) "Affectivity and Narrativity in Depression: A Phenomenological Study." *Medicine, Health Care and Philosophy* 20(1): 77–88.

Bortolan A. (2017b.) "Affectivity and Moral Experience: An Extended Phenomenological Account." *Phenomenology and the Cognitive Sciences* 16(3): 471–490.

Bowden H. (2012). "A Phenomenological Study of Anorexia Nervosa." *Philosophy, Psychiatry, & Psychology* 19(3): 227–241.

Bowden H. (2013). *A Phenomenological Study of Mania and Depression*. Durham theses, Durham University. Available at Durham E-Theses Online: http://etheses.dur.ac.uk/9456/ (accessed August 6, 2017).

Bowman G. (2006). *A Shape of My Own*. London: Penguin Books.

Brampton S. (2008). *Shoot the Damn Dog. A Memoir of Depression*. London: Bloomsbury.

Broome M. R. (2006). "Taxonomy and Ontology in Psychiatry: A Survey of Recent Literature." *Philosophy, Psychiatry, & Psychology* 13(4): 303–319.

Bruch H. (1978). *The Golden Cage: The Enigma of Anorexia Nervosa*. New York: Vintage Books.

Bruner J. (2004). "Life as Narrative." *Social Research* 71(3): 691–710.

Carel H. H. (2013). "Illness, Phenomenology, and Philosophical Method." *Theoretical Medicine and Bioethics* 34(4): 345–357.

Charon R. (2001). "Narrative Medicine: A Model for Empathy, Reflection, Profession, and Trust." *JAMA* 286(15): 1897–1902.

Colombetti G. (2009). "What Language Does to Feelings." *Journal of Consciousness Studies* 16(9): 4–26.

Cooper R. (2004). "What is Wrong with the DSM?" *History of Psychiatry* 15(1): 5–25.

Englebert J. and Stanghellini G. (2015). "La Manie et la Mélancolie comme Crises de l'Identité Narrative et de l'Intentionnalité." *L'Évolution Psychiatrique* 80(4): 689–700.

Frank A. W. (2000). "Illness and Autobiographical Work: Dialogue as Narrative Destabilization." *Qualitative Sociology* 23(1): 135–156.

Fuchs T. (2007). "Fragmented Selves: Temporality and Identity in Borderline Personality Disorder." *Psychopathology* 40: 379–387.

Fuchs T. (2013). "Depression, Intercorporeality and Interaffectivity." *Journal of Consciousness Studies* 20(7–8): 219–238.

Gallagher S. and Brøsted Sørensen J. (2006). "Experimenting with Phenomenology." *Consciousness and Cognition* 15(1): 119–134.

Gallagher S. and Zahavi D. (2012). *The Phenomenological Mind*, 2nd edn. New York: Routledge.

Goldie P. (2000). *The Emotions: A Philosophical Exploration*. Oxford: Clarendon Press.

Goldie P. (2012). *The Mess Inside. Narrative, Emotion, and the Mind*. Oxford: Oxford University Press.

Hardcastle V. G. (2003). "Emotions and Narrative Selves." *Philosophy, Psychiatry & Psychology* 10(4): 353–355.

Hawkins A. H. (1999). "Pathography: Patient Narratives of Illness." *Western Journal of Medicine* 171(2): 127–129.

Husserl E. (1973). *Experience and Judgment: Investigations in a Genealogy of Logic*, trans. J. S. Churchill and K. Ameriks. London: Routledge and Kegan Paul.

Husserl E. (1983). *Ideas Pertaining to a Pure Phenomenology and to a Phenomenological Philosophy. First Book. General Introduction to a Pure Phenomenology*, trans. F. Kersten. Dordrecht: Kluwer.

Husserl E. (1989). *Ideas Pertaining to a Pure Phenomenology and to a Phenomenological Philosophy. Second Book. Studies in the Phenomenology of Constitution*, trans. R. Roicewizy and A. Schuwer. Dordrecht: Kluwer.

Kidd I. J. and Carel H. (2017). "Epistemic Injustice and Illness." *Journal of Applied Philosophy* 34(2): 172–190.

Lamarque P. (2004). "On not Expecting Too Much from Narrative." *Mind & Language* 19(4): 393–408.

Legrand D. (2010). "Subjective and Physical Dimensions of Bodily Self-consciousness, and their Dis-integration in Anorexia Nervosa." *Neuropsychologia* 48(3): 726–737.

Merleau-Ponty M. (1945). *Phenomenology of Perception*, trans. C. Smith. London: Routledge and Kegan Paul.

Parnas J. and Henriksen M. G. (2016). "Mysticism and Schizophrenia: A Phenomenological Exploration of the Structure of Consciousness in the Schizophrenia Spectrum Disorders." *Consciousness and Cognition* 43: 75–88.

Pennebaker J. W. and Seagal J. D. (1999). "Forming a Story: The Health Benefits of Narrative." *Journal of Clinical Psychology* 55(10): 1243–1254.

Plath S. (1966). *The Bell Jar*. London: Faber & Faber.

Potter N. N. (2013). "Narrative Selves, Relations of Trust, and Bipolar Disorder." *Philosophy, Psychiatry, & Psychology* 20(1): 57–65.

Pugmire D. (2005). *Sound Sentiments: Integrity in the Emotions*. Oxford: Oxford University Press.

Radden J. (2008). "My Symptoms, Myself: Reading Mental Illness Memoirs for Identity Assumptions." In H. Clark (ed.), *Depression and Narrative: Telling the Dark*, pp. 15–28. Albany: SUNY Press.

Radden J. (2013). "The Self and Its Moods in Depression and Mania." *Journal of Consciousness Studies* 20(7–8): 80–102.

Radden J. and Varga S. (2013). "The Epistemological Value of Depression Memoirs: A Meta-analysis." In K. W. M. Fulford, M. Davies, R. G. T. Gipps, G. Graham, J. Z. Sadler, G.

Stanghellini, and T. Thornton (eds.), *The Oxford Handbook of Philosophy and Psychiatry*, pp. 99–115. Oxford: Oxford University Press.

Ratcliffe M. (2008). *Feelings of Being. Phenomenology, Psychiatry and the Sense of Reality.* Oxford: Oxford University Press.

Ratcliffe M. (2010). "Depression, Guilt and Emotional Depth." *Inquiry: An Interdisciplinary Journal of Philosophy* 53(6): 602–626.

Ratcliffe M. (2015). *Experiences of Depression: A Study in Phenomenology.* Oxford: Oxford University Press.

Ricoeur P. (1992). *Oneself as Another*, trans. K. Blamey. Chicago: University of Chicago Press.

Rosfort R. and Stanghellini G. (2009). "The Person in Between Moods and Affects." *Philosophy, Psychiatry, & Psychology* 16(3): 251–266.

Saks E. (2007). *The Center Cannot Hold.* New York: Hyperion.

Sass L. A. (1994). *The Paradoxes of Delusion: Wittgenstein, Schreber, and the Schizophrenic Mind.* Ithaca: Cornell University Press.

Schreber D. P. (2000). *Memoirs of My Nervous Illness*, trans. I. Macalpine and R. A. Hunter. New York: New York Review of Books.

Shapiro J. (2011). "Illness Narratives: Reliability, Authenticity and the Empathic Witness." *Medical Humanities* 37(2): 68–72.

Solomon A. (2001). *The Noonday Demon. An Anatomy of Depression.* London: Chatto & Windus.

Stanghellini G. (2004). *Disembodied Spirits and Deanimated Bodies: The Psychopathology of Common Sense.* Oxford: Oxford University Press.

Stanghellini G. (2013). "Philosophical Resources for the Psychiatric Interview." In K. W. M. Fulford, M. Davies, R. G. T. Gipps, G. Graham, J. Z. Sadler, G. Stanghellini, and T. Thornton (eds.), *The Oxford Handbook of Philosophy and Psychiatry*, pp. 321–356. Oxford: Oxford University Press.

Stanghellini G. and Rosfort R. (2013). "Borderline Depression. A Desperate Vitality." *Journal of Consciousness Studies* 20(7–8): 153–177.

Stein E. (2000). *Philosophy of Psychology and the Humanities*, trans. M. C. Baseheart and M. Sawicki. Washington: ICS Publications.

Strawson G. (2004). "Against Narrativity." *Ratio* 17(4): 428–452.

Styron W. (2001). *Darkness Visible.* London: Vintage.

Thompson T. (1995). *The Beast. A Reckoning with Depression.* New York: Putnam.

Woods A. (2011). "The Limits of Narrative: Provocations for the Medical Humanities." *Medical Humanities* 37(2): 73–78.

Zahavi D. (2003). *Husserl's Phenomenology.* Stanford: Stanford University Press.

Zahavi D. (2005). *Subjectivity and Selfhood. Investigating the First-Person Perspective.* Cambridge, MA: MIT Press.

Zahavi D. (2007). "Self and Other: The Limits of Narrative Understanding." *Royal Institute of Philosophy Supplement* 60: 179–202.

CHAPTER 96

PHENOMENOLOGICAL PSYCHOPATHOLOGY, NEUROSCIENCE, PSYCHIATRIC DISORDERS, AND THE INTENTIONAL ARC

GRANT GILLETT AND PATRICK SENIUK

INTRODUCTION

IN this article we reference common psychiatric disorders, with a particular eye toward depression and anxiety-related conditions (e.g. obsessive-compulsive disorder (OCD)) to flesh out an affinity between the early neuroscience of Hughlings-Jackson and the existential-phenomenology of Merleau-Ponty. We argue that the nature of some mental disorders is mischaracterized by neurobiological or psychological frameworks on the basis that they fail to capture the nuanced, affective relation that is evinced by an embodied-subject in the world (including others). In mental disorder this affective relation is susceptible to disturbance or "dis-integration," such that the meaning-making body-subject finds herself no longer "in touch" with the world. Consequently, one no longer finds (*Befindlichkeit*) that one is an effective self-in-the-world (Northoff 2016). For far too long mental disorders have been interpreted without an appreciation for the way in which a person incorporates, structures, and is structured by purposeful striving in his or her particular milieu.

Moreover, psychiatry's continued emphasis on pharmacological intervention neglects the brain as an active, engaged aspect of the body, which maintains healthy function through dynamic exchanges with the human life-world. Often, in explaining our psychological lives (as in propositional attitude psychology), the self is understood from the neck up, relying on the use of propositions, which are abstracted from speech and their neural substrates and it ignores the phenomenology of human experience, whereby the body-self is engaged in, and is intentionally *spread out* in the world, in both "normal" *and* pathological circumstances. We explore the way in which some mental disorders may be classified as affective-disturbances in that they disclose a disruption to the intentional arc's role in sustaining the dynamic interaction between body and world. This allows for a fruitful two-way exchange whereby phenomenology, through a focus on being and doing, deepens neuroscience, and is itself enhanced by neuroscientific findings.

Hughlings-Jackson, Evolution, and Dissolution

John Hughlings-Jackson (JHJ) linked higher mental life to the coordination and integration of sensorimotor functions in a highly evolved brain. He regarded the unique outcome of that integration, in a given human being, as the basis of subjectivity and the conscious self. Subjective activity drew on "impressions and movements of all parts of the body . . . in most complex . . . combinations . . . triply indirectly" (Hughlings-Jackson 1878: 29) to organize a holistic organismic response to a context. The "triply indirectly" refers to the *subsumption* and moderation of reflex-*like* connections (whereby inputs mechanistically elicit stereotyped outputs) between body and world. Higher levels included wide sources of information: exteroceptive, interoceptive, and intra-cerebral, including cortico-cortical, cortico-subcortical, and top-down connections to moderate human behavior and thought. The result is an integrated whole-body attunement between an organism and its context, dynamically maintained by normal adaptive activity. This attunement transcends an impoverished and untenable input–output (causal/functional) approach to the way in which a human inhabits his or her "world"; it transcends the particular view that mental states arise internally as a stage of elaborating perceptual inputs for ultimate translation into external action.

JHJ's understanding of human cognitive functions, including their neurological and psychiatric manifestations, was deeply informed by evolutionary thinking and rested on the continuity between human mental life and simpler sensorimotor routines evident in animals of all kinds (Hughlings-Jackson 1878). This sensorimotor engagement is also central in intersubjective relations and the inflection of behavior by the interpersonal resonance grounding experience of a "Self–other" (Merleau-Ponty 1964) dyadic system, a dynamic and responsive dyad with an inherent dynamism and flow of movement. In the early stages of life, a mutual sensibility gives rise to a "syncratic sociability," wherein the infant does not initially distinguish herself from others until "the objectification of the body intervenes to establish a sort of wall between me and the other: a partition . . . there is thus a correlative constitution of me and the other as two human beings amongst all others" (1964: 141). The objectifying partition potentially alienates a human subject from a primarily interactive source of the self as one-among-others.

Despite JHJ's predilection for sensorimotor descriptions, he rejected simple mechanistic (cause–effect) relationships between the nervous system and the mind, arguing that the relation should only be thought of as concomitance in which causal mechanisms—and the automaticity they seem to imply—are superseded so that the nervous system and mind are "the least automatic and the most imperfectly reflex centres" (Hughlings-Jackson 1887: 34). Instead, they are "unifying centres . . . whereby the organism *as a whole* is adjusted to the environment." In this metaphysical commitment JHJ undercuts any form of Cartesian interactionism between mind and body as distinct entities, and underscores a bodily (or sensorimotor) basis for the elaboration of the psychological self as a kind of coordination or integration of the whole. Merleau-Ponty's convergent critique of both empiricist and intellectualist explanations of conscious experience is equally a rejection of the view that the mind is *in* the brain, or that the mind can be said to be *in anything at all*, as a thing in itself. For Merleau-Ponty, consciousness is the body being subjective in its relations within itself and to the world; the mind is not a command center receiving input, which is then interiorized, reorganized, represented, and expressed as output via the nervous system's motor network. The body is not a locus of predictable behaviors causally elicited by stimuli (Merleau-Ponty 2012) alongside which representations have a quasi-ideal or abstract existence: "A behaviour [sketches] a certain manner of dealing with the world" (2012: 333) and inherently constitutes intelligence in that verbal articulation is seamlessly woven into all behavior and not merely into a distinct realm of "outputs."

This straightforward, but nuanced view interweaves human motivations into our practical relation to world, a relation in which the world solicits or makes demands upon the body, solicitations calling for embodied responses that constitute ourselves as intentional beings and the site from which our intentional threads reach out toward the world. Merleau-Ponty critiques psychological frameworks that invoke linear causal/ mechanistic explanations to make sense of human motivation, stating that the psychologist, as ostensible scientist, "*was himself,* in principle, that very fact that he was investigating. He was in fact this very representation of the body, this magical experience that he was now approaching with such indifference; he lived it at the same time he thought about it" (Merleau-Ponty 2012: 98; emphasis original). He thus rejects intentionality as an objectifying representation or stance toward ourselves as objects with certain properties and locates it in our dealings with things according to praxis, techniques, and self-delineating projects.

The affinity between the two thinkers is a vision of the human subject as a responsive, and engaged agent, who is coupled to her *situation*, and it rejects a theory in which sensory input data is translated into mental content and used to structure motor output (which Susan Hurley calls the cognitive sandwich model of cognition) (Hurley 1998). Their work also prefigures theories of embodied cognition, enactivism, and dynamical systems theories of brain function, offering tools for a more robust and neurally realistic characterization of mental disorders than those found in psychiatry's *Diagnostic and Statistical Manual,* 5th edition (DSM-5). More importantly, JHJ and Merleau-Ponty appreciate that conscious experience cannot be seen in representational or computational terms and that human subjectivity is holistic and fully engaged with a complex human world, features of which psychiatry's operationalized approach to diagnosis and underlying pathology often lose sight. In any situation, the body-subject necessarily engages the regions of perception, affect, cognitive-linguistic function, and motility in a unified, but appropriately distributed way, such that the demands of the situation are coped with skillfully and fit him or her for social life.

In the DSM-5, we find that one of the many criteria for depression is that it be clinically significant (APA 2013), a state that may be characterized precisely as an inability to no longer manage or cope with one's affective state in normal social life. However, the model upon which depression (and mental disorder in general) is conceptualized, is often partitioned along lines of functional and impersonal subsystems alienated from dynamic human functioning and it becomes problematic, largely because this dynamic functioning is (improperly) conceived of in relation to an internal or antecedent sets of causes which can go awry and may possibly be corrected.

JHJ claims that human bodies connect to the world according to "the latest developed and most elaborate part of a sensorimotor mechanism" (Hughlings-Jackson 1887: 36). Merleau-Ponty uses different terms and posits that this connection is a series of "intentional threads" (2012: 132) linking us to the world. Through them we establish a grip on our world where the senses and our active responses are coalesced (or gathered) under what he calls the "intentional arc" (2012: 137). Subjectivity and consciousness are often used interchangeably to capture an appreciation of the uniqueness of our human presence in the world as coordinated intentional beings. For JHJ, human subjectivity and consciousness are analyzed in terms of four functions: memory, reason, emotion, and will which we can approach in terms of a combination of bodily responses and "propositionising."

JHJ's analysis is deepened when we explore the idea of muscle memory, the role of bodily reactions in emotion, and the role of propositions in reasoning and human cognition ordering the incessant activity that a normal human being evinces. Propositions, central to the analysis of thought and language, lift human thought beyond the constraints on our animal cousins where intentionality just is clever means-end (or adaptive) activity. Propositions are abstractions from sentences about states of affairs in the world—"facts" (Wittgenstein 1975: § 1.11)—and are apprehended so as to be communicable to others (Foucault 2008: 34) and assessable as either true or false (Frege 1977: 4–5). But even sentence structure is closely tied to the neural correlates of episodes of perception and movement as discrete human acts in a domain of activity (Knott 2012). Words in sentences denote explicit contents of deeds attributable to only highly specialized and constrained kinds of action where identifiable objects and modes of acting can be discerned. In a similar way, we find that Merleau-Ponty's cognitive-linguistic region/dimension resonates with the "specialised" deed of propositional use so that, for Merleau-Ponty, not only is action primarily—and for the most part—initiated non-conceptually, but cognition itself is not a privileged plane of existence. Instead cognition comes to the fore in limit situations, where one's sedimented capacities for situational coping cannot navigate or manage a novel or unfamiliar situation. JHJ's four aspects of consciousness—memory, reasoning, emotion, and will—in fact converge with Merleau-Ponty's phenomenological analysis of four "existential" regions/dimensions: perceptual, cognitive-linguistic, affective, and motility (Mallin 1979) in analyzing embodied subjectivity.

Memory ought to be construed broadly rather than in terms of the popular stereotype of a video-like record of past events laid down as images in the brain and amenable to declarative recovery. Merleau-Ponty uses the term "sedimentation" (2012: 131) to convey a trace made by lived experience in a way that is more pliable, dynamic, and accommodating to situational ambiguity than declarative memory reports of episodes. Representational memory, according to Merleau-Ponty, favors certainty over ambiguity but sedimentation allows for the quasi-stability of the traces in our neural nets that rest on quasi-stable but subtly modifiable strengths of association patterns within the whole. The "snap shot" view depicts past experience in propositional terms apt to be deliberated about and acted upon so as to lead to a definite judgment or action, an intellectualizing abstraction that sees agency as enacting propositions capturing determinate, content-laden phenomena. But that account does not adequately or satisfactorily mesh with the development of perceptual, cognitive, and motor skills effectively linking us to our world in shifting ways. While an agent may recall ways in which a situation is similar to others, she can never give an explicit account of the infinite variety of similarities to and differences from other situations that may influence a response. By contrast, at the heart of sedimentation is a dynamic practical connection with the world and a "primordial affectivity" (Colombetti 2014) that manifests our fundamentally purposeful existence.

We are never indifferent to the world (*Umwelt*), even when passive, so that "the essence of any feature of the world is . . . indissociable from the reaction it calls forth in us" (Smith 2007: 19). Perception is therefore infused by affect which in turn structures one's possibilities for world-oriented action. It is continuously developed in ongoing articulations (or "laying down"), forming a series from our very first contact with the world up to and including the present, such that the multiple affinities and potential resonances of any given experience are temporally present, reflected in that sedimented history of situational coping, the success of which, however, need not elicit a positive habit or disposition. A neural structure incorporating that sedimentation is part of a more complex whole which must be integrated with other traces and translated into action on any given occasion to produce behavior (or even a settled train of thought). In fact, psychopathologies resistant to change may draw rigidity from bodily incorporation of ineffective or poor situational dealings in that habit creates disposition.

Time is implicit in Husserl's phenomenological analysis of cognition (Husserl 1960): retention (the effect of past encounters sufficiently like the present one) and protention (the way that one's current active engagement affects the future) link present experience to past events and the anticipation of what is to come by moulding perceptuo-motor cycles (Neisser 1976). Cognition is best thought of as a reflection of integrated and dynamic activity adapting the whole organism to a context rather than as an interposited domain of central processing between perception and action. Intentionality is therefore (essentially) perceptuo-motor activity arising in situations through sedimented traces activated as the agent is touched by the situation, moderated by other (possibly subtle) affordances (Chemero 2011) and intelligently enacted into experience and action. Merleau-Ponty reminds us that this integration is by a situated, symbolically aware, semiotic subject (1973: 50ff.) and that sedimentation creates structures embodying both retention and protention (Merleau-Ponty 1964) to encompass possibilities for the existential self. These arise from a human neural system as it melds bottom-up and top-down processes of neural structuration to enable the work of being-in-the-world-with-others (Thompson and Varela 2001). It therefore combines memory (reflecting sedimentation), will (the ability to give effect to thought), emotions evoked in us, and reasoning (our use of discursive abstractions and connections to order experience and organize behavior).

Emotions, as we now recognize, build on resonance with others (Singer et al. 2004; Fuchs and De Jaegher 2010) so they are inherently intersubjective and not just intrasubjective. As embodied integrated beings, we are shaped by forces acting within the discursive milieu of a primary social group (Freud 1986: 469) that shape human agents. We learn how to act in this milieu so that, as Nietzche has it, "psychology is the developmental theory of the will to power" (Nietzsche 1977: 35). Power, not cognition, is at the heart of this account, taking us *via* Foucault, directly to the body as an inscribed surface on which disciplines have effected a complex way of being and doing (Rabinow 1984: 56). Therefore discourse or reason incorporates the bottom-up and top-down effects of our human interactions on our sensori-motor processes which move us in diverse ways and inflect our thoughts and attitudes. That holism needs to inform our conceptions of mental disorder.

Reasoning and its abstract propositional structure organizes our thoughtful activity. Unambiguous communicability essential for reason and argument gives a subject access to a supra-individual mode of self-organization. For Kant, as for Aristotle, this is part of the activity of a natural and integrated whole—the embodied human being trained in judgment (or shaped by certain disciplines) in such a way as to potentiate wisdom and self-control in their inner and outer dealings with events (Kant 1978: 95). A neural focus implicates engaged, discursive, embodied, and multi-layered activity producing structures attuned to a world and primarily linked to action (despite the privileging of cognition in both rationalist and empiricist traditions). The neural correlates of self, and our external relations to the world and others, rest on dynamic balanced activity that allows adaptive patterns to emerge (Northoff 2016). These dynamics are both bound up with, and affect, intentionality; they are discernibly altered in psychiatric disorders such that a subject's grip on the world or her capacity affect them; they show the effects and require a kind of care only available if someone makes a space for recovery of equilibrium. A caring provision of and welcome into a space apt for recovery is a kind of hospitality or constrained giving of themselves by those who care.

JHJ argues that our cognitive nature is grounded in neural functions elaborated from sensorimotor interaction with the world as a human being exercises skills and enacted techniques of coping within his or her ongoing engagement with the world (Dreyfus 2014). For Merleau-Ponty, familiarity with certain forms of world-engagement are always imbued by affective tonality (or salience), which tacitly structures subjectivity as a general, bodily style. Ribot's "Le moi c'est une coordination" (Hughlings-Jackson 1887: 35), implicates active and holistic integration of multiple modes of acting and being affected by life (including affects implicit in symbolic and cultural realities) and it arises out of our being situated in the world and with others.

Neural network theory and enaction "within the net" of elaborated functions of the embodied self is the correlate of demonstrable disorders of function discernible in the neuroimaging of self-circuits. These circuits capture our purposeful and holistic embodied being-in-the-world (hence Damasio's "somatic markers") generated by evolutionary phylogeny and the distinctive ontogeny of human beings as intelligent, embodied, nodes of activity in a discursive and social world (Gillet and Haré 2013). Contemporary approaches to neuroscience of consciousness, social cognition (Saxe 2006), and neuroethics (Ellis 2010; Gillett and Franz 2016) support JHJ's conception of mental disorder as a dissolution of highly evolved neural function (the basis of mental processes), and evokes the idea of fragmentation or splitting of the self central to understandings of psychiatry from the nineteenth and early twentieth century (evident in terms like "schizoid" and "schizophrenia" applied to mental disorder). But this strand of evidence and more recent work on cerebral synchrony and the delicate balances between self and other excitation patterns in Cortical Midline Centers can be enlisted by those with an allegiance to the brain–body dualism that is contemporary Cartesian materialism. Losses of neural harmony or flow constitutive of a seamless psychosomatic mode of being are interpreted reductively by psychologies couched solely in terms of inner representational terms and can make invisible our grip on the world through the affective interplay of action, perception, and inner sense.

Cognitive states and events, as conceived in empiricist and rationalist orientations often embed the "cognitive sandwich" (Hurley 1998) view whereby perception is viewed as *input*, and action as *output*, rather than the focus being on what our bodies are doing in the world as directly coupled to it in ways that are then inflected by speech (or discourse more generally). Bodily interaction and hands-on problem-solving (often informed by the "offline," symbolic, and explicit representations) write into ourselves the praxis of a language (Merleau-Ponty 1973), and that praxis connects us to others through situated and engaged activity so that the thinking, feeling, body-subject develops a neural shape whereby (even if "triply indirectly") "the organism as a whole is adjusted to the environment" (Hughlings-Jackson 1887: 34). Such an active, integrated, psychosomatic, and intentional view of mental function is basic to a phenomenological understanding of neuroscience and mental disorder.

EVOLUTION, DISSOLUTION, AND BEING-IN-THE-WORLD-WITH-OTHERS

The thought that various mental disorders are different dissolutions of evolved neural function in the human life-world, lays bare the ethological complexity of embodiment and mental disorders. We all function more or less adequately in the world in terms of animal adaptation as creatures with, a more or less, unified mode of cognition (Kant 1978/ [1798]: 113). Kant was somewhat prescient insofar as he understood the "insane" to live in a subjective, inner world—perhaps fragmented—neither properly in touch with the *Umvelt* nor with others. An experience of alienation from place, from the shared and communicable embodied experience that most of us indwell (Kant 2012: 113) is, in phenomenological terms, an exclusion from a shared world in which one is able to present oneself familiarly, normally reflected in the very capacity to live, move, and enact one's being with ease. But, Kant overestimates the extent to which one retains his or her sense of understanding when one cannot act in a "real" world, a background upon which the body-subject, depending on the severity of the disorder, is no longer able "to *reckon* with the possible" (Merleau-Ponty 2012: 112; empashis original).

Both JHJ (1887) and Freud (1986) echo these Kantian and phenomenological themes as they distinguish mental disorder from disturbances of the neural function required for basic organismic integrity, at what we might call, an "animal" level. That primitive "fitness," which for Aristotle is part of *first nature*, can go awry at a more complex level when the world around one and one's own body, are "triply indirectly represented" (Hughlings-Jackson 1887: 32) with the aid of speech so that life incorporates the "collective reason of humankind" (Kant, 2012: 136). Being distanced from direct sensorimotor input arises from questioning the world within our ways of dealing with each other and incorporates wider symbolic information and so provides another joint at which subjectivity may become disrupted. Tomasello, discussing the complex social and semantic competencies mastered in human ontogeny, clearly identifies the multiperspectival character of the objective-reflective, normative domain that we construct to do this, which nevertheless remains tied to the actual sensorimotor, cooperative, and communicative activity that makes it possible (Tomasello 2014). The skills required to cope with that milieu relate our activity to *Sinn* or sense (Frege, Husserl, Merleau-Ponty, and Levinas) within the symbolic order rather than merely *Bedeutung* or reference. Whereas the latter is often analyzed in terms of causal/biological relations, or in terms of a natural or primitive information link between the thinker and the world (Evans

1982), Merleau-Ponty follows philosophical logic (Frege) and early phenomenology (particularly Husserl) by analyzing *Sinn* as resting on our language-related dealings with the world,
both individual and collective, and therefore implicates bodily expressions underpinning
the words and sentences we use to make sense of ourselves. The body, as a locus for *the* expression of self, thus has profound implications for embodiment and mental disorder that
cannot be exclusively linked to but that profoundly affect inner representations (in the mode
of some philosophy of mind).

Consider, for instance, a psychotic person who speaks articulately but what he or she
says has "disordered thought form and content" such that he or she assigns quite idiosyncratic content to life events and weaves them together in strange combinations. There may
be a superficial coherence, but the speech can seem to have little or no sense in terms of
actual dealings with a context (as in the dissociation between thought and life in Cotard's
delusion—*I am dead*).[1] Here we encounter instances of unusual affective-cognitive modes
of self-integration (I feel dead; I am not really part of the world; I do not belong here; I feel
as if somebody is putting thoughts into my head). In other syndromes we also observe affectively disordered self-location among others (I am being watched by the secret service;
my wife has been replaced by an imposter), as well as affectively enlarged self-evaluation (I
have committed the unforgivable sin; I am rotting away inside and it won't be long before it
is evident to all). Northoff discusses hallucinations—quasi-sensory experiences (there are
voices that speak to me) as imbalances between external arising and self-arising modes of
neural processing that wrongly locate sensory content and abstract it from lived-bodily engagement in idiosyncratic ways. In such cases symbolism and abstraction is read into an actual interaction with the world, used to shape re-re-representation and confounds the ability
of the subjective body to get on with life. A human life-world affected in this way becomes
full of contradictions and impasses from the mismatch between self-understanding and the
techniques of coping with situated human life. The often quite articulate use of words, in addition to the performance of many ordinary actions in psychosis, nevertheless illustrates a
high level of sensorimotor coordination that is impossible in neurological disorders such as
dyskinesia, dysarthria, or dysphasia.

However, the bodily attunement required for making sense of the world through thetic
acts of positing and acting in light of an intelligently negotiated and shared symbolic reality is
impaired. Cultural adaptation, and reason-responsive praxis are therefore severely affected
by an inability to engage in basic, often taken-for-granted, situations non-reflectively, in a familiar way, and unproblematically. The inhabited world and the experience of self therefore
become problematized in possibly unliveable ways. Merleau-Ponty holds that a hallucination is not a perception per se, but rather "reproduces the manner in which these realities affect me in my sentient or my linguistic being" (2012: 374). Similar to the Kantian formulation
of a private world we noted earlier, Merleau-Ponty contends that the hallucination, though
experienced within a common world, is not *of* the world: "it takes place in the individual
'landscape' . . . in order to carve out a private world within the common world, and always
runs into the transcendence of time" (2012: 357–358). On the other hand, in depression, self-
directed preoccupation and negative feelings may be exacerbated through hyperreflexivity
on account of the body's inability to go forward, to "decide" or act, a state arising from a

---

[1] For an excellent phenomenological discussion of Cotard's delusion see Ratcliffe (2008).

change in the body's ability to attune to affective world salience and respond. The perceptual "plenitude" or apodictic certainly of the world remains normal, yet the things *of* the world no longer affect us in the way characteristic of unreflective and concernful action. The inability to be solicited by the world is equally true of interpersonal relations which, in depression, quite often go awry; similarly, in obsessive-compulsive behavior, repeated hand-washing or rituals exemplify a "pathological" misdirecting thematization of intentionality that disrupts a normally seamless, dynamic, and good-enough engagement with the world. Having said that, in OCD (as well as in cases of schizophrenia), while a sense of owning some intentions rather than others is acknowledged, there are significant neural disruptions in self-function (Northoff 2016), such that the *willing* of the act is not experienced as one's own (Gallagher 2005; Gallagher and Zahavi 2008). Here the organic fusion of meaning and bodily activity, normally integrated and holistic, is fragmented. Such disintegration is not a breakdown in cognition or beliefs but in the whole organism's adjustment to an environment: "The normal subject," writes Merleau-Ponty, "does not revel in subjectivity, he flees from it, he is really in the world, he has a direct and naïve hold on time, whereas the hallucinating subject makes use of being in the world in order to carve out a private world within a common world" (2012: 358).

The dissolutions (JHJ) we call mental disorders disrupt the flow of sensorimotor activity and its re-re-representation (cognitive and social) exposing discontinuities not normally present. Thus a schizophrenic patient can speak words without the neurological impairments of dysphasia or dysarthria (apart, that is, from the extrapyramidal effects of medications) but may show disorders of thought form and content, making it hard to understand what is being said because thought is not in its normally seamless, dynamic, self-correcting relation to a world shared with others; in a word, the story is unable to be indwelt (*unheimlich*).

A very different disruption of psychosocial and neurocognitive functions is seen in a psychopath.[2] Such a person can act and think coherently and relate in an apparently normal manner to others so that both integrated animal function and propositionally directed social function definitely remains intact. Such a person might plausibly seem—especially in their own eyes—to be quite clever. But the psychopath lacks an adequate affective and comprehensive grasp of what matters to others so cannot be properly careful about interacting with them (Gillett 2009). The failure is not to identify or in some (partial) sense comprehend the feelings of others, it is rather in being properly affected by these experiences and therefore to treat others only as means to self-regarding ends. Sincere hospitality is lacking as there is no caring solicitude and self-giving to the other. This is a significant consideration in forging sustainable human relations in our complex psycho-socio-cultural world and normally moderates short-term, self-regarding, pay-off for actions. That dissolution of a fundamental ground of social intercourse distorts a person's being-in-the-world-with-others because it disables sensitivity to the fact that we are all creatures who *essentially* cohabit with others in an objective-reflective-normative domain, and take up a web of relationships where "I am because you are and you are because we are . . . by virtue of an interconnectedness" where "consequences for both the individual and society . . . are important" (Van Staden 2011: 15).

---

[2] Someone who has both the personality and behavioral features of the condition as standardly diagnosed.

We are, in short, normally creatures shaped by a discursive mirror comprised of imperatives and demands and meant to shape us for being-with-others in ways good-enough for our shared life together (Lacan 1977: 3, 106). This life is bodily and elaborated through the integration of sensorimotor function to shape a whole organism adjustment to the world in relation to which explicit construction is an abstraction from that part of human life where we are enmeshed in language games or discourse (a part that massively inflects the whole).

Affective disturbances commonly attributed to depression, schizophrenia, or personality disorders, arise within a slackened intentional arc, the function of which is to unite affect, perception, cognition, and motility such that the body is capable of answering, not only the world's solicitation to do things, but also the call of interpersonal relationships. In his lengthy essay on developmental psychology, Merleau-Ponty introduces the notion of syncratic sociabilty as a way to characterize our most basic childhood entwinement with others, persisting as the basic ontological description of intersubjectivity that permeates adult life. "The state of union with another," says Merleau-Ponty, "the dispossession of me by the other, are thus not suppressed by the child's arrival at the age of three years. They remain in other zones of adult life . . . what Piaget calls *displacement*" (1964: 155). Our childhood (in)capacity to cope with certain interpersonal situations may be "overcome at a certain level, [they have] yet (and perhaps never will be) overcome at a higher level" (1964: 155). A mental disorder must be viewed through disturbed affectivity, a domain of existence that makes possible our fundamental relation to others, whether it be bodily or "psychological." The skillful coping implicated in this relation is both sensorimotor and emotional (a touch here, a smile there). Hence, "the indistinction between me and the other does not inevitably reappear *except* in certain situations that for the adult are limiting situations but are quite important in his life" (Merleau-Ponty 1964: 154).

UNDERSTANDING DISORDER THROUGH NEUROPHENOMENOLOGY—A REPRISE

For human beings, the world is the background upon which a natural resonance germinates our primary intersubjectivity that implicitly conditions all our development (Trevarthen and Aitken 2001), including participation in discourse as beings of both flesh and word. Within this domain, the intentional arc (Merleau-Ponty 2012) traces the intelligent interaction whereby a human subject-agent is literally in-*tension* with the world of action according to distinct, but unified, domains of existence: "The intentional arc names the tight connection between body and world, such that, as the active body acquires skill, . . . 'stored', not as representations in the mind, but as dispositions to respond to the solicitations of situations in the world" (Dreyfus 2002: 367). The tightness of the intentional arc opens up for me a liveable space, not geometrically defined and translatable into visual representations, but sensorimotor—disclosing my body's relationship to itself and to situations "pregnant with meaning," perspectival entrées onto the world structured by my history of dealings with it. Ways of negotiating a particular bodily space are "sedimented" from my history (Vasterling 2003) so that my situated existence, as a body and its capacities internally organized by midline structures in the brain (Northoff 2016), is the biological basis on which I relate to the world through self–world circuits. Semantic modes of being and interpersonality are added, whereby I "read" the world and others in meaningful ways co-constructed with others (Tomasello 2014). This existence bears the traces of a unique personal development, affective intersubjectivity, and intercorporeality, and is jointly encoded in a neural synchrony organized into externally directed dynamic circuits of embodied activity.

Responding to the other in sustainable ways in that milieu is an ethological task requiring the development of skills that give rise to personal autonomy (Gillett 2012). The intentional arc therefore gathers into itself sensorimotor coupling between self and world, the dynamic internal flow of organism, and a normativity of the word as imperative (Lacan 1977: 106). Those aspects of human ethology locate me in an objective-normative-imperative domain interactively created as a world of value and self-worth which are therefore highly sensitive to our relations with others. In this way language delivers us to the doorstep of reason, truth, and the inner workings of "others" as a mature or "adultist" perspective (Merleau-Ponty 1968) which often fails to acknowledge that, prior to semantics, infants and children recognize that a gesture toward anything evinces a response from the adult, not only to that thing, but to an implicit demand from the child to be recognized, nurtured, educated, and empowered. Gestural meaning enlists anatomical structure and the flow of musculature, as bodily capacities, and the milieu of its engagement envelops us in the ontological truth of being-with, further underpinning all our later movements toward and away from things as things of this or that type themselves encountered amongst people who are there to enfold (not engulf), and create space for us to be body-subjects.

Consciousness and subjectivity result from the intentional arc and a tone that constantly strives to integrate (and balance, according to situational demands) memory, emotion, reasoning, and will so as to create the acts and interactions that make possible a lived story of being-in-the-world-with-others. Or better still, in commenting on the integration of interaction and reflection, Merleau-Ponty remarks: "I am never at one with myself. Such is the fate of a being who is born, that is, a being who once and for all was given to himself as something to be understood" (Merleau-Ponty 2012: 362). The lived story discloses meaning but also distances me from my dealings with the world allowing me to find solutions to situations underpinned by the ontogenetic evolution, from prepersonal to personal identity, whereby I speak through the person that comes into being as I relate to others. This is the basis of developed action and affect but also the basis of perplexity when the smoothly integrated flow of life and speech is disrupted. Its disordered formation yields an understanding of the phenomenology of mental disorder. The often vague signs and symptoms that constitute DSM-5 criteria sets do not lay bare for us the structures of dissolute lived-experience that constitute mental disorder, and therefore do not transparently relate to the neural organization that makes it possible for a person to engage with her practical world and its potential challenges. While the continued search for the biological or genetic basis of mental disorder should not be outright discounted, it is imperative that the categories from which research takes its starting point be conceptually apt. In listening to phenomenology, a completely different way of seeing disorders is revealed, with a clear focus on changes to structures of consciousness. If, as phenomenology contends, consciousness is not a "thing" but rather a type of experience (Husserl 2012), then, as we continue to explore the intersection of neuroscience and phenomenology, we should not look solely for causal connections, but instead, try to make sense of the rhythms of movement, the flow, the indwelling, and the cognitive techniques comprising a human capacity to self-organize amongst the world and worldly others: "My organism is not some inert thing, it itself sketches out the movement of existence" (Merleau-Ponty 2012: 86).

BIBLIOGRAPHY

APA. (2013). *Diagnostic and Statistical Manual of Mental Disorders: DSM-5.* Washington: American Psychiatric Publishing.

Chemero A. (2011). *Radical Embodied Cognitive Science.* Cambridge, MA: MIT Press.

Colombetti G. (2014). *The Feeling Body: Affective Science Meets the Enactive Mind.* Cambridge: MIT Press.

Dreyfus H. (2014). *Skillful Coping: Essays on the Phenomenology of Everyday Perception and Action.* Oxford: Oxford University Press.

Dreyfus H. L. (2002). "Intelligence Without Representation." *Phenomenology and the Cognitive Sciences* 1: 367–383.

Ellis R. D. (2010). "On the Cusp." In J. J. Giordano and B. Gordijn (eds.), *Scientific and Philosophical Perspectives in Neuroethics*, pp. 66–94. Cambridge: Cambridge University Press.

Evans G. (1982). *The Varieties of Reference.* Oxford: Clarendon Press.

Foucault M. (2008). *The Birth of Biopolitics: Lectures at the Collège de France, 1978–1979*, trans. G. Burchell. Basingstoke: Palgrave Macmillan.

Frege G. (1977). *The Logical Investigations*, trans. P. T. Geach. Oxford: Basil Blackwell.

Freud S. (1986). *The Essentials of Psycho-analysis*, trans. J. Strachey. London: Hogarth and the Institute of Psycho-Analysis.

Fuchs T. and De Jaegher H. (2010). "Understanding Intersubjectivity: Enactive and Embodied." In T. Fuchs, H. C. Sattel, and P. Henningsen (eds.), *The Embodied Self: Dimensions, Coherence and Disorders*, pp. 203–215. Stuttgart: Schattauer.

Gallagher S. (2005). *How the Body Shapes the Mind.* Oxford: Clarendon Press.

Gallagher S. and Zahavi D. (2008). *The Phenomenological Mind: An Introduction to Philosophy of Mind and Cognitive Science.* London: Routledge.

Gillett G. (2009). *The Mind and Its Discontents*, 2nd edn. Oxford: Oxford University Press.

Gillett G. (2012). "How Do I Learn To Be Me Again? Autonomy, Life Skills, and Identity." In L. Radoilska (ed.), *Autonomy and Mental Health*, pp. 233–251. Oxford: Oxford University Press.

Gillet G. and Haré R. (2013). "Discourse and Diseases of the Soul." In K. W. M. Fulford, et al. (eds.), *The Oxford Handbook of Philosophy and Psychiatry*, pp. 307–320. Oxford: Oxford University Press.

Gillett G. and Franz E. (2016). "Evolutionary Neurology, Responsive Equilibrium, and the Moral Brain." *Conscious and Cognition* 45: 245–250.

Hughlings-Jackson J. (1878). "On Affections of Speech from Disease of the Brain." *Brain* 1(3): 304.

Hughlings-Jackson J. (1887). "Remarks on Evolution and Dissolution of the Nervous System." *The British Journal of Psychiatry* 33(141): 25.

Hurley S. L. (1998). *Consciousness in Action.* Cambridge: Harvard University Press.

Husserl E. (1960). *Cartesian Meditations: An Introduction to Phenomenology*, trans. D. Cairns. The Hague: Martinus Nijhoff.

Husserl E. (2012). *Ideas: General Introduction to Pure Phenomenology*, trans. W. R. Boyce Gibson. London: Routledge.

Kant I. (1978/[1798]), *Anthopology from a Pragmatic Point of View*, trans. V. L. Dowdell. Carbondale: Southern Illinois University Press.

Kant I. (2012). *Anthropology from a Pragmatic Point of View*, trans. M. J. Gregor. The Hague: Martinus Nijhoff.

Knott A. (2012). *Sensorimotor Cognition and Natural Language Syntax*. Cambridge, MA: MIT Press).

Lacan J. (1977). *Écrits*, trans. B. Fink. New York: Norton.

Mallin S. B. (1979). *Merleau-Ponty's Philosophy*. New Haven: Yale University Press.

Merleau-Ponty M. (1964). "The Child"s Relations with Others.' In J. M. Edie (ed.), *The Primacy of Perception*, pp. 96–155. Evanston: Northwestern University Press.

Merleau-Ponty M. (1968). *The Visible and the Invisible*, ed. C. Lefort, trans. A. Lingis. Evanston: Northwestern University Press.

Merleau-Ponty M. (1973). *Consciousness and the Acquisition of Language*, trans. H. Silverman. Evanston: Northwestern University Press.

Merleau-Ponty M. (2012). *Phenomenology of Perception*, trans. D. A. Landes. Hoboken: Taylor and Francis.

Neisser U. (1976). *Cognition and Reality: Principles and Implications of Cognitive Psychology*. San Fransisco: W. H. Freeman.

Nietzsche F. W. (1977). *Beyond Good and Evil Prelude to a Philosophy of the Future*, trans. R. J. Hollingdale. Harmondsworth: Penguin Books.

Northoff G. (2016). *Neuro-Philosophy and the Healthy Mind: Learning from the Unwell Brain*. New York: W. W. Norton.

Rabinow P. (1984). *The Foucault Reader: An Introduction to Foucault's Thought*. London: Penguin Books.

Ratcliffe M. (2008). *Feelings of Being: Phenomenology, Psychiatry and the Sense of Reality*. Oxford: Oxford University Press.

Saxe R. (2006). "Uniquely Human Social Cognition." *Current Opinion in Neurobiology* 16(2): 235–239.

Singer T., et al. (2004). "Empathy for Pain Involves the Affective but not Sensory Components of Pain." *Science* 303(5661): 1157.

Smith A. D. (2007). "The Flesh of Perception." In T. Baldwin (ed.), *Reading Merleau-Ponty: on Phenomenology of Perception*, pp. 1–22. London: Routledge.

Thompson E. and Varela F. J. (2001). "Radical Embodiment: Neural Dynamics and Consciousness." *Trends in Cognitive Sciences* 5(10): 418–425.

Tomasello M. (2014). *A Natural History of Human Thinking*. Cambridge: Harvard University Press.

Trevarthen C. and Aitken K. J. (2001). "Infant Intersubjectivity: Research, Theory, and Clinical Applications." *Journal of Child Psychology and Psychiatry* 42(1): 3–48.

Van Staden C. W. (2011). "African Approaches to an Enriched Ethics of Person-centred Health Practice." *International Journal of Person-Centered Medicine* 1: 11–17.

Vasterling V. (2003). "Body and Language: Butler, Merleau-Ponty and Lyotard on the Speaking Embodied Subject." *International Journal of Philosophical Studies* 11(2): 205–223.

Wittgenstein L. (1975). *Tractatus Logico-philosophicus*, trans. D. F. Pears and B. McGuinness. London: Routledge.

CHAPTER 97

PHENOMENOLOGICAL PSYCHOPATHOLOGY OF NEURODIVERSITY

MARCO O. BERTELLI, JOHAN DE GROEF,
AND ELISA RONDINI

NEURODIVERSITY AND NEURODEVELOPMENTAL DISORDERS

THE term "neurodiversity" is commonly used to refer to neurodevelopmental disorders, which are considered a group of conditions with early onset, often before a child enters grade school, and are characterized by deficits that produce impairments of personal, social, academic, or occupational functioning. Deficits vary from very specific cognitive "functions" to more complex executive or relational skills. The term is sometimes used as an exclusive synonym for autism spectrum disorder and intellectual disability—which are the most prevalent neurodevelopmental disorders—but it actually includes many other clinical syndromes, such as attention deficit/hyperactivity disorder, specific learning disorders, or motor disorders.

INTELLECTUAL DISABILITY

The conceptualization of intellectual disability (also referred to here as ID) has always been controversial, as reflected by the several changes across its long history within the taxonomy of mental disorders. In fact, it is considered as a complex condition involving impairments of both mental and personal functions which are not easy to describe, such as intelligence, adaptive behavior, learning, and skills. These impairments occur in early developmental age and tend to persist across the life-span.

In spite of the complexity, issues concerning classification and diagnostic criteria are crucial for intellectual disability, since they have relevant implication for prevalence, intervention procedures, service provision, and outcomes.

Intellectual disability has been considered a relevant theme by World Health Organization (WHO) since it involves significant complexities surrounding the health construct, connected to the definition, classification, and operationalization of concepts such as health "condition," "status," and "domain" (Bertelli et al. 2016). Recently, beside the traditional categories of signs, syndromes, disorders, diseases, and discrete entities, WHO has considered other major groupings, such as "other conditions that require specific health care," "spectrum disorders," and "syndrome groupings," in any one of which intellectual disability could be included (WHO 2001). Furthermore, intellectual disability has also played a role in providing a global definition of concepts such as "autonomy," "well-being," "deficit," and "limitation in activities" and/or "restriction in participation," formerly "disabilities and handicaps" (Bertelli et al. 2016).

There is still no agreement on how intellectual disability should be considered. Experts of different disciplines, such as psychology, anthropology, and sociology have interpreted this condition in different ways and the issue whether ID should be regarded as a health condition, a disability, or a life condition remains unsolved (Bertelli 2015). In the tenth edition of the International Classification of Diseases (ICD-10; WHO 1992), intellectual disability is present with the name of "mental retardation," within the category of psychiatric conditions and impairments in intellectual functioning. On the other hand, in the International Classification of Functioning (ICF; WHO 2001) impairments in intellectual functions can also be placed in the group of body functions and intended as included in disability. Conversely, the American Association for Intellectual and Developmental Disorders (AAIDD) defines intellectual disability as a "disability," assembling a comprehensive description, classification, and systems of supports that concentrate principally on functions, adaptive behavior, and other personal needs. According to this definition, ID is a disability characterized by "significant limitations both in intellectual functioning and in adaptive behavior as expressed in conceptual, social, and practical adaptive skills" (Schalock et al. 2010) that occurs before age eighteen.

Considering intellectual disability only as a disability could entail its removal from ICD categories which are used across the world. Thus, canceling ID from the list of health conditions may have an impact on its visibility, on national and global policies, and on services available to this population. On the other hand, defining intellectual disability only as a health condition would contrast with the stands adopted by many governmental policies and worldwide organizations, and it would be criticized as a reductionist approach by many users and experts in the field (Salvador-Carulla et al. 2011). In defining intellectual disability as a health condition, important questions remain unsolved, for example, the large grouping within the health categorization where it should be placed, the age for onset, or the link between impairments in cognitive functions and behavioral skills.

The Section Psychiatry of Intellectual Disability of the World Psychiatric Association (WPA-SPID) conceptualized intellectual disability neither as a disease nor as a disability but as a meta-syndromic group of health conditions (diseases, disorders, and others), whose clinical entities are parallel to other meta-syndromic conditions such as Dementia, and may be related to a variety of specific aetiologies, ranging from genetic (e.g. fragile X syndrome) to nutritional (e.g. iodine deficiency), infectious (e.g. intra-uterine rubella), metabolic (e.g. phenylketonuria), or neurotoxic factors (e.g. fetal alcohol syndrome and heavy metal intoxications) (Salvador-Carulla et al. 2011). This group of developmental conditions is characterized by "a significant impairment of cognitive functions, which occurs early in the developmental age and is associated with limitations of learning, adaptive behavior and skills" (Salvador-Carulla et al. 2011).

In 2011, the WHO Working Group for the revision of ICD-10 extended this definition under the new term of "Intellectual Developmental Disorders" and endorsed a polysemic dimensional approach to distinguish between the clinical meta-syndromes and their functioning/disability counterpart. The first component, expressed by the term Intellectual Developmental Disorders, should have a place in the ICD, while the second, expressed by the term intellectual disability, perfectly suits the ICF model (Salvador-Carulla et al. 2011). This approach would best support the public health mission of the WHO and the provision of appropriate services and opportunities to people with intellectual disability (Salvador-Carulla and Saxena 2009).

AUTISM SPECTRUM DISORDER

The conceptualization of autism has also been controversial. Eugen Bleuler coined the term "autism" to define a type of schizophrenia described by individual "inward turning" into his/her own world which entails loss of contact with the external environment. The general theory of schizophrenia proposed by Bleuler is centred on the loss of interpretative and re-lational abilities as synthetically reported by 4A theory: inappropriate or flattened Affect, Ambivalence toward others, loosening of thought Associations, and Autism, which was described as "social withdrawal" and "preference for living in a fantasy world" (Bleuler 1911; 1950).[1]

According to Leo Kanner (1943), the fundamental symptom of autism was represented by the inability to relate to people and situations in the usual way from an early age. Autism is a disorder of social interaction which is characterized by a lack of interest in other people's emotions.

Kanner was the first to introduce the term of "Autistic Disturbances of Affective Contact," describing eleven children presenting social withdrawal, echolalia, repetitive behaviors, and temper tantrums when their routine was disrupted.

In 1944, Asperger referred to patients very similar to those described by Kanner using the term "Autistischen Psychopathen." Nevertheless, he observed three relevant differences, which are more fluent speech, higher level of learning skills, and problems in performing large movements but not fine gestures. Thus, Kanner's autism and Asperger's syndrome were identified as two distinct clinical forms with important common traits. At a later time, the term Asperger's syndrome started to be attributed to autistic individuals with relatively high Intelligent Quotient (IQ) scores.

Another differentiation was proposed by Lorna Wing, who distinguished three types of autism by the pattern of social interaction: confidential, passive, and strange. The first con-fidential type referred to individuals indifferent to other people, detached, characterized by the presence of motor stereotypes, good mechanical skills, good visual-spatial abilities,

---

[1] For further reflections on Bleuler's conception of autism see Gipps and de Haan, this volume.

and medium-severe cognitive impairments; the "passive" type described people with fewer symptoms that were detected later in life, and appeared to accept social approaches, to meet the gaze of others, and to become involved as a passive part of a game; the "strange" type was attributed to individuals who were a bit "naïve," but with good cognitive abilities.

In the 1950s and 1960s, autism was regarded as an early manifestation of schizophrenia and it was interpreted as an emotional disorder due to a pathological interaction between the parents and the child. For this reason, in the first edition of the Diagnostic and Statistical Manual of Mental Disorders (DSM) it was defined with the expression "schizophrenic reaction, childhood type" (APA 1952), whereas it was classified under the terms "childhood schizophrenia" (APA 1968) in the second edition of the manual.

It was during the 1970s that the scientific community started considering autism as a biological disorder with a high co-occurrence with mental retardation. The third edition of the DSM (APA 1980) emphasized the difference between autism and schizophrenia, presenting six diagnostic criteria for childhood autism, including absence of delusions, hallucinations, loosening of associations, and incoherence. Furthermore, DSM-III introduced the definition of pervasive developmental disorder, as a meta-syndromic group including clusters of symptoms sharing some main features but with some differences relevant for clinical identification and outcome, such as infantile autism, residual infantile autism, childhood onset pervasive developmental disorder, residual childhood onset pervasive developmental disorder, and atypical autism (APA 1980). Nevertheless, the ninth edition of the ICD continued for decades to consider autism as a sub-category of schizophrenia.

The current version of the DSM (DSM-5; APA 2013) merges the separate diagnostic categories of DSM-III-revised, DSM-IV, and DSM-IV-revised meta-syndromic groups into an unique condition named "autism spectrum disorder," characterized by different levels of symptoms intensity in two core domains defined as "deficits in social communication and social interaction" and "restricted repetitive behaviours, interests, and activities" (Achkova and Manolova 2014). To make diagnosis of autism spectrum disorder both components are required and symptoms must be present at an early developmental age, even if they might become completely evident only when social demands surpass the limited abilities.

DSM-IV and DSM-5 are held accountable for broadening the criteria for autism spectrum conditions which might have led to a progressive rise in prevalence rates (Wing et al. 2011). A recent trend to further enlarge the number of psychopathological features comprised in the autism spectrum disorder (Takara and Kondo 2014; Dell'Osso et al. 2015a, b) needs to be better evaluated for potential negative impact on research and clinical resources for the autism spectrum disorder core sub-type captured under the classical Kanner description and associated with lower personal functioning profiles and varying level of intellectual disability comorbidity, ascribed as a specifier in the DSM-5.

Although they pertain to two different constructs, autism spectrum disorder and intellectual disability often co-occur. The literature reports that 70% of people with autism spectrum disorder present some level of intellectual disability (Wilkins and Matson 2009; Noterdaeme and Wriedt 2010; Mefford et al. 2012) and another undetermined portion have some kind of impairment in specific cognitive functioning. On the other hand, around 30–40% of people with intellectual disability have an autism spectrum disorder or pervasive autistic features (Morgan et al. 2002; Cooper et al. 2007; Srivastava and Schwartz 2014).

The Neurodevelopmental Perspective

At present, the neurodevelopmental perspective is probably the most valued theoretical framework to explain the relationships between the different biological, psychological, and environmental systems. It answers an increased need of multi-level and multidisciplinary approaches to improve the scientific comprehension of mental disorders' etio-pathogenesis, prevention, and care planning.

Also the new DSM-5 embraced a developmental focus and introduced the new meta-structure of "Neurodevelopmental Disorders" (APA 2013), which has replaced the DSM-IV-TR section "Disorders usually first diagnosed in infancy, childhood, or adolescence" (APA 2000). As mentioned at the beginning of this chapter, this supra-ordinal group includes disorders which are apparently very different from each other, such as intellectual disability, autism spectrum disorder, attention-deficit/hyperactivity disorder, or motor disorders, but which may share etio-pathogenetic, risk, and clinical factors, such as neurodevelopmental genetic phenotype, abnormal neural circuit development, dysfunctions in cognition, learning, communication, and behavior, early emergence, continuing course, and co-occurrence (APA 2013; Bertelli 2015).

The neurodevelopmental perspective also provides an appropriate consideration of the way intellectual disability fades into normality, which is represented by borderline intellectual functioning (BIF), where the overall IQ reduction does not overcome the threshold of two standard deviations below the general population mean, as in intellectual disability. Borderline intellectual functioning is an extremely complex clinical entity, which has scarcely been studied and for which the scientific community has not reached even a minimum consensus on what the term should describe. In spite of these limits linked to the lack of terminological agreement, the prevalence of BIF is reported to be extremely high, ranging in the different studies between 12% and 18% of the population (Hassiotis et al. 2008; Seltzer et al. 2005; Emerson et al. 2010).

One of the most significant advances related to the neurodevelopmental perspective is the acknowledgment that disorders which have always been considered completely different to each other (e.g. intellectual disability, schizophrenia, bipolar disorder) may co-occur or represent variations of the same biological predisposition depending on the person's age or environment. It has increasingly been shown that copy number variants of many syndromes including intellectual disability are present also in many autism spectrum disorders and other psychiatric disorders such as schizophrenia, bipolar disorder, and major depressive disorder (Owen 2012; Bertelli 2015).

The Complex Vulnerability of Neurodiversity

It is widely proved that persons with intellectual disability or autism spectrum disorder present a higher vulnerability to mental and physical health problems than the general population (Bertelli et al. 2009).

Physical illnesses are reported to be around 2.5 fold higher (Cooper 1999; van Schrojenstein Lantman-de Valk et al. 2000; Dixon-Ibarra and Horner-Johnson 2014), with obesity, metabolic disorders (Pan et al. 2016), skeletal disorders, osteoporosis (Center et al. 1998), thyroid problems, cardiac disorders, sensory impairments (Kapell et al. 1998), and dementia (Janicki et al. 2000) being particularly frequent. People with intellectual disability also have a shorter life expectancy (Hollins et al. 1998; Puri et al. 1995).

The full range of mental health problems has been reported to be four times as prevalent as it is in the general population (Cooper et al. 2007), to appear earlier in life, and to persist across the life-span. The co-occurrence of autism spectrum disorder has been associated with a further increase in the prevalence of adjunctive mental health issues (Bradley et al. 2004; Noterdaeme and Hutzelmeyer-Nickels 2010), particularly in respect to attention-deficit/hyperactive disorder, mood disorders, eating disorders, and repetitive behaviors (Bradley et al. 2004; McCarthy 2007).

As mentioned earlier, the origin of such a high level of vulnerability lies within a complex interaction between biological, psychological, and social-environmental factors. Some of the most frequently reported biological factors are represented by genetic alterations, chronic physical disabilities, hypoactivity, unhealthy eating habits, inadequate personal hygiene, or pharmacological side effects (van Schrojenstein Lantman-de Valk et al. 2000). The risk of developing a psychiatric disorder was found to be dependent also on the severity of intellectual disability (at least for some disorders), and impairment of adaptive skills (Koskentausta et al. 2007).

Common psychological factors are lack of environmental mastery, low coping, communication deficits, and difficulties in self-determination, while the environmental influence is most frequently expressed by lack of satisfactory social relations and practical activities, inadequate living arrangements, repeated failures, or other negative life events and traumatic experiences (Raitasuo et al. 1997; Hastings et al. 2004; Hatton and Emerson 2004; Owen et al. 2004; Hamilton et al. 2005; Scott and Havercamp 2014; Rondini 2015).

A phenomenological description is provided here with reference to subjective, practical, and social experiences of persons with neurodevelopmental disorders, as reported in the literature (Gadamer 2010) and in the personal archives of the authors of the present chapter. This description, which includes thoughts on major existential issues, such as insight, time flow, mortality, and singularity is a kind of abstract of the life actuality as told by these persons. For us this process of interpretation can be conceptualized as a phenomenological reduction to the basic categories that structure our common human condition (Binswanger 1962).

THE SELF-EXPERIENCE OF BEING (NEURO)DIVERSE

The description of the self-experience of being neurodiverse is quite hard, mainly because of the difficulties some of these persons have in adequately communicating their own feelings and inner events. The shift from first-person to third-person perspective may determine a considerable depletion in the clinician's ability to understand, as mental states are subjective and direct access to them is probably the only way to get in touch with their complexity (Stanghellini 2003).

Beyond this noetic limit, the experience of being "neurodiverse" involves many other delicate issues. The first one refers to the act of comparing yourself with other persons, which often provokes "unheimlich" ("uncanny") feelings, because it affects the very foundations of our human nature (De Groef et al. 1999). This is particularly true when the comparison is influenced by the others' need to objectify the label of "disabled." The birth—or by extension the "diagnostic discovery"—of a child with a developmental disability shatters the dreams and the narcissistic project of the parents, as well as their perception of being-in-the-world and the way they experience time and life horizons. Another traumatizing character of the disability lies in the fact of the otherness being experienced too early, too intensely, and too radically. The usually slow pace of attuning dreamed reality to true reality needs more support and work.

In general, the meeting of two individuals with and without developmental disability obliges both of them to face a phenomenologically dual problem, which is the difficulty of identifying the impact that the disability has on the expressions of self-experiences.

The life of those with intellectual disability or autism spectrum disorder is punctuated by experiences which imply a considerable difficulty in defining the width of the atypicalness of their first-person givenness and their self-development across time. On the one hand there is the existential normative question: "Am I (still) a human being?" "Do I exist as a member of the humanity?"—or in contemporary jargon: "Am I included in society?"

> . . . Steven was the second of three children. Mary—his older sister with a physical handicap—died some time before. His parents' marriage was already in trouble and they were facing severe psychological difficulties. It meant that they had very little time left for Steven and he adapted to this, being seen as a "perfect quiet" baby. During a classic routine medical assessment, he was found to be affected by cerebral palsy. After having witnessed violence at home and after having been victim of attacks on himself, Steven was referred to me for psychotherapy. For several sessions he continued falling asleep. He stopped only when a safe contact with me was built up and I realized how sleeping could have been a protection for all the exhaustion he felt for being in the world. He suddenly opened his eyes and said "shut up". I thought that with these two of the very few words he ever said to me he was expressing the overcome from his secondary handicaps, his defences against preconceived meanings. After some further sessions, during which he showed a pitiful crying, he became more affectionate and responsive. He also stopped injuring himself. After two years of therapy his interaction skill was greatly improved, he started to react to what happened inside and outside the therapy room ("rain outside, "your tummy" gurgled, putting a hand to his ear as for increasing the sensitivity of the "outdoor"). He seemed to achieve a "psychological birth" and started to try to express himself toward existential themes. In Steven's case the wish for words to exist had developed only through the satisfaction perceived for being with me as a therapist able to bear the meaning of non-verbal communication.
>
> (Sinason 1992: 150–151)

The differentiation between "in"-clusion and "ex"-clusion is strongly related to the way normality and abnormality are conceptualized. The categorical classifications—even the psychopathological ones, which have been touched before—are based on a qualitative structural differentiation between normality and abnormality, while the daily experience of care providing seems to be more appropriately referred to a quantitative perspective of this differentiation. These different approaches also have ethical implications—the categorical one considers a person with neurodevelopmental disorders as a "humanly strange" individual, while the dimensional one remains focused on the suffering the person is experiencing, independently of how different he/she may appear. The intellectually disabled person makes us rethink the classical notions of norm, and places them in a larger ethical and facts-of-life frame. In short, understanding the phenomenon of "disability" is the ultimate psychopathological challenge for everyone involved.

On the other hand, "neurodiversity" is a phenomenon that confronts everyone within the core relational texture of the neurodiverse person—but mostly the neurodiverse person himself—with the hazards of a fundamentally disjointed time. The life horizon of the child and of his social context are under threat. All hopes and dreams remain literally "enveloped." The passage of time and the generational progression can slow down or even come to a halt (Ciccone 1999). Phenomenologically speaking the now appears as a perpetually frozen time of thwarted expectations and pent-up disappointments. This frozen time is the primary symptom of the trauma, as well as the ineffectual attempt to neutralize it.

Both these aspects of the traumatically threatened conditions of being-in-the-world for the disabled person and his parents form the "existential radical" which affects every domain of their life, and determines both their troubles and satisfactions. Declensions of this "radical" also manifest in the societal attribution of psychopathological character, as indicated by the terms used in the past to define ID, such as "mental retardation" or "feeble-mindedness."

This trauma casts a deep shadow on the relational history of the disabled person and his immediate *Mitwelt*, stresses his affective evolution, and enhances the risk of a problematic development of the indispensable separation and individuation. The disabled person increasingly develops a contactual ambivalence, which determines in turn an exaggerated attitude to accordance and concordance, and centripetally culminates in fusion and symbiosis with the main relational figure.

Also, this radical experience might well prove to be the *Verstehungsgrund* for the increased incidence of anxiety and depression on the one hand and the many behavioral problems on the other, the latter being a consequence of an insufficient attuning to the emotional functioning of intellectually disabled persons.

This allow us to comprehend that persons with neurodevelopmental disorders and their proxies wave between two phenomenological-psychiatric fundamental attitudes toward the way they get and keep in contact with others, as well as in their mood swings, namely between a manic and a depressive attitude. The manic attitude attempts to obliterate the handicap and tries every trick in the book to "solve" the disability. The depressive one on the contrary adopts a disillusioned relation with the disability which leads to sentences like "this is not the child we dreamed of," "we cannot even dream about this child anymore." Also the disabled child cannot allow himself to dream his own dream. For him and his proxies the dynamism of life threatens to shrivel to a static survival, bereft of any outlook.

They have to face the enormous psychic challenge of sidestepping both the pitfalls of manic denial and the depressive bleakness.

> Ali—a boy eight years old with a severe mental handicap—whose vocabulary was extremely simple "I Hulk," "I wake," "I angry," dramatically changed after having introduced bears, dolls and a clown in the therapy room. Suddenly he looked at the clown and he said "I sad," "It is not just my circumstar (his word for circumcision) that is sad" and . . . " I man now,"

"Everything all right". He lifted the clown to show me the happy face and then the sad face. . . . I said he was showing me that although he was saying everything was all right, he was sad because everything was not all right . . . ; "All right?" is very much a working-class version of "how are you?"

(Sinason 1992: 115–131)

Undoubtedly we can glean from the problematic histories of attachment some essential elements allowing us to understand that many people with an intellectual disability develop a damaged *self*, a fragile *self*, with a reduced narcissistic resilience. This raises the question of the extent to which they can overcome the intellectual disability and make their "own mind."

This perspective can help to understand why one of the main skills of many of those with intellectual disability is to adapt to what their parents and educators expect from them, and why on the contrary they have so much trouble dreaming their own dreams, going their own way, using the pathic verbs, *dare, can, may, want*, longing for their own rights, and becoming a sense-creating subject.

When an individual repeatedly experiences the feeling that he does not have control over many situations linked to internal, stable, and/or global qualities, he may generalize this experience to most circumstances in his life and develop a consciousness of being helpless. Once the helplessness is learned it leads to an expectation of adversity and the prediction of negative outcomes in future situations, which may determine in turn further cognitive and motivational deficits (Hassiotis et al. 2012).

Both from a theoretical approach and from clinical experience it becomes apparent that in the family history of a person with an intellectual disability the following five life themes are unconsciously and consciously at work at the same time (Korff-Sausse and Scelles 2017), and need to be treated, sometimes also in a therapeutic way:

1. the handicap itself as primary characteristic:
   "because I perceive myself as handicapped and not like the others, I emphasize my handicap or I behave as if it was not me" "May I become Jenny? Do you like me this way?" Indicating physically handicapped people: "they are handicapped."
2. the loss experience affecting it:
   "please don't go away and . . . ,"
3. the sense of dependency resulting from it:
   " . . . stay with me all the time and for ever" "Will you be my mum?" "When my mum dies I want to die also"
4. sexuality as source and transmission of life:
   "do you love me but I'm not allowed to have a relationship" "sexuality is something bad"
5. death and the fear of being killed as final symbols of finiteness:
   "I saw on the TV that they kill babies with Down syndrome" "They are afraid that I will have a baby" "Do you have children, are they also handicapped?"

A phenomenological support perspective needs, therefore, to focus on melting the frozen time perceived by the person with intellectual disability, which also represents the most effective way to start a process of empowerment. In effect this process implies a radical change of the existential perspective: from a timeless, static totalitarian "all or nothing" to a dynamic and hopeful "not yet" and "already," with a higher insight and a higher compliance for personal limits (see Barale et al. this volume).

EMOTIONAL AND SPIRITUAL LIFE

Scientific interest in the emotional skills of persons with intellectual disability or autism spectrum disorder is rapidly expanding, with the majority of studies addressing emotion recognition and showing a good capacity to reliably identify their own and other persons' emotions (Lindsay et al. 2004; Rose and West 1999; Sappok et al. 2016), particularly through facial expressions (Moore 2001). However, some authors identified some peculiarities in labeling specific emotions in comparison to the general population, as difficulties or advantages (Owen et al. 2001). Happiness has been repeatedly found to be more easily identified (Matheson and Jahoda 2005; Moore 2001; Owen et al. 2001; Wishart et al. 2007), while neutral faces raise higher issues (Moore 2001). There is some evidence that individuals with intellectual disability use a limited repertoire of coping strategies when emotionally aroused (Benson and Fuchs 1999), while a relationship between emotion recognition and aggression is controverted (Matheson and Jahoda 2005; Jahoda et al. 2006).

The spirituality of persons with intellectual disability has also attracted some attention in recent research. Nevertheless, the specific meaning of spirituality for people with intellectual disability and autism spectrum disorder still represents a relatively unexplored area, with little data on how such individuals see and live their own spirituality and how they express their spiritual needs (Zhang 2010).

This lack of attention comes from the common thought that a deep cognitive deficit prevents from developing and understanding immaterial life aspects.

Such investigations as there are into spiritual growth opportunities have repeatedly identified great limitations (Minton and Dodder 2003; Bertelli et al. 2011) caused by frequent expectation conflicts among care service providers and religious leaders, transportation problems, lack of support staff, and an insufficient tolerance toward some of the behaviors showed by people with neurodevelopmental disorders in the religious communities (Minton and Dodder 2003). Against old prejudices, recent neuroscientific acquisitions show that even people with the most severe intellectual disability have the potential to sense and develop an interior transcendent dimension. In fact, the emotional sphere of the human psyche, that is, the basis of spirituality, is defined as significantly distinct from the intellectual sphere, whose deficiencies determine the diagnosis of disability.

Some authors argue that rationality can even represent a limit for spirituality, providing descriptions of some extremely intense spiritual experiences in people with intellectual disability (Sulmasy 1997; Raji 2009).

According to some authors, the problem that spirituality requires a certain level of mental skills should be passed, even before being considered scientifically, through the application of prevalent philosophical-anthropological principles, which identifies spirituality as a fundamental and natural dimension in every human being regardless of the level of mental functions (Watts 2011).

In people with Down syndrome a feeling of spiritual well-being resulted in a general satisfaction toward life and other specific dimensions as self-control, building of positive relationships, acceptance of difficulties and life changes, internalization of existential meanings and aspects transcending individuality (Crompton and Jackson 2004). Recently, the connection between spirituality and quality of life was explained through the concept of "Spiritual Well-Being," which expresses how a spiritual dimension affects an individual's well-being and quality of life (Imam et al. 2009). Several studies identify spirituality as a dimension with a positive effect on the general well-being of people with intellectual disability or autism spectrum disorder (Coulter 2006; Büssing and Koenig 2010; Glicksman 2011; Liégeois 2014) and many aspects related to physical health, such as the absence of diseases (Selway and Ashman 1998; D'Souza R 2007) or the increase of life expectancy (WHO 2000).

Practical Experience

Practical experiences of people with neurodevelopmental disorders include several issues and difficulties they have to face in their daily lives. In fact, many people report finding routine activities difficult and say they need support with a variety of daily tasks such as cooking, shopping, getting around town, going to the cinema, using technology, managing money, finding a job, going to the doctor, or crossing the road. Some young adults with intellectual disability have been taught by their families or caregivers to do many tasks such as reading bus timetables or going shopping. Nevertheless, most of them find such daily activities challenging and need the help of caregivers.

According to the findings of a consultation conducted on behalf of the National Disability Authority (NDA) (Independent and Community Living: Focus Group Consultation Report; NDA 2010), grocery and clothes shopping is one area that presents difficulties for some people with intellectual disability, as we can see looking at some of the comments collected by the authors:

> I go shopping with my mam and if she tells me to go and get milk I go and give it to her. I know where everything is in the shop. Sometimes I go to the shop for a sandwich or a drink. I do shopping with my mam and sometimes on my own.
>> (NDA 2000: chapter 2.3, paragraph "Grocery shopping")

> I sometimes forget things in shops. On Sundays I get a newspaper for my nanny and my mam will write down the name of the paper that I have to get. I know how much it costs and the right change.
>> (NDA 2000: chapter 2.3, paragraph "Grocery shopping")

> I need someone with me if I was buying trousers. I buy what I want but sometimes they are not the right size. I get people to help me buy clothes . . . I can handle money ok. Staff are with me when I buy clothes.
>> (NDA 2000: chapter 2.3, paragraph "Shopping for clothes")

Getting around generally also entails a number of challenges for people with intellectual disability and low-functioning autism spectrum disorder. They may have difficulties in using public transport services, finding places in town, or crossing the road, as expressed in the words of some young adults (Independent and Community Living: Focus Group Consultation Report; NDA 2010):

> Sometimes I find it hard to cross the road. The cars go too fast and it is very dangerous not to cross at the lights. When I cross the road at traffic lights, sometimes I don't see things good and

> I can't see which way the cars are coming. If you get hit by a car, you are dead like.
>
> (NDA 2010: chapter 2.3, paragraph "Getting around")

> If you get lost in town you might not know where you are going. Me too. I got lost when I was young.
>
> (NDA 2010: chapter 2.3, paragraph "Getting around")

> When I go the cinema or anywhere I go in the car with my mam ... I have never taken a bus by myself and wouldn't like to ...
>
> (NDA 2010: chapter 2.3, paragraph "Getting around")

Moreover, some people with ID do not seem to like going out because of public attitudes they perceive, and avoid going to shops or dealing with locals in particular. They say that people "look at them funny" and "talk down to them."

Another major area of concern is living arrangements, which has been found to significantly impact on overall individual quality of life (Bertelli et al. 2013). Nevertheless, in this group issues related to housing may be particularly challenging due to difficulties specifically associated with the condition or to social disadvantages that people with ID often experience. The complexity of a person's vulnerability is often closely related to their living situations and levels of independence they have. For example, people with ID living in group home situations may have less possibility of choice, becoming more exposed to neglect or exploitation by staff or other decision-makers (https://communitydoor.org. au).

People with intellectual disability may have difficulties in accepting the high number of regulations operating in residential services, which they perceive as a restriction on their choices. In some cases, older people with intellectual disability feel that staff members do not treat them like adults, even though they acknowledge that staff are probably concerned with their safety (Independent and Community Living: Focus Group Consultation Report; NDA 2010). We can better understand this view by looking at the words of an adult with intellectual disability living in a residential service:

> You have to come in at this time and to have a bath when I don't want a bath. I want a bath tomorrow. The same with dinner—you have fish today but I don't want fish, I want steak. They take the kettle away at night (for safety) and you can't make tea before you go to bed ... There is too much safety at times. It has gone over the top. People should be allowed to make mistakes. There is too much control. You have to give people choices and be able to make mistakes.
>
> (NDA 2010: chapter 2.4, paragraph "Group housing")

Most of the younger adults with ID would like to live more independently away from their families and staff (Independent and Community Living: Focus Group Consultation Report; NDA 2010). They believe that living independently would allow them to have greater freedom to do what they want, to go where they want (provided it is safe), and to have their own space. Nevertheless, at the same time most of them feel they would require assistance with various daily routines.

> I would be a little bit worried living by myself. Sometimes the 23 bus doesn't go when it should. Sometimes I am lazy. I don't do much cooking. I love to cook but when I see my mam cooking I can see it is difficult.
>
> (NDA 2010: chapter 2.4, paragraph "Accommodation")

I would just like to have a housemate. I have three carers who come in and I do get time on my own but I would like more time on my own without staff coming and going. I feel it is not my house.

> (NDA 2010: chapter 2.4, paragraph "Accommodation")

I live out in independent living. I wash and cook myself. I don't have to wait for the staff to cook for me. I cook my own dinner and my own tea. I am able to do everything and I pay my own bills for the house. I have emergency response in case anyone comes to the door. It records to see who is outside. I am safe.....I live on my own. I love it.

> (NDA 2010: chapter 2.4, paragraph "Independent accommodation")

I want to live in an apartment, maybe close to where I live now in Donabate or maybe in Lusk or Balbriggan. I would like to live with my girlfriend.

> (NDA 2010: chapter 2.4, paragraph "Accommodation")

According to the findings of the above-mentioned consultation, when asked what they would do with €1,000, most people with intellectual and developmental disorders would like to go on holiday, give money to their families, and buy a house. One participant with complex physical and intellectual disability said he would just like to be respected, to perceive himself as important, and to be listened to when he expresses his opinion (NDA 2010).

Physical and mental health problems, unemployment, poor or inadequate education, social isolation, inappropriate or unsafe accommodation represent common risk factors for socio-economic disadvantage for many people with intellectual disability.

It is likely that the relation between economic disadvantage and intellectual and developmental disabilities is due in part to the health and social inequalities people with these conditions and their families experience. This relation seems to reflect two distinct processes. First, poverty is a risk factor for the development of these disorders, an effect which is mediated through the correlation between the socio-economic disadvantage and exposure to a number of environmental and psychosocial hazards. Second, families supporting a person with intellectual disabilities are at greater risk of experiencing poverty due to the financial and social impact of caring and the exclusion of people with intellectual disabilities from the working environment.

Practical experiences are more than just utilitarian activities, they represent a declension of an incarnate (gestaltung) inclusion, and have a relational implication. Carrying out practical tasks defines the extent to which a person with neurodevelopmental disorders expresses the intersubjective meaning of "doing," and the way he/she is in the world with others.

Social Experience

People with neurodevelopmental disorders say they like having friends but in fact many of them do not have friends outside their care facilities. Their social life is often limited to people and places where they feel safe and as a result most of their friendships are restricted to people they meet in the services and their families at home (WWILD Sexual Violence Prevention Association Inc. 2018). Due to their impaired social skills and their behavioral peculiarities, persons with intellectual disability may not be able to avoid or end social situations they perceive as negative and it seems that the relationships they establish are characterized by less intimacy and reciprocity than those of their peers without intellectual disability. Furthermore, their sexuality is likely to be limited. This has both historical and contemporary causes which are closely related to the eugenics arguments that were prevalent early this century and to prevailing attitudes toward people with intellectual disability which can compel them to have sexual intercourse secretly, increasing their risk of being victims of abuse (Johnson et al. 2001).

Sexual health is a vital but often neglected aspect of health care for people with neurodevelopmental disorders (Eastgate 2011). For decades, they were thought to be asexual, having no need for loving and fulfilling relationships with others. Individual rights to sexuality have been denied with negative consequences on their gender identity, friendships, self-esteem, body image, emotional growth, and social behavior (Joint Position Statement of AAIDD and The Arc 2013. Available at: https://aaidd.org).

In reality, young adults with mild intellectual disability seem to understand love very concretely, describing it as a combination of various positive feelings that produces happiness, peace of mind, and good mood (Mattila et al. 2017). They also perceived love as a fundamental part of their lives, with a crucial impact on overall well-being (Lee and Oh 2013). Young adults with ID connect love with precise personal experiences, understanding love in many ways. The behaviors they describe are mainly associated with daily interactions and attention paid to the partner, such as each supporting the other, tenderness, presence and attention, honesty, listening, and intimacy (Mattila et al. 2016; Lumley and Scotti 2001).

> Well, you can feel it when you fall in love. At least I do have the sensation that someone really cares. You can really know it, too, if the other one does not care, you can sense it.
>
> (Mattila et al. 2017: 300)

Specific social challenges are experienced at school and during other training and educational routes. A significant percentage of people with intellectual disability or autism spectrum disorder present serious communication impairments, and it is quite common for them to leave school without having achieved basic reading, writing, and math skills. They often need learning support and they are less likely to participate in school activities. These and other issues related to the school environment can significantly influence young people with intellectual disability the opportunity to benefit as they should from their educational experiences. Children and adolescents with intellectual deficits are often passive, submissive, and clumsy and, therefore, they are easier victims of abuse and bullying by peers. O'Connor and Fowkes (2000: 4) reported the words of one such individual:

> I knew there was something wrong with me. There were certain things I couldn't do in my head. Lots of students just thought I didn't want to go to school. They said things about me behind my back, things that really hurt then. They said I had brain damage. Would have hated to be at Special School because people would tease you, treat you like a fool. Sometimes I would be chased and bullied by two guys, verbally abused. I used to hide.

A lack of acceptance or experiences of discrimination in school were a major concern for them. Besides being the result of direct social experiences the negative impact of stigma may also influence their self-concept, leading to low levels of self-esteem. Whatever form discrimination takes, there has been consistent evidence that people with moderate to mild intellectual disabilities are aware of the stigmatized treatment that they experience (Beart, Hardy, and Buchan 2005).

> In school (elementary school), it was unhappy for us that they (classmates) saw us in strange ways. I didn't like it and felt embarrassed. Their stares made me feel like a monster!
>
> (Chen and Shu 2012: 246)

People with intellectual disability may sense stigmatized treatment throughout their lives and feel rejected by their peers (Zic and Lgric 2001; Cutts and Sigafoos 2001; Cooney, Jahoda, and Knott 2006). A particularly challenging time is the transition from school into employment. In fact, after leaving school many young people with intellectual disability have difficulties in finding a work or valued roles in their community, due to the negative social perception or confined social environment (Chappell, Goodley, and Lawthom 2001). The many challenging characteristics and behaviors that individuals with intellectual disability or autism spectrum disorder present can make them appear unsuitable for employment (Hendricks and Wehman 2009), with an additional negative impact on their social inclusion (Wilson et al. 2017) and psychological distress (Dagnan and Waring 2004).

Although it is commonly believed that people with ID receive a lot assistance from family members, service providers, or other organizations, in fact, many of them experience social isolation and exclusion.

> I'd like to have friends. It's really hard. I've tried lots of groups but none have worked out. I get really worried about if anyone is going to like me and if anyone is going to have things in common with me and it goes around in my mind and it's hard to decide to go, so a lot of times I don't.
>
> (O'Connor and Fowkes 2000: 5)

A great majority of people with neurodevelopmental disorders have limited resources to develop connections with others members of the community and to participate in community activities. As a result, they are often socially restricted to organizationally based social activities with other people with neurodevelopmental disorders (WWILD Sexual Violence Prevention Association Inc. 2018) and rely on support systems for developing and maintaining meaningful relationships within other contexts. Discrimination and prejudice against people with intellectual disability are often major challenges to their inclusion in the social networks of the community.

According to Abbott and McConkey (2006), people with intellectual disability themselves recognize various barriers to community inclusion, for example, not being accepted by other individuals or having limited opportunities for social exchange. A systematic review of the literature (Verdonschot et al. 2009) has identified a number of environmental factors which positively condition the participation of persons with intellectual disability in community activities. Some of these factors are decision-making opportunities, environmental stimulation, engagement of families, presence of services, social support, and positive personal attitudes.

People with intellectual disability are also more vulnerable to becoming victims of crime than the general population. This is probably due to the nature of their condition and the life circumstances in which they live which may make them extremely vulnerable to such experiences. French (2007) suggests that between 50 and 99% of people with intellectual and psychosocial impairments are subject to sexual assault in their lifetimes. The lack of meaningful and emotionally helpful relationships may increase their possibility of experiencing sexual assault through their search for companionship. An overwhelming majority of victims are women but men are also highly vulnerable to experiencing sexual assault

(Murray and Powell 2008). Moreover, sexual assault against people with intellectual disability is more likely to be repeated or violent (French 2007).

These attacks occur very often in familiar places and the perpetrator is generally a person known to the victim, such as another person with intellectual disability who frequents the same living or social environments, or service providers (e.g. teachers, caregivers, or support staff) (French 2007). According to Sobsey (1994), vulnerable people are made more vulnerable by the prevailing attitude of our society which teaches a person with disability to be compliant, especially toward authority figures.

EXPRESSING MENTAL HEALTH SUFFERING

In people with intellectual disability psychopathological suffering is usually much more difficult to identify than in the general population. Beside the "diagnostic overshadowing," which refers to the difficulty of distinguishing the adjunctive psychopathological symptoms from the observed or referred dysfunctions and behavioral alterations due to the basic condition of intellectual disability (Reiss et al. 1982; Reiss and Szyszko 1983; Deb et al. 2001; Jopp and Keys 2001), there are issues linked to the presentation of symptoms, which often is atypical, chaotic, intermittent, fluctuating, masked, mixed, or poorly defined.

The literature highlights a variety of factors that may determine these peculiarities, such as the developmental level, previous life experiences, and interpersonal, cultural, and environmental influences (Sovner 1986). Deficits in abstract thinking can limit introspective capacity and lead to difficulties in recognizing emotional symptoms, in defining one's own life experiences, and in communicating states of suffering (Sovner 1986; Cooper et al. 2003). People with intellectual disability can be passive and compliant due to a lower ability to tolerate stress and to a consequent anxiety-induced decompensation (Sovner 1986). People with more severe intellectual disability tend to express their psychic suffering exclusively through behavioral changes, including an increase in the severity or frequency of chronic maladaptive behaviors ("baseline exaggeration effect"; Sovner 1986; Sturmey and Ley 1990; Moss et al. 2000). Poor verbal expression abilities, impoverished social skills, and typical life experiences may also develop into "psychosocial masking" (Sovner 1986) that may lead to symptoms which do not seem as rich and defined as in the general population. An aspect that strongly characterizes the emotional dysregulation of many persons with intellectual disability is the neurovegetative vulnerability, with pains, organ dysfunctions, changes in circadian rhythms, and dystonia of the autonomic nervous system being very frequent (Costello and Bouras 2006).

The extent to which a behavioral change or problem can be interpreted as an expression of psychic suffering is a key question in psychopathology of intellectual disability. Some studies identified a relationship between problem behaviors and psychiatric disorders in people with intellectual disability (Emerson et al. 1999; Felce et al. 2009; Hemmings et al. 2006; Kishore et al. 2005; Moss et al. 2000; Rojahn et al. 2004), particularly strong in individuals with lower level of functioning (Felce et al. 2009), and some problem behaviors have been reported to be symptoms' equivalents of specific disorders (Hurley 2006), especially if accompanied by other observable symptoms of the same disorder, such as sleep alteration, considerable appetite changes, or neurovegetative dystonias (Charlot 2005). Other studies found no evidence of equivalence (Tsiouris et al. 2003) and maintained that problem and maladaptive behaviors should be interpreted as non-specific indicators of emotional distress rather than atypical symptoms (Rojahn and Meier 2009).

In spite of all this, psychological vulnerability of intellectual disability is a neglected topic in the mental health sector, particularly in adult psychiatry. Care needs often remain undetected and unmet (Baxter et al. 2006; Lindsay et al. 2006).

Many reasons have been identified for this lack of attention, including the above mentioned atypical presentation of symptoms and the diagnostic overshadowing with the manifestations of the neurodevelopmental disorder itself. However, the most relevant one is probably the assumption that the early neurodevelopmental impairment represents an untreatable neurological condition which significantly and definitely compromises the overall psychic functioning, so that there is not even the possibility of experiencing psychiatric suffering or at least of using any of the psychopathological knowledge acquired with the general population. Another major linked reason is a lengthy historiography of discrimination and stigma.

THE ISSUE OF UNITARY INTELLIGENCE

As mentioned earlier, intelligence reduction has a central role in the diagnostic criteria of intellectual disability in the current classification systems (WHO 2001; APA 2000; 2013). It is also very relevant for the differential diagnosis with autism spectrum disorder and between autism spectrum disorder sub-groups. In the DSM-5 intelligence is still defined in a very general way, as reasoning, problem-solving, planning, abstract thinking, judgment, academic learning, and learning from experience.

At present the assessment of intelligence is carried out exclusively through IQ measurement, although there is mounting evidence on that this often determines generic diagnostic labels and fails to capture individual variability in specific cognitive skills as well as the association with other variables of interest, such as genetic or biological factors.

Intelligence theories have evolved over the years, from unicomponential (g factor) or oligocomponential models, measuring individual performance on all cognitive tasks with a unique score, to more differentiated structures, with a combination of multiple specialized and interrelated cognitive functions, such as the Cattell-Horn-Carroll (McGrew 2005) or the "Planning, Attention, Simultaneous, and Successive" (Naglieri and Das 2002) models. At the same time, new instruments for measuring IQ level have been developed. Unfortunately, their utility in people with neurodevelopmental disorders is still questioned. The presence of the widely known floor effects and other measurements problems specific of this population limit the efficacy in capturing intellectual functioning, specifically of those with more severe impairment.

Research findings reveal that in people with intellectual disability the same IQ score can be related to very different cognitive weaknesses and strengths, also on the basis of ethiopathogenic factors (Simon 2010; Bertelli et al. 2014). As an example, persons with Down syndrome usually manifest impairments in specific areas of language, long-term memory, and motor performance, while showing relative strengths in visuo-spatial construction (Edgin et al. 2010). In contrast persons with Williams syndrome present deficits in attention, visuo-spatial construction, short-term memory, and planning (Tiekstra et al. 2009), while showing relative ability in auditory processing and concrete language (Thornton-Wells et al. 2010).

Furthermore, deficits in individual functioning, behavioral problems, and neuro-bio-psychological alterations associated with intellectual disability are reported in the literature to be more significantly correlated with the impairment of specific cognitive function rather than with overall IQ score (Bertelli et al. 2014).

The variability between and within cognitive phenotypes is also present in autism spectrum disorder. Of particular interest is the finding that in people with autism spectrum disorder low IQ scores are not necessarily a direct expression of an impairment of overall cognitive functioning, since they strictly correlate with anomalies of information processing, which in turn have pervasive effects on the overall intellectual functioning (Scheuffgen et al. 2000; Anderson 2008).

Despite this evidence, specific cognitive functions in people with neurodevelopmental disorders are still not given much attention, either in research or daily practice. Different terms are often used for the same functions, and vice versa. Also the differentiation between specific cognitive functions and executive functions is often uncertain. Studies are scanty and limited to working memory, orientation response, and attention switch (Bertelli et al. 2016). Thus, there is still no conceptual map or hierarchy of the cognitive functions and domains in neurodevelopmental disorders (Bilder et al. 2009). However, in people with intellectual disability a series of cognitive domains have been reported to be more significantly impaired than others, and include perceptual reasoning, working memory, processing speed, and verbal comprehension (Deary 2001; Holdnack et al. 2011).

The above-mentioned WHO Working Group for the revision of ICD-10 addressed this issue by proposing for conceptualization of intellectual disability within the ICD-11 the adoption of an articulated model of cognitive impairment, which might have relevant implications not only for education and services provision, but also for the general cultural attitude toward intellectual disability itself (Bertelli et al. 2018). This model juxtaposes a new concept of dimensional cognitive characterization with that of normal/subnormal intelligence and substitutes the measurement of IQ with the assessment of very specific cognitive functions and a contextualized description of consequent adaptive and learning difficulties. According to this approach, the clinical evaluation should aim to identify those cognitive dysfunctions that have the greatest negative impact in terms of behavior, adjustment, autonomy, and above all quality of life across the life-span (Bertelli 2016). A retesting during critical life periods would also be useful, as distinct cognitive developmental trajectories have been identified in different intellectual developmental disorders (Hodapp et al. 1991; Chapman and Hesketh 2000; Abbeduto et al. 2007) and cognitive losses overcome related to ageing, earlier and more frequently than in the general population.

Examples of neuropsychological tools used for revealing more complex profiles of cognitive functioning are KAIT—*Kaufman Adolescent and Adult Intelligence Test*, WCST—*Wisconsin Card Sorting Test*, and CAS—*Cognitive Assessment System*, for which simplified versions have been provided. Nevertheless, these tests are difficult to carry out on those with an intellectual disability or autism spectrum disorder. The complexity of these issues requires the use of neuropsychological measures progressively and promptly adapted to the various levels of severity of intellectual disability.

ADAPTIVE BEHAVIOR AND ATTUNEMENT
TO THE ENVIRONMENT

Adaptive behavior includes cognitive, social, and practical skills; it increases in complexity with developmental stages. For each age class, the appropriate levels of adaptive behavior are not exactly definable because they depend on the expectations of the environment (Jacobson and Mulik 1996). The scientific community agrees that adaptive behavior is a multidimensional construct, but there is no agreement about the nature or number of factors that should be considered for its definition (Schalock 1999; Thompson et al. 1999), although several pieces of research have been conducted to answer this question (Janicki and Jacobson 1986; Widaman et al. 1987; Bruininks et al. 1988), as well as to identify typical patterns of adaptive behavior in people with genetic syndromes including intellectual disability and autism spectrum disorder, such as Down syndrome (Loveland and Kelly 1991) or Fragile X syndrome (Dykens et al. 1993).

From a practical point of view, the assessment of adaptive behavior is based on the evaluation of individual daily performance in facing up to various situations in different life environments.

The DSM-5 and the forthcoming ICD-11 emphasizes the need to adopt standardized clinical evaluations for the diagnosis of intellectual disability, based on the severity of the impairment in adaptive behaviors rather than on the IQ score (APA 2013; WHO 2018). The three domains of main impact have been identified as conceptual (language, writing, reading, reasoning, and memory abilities), social (awareness of other people's thoughts and emotions, empathy, social judgment, interpersonal relationships), and practical (self-management, e.g. personal care, social responsibility, leisure activities, organization of school, and work tasks) (APA 2013). Most common assessment tools, such as the Vineland Adaptive Behavior Scales (Sparrow et al. 2005; Balboni and Pedrabissi 2003) or the Adaptive Behavior Assessment System (ABAS II; Oakland and Harrison 2008), detail these main domains in a variety of areas, including conceptual skills (i.e. arithmetic skills, knowing numbers, and shapes), communication (i.e. comprehension and use of written and oral language), daily living skills (i.e. self-care, home living, professional activities), socialization (i.e. interpersonal relationships, social problem-solving, recreational activities, respect of social norms, community use), health and safety (i.e. following safety rules, showing caution when needed, staying out of danger, and knowing when to get help), leisure (i.e. playing, hobbies, following rules in games, planning fun activities), self-direction (i.e. self-control, making choices, starting and completing tasks, following a routine, and following directions), and motor skills (both gross and fine).

The assessment of adaptive behaviors is particularly useful in planning and verifying individualized intervention programs and in monitoring rehabilitative progress; some phenomenologists argue that it may also be considered an operationalization of the level of attunement between the person and his environment (*Um-Mitwelt*) (Dōsen and De Groef 2015).

In the context of adaptive skills, the terms functioning and behavior are frequently used synonymously. Limited intellectual functioning affects social and emotional functioning. Many persons with intellectual disability function on an emotional and social level far below the average for their age. Impairments in functioning consist in lack of attainment of developmental and sociocultural standards for personal autonomy and social responsibility. Without continuing support, these deficits limit functioning in daily activities, such as communication, social participation, and autonomy, and in different areas, such as family, school, work, and community.

One of the problems with the functioning label is that it tends to focus almost exclusively on IQ and main abilities. However, this is a very narrow scope for neurodevelopmental disorders, which are by definition pervasive across all areas of a person's life, with high interindividual differentiation. There are persons with a considerable impairment of IQ and overall adaptation who have minimal difficulties with their everyday lives, while others who are labeled high functioning may be experiencing unemployment and friendlessness.

New Outcome for Life Experience

In recent years, scientific research has focused more on person-centred outcomes and quality of life. The latter in particular has repeatedly been defined as an essential component in the intervention planning and evaluation of intellectual disability and autism spectrum disorder, where the recovering of neuropsychic functions cannot be pursued as in other mental or physical conditions in the general population.

Quality of life evaluation aims at identify how the individual might achieve a satisfying life and be able to participate in society, take advantage of opportunities, and have the potential to make independent choices. According to this approach, the quality of life model consists in the identification of a way of living and not in the attainment of a specific goal (Bertelli and Brown 2006). The expression thus defines a multidimensional concept, involving several definitions and applications (Brown and Brown 2003; Schalock 2005; Verdugo et al. 2005; Bertelli and Brown 2006).

There is general agreement that quality of life measurement should be based on both qualitative and quantitative variables (Bertelli and Brown 2006; Cummins 2005), from both subjective and objective positions (Summers et al. 2005). For people with intellectual disability and autism spectrum disorder the most adequate models are the "whole-person" ones (Brown and Brown 2009), that refer to individual complexity and not specifically to areas of dysfunction. A very comprehensive approach is the one proposed by the Centre for Health Promotion of the University of Toronto (Brown et al. 1997), which includes nine areas applicable to every person's life to be defined for individual modulation by four dimensions: importance attributed, satisfaction perceived, self-determination, and opportunities. This last dimension refers to the opportunities a person has to develop importance and to experience satisfaction. The areas are organized in three major categories: Being (physical, psychological, and spiritual), Belonging (physical, social, and community), and Becoming (practical, leisure, and growth).

The quality of life model represents an excellent conceptual parameter in maintaining life projects of people with intellectual disability and autism spectrum disorder aligned with those of other people. In fact, this criterion is the sharing of the qualitative aspect of existence, independently of specific psychophysical conditions (Caldin 2014).

The quality of life model has been shown to have a number of positive implications for care and intervention in neurodevelopmental disorders, including alleviating the care-giver burden, support, health services, and health policies (Schalock et al. 2002). Despite this, an optimal implementation of the concept of quality of life into daily practices for the full range of cognitive impairments is yet to come, as well as a definition of its relationship with the non-reductionistic approach of the phenomenological tradition.

The phenomenological conceptualization of neurodiversity and the quality of life perspective share the same major conceptual premises, such as the centrality of the individual experience, the consideration of emic aspects of human life, or the "gestalted" (articulated) being-in-the-world-with-others (Fédida 1986; Fédida and Schotte 1991; De Groef 1997).

Conclusions

The term "neurodiversity" is commonly used to refer to neurodevelopmental disorders, which represents a group of life-span conditions with early childhood onset, characterized by impairments of conceptual, social, and practical adaptive skills. Among these, intellectual disability and autism spectrum disorder are the most common, connoted respectively by cognitive and socio-emotional difficulties.

The life of a "neurodiverse" person is punctuated by subjective, practical, and social experiences which imply a considerable difficulty in defining the width of the atypicalness of the first-person givenness and self-development over time. The daily being-in-the-world is much more challenging than for the neurotypical person, due to lack of environmental mastery, low coping abilities, communication deficits, and difficulties in self-determination, while the environmental influence is most frequently expressed by lack of satisfactory social relations and practical activities, inadequate living arrangements, repeated failures, or other negative life events and traumatic experiences. Existential issues, such as self-origin, insight, time flow, mortality, singularity, or transcendentality may be conceptualized as a phenomenological reduction to the basic categories that structure our common human condition. Nevertheless, this "neurodiverse" perspective seems to retain some relevant utilities for life skills that the neurotypical persons increasingly seem to lose in their chaotic and high performance-requiring lives. For instance, the *quality of life* approach, which was originally developed for persons with ID, may in fact benefit anyone wishing to define their relationship between personal attribution of importance and perception of satisfaction toward most emic areas of life.

Bibliography

Abbeduto L., Warren S. F., and Conners F. A. (2007). "Language Development in Down's Syndrome: From the Prelinguistic Period to the Acquisition of Literacy." *Mental Retardation and Developmental Disabilities Research Reviews* 13(3): 247–261.

Abbott S. and McConkey R. (2006). "The Barriers to Social Inclusion as Perceived by People with Intellectual Disabilities." *Journal of Intellectual Disabilities* 10: 275–286.

Achkova M. and Manolova H. (2014). "Diagnosis Autism—from Kanner 1—and Asperger to DSM-5." *Intellectual Disability—Diagnosis and Treatment* 2(2):112–117.

Anderson M. (2008). "What Can Autism and Dyslexia Tell Us About Intelligence?" *Quarterly Journal of Experimental Psychology* 61(1): 116–128.

American Psychiatric Association. (1952). *Diagnostic and Statistical Manual of Mental Disorders*, 1st edn. Washington, DC: Author.

American Psychiatric Association. (1968). *Diagnostic and Statistical Manual of Mental Disorders*, 2nd edn. Washington, DC: Author.

American Psychiatric Association. (1980). *Diagnostic and Statistical Manual of Mental Disorders*, 3rd edn. Washington, DC: Author.

American Psychiatric Association. (2000). *Diagnostic and Statistical Manual of Mental Disorders*, 4th edn., text rev. Washington, DC: Author.

American Psychiatric Association. (2013). *Diagnostic and Statistical Manual*, 5th edn. Washington, DC: Author.

Balboni G. and Pedrabissi L. (2003). *VABS-Vineland Adaptive Behavior Scales.* Firenze: Giunti O.S.

Baxter H., Lowe K., Houston H., Jones G., Felce D., and Kerr M. (2006). "Previously Unidentified Morbidity in Patients with Intellectual Disability." *The British Journal of General Practice* 56(523): 93–98.

Beart S, Hardy G., and Buchan L. (2005). "How People with Intellectual Disabilities View Their Social Identity: A Review of the Literature." *Journal of Applied Research in Intellectual Disabilities* 18: 47–56.

Benson B. A. and Fuchs C. (1999). "Anger-arousing Situations and Coping Responses of Aggressive Adults with Intellectual Disability." *Journal of Intellectual & Developmental Disability* 24(3): 207–214.

Bertelli M. (2015). "Mental Health and Intellectual Disability: Integrating Different Approaches in the Neurodevelopmental Perspective." *Advances in Mental Health and Intellectual Disabilities* 9(5): 217–221.

Bertelli M. (2016). "The 10th EAMHID International Congress: Integrating Different Approaches in the Neurodevelopmental Perspective—The Mental Health Care Evolution Timeline." *Advances in Mental Health and Intellectual Disabilities* 10(1): 1–5.

Bertelli M. and Brown I. (2006). "Quality of Life for People with Intellectual Disabilities." *Current Opinion in Psychiatry* 19: 508–513.

Bertelli M., Hassiotis A., Deb S., and Salvador-Carulla L. (2009). "New Contributions of Psychiatric Research in the Field of Intellectual Disability." In G. N. Christodoulou, M. Jorge, and J. E. Mezzich (eds.), *Advances in Psychiatry*, pp. 37–43 (Vol. 3). Athens: Beta Medical Publishers.

Bertelli M., Piva Merli M., Bianco A., Lassi S., La Malfa G., Placidi G. F., and Brown I. (2011). "A Battery of Instruments to aAsess Quality of Life (BASIQ): Validation of the Italian Adaptation of the Quality of Life Instrument Package (QoL-IP)." *Italian Journal of Psychopathology* 17: 205–212.

Bertelli M., Salvador-Carulla L., Lassi S., Zappella M., Ceccotto R., Palterer D., De Groef J., Benni L., and Rossi Prodi P. (2013). "Quality of life and living arrangements for people with intellectual disability." *Advances in Mental Health and Intellectual Disabilities* 7(4): 220–223.

Bertelli M. O., Salvador-Carulla L., Scuticchio D., Varrucciu N., Martinez-Leal R., Cooper S. A., Simeonsson R. J., Deb S., Weber G., Jung R., Munir K., Adnams C., Akoury-Dirani L., Girimaji S. C., Katz G., Kwok H., and Walsh, C. (2014). "Moving Beyond Intelligence in the

Revision of ICD-10: Specific Cognitive Functions in Intellectual Developmental Disorders." *World Psychiatry* 13(1): 93–94.

Bertelli M., Bianco A., Piva Merli M., and Salvador-Carulla L. (2015). "The Person-Centered Health Model in Intellectual Developmental Disorders/Intellectual Disability." *European Journal of Psychiatry* 29(4): 239–248.

Bertelli M. O., Salvador-Carulla L., and Harris J. (2016). "Classification and Diagnosis." In C Hemmings and N. Bouras (eds.), *Psychiatric and Behavioural Disorders in Intellectual and Developmental Disabilities*. Cambridge: Cambridge University Press.

Bertelli M. O., Cooper S. A., and Salvador-Carulla L. (2018). "Intelligence and Specific Cognitive Functions in Intellectual Disability: Implications for Assessment and Classification." *Current Opinion in Psychiatry* 31(2): 88–95.

Bilder R. M., Sabb F. W., Parker D. S., Kalar D., Chu W. W., Fox J., Freimer N. B., and Poldrack R. A. (2009). "Cognitive Ontologies for Neuropsychiatric Phenomics Research." *Cognitive Neuropsychiatry* 14(4–5): 419–450.

Binswanger L. (1962). *Grundformen und Erkenntnis menschlichen Daseins*. München/Basel: Ernst Reinhardt Verlag.

Bleuler E. (1911). *Dementia Praecox or the Group of Schizophrenias*. (Reprinted 1950). New York: International University Press.

Bradley E. A., Summers J. A., Wood H. L., and Bryson S. E. (2004). "Comparing Rates of Psychiatric and Behavior Disorders in Adolescents and Young Adults with Severe Intellectual Disability with and without Autism." *Journal of Autism and Developmental Disorders* 34(2): 151–61.

Bruininks R., McGrew K., and Maruyama G. (1988). "Structure of Adaptive Behavior in Samples with and without Mental Retardation." *American Journal on Mental Retardation* 3: 265–272.

Brown I., Renwick R., and Raphael D. (1997). *Quality of Life Instrument Package for Adults with Developmental Disabilities*. Toronto: Centre for Health Promotion, University of Toronto.

Brown I. and Brown R. (2003). *Quality of Life and Disability: An Approach for Community Practitioners*. London: Jessica Kingsley Publishers.

Brown I. and Brown R. (2009). "Choice as an Aspect of Quality of Life for People with Intellectual Disabilities." *Journal of Policy and Practice in Intellectual Disabilities* 6: 10–17.

Büssing A. and Koenig K. G. (2010). "Spiritual Needs of Patients with Chronic Diseases." *Religions* 1: 18–27.

Caldin R. (2014). "Educazione religiosa e disabilità." In F. Arici and R. Gabbiadini (eds.), *La risorsa religione e i suoi dinamismi. Studi multidisciplinari in dialogo* Milano: Franco Angeli.

Center J., Beange H., and McElduff A. (1998). "People with Mental Retardation Have an Increased Prevalence of Osteoporosis: A Population Study." *American Journal of Mental Retardation* 103: 19–28.

Chapman R. S. and Hesketh L. J. (2000). "Behavioral Phenotype of Individuals with Down's Syndrome." *Mental Retardation and Developmental Disabilities Research Reviews* 6(2): 84–95.

Chappell A. L., Goodley D., and Lawthom R. (2001). "Making Connections: The Relevance of the Social Model of Disability for People with Learning Difficulties." *British Journal of Learning Disabilities* 29: 45–50.

Charlot L. (2005). "Use of Behavioral Equivalents for Symptoms of Mood Disorders." In P. Sturney (ed.), *Mood Disorders in People with Mental Retardationm*, pp. 17–45. New York: NADD Press.

Chen C.-H. and Shu B.-C. (2012). "The Process of Perceiving Stigmatization: Perspectives from Taiwanese Young People with Intellectual Disability." *Journal of Applied Research in Intellectual Disabilities* 25: 240–251.

Ciccone A. (1999). *La transmission psychique inconsciente*. Paris: Dunod.

Cooney G., Jahoda A., Cumley A., and Knott F.(2006). "Young People with Intellectual Disabilities Attending Mainstream and Segregated Schooling: Perceived Stigma, Social Comparison and Future Aspirations." *Journal of Intellectual Disability Research* 50: 432–444.

Cooper S. A. (1999). "The Relationship Between Psychiatric and Physical Health in Elderly People with Intellectual Disability." *Journal of Intellectual Disability Research* 43: 54–60.

Cooper S. A., Melville C. A., and Einfeld S. L. (2003). "Psychiatric Diagnosis, Intellectual Disabilities and Diagnostic Criteria for Psychiatric Disorders for Use with Adults with Learning Disabilities/Mental Retardation (DC-LD)." *Journal of Intellectual Disability Research* 47(1): 3–15.

Cooper S. A., Smiley E., Morrison J., Williamson A., and Allan J. (2007). "Mental Ill-health in Adults with Intellectual Disabilities: Prevalence and Associated Factors." *British Journal of Psychiatry* 190: 27–35.

Costello H. and Bouras N. (2006). "Assessment of Mental Health Problems in People with Intellectual Disabilities." *Israel Journal of Psychiatry & Related Sciences* 43(4): 241–251.

Coulter D. L. (2006). "Presidential Address 2005: Peace-making is the Answer: Spiritual Valorization and the Future of Our Field." *Mental Retardation* 44(1): 64–70.

Crompton M. and Jackson R. (2004). *Spiritual Well-being of Adults with Down Syndrome*. Southsea, Hampshire: The Down Syndrome Education Trust.

Cummins R. A. (2005). "Moving from the Quality of Life Concept to a Theory." *Journal of Intellectual Disability Research* 49: 699–706.

Cutts S. and Sigafoos J. (2001). "Social Competence and Peer Interactions of Students with Intellectual Disability in an Inclusive High School." *Journal of Intellectual and Developmental Disability* 26: 127–141.

Dagnan D. and Waring M. (2004). "Linking Stigma to Psychological Distress: Testing a Social–Cognitive Model of the Experience of People with Intellectual Disabilities." *Clinical Psychology and Psychotherapy* 11: 247–254.

De Groef J. (1997). "Du sei wie Du, de l'amour et de la passion." *Le Coq-Héron* 145: 43–51.

De Groef J. and Heinemann E. (1999). *Psychoanalysis and Mental Handicap*. London: FAB.

Deary I. J. (2001) *Intelligence: A Very Short Introduction*. Oxford: Oxford University Press.

Deb S., Thomas M., and Bright C. (2001). "Mental Disorder in Adults with Intellectual Disability. 2: The Rate of Behavior Disorders Among a Community-based Population Aged Between 16 and 64 Years." *Journal of Intellectual Disability Research* 45(6): 506–514.

Dell'Osso L., Dalle Luche R., and Maj M. (2015a). "Adult Autism Spectrum as a Transnosographic Dimension." *CNS Spect* 9: 1–3.

Dell'Osso L., Dalle Luche R., Cerliani C., Bertelloni C. A., Gesi C., and Carmassi C. (2015b). "Unexpected Subthreshold Autism Spectrum in a 25-year-old Male Stalker Hospitalized for Delusional Disorder: A Case Report." *Comprehensive Psychiatry* 61: 10–14.

Dixon-Ibarra A. and Horner-Johnson W. (2014). "Disability Status as an Antecedent to Chronic Conditions: National Health Interview Survey, 2006–2012." *Preventing Chronic Disease* 30(11): E15.

Dosen A. and De Groef J. (2015). "What is Normal Behaviour in Persons with Developmental Disabilities?" *Advances in Mental Health and Intellectual Disabilities* 9(5): 284–294.

D'Souza R. (2007). "The Importance of Spirituality in Medicine and Its Application to Clinical Practice." *Medical Journal of Australia* 186(10): 57–59.

Dykens E. M., Hodapp R. M., Ort S. I., and Leckman J. F. (1993). "Trajectory of Adaptive Behavior in Males with Fragile X Syndrome." *Journal of Autism and Developmental Disorders* 23(1): 135–145.

Eastgate G. (2011). "Sex and Intellectual Disability: Dealing with Sexual Health Issues." *Australian Family Physician* 40(4): 188.

Edgin J. O., Pennington B. F., and Mervis C. B. (2010). "Neuropsychological Components of Intellectual Disability: The Contributions of Immediate, Working, and Associative Memory." *Journal of Intellectual Disability Research* 54(5): 406–417.

Emerson E., Moss S., and Kiernan C. K. (1999). "The Relationship Between Challenging Behavior and Psychiatric Disorders in People with Severe Intellectual Disabilities." In N. Bouras (ed.), *Psychiatric and Behavioral Disorders in Mental Retardation*, pp. 38–48. Cambridge: Cambridge University Press.

Emerson E., Einfeld S., and Stancliffe R. J. (2010). "The Mental Health of Young Children with Intellectual Disabilities or Borderline Intellectual Functioning." *Social Psychiatry and Psychiatric Epidemiology* 45(5): 579–587.

Fédida P. (1986). *Phénoménologie, Psychiatrie, Psychanalyse*. Paris: ed. G.R.E.U.P.P.

Fédida P. and Schotte J. (1991). *Psychiatrie et existence*. Collection Krisis. Grenoble: Millon.

Felce D., Kerr M., and Hastings R. P. (2009). "A General Practice-based Study of the Relationship Between Indicators of Mental Illness and Challenging Behaviour Among Adults with Intellectual Disabilities." *Journal of Intellectual Disability Research* 53(3): 243–254.

French P. (2007). *Disabled Justice: The Barriers to Justice for Persons with a Disability in Queensland*. Brisbane: Disability Studies and Research Institute for Queensland Advocacy Incorporated.

Gadamer H. G. (2010). *G.W. Bd. 1. Wahrheit und Methode. Grundzüge einer philosophicher Hermeneutik*. Tübingen: Mohr Siebeck.

Glicksman S. (2011). "Supporting Religion and Spirituality to Enhance Quality of Life of People with Intellectual Disability: A Jewish Perspective." *Journal of Intellectual and Developmental Disability* 49(5): 397–402.

Hamilton D., Sutherland G., and Iacono T. (2005). "Further Examination of Relationships Between Life Events and Psychiatric Symptoms in Adults with Intellectual Disability." *Journal of Intellectual Disability Research* 49: 839–844.

Hansen S. N., Schendel D. E., and Parner E. T. (2015). "Explaining the Increase in the Prevalence of Autism Spectrum Disorders: The Proportion Attributable to Changes in Reporting Practices." *JAMA Pediatrics* 169(1): 56–62.

Hassiotis A., Ukoumunne O. C., Byford S., Tyrer P., Harvey K., Piachaud J., Gilvarry K., and Fraser J. (2001). "Intellectual Functioning and Outcome of Patients with Severe Psychotic Illness Randomised to Intensive Case Management. Report from the UK700 Trial. *British Journal of Psychiatry* 178: 166–171.

Hassiotis A., Strydom A., Hall I., Ali A., Lawrence-Smith G., Meltzer H., Head J., and Bebbington P. (2008). "Psychiatric Morbidity and Social Functioning Among Adults with Borderline Intelligence Living in Private Households." *Journal of Intellectual Disability Research* 52(2): 95–106.

Hassiotis A., Serfaty M., Azam K., Martin S., Strydom A., and King M. (2012). *Manual of Cognitive Behaviour Therapy for People with Mild Learning Disabilities and Common*

Mental Disorders. London: Camden & Islington NHS Foundation Trust and University College.

Hastings R. P., Hatton C., Taylor J. L., and Maddison C. (2004). "Life Events and Psychiatric Symptoms in Adults with Intellectual Disabilities." *Journal of Intellectual Disability Research* 48: 42–46.

Hatton C. and Emerson E. (2004). "The Relationship Between Life Events and Psychopathology Amongst Children with Intellectual Disabilities." *Journal of Applied Research in Intellectual Disabilities* 17: 109–117.

Hemmings C. P., Gravestock S., Pickard M., and Bouras N. (2006). "Psychiatric Symptoms and Problem Behaviours in People with Intellectual Disabilities." *Journal of Intellectual Disability Research* 50(4): 269–276.

Hendricks D. R. and Wehman P. (2009). "Transition from School to Adulthood for Youth with Autism Spectrum Disorders: Review and Recommendations." *Focus On Autism And Other Developmental Disabilities* 24(2): 77–88.

Hodapp R. M., Dykens E. M., Ort S. I., Zelinsky D. G., and Leckman J. F. (1991). "Changing Patterns of Intellectual Strengths and Weaknesses in Males with Fragile X Syndrome." *Journal of Autism and Developmental Disorders* 21(4): 503–516.

Holdnack J. A., Zhou X., Larrabee G. J., Millis S. R., and Salthouse T. A. (2011). "Confirmatory Factor Analysis of the WAIS-IV/WMS-IV." *Assessment* 18(2): 178–191.

Hollins S., Attard M. T., von Fraunhofer N., and Sedgwick P. (1998). "Mortality in People with Learning Disability: Risks, Causes, and Death Certification Findings in London." *Developmental Medicine & Child Neurology* 40: 50–56.

Hurley A. (2006). "Mood Disorders in Intellectual Disability." *Current Opinion in Psychiatry* 19: 465–469.

Imam S. S., Abdul Karim N. H., Jusoh N. R., and Mamad N. E. (2009). "Malay Version Of Spiritual Well-Being Scale: Is Malay Spiritual Well-being Scale a Psychometrically Sound Instrument?" *The Journal of Behavioral Science* 4(1): 59–69.

Jacobson J. W. and Mulik J. A. (1996). "Definition of Mental Retardation." In American Psychological Association (ed.), *Manual of Diagnosis and Professional Practice in Mental Retardation*. Washington, DC: American Psychological Association

Jahoda A., Pert C., and Trower P. (2006). "Socioemotional Understanding And Frequent Aggression in People with Mild to Moderate Intellectual Disabilities." *American Journal on Mental Retardation* 111: 77–89.

Janicki M. P. and Jacobson J. W. (1986). "Generation Trends in Sensory, Physical, and Behavioral Abilities Among Older Mentally Retarded Persons." *American Journal on Mental Retardation* 90: 490–500.

Janicki M. P. and Dalton A. J. (2000). "Prevalence of Dementia and Impact on Intellectual Disability Services." *Mental Retardation* 38: 276–288.

Johnson K., Hillier L., Harrison L.,and Frawley P. (2001). *Living Safer Sex Lives. Final Report*. Melbourne: Australian Research Centre in Sex, Health and Society, La Trobe University, Melbourne.

Jopp D. A. and Keys C. B. (2001). "Diagnostic Overshadowing Reviewed and Reconsidered." *American Journal of Mental Retardation* 106(5): 416–433.

Kanner L. (1943). "Autistic Disturbances of Affective Contact." *Nervous Child* 2: 217–250.

Kapell D., Nightingale B., Rodriguez A., Lee J. H., Zigman W. B., and Schupf N. (1998). "Prevalence of Chronic Medical Conditions in Adults with Mental Retardation: Comparison with the General Population." *Mental Retardation* 36: 269–279.

Kishore M. T., Nizamie S. H., and Nizamie A. (2005). "The Behavioural Profile of Psychiatric Disorders in Persons with Intellectual Disability." *Journal of Intellectual Disability Research* 49(11): 852–857.

Korff-Sausse S. and Scelles R. (2017). *The Clinic of Disability. Psychoanalytical Approaches.* London: Karnac.

Koskentausta T., Iivanien M., and Almqvist F. (2007). "Risk Factors for Psychiatric Disturbance in Children with Intellectual Disability." *Journal of Intellectual Disability Research* 51(1): 43–53.

Lee E. K. O. and Oh H. (2013). "Marital Satisfaction Among Adults with Disabilities in South Korea." *Journal of Disability Policy Studies* 23: 215–224.

Liégeois A. (2014). "Quality of Life without Spirituality? A Theological Reflection on the Quality of Life of Persons with Intellectual Disabilities." *Journal of Disability & Religion* 18(4): 303–317.

Lindsay P. and Burgess D. (2006). "Care of Patients with Intellectual or Learning Disability in Primary Care: No More Funding So Will There Be Any Change?" *The British Journal of General Practice* 56(523): 84–86.

Lindsay W. R., Allan R., Parry C., Macleod F., Cottrell J., Overend H., and Smith A. H. W. (2004). "Anger and Aggression in People with Intellectual Disabilities: Treatment and Follow-up of Consecutive Referrals and a Waiting List Comparison." *Clinical Psychology & Psychotherapy* 11(4): 255–264.

Loveland K. A. and Kelly M. L. (1991). "Development of Adaptive Behavior in Preschoolers with Autism or Down Syndrome." *American Journal on Mental Retardation* 96(1): 13–20.

Lumley V. A. and Scotti J. R. (2001). "Supporting the Sexuality of Adults with Mental Retardation: Current Status and Future Directions." *Journal of Positive Behavior Interventions* 3: 109–119.

Matheson E. and Jahoda A. (2005). "Emotional Understanding in Aggressive and Nonaggressive Individuals with Mild or Moderate Mental Retardation." *American Journal on Mental Retardation* 110: 57–67.

Mattila J., Määttä K., and Uusiautti S. (2017). "Everyone Needs Love"—An Interview Study About Perceptions of Love in People with Intellectual Disability (ID)." *International Journal of Adolescence and Youth* 22(3): 296–307.

McCarthy J. (2007). "Children with Autism Spectrum Disorders and Intellectual Disability." *Current Opinion in Psychiatry* 20(5): 472–476.

McGrew K. S. (2005). "The Cattell-Horn-Carroll (CHC) Theory of Cognitive Abilities: Past, Present and Future." In P. Flanagan, J. L. Genshaft, and P. L. Harrison (eds.), *Contemporary Intellectual Assessment: Theories, Tests, and Issues*, 2nd edn, pp. 136–202. New York: Guilford Press.

Mefford H. C., Batshaw M. L., and Hoffman E. P. (2012). "Genomics, Intellectual Disability, and Autism." *The New England Journal of Medicine* 366: 733–743.

Minton C. A. and Dodder R. A. (2003). "Participation in Religious Services by People with Developmental Disabilities." *Mental Retardation* 41(6): 430–439.

Moore D. G. (2001). "Reassessing Emotion Recognition Performance in People with Mental Retardation: A Review." *American Journal on Mental Retardation* 106: 481–502.

Morgan C. N., Roy M., Nasr A., Chance P., Hand M., Mlele T., and Roy A. (2002). "A Community Study Establishing the Prevalence Rate of Autistic Disorder in Adults with Learning Disability." *Psychiatric Bulletin* 26(4): 127–129.

Moss S., Emerson E., Kiernan C. K., Turner S., Hatton C., and Alborz A. (2000). "Psychiatric Symptoms in Adults with Learning Disability and Challenging Behavior." *British Journal of Psychiatry* 177: 452–456.

Murray S. and Powell A. (2008). *Sexual Assault and Adults with a Disability: Enabling Recognition, Disclosure and a Just Response.* Canberra: Australian Institute of Family Studies.

Naglieri J. A. and Das J. P. (2002). "Practical Implications of General Intelligence and Pass Cognitive Processes." In R. Sternberg and E. Grigorenko (eds.), *The General Factor of Intelligence. How General is It?* pp. 55–84. New Jersey: Lawrence Erlbaum Associates.

National Disability Authority (NDA). (2010). Independent and Community Living: Focus Group Consultation Report; http://nda.ie/Publications/Social-Community/Independent-and-Community-Living-Focus-Group-Consultation-Report/Chapter-Two-The-views-and-experiences-of-people-with-intellectual-disabilities (l.a. 08/18/2018)

Newschaffer C. J., Croen L. A., Daniels J., Giarelli E., Grether J. K., Levy S. E., Mandell D. S., Miller L. A., Pinto-Martin J., Reaven J., Reynolds A. M., Rice C. E., Schendel D., and Windham G. C. (2007). "The Epidemiology of Autism Spectrum Disorders." *Annual Review of Public Health* 28: 235–258.

Noterdaeme M. A. and Hutzelmeyer-Nickels A. (2010). "Comorbidity in Autism Spectrum Disorders—II. Genetic Syndromes and Neurological Problems." *Z Kinder Jugendpsychiatr Psychother* 38(4): 67–72.

Noterdaeme M. A. and Wriedt E. (2010). "Comorbidity in Autism Spectrum Disorders—I. Mental Retardation and Psychiatric Comorbidity." *Z Kinder Jugendpsychiatr Psychother* 38(4): 257–266.

Oakland T. and Harrison P. (2008). *Adaptive Behavior Assessment System-II: Behavior Assessment System-II: Clinical Use and Interpretation.* New York: Elsevier.

O'Connor M. and Fowkes J. (2000). *Normal is Everyone: Some of Us Have a Learning Difficulty.* Nundah, Brisbane: Community Living Association Inc.

Owen M. J. (2012). "Intellectual Disability and Major Psychiatric Disorders: A Continuum of Neurodevelopmental Causality." *The British Journal of Psychiatry* 200(4): 268–269.

Owen A., Browning M., and Jones R. P. (2001). "Emotion Recognition in Adults with Mild–Moderate Learning Disabilities." *Journal of Learning Disabilities* 5: 267–281.

Owen D. M., Hastings R. P., Noone S. J., Chinn J., Harman K., Roberts J., and Taylor K. (2004). "Life Events as Correlates of Problem Behavior and Mental Health in a Residential Population of Adults with Developmental Disabilities." *Research in Developmental Disabilities* 25: 309–320.

Pan C. C., Davis R., Nichols D., Hwang S. H., and Hsieh K. (2016). "Prevalence of Overweight and Obesity Among Students with Intellectual Disabilities in Taiwan: A Secondary Analysis." *Research in Developmental Disabilities* 53–54: 305–313.

Puri B. K., Lekh S. K., Langa A., Zaman R., and Singh I. (1995). "Mortality in a Hospitalized Mentally Handicapped Population: A 10-year Survey." *Journal of Intellectual Disability Research* 39: 442–446.

Raitasuo J., Raitasuo S., Mattila K., and Mölsä P. (1997). "Deaths Anions Intellectually Disabled: A Retrospective Study." *Journal of Applied Research in Intellectual Disabilities* 10: 280–288.

Raji O. (2009). "Intellectual Disability." In C. Cook, A. Powell, A. Sims (eds.), *Spirituality and Psychiatry*, pp. 122–138. Glasgow: The Royal College of Psychiatrists.

Reiss S., Levtan G. W., and Szyszko J. (1982). "Emotional Disturbance and Mental Retardation: Diagnostic Overshadowing." *American Journal of Mental Deficiency* 86: 567–574.

Reiss S. and Syszko J. (1983). "Diagnostic Overshadowing and Professional Experience with Mentally Retarded Persons." *American Journal of Mental Deficiency* 87: 396–402.

Rojahn J., Matson J. L., Naglieri J. A., and Mayville E. (2004). "Relationships Between Psychiatric Conditions and Behavior Problems Among Adults with Mental Retardation." *American Journal of Mental Retardation* 109(1): 21–33.

Rojahn J. and Meier L. J. (2009). "Epidemiology of Mental Illness and Maladaptive Behavior in Intellectual Disabilities." In M. H. Robert (ed.), *International Review of Research in Mental Retardation*, pp. 38, 239–287). Amsterdam: Elsevier.

Rondini E. (2015). *Fattori socio-ambientali e disabilità intellettiva: studio di relazione in un'ottica dimensionale.* (Unpublished Thesis) University of Florence.

Rose J. and West C. (1999). "Assessment of Anger in People with Intellectual Disabilities." *Journal of Applied Research in Intellectual Disabilities* 12(3): 211–224.

Salvador-Carulla L. and Saxena S. (2009). "Intellectual Disability: Between Disability and Clinical Nosology." *Lancet* 374(9704): 1798–1799.

Salvador-Carulla L., Reed G. M., Vaez-Azizi L. M., Cooper S. A., Martinez-Leal R., Bertelli M., Adnams C., Cooray S., Deb S., Akoury-Dirani L., Girimaji S. C., Katz G., Kwok H., Luckasson R., Simeonsson R., Walsh C., Munir K., and Saxena S. (2011). "Intellectual Developmental Disorders: Towards a New Name, Definition and Framework for "Mental Retardation/Intellectual Disability" in ICD-11. *World Psychiatry* 10(3): 175–180.

Sappok T., Barrett B. F., Vandevelde S., Heinrich M., Poppe L., Sterkenburg P., Vonk J., Kolb J., Claes C., Bergmann T., Došen A., and Morisse F. (2016). "Scale of Emotional Development-Short." *Research in Developmental Disabilities* 59: 166–175.

Schalock R. L. (1999). "The Merging of Adaptive Behavior and Intelligence: Implication for the Field of Mental Retardation." In R. L. Schalock and D. L. Braddock (eds.), *Adaptive Behavior and Its Measurement*. Washington, DC: American Association on Mental Retardation.

Schalock R. L., Brown I., Brown R., Cummins R. A., Felce D., Matikka L., Keith K. D., and Parmenter T. (2002). "Conceptualization, Measurement, and Application of Quality of Life for Persons with Intellectual Disabilities: Report of an International Panel of Experts." *Mental Retardation* 40(6): 457–470.

Schalock R. L., Verdugo M. A., Jenaro C., Wang M., Wehmeyer M., Jiancheng X., and Lachapelle Y. (2005). "Cross-cultural study of quality of life indicators." *American Journal of Mental Retardation* 110(4):298–311.

Schalock R. L., Borthwick-Duffy S. A., Bradley M., Buntinx H. E., Coulter D. L., Craig E. M. P., Gomez S. C., Lachapelle Y., Luckasson R., Reeve A., Shogren K. A., Snell M. A., Spreat S., Tassé M. J., Thompson J. R., Verdugo-Alonso M. A., Wehmeyer M. L., and Yeager M. H. (2010). *Intellectual Disability: Definition, Classification, and Systems of Supports*, 11th edn. Washington, DC: American Association on Intellectual and Developmental Disabilities.

Scheuffgen K., Happé F., Anderson M., and Frith U. (2000). "High 'Intelligence,' Low 'IQ'? Speed of Processing and Measured IQ in Children with Autism." *Developmental Psychopathology* 12(1): 83–90.

Scott H. M. and Havercamp S. M. (2014). "Mental Health for People with Intellectual Disability: The Impact of Stress and Social Support." *American Journal on Intellectual and Developmental Disabilities* 119(6): 552–564.

Seltzer M. M., Floyd F., Greenberg J., Lounds J., Lindstromm M., and Hong J. (2005). "Life Course Impacts of Mild Intellectual Deficits." *American Journal of Mental Retardation* 110: 451–468.

Selway D. and Ashman A. F. (1998). "Disability, Religion and Health: A Literature Review in Search of the Spiritual Dimensions of Disability." *Disability & Society* 13(3): 429–439.

Simon T. J. (2010). "Rewards and Challenges of Cognitive Neuroscience Studies of Persons with Intellectual and Developmental Disabilities." *American Journal on Intellectual and Developmental Disabilities* 115(2): 79–82.

Sinason V. (1992). *Mental Handicap and the Human Condition. New Approaches from the Tavistock*. Free Association Books: London.

Sobsey D. (1994). *Violence and Abuse in the Lives of People with Disabilities: The End of Silent Acceptance?* Baltimore, MD: Paul H. Brookes.

Sovner R. (1986). "Limiting Factors in the Use of DSM-III Criteria with Mentally Ill/Mentally Retarded Persons." *Psychopharmacology Bulletin* 22(4): 1055–1059.

Sparrow S. S., Cicchetti D. V., and Balla D. A. (2005). *Vineland II Adaptive Behavior Scales*. Circle Pines, MN: American Guidance Service.

Srivastava A. K. and Schwartz C. E. (2014). "Intellectual Disability and Autism Spectrum Disorders: Causal Genes and Molecular Mechanisms." *Neuroscience and Biobehavioral Review* 46(2): 161–174.

Stanghellini G. (2003). "A Future for Phenomenology?" *Comprendre* 13.

Sturmey P. and Ley T. (1990). "The Psychopathology Instrument for Mentally Retarded Adults. Internal Consistencies and Relationship to Behaviour Problems." *British Journal of Psychiatry* 156: 428–430.

Sulmasy D. P. (1997). *The Healer's Calling: A Spirituality for Physicians and Other Health Care Professionals*. New York: Paulist Press.

Summers J. A., Poston D. J., Turnbull A. P., Marquis J., Hoffman L., Mannan H., and Wang M. (2005). "Conceptualizing and Measuring Family Quality of Life." *Journal of Intellectual Disability Research* 49: 777–783.

Takara K. and Kondo T. (2014). "Autism Spectrum Disorder Among First-Visit Depressed Adult Patients: Diagnostic Clues from Backgrounds and Past History." *General Hospital Psychiatry* 36(6): 737–742.

Thompson J. R., McGrew K. S., and Bruininks R. H. (1999). "Adaptive and Maladaptive Behavior: Functional and Structural Characteristics." In R. L. Schalock (ed.), *Adaptive Behaviour and Its Measurement*. Washington, DC: American Association on Mental Retardation.

Thornton-Wells T. A., Cannistraci C. J., Anderson A. W., Kim C. Y., Eapen M., Gore J. C., Blake R., and Dykens E. M. (2010). "Auditory attraction: activation of visual cortex by music and sound in Williams syndrome." *American Journal on Intellectual and Developmental Disabilities* 115(2):172–189.

Tiekstra M., Hessels M. G., and Minnaert A. E. (2009). "Learning Capacity in Adolescents with Mild Intellectual Disabilities." *Psychological Report* 105(1): 804–814.

Tsiouris J. A., Mann R., Patti P. J., and Sturmey P. (2003). "Challenging Behaviors Should Not Be Considered as Depressive Equivalents in Individuals with Intellectual Disability." *Journal of Intellectual Disability Research* 47: 14–21.

van Schrojenstein Lantman-De Valk H. M. J., Metsemakers J. F. M., Haveman M. J., and Crebolder H. F. J. M. (2000). "Health Problems in People with Intellectual Disability in General Practice: A Comparative Study." *Family Practice* 17: 405–407.

Verdonschot M. M. L., de Witte L. P., Reichrath E., Buntinx W. H. E. , and Curfs L. M. G. (2009). "Impact of Environmental Factors on Community Participation of Persons with an Intellectual Disability: A Systematic Review." *Journal of Intellectual Disability Research* 53(1): 54–64.

Verdugo M. A., Schalock R. L., Keith K. D., and Stancliffe R. J. (2005). "Quality of Life and Its Measurement: Important Principles and Guidelines." *Journal of Intellectual Disability Research* 49: 707–717.

Watts G. (2011). "Intellectual Disability and Spiritual Development." *Journal on Intellectual and Developmental Disabilities* 36(4): 234–241.

WHO—World Health Organisation (1992). *International Statistical Classification of Diseases and Related Health Problems—10th revision, ICD-10.* Geneva: World Health Organisation.

WHO—World Health Organisation (2000). *Ageing and Intellectual Disabilities—Improving Longevity and Promoting Healthy Ageing: Summative Report.* Geneva: World Health Organisation.

WHO—World Health Organisation (2001). *International Classification of Functioning, Disability and Health (ICF).* Geneva: World Health Organisation.

WHO—World Health Organisation (2018). *International Statistical Classification of Diseases and Related Health Problems—11th revision, ICD-11 Beta draft.* https://icd.who.int/dev11/l-m/en#/http%3a%2f%2fid.who.int%2ficd%2fentity%2f605267007 (l.a. 2/5/18)

Widaman K. F., Gibbs K. W., and Geary D. C. (1987). "Structure of Adaptive Behavior: I Replication Across Fourteen Samples of Nonprofoundly Mentally Retarded People." *American Journal of Mental Deficiency* 91: 348–360.

Wilkins J. and Matson J. L. (2009). "A Comparison of Social Skills Profiles in Intellectually Disabled Adults with and without ASD." *Behavior Modification* 33: 143–155.

Wilson N. J., Jaques H., Johnson A., and Brotherton M. L. (2017). "From Social Exclusion to Supported Inclusion: Adults with Intellectual Disability Discuss Their Lived Experiences of a Structured Social Group." *Journal of Applied Research in Intellectual Disabilities* 30: 847–858.

Wing L., Gould J., and Gillberg C. (2011). "Autism Spectrum Disorders in the DSM-V: Better or Worse than the DSM-IV?" *Research in Developmental Disabilities* 32(2): 768–773.

Wishart J. G., Cebula K. R., Willis D. S., and Pitcairn T. K. (2007). "Understanding of Facial Expressions of Emotion by Children with Intellectual Disabilities of Differing Etiology." *Journal of Intellectual Disability Research* 51: 551–563.

WWILD Sexual Violence Prevention Association Inc. (2018). How to Hear Me: A Resource Kit for Counsellors and Other Professionals Working with People with Intellectual Disability; https://communitydoor.org.au/service-delivery/disability/how-to-hear-me-a-resource-kit-for-working-with-people-with-intellectu-14 (l.a. 08/18/2018)

Zhang K. C. (2010). "Spirituality and Disabilities: Implications for Special Education." *Intellectual and Developmental Disabilities* 48(4): 299–302.

Zic A. and Lgric L. (2001). "Self-assessment of Relationships with Peers in Children with Intellectual Disability." *Journal of Intellectual Disability Research* 45: 202–211.

CHAPTER 98

THE BODILY SELF IN SCHIZOPHRENIA
From Phenomenology to Neuroscience

FRANCESCA FERRI AND VITTORIO GALLESE

THE BODY AND THE SELF

SEVERAL philosophers, psychologists, and neuroscientists suggested that the self is fundamentally shaped by the body (e.g.Baumaister 1999; Bermúdez, Marcel, and Eilan 1995; Gallese and Sinigaglia 2011; Tsakiris 2017). Hence, the *bodily self* would represent the most basic aspect of our self. Despite a wider range of body experiences likely participating in the constitution of the self, the most recognized contributions are from the sense of body ownership (i.e. the feeling that "my body" belongs to me (Gallagher 2000)) and the sense of agency (i.e. the feeling that "my actions" belong to me (Synofzik, Vosgerau, and Newen, 2008)). Psychologists and neuroscientists proposed that altogether these major dimensions of bodily self-awareness account for the multisensory and sensorimotor bases of the self.

Interestingly, the last several years have seen a tremendous growth in the study of anomalous body experiences in self-disorders, especially schizophrenia (Klaver and Dijkerman 2016). The conceptual framework behind this new empirical trend, which emerged after prolonged research focusing on higher-order cognitive functions (e.g. executive function, working memory), is provided by phenomenological psychopathology (Cermolacce, Naudin, and Parnas 2007; Fuchs and Schlimme 2009; Mishara 2007). The general idea is that schizophrenia is essentially characterized by deficits at the most basic level of self-experience, ipseity (Sass and Parnas 2003), which is rooted in bodily experience (Merleau-Ponty 1945; Piaget 1954). Consistent with this idea, several anomalies of the representations of the bodily self have been found not only in schizophrenia, but also in individuals with subclinical schizotypal personality. This evidence further supports the basic role of bodily-self disturbances in schizophrenia, as they seem to precede the onset of the illness. Moreover, it supports the idea that schizophrenia may exist on a dimensional continuum with normal experience (Kretschmer 1921).

The first part of this chapter will illustrate the most recent empirical evidence of anomalies of body experiences in schizophrenia and schizotypy. The second part of the chapter will propose a link between bodily-self disturbances and deficits in time-processing that have been shown in both populations.

What sorts of mechanisms underlie anomalies of body experiences in self-disorders? The third part of the chapter will tackle this issue by illustrating neural markers possibly associated with anomalies of time-processing and, as a consequence, with abnormal representations of the bodily self, in self-disorders. Specifically, we will illustrate how abnormal temporal patterns of the spontaneous brain activity may underlie deficits in the multisensory processes at the heart of the representations of the bodily self. Finally, we will refer to excitation/inhibition imbalance as a possible key to understanding the different neural markers of anomalies of bodily-self experiences in self-disorders.

PHENOMENOLOGICAL PHENOTYPES OF SCHIZOPHRENIA SPECTRUM DISORDERS

Abnormal experiences of self, or self-disorders, constitute a crucial schizophrenia spectrum phenotype (Parnas and Handest 2003; Sass and Parnas 2003). Self-disorders are thought to originate at the most "basic" level of self-awareness, that is, "ipseity" (Nelson, Parnas, and Sass 2014), which is rooted in bodily experiences (Merleau-Ponty 1945; Piaget 1954). Disturbances of bodily experiences seem to precede the onset of the illness (Nelson et al. 2009; Nelson, Thompson, and Yung 2012) and include, for instance, body alienation, loss of agency, and blurred body boundaries (Sass and Parnas 2003).

In recent years, there has been growing interest in the study of anomalous body experiences in schizophrenia spectrum disorders. The dimensions of the body awareness that have been most extensively investigated are the sense of body ownership, the sense of agency, and self–other boundary in the domain of touch.

Body Ownership in Schizophrenia

The *sense of body ownership* can be defined as the feeling that something is part of one's own body. Studies investigating body ownership in patients with schizophrenia used the rubber hand illusion (RHI) (Botvinick and Cohen 1998), which depends on the interaction between sensory inputs from three different modalities, namely vision, touch, and proprioception.

To elicit this illusion, the participant's real hand is hidden from view while a rubber hand is placed in front of her. The experimenter generally uses two paintbrushes to stroke synchronously the rubber hand and the participant's hidden hand. After a short period (about 30 seconds), most people have the experience that the rubber hand is their own hand and that it is the rubber hand that senses the touch of the paintbrush. In the control condition, the rubber hand and the participant's hidden hand are stroked asynchronously. Strength of the RHI has traditionally been measured in three ways. First, using introspective questionnaires that assess four dissociable components of the RHI experience, namely, embodiment of the rubber hand (with the agency, ownership, and location components), loss of the own hand, movement, and affect (Longo, Schuur, Kammers, Tsakiris, and Haggard 2008). Second, with the proprioceptive drift, that quantifies the feeling of relocalization of participant's hand toward the location of the rubber hand (Botvinick and Cohen 1998). Third, with skin conductance response. The RHI is typically measured on the basis of the difference between the ratings, or measures, after synchronous and asynchronous stimulation. Importantly, conclusions about the experience of ownership cannot be drawn from measuring proprioceptive drift alone, as recent studies indicate that a dissociation between subjective ratings and drift exists (e.g. Rohde, Di Luca, and Ernst 2011; Romano, Caffa, Hernandez-Arieta, Brugger, and Maravita 2015; Shimada, Fukuda, and Hiraki 2009).

People with schizophrenia have been shown to experience the RHI more strongly (Peled, Pressman, Geva, and Modai 2003) and faster (Peled, Ritsner, Hirschmann, Geva, and Modai 2000) than healthy controls, as indicated by self-report questionnaires. However, the authors of these studies only administered synchronous stimulation, thus providing only partial evidence of body ownership deficits in patients with schizophrenia. In a more recent study, Thakkar and colleagues (Thakkar, Nichols, McIntosh, and Park 2011) implemented both the synchronous and the asynchronous conditions and measured the illusion with both subjective (e.g. questionnaire) and objective (e.g. proprioceptive drift, autonomic responses) methods. With respect to the subjective measures, they found stronger RHI during synchronous stimulation in both healthy controls and patients. However, patients endorsed RHI-related perceptual effects more strongly than controls in both synchronous and asynchronous conditions. In regard to the objective measures, Thakkar and colleagues (Thakkar et al. 2011) found larger proprioceptive drift in the synchronous, as compared to the asynchronous, condition in patients with schizophrenia, but not in the control group. Finally, with respect to the autonomic measures, the authors did not find an effect of synchrony. Altogether, in agreement with previous investigations (Peled et al. 2003; Peled et al. 2000), the authors conclude embodiment of the RHI to be stronger in people with schizophrenia than in healthy controls. Interestingly, similar results have been found after inducing schizophrenia symptoms with ketamine, a noncompetitive N-methyl-D-aspartate agonist, in healthy volunteers (Morgan et al. 2011). Also in this case, subjective experience of RHI was greater under ketamine, compared to placebo, for both synchronous and asynchronous stroking. On the basis of prior evidence showing that RHI is associated with augmented gamma-band oscillations during synchronous visuo-tactile stimulation (Kanayama, Sato, and Ohira 2007, 2009), and that gamma-band oscillations are enhanced by acute ketamine administration (Hong et al. 2010), the authors suggested that during asynchronous stimulation, a ketamine-induced augmentation of gamma-band oscillation is likely sufficient to produce the illusion. As gamma oscillations are known to emerge from the coordinated interaction of excitation and inhibition (Buzsaki and Wang 2012), this explanation would particularly fit with the conceptualization of schizophrenia as a disorder associated with disturbances in excitation/inhibition balance (Uhlhaas and Singer 2015). See also the last part of this chapter on the neurobiological markers of abnormal temporal processing underlying bodily-self disorders.

Altogether, by showing the illusion also under asynchronous visuo-tactile stimulation, studies of sense of body ownership in schizophrenia suggest that patients are characterized by an increased cross-modal binding, which likely exceeds the temporal rules of multisensory integration (Costantini et al. 2016). Further support to this hypothesis, which however needs to be confirmed with more studies, comes from a study from our group (Ferri et al. 2014) that used a RHI induction procedure in which no synchronous/asynchronous visuo-tactile stimuli were delivered. In that study, multisensory integration was elicited only by anticipation of touch experience (see in (Ferri, Chiarelli, Merla, Gallese, and Costantini 2013), and people with schizophrenia showed weaker, rather than stronger RHI, compared to the healthy control group.

SENSE OF AGENCY IN SCHIZOPHRENIA

Another dimension of body awareness that has been extensively investigated in schizophrenia is the *sense of agency*, which refers to the feeling of being in control over one's own actions and their consequences. An interesting distinction has been drawn between the feeling of agency (FOA) and the judgment of agency (JOA) (Synofzik et al. 2008). The FOA refers to a non-conceptual feeling of being an agent, which is linked to low-level sensorimotor processes—that is, the FOA automatically registers agency or non-agency by tracking sensorimotor contingencies. Differently, the JOA refers to a higher-level conceptual judgment of agency, which arises in situations where we make explicit attributions of agency to the self or other—that is, the JOA is mainly based on causal attribution processes, rather than sensorimotor process (Gallagher 2000). Consistently with the distinction between FOA and JOA, measures of sense of agency can be implicit or explicit. In implicit experimental paradigms, participants are never asked to directly judge their agentic experience. Examples of implicit measures are the intentional binding (Haggard, Clark, and Kalogeras 2002; Moore and Obhi 2012) and the sensory attenuation (Blakemore, Smith, Steel, Johnstone, and Frith 2000; Blakemore, Wolpert, and Frith 2002). The intentional binding evaluates the reduction of the perceived time between a voluntary action and its effect (Haggard et al. 2002). Differently, the sensory attenuation measures the reduction in perceived intensity of sensory feedback of voluntary action, which is known to be lower than for passive movements (Blakemore, Frith, and Wolpert 1999; Blakemore, Goodbody, and Wolpert 1998). In explicit experimental paradigm, on the other hand, participants are directly asked to report something about their agentic experience. Examples of explicit measures are action recognition judgments, action monitoring tasks, and causal judgments during action recognition judgments (e.g. Farrer, Bouchereau, Jeannerod, and Franck 2008), participants make an action and observe some kind of feedback on a screen that, importantly, leaves uncertainty over the agent of the action. They are asked whose movement it is. Action monitoring tasks also use visual feedback about movements, but participants are required to make a judgment about the feedback itself (Synofzik, Thier, Leube, Schlotterbeck, and Lindner 2010). Finally, in causal judgment, participants have to judge how much they felt their action caused the outcome (e.g. Chambon, Moore, and Haggard 2015).

In schizophrenia, abnormal experiences of agency usually take the form of passivity symptoms (or delusions of control), with the patient feeling as though his or her actions are not under their control. Most interestingly, agency problems in people with schizophrenia concern not only high-level cognitive processes, like those revealed by action recognition tasks (Daprati et al. 1997). Indeed, patients already have problems with low-level sensorimotor processes, as revealed by intentional binding (Voss et al. 2010) and sensory attenuation (Blakemore et al. 2000) tasks, both suggesting that patients struggle predicting the sensory consequences of their actions.

In particular, it was demonstrated that people with schizophrenia show greater levels of intentional binding—that is, a bigger shift of the perceived time of voluntary action toward a subsequent tone—compared to controls. This suggested an enhanced, rather than reduced, sense of agency in patients (Haggard, Martin, Taylor-Clarke, Jeannerod, and Franck 2003). The relationship between intentional binding and sense of agency indicates a tight link between temporal processing of our actions and our sense of being the authors of these actions. This is also supported by evidence that key neurotransmitters that are altered in schizophrenia, such as dopamine and glutamate, are also implicated in timing (Meck 1996) and sense of agency (Moore et al. 2010; Moore et al. 2011). However, the nature and origins of the agency deficit in individuals with schizophrenia still need to be clarified.

A possible explanation could be based on the observation that, in healthy people, the shift in perceived time of action toward the outcome is partly linked to sensory prediction (Moore and Haggard 2008), as it occurs only when the outcome of the action is highly predictable. However, Voss et al. (2010) demonstrated that this predictive effect is absent in patients with schizophrenia, who show a shift in perceived time of action regardless of the predictability of the outcome. Furthermore, Graham-Schmidt et al. (2016) suggested more recently that the relationships between sensorimotor prediction and time shift perception in patients with schizophrenia might be further complicated by their passivity symptoms profile.

In sum, we still don't know how dysfunctions of time perception and processing (Thoenes and Oberfeld 2017) might affect motor planning, self-monitoring processes, and consequently sense of agency in patients with schizophrenia. Ultimately, by affecting the sense of self at such a basic and pre-reflective level, timing dysfunction might interfere also with the sensorimotor representation of the bodily self—that is, the immediate and implicit representation of oneself as a body with specific sensorimotor capacities (see Gallese and Ferri 2013, 2014) for reviews)—that is, likely linked to social deficit.

Self–Other Boundary in Schizophrenia: The Case of Touch

One of the novel contributions of neuroscience to psychopathology consisted in showing how much subjectivity and intersubjectivity be closely intertwined, allowing new light to be shed on the neurobiological mechanisms underpinning the link between the social deficits of patients with schizophrenia and their self-disorders. It should be added that so far, the exact nature and the dysfunctional neural mechanisms underlying social deficits in schizophrenia remain a topic of speculation. Research from our group has shown that by means of embodied simulation, conceived of in terms of neural reuse, that is, by mapping others' actions, emotions, and sensations onto one's own sensorimotor and visceromotor representations in bodily format of the same actions, emotions, and sensations, a pre-reflective, experiential understanding of others can be accomplished, so that others are conceived as other bodily selves (for a review, see Gallese and Ferri 2013, 2014).

However, in spite of shared representations generating vicarious experiences of others, a clear distinction between self and other is normally preserved. A brain imaging study from our group (Ebisch et al. 2013) revealed significant differences in posterior insular cortex between the participants with schizophrenia and the healthy individuals during the observation of affective social touch, either with a positive (caress) or with a negative (hit) valence. Reduced deactivation of posterior insular cortex in patients with schizophrenia when witnessing others' tactile experiences indicates a deficit in the pre-reflective suppression of self-oriented affective arousal. This suppression likely normally contributes to the differentiation between self and other during social interactions.

A further difference between patients with schizophrenia and healthy controls revealed by the study of Ebisch at al. (2013) consisted in the reduced activation of the ventral premotor cortex in the former group during first-person touch experience and touch observation. The lack of coherent, pre-reflective perception of bodily experiences, likely due to altered multisensory integration, as revealed by the hypofunction of the ventral premotor cortex in patients with schizophrenia, might lead to asymmetry in self–other relationship, accompanied by the blurring of the relationship and the distinction between self and other.

Bodily-Self Disturbances in Subclinical Schizotypy

Several bodily-self disturbances have been found not only in schizophrenia, but also in individuals with subclinical schizotypal personality traits (Asai, Mao, Sugimori, and Tanno 2011; Ferri, Ambrosini, and Costantini 2016; Germine, Benson, Cohen, and Hooker 2013; Kallai et al. 2015; Thakkar et al. 2011), as well as in individuals at ultra-high risk of psychosis (Madeira et al. 2016). This supports the idea that bodily-self disturbances may precede the onset of the illness and play a basic role in schizophrenia spectrum disorders.

Schizotypy is thought to reflect the subclinical expression of the symptoms of schizophrenia in the general population and to constitute a dynamic continuum ranging from personality variation to psychosis (Lenzenweger 2006; Raine 2006). Even if most schizotypes are not expected to develop psychosis, schizotypy is associated with heightened risk for the development of psychotic disorders (Kwapil, Gross, Silvia, and Barrantes-Vidal 2013). Indeed, substantial overlapping has been found between schizotypy and schizophrenia not only in terms of etiological factors—at the genetic, biological, and psychosocial levels (Barrantes-Vidal, Grant, and Kwapil 2015)—but also concerning a wide range of perceptual, cognitive, and motor impairments (Ettinger et al. 2015). However, the study of bodily self-dysfunction in schizotypy offers the advantage of preventing the psychological variables from being confounded by compensatory strategies, severity, distress, comorbidity, and therapy.

Abnormal sense of body ownership has been revealed also in schizotypy by the rubber hand illusion (Germine et al. 2013; Kallai et al. 2015; Thakkar et al. 2011). Participants with higher levels of schizotypy developed a stronger feeling that the rubber hand belonged to them. However, as with patients with schizophrenia (see earlier in the chapter), participants with higher levels of schizotypy showed increased proneness to the illusion also during asynchronous stimulation (i.e. when their own hand and the artificial hand were touched asynchronously). Moreover, positive (e.g. ideas of reference, magical thinking, unusual perceptual experiences) and negative schizotypy symptoms (social anxiety, constricted affect) (Raine 1991) in otherwise healthy individuals correlate with a greater susceptibility to illusions of body ownership during both synchronous and asynchronous conditions (Thakkar et al. 2011). In sum, studies of sense of body ownership in schizotypy, consistently with similar studies in schizophrenia, suggest that patients are characterized by an increased cross-modal binding. Moreover, such increased cross-modal binding likely exceeds the temporal rules of multisensory integration (Costantini et al. 2016) already in participants with high levels of schizotypal traits, as they show the illusion also under asynchronous visuo-tactile stimulation, like people with schizophrenia.

Evidence of agency disturbances in schizotypy is still inconclusive. Only one study investigated the sense of agency in highly schizotypal individuals (Asai and Tanno 2008). Participants were required to judge whether they felt they or someone else had generated a tone. The results showed that the high schizotypal individuals (n=10) had a weaker sense of self-agency than the low schizotypal individuals (n=8). However, given the small number of participants, the findings should be regarded as preliminary. Also, the fact that schizotypal people have a weaker sense of self-agency seems to contrast with evidence of stronger sense of self-agency in schizophrenia patients. Further studies on self-agency using the same tasks in both schizotypy, or other antecedents (e.g. ultra-high-risk state), and schizophrenia are warranted.

Bodily-Self Disturbances and Abnormal Temporal Binding of Multisensory Events

Body Ownership and Temporal Binding Window

Multisensory integration is generally regarded as a crucial component in coherent bodily self-representation and sense of body ownership. As noted above, the fact that both people with schizophrenia and schizotypal individuals show the rubber hand illusion also under asynchronous visuo-tactile stimulation suggests that abnormal sense of body ownership in both populations might specifically depend upon anomalous temporal binding of multisensory stimuli. Recent studies in patients with schizophrenia clearly support this hypothesis. Graham and colleagues (Graham, Martin-Iverson, Holmes, Jablensky, and Waters 2014) investigated body ownership in patients with schizophrenia with current, past, and no history of passivity symptoms. Instead of a rubber hand, they used a projected hand illusion, in which a live video image of the participant's hand is projected onto a video screen. The clinical sub-group with passivity symptoms continued to experience ownership over the projected hand during asynchronous stimulation (500 milliseconds delay). This may suggest that the temporal binding window, which allows integration of the bodily and external stimuli, is "wider" in patients with current passivity symptoms. Consequently, they experience stimuli that are further apart in time, as co-occurring.

In support of this hypothesis, we recently provided the first comprehensive evidence of a direct link between the individual susceptibility to the rubber hand illusion and the individual temporal binding window, measured as the timespan within which stimuli from different modalities are perceived as simultaneously occurring and, thus, perceptually bound. In particular, we showed that the larger the temporal binding window, the higher the level of asynchrony tolerated in the rubber hand illusion. In other words, the degree of temporal asynchrony necessary to prevent the induction of the rubber hand illusion depends upon the individuals' sensitivity to perceiving asynchrony during visuo-tactile stimulation (Costantini et al. 2016).

Agency and Temporal Binding Window

Other evidence suggesting that bodily-self disturbances on the schizophrenia spectrum might depend upon altered time-processing, especially a wider window of temporal binding, comes from studies on the sense-of-agency. People with schizophrenia seem to perceive events—that is, action and their consequences—as happening closer in time than they actually occurred. In other words, as reported earlier, these people show greater levels of intentional binding, which means enhanced sense-of-agency (Haggard et al. 2003). The tendency to bind events that are further apart in time may affect the ability to form causal mental relationships and a variety of other processes related to sensory-motor awareness and, consequently, self-recognition (Haggard et al. 2003). Despite there being enough empirical support to knowledge of abnormally wide temporal binding window in schizophrenia (Foucher, Lacambre, Pham, Giersch, and Elliott 2007; Martin, Giersch, Huron, and van Wassenhove 2013; Stevenson et al. 2017; Tseng et al. 2015) and schizotypy (Ferri et al. 2017), evidence of a direct link between the larger temporal binding window and the higher level of sense-of-agency is currently missing.

The temporal binding window has been measured in schizophrenia and schizotypy using simultaneity judgments (SJ) and temporal-order judgments (TOJ). In the SJ task two stimuli from different sensory modalities are presented either successively or simultaneously and the participant has to decide whether the onsets of the two stimuli were synchronous or asynchronous. The larger the simultaneity threshold, the lower the precision of the participant's judgments, the lower the temporal resolution of the sensory systems (Capa, Duval, Blaison, and Giersch 2014; Foucher et al. 2007; Lalanne, van Assche, and Giersch 2012; Martin et al. 2013; Schmidt, McFarland, Ahmed, McDonald, and Elliott 2011). In the TOJ task two different stimuli (e.g. a tone and a flash) are presented successively, and the participant has to indicate which stimulus was presented first (Capa et al. 2014). The larger the threshold that is sufficient to discriminate the temporal order of two stimuli, the worse is the temporal resolution of the sensory system (Hirsh 1959). The fact that a larger temporal binding window characterizes not only people with schizophrenia, but also individuals at higher risk (e.g. those with subclinical schizotypal personality traits), is consistent with the idea that abnormal temporal processing in these people might contribute to the development of bodily-self disturbance, which indeed are thought to precede the onset of psychosis and persist after remission of a frank psychotic episode (e.g. Raballo and Parnas 2011).

For the sake of completeness, we should mention here that temporal processing is not the only one temporal dimension altered in schizophrenia (Thoenes and Oberfeld 2017). Indeed, the fact that patients are less accurate than controls in estimating time duration across a wide range of tasks suggests that time perception is disturbed in schizophrenia (Ciullo, Spalletta, Caltagirone, Jorge, and Piras 2016). However, the potential relation between (i) deficit in time-processing (as revealed by, for instance, SJ and TOJ tasks) and time perception (as revealed by, for instance, time estimation tasks), and between (ii) altered time perception and bodily-self disturbance is currently under investigation.

Neurobiological Markers of Abnormal Temporal Processing Underlying Bodily-Self Disorders

We recently tested the hypothesis that spontaneous, or resting-state brain activity, may provide insight into an individual's propensity to integrate multisensory information over a wide or narrow temporal window (Ferri et al. 2017). We started from prior knowledge that spontaneous neural activity exhibits a rich temporal structure (He 2014; Murray et al. 2014) that affects the timescale over which brain regions process information from external stimuli (Honey et al. 2012; Stephens, Honey, and Hasson 2013). More specifically, we measured the temporal structure of spontaneous neural activity, and the temporal binding window, in healthy participants with lower to higher levels of schizotypy. As a measure of the temporal structure of spontaneous neural activity, we took the degree of the long-range temporal correlations (He, Zempel, Snyder, and Raichle 2010)—that is, an index of the regularity of brain activity patterns over time. This index is called the power law exponent (PLE) (He et al. 2010). Higher PLE values indicate stronger regularities of brain activity over time. We found lower PLE values predicting wider temporal binding windows in participants with higher levels of schizotypy (Ferri et al. 2017). These results were consistent with prior evidence of attenuated long-range temporal correlations in patients with schizophrenia (Nikulin, Jonsson, and Brismar 2012).

We further showed that interindividual differences in perceptual schizotypy, temporal binding window, and temporal structure of spontaneous brain activity were accounted for by the balance between excitatory (i.e. glutamatergic) and inhibitory (GABAergic) neurotransmissions. The individual excitation/inhibition balance was indexed by combining genetic information, about GABA and glutamate receptors genes, and neurochemical information, about the concentrations of GABA and glutamate in the brain. For participants that are already genetically shifted toward greater inhibition, higher concentrations of glutamatergic compounds were associated with higher values of PLE, narrower temporal binding window, and lower schizotypy. In contrast, for participants that are already genetically shifted toward greater excitation, higher concentrations of glutamatergic compounds were associated with lower PLE, wider temporal binding window, and higher schizotypy. This interaction pattern is consistent with recent studies, which describe the relationship between excitation/inhibition balance and information processing efficiency as an inverted U-shaped curve (Krause, Marquez-Ruiz, and Cohen Kadosh 2013). Indeed, higher concentrations of glutamatergic compounds in participants with an "excited" genetic background might worsen behavioral efficiency—for example, integration of events that are further apart in time—leading to disturbances of body ownership (i.e. higher proneness to body illusions) and agency (i.e. greater levels of intentional binding) and ultimately increase perceptual risk for schizophrenia.

Prior research on impaired excitation/inhibition balance in schizophrenia has mainly linked it to functional dysconnectivity patterns between and within brain networks (e.g. Rogasch, Daskalakis, and Fitzgerald 2014; Uhlhaas 2013). Given the relevance of resting state connectivity patterns between primary and multisensory brain regions to set the width of individuals' temporal binding window, it is possible to hypothesize that impaired excitation/inhibition balance causing dysconnectivity in schizophrenia might constitute another mechanism contributing to abnormal binding of multisensory events and, consequently, to bodily-self disturbances. Further studies testing this hypothesis are warranted.

CONCLUSIONS

Self-disorders are crucial elements in the psychopathology of schizophrenia. In this chapter, we focused specifically on bodily self-disorders—that is, disorders of the bodily representation of the self, such as the sense of body ownership and agency. We reported empirical evidence in support of the idea that both are likely linked to the temporal processing of multisensory stimuli, not only in schizophrenia but already in schizotypy. Most importantly, we put forward the hypothesis that, first, a wider temporal window of sensory integration may essentially contribute to bodily self-disorders in schizophrenia and schizotypy. Second, we suggested that abnormal temporal patterns of the spontaneous brain activity, associated with impairments in the excitation/inhibition balance, may represent an important neural mechanism underling abnormal sensory processing and consequently bodily self-disorders in schizophrenia and people at higher risk.

BIBLIOGRAPHY

Asai T. and Tanno Y. (2008). "Highly Schizotypal Students Have a Weaker Sense of Self-Agency." *Psychiatry and Clinical Neurosciences* 62(1): 115–119.

Asai T., Mao Z., Sugimori E., and Tanno Y. (2011). "Rubber Hand Illusion, Empathy, and Schizotypal Experiences in Terms of Self-Other Representations." *Conscious and Cognition* 20(4): 1744–1750.

Barrantes-Vidal N., Grant P., and Kwapil T. R. (2015). "The Role of Schizotypy in the Study of the Etiology of Schizophrenia Spectrum Disorders." *Schizophrenia Bullettin*, 41 Suppl 2: S408–416.

Baumaister R. (1999). "The Nature and Structure of the Self: An Overview." In R. Baumaister (ed.), *The Self in Social Psychology*, pp. 1–21. Philadelphia: Psychology Press.

Bermúdez J.-L., Marcel A., and Eilan N. (1995). *The Body and the Self*. Cambridge, MA: MIT Press.

Blakemore S. J., Goodbody S. J., and Wolpert, D. M. (1998). "Predicting the Consequences of Our Own Actions: The Role of Sensorimotor Context Estimation." *Journal of Neurosciences* 18(18): 7511–7518.

Blakemore S. J., Frith C. D., and Wolpert, D. M. (1999). "Spatio-Temporal Prediction Modulates the Perception of Self-Produced Stimuli." *Journal of Cognitive Neuroscience* 11(5): 551–559.

Blakemore S. J., Smith J., Steel R., Johnstone C. E., and Frith C. D. (2000). "The Perception of Self-Produced Sensory Stimuli in Patients with Auditory Hallucinations and Passivity Experiences: Evidence for a Breakdown in Self-Monitoring." *Psychological Medicine* 30(5): 1131–1139.

Blakemore S. J., Wolpert D. M., and Frith C. D. (2002). "Abnormalities in the Awareness of Action." *Trends in Cognitive Science* 6(6): 237–242.

Botvinick M. and Cohen J. (1998). "Rubber Hands "Feel" Touch that Eyes See." *Nature* 391(6669): 756.

Buzsaki G. and Wang X. J. (2012). "Mechanisms of Gamma Oscillations." *Annual Review of Neuroscince* 35: 203–225.

Capa R. L., Duval C. Z., Blaison D., and Giersch A. (2014). "Patients with Schizophrenia Selectively Impaired in Temporal Order Judgments." *Schizophrenia Research* 156(1): 51–55.

Cermolacce M., Naudin J., and Parnas J. (2007). "The 'Minimal Self' in Psychopathology: Re-Examining the Self-Disorders in the Schizophrenia Spectrum." *Consciousness and Cognition* 16(3): 703–714.

Chambon V., Moore J. W., and Haggard P. (2015). "TMS Stimulation Over the Inferior Parietal Cortex Disrupts Prospective Sense of Agency." *Brain Structure and Function* 220(6): 3627–3639.

Ciullo V., Spalletta G., Caltagirone C., Jorge R. E., and Piras F. (2016). "Explicit Time Deficit in Schizophrenia: Systematic Review and Meta-Analysis Indicate It Is Primary and Not Domain Specific." *Schizophrenia Bullettin* 42(2): 505–518.

Costantini M., Robinson J., Migliorati D., Donno B., Ferri F., and Northoff G. (2016). "Temporal Limits on Rubber Hand Illusion Reflect Individuals' Temporal Resolution in Multisensory Perception." *Cognition* 157: 39–48.

Daprati E., Franck N., Georgieff N., Proust J., Pacherie E., Dalery J., and Jeannerod M. (1997). "Looking for the Agent: An Investigation into Consciousness of Action and Self-Consciousness in Schizophrenic Patients." *Cognition* 65(1): 71–86.

Ebisch S. J., Salone A., Ferri F., De Berardis D., Romani G. L., Ferro F. M., and Gallese, V. (2013). "Out of Touch with Reality? Social Perception in First-Episode Schizophrenia." *Social Cognitive and Affective Neuroscience* 8(4): 394–403.

Ettinger U., Mohr C., Gooding D. C., Cohen A. S., Rapp A., Haenschel C., and Park S. (2015). "Cognition and Brain Function in Schizotypy: A Selective Review." *Schizophrenia Bullettin* 41 *Suppl* 2: S417–426.

Farrer C., Bouchereau M., Jeannerod M., and Franck N. (2008). "Effect of Distorted Visual Feedback on the Sense of Agency." *Behavioral Neurology* 19(1–2): 53–57.

Ferri F., Chiarelli A. M., Merla A., Gallese V., and Costantini M. (2013). "The Body Beyond the Body: Expectation of a Sensory Event Is Enough to Induce Ownership Over a Fake Hand." *Proceedings Biologica Sciences* 280(1765): 20131140.

Ferri F., Costantini M., Salone A., Di Iorio G., Martinotti G., Chiarelli A., Merla A., Di Giannantonio M., and Gallese V. (2014). "Upcoming Tactile Events and Body Ownership in Schizophrenia." *Schizophrenia Research* 152(1): 51–57.

Ferri F., Ambrosini E., and Costantini M. (2016). "Spatiotemporal Processing of Somatosensory Stimuli in Schizotypy." *Scientific Reports* 6: 38735.

Ferri F., Nikolova Y. S., Perrucci M. G., Costantini M., Ferretti A., Gatta V., Huang Z., Edden R. A. E., Yue Q., D'Aurora M., Sibille E., Stuppia L., Romani G. L., and Northoff G. (2017). "A Neural 'Tuning Curve' for Multisensory Experience and Cognitive-Perceptual Schizotypy." *Schizophrenia Bullettin*. 43(4): 801–813

Foucher J. R., Lacambre M., Pham B. T., Giersch A., and Elliott M. A. (2007). "Low Time Resolution in Schizophrenia Lengthened Windows of Simultaneity for Visual, Auditory and Bimodal Stimuli." *Schizophrenia Research* 97(1–3): 118–127.

Fuchs T. and Schlimme J. E. (2009). "Embodiment and Psychopathology: A Phenomenological Perspective." *Current Opinion in Psychiatry* 22(6): 570–575.

Gallagher I. I. (2000). "Philosophical Conceptions of the Self: Implications for Cognitive Science." *Trends in Cognitive Science* 4(1): 14–21.

Gallese V. and Sinigaglia C. (2011). "How the Body in Action Shapes the Self." *Journal of Consciousness Studies* 18(7–8): 117–143.

Gallese V. and Ferri F. (2013). "Jaspers, the Body, and Schizophrenia: The Bodily Self." *Psychopathology* 46(5): 330–336.

Gallese V. and Ferri F. (2014). "Psychopathology of the Bodily Self and the Brain: The Case of Schizophrenia." *Psychopathology* 47(6): 357–364.

Germine L., Benson T. L., Cohen F., and Hooker C. I. (2013). "Psychosis-Proneness and the Rubber Hand Illusion of Body Ownership." *Psychiatry Research* 207(1–2): 45–52.

Graham K. T., Martin-Iverson M. T., Holmes N. P., Jablensky A., and Waters F. (2014). "Deficits in Agency in Schizophrenia, and Additional Deficits in Body Image, Body Schema, and Internal Timing, in Passivity Symptoms." *Frontiers in Psychiatry* 5: 126.

Graham-Schmidt K. T., Martin-Iverson M. T., Holmes N. P., and Waters F. A. (2016). "When One's Sense of Agency Goes Wrong: Absent Modulation of Time Perception by Voluntary Actions and Reduction of Perceived Length of Intervals in Passivity Symptoms in Schizophrenia." *Consciousness and Cognition* 45: 9–23.

Haggard P., Clark S., and Kalogeras J. (2002). "Voluntary Action and Conscious Awareness." *Nature Neuroscience* 5(4): 382–385.

Haggard P., Martin F., Taylor-Clarke M., Jeannerod M., and Franck N. (2003). "Awareness of Action in Schizophrenia." *Neuroreport* 14(7): 1081–1085.

He B. J., Zempel J. M., Snyder A. Z., and Raichle M. E. (2010). "The Temporal Structures and Functional Significance of Scale-Free Brain Activity." *Neuron* 66(3): 353–369.

He B. J. (2014). "Scale-Free Brain Activity: Past, Present, and Future." *Trends in Cognitive Science* 18(9): 480–487.

Hirsh I. J. (1959). "Auditory Perception of Temporal Order." *Journal of the Acoustic Society of America* 3: 157–178.

Honey C. J., Thesen T., Donner T. H., Silbert L. J., Carlson C. E., Devinsky O., Doyle W. K., Rubin N., Heeger D. J., and Hasson U. (2012). "Slow Cortical Dynamics and the Accumulation of Information Over Long Timescales." *Neuron* 76(2): 423–434.

Hong L. E., Summerfelt A., Buchanan R. W., O'Donnell P., Thaker G. K., Weiler M. A., and Lahti A. C. (2010). "Gamma and Delta Neural Oscillations and Association with Clinical Symptoms Under Subanesthetic Ketamine." *Neuropsychopharmacology* 35(3): 632–640.

Kallai J., Hegedus G., Feldmann A., Rozsa S., Darnai G., Herold R., Dorn K., Kincses P., Csatho A., and Szolcsanyi T. (2015). "Temperament and Psychopathological Syndromes Specific Susceptibility for Rubber Hand Illusion." *Psychiatry Research* 229(1–2): 410–419.

Kanayama N., Sato A., and Ohira H. (2007). "Crossmodal Effect with Rubber Hand Illusion and Gamma-Band Activity." *Psychophysiology* 44(3): 392–402.

Kanayama N., Sato A., and Ohira H. (2009). "The Role of Gamma Band Oscillations and Synchrony on Rubber Hand Illusion and Crossmodal Integration." *Brain and Cognition* 69(1): 19–29.

Klaver M. and Dijkerman H. C. (2016). "Bodily Experience in Schizophrenia: Factors Underlying a Disturbed Sense of Body Ownership." *Frontiers in Human Neuroscience* 10: 305.

Krause B., Marquez-Ruiz J., and Cohen Kadosh R. (2013). "The Effect of Transcranial Direct Current Stimulation: A Role for Cortical Excitation/Inhibition Balance?" *Frontiers in Human Neuroscience* 7: 602.

Kretschmer E. (1921). *Körperbau und Charakter. Untersuchungen zum Konstitutionsproblem und zur Lehre von den Temperamenten*. Berlin: Springer.

Kwapil T. R., Gross G. M., Silvia P. J., and Barrantes-Vidal N. (2013). "Prediction of Psychopathology and Functional Impairment by Positive and Negative Schizotypy in the Chapmans' Ten-Year Longitudinal Study." *Journal of Abnormal Psychology* 122(3): 807–815.

Lalanne L., van Assche M., and Giersch A. (2012). "When Predictive Mechanisms Go Wrong: Disordered Visual Synchrony Thresholds in Schizophrenia." *Schizophrenia Bullettin* 38(3): 506–513.

Lenzenweger M. F. (2006). "Schizotaxia, Schizotypy, and Schizophrenia: Paul E. Meehl's Blueprint for the Experimental Psychopathology and Genetics of Schizophrenia." *Journal of Abnormal Psychology* 115(2): 195–200.

Longo M. R., Schuur F., Kammers M. P., Tsakiris M., and Haggard P. (2008). "What Is Embodiment? A Psychometric Approach." *Cognition* 107(3): 978–998.

Madeira L., Bonoldi I., Rocchetti M., Samson C., Azis M., Queen B., Bossong M., Perez J., Stone J., Allen P., Howes O. D., McGuire P., Raballo A., Fusar-Poli P., Ballerini M., and Stanghellini G. (2016). "An Initial Investigation of Abnormal Bodily Phenomena in Subjects at Ultra High Risk for Psychosis: Their Prevalence and Clinical Implications." *Comprehensive Psychiatry* 66: 39–45.

Martin B., Giersch A., Huron C., and van Wassenhove V. (2013). "Temporal Event Structure and Timing in Schizophrenia: Preserved Binding in a Longer 'Now.'" *Neuropsychologia* 51(2): 358–371.

Meck W. H. (1996). "Neuropharmacology of Timing and Time Perception." *Brain Research Cognitive Brain Research* 3(3–4): 227–242.

Merleau-Ponty M. (1945). *Phénomenologie de la Perception*. Paris: Gallinard.

Mishara A. L. (2007). "Missing Links in Phenomenological Clinical Neuroscience: Why We Still Are Not There Yet." *Current Opinion in Psychiatry* 20(6): 559–569.

Moore J. and Haggard P. (2008). "Awareness of Action: Inference and Prediction." *Conscious and Cognition* 17(1): 136–144.

Moore J. W., Schneider S. A., Schwingenschuh P., Moretto G., Bhatia K. P., and Haggard P. (2010). "Dopaminergic Medication Boosts Action-Effect Binding in Parkinson's Disease." *Neuropsychologia* 48(4): 1125–1132.

Moore J. W., Turner D. C., Corlett P. R., Arana F. S., Morgan H. L., Absalom A. R., Adapa R., de Wit S., Everitt J. C., Gardner J. M., Pigott J. S., Haggard P., and Fletcher P. C. (2011). "Ketamine Administration in Healthy Volunteers Reproduces Aberrant Agency Experiences Associated with Schizophrenia." *Cogn Neuropsychiatry* 16(4): 364–381.

Moore J. W. and Obhi S. S. (2012). "Intentional Binding and the Sense of Agency: A Review." *Consciousness and Cognition* 21(1): 546–561.

Morgan H. L., Turner D. C., Corlett P. R., Absalom A. R., Adapa R., Arana F. S., Pigott J., Gardner J., Everitt J., Haggard P., and Fletcher P. C. (2011). "Exploring the Impact of Ketamine on the Experience of Illusory Body Ownership." *Biological Psychiatry* 69(1): 35–41.

Murray J. D., Bernacchia A., Freedman D. J., Romo R., Wallis J. D., Cai X., Padoa-Schioppa C., Pasternak T., Seo H., Lee D., and Wang X. J. (2014). "A Hierarchy of Intrinsic Timescales Across Primate Cortex." *Nature Neuroscience* 17(12): 1661–1663.

Nelson B., Fornito A., Harrison B. J., Yucel M., Sass L. A., Yung A. R., Thompson A., Wood S. J., Pantelis C., and McGorry P. D. (2009). "A Disturbed Sense of Self in the Psychosis Prodrome: Linking Phenomenology and Neurobiology." *Neuroscience and Biobehavioral Reviews* 33(6): 807–817.

Nelson B., Thompson A., and Yung A. R. (2012). "Basic Self-Disturbance Predicts Psychosis Onset in the Ultra High Risk for Psychosis 'Prodromal' Population." *Schizophrenia Bullettin* 38(6): 1277–1287.

Nelson B., Parnas J., and Sass L. A. (2014). "Disturbance of Minimal Self (Ipseity) in Schizophrenia: Clarification and Current Status." *Schizophrenia Bullettin* 40(3): 479–482.

Nikulin V. V., Jonsson E. G., and Brismar T. (2012). "Attenuation of Long-Range Temporal Correlations in the Amplitude Dynamics of Alpha and Beta Neuronal Oscillations in Patients with Schizophrenia." *Neuroimage* 61(1): 162–169.

Parnas J. and Handest P. (2003). "Phenomenology of Anomalous Self-Experience in Early Schizophrenia." *Comprehensive Psychiatry* 44(2): 121–134.

Peled A., Ritsner M., Hirschmann S., Geva A. B., and Modai I. (2000). "Touch Feel Illusion in Schizophrenic Patients." *Biological Psychiatry* 48(11): 1105–1108.

Peled A., Pressman A., Geva A. B., and Modai I. (2003). "Somatosensory Evoked Potentials During a Rubber-Hand Illusion in Schizophrenia." *Schizophrenia Research* 64(2–3): 157–163.

Piaget J. (1954). *The Construction of Reality in the Child*. New York: Basic Books.

Raballo A. and Parnas J. (2011). "The Silent Side of the Spectrum: Schizotypy and the Schizotaxic Self." *Schizophrenia Bullettin* 37(5): 1017–1026.

Raine A. (1991). "The SPQ: A Scale for the Assessment of Schizotypal Personality Based on DSM-III-R Criteria." *Schizophrenia Bullettin* 17(4): 555–564.

Raine A. (2006). "Schizotypal Personality: Neurodevelopmental and Psychosocial Trajectories." *Annu Review of Clinical Psychology* 2: 291–326.

Rogasch N. C., Daskalakis Z. J., and Fitzgerald P. B. (2014). "Cortical Inhibition, Excitation, and Connectivity in Schizophrenia: A Review of Insights from Transcranial Magnetic Stimulation." *Schizophrenia Bullettin* 40(3): 685–696.

Rohde M., Di Luca M., and Ernst M. O. (2011). "The Rubber Hand Illusion: Feeling of Ownership and Proprioceptive Drift Do Not Go Hand in Hand." *PLoS One* 6(6): e21659.

Romano D., Caffa E., Hernandez-Arieta A., Brugger P., and Maravita A. (2015). "The Robot Hand Illusion: Inducing Proprioceptive Drift Through Visuo-Motor Congruency." *Neuropsychologia* 70: 414–420.

Sass L. A. and Parnas J. (2003). "Schizophrenia, Consciousness, and the Self." *Schizophrenia Bullettin* 29(3): 427–444.

Schmidt H., McFarland J., Ahmed M., McDonald C., and Elliott M. A. (2011). "Low-Level Temporal Coding Impairments in Psychosis: Preliminary Findings and Recommendations for Further Studies." *Journal of Abnormal Psychology* 120(2): 476–482.

Shimada S., Fukuda K., and Hiraki, K. (2009). "Rubber Hand Illusion Under Delayed Visual Feedback." *PLoS One* 4(7): e6185.

Stephens G. J., Honey C. J., and Hasson U. (2013). "A Place for Time: The Spatiotemporal Structure of Neural Dynamics During Natural Audition." *Journal of Neurophysiology* 110(9): 2019–2026.

Stevenson R. A., Park S., Cochran C., McIntosh L. G., Noel J. P., Barense M. D., Ferber S., and Wallace M. T. (2017). "The Associations Between Multisensory Temporal Processing and Symptoms of Schizophrenia." *Schizophrenia Research* 179: 97–103.

Synofzik M., Vosgerau G., and Newen A. (2008). "I Move, Therefore I Am: A New Theoretical Framework to Investigate Agency and Ownership." *Consciousness and Cognition* 17(2): 411–424.

Synofzik M., Thier P., Leube D. T., Schlotterbeck P., and Lindner A. (2010). "Misattributions of Agency in Schizophrenia Are Based on Imprecise Predictions about the Sensory Consequences of One's Actions." *Brain* 133(Pt 1): 262–271.

Thakkar K. N., Nichols H. S., McIntosh L. G., and Park S. (2011). "Disturbances in Body Ownership in Schizophrenia: Evidence from the Rubber Hand Illusion and Case Study of a Spontaneous Out-of-Body Experience." *PLoS One* 6(10): e27089.

Thoenes S. and Oberfeld D. (2017). "Meta-Analysis of Time Perception and Temporal Processing in Schizophrenia: Differential Effects on Precision and Accuracy." *Clinical Psychology Review* 54: 44–64.

Tsakiris M. (2017). "The Multisensory Basis of the Self: From Body to Identity to Others [Formula: see text]." *Quarter Journal of Experimental Psychology (Hove)* 70(4): 597–609.

Tseng H. H., Bossong M. G., Modinos G., Chen K. M., McGuire P., and Allen P. (2015). "A Systematic Review of Multisensory Cognitive-Affective Integration in Schizophrenia." *Neuroscience and Biobehavioral Reviews* 55: 444–452.

Uhlhaas P. J. (2013). "Dysconnectivity, Large-Scale Networks and Neuronal Dynamics in Schizophrenia." *Current Opinion in Neurobiology* 23(2): 283–290.

Uhlhaas P. J. and Singer W. (2015). "Oscillations and Neuronal Dynamics in Schizophrenia: The Search for Basic Symptoms and Translational Opportunities." *Bioogicall Psychiatry* 77(12): 1001–1009.

Voss M., Moore J., Hauser M., Gallinat J., Heinz A., and Haggard P. (2010). "Altered Awareness of Action in Schizophrenia: A Specific Deficit in Predicting Action Consequences." *Brain* 133(10): 3104–3112.

Name Index

Subject Index

dissociation 566, 568–72, 573
  borderline personality disorder 677
  disorders *see* dissociative disorders
  trauma 902–3
dissociative amnesia 570–1, 572
dissociative disorders
  dissociative identity disorder 571
  selfhood 470–1
  twilight state 423
disturbed cognitive/perceptual grip
    (schizophrenia) 599, 600, 605,
    609, 610–11
dopamine 411–12
dorsolateral prefrontal cortex (DLPFC), and
    eating disorders 716
Down syndrome 1087, 1094, 1096
dreams
  Boss 122
  Freud 122
  Heidegger 122
  loss of dreaming 451, 452
dressing apraxia 513
drowsiness 421
drug addiction 682–94
DSM *see Diagnostic and Statistical Manual of
    Mental Disorders*
dualism
  autonomy 375
  embodiment 367–8, 369, 371
duty 975–8
dysmorphophobia 515–16
dysphoria
  background 829, 830
  borderline personality disorder 665, 666–7,
    668, 669–73, 827–38
  pathways 828–30
  psychosis risk 843
  regulating 833
  situational 830–2

Early Heidelberg School 484, 487–91, 494–5,
    497–503
Early Recognition Inventory for the
    Retrospective Assessment of the Onset of
    Schizophrenia (ERIraos) 842
EASE (Examination of Anomalous Self
    Experiences) 945–8
  auditory–verbal hallucinations 794

depersonalization 604–5
  dimensional analysis 1025n
  dissociation 569, 570
  introspectionism 604–5
  normality 292
  panic disorder 605–6
  psychosis risk 842, 849
  schizophrenia 17, 598, 602–5, 607, 611–12,
    945–7, 948
eating behavior and disorders 529–37
  addiction 682
  as embodiment and identity
    disorders 710–23
  normality 292
  psychiatric ethics 983
  psychopathology 710–11, 715
  values 361
  see also anorexia nervosa; binge
    eating/binge eating disorder; bulimia
    nervosa
EAWE (Examination of Anomalous World
    Experiences) 612, 849, 948
echo contamination 523
echolalia 450, 451
  catatonia 521n, 523
echopraxia 523
education *see* clinicians, formation of
ego
  autism 739
  Binswanger 116
  depressive delusions 762–3
  mania 882, 887–8, 889
  paranoia 771, 772, 782, 785–6
  psychopathy 882, 887–8, 889
  Sartre 36
  schizophrenia 739
  schizophrenic autism 822
  self 301, 302, 303
  unconscious 316, 317, 321, 322, 323
eidetic reduction 251, 257–9, 278
eidetic understanding 953, 956–7
eidetic variation 376
eidos 13, 274
élan vital 143
  Bergson 106, 151
  Minkowski 106
elation 618
elderly, pathologizing of 53–5

Executive Dysfunction Hypothesis,
        autism 699, 705
exemplars 1024n
existential feelings 195, 195n, 197–8, 199, 201,
        202, 461–2
    grief 548–9n
    time 617–18
existentialism
    anxiety 476, 481
    Beauvoir 53
    emotion 307–8, 313
    Laing 182, 183–6, 188
    Merleau-Ponty 47–8
    phenomenology 212–13, 274
    trauma 900–2
existential phenomenology 186–7
existential psychiatry 183, 185
existential psychoanalysis 39–41
existentials 192–9, 202–3
experience
    emotion 309–10
    hermeneutical phenomenology 238–9,
        241–2, 243
    normality 284, 286, 288, 293
    perceptual articulation of, in autism 701–2
    personhood 336–7
    self 300, 301, 302
explaining
    clinicians, formation of 1010–11
    and understanding, distinction
        between 407–9, 412
explicationists 254–5, 257
extracampine hallucinations 731

fatigue 523
fear
    and anxiety, distinction between 478, 901
    Befindlichkeit 349
    Heidegger 195
    obsessions 579, 580
    phobias 577
feelings 309–11, 312, 477
    borderline personality disorder 678–9
    existential see existential feelings
    intentionality 327
    phenomenological approach 212–13
    types 477–8
fictional approaches to mental illness 987n

field observations 925
finger agnosia 514
finitude
    ethics of 904–5
    trauma 902–5
first-person accounts
    auditory–verbal hallucinations 796, 798
    autobiography 1053–64
    autonomy 377
    cognitive science 263–6
    consciousness 928
    depression and grief, similarities
        between 539–40
    existential feelings 461
    neurophenomenology 277, 279, 381
    phenomenology 942
    thought insertion 585, 586–7
flight of ideas 451, 452
focus groups 925
food restriction 530
formal thought disorder 450–4
fragile understanding 878–9
Fragile X syndrome 1096
fragility, strength of 981–4
freedom
    Blankenburg 158, 161, 162
    existentialism 184
    Ey 161
    Jaspers 101
    phenomenological approach 212, 213
    Ricoeur 74, 75
    Sartre 376–7
free variation 956, 1054n
frontal brain injury, and decision-making
        capacity 863, 865–6
fugue 570, 571
    twilight state 423

gender
    disorder of 553–4
    phenomenological approach 211
    role 555–6, 560
    terms relating to 557–8
gender dysphoria 552–65
    body image disturbance 529, 534
    DSM 993
gender identity 552, 553, 554–5, 559, 61
    disorder 993